second edition

Public Health in Canada 2.0

Kendall Hunt
publishing company

Wally J. Bartfay   Emma Bartfay

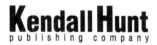

*This book is dedicated to the memory of "Lopa," Leung Kwong Chuen,
a very wise and talented man who will remain dear in our hearts forever.*

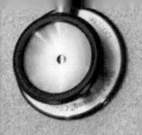

Table of Contents

Preface..*xvii*

Special Features and Learning Resources... *xxiii*

About the Authors...*xxv*

Chapter 1   Foundations and Essential Concepts for Public Health 1

Learning Objectives 1

Core Competencies Addressed in Chapter 1 2

Introduction 2

What is public health? 2

The Five Essential Pillars of Public Health 8

    Essential Pillar (i): Evidence-informed public health 8

    Essential Pillar (ii): Health Promotion and Prevention 15

    Essential Pillar (iii): Primary Health care 20

    Essential Pillar (iv): The 15 Social Determinants of Health 24

    Essential Pillar (v): Holistic Care Paradigm 30

The "Ripple Effect" in Public Health 32

Future Directions and Challenges 35

Summary 39

Critical Thinking Questions 40

References 41

**Chapter 2   Understanding the Concept of "Health": Its Evolution and
Definitions** 53

Learning Objectives 53

Core Competencies Addressed in Chapter 2 54

Introduction 54

A Brief History of Health 55

    Pre-historic Times 55

    Ancient Egypt 56

    Persians 57

    Traditional Chinese Medicine 58

    Ancient India 59

Ancient Greece..61

Ancient Rome..63

The Middle Ages..65

The Renaissance Period..69

Industrial Revolution Era..72

Public Health Activities in Canada: 1900–1950...75

The Emergence of Holistic Definitions of Health.. 80

1950s to Present...80

The Lalonde Report, 1974..81

Alma-Ata Conference, 1978...83

The Epp Report, 1986..83

Ottawa Charter for Health Promotion, 1986...84

The Jakarta Declaration (1997)..85

Bangkok Charter for Health Promotion in a Globalized World (2005)........86

Current developments in public health in Canada: 2000 and onwards....................... 87

Future Directions and Challenges.. 88

Summary.. 92

Critical Thinking Questions... 93

References.. 94

Chapter 3 **"Medicare" in Canada: History and Current Challenges**.................... **103**

Learning Objectives 103

Core Competencies Addressed in Chapter 3... 104

Introduction 104

Medicare 108

The Evolution of Health Services in Canada: A Brief History........................ 113

Pioneer Nurses...113

The Grey Nuns...113

Pioneer Surgeons and Physicians...114

Early Outbreaks and Epidemics...114

British North America Act (1867)...115

The Emergence of the Medical Model of Health 116

The Flexner Report (1910)..117

Medical Breakthroughs by Canadians 117

Shift from Home and Community to Hospital-based Health Services........................ 118

Redefining the Federal Governments Role in Health 120

Employment and Social Insurance Act (1935)..121

Marsh and Heagerty Reports (1943)..121

Saskatchewan's Pioneering Health Care Reforms.......................................122

National Health Grants Act (1948)...124

Hospital Insurance and Diagnostic Services Act (1957) 124

Medical Care Act (1966)...125

Federal Health Care Funding Arrangements 127

The Canada Health Act (1982) 130

Federal and Provincial/territorial Responsibilities Under the CHA 132

Chaoulli et al. Versus the Attorney General of Québec 136

Divergent Interpretations of the CHA 138

What is "medically necessary"? 138

Jake Epp's Letter 139

Diane Marleau's Letter 139

Penalties and Deductions 141

Rising Health Care Costs 142

Future Directions and Challenges 144

Summary 148

Critical Thinking Questions 150

References 151

Chapter 4   Indigenous Health in Canada 159

Learning Objectives 159

Core Competencies Addressed in Chapter 4 160

Introduction 160

Historical Perspectives 161

Indigenous Status 165

First Nations/Indian 166

Inuit 166

Métis 167

Indigenous Languages 168

Jesuit Missionaries and Residential Schools 168

Treaties and Reserves 170

Indian Act and Bill C-31 171

Social and Health Consequences of Colonization 172

Indigenous Perspectives of Health 174

Delivery of Health Services 176

Cultural Safety and Public Health 178

Major Current Health Issues 180

Mental Health Issues, Injuries, and Drownings 181

Gasoline Sniffing 181

Health of Indigenous Families 182

Sexually Transmitted Infections 184

Cardiovascular Disease and Diabetes 185

Future Directions and Challenges 187

Summary 188

Critical Thinking Questions 189

References 190

Chapter 5   **Essential Research Methods for the Practice of Public Health 199**

Learning Objectives 199

Core Competencies Addressed in Chapter 5 200

Introduction 200

Basic and Applied Research 201

Evidence-informed Public Health and Research 202

    Systematic Reviews 204

    Meta-analysis 205

    Meta-summaries and Meta-syntheses 206

The Research Process in Public Health 206

    Step I: Identification of a problem (Conceptualization phase) 207

    Step II: Review of the literature 208

    Step III: Formulate research questions or hypotheses..209

    Step IV: Design a study 211

    Step V: Ethical approval 222

    Step VI: Collect data (Empirical phase) 225

    Step VII: Data analysis (Analytical phase) 227

    Step VIII: Determine strengths and limitations of the findings 231

    Step IX: Dissemination and application of research findings 233

Knowledge Utilization in Public Health 233

Future Directions and Challenges 234

Summary 235

Critical Thinking Questions 236

References 237

Chapter 6   **Epidemiology: Essential Concepts for Public Health 243**

Learning Objectives 243

Core Competencies Addressed in Chapter 6 244

Introduction 244

Historical Developments in Epidemiology: A Brief Overview 246

    Hippocrates of Cos (460–377 BC) 246

    John Graunt (1620–1674) 247

    Thomas Sydenham (1624–1689) 248

    James Lind (1716–1794) 248

    Edward Jenner (1749–1823) 249

    William Farr (1807–1883) 251

    John Snow (1813–1858) 252

    Ignaz Philipp Semmelweis (1818–1865) 253

Twentieth-Century Developments in Epidemiology and Public Health 254

    Doll and Hill's Landmark Studies on Smoking and Lung Cancer 255

    Framingham Heart Study 256

Current Developments in Epidemiology and Public Health 256

Health Surveillance 257

Basic Concepts in the Epidemiological Approach 258

    The Epidemiological Triangle of Communicable Disease 258

    Agent 259

    Natural History of Disease 264

    Revised and Updated Epidemiological Triangle 265

Common Epidemiological Measures 271

    Disease Frequency 272

    Measures of Association 277

Future Directions and Challenges 280

Summary 283

Critical Thinking Questions 284

References 285

Chapter 7   **Human Responses to Disease, Illness, and Sickness 291**

Learning Objectives 291

Core Competencies Addressed in Chapter 7 292

Introduction 292

Nomenclature and the Common Classifications of Disease 294

    ICD-10 295

    DSM-V 295

What is Disease? 296

What is Illness and Stages of the Illness Experience? 297

    Stage I 297

    Stage II 298

    Stage III 299

    Stage IV 299

    Stage V 299

What is Sickness and the Sick Role? 299

The Five Disease Categories 301

What are Acute and Chronic Diseases? 303

What are Communicable and Noncommunicable Diseases? 305

Types of Immunity 308

    Antigenicity 310

    Acquired (Passive) Immunity 310

    Natural Immunity 310

    Active Immunity 310

    Herd Immunity 313

Common Modes of Disease Transmission 314

    Vertical and Horizontal Modes 314

    Airborne or Respiratory Mode of Transmission 315

    Fecal/Oral Mode of Transmission 315

    Waterborne Mode of Transmission 316

Community- and Hospital-Acquired Nosocomial Infections 316

    Parasitic Mode 318

    Vector-borne Mode 322

    Zoonotic Mode 325

Health Surveillance 327

    Active Surveillance...328

    Passive Surveillance 330

Reportable/Notifiable Disease Lists 333

Non-reportable/Notifiable Disease 334

Poisonings 336

    Poisonous Plants 337

    Pesticide Poisoning..337

    Food Safety and Poisonings..338

Injuries and Disabilities 340

Bioterrorism 341

Future Directions and Challenges 345

Summary.. 349

Critical Thinking Questions 350

References 351

Chapter 8   **Environmental and Occupation Health and Safety 365**

Learning Objectives 365

Core Competencies Addressed in Chapter 8 366

Introduction 366

What Is Global Warming and Climate Change? 369

    Greenhouse Effect...370

    International Frameworks and Protocols for Climate Change 371

How Does Global Warming and Climate Change Affect Human Health? 373

    Public Safety and Emergency Preparedness Legislation in Canada..................................375

    Emergency Management and Incident Management Systems 376

    Infectious Diseases..377

    Ozone Depletion and UV Radiation 379

    Air Quality and Pollution 379

    Sick-building Syndrome...382

    Water Quality and Pollution...383

What Is Toxicology? 389

Examples of Commonly Known Toxic Heavy Metals and Chemicals 393

    Mercury...393

    Lead...394

    Dichlorodiphenyltrichloroethane..395

    Bisphenol A...396

Canadian Legislation to Preserve and Protect the Environment 397

Work Environments and Occupational Health and Safety 400

Bernardino Ramazzini (1633–1714) 404

Percival Pott (1714–1788) 404

Alice Hamilton (1869-1970) 406

Occupational Health and Safety in Canada 406

Work-related Stress 410

Environmental and Occupational Risk Assessments for Public Health 414

Future Directions and Challenges 418

Summary 420

Critical Thinking Questions 421

References 421

Chapter 9   Global Health: A Primer 433

Learning Objectives 433

Core Competencies Addressed in Chapter 9 434

Introduction 434

What are the Millennium Development Goals? 437

What are the Sustainable Development Goals? 440

What is Globalization? 442

Common Global Burden of Disease Measures 450

Disability-adjusted life year 451

Healthy life years (HeaLY) lost measure 453

Health-adjusted life expectancy measure 453

Quality-adjusted life year 455

What are Neglected Tropical Diseases (NTDs)? 456

Global Spread of Infections 461

Future Directions and Challenges 463

Summary 465

Critical Thinking Questions 466

References 466

Chapter 10   Program Planning and Evaluation in Public Health 475

Learning Objectives 475

Core Competencies Addressed in Chapter 10 476

Introduction 476

Accessing and Developing Web-based Health Programs and Sites 477

What is Program Planning? 484

Strategic or Allocative Planning 485

Operational or Activity Planning 486

What is Program Evaluation? 487

What are the Types of Program Evaluations Conducted? 489

What is the Program Planning and Evaluation Process? 490

Step I 490

Step II 492

Step III 492

Step IV 495

Step V 495

Step VI 495

Step VII 496

Step VIII 496

What are Program Logic Models? 498

What is Health Services Research? 499

What is Outcomes Research? 500

Ethical Considerations for Public Health Professionals and Workers 502

Future Directions and Challenges 507

Summary 509

Critical Thinking Questions 510

References 510

Chapter 11   Current and Emerging Mental Health Issues in Canada 517

Learning Objectives 517

Core Competencies Addressed in Chapter 518

Introduction 518

What is mental health? 519

Mental Health Commission of Canada 519

School-based Mental Health Promotion 520

Mental Health First Aid Training in Canada 522

Major Theories Related to the Origins of Mental Illness and Disorders 522

(i) Supernatural theory 522

(ii) Psychogenic theories 524

(iii) Somatogenic theories 525

What is Stress? 529

General Adapation Syndrome Model 533

Physiological Responses to Stressors 534

(i) Nervous system 534

(ii) Endocrine system 535

(iii) Immune system 536

Personality-types and Stress 537

Coping and Managing Stressors 539

Positive coping and stress management techniques 540

Negative coping and stress management techniques 542

Public Health Caution Related to Natural Health Products and Stress 543

Major Mental Illnesses 544

Anxiety Disorders 545

Generalized Anxiety Disorder (GAD) 546

Obsessive Compulsive Disorder (OCD)..547

Post-Traumatic Stress Disorder (PTSD)..547

Panic Disorders 548

Phobias 549

Mood Disorders, Depression and Suicide 549

Depression 549

Bipolar disorder..550

Seasonal affective disorder...551

Suicide: A Canadian context 551

Schizophenia..552

Major Eating Disorders...553

Anorexia nervosa 554

Bulimia nervosa 555

Bing-Eating Disorder (BED) 555

Public Health Challenges Related to Eating Disorders.. 555

Future Directions and Challenges.. 556

Summary..559

Critical Thinking Questions 560

References 560

Chapter 12   Neurological Disorders: A Growing Public Health Challenge............573

Learning Objectives 573

Core Competencies Addressed in Chapter.. 574

Introduction 574

A Brief Overview of the Human Brain and Nervous System... 577

Traumatic Brain Injuries and Concussions 579

Glasgow Coma Scale...579

TBI's: A growing public health concern..580

Helmets for the prevention of TBIs and concussions example..582

Parkinson's Disease 583

Prevalence of Parkinson's Disease..584

Impact of Parkinson's Disease and Implications for Public Health................................584

Multiple Sclerosis 585

Amyotrophic Lateral Sclerosis... 587

Myasthemia Gravis.. 588

Huntington's Disease... 589

Dementia and Alzheimer's Disease 589

Direct and Indirect Health Care Costs Associated with Dementia....................................... 591

Future Directions and Challenges.. 595

Summary.. 597

Critical Thinking Questions 598

References 598

Chapter 13   Major Emerging and Re-emerging Infectious Diseases: A Canadian Perspective 605

Learning Objectives 605

Core Competencies Addressed in Chapter 606

Introduction 606

What are Infectious Diseases? 608

What is the Chain of Infection? 609

A Brief Overview of the Human Immune System 613

What are Emerging and Re-emerging Infectious Diseases? 615

Global Surveillance and Risk Assessments of EIDs and REIDs 618

Examing Major Emerging and Re-emerging Infectious Diseases from a Canadian Context 619

    Avian Influenza (Avian Flu or Bird Flu) 619

    Blastomycosis (Gilchrists disease) 622

    Chikungunya 623

    Ebola Virus Disease (EVD) 624

    Lyme Disease (Lyme Borreliosis) 628

    Sudden Acute Respiratory Syndrome (SARS) 631

    West Nile Virus (WNV) 632

    Zika Virus Infections 635

Future Directions and Challenges 638

Summary 640

Criticial Thinking Questions 641

References 641

Chapter 14   Major Noncommunicable Diseases: Current and Future Challenges...651

Learning Objectives 651

Core Competencies Addressed in Chapter 652

Introduction 652

Prevention of Noncommunicable Diseases in the 21st Century: Four Targeted Behavioural Risk Factors 654

    (i) Tobacco Use and Smoking 655

    (ii) Physical Inactivity and Sedentary Lifestyles 655

    (iii) Unhealthy Diet 657

    (iv) Harmful Use of Alcohol 658

Premature Mortality and HALE Trends in Canada 659

Chronic Disease Multi-morbidity in Canadians 661

Major NCDs: A Canadian Perspective 661

    (i) Cancer 661

    Is there a relationship between sugar consumption and cancer? 664

    Palliative, End-of-life Care (EOLC) and Community-based Hospice Services 665

    (ii) Cardiovascular Disease 666

    Ischemic Heart Disease 666

    Hypertension 667

    Stroke 667

(iii) Chronic Respiratory Diseases...668

Asthma 668

Chronic Objective Pulmonary Diseaes (COPD)...669

(iv) Diabetes (DM)..669

Insulin Metabolism..670

Prevalence of DM...670

Prediabetes..670

Impaired glucose tolerance and impaired fasting glycaemia 671

Type 1 DM 671

Type 2 DM 671

Gestational diabetes...672

Importance of Influenza Vaccinations for Clients with CRDs and CVD 672

Future Directions and Challenge 672

Summary...676

Criticial Thinking Questions..676

References 677

Appendix A: 36 Core Competencies (Public Health Agency of Canada) 683

Glossary of Key Terms...687

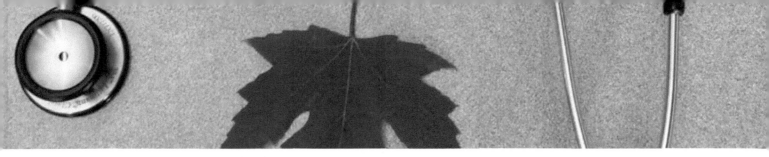

Preface

We define public health as a holistic and evidence-informed discipline that seeks to promote, maintain, and/or restore the health and quality of life of individuals, families, communities, and/or entire populations over the lifespan through health promotion and prevention and various primary health care initiatives, activities, policies, and/or legislations. We invite you to partake on an exciting learning journey related to public health theory, practice, and research in Canada. You will discover on your learning adventure that public health care professionals and workers provide essential health care services for the prevention, promotion, and restoration of health for diverse populations across the lifespan, which include public health nurses, physicians, epidemiologists, health promoters, and infection control specialists to name but a few. This book focuses on the unique contributions made by public health for preserving, preventing, and promoting the health and well-being of individuals, families, entire communities, and populations in Canada and globally. We contend that the art and science of public health embodies and consists of the following five essential pillars that form the foundations of this textbook: (i) Evidence-informed public health (EIPH), (ii) health promotion and prevention, (iii) primary health care, (iv) social determinants of health, and (v) the holistic care paradigm. The target audience for this textbook is upper level undergraduate and/or graduate students enrolled in community/public health sciences programs and professional programs (e.g., nursing, medicine, kinesiology, physiotherapy). The textbook may also be employed by instructors in the allied health sciences and social sciences.

We argue that when public health is doing their jobs effectively, then their collective efforts are often silent and invisible in nature to most. Public health professionals and workers often remark that many individuals do not understand, identify, or grasp what they do until something dramatic happens (e.g., bioterrorism, earthquake, environmental disaster, global pandemic) or goes wrong and their knowledge, training, problem-solving skills, and expertise are thrust into the forefront by the mass and social media. We note that nanotechnologies that seek to build biological machines on the molecular or subatomic scale, human genomics, stem cells, and other laboratory-based health care innovations that advance our understanding of human disease and their management often captures the interests of the mass and social media's and the awe of the general public. We must acknowledge that these noted innovations in science along with the services provided in acute care hospitals are undeniably critical. Nonetheless, they often pale in effectiveness to prevent disease, injury, or disability; or to maintain, promote, or restore health compared to most fundamental and rudimentary public health interventions (e.g., immunization), strategies (e.g., improvements in sanitation and water quality), or policies and legislations (e.g., tobacco and seat belt legislations).

Indeed, we tend to take it for granted that water taken from municipal water supplies in Canada is safe to drink and free of pathogens that can make us sick or even result in mortality. We do not worry about the safety of milk products sold commercially in Canada because of laws related to the need to pasteurize raw milk before it can be sold and consumed. The general public rarely worries about communicable diseases such as polio, tuberculosis, rabies, measles, rubella, smallpox, or diphtheria, which devastated millions of individuals around the world at the turn of the century. When they buckle up their seat belts in cars and put their children into car seats, they often don't realize the connection between public health and safety legislations that were derived from the best available scientific evidence. However, when dozens of individuals suddenly become ill as a result of eating some contaminated food (e.g., *E-coli* in burgers) in a local restaurant; develop a rash and experience shortness of breath due to exposure of some recent environmental chemical spill, or become severely ill or die as a consequence of some contagion such as sudden acute respiratory syndrome (SARS) or H5N1, then everyone looks to public health professionals and workers to investigate and find solutions to these noted health issues and concerns.

The stimulus for this textbook came from our collective experiences in teaching public health-related courses over several decades both at the undergraduate and graduate level, our programs of research, and inspiration from our students. Specifically, we were frustrated with a lack of current public health textbooks written from the uniquely Canadian perspective and experience. Moreover, the limited available pedagogical materials were often written from the outdated mechanistic medical-model of health perspective, which often fails to recognize or consider new evidence in light of holistic definitions of health and/or the social determinants of health. The *holistic health paradigm* incorporates the belief that human beings are more than the sum of their mind and body parts, but are dynamic and interrelated wholes that include their mind, body, spirit, culture, and environments. The *social determinants of health* encompass structural determinants and conditions of daily life that are responsible for a major part of health inequities between and within countries and include the distribution of power, income, goods and services by both genders; the circumstances of people's lives; access to health care services and education; employment and working conditions; and state of housing and various environmental factors.

EIPH involves a collaborative process between all stakeholders concerned for distilling and disseminating the best available evidence to inform public health policy and practice derived from research, practice, and/or personal experiences and needs. In fact, it may be argued that the *evidence* suggests that over three-quarters of "good health" is not achieved via direct episodic acute care health care services often provided in hospitals, but are the collective results of various lifestyle choices (e.g., decision not to smoke, exercise regularly, consume a diet low in saturated- and trans-fats, sugar, and sodium) and social determinants of health (e.g., level of education, poverty, social and economic status).

Health promotion activities enhance and/or reinforce the ability of an individual, family, group, community, or entire population to take control and maintain, improve, or restore their health and quality of life. *Prevention* entails actions, measures, interventions, programs, policies, and/or legislations, which seek to avert the development or progression of disease or possible harm, injury, disability, or death and improve, maintain, and/or restore health-related quality of life. The scope and levels of prevention have changed over the past few decades, and this textbook recognizes and describes the following five types: (i) primordial, (ii) primary, (iii) secondary, (iv) tertiary, and (v) quaternary.

In addition to the above, this textbook has been written based on the *primary health care approach*, which is a model that emphasizes the need for equity, accessibility, full participation by individuals and communities, the use of universally acceptable and affordable technologies and methods, sustainable development, and intersectoral collaboration. This model is based on practical, scientifically sound, and socially acceptable health care approaches and interventions which embrace the following five types of health care: (i) promotive, (ii) preventive, (iii) curative, (iv) rehabilitative, and (v) supportive/palliative. Hence, we felt it was imperative to teach our students about the need to adapt primary health care approaches in tackling current and emerging health care issues in Canada and globally. Accordingly, this textbook was written to fill this noted gap and provide students, educators, and practitioners in the public health sciences in Canada with an updated resource that addresses these noted shortcomings and deficiencies.

To our knowledge, there is no current public health textbook written from the uniquely Canadian perspective, especially one that promotes interdisciplinary professional collaboration, which we maintain is the very essence of public health practice. Indeed, public health care professionals and workers do not practice in isolation or in so-called "professional silos" in Canada or internationally. This textbook will provide you with the essential knowledge base and theoretical foundations that all public health care professionals and workers need to possess in order to provide safe and cost-effective EIPH services in Canada.

The Public Health Agency of Canada (PHAC) was established in response to the 2003 SARS crisis in Toronto, Ontario, and global pandemic. As a consequence of this pandemic and others that followed (e.g., avian flu, H1N1, West Nile virus), various reports have identified important deficiencies in the institutional capacity of our public health systems in Canada. These inquiries and various governmental agencies have outlined the current need to develop training programs for public health care professionals and workers. In fact, during the 1990s, there were only five university programs in public health and by September 2011, fifteen Canadian universities were offering MPH or MPH-type programs with as many as 500 new graduates annually. During the past decade, there has also been an explosion of undergraduate programs and schools in public health being offered across Canada due to increased public and student demands, and many of these programs did not exist just five years ago.

This book does not address practice mandates for specific public health care professionals (e.g., public health nurses, physicians, epidemiologists) per se, but advances the notion of interdisciplinary cooperation, practice, and research in a variety of public health settings. This book seeks to utilize current terms and concepts employed by governmental agencies, such as the PHAC and Health Canada, and those that are also utilized by international organizations such as the World Health Organization (WHO). This book also recognizes that regional, national, and international health programs often consist of a web of complex and interacting social determinants of health and well-being. Although individual health care programs or systems are not addressed for each specific provinces or territories, salient examples are provided throughout the chapters to illustrate core concepts and trends in public health that affect all Canadians across the lifespan.

This book consists of fourteen chapters that can be covered in its entirety in a single course or semester. Given that an instructor may choose to select specific chapters for their course(s) and that student's learning needs may vary, not all chapters may be required or reviewed. Hence, each chapter has been written in sufficient detail as "stand alone" chapters with ample explanations, definitions, examples, and complete references provided. Although certain chapters may be cross-referenced for greater information or details, each chapter provides sufficient information for the reader to be considered as a "stand alone" package per se. This is an important consideration because specific chapters may be chosen by instructors as a custom e-book package for their course.

Chapter 1 entitled *Foundations and Essential Concepts for Public Health* provides an overview of the art and science of public health, its scope of practice and various activities. An over of the 36 core competencies deemed essential for all public health professionals and workers by the PHAC is highlighted. A detailed discussion of the five essential pillars of public health is provided along with a discussion on how these pillars provide the reader with a conceptual vehicle and guide to meet the 36 core competencies is highlighted. A detailed discussion of the merits and benefits of EIPH versus evidence-based medicine or practice models are critically examined. The definitions of the five levels of prevention and examples of each are provided. We discuss the benefits, rationale, and need to adopt primary health care models in Canada to meet the health care needs of diverse populations across the lifespan in Canada. Lastly, we explore the so-called "ripple-effects" in public health across multiple levels and/or groups. For example, when a critical mass (e.g., 70%) of individuals have been immunized against a known contagion (e.g., measles), this can help protect all individuals in a given community or population via herd immunity.

Chapter 2 entitled *Understanding the Concept of "Health": Its Evolution and Definitions* provides a historical overview of how definitions of health have evolved overtime, and how current holistic definitions of health have evolved and are slowly replacing the outdated mechanistic medical model of health based on a growing body of evidence. We critically examine how the continued predominate directive of medical research for finding the specific causes and cures of diseases or so-called "magic bullet approach" has remained an enduring consequence of the unicausal laboratory-based medical model approach to health. We examine the national and global influences of the Lalonde Report (1974), which challenged this unicausal model of health and illness by examining four critical determinants of health: (i) human biology, (ii) environment, (iii) lifestyle, and (v) health care organization. We explore the influence of the 1978 Alma-Ata conference on holistic definitions of health and the idea that primary health care was declared as the major vehicle for reforming mechanistic medical models of health care that dominated health care systems globally. We also explore the impact of the 1986 Epp Report that expanding the definition of health to include a variety of sociopolitical and environmental determinants of health. We also examine the influence of various global conferences and charters including the Ottawa Charter for Health Promotion (1986), the Jakarta Declaration (1997), and the Bangkok Charter for Health Promotion in a globalized world (2005).

Chapter 3 entitled *"Medicare" in Canada: History and Current Challenges* provides a historical overview of health care practices in Canada and how social and political forces have shaped our current public health systems in Canada commonly referred to as "medicare." This chapter provides the reader with the evolution of public health care systems in Canada and provides an overview of major legislations (e.g., Medical Care Act 1966, Canada Health Act 1982). We also explore current challenges facing our publicly delivered public health care systems in Canada, which includes the growth of private for-profit clinics across Canada.

Chapter 4 entitled *Indigenous Health in Canada* addresses the issue of Indigenous health and well-being and the various health challenges these people face. We examine different Indigenous populations and cultures in Canada including First Nations, Métis, and Inuit peoples and the various health issues and challenges they face. For example, the growing incidence of obesity and type 2 diabetes due to changes in their traditional lifestyle and diet. We also examine the impact of colonization by westerners, the impact of the residential school system on Indigenous families, and the concept of "cultural safety" which is essential to practice in these communities.

Chapter 5 entitled *Essential Research Methods for the Practice of Public Health* details the critical link between research and EIPH practice by introducing the nine critical steps of the research process. In addition, salient research methodologies employed by qualitative, quantitative, and mix-methods researchers to advance public health theory and practice are highlighted. This chapter provides the reader with the critical background information necessary to read and comprehend published articles and reports that may utilize a variety of current research approaches and methods. Various examples and published reports are utilized throughout this chapter to reinforce and/or highlight key points and methodologies.

Chapter 6 entitled *Epidemiology: Essential Concepts for Public Health* addresses critical developments in epidemiological methods over time, and how it has influenced public health in Canada and abroad. Both the classical (composed of the agent, host, environment, and time), and the new and updated epidemiological triangle (composed of time, environment, individuals, and groups; environment, and determinants of health) are highlighted. This updated epidemiological triangle, unlike the traditional communicable disease triangle, is more comprehensive in nature and recognizes that alterations to health and well-being are often fluid in nature and more complex in reference to the environment, social determinants of health and/or associated risk factors, which can be both modifiable (e.g., inactivity, smoking, diet high in saturated fats) and nonmodifiable (e.g., genetic predisposition, gender) in nature. Indeed, although infectious diseases have been historically the leading causes of mortality and morbidity, they have been replaced by noninfectious chronic diseases such as heart disease and diabetes. In addition, the reader is introduced to core terms and concepts necessary to read and comprehend government public health reports, conference proceedings, and published studies, which employ a variety of epidemiological measures and approaches. Lastly, common epidemiological measures related to disease frequency (e.g., prevalence, incidence, attack rate, morbidity and mortality rates) and measures of association (e.g., relative risk, attributable risk, odds ratio) are presented in a user-friendly and nontechnical format.

Chapter 7 entitled *Human Responses to Disease, Illness, and Sickness* provides an overview of human responses to diseases, illness, and sickness and how definitions of these concepts involve social, political, and cultural norms, expectations, and traditions. We examine current global standards for classifying physical (e.g., ICD-10) and psychiatric disorders (e.g., DSM-V), disease classifications, along with their strengths and limitations. The five classical disease classification systems are highlighted and the common modes of disease transmission are explored with examples of each. This chapter also highlights the various types of immunity, how various diseases are tracked, and the various types of surveillance utilized by public health care officials in Canada and internationally. A discussion on bioterrorism and disaster planning and response, the various governmental agencies responsible for monitoring and intervening during a crisis are also highlighted.

Chapter 8 entitled *Environmental and Occupation Health and Safety* provides an introduction to environmental and occupational health and safety. We argue that the environment, be it one's living environment, climate, or work environment is a key social determinant of health and well-being. In concert with current evidence on the subject matter, we do not dichotomize the two but believe they are inseparable when viewed from a social determinant perspective on health. This is in concert with current national, provincial/territorial, and national definitions of health and our understanding of the critical role that one's environment plays in health outcomes for individuals, groups, communities, or entire nations. In addition, key concept and terms in the fields of toxicology are highlighted. Canadian legislations to protect the environment and workers (e.g., WHMIS), and various associated common environmental and occupational issues are also addressed in this chapter (e.g., climate change and global warming). We examine a variety of select environmental (e.g., lead, mercury, DDT) and occupational (e.g., work-related injuries and disabilities, work-related stress) health-related issues and concerns in Canada and globally. We introduce an easy to understand and implement six-step environmental and occupational risk assessment framework for public health.

Chapter 9 entitled *Global Health: A Primer* provides the reader with an introduction to global health and how it influences the health of Canadians across the lifespan. We argue that health should now be regarded as a global affair, as opposed to just regional or local issue per se. The student will be able to recognize and describe potential social, cultural, economic, and political factors affecting global health outcomes in terms of leading causes of mortality and morbidity in developed and developing countries and/or regions of the world. In addition, millennium development goals, concepts such as globalization and technology and their impact on health are highlighted. In addition, various common global burden of disease measures (e.g., HALE, HeaLy, QALYs,), neglected tropical diseases (e.g., malaria, leprosy, river blindness), and current and emerging health issues are discussed.

Chapter 10 entitled *Program Planning and Evaluation in Public Health* helps to consolidate the previous chapters by emphasizing the application of public health theory and various concepts covered in the previous chapters in regard to program planning and evaluation. Various types of program planning (e.g., strategic, operational) and evaluations (e.g., formative, process, summative) are described with salient examples of each provided. We introduce a user-friendly eight-step framework for program planning and evaluation in public health. We describe how program logic models may be utilized by public health care professionals and workers to assess the impact of public health programs in Canada and globally. We examine the importance of health services research and outcomes research in this field. Lastly, we explore various ethical considerations for public health professionals and workers in reference to program planning and evaluation and public health practice. Various ethical principles relevant to the practice of public health are explored. We argue that for public health ethics to contribute to effective program planning and evaluation, policy and practice, it must be understood in the context of an applied ethics that is relevant to all public health professionals, workers, and stakeholders concerned.

Chapter 11 entitled *Current and Emerging Mental Health Issues in Canada* examines major mental health issues and challenges facing Canadians across the lifespan. We begin with a discussion of what is mental health and examine public health challenges as outlined by the Mental Health Commission of Canada. The importance of school-based mental health promotion and mental health first-aid training is highlighted. We critical examine major theories related to the origins of mental illness (e.g., supernatural, psychogenic and somatogenic), the General Adaptation syndrome, the impact of stress on Canadians, and effective and ineffective coping mechanisms.

Chapter 12 is entitled *Neurological Disorders: A Growing Public Health Challenge*. We begin with an overview of the human brain and nervous system, which sets a necessary foundation for various neurological disorders. We examine the growing incidence of traumatic brain injuries and concussions, especially in contact sports like hockey and football, and provide an overview of major neurological disorders affecting Canadians (e.g., Parkinson's disease, ALS, dementia and Alzheimer's disease). We critically examine the growing direct and indirect health care costs (e.g., caregiver burden) associated with caring for clients with neurological disorders.

Chapter 13 is entitled *Major Emerging and Re-emerging Infectious Diseases: A Canadian Perspective*. We first discuss what are infectious diseases and examine the chain of infection from an epidemiological and public health perspective. We provide an overview of the human immune system and discuss how both global and national surveillance systems for the detecting and tracking of emerging and re-emerging infectious diseases. Lastly, we provide a critical overview of current major infectious diseases that are impacting or have the potential to impact Canadians (e.g., Avian Flu, West Nile virus, Zika virus).

Chaper 14 is entitled *Major Non-communicable Diseases: Current and Future Challenges*. We critically examine the following 4 targeted behavioural risk factors for the development of non-communicable diseases as outlined by WHO: (i) Tobacco and smoking; (ii) physical inactivity and sedentary lifestyles; (iii) unhealthy diet and (iv) harmful use of alcohol and their relevance from a Canadian context in terms of "best buy" public health actions. A discussion on chronic disease multi-morbidity in provided. Lastly, we critically examine the following 4 target major non-communicable diseases affecting Canadians, and examine the implications for public health: (i) Cancer; (ii) cardiovascular disease; (iii), chronic respiratory diseases, and (iv) diabetes.

The chapters are written in a concise and student-friendly format that outlines to the reader the specific learning objectives. Photos, diagrams, flowcharts, tables, and figures are integrated throughout the text to reinforce key concepts. Web-based resources provide the reader with additional links to credible websites to obtain additional information on a variety of concepts. Group activity-based learning boxes are integrated throughout each chapter to promote critical discussions, debates, critical thinking, and problem-solving related to a variety of issues. Research focus boxes in each chapter help to highlight and reinforce key concepts and themes and its critical link to EIPH. Chapter review exercises at the end of each chapter further help to consolidate and apply key concepts and themes in the chapter and to further engage students in critical thinking and problem-solving activities. At the end of each chapter, a summary of key concepts, definitions, and/or themes is provided for easy review by the student. Lastly, a glossary of key terms and critical thinking questions are provided which also assists students to master key definitions and concepts and to prepare for exams and assignments.

This book will appeal to educators and students in the public and allied health sciences and is intended to address current and emerging issues in public health in Canada and global influences (e.g., climate change, West Nile virus). This textbook is written in a concise yet user-friendly format that makes the material easy to access and comprehend by the reader. Specifically, this book is intended for upper level undergraduate and graduate students who are enrolled in professional and nonprofessional health sciences degree programs such as public and community health, medicine, nursing, epidemiology, and various allied health care professions (e.g., occupational and physiotherapy) that will work in a variety of community settings. Hence, this book in intended for a broad audience of public health care professionals and workers in the health sciences and students enrolled in general and professional health-related programs. Although this text is intended for students in the health sciences, it may also be utilized as a reference for students in the social sciences including those studying health sociology and health promotion and education. This book covers the essential history, concepts, current and emerging health care issues and challenges in public health facing Canadians across the lifespan, and addresses a variety of social determinants of health and well-being that will also appeal to these readers. We invite you to partake in this exciting learning journey related to public health theory and practice in Canada.

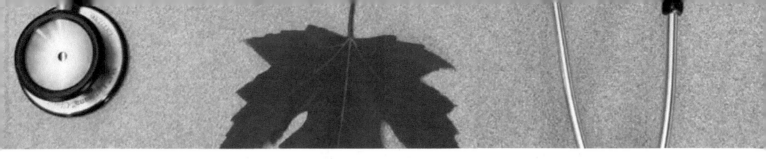

Special Features and Learning Resources

- **Learning objectives** are highlighted at the beginning of each chapter.
- **Web-based resource boxes** are integrated throughout the chapters in the text to help students and public health care professionals and workers find additional information on a variety of health-related concepts, topics, and practices and to assist with the completion of assignments.
- **A group activity-based learning boxes are integrated throughout the chapters and encourages** group thinking, negotiating and problem-solving approaches to a variety of public health issues. This feature allows students to apply theory and offer instructors with the opportunity to reinforce concepts by stimulating class discussions, group exercises, and Internet activities. The ability to work in groups and solve problems collectively is an essential skill for all public health workers and professionals in Canada.
- **Research focus boxes** features peer-reviewed articles and studies by Canadian and international researchers in public health on a variety of topics. The boxes are designed to encourage students and health care professionals to make the connections between current practice, theory, and research for EIPH.
- **Challenges and future directions** are highlighted at the end of each chapter. This section provides the reader with critical insights into future trends, issues, and challenges facing public health in Canada.
- **Group review exercise boxes** are presented near the end of each chapter to encourage students to apply theory, think critically, problem solve, and discuss current and emerging health care issues or problems. Instructors may choose to utilize these for assignments or to reinforce core concepts covered. The case studies involve Canadian and international film documentaries or investigative reports. We believe that today's students are visual learners and these documentaries help them to put a voice and context to various current and emerging public health issues.
- **Chapter summaries** are presented at the end of each chapter, which highlights key concepts in light of the learning objectives.
- **Critical thinking questions** are provided at the end of each chapter to encourage discussion, debates, and mastery of key terms and concepts.
- **Glossary of key terms** is provided to highlight key concepts and terms and to assist with the preparation of exams.

Pedagogical Features

- **Illustrations and flowcharts** are integrated throughout the text to highlight and reinforce concepts and theories covered.
- **Tables and graphs** are used to summarize key points, time lines, trends, and/or concepts covered in the various chapters.

- **Photographs and illustrations** are utilized to help reinforce core concepts and issues covered in the various chapters and provide the reader with insight into the many practice challenges and settings encountered in public health care in Canada. We believe that the students today are highly visualized learners.
- **References** are provided at the end of each chapter to facilitate access to the primary sources by instructors and students.

Instructor's Resources

- **Group activity-based learning boxes** are integrated throughout the chapters and encourage group thinking, negotiating and problem-solving approaches to a variety of public health issues. This feature allows students to apply theory and offer instructors with the opportunity to reinforce concepts by stimulating class discussions, group exercises, and Internet activities. The ability to work in groups and solve problems collectively is an essential skill for all public health workers and professionals in Canada. This feature may also be assigned by the instructor as individual assignments at their discretion.
- **Group review exercise boxes** are presented near the end of each chapter to encourage students to apply theory, think critically, problem solve, and discuss current and emerging health care issues or problems. Instructors may choose to utilize these for assignments or to reinforce core concepts covered. The case studies involve Canadian and international film documentaries or investigative reports. This feature may also be assigned by the instructor as individual assignments at their discretion.
- **Computerized test-bank** contains modifiable multiple-choice and short-answer questions and answers for each of the chapters. Users can also add their own questions. Instructors can also print out quizzes and tests in a variety of formats. Innovative electronic take-home testing (put on a disk) and Internet-based testing capabilities are perfect for distance education applications.
- **PowerPoint presentations** provide instructors with a vital resource for the core concepts and theories covered in each chapter. The presentations serve as a foundation on which instructors may customize their own unique presentations.

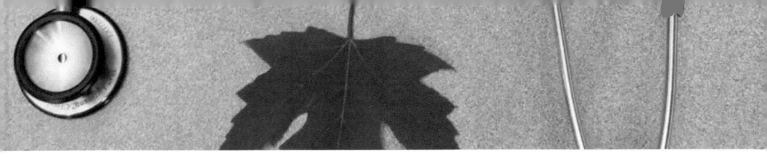

About the Authors

Dr. Wally J. Bartfay, RN, DEC, BA, BScN, MN, PhD

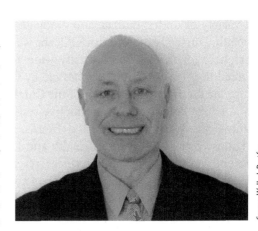

Source: Wally J. Bartfay.

Dr. Wally Bartfay's career in nursing spans more than thirty years, and he has practiced and taught nursing in four provinces in Canada and in a variety of settings including community health, mental health, medical-surgical nursing, and adult critical care and trauma services. Dr. Bartfay has taught nursing and health sciences in several institutions across Canada including Red River Community College in Winnipeg, the University of Western Ontario in London, Queen's University in Kingston, University of Windsor, and has been an associate professor in the Faculty of Health Sciences at the University of Ontario Institute of Technology (UOIT) in Oshawa since 2005. Dr. Bartfay has held various administrative positions in nursing and the health sciences, including the Director of the Cardiac Iron-overload Research Group (CIORG) at Queen's University in Kingston, Ontario, and Nursing Research Director at the University of Windsor. He was also the first Director of the Graduate Health Sciences program at UOIT. Dr. Bartfay is currently Director of the Bachelor of Allied Health Sciences and Bachelor of Health Sciences programs at UOIT.

Dr. Wally Bartfay began his career in the health sciences by first receiving his Diploma in Nursing Sciences from Dawson College (CEGEP) in Montréal, Québec. He subsequently obtained his Bachelor of Arts (BA) degree in health sociology from McGill University and his Bachelor of Science degree in Nursing (BScN) from Brandon University. He obtained his Masters of Nursing (MN) degree from the University of Manitoba with a specialization in community nursing and his Doctorate (PhD) from the Institute of Medical Science at the University of Toronto.

Dr. Bartfay has received several research grants as primary investigator or coinvestigator including grants from the Anemia Institute for Research and Education, Canadian Institute of Health Research (CIHR), Canadian Council of Cardiovascular Nurses, American Health Assistance Foundation, J. B. Bickell Foundation, and the Garfield Kelly Cardiovascular Research and Development Fund. He has over 150 publications including several peer-reviewed articles, conference proceedings, monographs, and chapters in books. He is the coauthor of the books *Public Health in Canada* (2014, Pearson) and *Community Health Nursing: Caring in Action* (2010, Nelson). Dr. Bartfay's work has appeared in national newspapers and other media and he serves as a reviewer for several nursing and other scientific journals.

Dr. Bartfay has been nominated for various teaching awards and is the recipient of various teaching awards including University of Windsor Male Teacher of the Year Award (2005); Faculty of Health Sciences Teaching Award, Queen's University (2003); and the Reddick Award for Excellence in Nursing Education, Queen's Nursing Society (2002). In addition, he is the recipient of various civil awards, including Air Canada's Honorary Flight Nurse Award for Humanitarian Emergency Services (1989) and the Meritorious Award for

Emergency Humanitarian Service (1989). He was also named to the Most Venerable Order of the Hospital of St. John of Jerusalem, Priory of Canada. Dr. Bartfay's current research interests include population and public health, noncommunicable chronic diseases, men in nursing, and the negative health effects associated with mobile information and communication technologies (ICTs) such as smartphone devices, tablets, and laptop computers.

Dr. Emma Bartfay, BSc, MSc, PhD

Dr. Emma Bartfay received her doctoral degree in Epidemiology from Western University in London, Ontario. She began her career as a research scientist at the Queen's Cancer Research Institute before joining academia in 2005 at the UOIT as an associate professor. Since then, she has developed and taught a variety of undergraduate and graduate courses in epidemiology and global health. During her tenure at UOIT, she was nominated by the Faculty of Health Sciences for the UOIT university-wide Teaching Excellence Award, and was called the "*most influential professor*" by student alumni. In addition to teaching, she is currently the Chair of the Curriculum Committee.

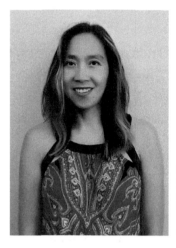

Source: Wally J. Bartfay.

Dr. Bartfay also has a productive research career, where she has received numerous research funding and awards. Most notably, she received the prestigious Ontario Ministry of Health and Long-Term Care (OMHLTC) Career Scientist Award in health services research through the Health Research Personnel Development Program open competition. As principal investigator, Dr. Bartfay has obtained many national peer-reviewed research grants from such national granting agencies as the CIHR, Canadian Health Services Research Foundation (CHSRF), Natural Sciences and Engineering Research Council of Canada (NSERC), the J. P. Bickell Foundation, the Clare Nelson Bequest Fund, and various internal grants to support her research.

Dr. Bartfay has accumulated over 100 publications, which includes international peer-reviewed journal publications, conference proceedings, chapters in books and monographs. She is also the coauthor of the book *Public Health in Canada* (2014, Pearson). Dr. Bartfay's work has appeared in national newspapers and other media, including a featured interview by the Elderbranch, a United State-based organization that acts as an information resource on matters related to the senior population, on her work in dementia care. Dr. Bartfay has also been invited and served on the editorial board and on review panel as well as reviewer for several peer-reviewed journals and research grant funding agencies, including the National Cancer Institute of Canada (NCIC). Dr. Bartfay's primary research interests include dementia care and gerontology. Most recently, she published a series of research articles in dementia diagnosis in high-impact international journals, including *Geriatric and Gerontology International, International Journal of Geriatric Psychiatry*, and *Public Health*. She is also passionate about global health issues, such as neglected tropical diseases and environmental health.

Dr. Bartfay is also an active member of the community where she contributes her expertise outside of academia. In the past, she has served on the Protocol Review Committee at the Windsor Regional Cancer Centre, the Scientific Advisory Committee at the Centre for Environmental Health of Ontario, and the Kingston, Frontenac, Lennox, and Addington Palliative Care Integration Project Evaluation Committee. Currently, she serves on the Steering Committee for the Age-Friendly Durham, a regional initiative funded by the Ontario Seniors' Secretariat. The purpose of this ongoing endeavor is to develop a plan to meet the needs of the residents and to address the challenges of the aging population in the region, based on the WHO framework of age-friendly community.

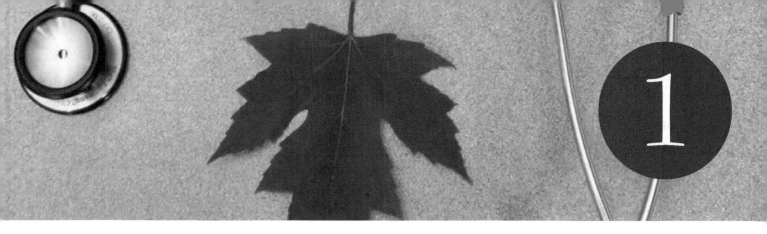

Foundations and Essential Concepts for Public Health

We cannot live only for ourselves. A thousand fibers connect us with our fellow men. And among those fibers, as sympathetic threads, our actions run as causes, and they come back to us as effects.

(Herman Melville, 1819–1891)

Learning Objectives

After completion of this chapter, the student will be able to:
- Define and describe the expanding contemporary definition of public health;
- Identify and describe the focus and major aims of public health in Canada;
- Discuss the importance of core competencies required by all public health professionals and workers in Canada;
- Describe and differentiate between the essential pillars of public health in Canada;
- List and describe the five essential pillars of public health;
- List and describe the limitations of evidence-based medicine (EBM) and practice;
- List and describe the benefits of evidence-informed public health (EIPH);
- List the nine steps of the research process and discuss its importance to the practice of public health;
- Identify and describe the five principles associated with the primary health care approach in Canada;
- Discuss how so-called *"ripple effects"* in public health may influence the health and well-being of individuals, groups, communities, or entire populations.

Core Competencies addressed in Chapter 1

Core Competencies	Competency Statements
1. Public Health Sciences	1.1, 1.2, 1.3, 1.4, 1.5
2. Assessment and Analysis	2.1, 2.2, 2.4, 2.5, 2.6
3. Policy and Program Planning, Implementation, and Evaluation	3.1, 3.2, 3.6, 3.7
4. Partnerships, Collaboration, and Advocacy	4.1, 4.2, 4.3, 4.4
5. Diversity and Inclusiveness	5.2
6. Communication	6.1, 6.2
7. Leadership	7.1, 7.2, 7.3, 7.4

Note: Please see the following document or web-based link for a detailed description of these specific competencies. Public Health Agency of Canada, *Core Competencies for Public Health in Canada: Release 1.1.* Ottawa, ON: Author, 2007. Web-based link: http://www.phac-aspc.gc.ca/core_competencies or http://www.phac-aspc.gc.ca/php-psp/ccph-cesp/pdfs/cc-manual-eng090407.pdf.

Introduction

We invite you to partake on an exciting learning journey related to public health theory, practice, and research in Canada. You will discover on your learning adventure that public health professionals and workers provide essential health care services for the promotion, preservation, and restoration of health for diverse populations across the lifespan. We focus on the unique contributions made by public health for improving the health and well-being of individuals, families, and entire communities. Public health is a critical and integral component of any functioning and comprehensive publicly funded health care system that seeks to promote and maintain health (Bartfay and Bartfay 2015; Schneider 2011; Turnock 2012). Public health and the various provincial and territorial health care systems in Canada share the common goal of attempting to maximize health and well-being and respond to actual or potential threats to the health and safety of their residents (Frank, et al. 2003). In this chapter, we shall present the five essential pillars of public health that embrace the concepts of: (i) Evidence-informed practice, (ii) health promotion and prevention, (iii) primary health care, (iv) 15 social determinants of health, and (v) the holistic health paradigm. Lastly, a discussion of the so-called "ripple effects" in public health shall be highlighted with salient examples, and how these effects may positively or negatively influence and impact on the health and quality of life of individuals, groups, communities, or entire populations.

What is Public Health?

The term "public health" often conjures up a variety of images and ideas by individuals in Canadian society and abroad. For some it means screening for communicable diseases, mass immunization programs, and legislation for healthy and safe work and public environments. For others, public health means the creation of governmental agencies, enforceable standards and legislations that ensure that we have safe food products and drinking water supplies, sustainable development, combatting the West Nile and Zika virus, and the safe disposal of toxic biological, chemical, and radioactive hazardous waste products. Finally, there are individuals who believe that public health means social justice and the empowerment of residents to make decisions and produce positive changes to improve their health-related quality of life. It may be argued that all of these perspectives are correct and valid from the current and expanding influences and mandate of public health in Canada (Butler-Jones 2001, 2012; Frank, et al. 2003; National Expert Commission Canadian Nurses Association 2012; Public Health Agency of Canada [PHAC] 2011). The primary aim of public health is to empower residents to make informed decisions and partake in interventions which seek to preserve, promote, and/or restore their health (Butler-Jones 2012; National Expert Commission Canadian Nurses Association 2012; PHAC, 2007).

Public health is defined as a holistic and evidence-informed discipline that seeks to promote; maintain, and/or restore the health and quality of life of individuals, families, communities, and/or entire populations over the lifespan through health promotion and prevention and various primary health care initiatives, activities, policies, and/or legislations (Bartfay and Bartfay 2015). Public health is also the art and science of "persuasion" for advancing and promoting the health of society at large. For example, public health professionals and workers have to utilize their personal skills (i.e., the art) to convince and encourage and persuade individuals to quit smoking, adopt a physically active lifestyle, and/or get their children immunized based the best available evidence (i.e., the science). The term **public** is employed in this chapter to denote health care services that are funded primarily via legislated tax-based or derived funds and processes. **Private**, by contrast, refers to *out-of-pocket* health care services that are paid for by an individual and/or private insurance plan or benefit (e.g., employee health benefits).

A **community** is defined as a permeable collection of citizens who interact with each other and their environment, and who share common traits, culture, qualities, features, social structures, and/or geographical boundaries (i.e., specific neighbourhoods) (Hitchcock, Schubert, Thomas and Bartfay, 2010). Members of the community gain their personal and social identity by sharing common beliefs, values and norms which have been developed by the community in the past and may be modified in the future. They also exhibit some awareness of their identify as a group or collective, and share common needs and a commitment to meeting them (WHO, 1988). **Community health** is a discipline within public health which concerns itself with the study and improvement of the health characteristics of communities that tend to focus on geographical areas or boundaries, rather than on populations with shared characteristics (Goldman, Brunnell and Posner, 2014; WHO, 2004).

Nanotechnologies that seek to build biological machines on the molecular or subatomic scale, human genomics, stem-cells, and other laboratory-based health care innovations that advance our understanding of human disease and their management often captures the imagination and awe of the public (Bartfay and Bartfay 2015). These innovations in science along with the services provided in acute care hospitals in various communities across Canada and globally are undeniably important. Nonetheless, these often pale in effectiveness to prevent disease and injury, or to maintain and promote health compared to the most rudimentary public health interventions, strategies, and policies (e.g., improvements in sanitation and water quality, mandatory seat belt legislations, food safety laws including the pasteurization of raw milk before sale) (McKeown 1976; Naidoo and Wills 2004; Rutty and Sullivan 2010). In fact, it has been estimated that some 75% of "good health" is the result of factors beyond episodic care provided in acute care hospitals (National Expert Commission Canadian Nurses Association 2012; Standing Senate Committee on Social Affairs, Science and Technology, Subcommittee on Population Health 2009). The reader is referred to Chapter 2 for a detailed discussion surrounding this essential concept.

For example, various global public health immunization initiatives and campaigns during the twentieth century has significantly decreased the incidence of various preventable communicable (a.k.a. infectious) diseases (e.g., smallpox, rabies, measles, mumps, rubella), and has saved millions of lives (Schneider 2011; Turnock 2012; World Health Organization [WHO] 2009). Immunization in the twenty-first century remains one of the most efficient and cost-effective public health programs to prevent the development and spread of various communicable diseases (e.g., smallpox, influenza, measles, mumps, rubella, tuberculosis, hepatitis A and B) in Canada and internationally (Jo Damazo and Bartfay 2010; PHAC 2012). In fact, every $1.00 spent on immunization results in a $16.00 health care cost saving or a return on investment (ROI) of 1500%. Nonetheless, infectious diseases continue to kill more than fourteen million people annually, and these deaths are primarily in developing and poorer regions of the world (Heymann 2008). Approximately 72% of the Canadian population in 2010 reported

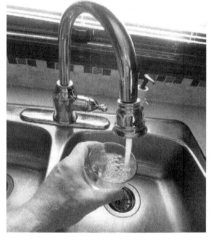

Source: Wally J. Bartfay

Photo 1.1 Access to a safe drinking water supply and proper sanitation is critical for health. Currently, 1.1 billion people around the world do not have access to a clean and safe water supply and 1:3 don't have access to a latrine or toilet (WHO/UNICEF 2015).

having received the influenza vaccination during the past two years, with the highest rates (91%) reported among seniors (Butler-Jones 2012). Similarly, in 2009, approximately 92% of two-year-olds in Canada were immunized against measles, mumps, and rubella; 83% against polio, and 77% against diphtheria (Laroche, et al. 2010).

Another major development in public health during the twentieth century for decreasing mortality and improving the health and quality of life for billions of individuals has been the realization that contaminated water supplies pose significant health risks (Schneider 2011; Turnock 2012). Indeed, ensuring a safe source of drinking water and an efficient sewage treatment infrastructure system for all residents in a community are vital components of all public health systems in Canada and internationally (Health Canada 2004; Quinlan and Dickinson 2002).

During the summer of 2000, the contamination of a community well with *E. coli 0157.57* bacteria in Walkerton, Ontario affected over 2,300 residents and resulted in seven deaths (Livernois 2002; O'Connor 2002). In 2001, an estimated 5,800 to 7,100 individuals (more than ½ of the city's population) in North Battleford, Saskatchewan were affected by an outbreak of the *Cryptosporidium* parasite due to a breakdown of the filtration system at the water treatment plant (Stirling et al., 2001). Moreover, the lack of a clean water supply and access to a proper sanitation system also significantly increases the risk for contracting schistosomiasis, trachoma,

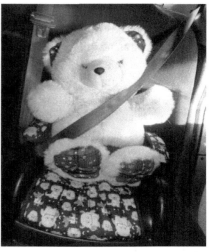

Source: Wally J. Bartfay

Photo 1.2 The introduction of mandatory seat-beat legislation as a public health intervention has had profound positive public health effects in terms of decreasing motor vehicle related injuries and deaths and associated health care costs over the past few decades (PHAC 2008a).

viral hepatitis, cholera, and dysentery. The Council of Canadians (2015) reports that as of January 2015, there were 1,838 drinking water advisories issued across Canada, including 169 advisories issued on First Nations Reserves across Canada.

In fact, seat belts were not common standard safety equipment in Canadian cars until the late 1960s, and the first law requiring mandatory seat belt use was passed in Ontario in 1976 (PHAC 2008a). By the late 1980s, all ten provinces and three territories in Canada had adopted similar legislations. Between 1975 and 2003, traffic fatalities decreased by over 50% in Canada, even though the number of cars on our roads increased significantly. It is notable that every $1.00 spent on road safety in Canada results in a $40.00 health care saving or an ROI of 3900%. We shall discuss the ripple effects associated with public health interventions and initiatives in greater detail below.

The PHAC was established in September, 2004 in response to the 2003 Severe Acute Respiratory Syndrome (SARS) outbreak in Toronto and global pandemic, which highlighted several deficiencies in our capacity to deal with such international public health issues. Dr. David Butler Jones was subsequently appointed as Canada's first Chief Public Health Officer (CPHO). The PHAC received Royal Accent by Parliament in December, 2006, which formally recognized the agency and the CPHO (PHAC 2006). This recognition also empowers the PHAC and the CPHO to introduce legislation in the interest of public health and safety. The establishment of the PHAC provides a mechanism to improve the coordination and collaboration between governmental and nongovernmental agencies (NGOs) in Canada and internationally; between the various levels of government; academia, and health researchers in various fields and disciplines. Figure 1.1 below is an organizational flowchart showing the organizational structure of the PHAC under the jurisdiction of the Minister of Health.

Currently, a variety of Canadian health centres, laboratories, and branches now report to the CPHO (PHAC 2006). These include:

- Centre for Emergency Preparedness and Response (CEPR)
- Infectious Disease and Emergency Preparedness (IDEP)

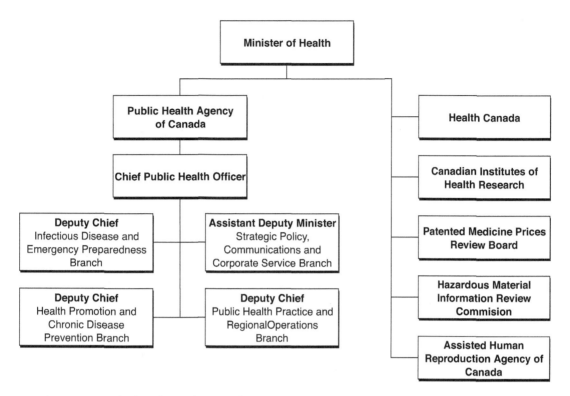

Figure 1.1 Organizational Flowchart Showing the Major Health Ministries, Institutes, Boards and Public Health Agencies in Canada

The organizational flowchart showing the roles of the Deputy Chief and the Assistant Deputy Minister who report to the CPHO. The CPHO and the PHAC reports to the federal Minister of Health.

- Laboratory for Foodborne Zoonoses
- Office of Public Health Safety
- National Microbiology Laboratory
- Pandemic Preparedness Secretariat

The PHAC also closely collaborates and shares critical health-related information, findings, and expertise with various international health agencies including the U.S. Centers for Disease Control and Prevention, European Centre for Disease Prevention and Control, and the World Health Organization.

The PHAC (2007) reports that there are critical values and principles for delivering public health to residents in Canada, which includes a commitment to equity, social justice, and sustainable development. **Social justice** is the entitlement of all Canadians to basic necessities, including adequate income and health protection and the acceptance of collective action, and an obligation to make such possible in our society (Bartfay and Bartfay 2015). This also encompasses the recognition of the importance of the health of individuals, groups, and entire communities and a respect for diversity, self-determination, empowerment of all, and active community participation.

Sustainable development encompasses environmental, economic, cultural, and socio-political sustainability for resource extraction and use by humans that seeks to meet current needs while being cognizant for the importance of preserving these limited and finite resources for use by subsequent future generations (Bartfay and Bartfay 2015).

"The link between sustainable development and public health is clear: improve human health and well-being to enable Canadians to lead economically-productive lives in a healthy environment while sustaining the environment for future generations" (PHAC 2011, 3).

The concept of sustainable development originated at the *United Nations Conference on Sustainable Development* in Rio in 2012. The objective was to produce a set of universally applicable goals that balances the three dimensions of sustainable development: (i) Environment; (ii) social, and (iii) economic (United Nations Development Programme [UNDP] 2015). The reader is referred to Chapter 9 for a detailed discussion of the eight *Millennium Development Goals* (MDGs) which originated in 2000, and the *2015: Time for Global Action Sustainable Development Goals* (SDGs) (UNDP 2015).

The *Federal Sustainable Development Strategy* (FSDS) became official legislation in 2008 and provides a legal framework for developing and implementing the FSDS by the PHAC by making environmental decision-making more transparent and accountable to the Parliament of Canada (PHAC 2011). The PHAC's Sustainable Development strategy and vision are guided by the following three principles (PHAC 2011, 4):

i.   Strengthen the capacity to improve and protect the health of Canadians and help to decrease pressures on our health care systems;

ii. Build an effective public health system that enables individuals to achieve and promote daily better health and well-being by promoting good health, preventing and controlling chronic diseases and injury, and protecting individuals from infectious diseases and other threats to their health (e.g., bioterrorism), and

iii. Reduce health disparities between the most advantaged and disadvantaged Canadians.

The PHAC seeks to accomplish this in five major ways. The first includes a long-term public health vision that incorporates a sustainable and healthy community's strategic outcome. The second is through an internal management structure which seeks to establish the capacity to provide leadership across the Agency to address priority issues, policies, programs, and initiatives. The third involves an external management structure that encourages interdepartmental working groups and committees to advance sustainable development for public health, and to introduce the notion that health should be viewed as a *"critical and viable outcome"* of sustainable development. The fourth requires integration with the Government's Core Expenditure, Planning, and Reporting System, which ensures that the activities of the PHAC are in concert with the FSDS goals, targets, and implementation strategies as mandated by law. The fifth component includes the application of analytical techniques which includes cost-benefit and multi-criteria analysis techniques, as well as the utilizing of science and evidence-informed approaches as the foundation for developing policies or other initiatives.

As part of your learning journey in public health, you will acquire the essential knowledge, theory, and foundations that all public health professionals and workers need to possess to provide safe and effective primary health care services. This chapter provides the reader with an introduction to essential concepts, practices, and effects associated with public health in Canada. An overview of the 36 core competencies deemed essential for all public health professionals and workers are highlighted (PHAC 2007). According to the PHAC (2007), public **health professionals** include physicians, nurses, public health inspectors, health promoters, epidemiologists, nutritionist, and dentist. **Public health workers** are regional or community-based health advocates who seek to promote health and well-being in its broadest form (Butler-Jones 2001; Naidoo and Wills 2004).

Public health professionals and workers practice in a variety of health care settings including rural and remote settings, urban settings, community health centres, schools, correctional settings, governmental and NGOs, environmental agencies, a variety of occupational and work settings, private homes, and community-based clinics (Bartfay 2010a; Community Health Nurses Association of Canada [CHNAC] 2003; PHAC 2007). The major roles of public health professionals and workers include, but are not limited to advocate, clinician, collaborator, consultant, case manager, educator, health promoter, policy developer, and researcher. We shall examine the diverse roles, settings, and populations in which public health professionals and workers provide health care services in Canada throughout this learning journal. Health care delivery systems, environments, population dynamics, and the various health care needs of our residents are changing at an unprecedented rate (Bartfay 2010a; Sullivan and Baranek 2002; Romanow 2002). Although we have made every attempt to provide up-to-date information regarding these developments in public health, it may not always be possible to provide current information about public health priorities, legislations, mandates, or protocols to be followed due to the dynamic and fluid nature of health in Canada and globally (e.g., the impact of the 2009–2010 H1N1 swine-flu pandemic on Canadians or banning of the chemical Bisphenol-A (BPA) in baby bottles by Health Canada in 2010). Consequently, we have provided the reader with web-based learning links and resources in each chapter of the book so that the most current information, public health protocols, or policy directives can be easily retrieved.

There have been a series of First Ministers Accords (e.g., 2000, 2003, 2004) in Canada, where a number of public health objectives and priority areas for health care funding have been identified (Dickinson 2009; National Expert Commission Canadian Nurses Association 2012). In fact, the Government of Canada has committed $21.1 billion over the next five years to the Canada Health and Social Transfer fund, including $800,000 to support the reform of primary health care services in Canada (Bartfay 2010a). To provide safe and cost-effective public

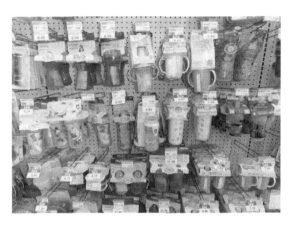

Source: Wally J. Bartfay

Photo 1.3 In September 2010, Canada became the first country in the world to declare *Bisphenol* A (BPA) a toxic substance used to harden plastic products including baby formula bottles because it is an endocrine disruptor which can mimic estrogen and may lead to negative health outcomes.

health services in Canada, all public health professionals and workers need to possess an essential knowledge and skills base (Butler-Jones 2012; Frank, et al. 2003; National Expert Commission Canadian Nurses Association 2012).

In the report entitled *Building the Public Health Workforce for the 21st Century*, the Federal/Provincial/Territorial Joint Task Group on Public Health Human Resources (Joint Task Force 2006) proposed the conception of a national framework to strengthen public health capacity. Consequently, the Federal/Provincial/Territorial Joint Task Group on Public Health Human Resources (Joint Task Group 2006; PHAC 2007) convened in January 2005 and drafted a set of core competencies for public health care workers and professionals in Canada. The Joint Task Group (2006) recommended that a pan-Canadian process be undertaken to review, validate, and/or modify these core competencies. These competencies were subsequently updated and revised in October, 2006 based on consultations, feedback, and recommendations from representatives of all levels of government in Canada, and various public health care practitioners (e.g., public health nurses, physicians, epidemiologists), agencies, and professional organizations (e.g., Canadian Medical Association, Canadian Nurses Association). This process resulted in the formulation of 36 core competencies deemed essential for all public health professionals and workers in Canada (see Appendix A). The reader is referred to the Web-based Resources Box below for a detailed list of each of these 36 core competencies with salient examples of each.

The PHAC (2007) asserts that the practice of public health embodies both an art and science, and that these noted core competencies help to define, describe, and standardize complex and multifaceted work performed by public health professionals and workers in diverse environments. These 36 core competencies are organized under the following seven broad categories: (i) Public health sciences; (ii) assessment and

Web-based Resource 1.1 The Public Health Agencies 36 Core Competencies Deemed Essential for All Public Health Care Professional and Workers

Learning Resource	Website
Public Health Agency of Canada These website details the 36 core competencies that are regarded as the essential knowledge base, skills, and attitudes necessary for the practice of public health in Canada. These competencies transcend the boundaries of specific disciplines and are independent of specific programs or topics.	http://www.phac-aspc.gc.ca/core_competencies

Web-based Resource 1.2 Canadian Community Health Nurses National Standards of Practice

Learning Resource	Website
Community Health Nurses Association of Canada (2003) This website details the standards for community health nursing practice in Canada which recognizes that caring is an essential and universal human need and that its expression in practice varies across diverse practice domains and cultures.	http://www.communityhealthnursescanada.org

analysis; (iii) policy and program planning, implementation, and evaluation; (iv) partnerships, collaboration, and advocacy; (v) diversity and inclusiveness; (vi) communication, and (vii) leadership. These interdisciplinary competencies currently provide the essential building blocks for providing safe and cost-effective primary health care services in Canada (Bartfay 2010a; Butler-Jones 2001, 2012). Interdisciplinary approaches in public health seek to build collaborative alliances and inter-sectoral partnerships at the community, regional, national, and/or international levels to maintain, promote, and/or restore health and quality of life. We further maintain that public health needs to *think globally and holistically about health based on the social determinants of health, but act locally"* (Bartfay and Bartfay 2015). We shall examine the holistic care paradigm and the social determinants of health in greater detail below.

The 36 core competencies further complement the current scope and practice of public health professionals and workers in the areas of health assessment, surveillance, disease and injury prevention, and health protection and health promotion (Advisory Committee on Population Health 2001; Joint Task Group 2006; PHAC 2007). There is a current effort to expand on these thirty-six noted competencies by developing discipline and profession specific competencies (e.g., epidemiologists, physicians, dentists, health promoters). For example, national standards of practice for community health nurses in Canada have already been developed and implemented (CHNAC 2003). The reader is referred to the Web-based Resource Box below for a detailed description of the competencies for community health nurses in Canada. The five interrelated standards for community health nursing are: (i) Promoting health, (ii) building individual and community capacity, (iii) building relationships, (iv) facilitating access and equity, and (v) demonstrating professional responsibility and accountability (CHNAC 2003).

The Five Essential Pillars of Public Health

The art and science of public health embodies and consists of the following five essential pillars (Bartfay and Bartfay 2015): (i) EIPH, (ii) health promotion and prevention, (iii) primary health care, (iv) 15 social determinants of health, and (v) the holistic care paradigm (Figure 1.2). Each of these pillars are connected and interrelated, and therefore it is argued that each must be present to meet the current and projected health care challenges facing Canadian's across the lifespan.

We also propose that the five essential pillars provide the reader with a conceptual vehicle and guide to meet the 36 core competencies deemed essential for all public health professionals and workers in Canada (PHAC 2007). If these essential pillars can be compared to the notes of a musical score, the knowledge, skills, beliefs, attitudes, proficiencies, and values that all public health professionals and workers must bring to their practice provide the tempo and personal interpretations of the musical score (Bartfay and Bartfay 2015). We shall examine each of these essential pillars in greater detail below.

Essential Pillar (i): Evidence-informed Public Health

According to the National Collaborating Centres for Public Health (NCCPH 2011, 1), **EIPH** "is the process of distilling and disseminating the best available evidence from research, practice and experience and using that

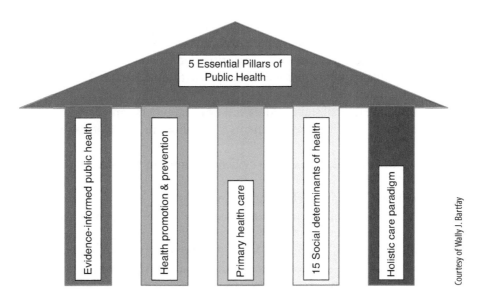

Figure 1.2 Conceptual Diagram of the Five Essential Pillars of Public Health

evidence to inform and improve public health policy and practice." During the past decade, there has been a growing consensus for the need to employ *evidence* to direct practice and policy directives in public health (Bowen and Zwi 2005; Ciliska, et al. 2008; Oxman, et al. 2007; Pach 2008; Rychetnik, et al. 2004). However, there has been little debate about what the evidence should be; how it should be appraised, and who is best to evaluate its relevance, context, and value in addressing diverse and complex health issues, settings, environments, and/or populations (Atkins et al. 2004; Guyatt et al. 2008; Jackson and Waters 2004; Pach 2008; Rychetnik et al. 2002). A common understanding is that evidence involves specific facts (actual or asserted), which is intended for use to support a specific viewpoint, goal, or conclusion. Furthermore, establishing what the *best available evidence* is requires judgment on its suitability and quality; formal debate, and consensus that it should be utilized by all stakeholders concerned for both public health practice and theory (Bartfay and Bartfay 2015).

For example, although a published study showing that a particular urban school-based intervention to decrease the incidence of childhood obesity has been reported to be effective in First Nations children, the results or outcomes achieved may not be applicable or transferable to other settings (e.g., schools located on reserves) or target populations (e.g., Inuit children, immigrants). Moreover, what should be done when the stakeholder's values disagree with the intervention selected by the public health care professional or worker? Should they attempt to persuade the stakeholder of the benefits of the intervention in question? Or should the stakeholder's preferences and values be accepted by the public health care professional and worker, and consequently suggest a different intervention based on the stakeholders unique values and preferences? In regards to the latter, clearly the best available evidence must be integrated with other factors such as values, standards, ethics, available resources, legislations, and financial considerations when justifying or considering the proposed intervention.

What is "evidence" in public health?

The term "evidence" employed in the scientific and public health literature has traditionally focused and referred to a single type of evidence by convention. That is to say, published peer-reviewed research studies. Hence, the evidence by its very nature has traditionally been contextually bound to the empirical literature, often privatized and individually interpreted (Bowen and Zwi 2005; Rycroft-Malone 2013). We argue that the nature of the evidence needs to be more fluid and inclusive in nature to be relevant to contemporary public health needs, mandates, and practice directives. This evidence may include, but is not limited to, published quantitative, qualitative, and mixed-design (hybrid) research reports from a variety of disciplines, current best-practice guidelines, legislations and policies, observations, and experiences, and both expert and lay opinions and perspectives for all stakeholders concerned. This evidence should be evaluated for its relevance and employed to identify possible interventions and priorities for action and program planning. We argue that evidence that is *significant, suitable, and applicable* should (Bartfay and Bartfay 2015):

i. Be transparent to ensure that all stakeholders and external others can examine what evidence was used to make decisions, as well as the judgments made about the evidence and its implications during the process;

ii. identify the strengths and limitations of the evidence being employed, including gaps in the available evidence at-hand;

iii. identify actual and/or potential benefits, harms, and costs;

iv. be sensitive to the specific context, environment, setting, and/or target population to which it is to be employed;

v. take into account the capacity, aptitude, and ability of individuals, families, groups, communities, or entire populations to critique, synthesize, comprehend, and utilize the evidence;

vi. recognize available community assets, limitations, and resources;

vii. consider conflicting or contradictory evidence as equally valid and potentially applicable;

viii. recognize cultural, moral, ethical, spiritual, financial, and political issues and values that may impact practice or policy decisions made; and

ix. take into account the ability and willingness of all stakeholders to mutually agree that the evidence being accessed, graded, and employed is, in fact, relevant to their unique health situation, goal, or need when planning and implementing various public health interventions, programs, or when formulating policies.

What are the Limitations of EBM and Practice?

The idea that practice in the health care professions should be based on published peer-reviewed empirical findings in the literature has its roots in EBM (Gibbs 2003; Sackett et al. 2000; Straus et al. 2005). **EBM** is defined as the conscientious, explicit, and judicious use of current best evidence in making decisions about the care of individual patients, and the practice of EBM means integrating individual clinical expertise with the best available external evidence from research studies (Davidoff et al. 1995; Grahame-Smith 1995; Sackett et al. 1996). Subsequently, the idea of employing published research investigations to guide clinical decision-making and practice has been adopted by various other health care professionals and public health over the past three decades (Atkins et al. 2013; Bowen and Zwi 2005; McCormack et al. 2013; Rycroft-Malone 2008). **Evidence-based practice (EBP)**, as the name implies, involves the critical appraisal and judicious use of published research studies in making decisions related to the care of individual patients (Nevo and Slonim-Nevo 2011; Sackett et al. 2000).

EBM and EBP encourages health care professionals and workers to conform to a five-step procedure: (i) Formulate a practice question; (ii) search for and retrieve the best published peer-reviewed scientific evidence available; (iii) critically grade and appraise the evidence; (iv) apply the findings and results; and (v) evaluate the clinical outcomes achieved in individual patients (Gibbs 2003; Sackett et al. 2000; Straus et al. 2005). Health care professionals need not, of course, conduct research themselves or gather the evidence themselves. Indeed, various empirically based investigations can easily be retrieved by searching a variety of electronic internet-based data bases (e.g., MEDLINE, PUBMED, CINAHL) or other bibliographic devices.

One of the major criticisms of EBM and EBP is that they often assume that randomized clinical trials (RCTs), meta-analyses, and systematic reviews provide the highest level of credible evidence by which to make decisions related to clinical practice or policies; whereas descriptive, observational studies, case reports, expert opinions, and those that employ qualitative (e.g., phenomenological, grounded theory) or mixed-design (hybrid) research methodologies or approaches are the weakest and least credible sources of evidence (Cullins, et al. 2005; Sawatzky-Dickson 2010). The reader is referred to Chapter 5 for a detailed description of these various research designs and approaches.

For example, let us suppose that a published statistically based meta-analysis shows that a certain public health intervention (e.g., immunization against seasonal flu) has the highest rates of success in cases of a certain kind (e.g., elderly living independently in their homes). Does this show that the *best available evidence* supports this type of intervention for all cases (e.g., children, young adults, clients with multiply chronic diseases)? Of course not! The best available evidence only suggests that the noted intervention (e.g., immunization) may potentially be applicable to similar target populations at best (e.g., elderly in nursing homes). We must always be cautious when applying correlational findings to causative outcomes in public health, no matter how highly significant or convincing the statistical data may be (Bartfay and Bartfay 2015). Some of the additional major limitations of the EBM and EBP models include the following (Bowen and Zwi 2005; McCormack et al. 2013; Nancarrow Clarke 2008; Nevo and Slonim-Nevo 2011; Rubin 2007; Rycroft-Malone 2008):

- It is often based on the mechanistic medical model of health.
- Not all research conducted is accessible because negative findings are often not published or considered applicable.
- Certain populations are often under-represented or studied (e.g., Indigenous populations, immigrants, the homeless, individuals with more than one chronic disease or condition).
- The process often lacks transparency in regards to what evidence was considered versus those that were not for decision-making, and who made these decisions per se.
- It ignores the unique characteristics, abilities, and personal assets of the health care professionals and the targeted stakeholders.
- It does not take into account the unique setting, environment, culture, finances available, politics and resources available, and contexts in which the evidence is to be evaluated and employed to guide practice or policies.
- Evidence in this context is often limited to published research reports only, which grades evidence solely on an artificial hierarchy based on the unique characteristics of the research approach utilized (i.e., quantitative, qualitative, or mixed-design) and the type of research design (e.g., RCT's, prospective cohort studies, case-control), as opposed to the specific research question, aims or goals addressed, and/or any consideration for the target population.
- Published research may not be representative of the best available evidence because of the time it takes to undertake and publish research findings.
- There is often a lack of theory-driven approaches considered, and
- researcher's funded by private-for-profit corporations (e.g., multi-national drug companies) or lobbyist may be restricted by the terms of grant to those that support the use of the intervention, device, and/or position statement financed by the company or specific lobby group in question.

What are the benefits of EIPH?

By comparison to EBM and EBP models for evidence, EIPH reflects the need to be context sensitive and considers the use of the best available evidence and knowledge from a variety of sources, disciplines, and stakeholders (Bartfay and Bartfay 2015). Considering the evidence within the unique context it is to be assessed and applied is critical for effective public health practice and policy making (Bowen and Zwi 2005; Rycroft-Malone 2008). The view of the health care professional or practitioner as the rationale agent capable of identifying, retrieving, appraising, and translating research evidence into individual practice has served as the core of EBM and EBP over the past three decades (Atkins et al. 2013; DiCenso, et al. 2005; Sackett et al. 1996). By contrast, EIPH involves a collaborative effort where public health professionals, workers, and affected stakeholders (e.g., target population, corporations, non-governmental organizations [NGO's], granting agencies, politicians) partake in a transparent process of determining what sorts of evidence are needed, and how it should be collected, appraised, synthesized, applied, and formally evaluated based on their unique needs, context, setting, and environments (Bowen and Zwi 2005; Ciliska, et al. 2010; McCormack et al. 2013; National Collaborating Centre for Methods and Tools 2012; Pach 2008). Hence, EIPH involves a mutual journey of decision-making between public health professionals and workers and the stakeholders for whom the interventions, actions, or policies are intended for. We also argue that for evidence to be adequate and meaningful as a basis for public health practice; then it must also be suitable as a basis for theory, since practice is and ought to be directed by social and scientific theories. The Research Focus Box below provides an example of a literature review spanning the years 1997 to 2007, which examined interventions and strategies to promote evidence-informed healthcare focusing on the role of change agencies.

A Model for Conducting EIPH

The *National Collaborating Centres for Public Health* at McMaster University in Hamilton, Ontario provides a seven-step model for conducing EIPH (Middlesex-London Health Unit 2013; NCCPH 2011). The first step of this process involves a clear definition of the issue, problem, or goal. This stage may be regarded as the program planning stage where all stakeholders mutually agree on the specific public health issue, problem, or goal they wish to address.

Program planning is defined as an organized and structured systematic decision-making process which attempts to meet specific primary health care aims or objectives through the application of currently available, and competing or needed resources in the future based on identified priorities or projected needs

---

Research Focus Box 1.1

A realist review of interventions and strategies to promote evidence-informed healthcare: A focus on change agency

Study Aim/Rationale:
To examine published literature related to change agency in its various forms as an intervention aimed to improve the effectiveness of the uptake of evidence. Facilitators, knowledge brokers, and opinion leaders are examples of change agency strategies employed to promote knowledge utilization in this context.

Methodology/Design:
A literature review spanning the years 1997 to 2007 was conducted to answer the following key question: What change agency characteristics work, for whom do they work, in what circumstances and why? Change agency was operationalized by the authors as roles that were aimed at effecting successful change in both individuals and organizations. A theoretical framework was developed through stakeholder consultation that formed the basis for the literature search. Working in small subgroups, team members independently themed the available data, and developed chains of inference to form a series of hypotheses related to change agency and its employment for knowledge utilization.

Major Findings:
A total of 24,478 electronic-based references were initially identified for search strategies. Preliminary screening of these potential sources and titles reduced the list of 196 potentially relevant peer-reviewed articles. Subsequently, a critical review of these potential articles resulted in a final list of fifty-two relevant sources. These findings add to the knowledge of change agency; how change agents' function, their individual characteristics, and how change agents affect evidence-informed health care. The findings also provide insight into how change agents influence the setting and their overall effect on knowledge utilization.

Implications for Public Health:
The findings highlight the importance of reflection on practice and the role of modeling. The findings from this study also highlight the complexity and diversity of the change agency literature; poor indexing of the literature, and a lack of theory-driven approaches. Particular issues such as how accessible the change agent is; their cultural compatibility, and their attitude to effectively mediate are highlighted.

Source: McCormack, B., J. Rycroft-Malone, K. Decorby, A. M. Hutchinson, T. Bucknall, B. Kent, A. Schultz, et al. "A Realist Review of Interventions and Strategies to Promote Evidence-Informed Healthcare: A Focus on Change Agency," *Implementation Science* 8, no. 1 (2013): 107. PMID: 240710732.

(Bartfay and Bartfay 2015). The establishment of health care needs or priorities may be situational (e.g., aging population trends in Canada), reactive (e.g., SARS), or predictive in nature (e.g., immunization against seasonal flu strains). Current trends in health system funding are making painfully clear that each public health intervention or program funded involves cost-benefit analysis outcomes and the prediction of its impact factor for public health. One of the major challenges facing public health is how to convince governments and officials for the need to invest in public health promotion initiatives and programs that seek to "prevent" the occurrence of negative health events or outcomes in the future (e.g., pandemic preparedness, health promotion programs to combat childhood obesity to decrease the likelihood of developing chronic disease such as heart disease or diabetes as adults). For example, only 7% of children and youth, or 9% of boys and 4% of girls in Canada, are currently meeting national recommended guidelines for physical activity comprised of sixty minutes of moderate to vigorous to intense activity daily (Active Healthy Kids Canada 2014; Statistics Canada 2013). A lack of physical activity has been linked to childhood obesity and development of various chronic noncommunicable diseases in adulthood (e.g., type 2 diabetes, certain forms of cancer, hypertension, heart disease, and stroke).

Quantitative questions regarding the effectiveness of possible public health interventions should consist of the following four elements: (i) **P**opulation, (ii) **I**ntervention, (iii) **C**omparison, and (iv) **O**utcome (PICO) (NCCPH 2011; Sawatzky-Dickson 2010). Whereas questions that are quantitative in nature and relate to exposure should include: **P**opulation; **E**xposure, **C**omparisons and **O**utcome (PECO). Questions that are qualitative in nature should identify the target **P**opulation and **S**ituation (PS).

The second step of this model involves searching for and locating evidence that best addresses the specific public health issue, problem, or goal identified. The reader is referred to the Web-based Resources Box below for examples of various forms of evidence that may be accessed by public health professionals and workers.

Web-based Resources 1.3

Learning Resource	Website
Canadian Best Practices Portal (PHAC) Created and managed by the PHAC, this portal contains a searchable database of community-based interventions which have been evaluated and shown to be effective. This portal also provides public health care professionals and workers with several helpful links and evidence-informed resources.	http://cbpp-pcpe.phac-aspc. gc.ca/
National Collaborating Centres for Public Health (November, 2011). What is evidence-informed Public Health? This website provides a definition of EIPH, describes why it should be implemented for public health practice and policy making, and outlines a seven-step model of EIPH.	http://www.nccmt.ca/eiph/
Middlesex-London Health Unit, (2013). Evidence-informed public health. This resource describes the types of evidence to be considered for public health practice and policy making and lists various helpful resources and databases.	https:www.healthunit. com/evidence-informed-public-health
TRIP Database TRIP is a clinical search engine designed to allow users to quickly and easily find and use high-quality research evidence to support their practice and/or care, which has been online since 1997.	http://www.tripdatabase. com/
World Health Organization (WHO)/Europe This portal provides the user with access to various health statistics and to detailed monitoring and assessment tools for key areas of health policy. These links also provide access to a broad range of information systems: from international comparisons of aggregate indicators to the results of detailed disease surveillance and the monitoring of specialized areas of health policy.	http://www.euro.who.int/ en/ data-and-evidence/ databases

The third step involves critically appraising the evidence collected in terms of its relevance or fit. Step four involves synthesizing the evidence and deciphering the "actionable messages" contained in the evidence as a whole. The fifth step involves adapting the information to the local context and situation. Once actionable messages have been derived, they can be tailed to ensure their relevance, suitability, and context for the specific stakeholders they are planned for. The sixth stage of this model consists of implementing the best available adapted evidence to create a change in public health practice, to deliver a new program or service, policy, and/or legislation. The final stage of this model consists of formally evaluating the effectiveness of your implementation efforts. The reader is referred to Chapter 10 for a detailed discussion on how to conduct formal and systematic program planning and evaluations in public health.

The importance of research in public health

In 2007, the federal government launched a national science and technology strategy entitled *Mobilizing Science and Technology to Canada's Advantage* with the objective of promoting research that addresses challenges in the health sciences and other areas (Health Council of Canada 2011; Science, Technology and Innovation Council 2009). Partnerships and collaborations are a key part of how these federal agencies and initiatives work in addressing health care challenges facing Canadians across the lifespan.

Research is of little value unless the findings are employed to improve public health practice, health outcomes, and health services access, delivery, and utilization. Public health care systems in Canada are being confronted by a variety of challenges. Public health professionals and policy makers are increasingly becoming responsive and accountable to the health care needs of our residents due to escalating costs, access to care issues, quality and the availability of health care resources and available funds (Bartfay 2010; Bartfay and Bartfay 2015). It is therefore critical that public health professionals and workers define their many contributions and the impact factor of these inventions in their communities by utilizing the research process effectively.

The **research process** consists of a series of steps and techniques used to structure a study and to gather, analyze, interpret, disseminate, and apply data and information in a systematic and formalized fashion (Bartfay and Bartfay 2015). Each step of the research process is logically linked to each other, as well as to the conceptual or theoretical foundations of the investigation (Burns and Grove 2007; Polit and Tatano Beck 2008). The nine steps of the research process are: (i) Identify a problem of concern; (ii) conduct a review of the available scientific literature; (iii) formulate clear research questions or hypotheses; (iv) design a study which addresses your research questions or hypotheses; (v) get ethical approval and funding for the study; (vi) collect data (qualitative, quantitative, or mixed-design); (vii) analyze the data; (viii) identify the strengths and limitations of the study; and (ix) disseminate (e.g., town hall meetings, conferences, publications) and apply the research findings (Bartfay and Bartfay 2015).

Qualitative research involves a holistic and subjective process used to describe and to promote a better understanding of human experiences and phenomena via the collection of rich narrative data, and to develop conceptual models and theories that seek to describe these experiences and phenomena (Bartfay and Bartfay 2015). For example, Porter (2005) conducted a qualitative study employing a phenomenological approach to evaluate the lived experiences of home care for elderly widows living in their communities. This investigation provides important insights into homecare services for the elderly and helps to facilitate an understanding of the growing problem of maintaining their independence in their homes and community.

Quantitative research is a formal, precise, systematic, and objective process in which numerical data are used to obtain information on a variety of health-related phenomenon of interest or concern (Bartfay and Bartfay 2015). For example, Olney (2005) conducted a quasi-experimental study to assess the effects of back massage taught by public health nurses to family members of hypertensive clients and its effect on blood pressure readings. The researcher found that ten minutes of back massage daily significantly decreased both systolic and diastolic blood pressure readings in these hypertensive clients.

Research provides the essential knowledge base that enables public health professionals' and workers to meet current and anticipated future public health care needs and challenges. For example, through a partnership between the PHAC and the Canadian Institutes of Health Research, the federal government committed $10.8 million over

---

Group Activity-based Learning 1.1

How can research contribute to the practice of public health?
The Group Activity-based Learning Box below highlights the importance of employing peer-reviewed research articles for the basis of current public health practice in Canada and abroad by various health care professionals and workers. Working in small groups of three to five students, discuss and answer the following questions:

1. Locate a current peer-reviewed article in the public health sciences on a topic of interest to you (e.g., immunizations, West Nile virus, growing obesity rates in youth, cyberbullying, food safety in Canada, etc.).

2. Discuss how the findings/outcomes of this research paper may be utilized to improve public health practice in your community?

---

a three period in 2009 to support a pan-Canadian influenza research network with the objective of strengthening Canada's capacity to prepare for a global influenza pandemic (Canadian Institutes for Health Research 2009; Health Council of Canada 2011). Research is also critical for linking public health theory, education, and practice in Canada and abroad. Public health professionals and workers need to be intelligent and critical consumers of published research investigations and government reports and participate in the research process at multiple levels.

Essential Pillar (ii): Health Promotion and Prevention

Health promotion and prevention is the second essential pillar of public health. The Public Health Agency of Canada defines the concept of **health promotion** as:

"The process of enabling people to increase control over, and to improve their health. It not only embraces actions directed at strengthening the skills and capabilities of individuals, but also action directed towards changing social, environmental, political and economic conditions so as to alleviate their impact on public and individual health". (PHAC 2007, 11–12).

Health promotion activities enhance and/or reinforce the ability of an individual, family, group, community, or entire population to take control and maintain, improve or restore their health and quality of life (McKenzie, et al. 2009; Naidoo and Wills 2004; Raphael 2010; Rootman et al. 2012). The *Ottawa Charter for Health Promotion* (WHO 1986) describes five key strategies for health promotion: (i) Build healthy public policy; (ii) create supportive environments; (iii) strengthen community action; (iv) develop personal skills; and (v) reorient health services. Priority areas include reducing inequalities in wealth and income distribution; strengthening communities by building alliances to improve unhealthy living conditions; supporting environments that promote healthy lifestyles, and promoting community development. The Charter notes that *health is created in the context of everyday life*, which includes *where people live, love, work, and play*. We believe that this is the most important concept that emerged out of the Charter. That is to say, health occurs within the context and situation of the environment in which we "live, love, work and play," as opposed to health care systems or acute care facilities. We argue that through various health promotion efforts, individuals, families, groups, and entire communities develop and foster a critical understanding of the determinants of health from a holistic perspective, while developing skills to maintain or improve their health related quality of life. Fran Baum of the *International Commission of the Social Determinants of Health* notes:

"The health promotion movement has the possibility of re-inventing itself in the twenty-first century to offer the holistic understanding of health, the skills, passion and commitment required to be the core of a social movement which advocates for new healthy, equitable and sustainable economic and social structures globally and within countries" (Baum 2008, 464).

Over the past four decades, we have learned that health is determined, achieved, maintained, and/or improved by a variety of interconnected factors and states of existence that must be examined from a holistic perspective. These go beyond access to acute episodic-types of health care to include a broad spectrum of social, political, cultural, and economic determinants (e.g., the association between lower incomes and poorer health outcomes) (National Expert Commission Canadian Nurses Association 2012; Standing Senate Committee on Social Affairs, Science and Technology, Subcommittee on Population Health 2009). These factors include such things as having an active lifestyle (as opposed to a sedentary one); eating a nutritious balanced diet (low in salt, fat, sugar, and processed foods); affordable housing; employment and working conditions; proper disposal of sanitary wastes, and access to clean and safe drinking water supplies, to name but a few. Other aspects of our lives such as where we live, how much support we get from family and friends, what we choose to eat, and our level of physical activity can all affect how healthy we are at different moments in time (Canadian Institute for Health Information [CIHI] 2007).

Section 3 of the Canada Health Act (CHA) supports the concept of health promotion including protective, promotive, and preventive health care services, although the specific methods of implementing and delivering health promotion services on a national level are not described in the Act (Government of Canada 1984). Moreover, the components of health promotion are currently not required in order for the ten provinces and three territories in Canada to conform to the criteria of the CHA or to qualify for federal transfer funds (Bartfay 2010b). Therefore, the extent to which each provincial or territorial government provide public health promotion services varies considerable in quality and quantity across Canada (Romanow 2002; Sullivan and Baranek 2002). The reader is referred to Chapter 3 for a detailed description of the CHA.

Healthy Cities Movement Example

The *Healthy Cities Movement*, which originated in Canada but has come to fruition in Europe, provides a salient example of a well-developed policy-oriented approach promoting health across the lifespan based on a holistic and ecological vision of health (WHO 2003; WHO Regional Office for Europe 2003). According to this vision of health, a healthy city is one that:

> " . . . is engaged in a process of creating, expanding and improving those physical and social environments and community resources which enable people to mutually support each other in performing all the functions of life and developing to their maximum potential" (Hancock and Duhl 1988, 41).

In Canada, the Healthy Cities Movement was initially known as the "Healthy Communities Movement" as an attempt to include municipal communities of all sizes (e.g., cities, towns) (O'Neill et al. 2012). This movement in Canada has been operating mostly as a set of provincial networks, as opposed to a unified pan-Canadian movement per se. In 2010, four networks of Healthy Communities were present in Acadian New Brunswick, Québec, Ontario, and British Columbia (Deplancke 2009; Hancock 2009). Although there are some variations, these four networks all rely on the principles promoted by the WHO; including the need for community participation, multi- and intersectorial partnerships, political commitment of local authorities, and implementation of healthy public policies (O'Neill et al. 2012). Although the provinces of Newfoundland, Nova Scotia, Manitoba, Saskatchewan, and Alberta were involved in the Healthy Communities movement or similar programs, they did not have formal networks in place to coordinate these efforts.

A *Healthy Cities* project consists of the following six key characteristics (Hancock and Duhl 1988; WHO 2003; WHO Regional Office for Europe 2003). The first involves a commitment to health based on a holistic understanding of this concept; where health can be created through cooperative efforts of individuals, families, and groups in the city or community. We shall explore the holistic care paradigm in greater detail below. The second entails political decision-making to promote public health. These include programs related to housing, the environment, education, and social programs and other known social determinants of health (SDH). The third component involves inter-sectoral action by which organizations (e.g., NGO's) working outside of the health sector can contribute to health. The fourth characteristic involves community participation in health through lifestyle choices, their use of health services, their views and perspectives on various health issues, and their active work and participation in community groups to promote health in their cities and communities. The fifth component requires the process of innovation to promote health and prevent the development of disease via inter-sectoral action that involves a constant search for new and creative ideas, methods, and solutions. The Healthy Cities projects create opportunities for innovation within a climate that supports change and innovation. The last critical component of the Healthy Cities Movement involves the development and implementation of healthy public policies. The various projects achieve their noted goals when homes, workplaces, schools, and other environments and components of the city or community become healthier settings in which to *"live, work, love and play."*

The Healthy Cities Movement has now grown beyond the borders of Canada and has become a vast international movement currently involving thousands of cities and communities on all major continents (O'Neill et al. 2012; De Leeuw 2009). The *Belfast Declaration* provides the latest insights related to the Healthy Cities Movement, which emphasizes the importance of building and fostering collaborative partnerships at all levels, and of good governance

Photo 1.4 Health Canada has enacted national legislation (i.e., primordial prevention) requiring that visible health warnings be placed all tobacco products sold in Canada to both discourage potential new smokers (i.e., primary prevention) from taking-up the highly addictive habit, and to persuade current smokers (i.e., secondary prevention) to quit smoking. Every $1.00 spent on tobacco prevention in Canada results in a $20.00 saving for health care or a return on investment (ROI) of 1900%.

(WHO 2003). Some of the specific priority areas of action include reducing inequalities and addressing poverty, assessing the impacts of various health-related policies, and taking an active role in shaping and implementing strategies which promote health across the lifespan. However, cities and communities cannot act alone or not be affected by external factors. Indeed, regional, provincial/territorial, and national governments along with other stakeholders (e.g., NGO's, business, and industry) must also be cognizant of the fact that various regional, provincial/territorial, or national policies may also have negative or positive health ripple effects on a local dimension. We must be cognizant of these external factors and acknowledge their mutual and interconnected relationships. We shall discuss the ripple effects in public health in greater detail below.

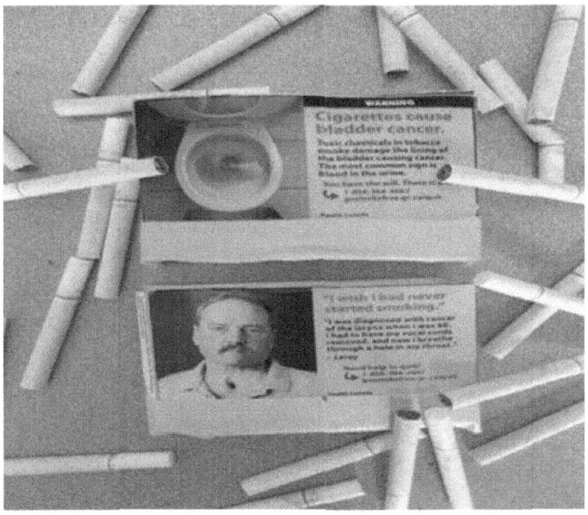

The Five Levels of Prevention

Prevention is defined as actions, measures, interventions, programs, policies, and/or legislations which seek to avert the development or progression of disease or possible harm, injury, disability, or death and improve, maintain, and/or restore health-related quality of life across the lifespan (Bartfay and Bartfay 2015). The scope and levels of prevention have changed over time, and there are currently five formally recognized levels of prevention (Bartfay and Bartfay 2015; Kuehlein et al. 2010; Porta 2008; Public Health Action Support Team 2011; Starfield, et al. 2008): (i) Primordial; (ii) primary; (iii) secondary; (iv) tertiary, and (v) quaternary. The reader is referred to Table 1.1 below which provides definitions for the five levels of prevention and examples of each.

The types and levels of prevention identified in the public and allied health literature have expanded over the past seven decades. A model comprised of three levels of prevention (i.e., primary, secondary, and tertiary) was first proposed by Leavell and Clark during the late 1940s from the Harvard and Columbia Schools of Public Health, respectively (Leavell and Clark 1958). Initially, prevention was influenced by the mechanistic medical model of health and therefore prevention activities focused on disease or pathological states only. For example, Clark and MacMahon (1967) defined prevention as "averting the development of a pathological state" and included all measures that "limit the progression of disease at any stage of its course." During this period, a distinction was made between medically based interventions that averted the occurrence of disease

Table 1.1 The Five Levels of Health Prevention

Level	Types	Definition	Examples
1	Primordial	Consists of conditions, actions, and measures that minimize hazards to health and that inhibit the emergence and establishment of process and factors known to increase disease, alterations to health, injury, and/or death.	– Legislation banning smoking in public places and the mandatory wearing of seat belts – Policies to reduce urban air pollution, including encouraging the planting of trees and the use of public transportation.
2	Primary prevention	Consists of preventative approaches and interventions that seek to avert the occurrence of alterations to health, and to prevent disease, injury or disabilities	– Immunization of a child with the measles, mumps, and rubella (MMR) vaccine. – Public and school-based health promotion program to encourage children to exercise and make healthy foods choices to help prevent childhood obesity.
3	Secondary prevention	Consists of activities that are aimed at early detection, diagnosis, and treatment of a condition, disease, or altered state of health, and consists of interventions which seek to stop or reverse further processes associated with this altered state of health and advocacy for accessible diagnostic and treatment services for vulnerable populations such as the elderly, Indigenous peoples, and homeless.	– Screening sexually active teenagers for the presence of sexually transmitted infections (STI's). – Vision screening of primary grade students by public health nurses in various school districts. – Isolation and quarantine to reduce the transmission of communicable agents and break the chain of infection. – Testing for hearing loss and advice concerning protection against noise in industrial workers. – Prophylaxis such as providing high risk pregnant women with the varicella-zoster immune globulin (VGIG) to protect her from acquiring varicella or lessen the symptoms if the disease occurs to protect the fetus in utero.
4	Tertiary prevention	Consists of activities that are aimed at preventing further deterioration or progress of an altered state of health or condition.	– Providing health education related to home-based monitoring of glucose levels and insulin administration for individuals with type 2 diabetes. – Providing exercise and physiotherapy to an individual recovering from a stroke. – Administering direct observed therapy (DOT) for prescribed medications for a client with tuberculosis (TB) by a public health nurse to reduce the risk of developing drug-resistant TB, which could place their family members, coworkers, or community at large at risk

(Continued)

Table 1.1 The Five Levels of Health Prevention (*Continued*)

Level	Types	Definition	Examples
5	Quaternary	Consists of a group of actions and measures which seek to prevent, monitor, decrease, and/or alleviate possible harm or adverse effects (a.k.a. iatrogenic effects) caused by health interventions, treatments, diagnostic procedures, medications and/or programs.	– Protecting vulnerable groups (e.g., uneducated, homeless, elderly) from over-diagnosis, being excessively medicated or other interventions that may result in negative alternations to health and safety (e.g., hospital acquired infections) via awareness educational sessions and workshops for health care professionals and stakeholders. – Banning of physical restraint devices in long-term nursing homes for the elderly residents with dementia to decrease associated anxiety and harm. – Avoidance of unnecessary screening and diagnostic procedures for bowel cancer in low risk individuals (e.g., no family history, aged 18 to 49 years).

(i.e., primary prevention); interventions that sought to halt or slowdown the progression of disease (i.e., secondary prevention), and those that attempted to limit the impact of impairments (i.e., tertiary prevention) (Clark and MacMahon 1967; Starfield et al. 2008). By the year 1978, the distinction between three levels of prevention had expanded to include primary prevention interventions which seek to promote health before the development of disease or injuries; secondary prevention activities that incorporated early detection of disease during the asymptomatic stages; and tertiary prevention that sought to arrest, reverse, or delay the progression of disease states, impairments, or conditions (Beaglehole, et al. 1993; National Public Health Partnership [NPHP] 2006; Nightengale, et al. 1978; Starfield et al. 2008).

During the past decade, primordial and quaternary prevention have been added to the levels of prevention. The term "primordial prevention" was first coined in 1978 by Strasser, who was the former Chief Officer of the Cardiovascular Division of the WHO (Strasser 1978). Primordial prevention involves actions and measures that seek to eradicate, eliminate, and/or minimize the impact of disease, injury, or disability and includes health policies and legislations (B.C. Ministry of Health 2013; Kindig 2011; Kuehleim et al. 2010; Public Health Action Support Team 2011). The term "quaternary prevention" was first coined Jamoulle and Rolande in 1995 at the *Wonca World Conference* in Hong Kong, and was based on the concept of "doing no harm" to the patient via excessive medical interventions or procedures, which included diagnosis and over treatments of medical conditions (Berleur et al. 1986; Kuehlein et al. 2010; Jamoulle and Roland 1995). The term has been expanded to now include iatrogenic interventions as well, which results from various health care interventions, procedures, programs, and/or policies. The term **iatrogenic** literally means "doctor generated," but it's definition has been expanded to include all adverse effects associated with diagnostic procedures, medical, surgical, nursing, or other allied health interventions, and the over prescription of medications (Elder and Davey 2002; Porter 2008; Mitty 2010; Vasilevskis et al., 2010). For example, Mitty (2010) reports that 65% of older residents in nursing homes are at risk for iatrogenesis resulting from adverse drug interactions, especially if they are also frail and have one or more geriatric syndromes.

Prevention remains a key component of various public health goals, activities, practices, and policies in Canada (Bartfay and Bartfay 2015). One of the major challenges facing Canadians in the next few decades will be to determine public health priorities related to prevention, and conceptualizing the concept of prevention as a set of mutually linked and connected primary health care activities that seek to improve, maintain, or restore quality of life over the lifespan.

For example, in 1969, a study by the *National Advisory Council for Fitness and Amateur Sport* found that the majority of Canadians were sedentary in nature, unfit and alarmingly uninterested in the health benefits associated with exercise (ParticipACTION 1969; Rutty and Sullivan 2010). As a result of this study, a federally funded national public health primary prevention initiative aptly coined "ParticipACTION" was launched in 1971 to promote active and healthy lifestyles with the aim of preventing health problems and chronic disease associated with inactivity, sedentary lifestyles and obesity (Thompson 2010; Rutty and Sullivan 2010). Federal cut backs resulted in the shut-down of this national public health primary prevention campaign in 2001. The program was reinstigated six years later in February 2007 due to alarming reports that over half of Canadians were overweight or obese and sedentary in nature (Canadian Society for Exercise Physiology 2012).

Current findings suggest that only 7% of Canadian children and youth are meeting the recommended guideline of at least sixty minutes of moderate to vigorous physical activity daily (Active Healthy Kids Canada 2014; Statistics Canada 2013). Between 1978/1979 and 2004, the combined prevalence of overweight and obese Canadians aged two to seventeen years increased from 15% to 26%, respectively. Moreover, 59% of Canadian adults are either overweight or obese. Notably, it is predicted that if the current trends continues, by the year 2040 up to 70% of adult Canadians will be either obese or overweight (Childhood Obesity Foundation 2015). The PHAC (2015) reports that 48% of Canadian adults report being inactive, meaning that their level of physical activity was not sufficient to meet the threshold of at least moderate activity. In fact, adults should be active for at least 2.5 hours per week to achieve health-related benefits, including weight control, decreased stress levels, and reductions in associated risks for developing various chronic noncommunicable diseases (e.g., heart disease, stroke, diabetes, certain cancers).

In July 2015, Rona Ambrose, the Minister of Health, announced funding of $2.5 million toward a pilot project to decrease the risk of chronic noncommunicable disease and increase active healthy living (PHAC 2015). In collaboration with the Government of British Columbia, the UPnGo with ParticipACTION pilot project encourages adults to take up the challenge to walk thirty minutes daily for twenty-three consecutive days, which is the time typically reported to develop new habits. We argue that to ensure "better health" for all individuals across the lifespan in Canada and globally requires a radical paradigm shift in thinking related to five levels of prevention based on the SDH; rather than on preventing specific target diseases or health conditions that have been the focus during the past five decades, especially in vulnerable populations (e.g., elderly, immigrants, Indigenous populations, the poor, and homeless) (Bartfay and Bartfay 2015).

Essential Pillar (iii): Primary Health Care

Primary health care is the third essential pillar for public health. We hear the term *"primary health care"* employed frequently in public health circles, but the concept is still poorly understood due in part to the confusion between the terms *"primary care"* and *"primary health care."* Simply put, **primary** care is what an individual receives when they visit their health care provider for advice or treatment of a disorder or ailment (Butler-Jones 2012; Dykeman 2012; National Expert Commission Canadian Nurses Association 2012). By contrast, the **primary health care approach** is defined as a model of health care that emphasizes equity, accessibility, full participation by individuals and communities, the use of universally acceptable and affordable technologies and methods, inter-sectoral collaboration, and is based on practical, scientifically sound and socially acceptable health care approaches and interventions which embrace the following five types of health care: (i) Promotive, (ii) preventive, (iii) curative, (iv) rehabilitative, and (v) supportive/palliative (Bartfay and Bartfay 2015).

Hence, offering public health care from a primary health care perspective means providing less fragmented and acute episodic care, and more continuous and ongoing care to manage complex health care issues and challenges facing Canadians. This includes the recognition for the need to become educated and involved about various social, political, cultural, and environmental issues that affect health. A major goal of primary health care in Canada is to build community capacity to achieve sustainable health through health promotion

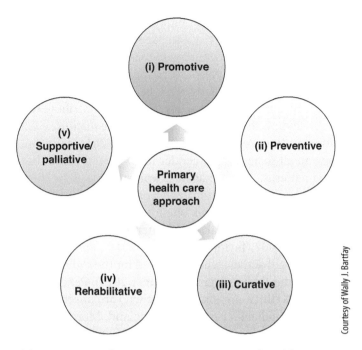

Courtesy of Wally J. Bartfay

Figure 1.3 The Primary Health Care Approach Encompasses Five Types of Health Care

efforts, as first detailed in the Ottawa Charter for Health Promotion (Frank and Smith 1999; WHO Health & Welfare Canada & CPHA 1986). Figure 1.3 above provides a conceptual representation of the five types of health care associated with the primary health care approach.

The term *"primary health care"* has traditionally been used interchangeably or confused with similar terms such as *"health promotion"* and *"prevention."* Accordingly, the WHO held a conference at Alma Ata in the former Soviet Union (U.S.S.R.) in 1978 to clarify and standardize the term globally. Delegates at this conference defined primary health care as follows:

> **"Primary health care** is essential care based on practical, scientifically sound and socially acceptable methods and technology made universally accessible to individuals, and families in the community through their full participation and at a cost that the community and country can afford to maintain at every stage of their development in the spirit of self-reliance and self-determination . . . It is the first level of contact of individuals, the family, and community with the national health system, bringing health care as close as possible to where the people live and work, and constitutes the first element of a continuing health care process." (WHO 1978, 21).

Hence, the primary health care approach embraces both a global philosophy of health care and a means of providing health care services that incorporate the principles of accessibility, public participation, the use of appropriate technologies, and inter-sectoral cooperation (Canadian Public Health Association [CPHA] 2001; Roger and Gallagher 2000; WHO 1978).

Accessibility

Accessibility is the first principle associated with the primary health care approach. To have accessibility by all to the five types of health care shown in Figure 1.3 above, health care should be universally available and accessible to all residents of Canada regardless of their income, social status, geographical location sex, or gender. It is important to note that although the terms sex and gender are often employed interchangeably in the mass and social medias, their meanings from the public health and scientific perspectives are quite different. The term **"sex"** is typically employed to refer to one's biological and physiological characteristics that distinguish males and females in binary terms, and incorporate multidimensional characteristics and traits such as hormones, genes, and one's anatomical makeup (Bartfay and Bartfay 2015). For example, women are more likely to development breast cancer (~99% of cases), in comparison to their male counterparts (~1% of cases).

By contrast, the term "**gender**" refers to an array of social, political, and/or culturally constructed roles, relationships, attitudes, personality traits, and characteristics, behaviours, values, and power structures between males and females (Bartfay and Bartfay 2015). A variety of factors contribute to the development of various gender-specific expectations including the mass and social medias, culture, secular societies and religious beliefs, and the political and educational establishments (Greaves 2011; Johnson, et al. 2007). Gender inequities and biases are pervasive in all societies and gender inequities influence health through, "among other routes, discriminatory feeding patterns, violence against women, lack of decision-making power, and unfair divisions of work, leisure, and possibilities of improving one's life" (Commission on Social Determinants of Health 2008, 16). Women in developing nations often have less opportunities to receive basic education and less job and career opportunities in comparison to their male counterparts due to social and cultural expectations (Reidpath and Allotey 2007; Taylor 2009; WHO 2012). For example, on October 9, 2012 Malala Yousafzai, a fifteen-year-old school girl activist who advocated for the right of girls to be educated in Pakistan, was brutally shoot in the head by the Taliban regime (Brenner 2013). Pakistan has five million children who should be in school, and two-thirds (three million) of those who are unschooled are girls. Ms. Yousafzai survived this brutal attack and received rehabilitative care in England. Moreover, she is the first child to ever be nominated for the Nobel Peace Prize and was granted honorary Canadian citizenship in 2013.

The **primary health care model** addresses the SDH and its services are centred on defined principles and values, and include health care services that are equitable, accessible, collaborative in nature, and based on the use of appropriate technologies and methods (Bartfay and Bartfay 2015). The **SDH** consist of various social measures believed to be associated with health and well-being and include income levels, education levels, job security, working conditions, adequate housing, food security, and the availability and access to health care services. We shall explore the SDH in greater detail below.

Public Participation

Public participation is the second principle associated with the primary health care approach. Individuals, groups, and entire communities are encouraged to participate in making decisions about their health; identifying health care priorities and trends, and consider the strengths and limitations of various approaches to address these needs and aspirations. This is critical in terms of planning and designing primary health care services, and for determining how they will be delivered. For example, most provincial and territorial health legislation in Canada focuses on the control of communicable diseases, although most preventable disabilities and death are currently attributed to chronic noncommunicable diseases (e.g., heart disease, stroke, diabetes) and injuries (e.g., motor vehicle, work-related) (Frank, Di Ruggiero, and Moloughney 2003; Butler-Jones 2012). Hence, current and emerging public health care priorities and trends need to be identified, debated, and prioritized accordingly. Public participation during this process also seeks to encourage effective planning and evaluation of primary health care services rendered.

Health Promotion and Primary Prevention

Health promotion is the third principle of the primary health care approach. The reader is referred to the section describing the second essential pillar of public health above entitled *Health Promotion and Prevention II*.

Use of Appropriate Technologies

The use of appropriate technologies is the fourth principle associated with the primary health care approach. In fact, the use of technology to complement and support primary health care initiatives has been expanding exponentially in the past decade in Canada. It has been estimated that 95% of youth are online every day in North America, and as of July 2010, Canada had the world's greatest number of Facebook users in proportion to its population; the United Kingdom was second, and the United States of America was third (CEFRIO 2010; O'Neill, 2012). Canadians are among the most active Internet users globally, and spend on average approximately 43.5 hours per week online, compared to the global average of 23.1 hours (Canadian Broadcasting Corporation [CBC] 2011). For example, the use of telehealth in Canada has grown by 35% annually in the past five years. The Health Council of Canada (2012) reports that there were 5,710 telehealth sites in use in 2010 in 1,175 communities nationally, which accounted for approximately 260,000 telehealth interventions, assessments, meetings, and consultations held between health care providers and their clients including an estimated 94,000 in rural and remote areas of Canada. Canadians on average have 4.5 electronic devices connected in their households; 52% watch television while using their mobile devices (e.g., smartphones, tablets), and 51% sleep with their mobile devices next to their bed, based on a national online survey conducted by Harris/Deima involving 1,009 individuals aged sixteen and over who owned a smartphone or tablet device (Christensen 2013; Rogers Communication 2013). The PHAC (2006) has developed a portal for knowledge exchange, which is highlighted in the Web-based Resources Box 1.4 below. This portal serves as a central access point for evidence-informed practice approaches for a variety of public health professionals and workers. This portal also serves as a vital vehicle for knowledge enhancement and exchange.

The use of appropriate technologies includes the recognition for the need to develop, deliver, and evaluate various innovative technologies and platforms (e.g., Facebook, Twitter, internet-based health promotion portals or websites, telehealth) for health across the lifespan. The technology and modes of care employed, however, should be in concert with the community or target population's social, cultural, and economic development. For example, the utilization of laptop computers for the documentation of assessments and interventions carried out by a group of home care nurses in Québec permitted them to increase time spent in direct care by 14%, and enabled the nursing team to make 780 more home visits per year (National Expert Commission Canadian Nurses Association 2012).

The consideration of alternatives to high-cost infrastructures, services, and technologies (e.g., massive brick-and-mortar water treatment plants, traditional health units, and clinics), where low-cost alternatives may be more feasible and cost-effective (e.g., UV-light filters on individual household water lines to kill harmful bacteria; mobile van health clinics, telehealth), need to be considered and evaluated (Bartfay and Bartfay 2015). For example, The Lu'ma Native Housing Society in Vancouver, British Columbia began a program in 2010 to provide free phone numbers and voice-mail to the homeless (Foster 2010; Paulsen 2010). This low-cost technology provides a cost-effective means to contract homeless individuals by various individuals in the community (e.g., public health nurses, case workers, prospective employers, family members, or loved ones), and for managing their appointments and affairs. Users have a password and can leave a personal greetings, messages, and voicemails. Moreover, the voicemail program allows various social and public health services to broadcast blanket messages to all users in their system (e.g., safety or extreme weather alerts, employment opportunities, free health care and screening services) (Foster 2010; Paulsen 2010).

Web-based Resources 1.4 The Canadian Best Practices Portal for Health Promotion and Chronic Disease Prevention

Learning Resource	Website
Canadian Best Practices Portal for Health for Health Promotion and Chronic Disease Prevention (PHAC 2006) This portal services for both knowledge exchange between various public health care professionals and workers related to evidence-informed approaches to manage and prevent variety of chronic diseases in Canada.	http://cbpp-pcpe.phac-aspc.gc.ca **or** http://www.phac.gc.ca/cbpp

Inter-sectoral Co-operation

The last principle of the primary health care approach involves inter-sectoral cooperation. This principle embraces the notion that public health professionals and workers do not practice in individual silos in the public health context, but work collaboratively to solve complex social–psychological, cultural, spiritual, and political issues associated with health in Canada and abroad. Indeed, health and well-being of individuals or entire communities are linked to a variety of SDH (e.g., poverty, income, job security, housing, nutrition). For example, a Human Resources and Skills Development Canada (2008) report identified the following five "high-risk" groups for low income between the years 2000 and 2006:

- Single parents with at least one child less than eighteen years of age;
- Single (unmarried) individuals between the ages of forty-five and sixty-four;
- Individuals with mental or physical disabilities that prevents them from being employed;
- Recent immigrants (within the past ten years) to Canada; and
- Indigenous peoples living off reserves.

Using Canadian Census data, Lee (2000) found that cities of over 500,000 individuals had the highest poverty rates and that Montréal was the city with the highest rates of poverty, followed by Vancouver and Winnipeg. Regional differences were also noted with Québec, the Atlantic provinces and Cape Breton having the highest incidence of individuals living in poverty. Poverty is strongly linked to homelessness and negative health outcomes in Canada and abroad. According to Human Resources and Skills Development Canada (2010), there were sixty-one communities in Canada that had significant social and health problems associated with homelessness that were receiving funding form the Homeless Partnering Strategy (HPS) to help address local issues and concerns.

The primary health care model embraces actions that are directed at strengthening the skills and capabilities of individuals, groups, and communities through intersectoral cooperation. This also includes actions or interventions directed toward changing social, environmental, political, and economic conditions so to alleviate their impacts on health (PHAC 2007). Furthermore, this approach is based on the principle of social justice for health promotion which entails the empowerment of residents or health care consumers to make informed decisions related to their health which is in harmony with their environment (Advisory Committee on Population Health 2001; CPHA 2001; McMurray 2007; Raphael 2004, 2009). Currently, many federal and provincial/territorial government services are divided into unique departments that function like independent silos. The primary health care approach, by contrast, requires contact at various levels and with a variety of governmental services including health, social development, public safety, justice, and education (Bartfay and Bartfay 2015). Services provided based on the primary health care approach take into account the SDH and associated principles (e.g., essential, accessible, equitable, collaborative, use of appropriate technologies). Hence, adoption of the primary health care approach increases responsibility for health to include not only provincial or territorial governments, but also individuals, groups, and entire communities.

For example, the Community Health Clinic (CHC) in Fredericton, New Brunswick is managed by the University of New Brunswick's Faculty of Nursing, and is based on a primary health care approach model (Dykeman 2012). This clinic provides a wide range of health and social services (e.g., outreach services in shelters, local soup kitchen, clothing bank, immigrant health care services, drug addiction services) based on an interdisciplinary approach and the clients are regarded as a respected member of the CHC health care team who provide community input into programs and needs assessments (Dykeman 2012).

Essential Pillar (iv): The 15 Social Determinants of Health

The fourth essential pillar of public health entails the 15 social determinants of health. At his address to the seventy-fifth World Health Assembly, the late Director General, Dr. Lee Jong-Wook, announced the creation of the Commission on Social Determinants of Health (WHO 2008). The WHO's establishment of the International Commission on the Social Determinants of Health has subsequently stimulated global public health interests and discussions on the societal factors that shape the health of individuals, families, groups, communities, and entire populations. We wish to highlight that two of the WHO commission's knowledge networks (Globalization and Health and Early Childhood Development) were centred in Canada, while Workplace Health also had significant Canadian representation. The Commission on Social Determinants of Health (2008) has adopted a holistic and global view of health which is in concert with those of the authors of this textbook. The **SDH** is defined as:

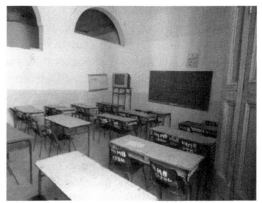

Source: Wally J. Bartfay

Photo 1.5 A classroom located in Havana, Cuba. Access to a basic education by both males and females is a critical social determinant of health.

"the structural determinants and conditions of daily life responsible for a major part of health inequities between and within countries. They include the distribution of power, income, goods and services, and the circumstances of people's lives, such as their access to health care, schools and education; their conditions of work and leisure; and the state of their housing and environment. The term "social determinants" is thus shorthand for the social, political, economic, environmental and cultural factors that greatly affect health status" (WHO 2008, 1).

Various SDH must be addressed to control and eliminate epidemics and pandemics that threaten entire populations, combat many disease-specific targets including the eight original global health-related MDG's and new seventeen SDGs (UNDP 2009, 2015). The reader is referred to Chapter 9 for a detailed discussion of the MDG's and SDGs. Most priority public health conditions globally share key elements including exposure to risks, disease vulnerability, access to care, and the consequences of disease (WHO 2008). The *Commission on the Social Determinants of Health* (2008, 3) recommended three key principles of action:

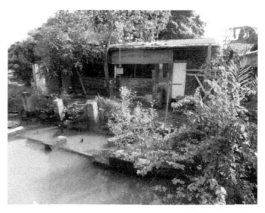

Source: Wally J. Bartfay

Photo 1.6 A squatter's home in Melaka, Malaysia. Access to basic and affordable housing and shelter is a critical social determinant of health globally.

i. Improve the conditions of daily life (i.e., the circumstances in which people are born, grow, live, work, and age);

ii. tackle the inequitable distribution of power, money, and resources (i.e., the structural drivers of those conditions of daily life globally, nationally, and locally); and

iii. measure the problem, evaluate action, expand the knowledge base, develop a workforce that is trained in the SDH, and raise public awareness.

The Lalonde Report (1974) was the first position document by an industrialized nation to acknowledge that the laboratory-based mechanistic medical model of health was inadequate, and that health was affected by four broad determinants: Human biology, environment, lifestyle, and health care organizations. The Department of Health and Welfare Canada commissioned the Canadian Institute for Advanced Research in 1987 to design and implement an initiative called the *Public Health Program* (Thompson 2010). The mandate of this program was to critically review the determinants of health, analyze their impact on the health status of Canadians across the lifespan, and assess the efficiency and effectiveness of health care systems in Canada. Their findings concluded that the determinants of health, as outlined in previous reports (e.g., Lalonde 1974; Epps 1986) and conferences (e.g., WHO international conference 1986), were in fact mutually linked and tied to a variety of factors (Thompson 2010).

Over time, Health Canada (2002a, 2002b) and the PHAC have expanded on these initial determinants of health to include a variety of sociopolitical and environmental factors such as one's gender, ethnicity, level of education, and socioeconomic status (Mikkonen and Raphael 2010; Muntaner, et al. 2012). For example, research has shown that individuals with a lower socioeconomic status (SES) have poorer health outcomes, in comparison to those with higher SES (Commission on Social Determinants of Health 2008; Health Canada 1994; Keating and Hertzman 1999; Raphael 2009, 2010). Similarly, a growing body of research has shown that those who are employed in lower echelon jobs or those who are unemployed experience significantly more anxiety, stress, depressive symptoms, health problems (e.g., cardiovascular disease), hospitalizations and mortality rates (Bartfay, Bartfay, and Wu 2013; Commission on Social Determinants of Health 2008; Ferrie 2004; D'Arcy 1986; Marmot et al. 1978).

At a 2002 national conference, held at York University in Toronto, more than four hundred public and social health researchers, policy expects, and community representatives gathered to review the state of the determinants of health in Canada by concentrating specifically on the SDH across the lifespan. The three major aims of the 2002 conference were to: (i) consider the state social or social determinants of health, (ii) explore the implications of these conditions for the health of all Canadians, and (iii) outline policy directions to improve the health of Canadian residents by influencing the quality of these determinants of health. This pivotal conference at York University in 2002 resulted in the first twelve key SDH listed in Table 1.2 below (Raphael 2009, 2010; Rootman, et al. 2012).

The 2002 conference in Toronto also formulated various short- and long-term public health goals and affirmed that all health care professionals and workers in Canada should be knowledgeable about how the SDH may influence health and well-being across the lifespan (Raphael 2002). Subsequently, Mikkonen and Raphael (2010) added *Race* and *Disability* to the list of SDH. Bartfay and Bartfay (2015) report that "*Access to and Appropriate Use of Technologies*" should also be considered critical in the new and technologically dependent millennium, bring the list to a total of 15 SDH. For example, it can be clearly argued that access to and the appropriate use of water treatment and sanitation technologies have had significant public health benefits in Canada and abroad. Conversely, having annual chest X-rays done for general screening of the public for lung cancer is not recommended and, in fact, be harmful to individuals due to exposure to unnecessary radiation. The reader is also referred to the section entitled "Use of Appropriate Technologies" under the third essential pillar of health for a discussion related to the beneficial applications of technology for public health.

Conversely, when "technology" is abused or improperly applied or utilized it can result in negative social, economic, mental, and/or physical health consequences. For example, *Internet Gaming Disorder* has been recently added to the appendix of the DSM-5, which is clearly a new public health challenge resulting from the inappropriate use of computer-based technologies and online Internet-based gambling sites (American Psychological Association [APA] 2013; Brand, et al. 2014). Similarly, the term "*Internet addiction*" (or Excessive/ Compulsive/ Problematic Internet Use [PIU]) has also appeared in various published international research reports over the past two decades (e.g., Gilbert, et al. 2011; Weinstein and Lejoyeux 2010; Young 2009). There is a growing body of empirical evidence to suggest that excessive use and/or abuse of mobile information and communication technologies (MICTs) (e.g., smartphones, tablets, laptops, iPods) and the Internet including social media (e.g., Twitter, Facebook, online gaming and gambling sites) may lead to a variety of negative social, economic, mental, and physical health outcomes. Indeed, various negative health outcomes associated

Table 1.2 The 15 SDH

(i) Indigenous status	(ix) Income and its distribution
(ii) Early life	(x) Social exclusion
(iii) Education	(xi) Social safety net
(iv) Employment and working conditions	(xii) Unemployment and employment security
(v) Food security	(xiii) Race
(vi) Gender	(xiv) Disability
(vii) Health care services	(xv) Access to and appropriate use of
(viii) Housing	technologies

with excessive MICTs use has been reported in the scientific literature including depression; anxiety and increased stress; social isolation; cyberbullying; cyber-crime; identify theft; pain and discomfort in the neck, shoulders, and wrist; sleep disturbances; and eye strain to name but a few (Cash et al. 2012; Gerr, et al. 2004; Ghori, et al. 2015; Morgan and Cotton 2003; Repacholi et al. 2012; Seitz et al. 2005; WHO 2013).

For example, dry eye disease (DED) is a growing public health concern in Canada and globally, which has been linked, in part, to prolonged exposures to video display terminals (VDTs) (Messmer 2015; Salomon-Ben Zeev, et al. 2014; Uchino et al. 2008). Prevalence rates range from 7% in the United States and Australia, 25% in Canada, and as high as 33% in Taiwan and Japan (Gayton 2009; Lin et al. 2005; Messmer 2015). Ghori and coworkers (2015) examined the prevalence of pain and discomfort in the neck, shoulder, hands, and wrists of 278 university students in Ontario, Canada aged seventeen to thirty-two years resulting from use of laptop computers and other mobile technologies with VDTs. The researchers found that 64.1% female and 45.7% of male university students surveyed experienced significant pain and discomfort in various areas of the body, as quantified via the Nordic Musculoskeletal Scale (Ghori, et al. 2015). We shall further illustrate the importance of examining the fifteenth SDH of "*Access to and Appropriate Use of Technologies*" with three recent and salient public health examples below: (i) Texting and associated dangerous behaviours, (ii) sexting and cyberbullying, and (iii) nomophobia.

(i) Texting and associated dangerous behaviours example

The use of *Short Messaging Texts* (SMT) or "texts" for short, have been growing exponentially during the past decade. In 2011 alone, Canadians sent on average 2,500 texts every second with a total number of texts exceeding 78 billion (The Canadian Press 2012). Moreover, the number of personal text messages sent every year has almost quadrupled since 2008 (The Canadian Press 2012). According to the Canadian Wireless Telecommunication Association (CWTA 2014), Canadians sent nearly 270 million text messages per day, or an average of ten messages per person per day in 2014, and there were approximately 27.9 million subscribers. Chomo (2014) reports that mobile traffic data will grow by an estimated 900% from 2013 to 2018 in Canada. In the United States, it is estimated that 60,000 pedestrian-related injuries and approximately 4,000 deaths are directly attributed to texting behaviours (Centers for Disease Control & Prevention WISQARS 2012), and over half of pedestrian-related traffic injuries globally (Naci, et al. 2009). In Canada, more than 85% of cellular and smartphone users admitted to using their phone at least on one reported occasion while driving, and more than 27% used their phones during half or more of their driving trips (Huang et al. 2010). Both Transport Canada and the Canadian Association of Emergency Physicians (CAEP) promote safe driving practices, which includes a ban on all hand-held MICTs including cellular phones and smartphones while operating a motor vehicle (Huang et al. 2010). In response to the growing public health concerns related to distracted driving, over fifty countries globally now have laws banning or limiting the use of MICTs such as cellular or smartphones. In Canada, six out of ten provinces currently have legislation as a form of primordial prevention, which prohibits the use of cellular or smartphones while operating a motor vehicle including Newfoundland and Labrador; Nova Scotia, Québec, Ontario, Saskatchewan and British Columbia. Other provinces and territories are considering implementing similar bans (Huang et al. 2010).

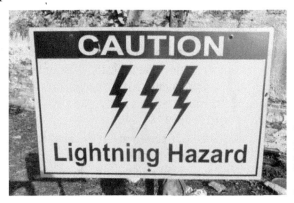

Source: Wally J. Bartfay

Photo 1.7 The likelihood of being hit by lightning during a storm is approximately 1 in 750,000. By comparison, individuals who send or read a text message while driving are 23 times more likely to be in a motor vehicle accident, in comparison to those who don't text and drive.

(ii) Sexting and cyberbullying example

The term "sexting" first appeared in dictionaries in 2012 (Mattey and Mattey Diliberto 2013; Merriam-Webster 2012). **Sexting** is defined as the act of sending sexually explicit images, which include pictures, photos, or videos via a MICT device. Several concerns have fueled the considerable attention paid to this new social behaviour by concerned parents, educators, law enforcement agencies, and public health professionals in the mass and social medias (e.g., Koppel and Jones 2010; Martinez-Prather and Vandiver 2014; Mitchell et al. 2012; Rice et al. 2012).

One of the major concerns is that individuals may be creating illegal child pornography and the potential for the exploitation of vulnerable youth. Another major concern is that individuals may be jeopardizing their reputation and/or futures by putting compromising or ineradicable images online that may be available to potential employers, academic institutions, and the general public at large. In 2014, a national survey of 5,436 Canadian students found that 15% of grade 11 students had sent a "sext," and 36% had received at least one "sext" (Steeves 2014). Male students (32%) were more likely than female students (17%) to receive a sext created specifically for them. Moreover, male students were more likely (26%) to forward a sext received, in comparison to their female counterparts (20%) (Steeves 2014).

On March 9, 2015, Bill C-13, the federal "*Cyber-bullying Act*," came into effect and was in response, in part, to the Rehtaeh Parsons and Amada Todd tragedies involving teen sexting and cyberbullying that received international media attention (Browne 2015; Library of Parliament 2014). Bill C-13, in essence, makes it a criminal offence for adults and children twelve years of age or older to share "*intimate images*" of anyone without their prior consent. Sexting of sexually explicit images is reported to currently involve a low percentage of youth, but still a considerable number exists to warrant this as a public health concern especially given the growing numbers of individuals who access and use MICTs on a daily basis globally.

(iii) Nomophobia example

Nomophobia is a relatively new term defined as the fear of being without a mobile phone or device; being beyond contact, or not being able to be in contact with or be connected to a mobile telecommunications provider (Bragazzi and Del Puente 2014; SecurEnvoy 2012a, 2012b; Spear King et al. 2010, 2014). The term *nomophobia* is a portmanteau or an acronym for "*no-mobile-phone phobia*," which was first coined during a study conducted in 2010 by the U.K. Post Office to investigate anxieties present in mobile phone subscribers (Elmore 2014; SecurEnvoy 2012a, 2012b). This study consisted of 2,163 cellular phone subscribers, and found that 58% of males and 47% of females suffer from this type of new phobia. Hence, nomophobia may be viewed as a modern-age technologically derived phobia and a by-product of the interaction between people and new technologies.

Individuals in Canada and abroad have become dependent on their MICTs more than ever, which in turn, may exacerbate feelings of anxiety caused by being out of mobile service provider contact, the Internet or WIFI. Indeed, several epidemiological investigations and surveys performed in different countries and cultures including Canada, United States, Brazil, India, England, Spain, Poland, Finland, Korea, and Japan suggest that nomophobia is universally widespread and a growing global mental public health concern for the new millennium associated with MICTs (e.g., Christensen 2013; Chóliz 2010, 2012; Dixit et al. 2010; Ha et al. 2008; Hong et al. 2012; King 2010; Krajewska-Kulak et al. 2012; Oksman and Turtianen 2004; Rogers Communication 2013; SecurEnvoy 2012a, 2012b; Spear King et al. 2014; Toda, et al. 2006; Yildirim 2014). Although nomophobia is not considered a mobile phone dependence or mobile phone addiction, it may become a comorbidity with problematic uses of MICTs. In fact, it is currently estimated that over twenty million (65%) Canadians suffer from nomophobia based on a national online survey conducted by Harris/Deima involving 1,009 individuals aged sixteen and over who owned a smartphone or tablet device (Christensen 2013; Rogers Communication 2013). We hypothesize that new negative social, economic, mental, and physical health outcomes will be identified in the decades to come as a result of various MICTs and other technologies (e.g., health care, pharmaceutical, industrial, mining, manufacturing) employed in Canadian society and abroad.

Examining the Limitations of the SDH

Various Canadian health care professionals and organizations have embraced these SDH and now view health as a critical resource and right for all citizens and residents (Mikkonen and Raphael 2010; Muntaner, Ng, and Chung 2012). For example, the CHNAC has declared in their standards of practice that "community health nurses consider health as a resource for everyday life that is influenced by circumstances, beliefs and the determinants of health" (CHNAC 2003, 10). However, we must acknowledge that one of the major limitations and criticisms of these determinants of health is that they imply that each of the determinants has equal weight or significance for influencing the health status of individuals. Indeed, there is a growing body of evidence to suggest that certain social and economic conditions (e.g., social and economic status) are, in fact, more influential determinants of health (Singh and Dickinson 2009; Raphael 2004, 2012).

For example, between the years 2008 and 2009 almost 67,000 Canadians required hospitalized resulting from a heart attack (a.k.a. myocardial infarction) (CIHI 2010b). Figure 1.4 above provides a breakdown of the Canadian population into five neighbourhood income levels. Notably, Canadians living in the least-affluent neighbourhoods were 37% (255 per 100,000) more likely to have a heart attack, in comparison to those living in the most affluent neighbourhoods (186 per 100,000) (CIHI 2010b). Interestingly, it has been estimated that if all socioeconomic groups in Canada had the same heart attack rate as those from the most-affluent and wealthy neighbourhoods, the overall rate of hospitalized heart attacks would have decreased by approximately 16%, or the equivalent of about

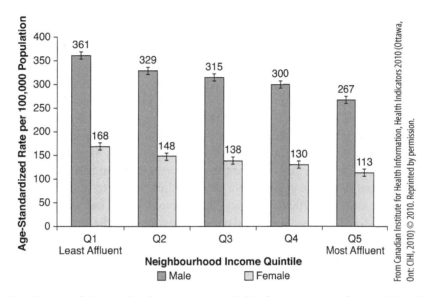

Figure 1.4 Age-Standardized Rates of Hospitalized Acute Myocardial Infarction Events by Neighbourhood Income Quintile and Sex, Canada, 2008–2009

Note: Population by income quintile for 2008–2009 was projected using 2001 and 2006 Canadian census data. I represents 95% confidence intervals.

Web-based Resources 1.5 The SDH

Learning resource	Website
Commission on Social Determinants of Health (CSDH 2008). Closing the gap in a generation. Health equity through action. Geneva, Switzerland: WHO ISBN 978 92-4 1563703. This is the final report of the CSDH. Various SDH are critically examined from a global health perspective.	http://www.usask.ca/sph/documents/Resources/ WHO%20Commission%20on%20Social%20 Determinants%20of%20Health.
Public Health Agency of Canada: The social determinants of health. This document provides an overview of the SDH and their implications for developing health policies and the role of the public health sector.	http://www.phac-aspc.gc.ca/ph-sp/phdd/overview_ implications/01_overview.html

10,400 hospitalized heart attacks. Moreover, this would represent an estimated potential savings in hospital costs of approximately $100 million per year, not including physician fees (CIHI 2010b). As one can see from this example, where one resides in Canada in reference to their wealth and affluence, has significant health implications for their residents. Add to your knowledge of the SDH by accessing the Web-based Resources Box below.

Essential Pillar (v): Holistic Care Paradigm

The fifth essential pillar encompasses the holistic care paradigm of public health. The **holistic care paradigm** incorporates the belief that human beings are more than the sum of their mind and body parts, but are dynamic and interrelated wholes that include their mind, body, spirit, culture, and environments (see Figure 1.5 below) (Bartfay and Bartfay 2015). A **paradigm** in this context is defined as a specific worldview or perspective; a way of thinking, and/or methodology which guides practice in the health sciences. In the Canadian context of public health practice, providing holistic care to individuals, families, groups, communities, or entire populations is based on the principle of social justice, in which the public health professional or worker brings an awareness of equity and the fundamental rights of all residents to accessible, competent practice and the essential SDH (Bartfay and Bartfay 2015). These SDH are broad based and holistic in nature and include individual biology and genetic endowment, health behaviours, lifestyles, social and economic factors including income, education, food security, social exclusion, housing shortages, social support networks, education, employment and working conditions, social and physical environments, personal health practices and coping skills, access to health care services, gender, and culture (Health Canada 2002; Raphael 2003). Figure 1.5 belowprovides the reader with a conceptual representation of the holistic care paradigm for public health in Canada.

For example, poverty has been described as the most critical global SDH, since it often serves as a decisive factor to other essential factors (e.g., adequate food, shelter, access to affordable medicines and health care services) (Birn, Pillay, and Holtz 2009; Jacobsen 2008; Skolnik 2012). **Extreme poverty,** defined as individuals who live on less than $1.75 (Canadian) per day, is a growing Canadian and global concern (Deviney 2013; Skolnik 2012; UNDP 2009). This $1.75 figure includes all food, water, shelter, energy, medications, and other associated health costs per day. Poverty in Canada affects over three million individuals (13.3% of the total population), including over 600,000 children (Ontario Association of Food Banks 2008). In fact, 882,188 individuals in Canada used food banks in 2012 and 38.4% of users were children and youth (Food Banks Canada 2012), and 150,000 Canadians were living on the street (Salvation Army 2011). During March of 2014 alone, 841,191 individuals across Canada used a food bank, and 37% of these were children (Patel 2014).

According to a recent report examining child poverty in the world richest industrialized nations by UNICEF (2012), Canada's poverty rate was 13.3% (a middle ranking). By comparison, the child poverty rate

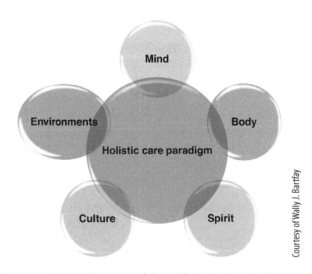

Figure 1.5 Conceptual Model of the Holistic Care Paradigm.

in Iceland was 4%; 8.51% in Germany; 10.9% in Australia; 12.1% in the United Kingdom; 17.1% in Spain, and 23.1% in the United States (UNICEF 2012). Most concerning is that Canada is currently ranked 27 out of 29 rich countries on the dimension of health and safety; 16 out of 29 in terms of behaviours and risks; 15 out of 29 in reference to maternal well-being; 14 out of 29 in regards to education, and 11 out of 29 in terms of housing and the environment (UNICEF Canada 2013). Currently, 1 in 7 or 4.8 million residents in Canada live in poverty; 1 in 10 cannot fill out a required prescription medication due to inadequate funds, and over 200,000 individuals live in extreme poverty (Canada Without Poverty 2015).

Moreover, the 2008 global economic recession has resulted in negative ripple effects in terms of the availability finances for public health services and government funded health research initiatives in various countries and regions around the world (e.g., Africa, Australia, European Union, and North America).

A commissioned survey by the British Broadcasting Corporation (BBC) World Service (2013) involving more than 25,000 subjects in twenty-three countries globally found that extreme poverty (77%) was reported to be a more serious problem than climate change (58%), terrorism (59%), the spread of human diseases (59%), or the environment and concerns related to pollution (64%). Food prices have also been increasing globally resulting in increased states of hunger and associated extreme poverty. Indeed, there are an estimated 1.02 billion people who are malnourished and living in poverty; including an estimated 642 million in Asia, 265 million in sub-Saharan Africa, and fifteen million undernourished people are now living in high-income countries which represent an alarming increase of 50% in comparison to 2003 levels (Food and Agriculture Organization [FAO] 2009).

The concept of care in the health sciences has been described as both a noun and a verb (Bartfay 2010a; Bartfay and Bartfay 2015). The holistic care paradigm expands the notion of a duality of the mind and body to one that acknowledges the simultaneous and continuous interaction of the person with health and their environment (Gorden 2005; Scotto 2003; Swanson, 1999; Watson and Lea 1997; Gaut, 1993). The holistic care perspective encompasses the belief that human beings are more than the sum of their mind and body parts, but consist of dynamic and interrelated wholes that include the mind, body, spirit, culture, and sociopolitical and physical environments (Bartfay 2010a).

Morse et al. (1991) conducted a meta-analysis of thirty-five separate theories and conceptual definitions of caring. The following five epistemological perspectives emerged from their analysis: (i) A human trait, which proposes that caring is an innate trait which is essential to the human experience; (ii) a moral imperative or ideal, which serves as the basis for health-related actions and interventions; (iii) an affect, which implies that caring entails feelings or an emotional involvement with health care consumers that requires empathy on behalf of health care professionals and workers; (iv) an interpersonal relationship; and (v) a therapeutic intervention (Morse et al. 1991).

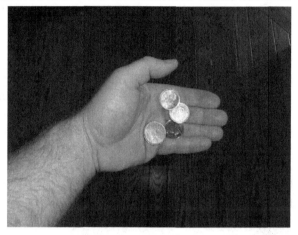

Source: Wally J. Bartfay

Photo 1.8 Poverty is a major social determinant of health. Extreme poverty in Canada is defined as those having to live on less than $1.75 per day. This includes the costs for all food, water, shelter, energy, medications, and other associated costs per day.

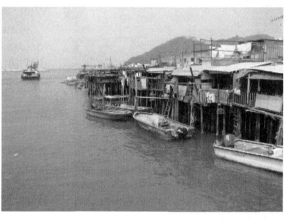

Source: Wally J. Bartfay

Photo 1.9 A squatter settlement in Hong Kong. It is now estimated that between 55 and 90 million individuals are living in extreme poverty conditions worldwide, as a consequence of the 2009 global economic crisis (UNDP 2009).

Taken together, it may be argued that all of these viewpoints are relevant to the practice of public health. Currently, there is no universally accepted or employed definition of holistic care in Canada. Nonetheless, it may be argued that the holistic care paradigm remains a cornerstone for providing culturally appropriate, safe, and cost-effective primary health care services and interventions in Canada. Holistic care provides a mechanism by which public health professionals and workers can enable, support, and facilitate individual, family, group, community, or population-based health care interventions or initiatives that encompass the principles of primary health care (Canadian Nurses Association 2000; CPHA 2001; Romanow 2002).

We also acknowledge and recognize the interdependence between human health and the health of global ecosystems (Birn, Pillay, and Holtz 2009; Jacobsen 2008; Skolnik 2012). The World Health Organization notes, for example, that global warming is associated with approximately 150,000 deaths annually and five million associated illnesses, and these numbers are predicted to double by 2030 (West 2015; Wilson 2007). Moreover, global climate changes have been linked to a growing number of infectious diseases, floods, heat waves, and hurricanes. Flooding as a result of coastal storm surges will affect the lives of up to two hundred million people globally by 2080 (West 2015). A 2005 flood in Alberta, for example, affected more than fourteen communities, resulted in the evacuation of over 7,000 residents, damaged over 4,000 homes and caused the death of two individuals (Public Safety & Emergency Preparedness Canada 2005). More recently, on June 20, 2013, Alberta experienced heavy rainfalls that resulted in catastrophic flooding along the Bow, Elbow, Highwood, Red Deer, Sheep, Little Bow, and South Saskatchewan rivers and tributaries (Davison and Powers 2013; Government of Alberta 2013a, 2013b, and 2013c). A total of thirty-two states of local energy were declared and twenty-eight emergency operation centres were activated as flood waters rose and entire communities had to be evacuated. For example, in Canmore, a town located in Alberta's Rockies, over 220 millimeters (or 8.7 inches) fell in a period of 36

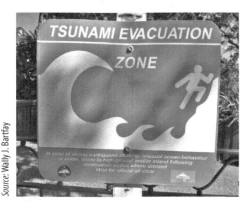

Source: Wally J. Bartfay

Photo 1.10 A tsunami evacuation sign informating individuals where to evacuate in the event of an earthquake in New Zealand. Emergency and diaster preparedness are critical components of public health. On February 22, 2011, and earthquake devasted the city of Christchurch, New Zealand, which resulted in the death of 185 people and several thousands were injured. This was one of thousands of earthquakes experienced in the region since September 4, 2010.

hours, nearly half of the town's annual rainfall (Alberta Environment and Sustainable Resource Development 2013). As a consequence of 2013 Alberta floods, over 100,000 people were displaced from their homes and businesses, four people were confirmed dead as a direct result of the flooding, and the damage to homes, businesses, public infrastructures and the economy was estimated to be between $3 to $5 billion for the region (Canadian Broadcasting Corporation 2013; White 2013; Williams and Haggett 2013).

Similarly, natural (e.g., earth quakes, tsunamis, volcanoes) and man-made disasters (e.g., 1986 Chernobyl nuclear accident, 2010 BP Gulf of Mexico oil spill) can have negative impacts on the health, safety, and well-being of individuals, communities, or entire regions. For example, the 2004 tsunamis that hit the costs of India, Thailand, Indonesia, and surrounding areas caused billions of dollars of damage and the death of 280,000 victims (Landsman 2005). Accordingly, we believe that it is no longer possible to examine health from the local, regional, provincial/territorial, or national perspective only. We must also embrace health from a global perspective (PHAC 2007; WHO 1998). The emergence of West Nile virus, SARS, Avian Flu, and the H1N1 Swine Flu influenza in Canada are recent examples of how quickly diseases can spread across international borders, and the global public health challenges we face in their surveillance and management (Campbell 2006; Quinlan and Dickinson 2009).

The "Ripple Effect" in Public Health

A **ripple effect** in public health is defined as a public health situation, interaction, or intervention and is similar to the ever expanding ripples across a static body of water when an object is dropped into it where an effect from an initial state can be followed incrementally (Bartfay and Bartfay, 2015). These public health situations, interactions, or interventions can directly or indirectly affect and impact individuals, groups, or entire communities. Figure 1.6 below provides a conceptual diagram representing the ripple effects produced in the public health context. Although the practice of public health has traditionally only focused on broad populations per se (Orme et al 2007; Scriver and Garman 2007), this has expanded in recent decades as a result of our understanding related to the dynamic nature of health and evolving definitions surrounding the concept of health (Bartfay 2010b; PHAC 2007; World Health Organization and Health and Welfare Canada and the Canadian Public Health Agency [CPHA], 1986). A growing body of research has confirmed that an individual's health-related behaviours and/or practices can also profoundly affect the health and well-being of other members of society, including their family members (e.g., effects of alcohol or smoking on the fetus) (Stade et al. 2006); coworkers or employees (e.g., unsafe handling of hazardous chemicals) (Hales and Lauzon 2007); entire communities (e.g., contamination of water supply with *E. coli*) (Ali 2004; O'Conner 2002), or society at large (e.g., bioterrorism) (Goodwin Veenema 2007; PHAC 2001).

In fact, it may be argued that the health of the public influences and affects us on multiple levels including the individual, family or group, and the community or population levels. Indeed, we are the "*public*" and it is our health and wellness that is affected either positively or negatively by the actions and behaviours of our residents in society (e.g., unwanted exposure of patrons or employees to toxic second hand smoke in restaurants or bars). The behaviours, actions, and/or practices at the individual level of origin, or their lack of, can have a negative or positive "*ripple health effect*" at the family or group level and/or the community or population level as well. For example, during the summer of 2000, human error resulted in the contamination of the community water supply with the potentially deadly *E. coli 0157:57* in Walkerton, Ontario (Ali 2004; O'Conner 2002). More than 2,300 residents became seriously ill, seven died, and the economic impact was estimated to be in excess of $64.5 million (Sullivan 2004).

Conversely, the actions or behaviours of a single individual can have positive ripple effects at the family or group levels and/or the community or group levels. For example, the Hungarian-born physician Ignaz Philipp Semmelweis (1818–1865) performed the first preventive clinical trial to establish the importance of proper hand washing to prevent the spread of infections in the first obstetric ward of the Allgemeines Krankenhaus in Vienna in 1846 (Gallin and Ognibene 2007). From 1841 to 1846, Semmelweis observed that the maternal mortality rate from puerperal sepsis or "childbed fever" ranged from 10% to 50% in the First Maternity Division of the Vienna General Hospital. Conversely, the mortality rate was only 2% to 3% on the Second Division, where the births were attended by midwives, as opposed to physicians or medical students.

In 1847, his fellow physician and friend, Jakob Kolletschka, died after receiving a small cut on his finger while performing an autopsy on one of the victims of childbed fever. Although cuts were common during

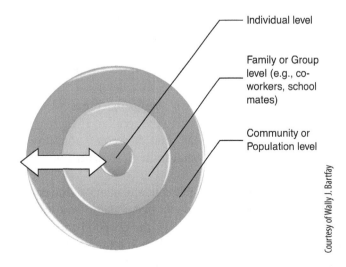

Figure 1.6 Conceptual Diagram of the "Ripple Effect" in Public Health

autopsies, Semmelweis deduced that Kolletschka exhibited clinical symptoms characteristic of childbed fever. In addition, he observed that midwives did not perform frequent vaginal examinations and had no contact with infected cadavers, whereas medical students and physicians did. Although the germ theory of disease causation has not yet been established, he deduced that childbed fever was:

> "caused by conveyance to the pregnant women of putrid particles derived from living organisms, through the agency of examining fingers" (cited in Gallin and Ognibene 2007, 7).

Consequently, Semmelweis insisted that all medical students and physicians scrub their hands vigorously with a chlorinated lime solution before entering the maternity ward to attend to their patients. From 1847 to 1848, the mortality rate on the First Maternity ward dramatically decreased from 9.92% to 1.27%. Hence, the actions or behaviours of a single individual, such as proper handing, can have major positive ripple health effects at the family or group levels and/or community or population levels. In addition to proper hand washing practices, the methods employed to dry one's hands also needs to be considered from the public health perspective. For example, evidence suggests that reusable towels on rolls are less desirable in comparison to air-based hand dryers, which may result in the transmission of person-to-person transfer of bacterial, viruses, or fungi (Huang, et al. 2012; Snelling, et al. 2011).

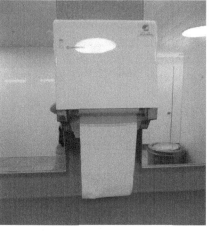

Source: Wally J. Bartfay

Photo 1.11a A reusable roll-type of hand towel is a potential source of harmful bacterial, viruses, and fungi.

Semmelweis' work was widely ignored by the medical community until the discovery of microbes as causative agents of disease by Louis Pasteur (1822–1895) late in the nineteenth century. Subsequently, Semmelweis was posthumously vindicated and sterile techniques were gradually introduced into medical and nursing practice to prevent the spread and development of microbes in hospitals, homes, and communities. Currently, community-acquired *Staphylococcus aureus* (CA-MRSA) infections, for example, remains a major public health challenge for children in daycare centres and schools, military personnel, athletes, sex-trade workers, and those serving time in correctional facilities in Canada (Allen 2006; Jo Damazo and Bartfay 2010).

The behaviours, actions, and/or practices at the family or group level of origin, or their lack, can also have a negative or positive ripple effect at the individual and/or community or population levels. For example, in August 2008, the Maple Leaf Food plant in Toronto, Ontario stopped production due to a national outbreak of listeriosis, which resulted in the death of twenty individuals and several suspected cases due to two contaminated deli meat slicing machines (Bouzane and Wylie 2000). This outbreak resulted in the recall of 191

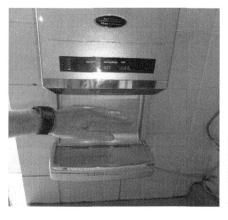

Source: Wally J. Bartfay

Photo 1.11b An air blown hand-dryer with UV light significantly decreases the risk of spreading unwanted germs from person-to-person.

deli meat products sold across Canada over fears that they could contain meat tainted with the potentially deadly gram-positive *Listeria monocytogens* bacterium (Canadian Food Inspection Agency [CFIA] 2008; Ramaswamy and Cresence 2007).

In 2008, the CFIA also issued warnings for possible contamination of food products with listeria including mushrooms from Ravine Mushroom Farms Inc. in Woodbridge, Ontario and Ivanhoe Cheese Inc., based in Madoc, Ontario (Bouzane and Wylie 2008). In September 2011, the US Food and Drug Administration recalled 300,000 cases of cantaloupe grown on the Jensen Farm in Colorado after linking it to a listeria outbreak which caused seventy-two illnesses and thirteen deaths. Marchione (2011) argues that no food will ever be completely free of risk even if the government quadrupled food inspections and this was, in fact, the nineteenth outbreak involving a melon since the year 1984. It is notable that this was the first caused by listeria bacteria that actually likes to be in the refrigerator and thrives at these low temperatures (5° to 7° Celsius).

The September 2012 *E. coli*-contaminated beef scandal from the XL beef processing plant in Brooks, Alberta, is a recent example of how human error, the failure to follow protocols and the many challenges industry and the CFIA face in assuring that our food supplies are safe for human consumption (CFIA 2013; PHAC, 2012). This outbreak of *E. coli* 0157:H7 in beef products lead to eighteen confirmed human cases, including eight in Alberta, six in Québec, three in British Columbia, and one in Newfoundland and Labrador. This incident not only affected Canadians, but alerts and recalls were extended beyond our bounders to the United

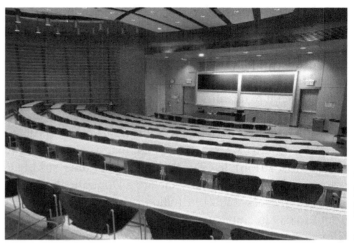

Source: Wally J. Bartfay

Photo 1.12 A critical mass of highly trained and educated public health professionals and workers will be needed in the next few decades to address major health challenges faced by Canadians across the lifespan.

States and Hong Kong in October, 2012. Hence, contamination at a single meat processing plant can have profound negative ripple effects across provinces and territories and also across international borders.

Canadians are also vulnerable to negative health effects at the community and/or population levels of origin. For example, the global pandemic known as "Severe Acute Respiratory Syndrome" (SARS) first emerged in China in 2002, and quickly spread globally. During the spring of 2003, SARS reached Toronto and killed 44 people and 375 were severely ill in Ontario over a period of only five months (Campbell 2006; Naylor 2003). A total of 8,098 people worldwide became sick during the 2003 SARS pandemic.

Future Directions and Challenges

These current events described above that have resulted in mortality and altered states of health for our residents, highlight the critical need to strengthen and cultivate our public health care systems in Canada (Bartfay 2010a; Bartfay and Bartfay 2015). These systems in Canada exists to safeguard, maintain, and improve the health of our residents and citizens across the lifespan. Great progress has been made in the past century, but many challenges still remain.

Masse and Moloughney (2011) report that during the 1990s, there were only five programs in public health in Canada and by September 2011, fifteen Canadian universities were offering Masters of Public Health (MPH) or MPH-type programs with as many as five hundred new graduates annually. During the past decade, there has also been an explosion of undergraduate programs in public health being offered across Canada. For example, in Ontario alone, there is the University of Ontario Institute of Technology public health program, Ryerson University, University of Toronto, McMaster University, Queen's University, University of Western Ontario, and Brock University. These programs were established because of increased public and student demands and many did not exist just five years ago. In addition, various universities have established specialized schools of public health including the University of Victoria, University of British Columbia, University of Alberta, University of Saskatchewan, Ryerson University, University of Toronto, and the University of Montréal (Massee and Moloughney 2011). Many of these schools are now offering both undergraduate and graduate programs in public and community health.

The second major challenge facing public health in Canada is our continued reliance on antiquated models of funding public health care systems and services in Canada. When Medicare was first conceived in Canada more than fifty years ago, it was based on the publicly insured episodic-care physician-led model of health centred primarily in acute care hospitals and clinics (Armstrong and Armstrong 2003; Health Council of

Canada 2010; Soroka and Mahon 2012; Wilson 2002). This current model is very costly, and ultimately is not meeting the complex public health care challenges faced by residents in Canada and abroad (e.g., poverty, income, having multiply chronic diseases or disabilities). With the exception of Ontario whose public health services are cost-shared on a 50:50 basis with their municipalities, all provinces and territories are responsible for funding their own public health services.

It is difficult to quantify how much of tax payer's money is actually spent directly on public health activities in Canada because estimates are often confounded by the inclusion of substantial administrative costs for the provincial and territorial health Ministries (Frank, Di Ruggiero, and Moloughney 2003). Nonetheless, we do know that health care accounts for approximately 40% of the total provincial/territorial budgets (CIHI 2013, 2014, 2015a, 2015b). In 1975, the cost of providing our Medicare systems in Canada was $12.2 billion, which represented about 7% of our total Gross Domestic Product (GDP). By 2015, our national health care expenditure was in excess of $219.1 billion ($6,105 per person, or 10.9% of GDP) (CIHI 2015a). The costs ranged from $14,059 in Nunavut to $5,665 in Québec. The top three drivers for health care costs were: (i) Hospitals (29.5%); In 2016, health care spending rose to $228.1 billion or $6,299 per Canadians, which represented 11.1% of our nation's GDP (CIHI, 2016). It is notable that spending for acute care hospitals accounted for the largest share of total health spending by the public sector (37.7% or $86 billion). (ii) drugs (15.7%), and (iii) payments to physicians (15.5%) (CIHI 2015a, 2015b). Notably, public health and all of its associated activities (e.g., health promotion and prevention campaigns and programs) accounted for only 5.5% of total health expenditures in 2015. Based on budget data from Ontario, Canada's most populated province, only 2.3% of the provincial health budget went into public health services and programs (Frank, Di Ruggiero, and Moloughney 2003). Predictions for a weaker economic growths over the next decade, combined with fiscal deficits and less savings from debt service charges, will have a dampening and negative effect on health care services in general, including those funds currently allocated for public health (CIHI 2015a).

In addition to the above, the current health care spending models and trends in Canada brings into question the sustainability of these funding schemes. For example, the development of chronic noncommunicable diseases (e.g., heart disease, diabetes, arthritis, Alzheimer's disease) and disabilities increases with age. In fact, noncommunicable diseases currently account for approximately 89% of all associated deaths in Canada, and chronic illnesses and disabilities are major drivers of health-care costs and lost productivity for our nation (National Expert Committee Canadian Nurses Association; WHO 2011). Given that the number of seniors in Canada is expected to reach 6.7 million in 2020 and 9.2 million in 2041 (PHAC 2008b; CIHI 2015a, 2015b), this will continue to place increased stress and burden on our already strained public health care systems. As of July 1, 2014, 15.7% (nearly 1:6) of Canada's population (N = 35,540,400) was aged 65 years or older (Statistics Canada 2014). This was the first time that the number of young Canadians was lower than the proportion of older Canadians. Specifically, 4.6 million Canadians were aged 15 to 24 years, compared to 4.7 million aged 55 to 64 years (Statistics Canada 2014). In 2015, the average health care cost for a senior aged 65–69 years was $6,298; $8,384 for a senior aged 70–74; $11,578 for a senior aged 75–79 years, and $20,917 for a senior 80 years or more (CIHI 2015a, 2015b). Hence, given our current lack of focus on primary health care models of health, which embrace concepts such as health promotion and prevention across the lifespan that seek to maintain health and prevent the development of chronic diseases, injuries, and disability, our current episodic and acute care funded hospital-driven models of care are simply not viable or sustainable (Adams et al. 2008; Order of Nurses of Québec 2012; Soroka and Mahon 2012).

The third major challenge is to convince governments and authorities for the need to develop, embrace, and fund primary health care systems of delivery in Canada. There is an urgent need for funding on all levels of government to support the delivery of safe and cost-effective evidence-informed public health services delivered through strong primary health care networks, with interdisciplinary teams of public health professionals and workers collaboratively working together to increase access for all individuals across the lifespan (Adams et al. 2008; Order of Nurses of Québec 2012; Starfield 2011).

"Our focus on acute treatment makes family physicians gatekeepers, and their training is to send patients for specialized diagnostics and treatment, which in recent years have often been offered in hospitals and other institutions. We cannot break out of the cycle of sickness-doctor-acute care until we make the choice to fund differently and reinforce the shift to team-based community care with plans for more accountability for health spending—including monitoring treatments and outcomes" (National Expert Commission Canadian Nurses Association 2012, 28).

The antiquated medical-model of health, unfortunately, has also served as the basis for the development of the CHA (1982), which is characterized by physician and hospital-based health care and diagnostic services (Armstrong and Armstrong 2003; Bartfay 2010c; Bartfay and Bartfay 2015; Health Canada 2003). Experiences in Canada and abroad has generally indicated a lack of commitment by federal and provincial/territorial governments to change these outdated models of health care delivery and funding, until we are faced with a national crisis (e.g., SARS, H1N1, bioterrorism). It is noteworthy that approximately 75% of good health maintained or achieved is the result of factors (e.g., lifestyles, diet, sanitation, clean water supplies) beyond direct episodic acute care that is often delivered in hospitals (National Expert Commission Canadian Nurses Association 2012; Standing Senate Committee on Social Affairs, Science and Technology, Subcommittee on Population Health 2009). Frank, Di Ruggiero, and Moloughney (2003, 31) argue that a strong national public health system needs to be clearly defined and developed because:

- Infectious (communicable) diseases and other threats (e.g., bioterrorism) do not respect political boundaries (provincial/territorial or international);
- there is a critical need for common standards of public health to provide a mechanism for sharing information and for making comparisons;
- to provide potential efficiencies in the system and avoid the duplication of public health services or initiatives (e.g., skills trainings, research, information management); and
- be positioned to lead a systematic approach to promote health, and to prevent injuries and disease.

Moreover, there is a growing recognition in Canada and abroad that health is not only influenced by one's biology or genetic makeup, but is also impacted by a variety of social, political, economic, and environmental determinants of health (WHO 1986, 2000, and 2005). Hence, there is a need to develop national and provincial/territorial legislations that recognize the SDH and the need to fund public health care services provided by a variety of public health professionals and workers in diverse settings (e.g., homes, schools, community clinics). We argue that legislation plays a key role in defining roles, expectations, mandates, and establishing standards for the delivery of primary health care services. Indeed, there is also a need to update and/or develop public health legislations to give Health Canada, the Public Health Agency of Canada, and/or other health authorities and ministries the authority to act quickly and decisively in the event of an actual or potential national health threat or emergency (e.g., bioterrorism, pandemic). For example, most provisions of the *Quarantine Act* date back to 1872 when it was first conceived to deal with pandemics such as the plaque in Canada. This legislation does not clearly identify the federal government's public health mandate in reference to the Quarantine Act, nor its specific roles and responsibilities (Bartfay 2010c; Schabas 2007).

There is also an emerging acknowledgement between the various levels of government in Canada that more resources will be required for our public health care systems in the next few decades (Quinlan and Dickinson 2009). The primary goal of primary health in Canada is to build community capacity to achieve sustainable health and well-being of our residents through health promotion efforts, as first outlines in the Ottawa Charter for Health Promotion (PHAC 2007; WHO, Health and Welfare Canada and CPHA, 1986). We argue that if Canada were to truly embrace and adopt a primary health care model for providing public health services and delivery, the responsibility for health would be expanded to include individuals, groups, their communities, and their governments, as opposed to just provincial and territorial departments of health (Adams et al. 2008; Dykeman 2012; Starfield 2011). To embrace a true primary health care model will require us to work in collaboration with a variety of government departments and services including health, public safety, justice, social development, and education to name but a few.

Although the term *"primary health care"* has been employed for over a decade now, this form of open collaborative communication is still in its infancy in many regions of Canada. We need to promote a better widespread understanding of the principles of primary health care and the determinants of health to ensure this model of public health becomes the dominant model of care across Canada. In several regards, the province of Québec has the most comprehensive and developed public health system in Canada that is characterized by comprehensive public health legislation; clearly articulated and operationalized core function expectations; the encouragement of intersectorial partnerships for health; and investments in the development of a public health workforce, which includes educational investments, training, and unique remuneration schemes for public health specialists (Frank, Di Ruggiero, and Moloughney 2003; Order of Nurses of Québec 2012). The practice of public health in Canada must continue to embrace and foster health promotion strategies and interventions that seek to facilitate the ability of individuals, families and groups, and entire communities and populations to prevent, enhance, maintain, or restore health across the lifespan. Public health professionals must work and development partnerships with local, national, and international governmental and nongovernmental health care agencies that seek to promote and preserve the health of all residents globally.

Finally, more research and systematic reviews of the empirical literature related to public health are urgently needed to evaluate the effectiveness of various public health practices, policies, interventions, legislations, delivery systems, and services (Butler-Jones 2012; Frank, Di Ruggiero, and Moloughney 2003; National Expert Commission Canadian Nurses Association 2012). Although only a few public health professionals and workers will direct programs of research, all will need to participate in research, critically read and review research findings, and apply the best available evidence to their practice of public health. There is a growing need to assess and determine the actual outcomes of public health interventions and policies and their impact factor. There is little information available on the functioning of Canada's public health systems, given that there is currently no accepted list of expected system functions or outcome measures for health promotion (Butler-Jones 2012; Frank, Di Ruggiero, and Moloughney 2003). Indeed, it is difficult to discuss, measure, and improve on existing public health care systems in Canada when these systems and their functions are not clearly defined. For example, performance measures could be developed and included for assessments involving infrastructure elements (e.g., public health workforce development and training). This would provide a mechanism to monitor progress, identify deficiencies and priorities in public health systems requiring greater attention locally, regionally, nationally, and globally.

Group Review Exercise "Superbug Resistance in Poultry Sold to Canadians' in Supermarkets"

Overview of this investigative documentary

Canadians are becoming increasingly resistant to antibiotics (Abs) due to a variety of factors including incorrect use and over prescription of antibiotics, mutation of strains, inappropriate or ineffective infection control, and prevention regimes and current agricultural practices. The latter includes the routine use of antibiotics by Canadian farmers for their animals and is based on the belief that they can prevent infection, improve the health of their animals, and increase production. Nonetheless, traces of these antibiotics remain in the animal and are later consumed by humans. A growing number of individuals in Canada and abroad are getting sicker and are taking longer to get well due to Abs.-resistance. Consequently, it is becoming increasingly necessary to administer antibiotics through an IV in a clinic or hospital because the usual drugs in pill form are becoming increasingly ineffective against these bacterial acquired infections.

In this Canadian Broadcasting Corporation (CBC), investigative television documentary by *"Marketplace,"* the team tested hundred samples of fresh unfrozen chicken, which were purchased at major supermarkets across Canada. The team tested both conventionally grown poultry and those farmed organically. The results may surprise you and the implications for public health are startling in nature.

Instructions:
This assignment may be done alone, in pairs, or in groups of up to five people (note: if you are doing this assignment in pairs or groups, please only submit one hard or electronic copy to your instructor). The assignment should be typewritten and no more than four to six pages maximum in length (double-spaced please). View the documentary entitled *"Superbugs in the supermarket,"* which aired on CBC-TV investigative program Marketplace. See link: http://www.cbc.ca/marketplace/2011/superbugsinthesupermarket/
View this documentary and take detailed notes during the presentation.

   i. Provide a brief overview of the salient points in this investigative documentary and the research methodology employed to reach their current conclusions.
  ii. Which governmental and nongovernmental agencies were alerted to the findings from this investigation? What are their roles in protecting the health and well-being of Canadian population.
 iii. Discuss the public health implications of this investigative documentary in terms of current agricultural practices in Canada and its actual and/or potential *"ripple effects"* on human health and well-being.

Summary

- Public health is considered both an art and science.
- Public health is a holistic and evidence-informed discipline that seeks to promote, maintain, and/or restore the health and well-being of individuals, families, communities, or entire populations over the lifespan through primary health care initiatives and interventions.
- Primary health care encompasses five types of health care: (i) promotive; (ii) preventive; (iii) curative; (iv) rehabilitative, and (v) supportive/palliative.
- The primary aim of public health is to empower citizens to make informed decisions and partake in interventions related to their health and care.
- A total of 36 core competencies deemed essential for all public health professionals and workers in Canada have been identified and are organized under the following seven broad categories: (i) Public health sciences; (ii) assessment and analysis; (iii) policy and program planning, implementation, and evaluation; (iv) partnerships, collaboration, and advocacy; (v) diversity and inclusiveness; (vi) communication; and (vii) leadership.
- These core competencies help to provide a common language and means to define, describe, and standardize complex work by a variety of public health professionals and workers in complex environments, and provide the essential skills and knowledge base to provide safe and cost-effective public health services in Canada.
- The five essential pillars of public health are: (i) Evidence-informed public health; (ii) health promotion and prevention; (iii) primary health care; (iv) social determinants of health; and (v) holistic care paradigm.
- Each of these pillars are connected and interrelated and each must be present to meet current and projected health care challenges facing Canadians across the lifespan.
- The five principles of the primary health care approach include: (i) Accessibility, (ii) public participation, (iii) health promotion, (iv) use of appropriate technologies, and (v) intersectoral cooperation.
- The research process consists of a series of nine steps used to structure a study and to gather, analyze, interpret, disseminate, and apply data and information in a systematic and formalized fashion.
- The ripple effect in public health was defined as any public health situation, interaction, or intervention that is similar to the ever expanding ripples across a static body of water when an object is dropped into it where an effect from an initial state can be followed incrementally.

- For example, we learned that improper handwashing by an individual can have negative ripple effects at the group or community level due to the transmission of pathogens into their immediate environments.
- There is currently a growing recognition in Canada and abroad that health is not only influenced by one's biology or genetic makeup, but is also impacted by a variety of social, cultural, political, economic, and environment determinants of health.

Critical Thinking Questions

1. Identify and describe some examples from your own community where public health interventions, programs, or policies has empowered individuals, families, groups, or the entire community toward achieving and preserving a healthier community?

2. Is poverty a "cause" of poor health in your community, or is poor health a "cause" of poverty? How would different perspectives regarding this question influence public health policy or practice in your community?

3. Compare the major public health achievements during the twentieth century presented in this chapter. Which of these accomplishments, in your opinion, has had the greatest impact on health and well-being of Canadians during the twenty-first century? Justify your selection.

4. Population trends and projections in Canada suggest that the life expectancy will continue to increase during the first half of the twenty-first century. What effect will this increased life expectancy have on public health needs, resources, and costs?

5. Debate the merits and needs for the formulation and implementation of national public health legislations that would provide standardized expectations and services in the ten provinces and three territories across Canada. What are the current barriers to make this a reality and how can we overcome them?

References

Active Healthy Kids Canada. *2014 Report Card on the Physical Activity of Children and Youth: Is Canada in the Running?* Toronto, ON: Author, 2014. Accessed November 15, 2012. http://dvqdas9jty7g6.cloudfront.net/reportcard2014/AHKC_2014_ReportCard_ENG.pdf.

Adams, J., R. Bakalar, M. Roroch, K. Knecht, E. Mounib, and N. Stuart. *Healthcare 2015 and Care Delivery. Delivery Models Refined, Competencies Defined.* Somers, NY: IBM Institute for Business Values, 2008.

Advisory Committee on Population Health. *Survey of Public Health Capacity in Canada. Highlights Report to the Federal, Provincial, Territorial Deputy Ministers of Health.* Ottawa, ON: Health Canada, 2001.

Alberta Association of Registered Nurses. "Entry-to-practice Competencies." Accessed September 25, 2007. http://www.nurses.ab.ca/publications/papers.html.

Alberta Environment and Sustainable Development. *Precipitation Map: June 19-22, 2013.* Calgary, AB: Author, 2013. Accessed July 25, 2013. http://environment.alberta.ca/forecasting/data/precipmaps/event/pdf.

Allen, U. A. "Public Health Implications of MRSA in Canada." *Canadian Medical Association Journal* 175, no. 2 (2006): 161–62.

Ali, S. H. "A Socio-ecological Autopsy for the *E. coli* 0157:H7 Outbreak in Walkerton, Ontario, Canada." *Social Science and Medicine* 58 (2004): 2601–12.

American Psychological Association (APA). *Diagnostic and Statistical Manual of Mental Disorders,* 5th ed. Washington, DC: APA, 2013.

Armstrong, P., and H. Armstrong. *Wasting Away: The Undermining of Canadian Health Care,* 2nd ed. Don Mills, ON: Oxford University Press, 2003.

Arthur, D. M., D. M. Wright, and K. M. Smith. "Women and Heart Disease: The Treatment may End but the Suffering Continues." *Canadian Journal of Nursing Research* 33, no. 3 (2001): 17–29.

Atkins, D., D. Best, P. A. Briss, M. Eccles, Y. Falck-Ytter, S. Flottorp, G. H. Guyatt, et al. "Grading Quality of Evidence and Strength of Recommendations." *British Medical Journal* 328, no. 7454 (2004): 1490–5002.

Atkins, L., J. A. Smith, M. P. Kelly, and S. Michie. "The Process of Developing Evidence-based Guidance in Medicine and Public Health: A Qualitative Study of Views from the Inside." *Implementation Science* 4, no. 8 (2013): 101–08. PMID: 24006933.

Bartfay, W. J. "Introduction to Community Health Nursing in Canada." In *Community Health Nursing: Caring in Action,* edited by E. Hitchcock, P. E. Schubert, S. A. Thomas, and W. J. Bartfay, 1st Canadian ed. 1–10. Toronto, ON: Nelson Education, 2010a.

Bartfay, W. J. "Perspectives on Health and its Promotion and Preservation. In *Community Health Nursing: Caring in Action,* edited by J. E. Hitchcock, P. E. Schubert, S. A. Thomas, and W. J. Bartfay, 1st Canadian ed., 98–116. Toronto, ON: Nelson Education, 2010b.

Bartfay, W. J. "Canada's Health Care System: History and Current Challenges." In *Community Health Nursing: Caring in Action,* edited by J. E. Hitchcock, P. E. Schubert, S. A. Thomas, and W. J. Bartfay, 1st Canadian ed., 23–41. Toronto, ON: Nelson Education, 2010c.

Bartfay, W. J., E. Bartfay, and Wu Terry. "Impact of the Global Economic Crisis on the Health of Unemployed Autoworkers." *Canadian Journal of Nursing Research* 45, no. 3 (2013): 66–79.

Bartfay, W. J. and E. Bartfay. *Public Health in Canada.* Boston, MA: Pearson Learning Solutions, 2015.

Baum, F. "The Commission of the Social Determinants of Health: Reinventing health Promotion for the Twenty-first Century?" *Critical Public Health* 18, no. 4 (2008): 457–66.

B.C. Ministry of Health. *Preventive Interventions.* Vancouver, BC: Author, 2013. Accessed October 17, 2013. http://www.health.gov.bc.ca/public-health/strategies/preventive-interventions/.

Beaglehole, R., R. Bonita, and T. Kjellstrom. *Basic Epidemiology.* Geneva, Switzerland: World Health Organization, 1993.

Birn, A. M., Y. Pillay, and T. H. Holtz, eds. *Textbook of International Health: Global Health in a Dynamic World.* New York: Oxford University Press, 2009.

Bouzane, B., and D. Wylie. *Slicing Machines Likely Listeria Source: Maple Leaf.* CanWest News Services, 2008. Accessed June 1, 2010. http://www.canada.com/windsorstar/news/sotry.html?id=d5428eb-aaa2-4b3a-af40-c67.

Bowen, S., and A. B. Zwi. "Pathways to "Evidence-informed" Policy and Practice: A Framework for Action." *PLoS Medicine* 2, no. 7 (2005): 1–6. doi:10.1371/journal.pmed.0020166.

Bragazzi, N. L., and G. Del Puente. "A Proposal for Including Nomophobia in the New DSM-V." *Psychological Research and Behavioral Management* 7 (2014): 155–60. doi:10.2147/PRBM.S41386.

Brand, M., K. S. Young, and C. Laier. "Prefrontal Control and Internet Addiction: A Theory Model and Review of Neuropsychological and Neuroimaging Findings." *Frontal Lobe Human Neuroscience* 8 (2014): 375–90. doi:10.3389/fnhum.2014.00375.

Brenner, M. The Target. Vanity Fair, 2013. Accessed June 13, 2013. http://www.vanityfair.com/politics/2013/04/malala-yousafzai-pakistan-profile.

British Broadcasting Corporation (BBC) World Service. *Annual Global Poll.* London, England: Globe Scan Press and BBC World Service, 2013. Accessed July 17, 2013. http://www.globescan.com/news-archieves/bbcWorldSpeaks-2010/.

Browne, R. "How Safe is Sexting?" Toronto, Ontario: MacLeans Magazine, February 6, 2015. Accessed April 2, 2015. http://www.macleans.ca/tag/sexting/.

Burns, N., and S. K. Grove. *Understanding Nursing Research: Building an Evidence-based Practice.* 4th ed. Philadelphia, PA: Saunders/ Elsevier, 2007.

Butler-Jones, D. *The Chief Public Health Officer's report on the state of public health in Canada.* Ottawa, ON: Her Majesty the Queen in Right of Canada, 2012. Cat. No. HP2-10/2012E, ISSN: 1917-2656. Accessed June 10, 2013. http://publichealth.gc.ca/CPHOreport.

———. "The Future of Public Health in Canada." Canadian Public Health Association Board of Directors Discussion Paper. Ottawa, ON: Canadian Public Health Association, 2001.

Campbell, A. *The SARS Commission-Spring of fear. Final report.* Ontario Ministry of Health and Long-Term Care, 2006. Accessed April 17, 2008. http://www.health.gov.on.ca/english/public/pub/ministry_reports/campbell06/online_rep/index.html.

Canada Without Poverty. *General: Basis statistics about the realities of poverty faced by Canadians.* Ottawa, ON: Author, 2015. Accessed October 22, 2015. http://www.cwp-csp.ca/poverty/just-the-facts/.

Canadian Association of Schools of Nursing. *CASN Research Mandate and Goals Discussion Paper,* n.d. Accessed April 2, 2008. http:www.causn.org/research/casn_research_mandate.htm.

Canadian Broadcasting Corporation (CBC). *4 Feared Dead from Alberta Floods.* Toronto, ON: Author, 2013. Accessed July 25, 2013. http://www.cbc.ca/news/Canada/Calgary/story/2013/06/21/alberta-flooding-calgary-canmore-high-water.html.

Canadian Institute for Health Information. (CIHI, 2016). *National Health Expenditures: How Much Does Canada Spend on Health Care?* Ottawa, Ontario: CIHI. Retrieved April 14, 2017, http://www.cihi.ca/en/nhex2016-topic1.

———. *Canadians Lead World in Internet Use: A Report.* Toronto, ON: CBC, 2011. Accessed October 21, 2015. http://www.cbc.ca/news/technology/canadians-lead-world-in-Internet-use-report-1.1063588.

Canadian Food Inspection Agency. *CFIA Investigation into the XL Food Inc. (E. coli 0157:H7).* Ottawa, ON: Government of Canada, 2013. Accessed June 13, 2013. http://www.inspection.gc.ca/food/information-for-consumers/food-safety-investigations/xl-foods/eng/1347937722467/1347937818275.

———. *Food Safety Facts on Listeria: Listeria Investigation and Recall-2008.* Ottawa, ON: Government of Canada, 2008. Accessed June 1, 2010. http://www.inspection.gc.ca/english/casn_research_mandate.htm.

Canadian Institute for Health Information (CIHI). *Canada's Health Care Spending Growth Slows. Provincial and Territorial Government Health Expenditures Expected to Grow 3.1%, Lowest Since 1997.* Ottawa, ON: CIHI, 2013. Accessed June 13, 2013. http://www.cihi.ca/cihi-ext-portal/internet/en/document/spending+and+health+workforce/spending/release_30oct12.

———. *More Doctors, Higher Spending: Data Sheds Light on Trends in the Physician Workforce.* Ottawa, ON: CIHI, 2015b.

———. National Health Expenditure Trends, 1975 to 2015. Ottawa, ON: CIHI, 2015a. Accessed November 10, 2015. https://www.cihi.ca/en/spending-and-health-workforce/spending/canadas-slow-health-spending-growth-continues.

———. *National Health Expenditure Trends, 1975 to 2014.* Ottawa, ON: Author, 2014. Accessed October 22, 2015. https://secure.cihi.ca/estore/productSeries.htm?pc=PCC52.

Canadian Institutes for Health Research. "2010 Health Indicators Report." Ottawa, ON: Author, 2010. http://www.cihi.ca.

———. *Government of Canada Announces Funding for Research to Further Protect Canadians from the H1N1 Flu Virus (news release).* Ottawa, ON: Author, 2009. www.cihr-irsc.gc.ca/e/39485.html.

Canadian Nurses Association (CNA). *Evidence-based Decision-making and Nursing practice*, 1998. Accessed April 15, 2008. http://www.cna-nurses.ca.

Canadian Nurses Association (CNA). *Fact Sheet. The Primary Health Care Approach*. Ottawa, ON: CNA, 2000.

Canadian Public Health Association (CPHA). *The Future of Public Health in Canada*. Ottawa, ON: CPHA, 2001.

Canadian Public Health Association, World Health Organization. *Ottawa Charter for Health Promotion*. Ottawa, ON: Health and Welfare Canada, 1986.

Canadian Society for Exercise Physiology. *Canadian Physical Activity Guidelines 2012: Background Information*. Ottawa, ON: Author, 2012. Accessed September 13, 2013. http://www.csep.ca/english/view.asp?x=587.

Canadian Wireless Telecommunication Association (CWTA). *Facts and Figures. Wireless Phone Subscribers in Canada*. Ottawa, ON: CWTA, 2014. Accessed April 2, 2015. http://cwta.ca/facts-figures/ and http://cwta.ca/wordpress/wp-content/uploads/2011/08/SubscribersStats_en_2014_Q3-1.pdf.

Cash, H., C. D. Rae, A. H. Steel, and A. Winkler. "Internet Addiction: A Brief Summary of Research and Practice." *Current Psychiatry Reviews* 8, no. 4 (2012): 292–98.

CEFRIO. *L'explosion des médias sociaux au Québec*. Netendance 2010, 1.4. QC, 2010. Accessed October 17, 2013. http://www.cefrio.qc.ca/fileadmin/documents/Publication/NEWendances-Vol1-.pdf.

Centers for Disease Control & Prevention WISQARS. *Web-based Injury Statistics Query and Reporting System (WISQRS)*. Atlanta, GA: Author, 2012. Accessed May 14, 2015. http://www.cdc.gov/ncipe/wisqars/

Childhood Obesity Foundation. Statistics. VGH Hospital Campus, Vancouver, BC, 2015. Accessed November 10, 2015. http://childhoodobesityfoundation.ca/what-is-childhood-obesity/statistics/.

Chóliz, M. *Mobile Phone Addiction in Adolescence: Evaluation and Prevention of Mobile Addiction in Teenagers*. Saarbrucken, Germany: Lambert Academic Publishing, 2010.

Chóliz, M. "Mobile-Phone Addiction in Adolescence: The Test of Mobile Phone Dependence (TMD)." *Progress in Health Sciences* 2, no. 1 (2012).

Chomo, M. *Communications Monitoring Report*. Ottawa, ON: Canadian Wireless Telecommunications Association, 2014.

Christensen, S. 20 Million Canadian Suffer from Nomophobia Rogers says, and This is just the Beginning. *Techvibes*,2013. Accessed October 21, 2015. http://www.techvibes.com/blog/canadians-suffer-from-nomophobia-2013-01-02.

Ciliska, C., H. Thomas, and C. Buffet. *An Introduction to Evidence-informed Public Health and a Compendium of Critical Appraisal Tools for Public Health Practice*, 2008. Accessed October 8, 2013. http://www.nccmt.ca/pubs/eiph_backgrounder.pdf.

Commission on the Social Determinants of Health. *Closing the Gap in a Generation. Health Equity through Action on the Social Determinants of Health*. Geneva, Switzerland: World Health Organization, 2008.

Community Health Nurses Association of Canada (CHNAC). *Canadian Community Health Nursing Standards of Practice*. CHNAC, 2003. Accessed March 23, 2008. http://www.communityhealthnursescanada.org.

Cradduck, G. R. "Primary Health Care Practice." In *Community Nursing: Promoting Canadian's Health*, 2nd ed., edited by M. Stewart, 352–269. Toronto, ON: W. B. Saunders, 2000.

Cullins, S., T. Voth, A. DiCenso, and G. Guyatt. "Finding the Evidence." In *Evidence-based Nursing: A Guide to Clinical Practice*, 20–43. St. Louis, MO: Elsevier/Mosby, 2005.

Damazo, R., and W. J. Bartfay. "Communicable Diseases: Current Perspectives and Challenges." In *Community Health Nursing: Caring in Action*, 1st Canadian ed., 191–215. Toronto, ON: Nelson Education, 2010.

Davidoff, F., B. Haynes, D. Sackett, and R. Smith. "Evidence-based Medicine: A New Journal to Help Doctors Identify the Information They Need." *British Medical Journal* 310 (1995): 1085–86.

Davison, J., and L. Powers. *Why Alberta's Floods Hit so Hard and Fast*. Toronto, ON: Canadian Broadcasting Corporation, 2013. Accessed July 25, 2013. http://www.cbc.ca/news/Canada/Calgary/story/2013/06/21/f-alberta-floods.html.

De Leeuw, E. "Evidence for Healthy Cities: Reflection on Practice, Methods, and Theory." *Health Promotion International* 24, no. S1 (2009): i19–i36.

Deplancke, E. *Healthy Communities Report: A Report on Healthy Communities Initiatives in Canada and Around the World and How to Apply these Strategies in Haldimand and Norfolk Counties*. Ontario, Canada: Haldimand-Norfolk Health Unit, 2009.

Deviney, E. Could you live on $1.75 a day? *The Huntington Post*, 2013. Accessed July 25, 2013. http://www.huntington-post.ca/tag/extreme-poverty-canada.

Dickinson, H. D. "Health Care and Health Reforms: Trends and Issues." In *Health, Illness, and Health Care in Canada*, edited by B. Singh Bolaria, and H. D. Dickinson, 4th ed., 23–41. Toronto, ON: Nelson Education, 2009.

DiCenso, A., D. Ciliska, and G. Guyatt. *Evidence-based Nursing: A Guide to Clinical Practice*. St. Louis, MO: Elsevier Mosby, 2005.

Dixit, S., H. Shukla, A. Bhagwat, A. Bindal, A. Goyal, A. K. Zaidi, and A. Shrivastava. "A Study to Evaluate Mobile Phone Dependence among Students of a Medical College and Associated Hospital of Central India." *Indian Journal of Community Medicine* 35, no. 2 (2010): 339–41. doi: 10.4103/0970-0218.66878.

Dykeman, M. "Primary Health Care Leads to Better Health." *The Canadian Nurse* 108, no. 7 (2010): 52.

Edwards, N., K. Benjamin, and D. Lockett. "Environmental Hazards and Falls Prevention: Defining a New Research Agenda." Poster presented at the 2006 Australian Public Health Association conference, Sydney, Australia, September 25–27, 2006.

Edwards, N., L. MacLean, A. Estable, and M. Meyer. *Multiple Interventions Program Recommendations for Mandatory Health Program and Services Guidelines Technical Review Committee*. Ottawa, ON: Community Health Research Unit, University of Ottawa, 2006.

Elder, N.C., and S. M. Dovey. "Classification of Medical Errors and Preventable Adverse Events in Primary Care: A Synthesis of the Literature." *Journal of Family Practice* 51, no. 11 (2002): 927–32.

Elmore, T. (2014). "Nomophobia: A Rising Trend in Students." *Psychology Today*, Narcross, GA: Growing Leaders Inc., 2014. Accessed April 8. https://www.psychologytoday.com/blog/artificial-maturity/201409/nomophobia-rising-trend-in-students.

Food and Agriculture Organization (FAO). *The State of Agricultural Commodity Markets: High Food Prices and the Food Crisis-experiences and Lessons Learned*. Rome: FAO, 2009.

Food Banks Canada. *Hungercount 2012. A Comprehensive Report on Hunger and Food Bank Use in Canada, and Recommendations for Change*. Toronto, ON: Author, 2012.

Foster, J. "Phonelines are Lifelines." 2010.Accessed June 5, 2013. http://www.tenants.bc.ca/ckfinder/userfiles/files/CVM%20-%2020Phonelines%20are%20Lifelines.pdf.

Frank, J., E. Di Ruggiero, and B. Moloughney. *The Future of Public Health in Canada: Developing a Public Health System for the 21st Century*. Ottawa, ON: Canadian Institute of Health Rearch, 2003. Accessed June 10, 2013. http://www.cihr-irsc.gc.ca/e/19573.html.

Frank, F., and A. Smith. *The Community Development Handbook: A Tool to Build Community Capacity*. Ottawa, ON: Human Resources Development Canada, 1999.

Gallin, J. E., and F. P. Ognibene. *Principles and Practice of Clinical Research*. 2nd ed. New York: Elsevier, 2007.

Gaut, D. A. "A Vision of Wholeness for Nursing." *Journal of Holistic Nursing* 11, no. 2 (1993): 164–71.

Gayton, J. L. "Etiology, Prevalence, and Treatment of Dry Eye Disease." *Clincal Opthalmology* 3 (2009): 405–12.

Gerr, F., M. Marcus, and C. Monteilh. "Epidemiology of Musculoskeletal Disorders among Computer Users: Lessons Learned from the Role of Posture and Keyboard Use." *Journal of Electromyomyography and Kinesiology* 14, no. 1 (2004): 25–31.

Ghori, A., W. J. Bartfay,* E. Bartfay, and O. Sanchez. "Exposure to Electronic Video Display Terminals and Associated Neuromuscular Pain and Discomfort in Male and Female Undergraduate University Students." *Health Tomorrow: Interdisciplinarity and Internationality* 3, no. 1 (2015): 105–26. http://ht.journals.yorku.ca/index.php/ht/article/view/40191/36376.

Gibbs, L. E. *Evidence-based Practice for Helping Professions*. Pacific Grove, CA: Brooks/Cole, 2003.

Gilbert, R. L., N. A. Murphy, and T. McNally. "Addiction to the 3-dimensional Internet: Estimated Prevalence and Relationship to Real World Addictions." *Addiction Research and Theory* 19 (2011): 380–90.

Goldman, R. A., Brunnell, R., and Posner, S. F. (October, 2014). What is "community health"? Examining the meaning of an evolving field in public health. *Preventative Medicine*, 67 (Supplement 1): S58–S61.

Goodwin Veenema, T. *Disaster Nursing and Emergency Preparedness for Chemical, Biological, and Radiological Terrorism and Other Hazards*. 2nd ed. New York: Springer Publishing, 2007.

Gorden, S. *Nursing Against the Odds. How Health Care Cost Cutting, Media Stereotypes, and Medical Hubris Undermine Nurses and Patient Care*. Ithica, NY: ILR Press, 2005.

Government of Alberta. *Affected Communities. Rainfall-impacted Areas.* Calgary, AB: Author, 2013a. Accessed July 25, 2013.http://alberta.ca/rainfall-impacted-areas.cfc/.

———. *2013 Alberta Flood Recovery: Your Community.* Calgary, AB: Author, 2013b. Accessed July 25, 2013. http://alberta.ca/rainfall-impacted-areas.cfm/.

———. *Update 5: Government Continues to Respond to Flood Emergency.* Calgary, AB: Author, 2013c. Accessed July 25, 2013. http://alberta.ca/can/201306/3439971DE6A21-FD13-B8D7-01FE9183DB16ACAC.html.

Government of Canada. *House of Commons: An Act Relating to Cash Contributions by Canada in Respect of Insured Health Services Provided under Provincial Health Care Insurance Plans and Amounts under Provincial Health Care Insurance Plans and Amounts Payable by Canada in Respect to Extended Health Care Services and to Amend and Repeal Certain Acts in Consequence Thereof (The Canada Health Act).* Ottawa, ON: Author, 1984.

Grahame-Smith, D. "Evidence Based Medicine: Socratic Dissent." *British Medical Journal* 310 (1995): 1126–27.

Greaves, L. "Why Put Gender into Health Research?" In *Designing and Conducting Gender, Sex and Health Research,* edited by J. L. Oliffe, and L. Greaves, 3–13. Thousand Oaks: Sage Publications, Inc., 2011.

Guyatt, G. H., A. D. Oxman, R. Kunz, G. E. Vist, Y. Falck-Ytter, H. J. Schunemann, and GRADE Working Group. "GRADE: What is "Quality of Evidence" and Why Is it Important to Clinicians?" *British Medical Journal* 336, no. 7651 (2008): 995–98.

Ha, J. H., B. Chin, D. H. Park, S. H. Ryu, and J. Yu. "Characteristics of Excessive Cellular Phone Use in Korean Adolescents." *Cyberpscyhology and Behavior* 11 (2008): 783–84.

Hales, D., and L. Lauzon. *An Invitation to Health.* 1st Canadian ed. Toronto, ON: Thomson Nelson, 2007.

Hancock, T. *Act Locally: Community-based Population Health Promotion. Report for the Canadian Sub-committee on Population Health.* Ottawa, ON: Canadian Sub-committee on Population Health, 2009.

Hancock, T., and L. Duhl. *Healthy Cities: Promoting Health in the Urban Context. WHO Healthy Cities Paper 1.* Copenhagen: FDAL, 1988.

Health Canada. *Canada Health Act: Frequently Asked Questions.* Ottawa, ON: Government of Canada, 2003. Accessed June 13, 2013. http://www.hc-sc.gc.ca/medicare/FAQ/htm.

———. *Guidelines for Canadian Drinking Water Quality: Supporting Documents.* Ottawa, ON: Author, 2004. Accessed June 1, 2010. http://www.hc-sc.gc.ca/ewh-semt/pubs/water-eau/doc_sup-appui/index_e.html.

Health Council of Canada. *Decisions, Decisions: Family Doctors As Gatekeepers to Prescription Drugs and Diagnostic Imaging in Canada.* Toronto, ON: Author, 2010.

———. *Progress Report 2011: Health Care Renewal in Canada.* Toronto, Ontario: Author, 2011. information@health-councilcanada.ca.

———. *Progress Report 2012: Health Care Renewal in Canada- Fact Sheet.* Toronto, ON, 2012. Accessed June 13, 2013. http://www.healthcouncilcanada.ca/rpt_det.php?id=377.

Heymann, D. L. *Control of Communicable Diseases Manual: An Official Report of the American Public Health Association.* 19th ed. Washington, DC: American Public Health Association, 2008.

Hinshaw, A. S. "Nursing Knowledge for the 21st Century: Opportunities and Challenges." *Journal of Nursing Scholarship* 32, no. 2 (2000): 117–23.

Hitchcock, J. E., Schubert, P. E., Thomas, S. A. and Bartfay, W. J. (2010). *Community health nursing: Caring in action (1st Canadian edition).* Toronto, ON: Pearson's. (ISBN: 13-978-0-17-644103-6).

Hong, F. Y., S. I. Chiu, and D. H. Huang. "A Model of the Relationship between Psychological Characteristics, Mobile Phone Addiction and Use of Mobile Phones by Taiwanese University Female Students." *Computers and Human Behaviour* 28, no. 6 (2012): 2152–58.

Huang, C., W. Ma, and S. Stack. "The Hygienic Efficacy of Different Hand-drying Methods: A Review of the Evidence." *Mayo Clinical Proceedings* 87, no. 7 (2012): 791–98. doi:10.1016/j.mayocp.2012.02.019.

Huang, D., A. K. Kapur, P. Ling, R. Purssell, R. J. Henneberry, C. R. Champagne, V. K. Lee, and L. H. Franescutti. "CAEP Position Statement on Cellphone Use while Driving CAEP Position Statements." *Canadian Journal of Emergency Medicine (CJEM)* 12, no. 4 (2010): 365–70.

Human Resources and Skills Development Canada. *Low Income in Canada: 2000-2006 Using Market Basket Measures,* 2008. Accessed June 5, 2013. http://www.servicecanada.gc.ca/eng/cs/sp/sdc/pkrf/publications/research/SP-630-06-06/page06.shtml.

———. *The Homeless Partnering Strategy*, 2010. Accessed June 5, 2013. http://www.hrsdc.gc.ca/eng/homelessness/index.shtml.

Jackson, N., and E. Waters. "The Challenges of Systematically Reviewing Public Health Interventions." *Journal of Public Health* 26 (2004): 303–07.

Jacobsen, K. H. *Introduction to Global Health*. Toronto, ON: Jones and Bartlett Publishers, 2008.

Jamoulle, M., and M. Roland. *Quaternary Prevention*. Wonca Classification Committee, Hong Kong. Bruxelles, Belgium: Research group, Fédération des Maisons Médicales, Ch.de Waterloo 255/12 B-1060, 1995. Accessed October 17, 2013. http://www.ph3c.org/PH3C/docs/27/000103/0000261.pdfJo.

Johnson, J. L., L. Greaves, and R. Repta. "Better Science with Sex and Gender: Facilitating the Use of Sex and Gender-based Analysis in Health Research." *International Journal for Equity in Health* 8, no. 14 (2009): 8–15.

Joint Task Group. *Federal/Provincial/Territorial Joint Task Group on Public Health Human Resources. Building the Public Health Workforce for the 21ˢᵗ Century*. Ottawa, ON: Author, 2006.

Kindig, D. *Have You Heard of "Primordial Prevention"?* Blog in Population Health Basics, 2011. Accessed October 17, 2013. http://www.improvingpopulationhealth.org.blog/2011/05/primoridial_prevention.html.

King, A. L., A. M. Valenca, and A. E. Nardi. "Nomophobia: The Mobile Phone in Panic Disorder with Agoraphobia. Reducing Phobias or Worsening of Dependence?" *Cognitive and Behavioural Neurology* 23, no. 1 (2010): 52–54. doi: 10.1097/WNN.0b013e3181beabc.

King, A. L. S., A. M. Valença, A. C. Silva, F. Sancassiani, S. Machado, and A. E. Nardi. "'Nomophobia': Impact of Cell Phone Use Interfering with Symptoms and Emotions of Individuals with Panic Disorder Compared with a Control Group." *Clinical practice and epidemiology in mental health: Clinical Practice and Epidemiological Mental Health* 10 (2014): 28–35. doi: 10.2174/174501790141001002.

Koppel, N., and A. Jones. "Are "Sext" Messages a Teenage Felony or Folly?" *Wall Street Journal—Eastern Edition* 256, no. 47 (2010): D1–D2. Accessed May 12, 2015. http://www.wsj.com/articles/SB10001424052748703447004575449423091552284.

Krajewska-Kulak, E., W. Kulak, A. Stryzhak, A. Szpakow, W. Prokopowicz, and J. T. Marcinkowski. "Problematic Cell Phone Use among the Polish and Belarusian University Students, a Comparative Study." *Progress in Health Sciences* 2, no. 1 (2012): 45–50.

Kuehlein, T., D. Sghedoni, G. Visentin, J. Gérvas, and M. Jamoule. "Quaternary Prevention: A Task of the General Practitioner." *Primary Care* 10, no. 18 (2010): 350–54.

Landsman, L. Y. *Public Health Management of Diseases. The Practical Guide*, 2nd ed. Cornell University Press New Office, 2005.

Laroche, J., A. Frescura, and L. Belzak. *Results From the 2006 and 2009 Childhood National Immunization Coverage Surveys*. Presentation at the 9th Canadian Immunization Conference. Immunization: A Global Challenge for the 21st Century, Québec City, QC, 2010.

Lee, K. *Urban Poverty in Canada: A Statistical Profile*. Ottawa, ON: Canadian Council on Social Development, 2000.

Leeseberg Stamler, L., B. Thomas, K. Lafrenier, and R. Charbonneau-Smith. "Women's Perceptions of Breast Cancer Screening and Education Opportunities in Canada." *Canadian Nurse* 97, no. 9 (2001): 23–27.

Leininger, M. *Culture Care Diversity and Universality: A Theory of Nursing*. New York, NY: National League for Nursing Press, 1991.

Lemire Rodger, G. "Canadian Nurses Association." In *Realities of Canadian Nursing: Profession, Practice and Power Issues*, 2nd ed., edited by M. McIntye, E. Thomlinson, and C. McDonald, 133–51. Baltimore: Lippincott Williams & Wilkins, 2006.

Leavell, H., and E. Clark. *Preventive Medicine for the Doctor in His Community: An Epidemiologic Approach*. New York: McGraw-Hill, 1958.

Leung, M. *Typical Family Will Pay More than $11K for Health Care in 2014: Fraser Institute*. Toronto, ON: CTV News Canada, 2014. Accessed October 22, 2015. http://www.ctvnews.ca/health/typical-family-will-pay-more-than-11k-for-health-care-in-2014-fraser-institute-1.1897266.

Library of Parliament. *Bill C-13. Protecting Canadians from On-line Crime Act. An Act to Amend the Criminal Code, the Canada Evidence Act, the Competition Act and the Mutual Legal Assistance in Criminal Matters Act*. Ottawa, ON: Government of Canada, 2014. Accessed April 13, 2015. https://openparliament.ca/bills/41-2/C-13/.

Lin, P. Y., C. Y. Cheng, W. M. Hsu, S. Y. Tsai, M. W. Lin, J. H. Liu, and P. Chou. "Association between Symptoms and Signs of Dry Eye among an Elderly Chinese Population in Taiwan: The Shihpai Eye Study." *Investigative Ophthalmology and Visual Science* 46, no. 5 (2005): 1593–98.

Livernois, J. *The Walkerton Inquiry Commissioned Paper 14: The Economic Costs of Walkerton Water Crisis.* Ottawa, ON: Ontario Ministry of the Attorney General, Queen's Printer for Ontario, 2002. Accessed June 13, 2013. http://www. uoguelph.ca~live/WICP-14-Livernois1.pdf.

LoBiondo-Wood, G., J. Haber, C. Canmerson, and M. D. Singh. "The Role of Research in Nursing." In *Nursing Research in Canada: Methods, Critical Appraisal, and Utilization,* 1st Canadian ed., edited by G. LoBiondo-Wood, and J. Haber, 5–27. Toronto, ON: Elsevier Mosby, 2005.

Nancarrow Clark, J. *Health, Illness, and Medicine in Canada,* 5th ed. Toronto, ON: Oxford University Press, 2008.

National Collaborating Centre for Methods and Tools. "A Model for Evidence-informed Decision-making in Public Health." Fact sheet, 2012. Accessed October 15, 2013. http://www.nccmt.ca/pubs/FactSheet_EIDM_EN_WEB.pdf.

National Collaborating Centres for Public Health (NCCPH). "What is Evidence-informed Public Health?" Fact sheet, 2011. Accessed October 12, 2013. http://www.nccmt.ca/eiph/.

National Expert Commission Canadian Nurses Association. *A Nursing Call to Action. The Health of Our Nation, the Future of Our Health System.* Ottawa, ON: Canadian Nurses Association, 2012. Accessed June 10, 2013. http://www. can-aiic.ca/expertcommission/.

Manitoba Health. *The Role of the Public Health Nurse within the Regional Health Authority.* Winnipeg, MB: Community Health Assessment Unit and Manitoba Health, 1998. http://www.gov.mb.ca/health.

Marchione, M.. "Killer Cantaloupe, Scary Sprouts—What to Do?" *The Associated Press,* 2011. Accessed September 29, 2011. http://news.ca.msn.com/health/killer-cantaloupe-scary-sprouts-what-to-do-42.

Martinez-Prather, K., and D. M. Vandiver. "Sexting among Teenagers in the United States: A Retrospective Analysis of Identifying Motivating Factors, Potential Targets, and the Role of Capable Guardian." *International Journal of Cyber Criminology* 8, no. 1 (2014): 21–35.

Masse, R., and B. Molughney. "New Era for Schools and Programs of Public Health in Canada." *Public Health Reviews* 33, no. 1 (2011): 277–88.

Mattey, B. and G. Mattey Diliberto. "Sexting—It's in the Dictionary." *National Association of School Nurses (NASN)* 28, no. 2 (2013): 94–99.

McCormack, B., Rycroft-Malone, J., Decorby, K., Hutchinson, A. M., Bucknall, T., Kent, B., Schultz, A., et al. "A Realist View of Interventions and Strategies to Promote Evidence-informed Healthcare: A Focus on Change Agency." *Implementation Science* 8, no. 8 (2013): 107–14.

McKenzie, J. F., B. L. Neiger, and R. Thackeray. *Planning, Implementing, and Evaluating Health Promotion Programs: A Primer,* 5th ed. Toronto, ON: Pearson Benjamin Cummings, 2009.

McKeown, T. *The Role of Medicine: Dream, Mirage or Nemesis?.* London, England: Nuffield Provincial Hospital, 1976.

McMurray, A. *Community Health and Wellness: A Socio-ecological Approach.* Toronto, ON: Mosby/Elsevier, 2007.

Merriam-Webster. *Merriam-Webster Dictionary.* Springfield, MA: Author, 2012. Accessed October 24, 2015. http://www. merriam-webster.com/.

Messmer, E. M. "The Pathophysiology, Diagnosis, and Treatment of Dry Eye Disease." *Deutsches Arzteblatt International* (January 2015). doi:10.3238/arztebl.2015.0071.

Mhatre, S.L., and R. Deber. "From Equal Access to Health Care Equitable Access to Health: Review of Canadian Provincial Commissions and Reports." *International Journal of Health Services* 22, no. 4 (1992): 645–68.

Middlesex-London Health Unit. *Evidence-informed Public Health.* Middlesex-London, ON: Author, 2013. Accessed October 12, 2013. http://www.healthunit.com/evidence-informed-public-health.

Mitchell, K. J., D. Finkelhor, L. M. Jones, and J. Wolak. "Prevalence and Characteristics of Youth Sexting: A National Study." *Pediatrics* 129, no. 1 (2012): 1–8. doi:10.1542/peds.2011-1730.

Mitty, E.. "Iatrogenesis, Frailty, and Geriatric Syndromes." *Geriatric Nursing* 31, no. 5 (2010): 368–74. doi:10.1016/j. gerinurse.2010.08.004.

Morgan, C., and S. R. Cotton. "The Relationship between Internet Activities and Depressive Symptoms in a Sample of College Freshman." *Cyberpsychology & Behaviour: The impact of the Internet, multimedia and virtual reality on behaviour and society* 6, no. 2 (2003): 133–38.

Morse, J. M., J. Botorff, W. Neander, and S. Solberg. "Comparative Analysis of Conceptualizations and Theories of Caring." *Image: Journal of Nursing Scholarship* 23, no. 2 (1999): 119–26.

Mussalem, H. K. "Professional Nurse's Associations." In *Canadian Nursing Faces the Future*, 2nd ed., edited by A. J. Baumgart, and J. Larsen, 495–518. Toronto, ON: Mosby, 1992.

Naci, H., D. Chisholm, and T. D. Baker. "Distribution of Road Traffic Deaths by Road User Group: A Global Comparison." *Injury Prevention* 15 (2009): 55–59. doi:10.1136/ip.2008.018721.

Naidoo, J., and J. Wills. *Health Promotion: Foundation for Practice*. 2nd ed. Toronto, ON: Bailliere Tindall/Elsevier Limited, 2004.

National Expert Commission Canadian Nurses Association. *A Nursing Call to Action: The Health of Our Nation, the Future of Our Health System*. Ottawa, ON: Canadian Nurses Association, 2012.

National Public Health Partnership (NPHP). *The Language of Prevention*. Melbourne, Australia: NPHP, 2006.

Naylor, D. *Learning from SARS: Renewal of Public Health in Canada: A Report of the National Advisory Committee on SARS and Public Health*. Ottawa, ON: Health Canada, 2003.

Nevo, I., and V. Slonim-Nevo. "The Myth of Evidence-based Practice: Towards Evidence-informed Practice." *British Journal of Social Work* 1–22. doi:10.1093/bjsw/bcq149.

Nightengale, E. O., M. Cureton, and V. Kalmar. *Perspectives on Health Promotion and Disease Prevention in the United States*. Washington, DC: Institute of Medicine, National Academy of Science, 1978.

O'Connor, D. R. *Walkerton Commission of Inquiry Reports: A Strategy for Safe Drinking Water*. Toronto, ON: Ontario Minister of the Attorney General, 2002. Accessed June 13, 2013. http://www.attorneygeneral.jus.gov.on.ca/English/about/pubs/walkerton/.

Office of Nursing Policy—Health Canada. *Key Policy Directions 2002-2003*, 2003. Accessed April 7, 2008. http://www.hc-sc.gc.ca/onp-bpsi/english/about_us/priorities.html.

Olney, C. M. "The Effect of Therapeutic Back Massage in Hypertensive Patients: A Preliminary Study." *Biological Research for Nursing* 7, no. 2 (2005): 98–105.

Oksman, V., and J.Turtianinen. "Mobile Communication As a Social Stage. The Meaning of Mobile Communication among Teenagers in Finland." *New Medicine and Sociology* 6, (2004): 319–39.

O'Neill, M., P. Simard, N. Sasseville, J. Mucha,B. Losier, and M. Niquette. "Promoting Health through the Setting Approach." In *Health Promotion in Canada: Critical Perspectives on Practice*, edited by I. Rootman, S. Dupéré, A. Pederson, and M. O-Neill, 171–92. Toronto, ON: Canadian Scholar's Press International, 2012.

Order of Nurses of Québec. *How Much Longer until Adequate Funding is Provided for Community Nursing Services?* Montréal, QC: Author (In French), 2012. Accessed June 3, 2013. http://www.oiiq.org/node/7371.

Orme, J., J. Powell, P. Taylor, and M. Grey. *Public Health for the 21st Century: New Perspectives on Policy, Participation and Practice*. 2nd ed. New York: Open University Press, 2007.

Ontario Association of Food Banks. *The Costs of Poverty: An Analysis of the Economic Costs*. Toronto, ON: Author, 2008.

Oxman, A. D., J. N. Lavis, and A. Fretheim. "Use of Evidence in WHO Recommendations." *The Lancet* 369, no. 9576–9578 (2007): 1883–89.

Pach, B. *What Is the "Evidence" in Evidence-based Public Health? Pathways to Evidence Informed Public Health Policy and Practice*. Toronto, ON: Ontario Public Health Libraries Association (OPHL) Foundation Standard Workshop, 2008.

Patel, A. *Canada Food Bank Use Increases Across the Country: Report*. Toronto, ON: The Huntington Post Canada, 2014. Accessed October 22, 2015. http://www.huffingtonpost.ca/2014/11/04/canada-food-bank-use-2014_n_6101004.html.

ParticipACTION. *The ParticipACTION Archive Project*. Ottawa, ON: Government of Canada. Accessed May 15, 2013. http://www.usask.ca:80/archieves/participation/English/impact/index.html.

Paulsen, M. "Giving Voice(mail) to the Homeless." 2010. Accessed June 5, 2013. http://thetyee.ca/Blogs/TheHook/Housing/2010/04/30/Giving-voicemail-to-the-homeless/.

Polit, D. F., and C. Tatano Beck. *Nursing Research: Generating and Assessing Evidence for Nursing Practice*. New York: Wolters Kluwe/Lippincott Williams & Wilkins, 2012.

Porta, M. *A Dictionary of Epidemiology*. 5th ed. Toronto, ON: Oxford University Press, 2008.

Porter, E. J. "Older Widows' Experiences of Home Care." *Nursing Research* 54, no. 5 (2005): 296–303.

Public Health Action Support Team. *Epidemiological Basis for Preventive Strategies*. England, UK, 2011. Accessed October 18, 2013. http://www.healthknowledge.org.uk/public-health-textbook/research-methods/1c-health-c.

Public Health Agency of Canada (PHAC). *Act to Establish Public Health Agency Outcomes into Force*, 2012. Accessed April 19, 2008. http://www.phac-aspc.gc.ca/media/nr-rp?2006/2006_11_e.html.

———. "Bioterrorism and Public Health." *Canada Communicable Disease Report*, 27, no. 4. (2001).

———. *Canada's Aging Population. Division of Aging Seniors*. Ottawa, ON: PHAC, 2008b. Accessed June 13, 2013. http://www.phac-aspc.gc.ca/seniors-aines/publications/public/various-varies/papier-fed-paper/index-eng.php.

———. *Canadian Iimmunization Guide*. Ottawa, ON: Author, 2012. Accessed June 11, 2013. http://www.phac-aspc.gc.ca/publicat/cig-gci/.

———. *Core Competencies for Public Health in Canada: Release 1.1*. Ottawa, ON: Author, 2007.

——— *Government of Canada Invests in Project Promoting Walking to Prevent Chronic Disease*. Ottawa, ON: Government of Canada and PHAC, 2015. Accessed October 21, 2015. http://news.gc.ca/web/article-en.do?nid=1013839&tp=1.

———. *Planning for a Sustainable Future. The Public Health Agency of Canada's Departmental Sustainable Development Strategy 2011-2014*. Ottawa, ON: Office of Sustainable Development-Public Health Agency of Canada, 2011.

———. *Public Health Notice: E. coli 0157 Illness Related Beef*. Ottawa, ON: PHAC, 2012. Accessed June 13, 2013. http://www.phac-aspc.gc.ca/fs-sa/phn-asp/ecoli-1012-eng.php.

———. *The Chief Public Health Officer's Report on the State of Public Health in Canada-2008—Chapter 2*. Ottawa, ON: PHAC, 2008a. Accessed June 26, 2010. http://www.phac-aspc.gc.ca/publicat/2008/cphorsphc-respcacsp/cphorsphc-respcacsp)5B-2.

Public Safety and Emergency Preparedness Canada. *Canada Disaster Database*, 2005. Accessed June 10, 2010. http://www.psepc-sppcc.gc.ca/res/em/cdd/search-en.asp.

Quinlan, E., and H. D. Dickinson. "The Emerging Public Health System in Canada." In *Health, Illness, and Health Care in Canada*. 4th ed., edited by B. Singh Bolaria, and H. D. Dickinson, 42–55. Toronto, ON: Nelson Education, 2009.

Ramaswamy, V., and V. M. Cresence. Listeria: Review of Epidemiology and Pathogenesis. *Journal of Microbiology, Epidemiology and Infections*, 40, (2007): 4–13.

Raphael, D. *Health Promotion and Quality of Life in Canada. Essential Readings*. Toronto, ON: Canadian Scholars Press, Inc., 2010.

———. ed. *Social Determinants of Health*. 2nd ed. Toronto, ON: Canadian Scholars Press, Inc., 2009.

———. ed. *Social Determinants of Health: Canadian Perspectives*. Toronto, ON: Canadian Scholars Press, Inc., 2004

Reidpath, D. D., and P. Allotey. "Measuring Global Inequity." *International Journal for Equity in Health* 6, no. 16. doi:10.1186/1475-9276-6-16.

Repacholi, M. H., M. Lerchl, M. Rossli, A. Sienkiewicz, A. Auvinen, J. Breckenkamp, G. d'Inzeo, et al. "Systematic Review of Wireless Phone Use and Brain Cancer and Other Health Tumors." *Bioelectromagnetics*, 33, (2012): 187–206. doi:10.1002/bem/20716.

Rice, E., H. Rhoades, H. Winetrobe, M. Sanchez, J. Montoya, A. Plant, and T. Kordic. "Sexually Explicit Cell Phone Messaging Associated with Sexual Risk among Adolescents." *Pediatrics* 130 (2012): 667. doi:10.1542/peds.2012-0021.

Roger, G.L., and S. M. Gallagher. "The Move Toward Primary Health Care in Canada: Community Health Nursing from 1985 to 2000." In *Community Nursing: Promoting Canadian's Health*. 2nd. ed., Edited by M. J. Stewart, 35–55. Toronto, ON: W. B. Saunders, 2000.

Rogers Communication. *Rogers Innovation Report Infographic 2013*. Toronto, ON: Author, 2013. Accessed October 21, 2015. http://redboard.rogers.com/rogers-innovation-report-infographic-2013/.

Rootman, I., S. Dupéré, A. Pederson, and M. O'Neil. *Health Promotion in Canada. Critical Perspectives on Practice*. 3rd ed. Toronto, ON: Canadian Scholars Press, Inc., 2012.

Romanow, R. J. *Building on Values: The Future of Health Care in Canada*, 2002. Accessed June 5, 2010. http://www.hcsc.gc.ca/english/care/romanow/hcc0086.html.

Rubin, A. "Improving the Teaching of Evidence-based Practice: Introduction to the Special Issue." *Research on Social Work Practice* 17 (2007): 541–47.

Rutty, C., and S. C. Sullivan. *This is Public Health: A Canadian History*. Ottawa, ON: Canadian Public Health Association, 2010. Accessed September 13, 2013. http://www.cpha.ca/uploads/history/book/History-book-print_ALL_e.pdf.

Rychetnik, L., M. Frommer, P. Hawe, and A. Shiell. "Criteria for Evaluating Evidence on Public Health Interventions." *Journal of Epidemiology and Community Health* 56 (2002): 119–27.

Rycroft-Malone, J. "Evidence-informed Practice: From Individual to Context. *Journal of Nursing Management* 16, no. 4 (2008): 404–08. doi:10.111/j.1365-2834.2008.00859.x.

Sackett, D. L., W. M. C. Rosenberg, J. A. Muir Gray, R. B. Haynes, and W. C. Richardson. "Evidence-based Medicine: What It Is and What It Isn't." *British Medical Journal* 312 (1996): 71–72.

Sackett, D. L., S. E. Straus, W. S. Richardson, W. Rosenberg, and R. B. Haynes. *Evidence-based Medicine: How to Practice and Teach EBM*. 2nd ed. New York: Churchill Livingstone, 2000.

Salomon-Ben Zeev, M., D. D. Miller, and R. Latkany. "Diagnosis of Dry Eye Disease and Emerging Technologies." *Clinical Ophthalmology* 8 (2014): 581–90. doi:10.2147/OPTH.S45444.

Salvation Army. *Canada Speaks. Exposing Myths About the 150,000 Canadians Living on the Street*. Toronto, ON: Author, 2011.

Sawatzky-Dickson, D. *Evidence-informed Practice Resource Package*. Winnipeg, MB: Winnipeg Regional Health Authority, 2010.

Schneider, M. J. *Introduction to Public Health*. 3rd ed. Toronto, ON: Jones and Bartlett Publishers, 2012.

Scotto, C. J. "A New View of Caring." *Journal of Nursing Education* 42, no. 7 (2003): 289–91.

Scriver, A., and S. Garman. *Public Health: Social Context and Action*. New York: Open University Press, 2007.

SecurEnvoy. "Could You Live without Your Cellphone?" SecurEnvoy, 2012a. Accessed April 8, 2015. http://www.securenvoy.com/blog/2012/05/23could-you-live-without-your-cellphone/.

———. *66% of the Population Suffer from Nomophobia the Fear of Being without Their Phone*, 2012b. Accessed May 12, 2014. http://www.securenvoy.com/blog/2012/02/16/66-of-the-population-suffer-fromnomophobia-the-fear-of-being-without-their-phone/.

Seitz, H., D. Stinner, T. Eikmann, C. Herr, and M. Roosli. "Electromagnetic Hypersensitivity (EHS) and Subjective Health Complaints Associated with Electromagnetic Fields of Mobile Phone Communication—A Literature Review Published between 2000 and 2004." *Science Total Environ* 349 (2005): 45–55. doi:10.1016/j.scitotenv.2005.05.009 pmid:15975631.

Schabas, R. "Is the Quarantine Act Relevant?" *Canadian Medical Association Journal* 176, no. 13 (2007). doi:10.1503/cmaj.070130.

Skolnik, R. *Global Health 101*. 2nd ed. Mississauga, ON: Jones & Bartlett Learning Canada, 2012.

Snelling, A. M., T. Saville, D. Stevens, and C. B. Beggs. "Comparative Evaluation of the Hygienic Efficacy of an Ultra-rapid Hand Dryer vs Conventional Warm Air Hand Dryers. *Journal of Applied Microbiology* 110, no.1 (2011): 19–26. doi:10.111/j.1365-2672.2010.04838.x.

Soroka, S., and A. Mahon. *Analysis of the Impact of Current Health Care System Funding and Financing Models and the Value of Health and Health Care in Canada. Part III*. Ottawa, ON: Canadian Health Services Research Foundation and Canadian Nurses Foundation, 2012.

Spear King, A. L., A. M. Valenca, A. C. Silva, F. Sancassiani, S. Machado, and A. E. Nardi. "Nomophobia": Impact of Cell Phone Use Interfering with Symptoms and Emotions of Individuals with Panic Disorder Compared with Control Group." *Clinical Practice and Epidemiological Mental Health* 10 (2014): 28–35. doi:10.2174/1745017901410010028.

Stade, B., W. J. Ungar, B. Stevens, J. Beyene, and G. Koren. "The Burden of Prenatal Exposure to Alcohol: Measurement of Cost." *Journal of FAS International* 4 (2006): 1–14.

Standing Senate Committee on Social Affairs, Science and Technology, Subcommittee on Population Health. *A Healthy, Productive Canada: A Determinant of Health Approach*. Ottawa, ON: Author, 2009. Accessed October 7, 2013. http://www.parl.gc.ca/Content/SEN/Committee/402/popu/rep/rephealth1jun09-e.pdf.

Starfield, B. "Politics, Primary Healthcare and Health: Was Virchow Right?" *Journal of Epidemiology and Community Health* 65 (2011): 653–55.

Starfield, B., J. Hyde, J. Gervas, and I. Health. "The Concept of Prevention: A Good Idea Gone Astray?" *Journal of Epidemiology and Community Health* 62 (2008): 580–83. doi:10.1136/jech.2007.071027.

Statistics Canada. "Canada's Population Estimates; Age and Sex 2014." Ottawa, ON: Author, 2014. Accessed November 10, 2015. http://www.statcan.gc.ca/daily-quotidien/140926/dq140926b-eng.htm.

————. *Physical Activity Levels of Canadian Children and Youth, 2007 to 2009.* Ottawa, ON: Author, 2013. (Report 82-625-X). Accessed November 10, 2015. http://www.statcan.gc.ca/pub/82-625-x/2011001/article/11553-eng.htm.

————. *2011 Census: Population and Dwelling Counts.* Ottawa, ON: Author, 2012. Accessed June 13, 2013. http://www.statcan.gc.ca/pub/91-003-x/91-003-x2007001.eng.pdf.

Steeves, V. "Media Smarts. Young Canadians in a Wired World. Sexuality and Romatic Relationships in the Digital Age." Ottawa, ON: Media Smarts, 2014. Accessed April 2, 2015. http://mediasmarts.ca/sites/mediasmarts/files/pdfs/publication-report/full/YCWWIII_Sexuality_Romantic_Relationships_Digital_Age_FullReport_0.pdf.

Stirling, R., J. Aramini, A. Ellis, G. Lim, R. Meyers, M. Fleury, and D. Werker. "Waterborne Cryptosporidiosis Outbreak, North Battleford, Saskatchewan, Spring 2001." *Canadian Communicable Disease Reports* 27, no. 22 (2001): 185–92.

Strasser, T. "Relections on Cardiovascular Disease." *Interdisciplinary Science Reviews* 3 (1978): 225–30.

Straus, S. E., W. S. Richardson, P. Glasziou, and R. B. Haynes. *Evidence-based Medicine: How to Practice and Teach EBP.* 3rd ed. New York: Churchill Livingston, 2005.

Skolnik, R. *Global Health 101.* (2nd ed. Mississauga, ON: Jones & Bartlett Learning Canada, 2012.

Sullivan, P. *Safety of Drinking Water Remains a Crucial Health Issue. CMA President Says.* Canadian Medical Association, 2004. Accessed May 2, 2008. http://www.cam.ca/index.cfm/ci_id/10013192/la_id.1.html.

Sullivan, T., and P. Baranek. *First Do No Harm: Making Sense of Canadian Health Reform.* Toronto, ON: Malcolm Lester & Associates, 2002.

Swanson, K. M. "What is Known About Caring in Nursing Science: A Literary Meta-analysis." In *Handbook of Clinical Nursing Research*, edited by A. S. Hinshaw, S. L. Feetham, and J. L. F. Shaver, 31–60. Thousand Oaks, CA: Sage Publications, 1999.

Taylor, S. "Wealth, Health and Equity: Convergence to Divergence in the Late 20th Century Globalization." *British Medical Bulletin* 91 no. 1 (2009): 29–48.

The Canadian Press. "Text Messaging Canadians Sent on Average 2,500 Texts Every Second in 2011, Total of 78 Billion." Ottawa, ON: Author, 2012. Accessed April 2, 2015. http://www.huffingtonpost.ca/2012/04/13/text-messaging-canada_n_1424730.html?.

The Council of Canadians. *Report on Notice for Drinking Water Crisis in Canada.* Bank Street, Ottawa, ON: Author, 2015. Accessed October 15, 2015. http://canadians.org/drinking-water.

Thompson, V. D. *Health and Health Care Delivery in Canada.* Toronto, ON: Mosby/Elsevier, 2010.

Toda, M., K. Monden,, K. Kubo, and K. Morimoto. "Mobile Phone Dependence and Health-related Lifestyle of University Students." *Sociological Behavioral Perspectives* 8, no. 2 (2006): 121–30.

Turnock, B. J. *Public Health: What It Is and How It Works*, 5th ed. Toronto, ON: Jones & Bartlett Publishing, 2012.

Uchino, M., N. Yokoi, Y. Uchino, M. Dogru, M. Kawashima, and A. Komuro. "Prevalence of Dry Eye Disease and Its Risks Factors in Visual Display Terminal Users: The Osaka Study." *American Journal of Ophthalmology* 2013. doi:10.1016/j.ajo.2013.05.040.

UNICEF Canada. *UNICEF Report Card 11: Child Well-being in Rich Countries.* Toronto, ON: Author, 2013. Accessed July 25, 2013. http://www.unicef.ca/en/discover/article/child-well-being-in-rich-countries-a-comparative-overview.

UNICEF. Innocenti Research Centre. *Innocenti Report Card 10: Measuring Child Poverty. New League Tables on Child Poverty in the Worlds Rich Countries.* Florence, Italy: Author, 2012.

United Nations Development Program (UNDP). "A New Sustainable Development Agenda." New York: United Nations, 2015. Accessed October 25, 2015. http://www.undp.org/content/undp/en/home/mdgoverview.html.

————. *The Millennium Development Goals Report 2009.* New York: United Nations, 2009.

Vasilevskis, E. E., E. W. Ely, T. Speroff, B. T. Pun, L. Boehm, and R. S. Dittus. "Reducing Iatrogenic Risks: ICU-acquired Delirium and Weakness—Crossing the Quality Chasm." *Chest* 138, no. 5 (2010): 1224–33. doi:10.1378/chest.10-0466.

Watson, R., and A. Lea. "The Caring Dimension Inventory (CDI): Content, Validity, Reliability, and Scaling." *Journal of Advanced Nursing* 25 (1997): 87–94.

Weinstein, A., and M. Lejoyeux. "Internet Addiction or Excessive Internet Use." *American Journal of Drug, and Alcohol Abuse* 36 (2010): 277–83.

West, L. "Global Warming Leads to 150,000 Deaths Every Year. Infectious Diseases and Death Rates Rise Along Global Temperatures." *About News*, 2015. Accessed December 8, 2015. http://environment.about.com/od/globalwarmingandhealth/a/gw_deaths.htm.

White, R. *Good Samaritan killed in ATV Crash while Attempting to Check Flood Damage to Neighbour's Home*. Calgary, AB: CTV News, 2013. Accessed July 25, 2013. http://Calgary.ctvnews.ca/good-smaritan-killed-in-atv-crash-whie-attempting-to-check-flood-damage-to-neighbour-s-home-1.1338585.

Williams, N., and S. Haggett. "Floods Shut Down Canada's Oil Capital, Four to Five may be Dead." *Reuters*, June 21, 2013. Accessed July 25, 2013. http://ca.news.yahoo.com/floods-canadas-oil-capital-calgary-force-75-000-151201622.html.

Wilson, R. *The Canadian Medicare System—An Overview*. Pulmonary Hypertension Central, 2002. Accessed June 10, 2013. http://www.phcentral.org.feature/110102wilson.html

Wilson, J. "Facing an Uncertain Climate." *Annuals of Internal Medicine* 146, no. 2 153–56.

Wood, J. "Harper, Redford Promise Help." *Calgary Herald*, June 22, 2013, A5.

World Health Organization. (1998). Health promotion glossary. Geneva, Switzerland. Author.

World Health Organiztion. (2004). A *glossary of key terms for community care services for older persons*. Geneva, Switzerland. Author.

World Health Organization and UNICEF. *WHO/ UNICEF Joint Monitoring Programme for Water Supply and Sanitation. Progress on Drinking Water and Sanitation*, 2015 update. Geneva, Switzerland: Author, 2015.

World Health Organization (WHO). *Belfast Declaration for Healthy Cities*. Geneva, Switzerland. WHO, 2003. Accessed October 15, 2013. http://www.euro.who.int/document;Hcp/Belfast_DEC_E.pdf.

———. *Commission on Social Determinants of Health. Report by the Secretariat. Executive Board 124th Session Provisional Agenda Item 4.6 (EB124/9)*. Geneva, Switzerland: WHO, 2008.

———. *Communicable Diseases: Highlights of Communicable Disease Activities, Major Recent Achievements*. Switzerland, Geneva: Author, 2009. Accessed June 13, 2013. http://www.searo.who.int/EN/Se;ction10.htm.

———. *Health Promotion Glossary*. Geneva, Switzerland: Author, 1998.

———. *Millennium Development Goals: Progress Towards the Health-related Millennium Development Goals* (Fact sheet No. 20). Geneva, Switzerland: WHO, 2012.

———. *NCD Country Profiles, 2011 Canada*. Geneva, Switzerland: Author, 2011. Accessed June 13, 2013. http://www.who.int/nmh/countries/can.en.pdf.

———. *Primary Health Care: Report on the International Conference on Primary Health Care, Alma Ata, USSR, September 6–12, 1978*. Geneva, Switzerland: WHO, 1978.

———. "Systematic Review of the Health Effects of Exposure to Radiofrequency Electromagnetic Fields from Mobile Phone Base Stations by Martin Roosli, Patrizia Frei, Elelyn Mohler and Kerstin Nug." *Bulletin of the World Health Organization* 88 877–96F. doi:10./2471/BLT.09.071852.

———. *The Bangkok Charter for Health Promotion in a Globalized World*. Geneva, Switzerland: WHO, 2005.

———. *The World Health Report*. Geneva, Switzerland: WHO, 2000.

World Health Organization and Health and Welfare Canada & the Canadian Public Health Agency. "Ottawa Charter for Health Promotion." *Canadian Journal of Public Health* 77, no. 12 (1986): 425–30.

World Health Organization Regional Office for Europe. *Healthy Cities: Books and Published Technical Documents*. Geneva, Switzerland: WHO, 2003. Accessed October 15, 2013. http://www.euro.who.int/healthy-cities/publications/20030206_3.

Yildirim, C. "Exploring the Dimensions of Nomophobia: Developing and Validating a Questionnaire Using Mixed Methods Research." Graduate Theses and Dissertations. Paper 14005. Anes, Iowa: Iowa State University, 2014. Accessed April 8, 2015. http://lib.dr.iastate.edu/cgi/viewcontent.cgi?article=5012&context=etd.

Young, K. "Understanding On-line Gaming Addiction and Treatment Issues for Adolescents." *American Journal of Family Therapy* 37 (2009): 355–72.

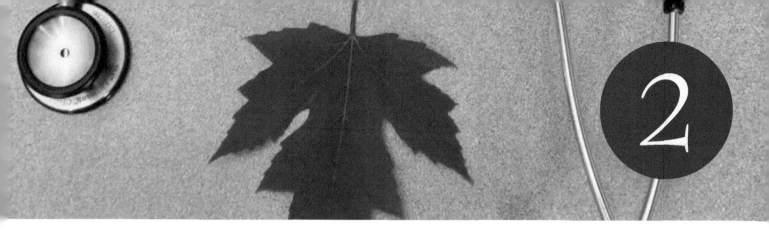

Understanding the Concept of "Health": Its Evolution and Definitions

Those who dwell among the beauties and mysteries of the Earth are never alone or weary of life.
—Rachel Carson, 1907–1964

Learning Objectives

After completion of this chapter, the student will be able to:
- list and critically examine historical events and forces that have shaped definitions of what health is and how it is believed to be maintained, achieved, restored and promoted;
- describe physical, biochemical, socio-political, cultural, spiritual, and environments factors that can both negatively and positively affect the health of individuals, families, groups, and entire communities;
- describe three strengths and limitations of the medical model of health;
- describe how current holistic definitions of health have evolved based on research related to the social determinants of health; and
- describe the role of public health care professionals and workers in maintaining, achieving, restoring and promoting the health and well-being of Canadian residents and citizens across the lifespan.

Core Competencies addressed in Chapter 2

Core Competencies	Competency Statements
1.0 Public Health Sciences	1.1, 1.2, 1.4, 1.5
2.0 Assessment and Analysis	2.1, 2.2., 2.4, 2.5, 2.6
3.0 Policy and Program Planning, Implementation, and Evaluation	3.1, 3.2, 3.3, 3.6
4.0 Partnerships, Collaboration, and Advocacy	4.1, 4.3, 4.4
5.0 Diversity and Inclusiveness	5.1, 5.2
6.0 Communication	6.1, 6.2
7.0 Leadership	7.1, 7.2, 7.3, 7.4

Note: Please see the following document or web-based link for a detailed description of these specific competencies (Public Health Agency of Canada, 2007).

Introduction

The concept of "health" may be regarded as a ubiquitous and dynamic term with diverse interpretations, contexts and meaning to individuals in different cultures and across the lifespan (Bartfay 2010a, Bartfay and Bartfay 2015). For some, being healthy simply means the absence of acute or chronic disease. By contrast, individuals living with a chronic communicable (e.g., HIV) or non-communicable disease (e.g., type I diabetes mellitus) may regard themselves as being healthy. For others, health means a positive sense of soundness, wholeness, and wellness between one's psychological, spiritual, socio-political, environmental, and biological states of being. For others, health is a viewed as a positive resource and basic human right for all global citizens. Indeed, there is currently no universally employed or accepted and unwavering standardized definition of health for all concerned.

In fact, it may be argued that **health** is not a single state or goal, but a process that involves various interconnected and interdependent factors and dynamic states of existence across the lifespan (Bartfay and Bartfay 2015). Health is not a single lineal destination, but a dynamic and complex interactive journey through one's physical, biochemical, socio-political, cultural, and spiritual environments.

Our understanding of the concept of health and the evolution of various definitions of this state of existence over time, is closely associated and interwoven with the history of agricultural societies and the development of various civilizations; the growth of religious practices and beliefs; shamanism, and other healing practices; pharmacy; medicine, nursing, and developments in public health. The word *health* is derived from the old Anglo-Saxon word "haelth" which is derived from the proto-Germanic word *hailitho* referring to a general state of mental and physical soundness or wholeness, and the old English word "haelan" meaning to heal (Harper 2013; Thompson 2010). However, the meaning of this word has evolved overtime due to a better understanding of a variety of factors and determinants which can either negatively (e.g., smoking, genetic pre-disposition to breast cancer) or positively (e.g., exercise, diet low in saturated and trans fats) affect this state of existence.

Accordingly, in this chapter, we shall attempt to collectively examine how these influences and factors have collectively shaped our current understanding of this critical concept. Indeed, it is critical for all public health professionals and workers to first have a clear understanding of what the concept of health entails if their mandate is to preserve, promote, and/or restore the health of individuals, families, groups, communities, or entire populations. Accordingly, we shall survey evidence-informed holistic definitions of health and how they influence current Canadian public health care policy and practice directives. We shall also examine how the dominant mechanistic medical model of health has evolved overtime, and its influence on our current public health

---

Group Activity-based Learning Box 2.1

What exactly does the concept of "health" mean to you?

The Group Activity-Based Learning Box 2.1 is designed to stimulate classroom discussions and debate related to the concept of health; what it means to you currently, and how it is maintained and promoted. Working in small groups of three to five students, discuss and answer the following questions:

1. How would your group define health?

2. How does your group's definition of health compare and/or contrast with other definitions of health in your class?

3. What factors and behaviours does your group believe are important for contributing to the health of Canadians across the lifespan?

4. How do these factors and behaviours compare and/or contrast with other groups?

5. Based on your group's definition of health, can an individual with a chronic communicable disease (e.g., HIV, hepatitis B) and/or non-communicable disease (e.g., diabetes, heart disease, arthritis, bipolar disorder) be healthy? Why or why not?

---

care systems in Canada. Lastly, we shall highlight the many Canadian influences that have helped to shape this dynamic and evolving holistic concept of health from the growing global perspective and need.

A Brief History of Health

This section provides a brief historical account of our understanding of the concept of health from pre-historic times to current times. Although a description of all major social, cultural, political, religious, and scientific influences is beyond the scope and purpose of this chapter, we shall examine critical historical milestones and reflect on their legacy and continued importance. We shall examine how the mechanistic medical model of health has come to dominate societal perspectives of what health is and how it should be delivered since the turn of the twentieth century. Lastly, we shall highlight and examine major Canadian contributions made during the twenty-first century to recent developments in our understanding of holistic definitions of health based on various SDH, and their impact from a global perspective. The term **social determinants of health (SDH)** is defined as the structural determinants and conditions of daily life responsible for a major part of health inequities between and within countries (e.g., distribution of power, income, access to health care, education, work and leisure, state of their housing, and environment) (World Health Organization (WHO) Commission on Social Determinants of Health 2008). Hence, the term social determinants may be regarded as shorthand for the various social, political, economic, environmental, spiritual, and cultural factors that affects the health of individuals, families, groups, or entire communities across the lifespan (Baum 2008; Mikkonen and Raphael 2010; Raphael 2010; Rootman et al. 2012).

Pre-historic Times

Based on archaeological evidence, the establishment of settled permanent communities first occurred during the Neolithic period of the eighth millennium BCE in the Near East, and then spread to northern parts of Europe during the fourth millennium BCE (Hanlon and Pickett 1984; Polgar 1964). There is evidence to demonstrate that these early societies employed a variety of health-related interventions including banishment and isolation of individuals with overt signs of disease; voodoo and other forms of psychosomatic medicine, and fumigation (Hanlon and Pickett 1984).

Both men and women in these early societies functioned as health care providers who were often trained priests, priestesses, shamans, or so called "witch doctors." These primitive health care providers sowed the seeds for all future forms of health care and therapeutics including medicine, nursing, midwifery, and pharmacology (Bartfay and Bartfay 2015). As the caste of healers developed, a distinct class of practitioners became associated with this trade (Donahue 1996; Hanlon and Pickett 1984). These individuals were often women of the tribe who applied treatments, ascertained certain qualities of drugs, learned how to decrease a fever and became skillful in dressing wounds.

The worship of nature became a logical vehicle upon which primitive agricultural societies based their healing practices, mythologies, and religious

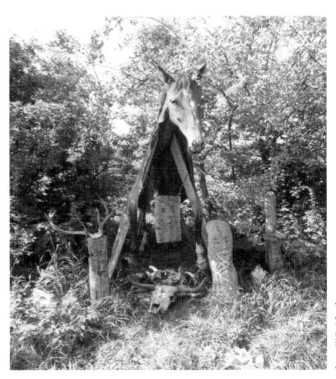

Source: Wally J. Bartfay

Photo 2.1 A replica of an ancient Viking/ Norse temple with various deities based on powerful animals and/or nature.

practices (Bartfay 2010a; Bartfay and Bartfay 2015). The belief in evil spirits, angry gods or deities as the root cause of all ill health and disease first emerged during this period (Goodnow 1942; Nutting and Dock 1937). Accordingly, religious leaders were often given the responsibility for organizing worship for healing, and were also given the responsibility for administering care to the ill and injured by seeking divine aid and knowledge on how to prevent and cure illness and disease.

Ancient Egypt

For more than 3,000 years, the Egyptians were ruled by kings called "pharaohs" who established a remarkable civilization along the banks of the Nile River (Jackson 2011; Porter 1997, 2011; Renouard 2010). Like pre-historic societies, some of the beliefs related to health and disease of these ancient Egyptians were based on mythology and spirituality. For example, "Bes" was an ancient Egyptian god with the mandate of frightening away evil spirits associated with disease and illness in society. In the old kingdom, Bes was shown to be associated with fertility, circumcision, and various harvest rituals. By the middle kingdom, he had evolved into a guardian of the home, infants, and new mothers and was a protector of pregnant women. Nonetheless, their knowledge of disease and states of health were increasingly based on empirical observations of human anatomy, clinical diagnosis, and medical interventions (e.g., surgery, pharmacological preparations) (Bartfay and Bartfay 2015). Notably, several ancient papyri scrolls were discovered in the dry sands of Egypt, which contain one of the most complete examples of ancient beliefs related to health and health care practices (Breasted 1930; Nunn 2002).

According to Edwards (1892), the finest example was the celebrated Ebers papyrus, which was bought at Thebes by Dr. Ebers in 1874. The papyrus is 110 pages total, and each page consists of approximately twenty-two lines of bold hieratic writings which has been described as an *Encylopaedia of Medicine* as known and practiced by the Egyptians of the eighteenth dynasty.

Several of these scrolls were subsequently located and named after their discoverers including the Brugsch, Ebers, Kahun, Smith, Hearst, Berlin, and London papyri scrolls (Berdoe 1893; Breasted 1930; Edwards 1892; Nunn 2002). For example, the Papyrus Ebers provides detailed written evidence regarding their anatomical knowledge of the human body, its various organs, and vessels:

> 46 vessels go from the heart to every limb, if a doctor places his hand or fingers on the back of the head, hands, stomach, arms or feet then he hears the heart.
>
> (Retrieved June 10, 2010 from http://www. historylearningsite.co.uk/a-history-of-medicine/ ancient-egyptian-medicine/)

Interestingly, these scrolls reveal that health and disease were attributed to both natural causes and to supernatural causes. The physician and healer Imhotep (circa 2900–2800 BCE) is often credited as being the founder of Egyptian medicine during the third dynasty and is believed to be the original author of the Edwin Smith Papyrus, which may date to as early as 3000 BCE (Breasted 1930; Bryan 1930; Nunn, 2002). Imhotep was the physician to King Zozer who was also a renowned surgeon, a temple priest, magician, and an architect for one of the Pharaohs temples. He was so successful that the ancient Egyptians elevated him to the rank of the Egyptian god of medicine and healing. The earliest known surgeries were performed in Egypt around 2700 BCE, and are detailed in the Smith Papyrus. Public medical institutions, referred to as "Houses of Life," were established in ancient Egypt by the first dynasty (Donahue, 2006; Nunn, 2002). Interestingly, by the time of the nineteenth dynasty, some workers in ancient Egypt enjoyed benefits including medical insurance, pensions, and sick leave.

Persians

By approximately 500 BCE, the Egyptians were conquered by the Persians from present day Iran (Jackson 2011; Porter 1997, 2011; Renouard 2010; Shryock 1959). The Persians adapted many aspects of ancient Egyptian culture and their health care practices. The Persians were also the first to introduce the sacred elements of fire, earth, and water, which latter served as the basis for alchemy. Alchemy, which was concerned with the transmutation of base metals into gold, later evolved into the present day science of chemistry (Bartfay and Bartfay 2015).

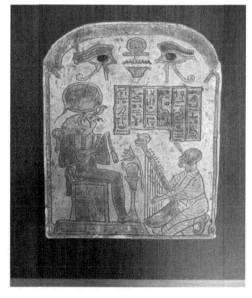

Source: Wally J. Bartfay

Photo 2.2 The Stele of Horus (Egypt–New Kingdom Era). This plaque portrays a sick man who sings a lament on a harp to the seated god Horus, son of Osiris and the goddess Isis. Horus was worshipped for centuries as the god of healing. At the top, we see the "Eye of Horus," which has come down over the centuries to represent the Rx sign commonly see on prescriptions today.

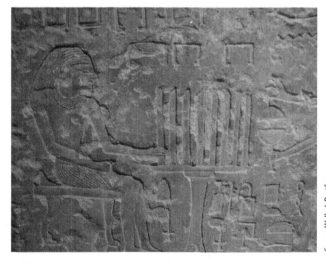

Source: Wally J. Bartfay

Photo 2.3 Egypt is one of the best known and documented ancient civilizations dating to as far back as 3000 BCE, with extensive written records employing, cravings, hieroglyphics, and papyri scrolls with ink.

The Emperor Darius of Persia is credited as being the first to establish a royal or governmental-funded medical centre in history (Donahue 1996; Risse 1990). Darius renovated an old school to be utilized for the training of priest–physicians, which was largely modeled after ancient Egyptian medical practices. Nutting and Dock (1937) reported that three types of health care practitioners emerged from this medical centre: (a) Those who healed by the use of exorcism and incantations; (b) those who used various plant-based herbal remedies, and (c) those who healed using the knife (scalpel) for various surgical interventions.

The Iranian born Muhammad Idn Zakariya Al-Razi (or Rhazes, 865–925 CE), became the first person to describe in detail smallpox and measles (Martin-Aragus et al. 2002). His *Comprehensive Book of Medicine*, provided useful insights into many diseases and was very influential in European medical schools.

Abu-al-Qasim (Abulcasis) wrote the influential thirty volume medical encyclopaedia entitled *Kitab al-Tasrif* (1000 CE), and is also credited by

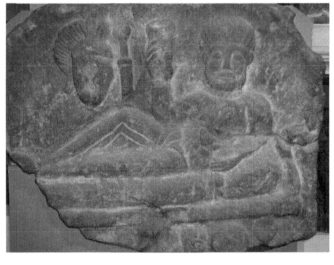

Source: Wally J. Bartfay

Photo 2.4 A carving of Persian healer administering a decoction made from medicinal plants to his client lying in bed. The Vendidad, one of the surviving texts of the Zend-Avesta (1500 and 1200 BCE), distinguishes three kinds of healing: (a) those performed by the knife (surgery) (b) those achieved through the ingestion or application of herbs and plants, and (c) those achieved through divine hymns or incantations.

some scholars as being the father of modern surgery (Martin-Araguz et al. 2002; Saad et al. 2005). Ibn al-Haytham (Alhacen) made important advances in eye surgery and he is credited as being the first to correctly explain the process of sight and visual perception in his work entitled *Book of Optics* (1021 CE) (Saad et al. 2005).

Traditional Chinese Medicine

The philosophy of traditional Chinese medicine was derived from both empirical observations of disease and illness by Taoist healers and physicians, and the belief that individual human experiences express causative factors in their environment (Jackson 2011; Porter 1997, 2011; Renouard 2010; Unschuld 2003; Wujastyk 2003; Zysk 1998).

Health and ways to achieve and maintain this state in ancient China is perhaps one of the first to focus on "holistic health," meaning the whole person, which also incorporated the prevention of illness and disease (Bartfay 2010a; Donahue 1996; Lyons and Petrucelli 1978; Unschuld 2003). Accordingly, health was defined as a state of harmony between the universe and the individual, and was achieved through the equilibrium of nature's energy dualities of *yang* (male principle) and yin (female principle) (Bartfay 2010a; Bartfay and Bartfay 2015). The yin force is described as being negative, cold, moist, weak, and lifeless. Conversely, the yang force is described as being positive, warm, dry, strong, and, full of life and light. The Chinese emperor "Fu His" (2900 BCE) created the *pa kua* symbol

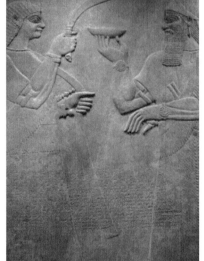

Source: Wally J. Bartfay

Photo 2.5 Interestingly, the distinction between medicine and pharmacy as separate and distinct fields and professions occurred in 754 CE, when the first drugstores opened in Baghdad, Iraq (Hadzovic 1997; Syed 2003).

which consists of yang and yin lines combined in eight separate trigrams that characterize all the yin-yang conditions (Donahue 1996; Porter 1997, 2011;Unschuld 2003).

The ancient Chinese also believed that alterations to health or the presence of disease could be caused by evil spirits, demons and/or animistic forces. Charms were often used to help ward-off evil spirits and forces associated with altered states of health (Lyons and Petrucelli 1978; Porter 1997, 2011; Unschuld 2003). The charms were often transcribed onto paper, burned in a fire, and the ashes drunk in a form of a decoction or tea. Evil spirits could also be frightened off by loud noises (e.g., cymbals, drums, trumpets, fire crackers, and other loud noise makers).

The use of numerous plant-based extracts and herbal remedies were also employed to treat alterations to health. The Red Emperor, Shen Nung (Hung Ti), for example, wrote the famous herbal compendium known as the *Pen Tsao* This compendium detailed the carefully investigated and clinically evaluated effects of 365 plant based medications on clients (Donahue 1996).

Shen Nung is also credited as being the first to have compiled and drawn detailed acupuncture charts for preventing and treating various ailments (e.g., pain, headaches, circulatory, and digestive problems). There is empirical evidence which has documented many clinical and health related benefits associated with the ancient Chinese practice of acupuncture. For example, various carefully designed randomized clinical trials (RCTs) have documented the effectiveness of true acupuncture for the control of pain versus sham (placebo) acupuncture (Sodipo, Gilly, and Pauswer 1981; Vickers et al. 2012; Watawaba et al. 1978). In fact, it has been demonstrated that acupuncture treatment results in the release of endorphins into the circulatory system, which are morphine-like substances that block pain receptors.

Ancient India

The Atharvaveda, a sacred text of Hinduism dating from the Early Iron Age, is regarded as the first

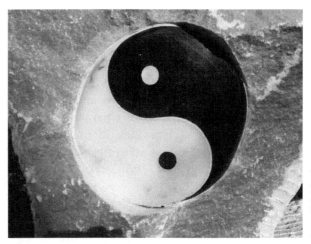

Source: Wally J. Bartfay

Photo 2.6 The Yin-yang symbol representing the state of harmony between an individual and the universe, is critical to the achievement of health in traditional Chinese medicine and healing practices.

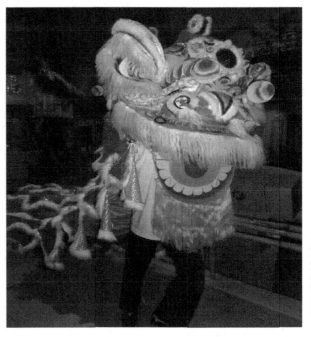

Source: Wally J. Bartfay

Photo 2.7 The Chinese dragon often seen during ceremonies and accompanied by clashing cymbals and firecrackers to ward off evil spirits and demons. These practices remain a vital component of many present day Chinese celebrations and festivals (e.g., Chinese weddings, New Year celebrations).

known medical text in India (Wujastyk 2003; Zys 1998). Ancient Indian medicine was based partially on practices of exorcism of demons and magic, in addition to the use of plant-based pharmaceuticals and surgical procedures (Porter 1997, 2011; Wujastyk 2003; Zysk 1998). For example, ancient Hindu physicians often employed plants with somatic and hypnotic properties including *Cannabis Indica, hyposcyamus,* and *henbane* in their practice. The scholarly system of Indian medicine known as *Ayurveda*, originated in post-Vedic India, and its two most famous medical texts belong to the schools of Charaka (or Charaka Samhita) (circa 300 BCE) and Sushruta Samhita (or Susrutasnhita) (third and fourth century CE) (Wujastyk 2003; Zysk 1998).

Operations, such as tonsillectomies, were often performed in India, and which remained unfamiliar to the later Greek and Roman surgeons (Donahue 1996). Furthermore, approximately 125 surgical instruments were employed by Hindu surgeons who performed operations such as amputations, excised tumors, repaired hernias and harelips, removed bladder stones, couched cataracts, reconstructed noses damaged in battle, and delivered infants by caesarean section (Bartfay and Bartfay 2015). *Ayurveda* is derived from the Sanskrit word that means "knowledge of life and longevity," and is based on the principles and rhythms found in nature (e.g., one's pulse). The normal length for the training of practitioners of Ayurvedic medicine was seven years, and the teaching of relevant subjects (e.g., surgery, obstetrics) were interwoven with hands-on experiences (Wujastyk 2003; Zysk 1998).

The emergence of the first hospital-like structures termed *xenodocheions* (or xendochiums) meaning *House of God*, occurred in pre-Christian India (800–600 BCE) and then in Europe (Dock 1932; Kelly 1975). There is no question based on the recorded historical evidence that hospitals of some sort were built during this period as centres for providing health care services to their citizens, and were staffed primarily by male health care providers including nurses, physicians, and priests (Donahue 1996; Jackson 2011; Renouard 2010; Shryock 1959). Shryock (1959) notes that during this time, it was regarded as more economical in nature to gather all classes of so-called *unfortunates* into one institution known as a

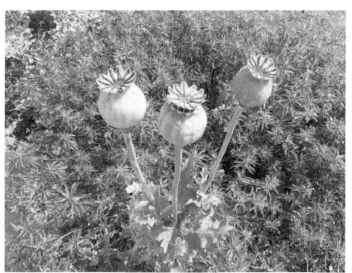

Source: Wally J. Bartfay

Photo 2.8 Historically, opium derived from these poppies (*Papaver somniferum* L. and *Papaver bracteatum)* have been used medicinally primarily as an analgesic for pain relief and to induce sedation in clients. Poppy extracts have also been used in traditional Chinese medicines as smooth muscle relaxants, making them potentially useful in the treatment of diarrhea and abdominal cramping and prescribed as an antitussive.

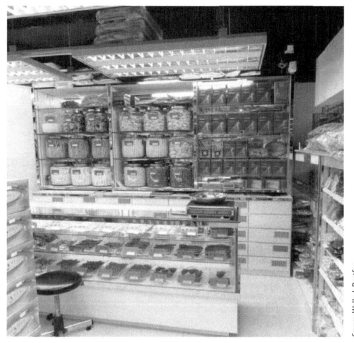

Source: Wally J. Bartfay

Photo 2.9 A traditional Chinese pharmacy in Hong Kong, which employs an assortment of carefully selected and weighed plants, herbs, and animal products in the preparation of medicines to treat a variety of ailments, conditions and diseases, and to restore harmony between an individual and nature.

xenodocheion, which was the ancestor of the modern hospital as well as most other types of charitable institutions.

Ancient Greece

The Greeks had a rich culture and mythology comprised of various gods of the earth and underworld, and special healing agents including snakes and symbols were integrated in medicine and other healing practices (Donahue 1996; Lyons and Petrucelli 1978; Porter 1997, 2011). *Apollo,* who was the son of Zeus and Leto, was the god of medicine and healing, whether through himself or mediated through his son Asclepius. Apollo was also portrayed in ancient Greece as a god who could bring ill-health and deadly plague when angered. He was also known as the god of music, poetry, art, oracles, archery, sun, light, and knowledge to the ancient Greeks.

The Greek scientist and philosopher *Thales* (approximately 640–546 BCE) is credited as being the first to use science, as opposed to religion, meta-physical reasons and/ or mythology, to explain natural processes and the universe. Later, *Aristotle* (384–322 BCE) had a profound influence on health care and medicine in Greece and abroad, and he also laid the foundations for biology and comparative anatomy. The first known Greek school of medicine opened in Cnidus in 700 BCE on the Carian Chersonese, located on the southwest coast of Anatolia. The city was an important commercial centre, and also the site of the observatory of the astronomer *Eudoxus. Alcmaeo*n, author of the first anatomical compilation in Greece, worked at this school in Cnidus, and it was here that the practice for the need of careful observation and empirical monitoring of clients was first established.

It is quite apparent, however, that the ancient Greeks incorporated many Egyptian-derived substances, plants and herbal preparations into their own pharmacopoeia. This influence became even more pronounced after the establishment of a school of Greek medicine in 330 BCE in Alexandria, Egypt, which was known as the "Empirical School." In keeping with the Greek philosophy, *Aristotle*, the tone of the scientific and medical research conducted at the medical school in Alexandria was very open-minded and empirically or observation based. This medical school also attracted the best physicians and medical scholars from Greece, and became instrumental in the transmission of Greek medicine to Rome after the Roman conquest of Egypt. As a consequence of *Alexander's the Great* conquests, Arab, Turkish, and Persian peoples of the Middle East were exposed to the medical teachings and philosophies of the Greeks.

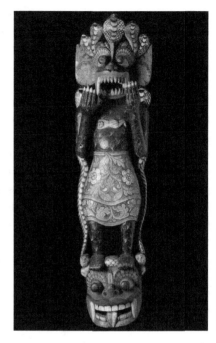

Photo 2.10 An example of a curing and healing mask from Sri Lanka, Asia, which was carried during special rituals performed to please the demon gods and cure sick villagers. This mask represents the "sickness demon" with his eight servant demons that each represents a different disease or condition.

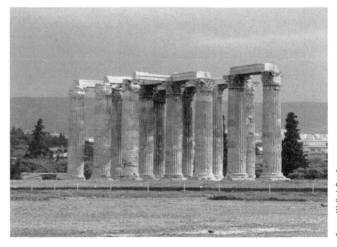

Photo 2.11 Ancient Greece was made up of many independent city states and temples to worship the gods. Originally, Ancient Greeks believed that illnesses and disease were "divine punishments" and that healing was a "gift from the Gods." However, by the fifth century BCE, there were attempts to identify the material causes for illnesses and disease via scientific enquiry, which led to a movement away from spiritual causes or angry gods.

Hippocrates of Cos (Kos) (460–370 BCE) was one of the first to employ case histories to describe various ailments, treatment outcomes, and complications in a collective work entitled the *Epidemics* (Donahue 1996; Lyons and Petrucelli 1978). Case histories are still utilized today by various health care professionals (e.g., physicians, nurses) for clinical practice and research purposes. Hippocrates was also one of the first to teach his students and fellow health care providers that ill health or disease, did not result from the work of evil spirits, demons, or gods, but resulted as a consequence of a break in a law of nature or the universe (Bartfay 2010a; Bartfay and Bartfay 2015; Swanson and Albrecht 1993). Consequently, public health care and medicine focused on "cure" as opposed to prevention for the first time in recorded history. Figure 2.1 is a conceptual representation of the four body humours of disease causation, as described by Hippocrates, based on the belief that the health was achieved by maintaining a balance between the four body humors identified as: (a) Phlegm (phlegma); (b) yellow bile (khole); (c) black bile (melagkholikos), and (d) blood (sanguineus) (Aschengrau and Seage 2003; Lyons and Petrucelli 1978).

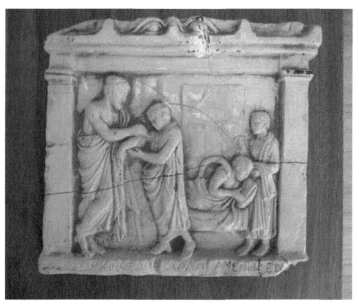

Source: Wally J. Bartfay

Photo 2.12 This votive relief shows Archinos (or Amphiaraus)—the legendary king of Argos, seer and the chthonian god of healing, appears as a healer–priest who supports himself with a staff while tending to the wounded arm of a client. Ceremonies performed in the Aesculapian Temple of Sanatoria featured holy snakes that were apparently trained to "lick the ailing parts of the sick" while soft music was played to lament them. *Popona*, was a special "snake biscuit" sold to sick clients who fed it to serpents in the hope of being healed. The Greek symbols of the staff and serpents have come down over the centuries to epitomize medicine.

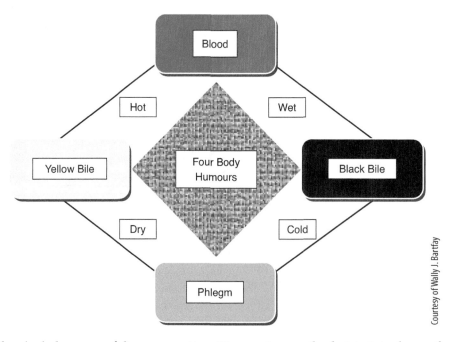

Courtesy of Wally J. Bartfay

Figure 2.1 The four body humours of disease causation. Hippocrates was the first to introduce a theory of disease causation that revolved around the belief of an imbalance in the four body humours. Remarkably, his theory was taught to medical students around the world for over 2000 years following its conception.

For example, if a client had a fever, he would treat it with cold. Likewise, individuals who were weak were prescribed exercise to build up their muscles. This is a critical milestone in the evolution of our understanding of health and its definition based on natural causes, as opposed to those associated with supernatural forces that could not be controlled or manipulated by mortal man.

The *Hippocratic Corpus* remains an important collection, comprised of approximately 70 volumes from ancient Greece (Jackson 2011; Porter 2011; Renouard 2010). Many of his detailed descriptions, symptomatology, clinical findings, surgical treatments, and prognosis remain relevant to present day health care professionals such as physicians and nurses (e.g., thoracic empyema). He was the first to categorize illnesses such as acute, chronic, endemic, and epidemic and employ the terms exacerbation, relapse, resolution, crisis, paroxysm, peak, and convalescence to medical practice. Hippocrates was also the first recorded chest surgeon and is famous for being the first to describe clubbing of the fingers as an important clinical symptom associated with heart disease, respiratory disorders, and lung cancer. In fact, clubbed fingers are still often clinically referred to as "Hippocratic fingers." Interestingly, many medical students upon graduation still take the Hippocratic Oath, which emphasizes the *cure* directive of medical practice geared towards single client outcomes and directives, as opposed to groups, communities, or entire populations (Bartfay 2010a; Bartfay and Bartfay, 2015).

Ancient Rome

Rome was founded in 753 BCE, and in 510 BCE, the city had officially become a republic (Jackson 2011; Porter 2011; Renouard 2010). The Roman Empire reached its greatest extent in AD 117 and enjoyed approximately 300 years of prosperity. The Romans borrowed and adapted a great deal from the ancient Greeks, who first came into contact with them in approximately 500 BCE.

Claudius Galen (131–201 BCE) was a famous Greek physician who studied at the medical school in Alexandria, Egypt, and went to Rome to seek his fame and fortune (Davis and Park 1984; Dear 2001). At the age of twenty-eight, he became a surgeon to the gladiators and revived the methods favoured by Hippocrates including his theory of the four humours. Galen was also the first to demonstrate that blood alone filled arteries, not air as previously thought, and that a surgeon could stop the bleeding from a vessel if he applied pressure to it with his fingers (Davis and Park 1984).

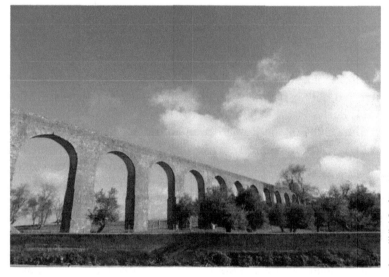

Source: Wally J. Bartfay

Photo 2.13 Roman aqueducts were carefully designed and engineered to carry fresh water supplies from great distances away based on gravity and incline sloping, and many are still in use today in various European cities and towns.

The Romans believed that altered states of health and disease were caused by natural sources, especially bad water supplies and raw sewage. Accordingly, they became experts at draining swamps and marshes to rid them of malaria-carrying mosquitoes. Julius Caesar, for example, drained the Codetan Swamp and planted a forest in its place.

Care should be taken where there are swamps in the neighbourhood, because certain tiny creatures which cannot be seen by the eyes breed there. These float through the air and enter the body by the mouth and nose and cause serious disease.

(Marcus Varro, Retrieved June 10, 2010 from http://www.historylearningsite.co.uk/medicine_in_ancient_rome.html)

The Romans were outstanding engineers who built long and elaborate aqueducts and viaducts to bring fresh water into their towns and cities for drinking, toilets, and for the many baths they constructed (Jackson 2011; Porter 2011; Renouard 2010). Roman houses were also equipped with toilets and several public toilets were also built. By 315 BCE, Rome had an estimated 150 public toilets which were flushed clean by continuous running water from the aqueducts. The Romans also valued personal hygiene and several baths were built throughout their Empire, which were used by both the rich and poor alike. For example, one of the most famous of these Roman baths is located in City of Bath in England (aka *Aquae Sulis* by

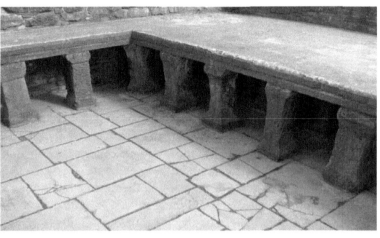

Source: Wally J. Bartfay

Photo 2.14 Ruins from an ancient Roman hypocaust in Chester, England (circa 75 AD). Roman houses and baths were often heated by an elaborate hypocaust, or central heating system, that diverted hot air form burning fire pits which provided heat under ceramic floors and into the cavities of specially designed hollowed walls.

the Romans). Roman buildings and baths were heated by a hypocaust, or central heating systems that diverted hot air from burning fire pits up under the ceramic floors and into the cavities of walls (Jackson 2011; Porter 2011; Renouard 2010).

The genius of the Romans was not in the establishment of rationale or scientific medicine per se, but in their colossal engineering feats involving public sanitation and drains; aqueducts; roads; the draining of marshes infested with mosquitoes; systems of central heating for buildings and homes; proper cemeteries, and public baths (Lyons and Petrucelli 1978; Nutting and Dock 1937). The Romans were also the first to employ public physicians to provide care to their citizens in surrounding towns and villages. They also provided care to the poor and were permitted to charge a fee to the state for those who could not pay for their health care services provided (Swanson and Albrecht 1993). Moreover, several Roman families paid an annual tax or user fee for health care services. In fact, it may be argued that the concept of a national public health care system first originated in ancient Rome (Bartfay 2010a; Bartfay and Bartfay 2015).

Swanson and Albrecht (1993) report that in ancient Rome, a prototype of a health maintenance organization or group practice emerged, where several families paid an annual fee. In addition, hospitals, a variety of surgical procedures and infirmaries for slaves as well as long-term nursing home-type structures appeared during this period. A hospital was established by a wealthy Christian women known as *Fabiola* in the fourth century in Rome, and this model was repeated throughout medieval times (Swanson and Albrecht 1993). In fact, the Roman's believed that everyone in their Empire was entitled to good health, and therefore the Romans were the first civilization to introduce a programme of public health for all their citizens regardless of their age, wealth, or social status. The Romans considered that a healthy mind equalled a healthy body, and that individuals should devote time each day to exercise and keeping fit (Hortmanshoff et al. 2004; Lyons and Petrucelli 1978; Nutting and Dock 1935). Paradoxically, this remains a major challenge in Canada today with the growing number of children and adults who are sedentary by nature.

The Romans were the first to document various occupational health hazards, and devised interventions to help limit injury or death for vulnerable workers (Rosen 1958). For example, the Romans paid particular attention to the health of miners who were at risk of suffocation from toxic fumes, miner's lung, traumatic amputations and premature death. Accordingly, one of the earliest mentions of safety equipment involves the use of bags, sacks, and masks made from the membranes of various animals and bladder skins to help protect the lungs of Roman miners. Mining remains one of the most dangerous occupations globally accounting for approximately 12,000 preventable deaths annually (Shaw Media 2011). For example, between the years 2006 and 2009, eighty workers died in Canada's mining, quarrying, and petroleum industries. By comparison, thirty-four deaths occurred in the United States and 2,631 deaths occurred in China (Shaw Media 2011). Donahue (1996) notes that the Romans were also advanced in military medicine and hospitals, and provided first aid on the battlefields and field ambulance services for their soldiers. The Romans also invented numerous surgical instruments including the surgical needle, cross-bladed scissors, and specula's and forceps for delivery of infants.

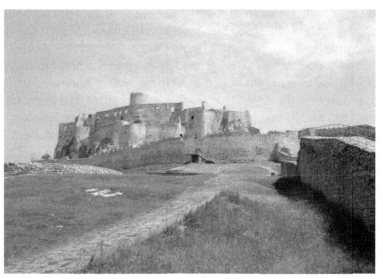

Source: Wally J. Bartfay

Photo 2.15 The Middle Ages is characterized as a period of intense, powerful and rapid growth in the belief for supernatural or meta-physical causes of diseases and illness; the rise of political power and influence of the Catholic Church in Europe, and numerous military conflicts between rival regions and countries.

The Middle Ages

The Middle Ages represents the time period between the fall of the Roman Empire (476 CE) to the fall of Constantinople (1453 CE). Following the collapse of the Roman Empire, health care became progressively more localized in nature on the European continent, and folk medicine supplemented what remained of the medical knowledge of antiquity (Jackson 2011; Porter 1997, 2011; Renouard 2010). During the Middle Ages, the domination of health care and society in Europe by the Catholic Church was practically unchallenged (Neuburger 1910; O'Lynn 2007). Folklore cures and potentially poisonous metal-based compounds (e.g., mercury, arsenic, lead) were popular treatments for many ailments and conditions.

Due to population growth in Europe, the occurrence of communicable diseases such as smallpox; measles; diphtheria, and the bubonic plague characterize this period (James 2003; Rosen 1958). During the reign of the Roman Emperor Justinian (527–565 CE), bishops were given authority over all hospitals. Consequently, the number of charitable hospitals and shelters increased dramatically in the empire, as did the number of religious orders founded to care for the sick and the poor (Bartfay and Bartfay 2015). For example, St. Ephrem served as a deacon in Edessa (located in present-day Turkey) in 350 CE at the time of a serious plague outbreak.

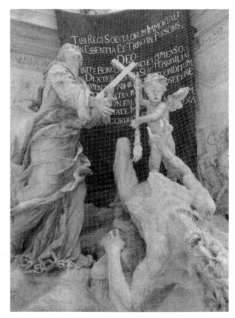

Source: Emma Bartfay

Photo 2.16 A plague memorial in Vienna, Austria. During the fourteenth century in Eurasia, an estimated 75 to 200 million people died as a consequence of the "Black Death" (aka Bubonic plague). It is estimated that over 1,200 victims died daily in Vienna alone at the height of the pandemic.

He collected money from wealthy patrons in the town and bought 300 beds, which he installed in public porticoes and galleries to care for the sick. Ephrem visited the sick daily and administered nursing care to many of the clients himself (O'Lynn 2007).

The Middle Ages is characterized by an amplified belief in supernatural or meta-physical causes of disease, illness, and alterations to health, and the growth of religious nursing orders to administer health care services to residents in the region (Bartfay and Bartfay 2015). It is interesting to note that significantly more male deacons and monks practiced nursing during the Byzantine Empire (Later Roman—fourth century CE), in comparison to female deaconesses and nuns (Bullough 1993; Pelley 1964). For example, the Parabolani brothers (circa 300 CE) of eastern Rome were an early organization of male nurses whose name literally means *those who risk their lives by coming into contact with the sick* (Donahue 1996). It is believed that this brotherhood originated as a consequence of the *Black Plague*, which devastated entire populations of the Mediterranean basin and many parts of Europe. A non-military nursing order known as the Brothers of St. Anthony cared for victims of the disfiguring skin disease erysipelas, which was later renamed St. Anthony's fire after the brotherhood (Bartfay 2010a; Evans 2004). Erysipelas is a superficial cellulitis that classically occurs on the cheeks of the victim, although it can occur anywhere on the body or extremities. It is caused by *β-hemolytic streptococcus* (i.e., streptococcal infection) and occurs predominantly in infants and in adults greater than thirty years of age (Bartfay and Bartfay 2015). The church also took over the care of victims of leprosy, and employed hygienic codes from Leviticus in the Bible and established isolation communities and leper houses known as "leprosaria" (Swanson and Albrecht 1993).

A critical mass of individuals is required to maintain a disease in endemic proportions (Bartfay and Bartfay 2015). The sexually transmitted infection (STI) syphilis, for example, originated as a non-venereal disease and evolved into one as a result of increased population densities (Hudson 1965). Similarly, it has estimated that approximately one million individuals are required to sustain measles at an endemic level in a given population (Cockburn 1967). With population expansions and crowding in various cities and towns in Europe, came additional public health challenges in relation to the domestication of animals, food availability and supplies, irrigation, and sanitation demands (Polgar 1964; Rosen 1958).

For example, pollution has been known as a public health menace since biblical times. In Exodus, it was reported that all the water in the river stank. Leviticus contains the first written hygienic codes formulated by the Hebrews which dealt with laws governing both personal and community hygiene measures including disinfecting, controlling contagions, and sanitary practices including the protection of water and food supplies (Swanson and Albrecht 2003). Medical historians report that the Catholic Church was greatly influenced by the Five Books of Moses, which contain various health related laws and rituals, including the isolation of infected individuals (Leviticus 13:45–46); the importance of washing one's hands after handling a corpse (Number 19:11–19), and the need to bury human excrement away from one's dwelling (Deuteronomy 23:12–13) (Swanson and Albrecht 1993; Neuburger 1910).

The Middle Ages is further identified by historians as the period of the so-called "Holy Crusades" (Green and Ottoson 1994; Nutting and Dock 1937). The crusades were of great significance to the development of health services provided by trained individuals because they lead

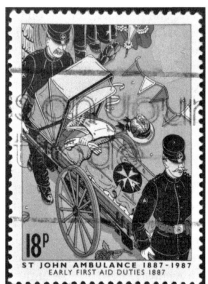

Photo 2.17 St. John's Ambulance Service of Canada. St. John Ambulance Foundation is an international humanitarian organization that currently provides courses in first aid, CPR, and occupational health and safety training to name but a few of its community-based services. Interestingly, it's charitable origins date back to 11th century where monks first established a hospital in Jerusalem, and which subsequently developed into a religious and military order with its brothers and sisters (commonly known as Hospitallers of St John or Knights Hospitallers) providing care to the poor and sick of any faith.

to an eventual decline in monasticism; further developments in medicine; the establishments of charitable hospitals on the European continent, and the establishment of various military nursing orders (Bartfay and Bartfay 2015; Frank 1953).

The crusades also served as a rallying point for the formation of a variety of military nursing orders including the Knights Hospitallers, Knights of St. John of Jerusalem, and the Teutonic Knights (Bullough and Bullough 1993; Dock and Stewart-Maitland 1932; Kalisch and Kalisch 1986). It is noteworthy that these nursing orders were also the first recorded field nurses, which is a specialized form of public health nursing that provides care to a community of military personnel as well as injured civilians as a consequence of war or conflicts (Bartfay 2010b; Bartfay and Bartfay 2015; Nutting and Dock 1937). The Knights of St. John were also the only historically documented military nursing order to provide care to the mentally ill. During the industrial revolution during the 19th century, members of the British Order wanted decided to train ordinary people in first aid so accident victims could be treated promptly on location, and in 1877 they set up St. John Ambulance service was formally established (St. John Ambulance Foundation, 2018P. Classes were set-up to train workers and other concerned civilians across the country, particularly in workplaces and areas of heavy industry, but also in villages, seaside towns and middle class working neighbourboods. There were originally three charitable Foundations of the modern Order: (i) The St John of Jerusalem Eye Hospital Foundation (established in 1882); (ii) St John Ambulance Association, which was concerned with training the public in first aid (established in 1877), and (iii). And St John Ambulance Brigade, which provided first aid care to the public, which had its origins 1873, and became a Foundation in 1887. The St. John Ambulance Association and St. John Ambulance Brigade were amalgamated in 1974 to form the current charitable organization collective known as the "*St John Ambulance Foundation*" (St. John Ambulance Foundation, 2018)." As part of their nursing legacy today, the British order of the Knights of St. John established the famous St. John's Ambulance Service during World War I (Bedford and Holbeche 1902; Hume 1940). This service continues to provide emergency public health services and classes in first aid and cardiopulmonary resuscitation (CPR) to individuals in many countries, including Canada.

During the twelfth century, the term *xenodocheia* (or xendochium) had disappeared and was replaced by the modern term *hospital*, a creation of the Knights Hospitallers for these health care institutions (Bullough 1994; Nutting and Dock 1937). The Knights Hospitallers were a military nursing order that were given official recognition by Pope Celestin III in 1113 AC for the public health services they provided to the sick and poor, and for establishing various hospitals throughout Europe (Bullough and Bullough 1993; Davis and Bartfay 2001; Kelly 1975).

Subsequently, during the thirteenth century, a more modern type of secular hospital was sanctioned by Pope Innocent III, where nursing care was provided almost entirely by men in these medieval hospitals (Bullough and Bullough 1993; Davis and Bartfay 2001). Pope Innocent III encouraged the development of hospitals throughout Europe. Hospitals were erected principally to care for the poor who were sick, although they also served

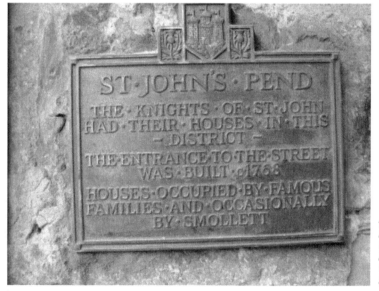

Source: Emma Bartfay

Photo 2.18 A plaque commemorating the location of houses for the order of the Knights of St. John in Edinburgh, Scotland. Various military nursing knights provided care to the wounded on the battlefields, protected those who could no longer defend themselves and were, in fact, the first documented public health nurses to provide care to individuals afflicted with leprosy in the world (Bartfay 1996, 2007; Bartfay and Bartfay 2015).

as orphanages, hospices for travelers, and almshouses (Bartfay 2010a; Donahue 1996). In fact, these hospitals were regarded as a place to keep, as opposed to cure clients per se. The cure directive which dominates modern acute care hospitals in Canada and elsewhere did not evolve until the late nineteenth century.

During the fourteenth century, approximately twenty-five million people died as a consequence of the bubonic plague (Black Death), which migrated from Asia to Africa, then spread through Crimea, Turkey, Greece, Italy, and up through the European continent (Green and Ottoson 1994; Swanson and Albrecht 1993). The Black Death arrived in Europe via twelve trading ships from central Asia, docked in Italian seaports, and then rapidly spread throughout the continent. Green and Ottoson (1994) provide some idea of the devastation of the pandemic by recanting the mortality rates in the following cities in Europe: Paris, 50,000; Seine, 70,000; Marseilles, 16,000 in just one month and Vienna; 1,200 daily victims, and in England two million died which represents half the population of the entire country at the time. The Italian writer Boccaccio reported that there was a terrible outbreak of the plague in Florence in 1348, where pity and humanity were forgotten by the residents and families deserted their sick. The Black Death was, in fact, caused by a flea infected with the bacterium *Yesinia pestis*, which could be carried by rats (Bartfay 2010a; Bartfay and Bartfay 2015).

During this period, epidemics and pandemics were attributed to various natural causes including toxic fumes and gases known as *miasmas* (or miasis) (e.g., swamp gases); comets, drought, and crop failures; severe storms, urban crowding, and poor sanitation (Bartfay 2010a; Bartfay and Bartfay 2015). During the fourteenth century, it was also widely known that infections could be spread through the contact of infected victims. Accordingly, cities and towns often engaged in various public health initiatives to help and control the spread of epidemics and disease, including limiting travel in their jurisdictions and various isolation and quarantine practices. **Isolation** is defined as the separation of an infectious individual for a defined period of time (e.g., 30 days) to prevent or limit the direct or indirect transmission of an infectious agent (Bartfay and Bartfay 2015). **Quarantine** is defined as the restriction of activities of individuals who remain diseased or symptom free but who have been exposed to an infectious agent (Bartfay and Bartfay 2015).

For example, in 1377 at Rogussa it was ruled that travelers from plague areas should stop at designated places and remain there free of disease for two months before being allowed to enter the city. Technically, this is the first official quarantine method on record (Green and Ottoson 1994). In 1383, Marseilles passed the first quarantine law and erected the first official quarantine station in Europe. In the City of Venice, the local government appointed three guardians of public health who promptly denied entry to the city of infected or suspected travelers, ships and freight in 1374. In 1403, a quarantine of forty days was imposed on anyone suspected of having the disease in many regions in Europe (Green and Ottoson 1994).

Interestingly, Canada established its first official quarantine laws in 1720 due to an outbreak of bubonic plague, which was carried to our shores by rat infected ships from the Mediterranean (Bartfay 2010a; Swan 1966). An estimated 20,000 settlers died as a consequence of a cholera epidemic of 1832 in Upper and Lower Canada (PHAC 2008a). The Lower Board of Health created a quarantine station on Grosse Île located along the shores of the St. Lawrence River, for new settlers to Canada.

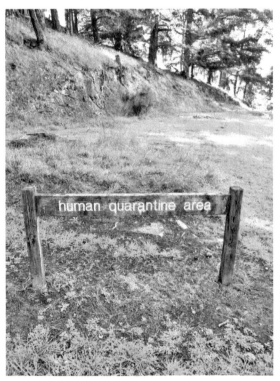

Source: Photo by Wally J. Bartfay

Photo 2.19 Sign marking the site of a former human quarantine station. Quail Island (*Ōtamahua* in Māori, sometimes also known as *Te Kawakawa*) is a small uninhabited island within Lyttelton Harbour in the South Island of New Zealand, close to Christchurch. The island was turned into a quarantine station in 1875, and later into a small leper colony from 1907–1925, and was also used as a hospital during the influenza epidemic of 1907.

The quarantine directive was reinforced by the military to prevent the spread of cholera into Upper and Lower Canada (PHAC 2008a).

The practice of isolating or quarantining individual remains as a common public health intervention today to both, contain and limit the spread of a known or suspected infectious agent. For example, during 2003, severe acute respiratory syndrome (SARS) pandemic, both suspected and known victims of this contagion were isolated and quarantined, and cross-border travel to the United States and abroad were also restricted to prevent its spread (Campbell 2006; Naylo, 2006). A total of 8,098 people worldwide became sick during the 2003 SARS pandemic. In Canada, the federal government is responsible for the instigation of quarantine laws as detailed in section 91 of the British North American Act (aka Constitution Act, 1982) (Van Loon and Whittington 1976).

The Renaissance Period

The Renaissance Period is marked by the fall of Constantinople in 1453 CE to 1600 CE (Bartfay 2010a; Green and Ottoson 1994). This Renaissance period produced various distinguished scholars and scientists including Copernicus, DaVinci, Galileo, and Versalius, to name but a few. *Leonardo DaVinci*, for example, was one of the first individuals to dissert the human body, which was considered taboo by the Catholic Church in Europe during the fifteenth century. DaVinci often secretly dissected corpses at night, and produced detailed anatomical drawings of which more than 750 are still in existence today including those of the skeletal, muscular, nervous and vascular systems (Lyons and Petrucelli 1978).

Fracas Toro (1478–1553), a physician from Verona, is credited as being the first to theorize that tiny microorganism caused ill health or disease in 1546 (Green and Ottoson 1994). It is interested to note that Francastoro envisioned these tiny disease-causing microorganisms before the discovery of the microscope and the germ theory of disease causation, as later detailed by Louise Pasteur (1822–1895) and Robert Koch (1849–1910) (detailed below). Fracas Toro was also the first to note that syphilis could be transmitted from an individual to another as a consequence of sexual intercourse. The name *Syphilis* comes from the poem by Fracastoro entitled *syphilis sive morbus gallicus,* which is about a shepherd boy named Syphilis, who by angering the sun god of Haiti, bought upon himself the dreaded infection. The poem also suggests mercury and guaiaco as a treatment for this STI.

On June 15, 1520, Pope Leo X informed *Martin Luther,* that he would be excommunicated from the Catholic Church unless he recanted forty-one sentences from his controversial writings, including the Ninety-Five Theses, which criticized elements of the Catholic Church and its faith (Donahue 1996; Loades 1990). Despite these threats from the Pope, Luther did not back down from his beliefs and continued to criticize and attack the corruption present in the Catholic Church headed by the Pope. As a result of his continued defiance, Luther was excommunicated from the church on January 3, 1521. Consequently, a revolt and rebellion swept across the European continent, and these individuals were subsequently called "Lutherans" and "Protestants," meaning those who protested against the corrupt Catholic Church and Pope Leo X. Within a few years, Denmark, Norway, Sweden

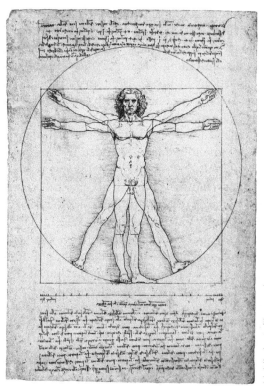

Jakub Krechowicz/Shutterstock.com

Photo 2.20 Leonardo DaVinci was the first to describe the human body as a "beautiful living machine." This remains a critical milestone in our evolution of the concept of health because it served as the foundation for the mechanistic medical model of health, which continues to dominate our publicly funded health care systems in Canada today (Bartfay and Bartfay 2015).

and Germany had declared themselves to be Lutheran. Although the Protestant Revolt did not have any major effects on charitable hospitals in countries that remained under Catholic rule, the majority of hospitals run by Catholic religious orders were closed or confiscated by the Protestant rebels. This had significant implications for the sick and the poor who were driven-out of these institutions for the sick and poor (Donahue 1996). The most notable chaos that resulted from these reforms and protests against the Catholic Church and the authority of the Pope occurred in England under the rule of *King Henry VIII* (Tudor). King Henry VIII appointed himself the head of the Church of England and confiscated the property of more than 600 Catholic charitable endowments (Donahue 1996; Loades 1990). Consequently, the care received by the sick and poor quickly deteriorated because formally educated and trained nurses in these once Catholic charitable establishments were replaced by untrained lay attendants or uneducated nurses (Bartfay 2010a).

Women in England were recruited from all sources to fill the nursing ranks, which included drunks, social undesirables, and prostitutes. The majority of these were illiterate, rough, and ill-qualified and trained women who were assigned nursing duties in lieu of serving jail sentences. In fact, when a woman in England could no longer earn a living from gambling or prostitution, she might consider becoming a nurse (Donahue 1996). There was little or no organizations in these institutions as a consequence of these dramatic reforms and no one with any credible social standing would consider becoming a nurse. Fortunately, the reputation of nurses in England was revised during the Victorian Era of the nineteenth century due to reforms instigated by Florence Nightingale and her contemporaries.

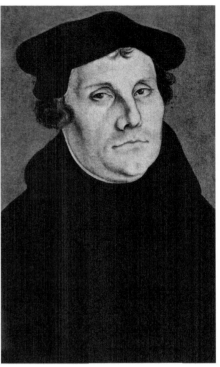

Photo 2.21 Oil painting of Martin Luther by Lucas Cranach den Ældre. The year 1517 marks the beginning of the *Reformation* or the *Protestant Revolt* against the authority of Pope Leo X and patriarchal rule by the Catholic Church in Europe.

During the sixteenth and seventeenth centuries, we observe the beginnings of the so-called *mechanistic medical model of health* (Brike and Silvertown 1984; Capra 1982; Lyons and Petrucelli 1978; McKeown 1976). Similar to DaVinci's description, William Harvey (1578–1657) also viewed the human body as a *living biological machine* when he detailed how that heart and circulatory systems correctly functioned. However, this biological machine remained disconnected from one's environment, mind, or spirit (Bartfay 2010a). Indeed, there was an increasing opinion and clinical view that various body components or systems (e.g., neurological, circulatory, digestive) were interconnected, yet one could diagnosis specific malfunctions and diseases and treat them separately based on the specific body component or system effected. The purpose of medicine was redefined to entail the correct diagnosis and treatment of the defective or malfunctioning component or system of the biological human machine that resulted from disease or illness (Brike and Silvertown 1984; Capra 1982).

Thomas Sydenham (1624–1689) argued that this mechanistic medical model of health should be employed for treating clients and the need to develop medical specialist with the appropriate expertise in diagnosing and managing defective body systems or components (e.g., heart, lungs, digestive system) (Capra 1982; Donahue 1996). This perspective is analogous to the repair of a defective gear in a machine such as a clock, or the replacement of water or an oil pump in a car. Consequently, the mechanistic medical model for health has resulted in the establishment of a variety of specialized fields in medicine and hospital units or wards that cater to these specific body systems. In fact, we now have specialist for the mind (psychiatrists); the kidneys (nephrologists); our digestive system (gastroenterologists); the heart (cardiologists); our immune system (immunologists), and our skin (dermatologists), to name but a few.

The adoption of the medical model of health is a critical milestone in the historical evolution of the concept of health because it viewed alterations to one's health as simply defects in some biological component or system that needed repair that could be achieved through medical interventions (e.g., surgery, medications). It is also a critical turning point because it further distinguished and defined health via body components, and the call to develop medical specialist to better diagnosis and treat each of these defective parts or systems. Hence, health from the mechanistic medical model paradigm was based on the notion that an individual was deemed "healthy" provided that they were disease free and that each body system or component was functioning optimally (Armstrong and Armstrong 2001; Birke and Silvertown 1984; Capra 1982; Illich 1975). A **paradigm** is defined as a specific worldview or perspective, way of thinking, and/or methodology which guides practice in the health sciences (Bartfay and Bartfay 2015). Moreover, the mechanistic medical model paradigm of health remains central to the organization of specialized acute care hospital units (e.g., cardiac, obstetrical, neurological) in Canada and globally (Bartfay and Bartfay 2015).

The medical model of health care delivery has also provided a mechanism for institutions such as hospitals in Canada to calculate or determine the amount of work time required for other allied health care professionals (e.g., nurses, physiotherapists) and workers (e.g., orderlies, x-ray technicians) on the basis of the specific part being repaired and/or replaced (e.g., heart valve, new knee). In fact, our current publicly funded health care systems in Canada have been compared to piecework payments in manufacturing industries, in which workers are paid for each component produced (Armstrong and Armstrong 2003; Armstrong et al. 2001).

In the widely quoted and influential book entitled *The Role of Medicine: Dream, Mirage or Nemesis?* Thomas McKeown (1976) critically examines the validity of the mechanistic medical model of health which is rarely stated explicitly, but which medical activities and directives today continue to be largely dependent on. Specifically, that the concept of health based on the medical model paradigm is essentially derived from a mechanistic approach based on the understanding of the structure and function of human body parts and systems and disease processes which affect them directly.

Medical services is dominated by the image of the acute hospital where the technological resources are concentrated, and much less attention is given to environmental and behavioural determinants of disease, or to the needs of sick people who are not thought to provide scope for investigation or therapy.

—McKeown 1976, p. 6

The medical model of what health is and how it is to be achieved, promoted, or restored remains the dominant paradigm in Canada and the basis for the Canada Health Act passed by Parliament in 1982 (Bartfay 2010a; Bartfay and Bartfay 2015; Government of Canada 1984). In fact, funding transfer payments to the various provinces and territories by the federal government, as detailed in the Canada Health Act (1982), is based on "medically necessary" physician services (Bartfay 2010a; Government of Canada 1984). In addition, the medical model paradigm of health was central to the evolution of our Medicare systems and how health care continues to be largely funded and delivered in Canada (Frank, Di Ruggiero, and Moloughney 2003; National Expert Commission Canadian Nurses Association 2012). We shall examine the limitations of the medical model of health and examine the need to adopt more holistic models based on primary health care models in greater detail below.

Our publicly insured (tax-based) health care systems in Canada have been largely conceived on the basis of a medical model of health that is largely delivered in acute care hospitals and are physician driven (Bartfay 2010a; Bartfay and Bartfay 2015). In fact, physicians remain the primary referral agents for access to a variety of health care services in Canada. Indeed, physicians may be regarded as "gate keepers" to specific diagnostic procedures and laboratory-based tests; other medical specialists (e.g., cardiologists, neurologists, orthopedic surgeons), and to various health care services (Browne, Birch, and Thabane 2012; National Expert Commission Canadian Nurses Association 2012; Soroka and Mahon 2012). Physicians in many parts of the world and in Canada are still optimally in charge of making diagnoses, administering treatments and cure. Furthermore, the cutbacks in health care funding over the past four decades have resulted in an increasing focus on quick treatments and cure by politicians and policy makers, thus ensuring that physicians remain at the centre of acute care institutions (Armstrong and Armstrong 2003; Bartfay and Bartfay 2015).

No discussion of "better value" for dollars spent in our publicly funded health-care system can be complete without addressing the question of how we pay care providers…an acute, treatment model drives Canada's system, where the physician acts as gatekeeper to specialized diagnostic and treatment-often offered in hospitals. Yet evidence shows that this model is insufficient to meet current and future health and wellness care needs of Canadians.

—National Expert Commission Canadian Nurses Association 2012, p. 28

The reader is referred to Chapter 3 for a detailed discussion related to the Canada Health Act and the challenges facing our publicly funded health care systems based on the medical model of health in the new millennium.

Industrial Revolution Era

The eighteenth and nineteenth centuries are characterized by various technological and scientific discoveries, which were often fuelled by the causative medical model of health (Bartfay 2010a; Madigan and Martinko 2006). For example, Pasteur discovered how viruses were attenuated, developed an effective treatment for rabies, and discovered the process of pasteurizing milk to kill harmful bacteria along with Claude Bernard. A wide variety of germs that are sometimes present in raw milk, can make individuals very ill including bacteria (e.g., *Brucella*, *Campylobacter*, *Listeria*, *Mycobacterium bovis* (a causative organism of tuberculosis [TB]), *Salmonella*, Shiga toxin-producing *Escherichia coli* (e.g., *E. coli* O1570, *Shigella*, *Yersinia*), parasites (e.g., *Giardia*), and viruses (e.g., norovirus) (British Columbia Centre for Disease Control 2013; Centers for Disease Control and Prevention 2006).

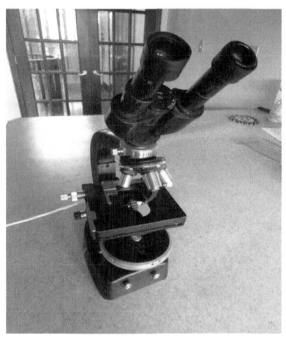

Source: Wally J. Bartfay

Photo 2.22 Louis Pasteur (1822–1895) brought about a revolution in medicine when he linked tiny microorganisms which could be seen only under the microscope, with certain communicable diseases and confirmed the germ theory of disease causation. This theory eventually replaced Hippocrates' 2,000-year-old theory of the four body humours previously taught to medical students.

Selling unpasteurized milk in Canada has been prohibited under the Food and Drug Regulations Act (section B.08.002[1]) since 1991. In addition, several provinces have similar legislation that prohibits the sale or distribution of raw milk products. For example, Ontario's Health Protection and Promotion Act, subsection 18(1) reads: "No person shall sell, offer for sale, deliver or distribute milk or cream that has not been pasteurized or sterilized in a plant that is licensed under the Milk Act or in a plant outside Ontario that meets the standards for plants licensed under the Milk Act" (Government of Ontario 2011).

Robert Koch (1849–1910) discovered the tubercle bacillus in 1882 as the cause of TB and also the cholera bacillus in 1883. Koch was subsequently awarded the Nobel Prize in Medicine in 1905 for his work. Pasteur and Koch collectively founded the scientific field of bacteriology, which has helped to further establish the dominance of the laboratory-based single-agent causative medical model of health in the nineteenth and twentieth centuries (Madigan and Martinko 2006).

Joseph Lister (1827–1912) revolutionized surgery by decreasing the incidence of post-operative infections through the use of a mild carbolic acid solution sprayed during surgical procedures. Donahue (1996) reports that by the middle of the nineteenth century, several clinical diagnostic instruments such as the thermometer and stethoscope along with diagnostic tools such as x-rays became important adjuncts to the practice of medicine in North America and Europe. The introduction of ether and chloroform as general anesthetics greatly advanced surgical outcomes and practices. In addition, the science of bacteriology had become the basis of modern medical practice and surgery.

The eighteenth and nineteenth centuries are also characterized by increased mechanization and the growth and expansion of industry termed the "Industrial Revolution" (Hanlon and Pickett 1984; Swanson and Albrecht 1993). During this period, the health and lives of the poor, including children, were often sacrificed for industrial profit and gains. For example, local parishes in England were often given the responsibility for providing relief for the poor under the so-called *Elizabethan Poor Law* (Swanson and Albrecht 1993). In essence, these were workhouses for the poor which often included orphaned and poor children who were wards of the parish. These children were often required to labour for long hours with limited food and shelter or other comforts of home. Individuals with affluence and status were predominately treated in their own homes by physicians or private duty nurses; whereas the less affluent and poor were cared for in hospitals. Hence, the subsequent deterioration in the condition and reputation of Protestant run hospitals in Europe during this time is undeniable (Bartfay 2010a; Bartfay and Bartfay 2015).

A number of humanitarian leaders, however,

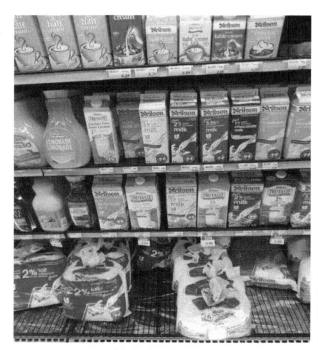

Source: Wally J. Bartfay

Photo 2.23 Pasteurization of all milk products in Canada is a form of both primordial and primary preventions for public health. In fact, an individual who consumes contaminated raw milk may develop severe or even life-threatening diseases, such as Guillain-Barré syndrome resulting in paralysis and hemolytic uremic syndrome, which can result in kidney damage or failure, stroke and even death.

emerged to reform these practices and institutions. For example, the English philanthropist *John Howard* (1727–1789) wrote detailed reports on the conditions of various public institutions including hospitals, asylums, and prisons (Donahue 1996; Lyons and Petrucelli 1978). These reports were highly significant in improving the health conditions of these public institutions, including the necessity for fresh air, cleanliness, and compassion for those less fortunate in the eighteenth century. The following account provides the reader with an example of the deplorable conditions and treatments by Howard:

> One ward is for clients dangerously sick or dying; another for clients of the middle rank of life; and the third for the lower and poorer sort of clients. In the last ward (which is the largest) there are four rows of beds; in the others, only two. They were so dirty and offensive as to create the necessity of perfuming them; and yet I observed that the physicians, in going his rounds, was obliged to keep his handkerchief to his face…These were served by the most dirty, ragged, unfeeling and unhuman persons I ever saw. I once found eight or nine of them highly entertained with a delirious dying client. The governor told me that they had only twenty-two servants, and that many of them were debtors or criminals, who had fled thither for refuge.

—Howard 1791, pp. 58–60

Similarly, *Elizabeth Gurney Fry* (1780–1845) advocated for improving the health and living conditions of women prisoners in England (Bartfay 2010a). Fry also established a society for visiting nurses first known as the *Society of Protestant Sisters of Charity* in 1840, and which later become known as the *Institute of Nursing Sisters*. These public health nurses provided private home based nursing services to individuals of all social classes and standings in England (Donahue 1996; Swanson and Albrecht 1993). This is an important historical milestone for our understanding of how various social determinants (e.g., education, poverty, homelessness) affect health. The reader is referred to Chapter 1 for a detailed description of our current understanding of the SDH. The Research

Focus Box 2.1 provides an overview of a mixed-design study which examined the health care needs and resources being accessed in their communities by women who were recently released from a correctional institution.

The Industrial Revolution period is also marked by the scientific study of medicinal plants and herbal remedies for clinical applications. Perhaps one of the best examples involves the use of the elegant Foxglove plant (aka Lady's Glove, Virgin's Glove) or *Digitalis purpurea* in Latin for the treatment of dropsy, a symptom of congestive heart failure (Aikman 1977; Grieve 1931; Weiner 1980).

Withering devoted ten years to investigating the medicinal properties of this plant and the noted clinical outcomes for each of the 163 clients that he treated. He also worked out the safe dosage range for prescribing this herbal remedy to his clients (i.e., 1–3 g of the powdered green leaves twice daily) that he knew to be highly dangerous and sometime lethal in higher dosages. He published his findings in his classic treatise, *An Account of the Foxglove and Some of its Medical Uses*. Foxglove contains a glycoside which has been used as a stimulant in acute circulatory failure, as a diuretic, and as a cardiac tonic in chronic heart disorders for over 200 years now (Aikman 1977; Grieve 1931;

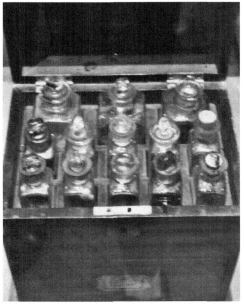

Source: Photo by Wally J. Bartfay

Photo 2.24 An ancient portable medicine chest. A significant amount of plant-based medications and remedies were employed during the 18th and 19th centuries.

Research Focus Box 2.1

Health care needs of women immediately post-incarceration: A mixed methods study

Study Aim/Rationale: The aim of this study was to assess the health status of women who were recently incarcerated in a prison and explore their health care needs and resources being accessed immediately following their release.

Methodology/Design
A mixed-methods study design was employed by the researchers, which consisted of a: (i) a quantitative survey in phase I of the investigation; and (ii) qualitative interviewing in phase II. In phase I, data were collected on demographics, health history, health status, and health-promoting behaviours. In the second phase, semi-structured interviews were used. The inclusion criteria included that all participants be at least eighteen years of age and had to be released from a prison in the last twelve months. Thirty-four women participated in phase I, and eleven women took part in phase II of the investigation.

Major findings
The results from this investigated showed that women who were recently discharged from a correctional institution had below average health status, in comparison to the general population. The major health issues identified by participants were associated with the lingering effects of being incarcerated, including recovery from substance abuse as a major health concern; mental health issues; routine health promotion and maintenance, and social and environmental barriers to accessing care.

Implications for public health
This study suggests that women discharged from correctional institutions have significant and complex health care needs. This period of transition appears to be an opportune time to offer support, services, and other health-promoting interventions by public health care professionals and workers.

Source: Colbert et al. (2003).

Weiner 1980). It has been estimated that over 400 different kinds of cardio-active glycosides have already been isolated from the plant kingdom alone.

Public Health Activities in Canada: 1900–1950

Public health activities in Canada during the early part of the twentieth century continued to be largely unco-ordinated and unorganized in nature, and were mostly in response to infectious outbreaks (PHAC 2008a; Rutty and Sullivan 2010). For example, the City of Toronto was the first to hire a civic nurse in 1907 to provide public health services including health education in the home of individuals diagnosed with TB (Bartfay 2010b; Royce 198; Rutty and Sullivan 2010). Subsequently, the City of Montréal hired a nurse from the Victorian Order of Nurses to provide health education for individuals infected with TB (Gibbon 1947).

Public health activities also increased in response to Canadian sol-diers who were returning from the First World War (1914–1918), and who were exposed to the Spanish influenza pandemic of 1918–1919 (PHAC 2008a; Quinlan and Dickinson 2009). Once former Canadian soldiers were at home, the Spanish flu virus quickly spread across Canadian cities, and even affected remote and isolated communities. The Spanish flu pandemic killed an estimated fifty to one hundred mil-lion individuals worldwide, including approximately 50,000 Canadians.

The Canadian Public Health Association (CPHA), which was first a voluntary association comprised of concerned medical and other allied health care professionals, held their first meeting on October 12, 1910 in Ottawa to discuss public health concerns that were affecting commu-nities across Canada (Rutty and Sullivan 2010). The CPHA held its first annual conference in December, 1911 at McGill University in Montréal. The importance of this voluntary association in addressing public health concerns is evidenced by the fact that the Prime Minister of Canada, the Governor General, and the Premier of Québec were all in attendance. One of the major agenda items of this conference was to develop a comprehen-sive public health plan for the prevention, control, and eradication of TB. The CPHA also played a major role in advocating for the creation of the Department of Health in 1919 (PHAC 2008a). This department retained functions related to quarantine and food and drug standards, but its role was expanded to include the promotion of child welfare and the imple-mentation of public health campaigns against STI and TB. During this time period, cities such as Toronto and Montréal began to pasteurize milk against bovine TB and towns such as Peterborough, began using chlorina-tion to disinfect their public drinking water supplies (PHAC 2008a).

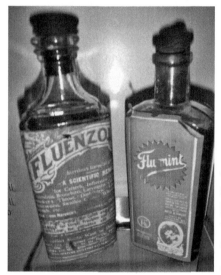

Source: Photo by Wally J. Bartfay

Photo 2.25 Examples of clinically unproven and ineffective flu rememdies sold. The 1918 Spanish flu pandemic, also known as the" La Grippe", was an unusu-ally deadly influenza pandemic, the first of the two pandemics involving H1N1 influ-enza virus. The surveillance and tracking of infectious (i.e., communicable) diseases nationally and globally remains a public health challenge and priority.

Additional public health developments during the early part of the twentieth century in Canada included school-based immunization programs against smallpox and diphthe-ria, and the appointment of nurses by school boards to monitor the health and wellness of children. The first public health nurses in Canada were appointed in 1909 in Hamilton and 1910 in Toronto (Bartfay 2010b; Ross-Kerr 2003). *Lina Rogers* (Struthers—married name) who was appointed to the School Nursing Service of the Toronto Board of Education, achieved international recognition for her work correlating the absence of children from school with a lack of health care (Gibbon and Mathewson 1947). Roger's wrote the first textbook for school nurses in 1917 entitled *The School Nurse: A Survey of the Duties and Responsibilities of the Nurse in Maintenance of Health and Physical Perfection and the Prevention of Disease among School Children.* Roger's and her assistant often had to improvise when administering nursing care to students in schools. For example, radiators and window sills often served as dressing tables to address wounds (e.g., from rat bites), and a discarded high chair doubled as a treatment table for treating eye infections (e.g., conjunctivitis). They also identified children with disabilities (e.g., vision or hearing problems) that made learning a challenge for them in the classroom. A contagious condition such as TB would still cause a student's dismissal from the classroom, but Roger's and her assistant followed-up with family visits and used the time to teach about hygiene and prevention to parents and guardians. Comprehensive school-based primary health programs and initiatives delivered in communities' remains an internationally recognized framework that supports improvements in both educational and health outcomes in a planned, integrated, and holistic fashion (Murray et al. 2007; National Expert Commission Canadian Nurses Association 2012; Stewart-Brown 2006).

Following the First World War, the Canadian Red Cross Society was fundamental in establishing one-year post-graduate certificate in public health nursing programs offered at various universities across Canada (Canadian Red Cross Society 1962). These programs were available at the University of British Columbia, University of Western Ontario, University of Toronto, McGill University, and Dalhousie University (Bartfay 2010b). These public health nurses received training in both disease prevention and the delivery of home-based health care services to a variety of individuals across the lifespan affected with illness or disease. In 1927, the School of Hygiene at the University of Toronto was also founded to provide post-graduate training for a range of public health professionals. It is notable how instrumental voluntary organizations such as the Canadian Red Cross Society and the CPHA, have been in shaping the current public health fabric in Canada (Bartfay 2010b; Bartfay and Bartfay 2015).

The health of Canadians was dealt a serious blow during the Great Depression of the 1930s that resulted in the collapse of many industries in cities and towns, and several farmer's and individuals lost their homes and livelihoods (PHAC 2008a). The Great Depression was subsequently followed by the Second World War (1939–1945). Infectious diseases, such as polio, remained as a serious threat to the health and well-being of Canadians. Following World War II, public health services remained minimal in smaller towns and communities, and the majority of the Medical Officers of Health (MOHs) in larger urban centres often lacked formal training in public health and worked on a part-time basis only (Rutty and Sullivan 2010).

In 1939, Ian MacKenzie, the Minister for the Department of Pensions and National Health, wrote a letter to Prime Minister King urging that unemployment and health insurance can be introduced as a war measures initiative along with the need to develop a national health care system for all returning soldiers and sailors (Taylor 1987). MacKenzie's arguments were strengthened by the fact that several allied countries (e.g., England, Australia) were already developing these programs. He subsequently hired Dr. J. J. Heagerty as the Director of Public Health Services to formally develop a proposal for health insurance (Storch 2006; Taylor 1987, 1973). Dr. Heagerty strategically consulted with his provincial counterparts and established the Inter-Departmental Advisory Committee on Health Insurance. During the same period, Leonard Marsh was serving as a consultant to the federal government and was involved with the Committee on Postwar Reconstruction in 1944–1945. Marsh's tabled a report entitled *Report on Social Security for Canada* in which he outlined the need to develop a post-war welfare state in Canada (Storch 2006; Taylor 1987, 1973). The work of Heagerty and Marsh reflected national post-war idealisms, and subsequently served as blueprints for the development of various health and social insurance programs in Canada (Bartfay 2010c; Bartfay and Bartfay 2015). Furthermore, these reports planted the seed in Canadian society and idealism that the concept of health was much more than the absence of disease, but was also influenced by a variety of environmental and SDH.

Following World War II, Canada prospered as a nation and the general health and well-being of our citizens and residents improved. The post-war economic boom resulted in new jobs and increasing affluence for Canadian families. By 1950, mortality rates decreased by one-quarter in comparison to those of 1921 (9 per 1,000 compared with 12 per 1,000) (PHAC 2008a). It is noteworthy that employment remains a critical social determinant of health in Canada and globally. A variety of national and social programs were also introduced, including the *Canada Pension Plan* (CPP) and the *Old Age Security* (OAS) plan, which positively affected the health and well-being of seniors.

In 1948, the Government of Canada established the *National Health Grants Program* which served as a major stimulus for the development of basic public health infrastructures and programs in the provinces over the next three decades (PHAC 2008a). The program consisted of grants-in-aid to the provinces for general public health initiatives including the formulation of provincial health plans, TB control, mental health, cancer control, child and maternal health and the training of health care professionals (e.g., physicians and nurses). Access to acute care hospital services were also guaranteed through the introduction of legislation including the Hospital Insurance and Diagnostic Services Act (1957) and the Medical Care Act (MCA 1966) (Falk-Rafael and Coffey 2005; Government of Canada 2002; Rachlis and Kushner 1994).

It is noteworthy that these funding schemes were based on an episodic acute care medical model of health dominated and driven by physicians for the past fifty years (Browne et al. 2012; National Expert Commission Canadian Nurses Association 2012; Soroka and Mahon 2012). Based on this model, physicians acted as "gate keepers" for referrals and access to various diagnostic and laboratory-based tests (e.g., x-rays, blood tests, electrocardiograms); were responsible for writing all prescriptions filled by pharmacists; made referrals to access the services of other medical specialists (e.g., cardiologists, neurologists, orthopedic surgeons), and ordered and directed specialized care performed by other health care professionals or workers (e.g., wound dressing changes performed by nurses, specific exercises performed by physiotherapists after a stroke). The 1964 Royal Commission on Health Services recommended:

> That as a nation, we now take the necessary legislative, organizational and financial decisions to make all the fruits of health sciences available to all our residents without hindrance of any kind—there can be no greater challenge to a free society of free men.
>
> —PHAC (2008a)

It was not until the early part of the current century that we observe acute care hospitals evolving into the more familiar highly specialized sites for treating clients across the various social classes. This was largely due to the high cost of medical diagnostic equipment and technologies (e.g., x-rays, diagnostic laboratory-based blood tests). Indeed, the average physician could not afford these newly discovered diagnostic and treatment technologies for their individual private offices (Storch 2006). By 1955 there were 1,216 hospitals in Canada (Armstrong and Armstrong 2003). Hence, hospitals became the logical site for physicians and other health care professionals to access these new technological tools of their trade developed as a consequence of the laboratory-based medical model of health.

It is notable that prior to World War II, the majority of nurses in Canada (approximately 60%) worked as public health nurses or were self-employed in private homes (Baumgart and Wheeler 1992; Canadian Nurses Association 1996). Similarly, Coburn (1988) reports that during the 1930s, only twenty-five percent of all nurses worked in hospitals. This number increased to over sixty-five percent by the early 1950s, and by the year 1989, approximately eighty-five percent were of all nurses in Canada were practicing in publicly insured hospitals (Canadian Institute for Health Information 2006). Add to your knowledge of the history of nursing and how the profession has contributed to reforming our current understanding and definitions of health by accessing the Web-based Resource Box 2.1.

Web-based Resource Box 2.1   History of Nursing

Learning Resource	Website
AMS Nursing History Research Unit This website provides various historical facts and links to vital resources related to historical developments, legislations and practice mandates for nurses in American and abroad.	http://www.health.uottawa.ca/nursinghistory
BCE History of Nursing Group This website concentrates on the history of nursing in British Columbia, but also provides historical facts and data from other Canadian-based resources related to nursing.	http://www.bcnursinghistory.ca
Canadian Association for the History of Nursing This website provides access to historical developments in the profession of nursing from both Canadian and international perspectives and influences.	http://www.cahn-achn.ca

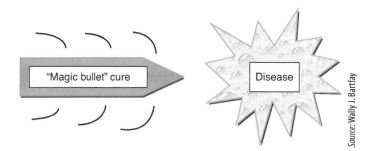

Source: Wally J. Bartfay

Figure 2.2 Conceptual diagram showing the unicausal model of disease origin and cure. The continued predominate directive of medical research for finding the specific causes and cures of disease, or so-called "magic bullet" cure approach, has remained an enduring consequence of the unicausal laboratory-based medical model of health.

Challenges to this unicausal laboratory-based medical approach to achieving health included the nineteenth century German physician and hygienist Max von Pettenkofer (Swanson and Albrecht 1993). Von Pettenkofer boldly challenged his contemporaries and the dominate unicausal germ theory of disease origin by swallowing a large quantity of the *cholera bacillus* in front of his students. Hence, he directly challenged the validity of this unicausal model of disease by not contracting cholera or dying as a consequence of his radical experiment (Hume 1927).

Figure 2.2 provides the reader with a conceptual diagram of the unicausal laboratory-based medical model of health (Bartfay and Bartfay 2015). Based on this perspective, once the exact cause of the disease is discovered in the laboratory, unique cures (e.g., antiviral agent, antibiotic, gene therapy) can be developed to produce or restore optimal health. Ironically, corporate based fund raising efforts (e.g., CIBC's or Sear's run for the cure for cancer) in Canada continue to socially reinforce the dominance of this unicausal medical model of health in our society via the emphasis and preferential funding for laboratory-based research programs and grants to find the causes and associated cures for various diseases (Bartfay and Bartfay 2015). One of the major limitations of the unicausal medical model paradigm of health is that it fails to consider complex environmental interactions or multifactorial determinants of health that can lead to negative health outcomes. For example, there is no "magic bullet" cure (e.g., antiviral agent, antibiotic, gene therapy) for children who live in poverty; are physically and psychologically abused, and suffer from malnutrition. Similarly, there is no "magic bullet" cure for an adult with type 2 diabetes who is morbid obese; smokes a pack of cigarettes daily; leads a sedentary lifestyle, and makes poor dietary choices (Bartfay and Bartfay 2015). In fact, there is no magic bullet cure for a single noncommunicable disease (e.g., diabetes, heart disease, stroke, COPD, rheumatic arthritis, ALS, Alzheimer's disease, bi-polar disorder, schizophrenia), because their causes, associated risk factors and social determinants of health, are deemed multifactorial in nature.

In his widely quoted work entitled *Medical Nemesis: The Expropriation of Health,* Ivan Illich (1975) argues that the medicalization of health is a monopoly that has only served their interest of physicians since the turn of the century. Nonetheless, the concept of *medicalization* was first introduced by Zola (1972) who defined it as a social process whereby various psychosocial aspects of human daily life are progressively and deliberately understood in terms of health and illness.

For example, homosexuality was historically regarded as a social deviance that was consequently defined and categorized via medical terms and clinical standards at the turn of the present century, which in-turn required diagnosis and treatment by physicians (Conrad and Schneider 1985). Specifically the influential American Psychiatric Association (APA) first listed homosexuality in the Diagnostic and Statistical Manual (DSM-I) as a sociopathic personality disturbance in 1952 (McCommon 2006; Spitzer 1981). It is notable that the DSM (version V now) has been translated into various languages and continues to be the "gold standard" for making diagnosis by psychiatrists and clinical psychologists. In 1968, the DSM II removed homosexuality from the sociopathic list and re-categorized it with other sexual deviations. It was finally removed and decategorized as a sexual deviation from the DSM in 1973 (McCommon 2006; Spitzer 1981). Hence, it has been argued that the practice of medicine was seen as a means of social control and dominance for homosexuals in North America and abroad (Conrad and Schneider 1985; Illich 1975).

Currently in Canada, homosexuality is not regarded as a "disease" per se requiring diagnosis and treatment by physicians, but a sexual preference and lifestyle choice (Bartfay and Bartfay 2015). Nonetheless, the international gay, lesbian, and bisexual communities continue to face discrimination in many parts of the world based on the criminalization of homosexuality as a continued means of social control by politicians and policy makers. For example, the Russian Parliament under the leadership of President Vladimir Putin has passed a law in 2013 criminalizing the "propaganda of non-traditional sexual relations" (Kordunsky 2013). Homosexuality also remains criminalized in seventy-six countries around the world including Afghanistan, thirty-eight states in sub-Saharan Africa, Barbados, Belize, Burundi, Cameron, Egypt, Iran, Jamaica, Lebanon, Malaysia, Mauritania, Morocco, Papua New Guinea, Tonga, Trinidad, Shi Lanka, United Arab Emirates, Qatar, and Yemen, to name but a few (Bay Windows 2010; Kordunsky 2013; Saner 2013). Moreover, there are several countries with the death penalty associated with homosexuality including Iran, Saudi Arabia, Sudan, Yemen, Nigeria, and Somalia.

McKeown (1976) argues that the predominant influences that have resulted in improvements in health during the past three centuries were not linked to the practice of medicine per se, but attributed to improvements in diet and nutrition (e.g., food safety); the environment (e.g., safe water supplies, sewage disposal); behavioural changes (e.g., smoking cessation, exercise), and reproductive practices which limited population growth. McKeown (1981) further disputes the validity and true impact of the unicausal germ theory of disease causation for improving the overall health of individuals and communities. For example, although Koch identified the *tubercle bacillus* as the cause of TB in 1882, no effective treatments were available until the antibiotic streptomycin was discovered sixty-five years later in 1947. However, by the time this antibiotic agent was discovered, mortality rates were only a fraction of what they were during the nineteenth century. Hence, improved survival rates and decreased mortality rates could not be linked directly to the discovery of streptomycin and its ability to rid clients of the *tubercle bacillus*, but were in fact largely attributed due to improvements in public sanitation, improved nutritional status of individuals, improved living conditions, and other SDH (Bartfay 2010a; McKeown 1981; Rutty and Sullivan 2010).

Interestingly, the 1842 British report entitled *The Sanitary Conditions of the Labouring Population of Great Britain* concluded that clean drinking water, sewers and adequate housing for their residents were essential to prevent the spread of infectious disease (PHAC 2008a). This report led to the establishment of the first Public Health Act in the United Kingdom in 1848. Similarly, the 1900 *Annual Report of the Provincial Board of Health for Ontario* concluded that there has been a remarkable decline in mortality associated with communicable diseases by the turn of the century, which were largely attributed to improvements in drinking water quality, sanitation measures put in place and public infrastructures such as proper sewers (PHAC 2008a).

Similarly, Naidoo and Wills (2000) argue that the overall contributions of mechanistic medical model of health for reducing mortality globally has been minor, in comparison with those related to improvements made to environmental conditions such as clean drinking water supplies, proper sanitation, adequate nutrition, and housing. In fact, it is estimated that approximately seventy-five percent of "good health" maintained or achieved is the result of factors (e.g., lifestyle choices, clean water supplies, proper sanitation, legislations such as the mandatory pasteurization of milk in Canada) that are beyond direct episodic acute care that is often delivered in hospitals (National Expert Commission Canadian Nurses Association 2012; Standing Senate Committee on Social Affairs, Science and Technology, Subcommittee on Population Health 2009). These health factors and determinants are critical to highlight in terms of our current understanding and definitions of health and how it is achieved, maintained, restored, and promoted across the lifespan.

Add to your knowledge of the history of medicine and the development of the mechanistic medical model of health by accessing the Web-Based Resource Box 2.2.

Web-based Resource Box 2.2 History of Medicine and the Development of the Mechanistic Model of Health

Learning Resource	Website
Canadian Society for the History of Medicine (CSHM) This website promotes the history of health and medicine in all its facets from a multi-disciplinary perspective.	http://cshm-schm.ca/
History learning site—History of Medicine This website provides an overview of major historical developments in the evolution of medical practice and other major developments in medicine including the germ theory.	http://www.historylearningsite.co.uk
International Society for the History of Medicine (ISHO) This international society provides the dissemination of historical facts, timelines, and research related to the history of medicine and surgery from an international perspective.	http://www.uia.be/s/or/en/1100042324

The Emergence of Holistic Definitions of Health

1950s to Present

The post–World War I and World War II era of health care in Canada and abroad continued to be dominated by the mechanistic medical model of health, with the emphasis on diagnosis, treatment, and cure of communicable (infectious) disease, as opposed to consideration for complex and compounded multiple health conditions, chronic diseases, or disabilities (Bartfay and Bartfay 2015). The Government of Canada appointed Justice Emmett Hall in 1965 to chair a Royal Commission on Health Services (Bartfay 2010c). The mandate of this Royal Commission was to carefully examine the existing public health care systems in Canada and report on their overall effectiveness (Hall 1980).

The Canadian Nurses Association (CNA 1980) responded to the Hall's Commission request for input by health care professionals with its influential document entitled *Putting Health Back into Health Care*. This document made several critical recommendations, including that: (a) Existing hospital and medical insurance programs be revised to stimulate the development of primary health care services in Canada; (b) improve preventive, diagnostic, and ambulatory-community-based points of entry into the health care systems; (c) that qualified health care professionals and workers be better utilized by the public health care system, and (d) changes to provincial legislation be revised to allow qualified nurses and other health care professionals to undertake health services currently only performed by physicians (CNA 1980).

The Hall Commission served as an impetus for a series of discussions between the Government of Canada and the provincial and territorial governments regarding the need for a national publicly insured health care system. Consequently, the MCA (1966) was passed by Parliament in 1966 with support by all major federal political parties, and implemented in 1968 (Bartfay 2010c). Hence, the publicly funded national Medicare system that we know today was effectively created with the passage of the MCA. In 1972, our national publicly funded Medicare program was finally instituted when all provinces and territories agreed to enlist with the plan. Nonetheless, this national Medicare program was directly primarily towards acute-care hospital and physician-driven health care services, despite lobbying efforts by the CNA and other health care professionals (Bartfay 2010c; Bartfay and Bartfay 2015). Currently, each province and territory in Canada is responsible for delivering its own public health care system, with independently negotiated health transfer funds from the federal government to help to cover the associated costs. The fee-for-service acute care model driven by physicians who act as gatekeepers to various diagnostic and health care services continues to dominate our current publicly funded health care systems in Canada (Browne, Birch, and Thabane 2012; Soroka and Mahon 2012).

We know that while this model suited doctors and most Canadians when Medicare was first introduced, times have changed. That model – delivered so often in and around hospitals – is very costly, and ultimately inefficient, way to meet the needs of Canadians now. This is one reason why we propose the funding of an integrated primary health-care model and urge governments to undertake the work needed to do this.

—National Expert Commission Canadian Nurses Foundation 2012, p. 29

The Lalonde Report, 1974

By the mid-1970s, a renewed interest in primary health care and health promotion had occurred almost simultaneously in several industrialized western countries including Canada, the United States, Great Britain, Germany, France, and Australia (Green and Ottoson 1994). In 1974 Marc Lalonde, the Federal Minister of Health, was the first to acknowledge the fact that our publicly insured health care systems in Canada were dominated by the outdated medical model of health (Bartfay 2010c). Lalonde was the first Minister of Health to also view the concept of health as resource that is influenced by a broad range of factors, rather than by only biological processes in his document entitled New Perspective on the Health of Canadians, which is informally known as the *Lalonde Report* (Lalonde 1974). Moreover, this landmark document is considered as the first report by a major industrialized nation to formally acknowledge that health is determined by more than just biological factors, but also other determinants of health based. This is a critical milestone in our understanding of the concept of health and its definition because it was the first official document by a developed nation in the world to recognize the link between health and a variety of SDH based on the best available scientific evidence to date from a variety of disciplines.

Hence, the Lalonde Report (1974) challenged the unicausal medical model of health and illness by introducing four critical determinants that were evidence-informed and shown to be associated with influencing the health of Canadians across the lifespan:

1. *Human biology*—Comprised of both physical and mental elements.
2. *Environment*—Comprised of all elements related to health that are regarded as external to one's body.
3. *Lifestyle*—Comprised of elements which an individual had control over, such as self-imposed behaviours.
4. *Health care organization*—Consists of access to health care services by all residents within a given community.

The Lalonde Report (1974) recommended that all levels of government should be actively involved in health promotion and be responsible for any associated increase in costs associated with the delivery of health care services to their citizens and residents across the lifespan. Health promotion activities enhance and/or reinforce the ability of an individual, family or group, community, or entire population's capacity to promote, maintain or restore their health and wellness (Raphael 2010; Rootman et al. 2012). Lalonde (1974) argued that the individual's lifestyle choices and behaviours (e.g., smoking, inactivity, impaired driving) had direct consequences on health, and that various levels of government and community organizations should work collaboratively to promote healthy lifestyle choices, along with the need to conduct ongoing research to validate health outcomes achieved. For example, for every $1.00 invested towards tobacco prevention programs in Canada results in a health care saving of $20.00, or a return on investment (ROI) of 1900%. The concept of health promotion currently includes a synthesis of five levels of prevention: (a) Primordial; (b) primary; (c) secondary; (d) tertiary, and (e) quaternary (British Columbia Ministry of Health 2013; National Public Health Partnership 2006; Porta 2008; Public Action Support Team 2011). The reader is referred to Chapter 1 for a detailed description of the five levels of prevention and examples of each (Figure 2.3).

Shortly after the release of this report, a population-based approach to health promotion and health care was gradually introduced to all levels of government in Canada (Rootman et al. 2012; Thompson 2010). According to the PHAC (2007), health promotion in Canada is perceived as a process that permits individuals to increase control over, maintain and/or improve their health. This process of health promotion embraces actions directed at strengthening the skills and capabilities of individuals across the lifespan. It also includes actions directed towards changing and improving social, environmental, political, and economic conditions so as to positively advance their impact on public and individual health (PHAC 2007). Add to your knowledge of the Lalonde Report (1974) by accessing the Web-Based Resource Box 2.3.

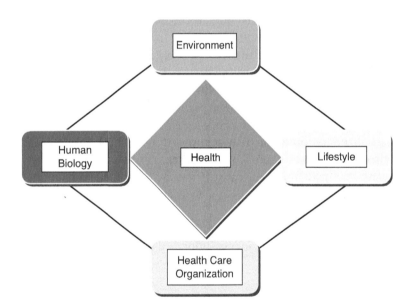

Figure 2.3 Conceptual diagram showing the four critical determinant of health as outlined by the Lalonde Report (1974). The Lalonde Report (1974) was the first evidence-informed report by a developed nation to challenge the mechanistic medical model of health by introducing four critical determinants of health.

Source: Adapted from Lalonde (1974).

Web-based Resource Box 2.3 The Lalonde Report

Learning Resource	Website
Lalonde (1974) This document is empirically based and highlights how our understanding of the concept of health has evolved based on critical determinants of health over the lifespan.	http://www.hc.sc.gc.ca/hcs-sss/com/fed/Lalonde-eng.php

In 1969, a study by the *National Advisory Council for Fitness and Amateur Sport* found that the majority of Canadians were sedentary in nature, unfit and alarmingly uninterested in the health benefits associated with exercise (ParticPATION 1969; Rutty and Sullivan 2010). As a result of this study, a federally-funded national public health initiative aptly coined "ParticiPACTION" was launched in 1971 to promote active and healthy lifestyles with the objective of preventing health problems and chronic disease associated with inactivity (Thompson 2010; Rutty and Sullivan 2010). Federal cut-backs resulted in the shut-down of this national public health promotion campaign in 2001. The program was re-instigated in February 2007 due to alarming reports that over half of the Canadians were overweight or obese and sedentary in nature.

Alma-Ata Conference, 1978

The Lalonde Report's (1974) new definition of health and emphasis on health promotion was embraced by many nations around the world and the WHO, which now viewed embraced the importance of health promotion to preserve and promote the health of their citizens (Bartfay and Bartfay 2015). Hence, the Lalonde Report (1974) was viewed as a futuristic and ground-breaking evidence-informed document by many nations around the world (Bartfay 2010a; Thompson 2010). In September 1978, the WHO convened the Alma-Ata Conference on Primary Health Care in Kazakhstan (located in the former Soviet Union) to address the need for global cooperation on a variety of health related issues and health care reforms. The adapted motto for this international conference was *Health for all by the Year 2000*, which emphasized the desire to reduce global inequities in health through the adoption of primary care initiatives (WHO 1978).

It is noteworthy that the Lalonde Report (1974) was the driving force behind the signing of the Declaration of Alma Ata by 134 nations at this international conference on primary health (Bartfay 2010a). This Declaration urged governments globally to take immediate action to protect and promote the health of all individuals across the lifespan. In fact, primary health care was seen as the major vehicle for reforming the mechanistic medical model of health that dominated health care systems globally (Ottoson and Green 1999). Add to your knowledge of the Declaration of Alma-Ata and its significance in the evolution of the definition of health from the laboratory-based mechanistic medical model of health to more holistic definitions of health based on various determinants of health derived from the best available evidence to date in the Web-Based Resource Box 2.4.

The Epp Report, 1986

The national public health document entitled *Achieving Health for All: A Framework for Health Promotion* was released in 1986 by the Federal Minister of Health, Jake Epp, and is informally known as the *Epp Report* (Epp 1986). The Epp Framework (1986) was based largely on the Lalonde Report (1974), but expanded on his definition of health promotion by including a wide range of socio-political and environmental determinants of health (Bartfay 2010a; Mikkonen and Raphael 2010; Muntaner et al. 2012). The report focused on the following three key areas and stated that governments needed to be more active in

Web-Based Resource Box 2.4 Alma-Ata Declaration on Health

Learning Resource	Website
Declaration of Alma-Ata: International Conference on Primary Health Care, Alma-Ata, USSR, September 6–12, 1978 (WHO 1978). This website highlights the Alma-Ata Conference 10 point declaration on primary health care.	http://www.who.int/publications/ almaata_declaration_en.pdf

providing support to groups and agencies within the community to engage in health promotion activities (Thompson 2010):

1. Survey the health status of disadvantaged groups and reduce inequities by enhancing the ability of individuals to cope.
2. Enhance detection and the management of chronic disease in Canada.
3. Identify diseases that were largely preventable in nature, and focus on the prevention of these diseases.

The Epp Report (1986) argued that primary health care initiatives must be supported at a variety of levels and stakeholders including various levels of government, local groups and employers. The report also cautioned against the limitations of focusing only on individual lifestyle choices or risk factors associated with the development of chronic disease in Canadian populations (e.g., link between smoking and heart disease, or lung cancer). This report was the first to caution against blaming the victim and criticizing lifestyle risk factor strategies that focused solely on individuals (e.g., smoking cessation programs) without consideration for additional broad determinants of health (Bartfay 2010a). Add to your knowledge of the *Epp Framework for Health Promotion* by accessing the Web-Based Resource Box 2.5.

Ottawa Charter for Health Promotion, 1986

The Epp Framework (1986) was released in November 1986 at First International Conference on Health Promotion by the WHO held in Ottawa, Ontario (CPHA, Welfare Canada and WHO 2006; PHAC 2001a). This international WHO conference was convened to review and expand on the proposals put forward at the Alma-Ata conference and to determine the progress that has been achieved to date in meeting these global objectives. At the conference, both Lalonde's (1974) and Epp's (1986) definitions of health were embraced and broadened to include a variety of health prerequisites including peace, education, a stable ecosystem, sustainable resources, shelter, food, income and employment, and social justice and equity (CPHA, Welfare Canada and WHO 2006; PHAC 2001a). The Ottawa Charter outlined five broad strategies for global health promotion (Raphael 2010; Rootman et al. 2012):

1. Build healthy public policies;
2. Create supportive environments;
3. Strengthen community actions;
4. Develop personal skills, and
5. Re-orientate health services. Add to your knowledge of the Ottawa Charter for Health Promotion (1986) by accessing the Web-Based Resource Box 2.6.

The 1986 WHO international conference was also instrumental in reinforcing the idea that the medical model of health, and the delivery of health care services based on this model, were inadequate to currently address the health challenges facing diverse populations across the lifespan globally. An alternative

Web-based Resource Box 2.5 The Epp Framework for Health Promotion

Learning Resource	Website
Epp (1986).	http://www.frcentre.net/library/AchievingHealthForAll.pdf

Web-based Resource Box 2.6   Ottawa Charter for Health Promotion

Learning Resource	Website
PHAC (2001a).	http://www.phac-aspc.gc.ca/ph-sp/docs/charter-char-tre/pdf/charter.pdf or http://www.who.int/hpr/NPH/docs/ottawa_charter_hp.pdf

view to the mechanistic medical model of health is termed the "holistic view" (Naidoo and Wills 2000; Edelman and Mandle 1994). Health from this perspective directly challenges the laboratory-based mechanistic medical model which asserts that alterations to health results from a biological breakdown of a component of the human body that result from disease (Bartfay and Bartfay 2015). Although there are numerous definitions of health based on this holistic perspective, one of the first global definitions advanced was by the WHO which defined this concept as "a state of complete physical, mental, and social well-being, not merely the absence of disease and infirmity" (WHO 1948, p. 100). In 1986 at the Ottawa Conference, WHO revised this definition by incorporating a socio-ecological component that recognized the inextricable links between the individual and their environment. Accordingly, the definition of **health** was revised to include:

…the ability to identify and to realize aspirations, to satisfy needs, and to change or cope with the environment. Health is therefore a resource for everyday life, not the objective of living. Health is a positive concept emphasizing social and personal resources, as well as physical capacities.

—Canadian Public Health Association, and WHO 1986, p. 426

The holistic view of health identifies the relationship between an individual's internal and external environments, and that health is an asset, human resource and basic human right. Although this revised holistic definition has been criticized for being too broad, for concentrating too much on a condition of health rather than a process, and for being impossible to achieve by many, it nevertheless has become the most widely quoted definition of health globally (Bartfay 2010a; Bartfay and Bartfay 2015).

Variations of the above mentioned definition of health by WHO have now been adopted by all the provincial and territorial ministries of health in Canada. Indeed, there appears to be a general consensus on what determines a state of health and well-being in Canada, as evidenced by the consensus statement reached at the *National Forum on Health* in 1997:

We have known for some time that the better off people are in terms of income, social status, social networks, sense of control over their lives, self-esteem and education, the healthier they are likely to be…. We know that there is a gradient in health status, with health improving at each step up the slope of income, education and social status.

—National Forum on Health 1997, p. 15

The Jakarta Declaration (1997)

In July of 1997, a conference on the need to strengthen global health promotion efforts was held in Jakarta, Indonesia (Shah 2003; Naidoo and Wills 2000). This conference entitled *New Era: Leading Health Promotion into the 21st Century in Jakarta* advanced the notion that various prerequisites for health were required including: peace; shelter; education; social security, and relations; income, nutrition; sustainable resources, and ecosystems; social justice, and respect for human rights including equality and the empowerment of women (WHO 1997). The Jakarta Declaration extended on the major strategic areas for health promotion first described in the Ottawa Charter (1986) by identifying the following five global health priority areas:

1. Promote social responsibility for health, including policies and practices that protect the environment, resources and individuals from harm or degradation.
2. Increase investments for health development and equality, especially for children, the elderly, Indigenous peoples, and marginalized populations.
3. Strengthen existing partnerships and explore the potential for new partnerships between various sectors, levels of government, and society at large.
4. Increase community capacity and empowerment of the individual.
5. Securement of infrastructures for health promotion, which include government organization, educational institutions, and the private sector (WHO 1997).

The Jakarta Declaration recognized that infectious diseases and mental health were two areas that required urgent global attention and prompt responses. The Declaration also acknowledged for the first time that various socio-economic and environmental factors also have major impacts on the health and well-being of citizens globally (WHO 1997). Transitional factors, such as the integration of the global economy, the stability of financial markets and trade, and access to mass and social medias, and communication technologies also have significant impact on health, as does environmental degradation due to the irresponsible use of natural resources (Shah 2003). Advocating, mediating, and enabling were identified as major strategies for engaging in health promotion.

Bangkok Charter for Health Promotion in a Globalized World (2005)

The *Bangkok Charter for Health Promotion in a Globalized World* is an international agreement reached among participants at the sixth Global Conference on Health Promotion held in Bangkok, Thailand in August 2005 (de Leeuw, Cho Tang, and Beaglehole 2007; WHO 2013). The global health promotion charter acknowledges the health inequalities between developed and developing nations; changing trend of communication including the internet and consumption in a globalized world; the growth of urbanization in developing regions of the world, global environmental changes (e.g., global warming, severe weather), and increased global trade and commercialization. The following five key areas of action for a healthier world are highlighted in the Charter (WHO 2013):

1. **Partner and build alliances** with private, non-private, non-governmental, or international organizations to create sustainable actions.
2. **Invest in sustainable policies**, actions and infrastructure to address the determinants of health.
3. **Build capacity for policy development**, health promotion practice and health literacy.
4. **Regulate and legislate** to ensure a high level of protection from harm and enable equal opportunity for health and well-being.
5. **Advocate health** based on human rights and solidarity.

The Bangkok Charter provides a critical link between foreign policies and the global practices related to health promotion and provides leadership and targeted areas for health promotion on an international scale. Moreover, the Charter identifies specific actions, commitments and pledges required to address the determinants of health in a globalized world through health promotion efforts. The reader is referred to Chapter 9 for a detailed discussion on current and emerging global health issues and concerns.

This link has been strengthened by the recent UN reform proposals to elevate public health as a foreign policy priority to support the four governance tasks served by foreign policy: security, economic well-being, development and human dignity. The emergence of health as a domain for foreign policy presents opportunities and risks for health promotion that can be managed by emphasizing that public health is a public good that benefits all those governance tasks.

—de Leeuw, Cho Tang, and Beaglehole 2007, p. 2

More recently, Canada hosted the nineteenth International Union for Health Promotion and Education World Conference in 2007 in Ottawa entitled *Health Promotion Comes of Age: Research, Policy and Practice for the 21st Century* (PHAC 2008a). This conference provided an opportunity to reaffirm the commitment and vision of the Ottawa Charter (1986) and the Bangkok Charter (2005), and it also provided an opportunity to look at the future and enhance the building of national and international partnerships and intersectoral collaborations for health promotion and research.

Current Developments in Public Health in Canada: 2000 and Onwards

The Canadian Institutes of Health Research (CIHR) Act was passed by Parliament in 2000, establishing the CIHR with a new and bold vision to transform health research in Canada based on international standards of excellence. The CIHR's vision and mandate clearly distinguished it from its predecessor, the Medical Research Council (Rutty and Sullivan 2010). Specifically, passage of the CIHR Act formally recognized the value of engaging in interdisciplinary and integrative health research that recognized the continued importance of laboratory-based biomedical and clinical research, but expanded it to include the importance of the health of populations across the lifespan, health services, health systems, and societal, cultural and environmental influences on health. As a part of the transformation, thirteen separate virtual institutes were created including the internationally unique Institute of Population and Public Health (IPPH).The IPPH's current mission for the years 2009 to 2014 and strategic research priorities are in concert with several global calls to reduce health inequities within and between countries and to develop and evaluate effective health policies and programs that lead to population-based health improvements and the promotion of health equity (IPPH 2009).

The second major development that has greatly influenced the scope and mandate of public health is related to the 2003 Severe Acute Respiratory Syndrome (SARS) pandemic. The first Canadian outbreak of SARS was linked to a female returning from a vacation in Hong Kong in May, 2003 (Health Canada 2008; Naylor 2003, Varia et al. 2003). As of September 5, 2003, there were 438 cases of SARS reported in Canada and eighty-five percent of these cases were in Ontario and the Greater Toronto Area (GTA) (Health Canada 2008; Varia et al. 2003). As a consequence of the SARS pandemic, forty-four individuals died, over 400 became seriously ill, and approximately 25,000 individuals in the GTA were placed under quarantine, and the WHO issued travel warnings to Canada. Moreover, the economic costs associated with the SARS pandemic for Toronto alone were estimated to be $35 million per day (Rutty and Sullivan 2010).

Dr. David Naylor's (2003) inquiry into the SARS crisis in Canada lead to the report entitled *Learning from SARS: Renewal of Public Health in Canada*, which highlighted several deficiencies in our public health capacities to manage such a crisis. Moreover, Naylor's (2003) strongly recommended that the federal government establish an independent agency for public health to co-ordinate and more effectively manage public health crisis such as SARS. Subsequently, the PHAC was established in September, 2004 and confirmed by Parliament in December, 2006 by the PHAC Act (PHAC 2006; Rutty and Sullivan 2010). The Act also recognized and empowered our first Chief Public Health Officer (CPHO), Dr. David Butler-Jones, to introduce legislation in the interest of public health and safety. Currently, a variety of Canadian health centres, laboratories and branches report to the CPHO including the Centre of Emergency Preparedness and Response; Infectious Disease and Emergency Response; Laboratory for Foodborne Zoonoses; Office of Public Health Safety; National Microbiology Laboratory, and the Pandemic Preparedness Secretariat (PHAC, 2006). The PHAC also shares expertise, critical health related information, and collaborates closely with various international health agencies such as the WHO, European Centre for Disease Prevention and Control, and the Centers for Disease Control and Prevention.

The SARS pandemic, amongst other crisis (e.g., 2000 Walkerton *E-coli* water crisis; 2005 H5N1 pandemic; 2008 Maple Leaf deli meat national listeria outbreak, 2010 federal ban on bisphenol A [BPA] for plastic bottles) has resulted in growing public interest in public health during the past decade. This is reflected in the growth of schools and programs in community and public health in Canada. In fact, during the 1990s there were only five programs in public health in Canada and by September 2011, fifteen universities were providing Masters of Public Health (MPH) or similar programs in community health. There has been an explosion of undergraduate programs in public health including Brock University, Ryerson, McMaster University, Queen's University, University of Western Ontario, University of Alberta, University of British Columbia, Université de Montréal, University of Saskatchewan, the University of Ontario Institute of Technology, University of Victoria, to name but a few. Many of these universities are now offering both undergraduate and graduate training opportunities in public and/or community health (Masse and Moloughney 2011). These programs are critical for developing a critical mass of public health professionals and workers in Canada to address current and emerging health issues across the lifespan, and for creating a cadre of individuals who will exert positive health ripple effects for decades to come (PHAC 2012; Rutty and Sullivan 2010).

Add to your knowledge of the history of public health in Canada by accessing the following resources.

Web-based Resource Box 2.7 History of Public Health in Canada

Learning Resource	Website
City of Toronto Archives, Infectious Idea: 125 years of PublicHealth in Toronto. City of Toronto Archives (1998–2013). This website showcases an exhibition celebrating 125 years of public health in Toronto through archival photographsand documents from 1883 to present.	http://www.toronto.ca/archives/public-An health/index.htm
Public Health Agency of Canada. (2008). The Chief Public Health Officer's Report on The State of Public Health in Canada in 2008. Canada's Public Health History Chapter 2. Ottawa, ON: Author. This websites provides the reader with a brief historical overview of the history of public health in Canada from the 1830s to the 2000s and major developments.	http://www.phac-aspc.gc.ca/cph-orsphc- respcacsp/2008/fr-rc/cphorsphc-respcacsp05b-eng…
Rutty and Sullivan (2010). An excellent resource which details the history of public health in eight chapters from Confederation in 1867 to the Epp Report in 1986.	http://www.cpha.ca/uploads/history/book/History-book-print_ALL_e.pdf

Future Directions and Challenges

Both our understanding and definitions related to the concept of health has evolved dramatically over the centuries. Currently, there is a growing recognition globally that health is not only affected by one's biology, but is influenced by a variety of SDH (Health Canada 2002; PHAC 2007; Raphael 2004, 2010; Rootman et al. 2012; Singh and Dickinson 2009). Because public health issues and threats often transcend political or international borders (e.g., bioterrorism, H1N1 Swine flu pandemic; migration of the West Nile Virus into Canada; Mad Cow Disease; air pollution), one of the major challenges we face is the need to consider health from both national and global perspectives when planning primary health care initiatives and interventions (Edwards 2001; Hodge et al. 2002; McDade and Franz 1998;Watson 2007). A recent study commissioned by the World Economic Forum estimated that cancer, diabetes, mental illness, heart disease, and respiratory illnesses could cost the global economy more than $47 trillion (US) due to lost productivity due to illness over the next twenty years (Bloom et al. 2011).

Undoubtedly, health is perceived by many to be a desirable yet dynamic process that can be positively or negatively affected by an array of internal and external factors (e.g., global economic downturns, pandemics, tornado's, floods, contaminated water or food supplies) (Hodge et al. 2002; Edwards 2001; D'Arcy 1986). In order to practice safely and effectively, public health care professionals and workers must be knowledgeable and vigilant regarding actual or potential threats to the health and well-being of our residents. Instead of having health care professionals such as physicians and registered nurses responsible for identifying public health problems of concern, individuals are now being encouraged to empower themselves and to define health issues they perceive as relevant in Canadian society (Butler-Jones 2012; PHAC 2007). Public health in Canada requires commitments to the valued ideals and beliefs in our society related to equity, social justice, and sustainable development, recognition of the importance of the health of entire communities as well as the individual, and respect for diversity, self-determination, empowerment, and community participation (PHAC 2007; Rootman et al. 2012).

The second major challenge is to develop national standards of health that clearly define and regulate primary health efforts that embrace health promotion and the five levels of prevention (British Columbia Ministry of Health 2013; National Public Health Partnership 2006; Porta 2008; Public Action Support Team 2011). For example, although Section 3 of the Canada Health Act (CHA) supports the concept of health promotion, which includes protective, promotive, and preventative services, the specific methods or strategies for delivering public health promotion services on a national basis are not described in the Act (Government of Canada 1984). Unfortunately, the CHA was devised to limit its focus on medically necessary physician and dental-surgical publicly insured acute health care services that are primarily hospital-based as opposed to those which embrace the primary health care model that encompasses health promotion and holistic definitions of health (Bartfay 2010a; Bartfay and Bartfay 2015). In addition, it is also regrettable that the components of health promotion are not required in order for the ten provinces and three territories to meet their obligations surrounding the five founding criteria's of the CHA to qualify for health transfer payments from the federal government (Government of Canada 1984). The reader is referred to Chapter 3 for a detailed discussion of the CHA and how public health care services are financed in Canada. The extent towards which the various provinces and territories in Canada provide public health promotion services to their residents varies considerably in quality and quantity across Canada (Romanow 2002; Sullivan and Baranek 2002). Hence, there is a need to create new legislations and standards of health care to replace these outdated and costly medical models of health with more cost efficient and effective holistic primary health models of care (Adams et al. 2008; Frank, Di Ruggiero, and Moloughney 2003; National Expert Commission Canadian Nurses Association 2012; Soroka and Mahon 2012; Starfield 2011).

The third major challenge is to identify health priorities in Canada (Bartfay and Bartfay 2015). Although communicable (infectious) diseases such smallpox, TB, measles, and polio were the leading causes of mortality during the nineteenth and twentieth centuries, they have been replaced by complex non-communicable chronic diseases and disabilities (Rutty and Sullivan 2010). In fact, non-communicable disease are responsible for eighty-nine percent of all deaths in Canada, and chronic illness and disabilities are major drivers of healthcare costs and lost productivity for our nation (National Expert Committee Canadian Nurses Association 2012; WHO 2011). Moreover, more than forty percent of Canadian adults report having at least one of the following seven common health conditions: Arthritis; cancer; emphysema, chronic obstructive pulmonary disease (COPD); diabetes; heart disease; hypertension, or a mood disorder (Canadian Academy of Health Sciences 2010). Many of these conditions are amenable to healthy public policies, preventive care, and treatments that focus on monitoring and maintenance of health from a holistic perspective.

Total health care spending continues to rise in Canada, due in part to a lack of coordinated national and provincial/territorial public health promotion efforts and strategies, which seek to promote and support the need for active and healthy lifestyles to help curb the growing incidence of various chronic non-communicable diseases (e.g., type 2 diabetes, heart disease, stroke). For example, a startling ninety percent of Canadians are aware that cardiovascular disease is preventable, but the vast majority do not appear to be aware of the associated lifestyle risk factors (e.g., diet high in saturated and transfats, excessive dietary salt intake, inactivity, smoking) (PHAC 2008b; MacDonald et al. 1992). Moreover, between 1985 and 2001, the number of obese Canadians almost tripled from 5.6% to 14.9% (Hales and Lauzon 2007), and physical inactivity has been shown to cost our publicly insured health care systems in excess of $2.1 billion annually (Katzmarzyk et al. 2000). The PHAC (2015) notes that currently, forty-eight percent of Canadian adults report being inactive, meaning that that their level of physical activity were not sufficient to meet the threshold of at least moderate activity. Moreover, evidence shows that as much as half of the decline in the ability to perform usual activities of daily living between the ages of 30 and 70 is the result of an inactive lifestyle (PHAC 2015).

This trend related to inactivity and the growing number of Canadians who are overweight or obese is continuing. In fact, more than half of adult Canadians are inactive and only nine percent of children and youth (aged 5–19 years) meet the recommendations in *Canada's Physical Activity Guide for Children and Youth* (Canadian Fitness and Lifestyle Research Institute 2007, 2005; Canadian Society for Exercise Physiology 2012). Regular physical activity actually helps to prevent chronic diseases and premature death. Moreover, individuals who are physically active tend to be significantly healthier in comparison to their sedentary counterparts.

The fourth major challenge is to have politicians, policy makers and public health care professionals and workers embrace holistic definitions of health based on the SDH. This also encompasses a willingness to reform our health care systems and embrace holistic primary health care models of delivery (Browne et al. 2012; Mikkonen and Raphael 2010; Muntaner et al. 2012). Simply stated, our current outdated medical model of health is costly, not sustainable from a tax-base perspective, and is not able to meet the diverse health challenges facing Canadians in the new millennium (Adams et al. 2008; Soroka and Mahon 2012; Starfield 2011).

For example, in 2015, our national health care expenditure was in excess of $219.1 billion, compared with only $12.2 billion in 1975 (CIHI 2010a; CIHI 2015a, 2015b). This 2015 figure translates into $6,106 per person or 10.9% of Canada's entire GDP (CIHI 2015a, 2015b). Bunker, Frazier and Mosteller (1994) have estimated that during the past century, a total of only five of the thirty years (16.7%) related to one's life expectancies can be credited to medical practice alone.

In Canada, this is despite the fact that ninety-five percent of health care expenditures are spent on physician- and/or hospital-driven acute care health services, whereas less than five percent are spent on public health promotion efforts (Brown et al. 1992; CIHI 2015a; Frank, Di Ruggiero, and Moloughney 2003). In fact, acute care hospital-based health care services continue to account for the largest component accounting for 29.5% of health care expenditures in 2015 (CIH 2015ab). Payments to physicians represent Canada's third-largest share of health care expenditures, accounting for approximately 15.5% of health care expenditures in 2015. CIHI (2015a, 2015b) reports that total payments to physicians increased almost six percent in 2014, reaching a record total of $24.1 billion. Total health expenditures reached $228.1 billion (or 11.1 % of GDP) in 2016, represented a 2.7% in comparison to 2015 figures (CIHI 2016). Total health care spending per Canadian was approximately $6,299. It is notably that spending for acute care hospital services accounted for the largest share of total health spending at 37.7%, or $86 billion (CIHI 2016).

We argue that these elevated costs are associated, at least in part, with a decreased emphasis on home and community-based health care services and primary health promotion initiatives and programs nationally (Bartfay and Bartfay 2015). There is also a growing need to encourage research to validate the cost savings and effectiveness of primary health care models based on the SDH (Browne et al. 2012; Butler-Jones 2012; Muntaner et al. 2012).

Group Review Exercise "MS Wars"

About this investigative documentary
Multiple sclerosis (MS) is a debilitating disease, and there is currently no known cure in Canada or abroad. The effects of MS are cruel and include fatigue, progressive loss of muscle control, increasing debility and decreasing quality of life. *MS Wars* is a CBC documentary that explores the science, scientific controversies, and human drama around a novel experimental treatment called *Liberation Therapy* (AKA chronic cerebrospinal venous insufficiency or CCSVI). This treatment was first detailed and pioneered by the scientist Dr. Paolo Zamboni in Northern Italy in 2009. A small research paper by Dr. Zamboni was released online

before it was published in the traditional journal print-format. Immediately, this new experimental intervention for MS was circulating globally via various social media circles, and created a sudden explosion of interest and attention by MS clients, their loved ones looking after them, and health care professionals and researchers. This documentary explores the concept of health, personal values and meanings surrounding this concept, and how it is believed to be achieved or obtained by clients suffering from this chronic disease with currently no known cure.

The scientific community has developed research protocols (e.g., RCTs), processes and socio-political systems regarding how health research should be conducted and how they provide *evidence-informed care* in their clinical practices. These protocols, processes, and systems have been entrenched in the way public health care researchers and providers go about doing their business for centuries. But, this time, the traditional health research system is being challenged by two factors: hope, and the power of the internet and social media as a means of communicating health-related information and treatments. This documentary explores how the internet has spurred a global social network movement that is changing and challenging traditional physician/client relationships and the repercussions for research and public health in Canada. A few Canadian clinics began to look into this noted clinical intervention, but the Canadian public health establishment (aka Medicare in the provinces and territories) were reluctant to proceed with an unproven treatment that had not followed the proper traditional and socially embedded research protocols and required RCTs required by the public health scientific community. With an increasing number of clients electing to get the treatment in private clinics or abroad, video testimonies and other forms of anecdotal evidence soon began to appear on the internet showing miraculous improvements to the health related quality of lives of these clients. Many began travelling out of the country for the procedure paying for their own treatment—often without telling their physicians.

Instructions

This assignment may be done alone, in pairs or in groups of up to five people (note: if you are doing this assignment in pairs or groups, please submit only one hard or electronic copy to the instructor).

- The assignment should be type-written and not more than four to six pages maximum in length (double-spaced please).
- View the documentary entitled *MS Wars: Hope, Science, and the Internet* which aired on Thursday August 30, 2012 on CBC-TV and on Thursday September 6 on CBC News Network.
- See link: http://www.cbc.ca/natureofthings/episode/ms-wars-hope-science-and-the-internet.html or http://www.cbc.ca/player/Shows/Shows/The+Nature+of+Things/2011-12/ID/2196927676/
- View this documentary and take detailed notes during the presentation.

  i. Provide a brief overview of the salient points in this documentary.
  ii. Comment on who is ultimately responsible for their own health? The individual afflicted with the disease or disorder or health care professionals?
  iii. Can an individual with a chronic debilitative disease such as MS ever be healthy? Discuss why or why not.
  iv. Highlight some of the negative and positive ripple effects related to this controversial experimental treatment for MS as part of the client's quest to be healthy based on their unique values and meanings related to this concept.
  v. Briefly discuss how social media, public opinion and the internet can affect the mandate of provincial/territorial public health officials or governments via political lobbying and pressure.

Summary

- The concept of health and the evolution of various definitions of this state of existence over time, is interwoven with the history of agricultural societies and the development of various civilizations; the growth of religious practices and beliefs; shamanism and other healing practices; pharmacy; medicine, nursing, and developments in public health.
- Health is a ubiquitous and dynamic term with diverse interpretations and meanings to individuals in different cultures across the lifespan.
- Health is not a single state or goal, but a process that involves various interconnected and interdependent factors and dynamic states of existence.
- The worship of nature became a logical vehicle upon which primitive agricultural societies based their healing practices, mythologies, and religious practices because it directly influenced their prosperity and survival.
- Hippocrates (460–370 BCE) is regarded as the father of modern empirical or rationale medicine and was the first to dismiss the belief that disease or states of ill health were caused by angry spirits, demons, or deities, but resulted as a consequence of a break in the laws of nature.
- The Romans believed that altered states of health and disease were caused by natural sources, especially bad water supplies and raw sewage. Hence, they became experts at draining swamps and marshes associated with malaria for example, and built extensive aqueducts, public toilets, and proper cemeteries for their deceased.
- Romans believed that everyone in their Empire was entitled to good health, and were the first civilization to introduce a programme of public health for all their citizens regardless of their age, occupation, or wealth.
- During the Byzantine Empire (later Roman period—fourth century CE), significantly more male deacons and monks practiced nursing in community settings and charitable institutions, in comparison to female deaconesses and nuns.
- During the Middle Ages, various military nursing orders of knights (e.g., Teutonic Knights, Knights of St. John, Knights Hospitallers) provided care to the wounded on the battlefields during the Crusades abroad, protected those who could not defend themselves, and were the first documented public health nurses to provide care to individuals afflicted with leprosy in the world.
- The association between physicians and hospitals as places of practice, first occurred during the middle ages where they were called upon to make in-house diagnosis or to treat clients.
- During the sixteenth and seventeenth centuries, we observed the beginning of scientific investigations to explain the mechanistic functioning of the human body.
- Health from this perspective has evolved into the so-called laboratory-based mechanistic "medical model" which attributes alterations to health as malfunctioning biological components resulting from disease processes.
- Louis Pasteur (1822–1895) brought about a revolution in medicine when he linked tiny microorganisms with the development of disease and confirmed the unicausal germ-theory of disease origin.
- The modern era of health care has been dominated by the laboratory-based mechanistic medical model of health, with the emphasis on diagnosis, treatment and cure of disease as opposed to health promotion and prevention.
- During the turn of the last century, hospitals evolved into primary centres for accessing health care services due to the growing use and application of diagnostic medical technologies (e.g., x-rays) that physicians could not afford in private practice settings.
- This also resulted in a growing demand and need for nurses in hospitals and a dramatic decline in the number of home and public health nurses in Canada.
- Developments in public health during the early part of the twentieth century in Canada included school-based immunization programs against smallpox and diphtheria, and the appointment of nurses by school boards to monitor the health and wellness of children.

- In 1948, the Government of Canada established the National Health Grants Program, which served as a stimulus for the development of basic public health infrastructures and programs in the provinces over the next three decades.
- These programs consisted of grants-in-aid to the provinces to help fund the education and training of physicians and nurses, TB control, mental health, cancer control, and child and maternal health programs.
- The document known as the Lalonde Report (1974) challenged the unicausal medical model of health and illness by introducing the following four critical determinants of health: Human biology; environment; lifestyle, and health care organizations.
- In 1986, Jake Epp expanded on Lalonde's Report (1974) by extending the definition of health promotion to include a wide range of socio-political and environmental determinants of health.
- The Ottawa Charter for Health Promotion (1986) outlined five broad global strategies to achieve global health promotion and challenged the unicausal medical definition of health and associated care delivery models.
- Although this definition has been criticized for being too broad in nature, for concentrating too much on a condition of health rather than a process, and for being impossible to achieve by many, it remains the most widely quoted definition of health globally that has Canadian origins.

Critical Thinking Questions

1. Construct your own unique definition of health and see how it contrasts with the definition of health provided in this chapter and the WHO's (1978) definition. What are the similarities and differences in comparison to your own definition of health?
2. As a public health care professional or worker, what questions and criteria would you employ to assess the health of specific individuals versus those of families, groups, communities, or entire populations? How do your questions and criteria vary and how would your assess the effectiveness of targeted primary health interventions, strategies, or policies?
3. Select a determinant of health that you believe is most important for positively influencing the health and well-being of residents in your community. Why did you choose this determinant and what evidence is there to suggest that it is the most important determinant per se? How would you employ this evidence to shape public health policies or practice in your community?

References

Adams, J., R. Bakalar, M. Boroch, K. Knecht, E. Mounib, and N. Stuart. *Healthcare 2015 and Care Delivery. Delivery Models Refined, Competencies Defined.* Somers: IBM Institute for Business Value, 2008. Accessed August 15, 2013. http://www-03.ibm.com/industries/ca/en/healthcare/files/hc2015_full_report_ver2.pdf.

Aikman, L. *Nature's Healing Arts: From Folk Medicine to Modern Drugs.* Washington, DC: National Geographic Society, 1977.

Armelagos, G. K., and J. R. Dewey. "Evolutionary Response to Human Infectious. Disease." In *Health and the Human Condition*, edited by M. H. Logan and E. E. Hunt, 101–107. North Scituate: Duxbury Press, 1978.

Armstrong, P., and H. Armstrong. *Wasting Away: The undermining of Canadian Health Care.* 2nd ed.. Don Mills, ON: Oxford University Press, 2003.

Armstrong, P., H. Armstrong, and D. Coburn. *Unhealthy Times: Political Economy Perspectives on Health and Care.* Don Mills: Oxford University Press, 2001.

Aschengrau A., and G. R. Seage III. *Essentials of Epidemiology in Public Health.* Toronto: Jones and Bartlett Publishers, 2003.

Barrett, P. *Science and Theology Since Copernicus: The Search for Understanding.* New York: Continuum International Publishing Group, 2004.

Bartfay, W. J. "A Masculinist" Historical Perspective of Nursing." *Canadian Nurse 92*, no. 2 (1996): 17–19.

Bartfay, W. J. "Men in Nursing in Canada: Past, Present and Future Perspectives." In *Men in Nursing History, Challenges, and Opportunities*, edited by C. E. O'Lynn and R. E. Tranbarger, 205–18. New York: Springer Publishing Company, 2007.

Bartfay, W. J. "Perspectives on Health and its Promotion and Preservation." In *Community Health Nursing: Caring in Action,* edited by J. E. Hitchcock, P. E. Schubert, S. A. Thomas, and W. J. Bartfay, 89–116. Toronto: Nelson Education, 2010a.

Bartfay, W. J. "Introduction to Community Health Nursing in Canada." In *Community Health Nursing: Caring in Action,* edited by J. E. Hitchcock, P. E. Schubert, S. A. Thomas, and W. J. Bartfay, 1–22. Toronto: Nelson Education, 2010b.

Bartfay, W. J. "Canada's Health Care System: History and Current Challenges." In *Community Health Nursing: Caring in Action,* edited by J. E. Hitchcock, P. E. Schubert, S. A. Thomas, and W. J. Bartfay, 23–41. Toronto: Nelson Education, 2010c.

Bartfay, W. J., and E. Bartfay. *Public Health in Canada.* Boston: Pearson Learning Solutions, 2015.

Baum, F. "The Commission on the Social Determinants of Health: Reinventing Health Promotion for the Twenty-first Century?" *Critical Public Health 18*, no. 4 (2008): 457–66.

Baumgart, A. J., and Wheeler, M. M. "The Nursing Workforce in Canada." In *Canadian Nurses Face the Future*, edited by A. J. Baumgart and J. Larsen, 45–69. Scarborough: Mosby-Year Book, 1992.

Bay Windows. *ILGA: 76 Countries Ban Gay Sex, 7 have Death Penalty,* 2010. Accessed August 16, 2013. http://deathpenaltynews.blogspot.ca/2010/06/ilga-76-countries-ban-gay-sex-7-have.html.

Bedford, W. K. R., and Holbeche, R. *The Order of the Hospital of St. John of Jerusalem.* London: Robinson and Company, 1902.

Berdoe, E. *The Origin and Growth of the Healing Art.* London: Swan and Company, 1893.

Bhishagratna, K. K. L. *The Sushrutra Samhita.* Translated by J. N. Bose. Calcutta, 1907.

Bloom, D., E. Cafiero, E. Jane-Llopis, S. Abraham-Gessel, L. Bloom, S. Fathima, A. Feigl, T. Gaziano, M. Mowafi, A. Pandya, K. Prettner, L. Rosenberg, B. Seligman, A. Z. Stein, and C. Weinstein. *The Global Economic Burden of Noncommunicable Diseases.* Geneva: World Economic Forum, 2011. Accessed August 16, 2013. http://www.weforum.org/reports/global-economic-burden-non-communicable-diseases.

Breasted, J. H. *The Edwin Smith Surgical Papyrus.* Boston: University of Chicago Press, 1930.

Brike, L., and J. Silvertown. *More than the Parts: Biology and Politics.* London: Pluto Press, 1984.

British Columbia Centre for Disease Control. *Raw Milk.* Vancouver: Author, 2013. Accessed August 30, 2013. http://www.bccdc.ca/foodhealth/dairy/Raw+Milk.htm.

British Columbia Ministry of Health. *Core Public Health Functions. Preventive Interventions.* Vancouver: B.C. Government, 2013. Accessed September 21, 2013. http:www.health.gov.bc.ca/public-health/strategies/preventive-interventions/

Brown, R., J. Corea, B. Luce, A. Elixhauser, and S. Sheingold. "Effectiveness in Disease and Injury Prevention–Estimated National Spending on Prevention—United States, 1988." *Morbidity and Mortality Weekly* 41, no. 29 (1992): 529–31.

Browne, G., S. Birch, and L. Thabane. *Better Care: An Analysis of Nursing and Health Care System Outcomes*. Ottawa: Canadian Health Services Research Foundation and Canadian Nurses Association, 2012.

Bryan, P. W. *The Papyrus Ebers*. London: Geoffrey Bles, 1930.

Bullough, V. L. "Men in Nursing." *Journal of Professional Nursing* 10, no. 5 (1994): 267.

Bullough, V. L., and B. Bullough. "Medieval Nursing." *Nursing History Review* 10, no. 1 (1993): 89–104.

Bunker, J. P., S. H. Frazier, and F. Mosteller. "Improving Health: Measuring Effects of Medical Care." *Millbank Quarterly* 72 (1994): 225–258.

Butler-Jones, D. *The Chief Public Health Officer's Report on the State of Public Health in Canada*. Ottawa: Her Majesty the Queen in Right of Canada, 2012.

Campbell, A. *The SARS Commission-Spring of Fear*. Final Report. Ontario Ministry of Health and Long-Term Care, 2006. Accessed April 17, 2008. http://www.health.gov.on.ca/english/public/pub/ministry.

Canadian Academy of Health Sciences. *Transforming Care for Canadians with Chronic Health Conditions*. Ottawa: Author, 2010. Accessed August 16, 2013. http://www.dfcm.utoronto.ca/Assets/DFCM+Digitial+Assets/CAHS+Transforming+Care+for+Canadians+with+Chronic+Health+Conditions.pdf.

Canadian Fitness and Lifestyle Research Institute. *Kids CAN PLAY!* Ottawa: Author, 2007. Accessed June 29, 2010. http://www.cflri.ca/eng/programs/canplay/documents/kidsCANPLAY_b1.pdf.

Canadian Fitness and Lifestyle Research Institute. *2005 Physical Activity and Sport: Encouraging Children to be Active*, 2005. Accessed June 29, 2010. http://www.cflri.ca/eng/statistics/surveys/documents/PAM2005.pdf.

Canadian Institute for Health Information. *Workforce Trends of Registered Nurses in Canada*: Ottawa: Author, 2006. Accessed June 23, 2010. http://www.cihi.ca.

Canadian Institute for Health Information. *Health Care in Canada, 2006*. Ottawa: Canadian Institute for Health Information, 2007.

Canadian Institute for Health Information. *National Health Expenditure Trends 1975–2009*. Ottawa: Author, 2010a.

Canadian Institute for Health Information. *2010 Health Indicators Report*. Ottawa: Author, 2010b.

Canadian Institute for Health Information. *Canada's Health Care Spending Growth Slows. Provincial and Territorial Government Health Expenditures Expected to grow 3.1%, Lowest Since 1997*. Ottawa: Canadian Institute for Health Information, 2013. Accessed June 13, 2013. http://www.cihi.ca/cihi-ext-portal/internet/en/document/spending+and+health+workforce/spending/release_30oct12.

Canadian Institute for Health Information. *National Health Expenditure Trends, 1975 to 2014 Report*. Ottawa: Canadian Institute for Health Information, 2014. Accessed November 10, 2015. https://secure.cihi.ca/estore/productSeries.htm?pc=PCC52.

Canadian Institute for Health Information. *National Health Expenditure Trends, 1975 to 2015*. Ottawa: Canadian Institute for Health Information, 2015a. Accessed November 10, 2015. https://www.cihi.ca/en/spending-and-health-workforce/spending/canadas-slow-health-spending-growth-continues.

Canadian Institute for Health Information. (CIHI 2016). *National health expenditures: How Much Does Canada Spend on Health Care?* Ottawa, Ontario: CIHI. Retrieved April 14, 2017, http://www.cihi.ca/en/nhex2016-topic1.

Canadian Institute for Health Information. *More doctors, Higher Spending: Data Sheds Light on Trends in the Physician Workforce*. Ottawa: Canadian Institute for Health Information, 2015b.

Canadian Nurses Association. *Putting "health" Back into Health Care. Submission to the Health Services Review'79*. Ottawa: Author, 1980. Accessed June 22, 2010. http://206.191.29.104/_frames/policies/policiesmainframe.htm.

Canadian Nurses Association. *On Your Own: The Nurse Entrepreneur*. Ottawa: Author, 1996. Accessed June 23, 2010. http://www.cannurses.ca/pages/issuestrends/nrgnow/OnYourOwnEntrepreneur_September1996.pdf.

Canadian Public Health Association, Welfare Canada, and World Health Organization. *Ottawa Charter for Health Promotion. Charter Adopted at the Move Towards a New Public Health International Conference on Health Promotion, 17–21 November, 1986*. Ottawa: Health and Welfare Canada, 2006. Accessed June 26, 2010. http://www.who.int/hpr/NPH/docs/ottawa_charter_hp.pdf.

Canadian Red Cross Society. *The Role of One Voluntary Organization in Canada's Health Services: A Brief Presented to the Royal Commission on Health Services on Behalf of the Central Council of the Canadian Red Cross Society*. Toronto: Author, 1962.

Canadian Society for Exercise Physiology. *Canadian Physical Activity Guidelines2012: Background Information*. Ottawa: Author, 2012. Accessed September 13, 2013. http://www.csep.ca/english/view.asp?x=587.

Capra, F. *The Turning Point: Science, Society, and the Rising Culture*. New York: Simon and Schuster, 1982.

Cek, C. L. "The Father of Medicine, Avicenna, in our Science and Culture: Abu Ali Ing Sina (980–1037)." *Becka Journal* 119, no.1 (1980): 17–23.

Centers for Disease Control and Prevention. *Raw Milk Qquestions and Answers*. Atlanta: Author, 2006. Accessed June 08, 2010. http://www.cdc.gov/ncid/vcjd/index/html.

Centers for Disease Control and Prevention. *BSE (bovine spongiform Encephalopathy, or MadCow Disease*. Atlanta: Author, 2007a. Accessed June 08, 2010. http://www.cdc.gov/ncidod/dvrd.bse.

Centers for Disease Control and Prevention. *vCJD (variant Creutzfeld Jakob disease)*. Atlanta: Author, 2007b. Accessed June 08, 2010. http://www.cdc.gov/ncid/vcjd/index/html.

Christman, L. P. Men in Nursing. In *Annual Review of Nursing Research,* edited by J. L. Fitzpatrick, R. L. Taunton, and J. Q. Benolie, 193–205. New York: Springer Publishing Company, 1988.

Colbert, A. M., L. K. Sekula, R. Zoucha, and S. M. Cohen. "Health Care Needs of Women Immediately Post-incarceration: A Mixed Methods Study." *Public Health Nursing* 30, no. 5 (2003): 409–19. doi:10.1111/phn.12034.

Cockburn, T. A. *Infectious Diseases: Their Evolution and Eradication*. Springfield: Charles C. Thomas, 1967.

Community Health Nurses Association of Canada. *Canadian Community Health Nursing Standards of Practice*, 2003. Accessed June 27, 2010. http://www.communityhealth-nursescanada.org.

Conrad, P., and J. W. Schneider. *Deviance and Medicalization: From badness to Sickness*. Columbus: Merrill, 1985.

D'Arcy, C. "Unemployment and Health: Data and Implications." *Canadian Journal of Public Health* 77, no.1 (1986): 124–31.

Davis, M. T., and W. J. Bartfay. Men in Nursing: An Untapped Resource. *Canadian Nurse* 97, no.5 (2001): 14–18.

Davis, G. P. Jr., and E. Park. *The Heart: The Living Pump*. Toronto: Torstar Books, 1984.

Dear, P. *Revolutionizing the Sciences: European Knowledge and its Ambitions, 1500–1700*. Princeton: Princeton University Press, 2001.

Dock, L. L., and I. Stewart-Maitland. *A short History of Nursing: From the Earliest Times to the Present day*. 3rd ed. New York: G.P. Putnam's Sons, 1932.

Donahue, P. *Nursing: The finest Art*. Toronto: Mosby Company, 1996.

Edelman, C. L., and C. L. Mandle. *Health Promotion Throughout the Lifespan*. Toronto: Mosby, 1994.

Edwards, P. "Climate Change: Air Pollution and your Health." *Canadian Journal of Public Health* 92, no. 3 (2001): I1–I12.

Edwards, A. B. *Pharaohs, Fellahs, and Explorers*. New York: Harper and Brothers, 1892.

Epp, J. *Achieving Health for All: A Framework for Health Promotion*. Ottawa: Health and Welfare Canada, 1986.

Falk-Rafael, A., and Coffey, S. "Financing, Policy, and Politics of Health Care Delivery." In *Community Health Nursing: A Canadian Perspective*, edited by L. Lesseberg Stamler and L. Yiu, 17–34. Toronto: Pearson Prentice Hall, 2005.

Ferrie, J. E. *Work, Stress and Health: The Whitehall II Study*. London: Public and Commercial Services Union on Behalf of the Council of Civil Service Unions/Cabinet Office, 2004. Accessed June 26, 2010. http://www.ucl.ac.uk/whitehallII/findings/Whitehallbooklet.pdf.

Frank, C. M. *The Historical Development of Nursing*. Philadelphia: Saunders Company, 1953.

Frank, J., E. di Ruggiero, and B. Moloughney. *The Future of Public Health in Canada: Developing a Public Health System for the 21st Century*. Ottawa: Canadian Institute of Health Research—Institute of Population and Public Health, 2003.

Gibbon, J. M. *The Victorian Order of Nurses for Canada: 50th Anniversary, 1897–1947*. Montréal: Southam Press, 1947.

Gibbon, J. M., and M. S. Mathewson. *Three Centuries of Canadian Nursing*. Toronto: Macmillan, 1947.

Goodnow, M. *Nursing History*. Philadelphia: W.B. Saunders Company, 1942.

Government of Canada. *A Brief History of the Canada Health and Social Transfer (CHST)*. Ottawa: Department of Finance, 2002. http://www.fin.gc.ca/FEDPROV/hise.html.

Government of Canada. *House of Commons: An Act Related to Cash contributions by Canada in Respect of Insured Health Services Provided Under Provincial Health Care Insurance Plans and Amounts Payable by Canada in Respect to Extended Health Care Services and to Amend and Repeat Certain Acts in Consequence thereof (The Canada Health Act)*. Ottawa: Author, 2004.

Government of Ontario. *Health Protection and Promotion Act. R.S. O. 1990, Chapter H.7* (last amended 2011). Toronto: Author, 2011. Accessed August 30, 2013. http://www.e-laws.gov.on.ca/html/statutes/english/elaws_statutes_90h07_e.htm.

Green, L. W., and J. M. Ottoson. *Community Health.* 7th ed. Toronto: Mosby, 1994.

Green, L. W., and M. J. Ottoson. *Community Health and Population Health.* Toronto: McGraw-Hill, 1999.

Grieve, M. *A Modern Herbal: The Medicinal, Culinary, Cosmetic and Economic Properties, Cultivation and Folk-lore of Herbs, Grasses, Fungi, Shrubs and Trees with all Their Modern Scientific Uses.* Vol. 1. Toronto: Jonathan Cape Ltd, 1931.

Hadzovic, S. "Pharmacy and the Great Contribution of Arab-Islamic Science to its Development." *Medical Achieves* 51, no. 1–2 (1997): 47–50.

Hales, D., and L. Lauzon. An Invitation to Health. 1st ed. Toronto: McGraw-Hill, 2007. Hall, E. M, (1980). *Canada's national-provincial health programs in the 1980s: A commitment for renewal.* Ottawa: Department of National Health and Welfare.

Hanlon, J. J., and G. E. Pickett. *Public Health Administration and Practice.* 8th ed. St. Louis: Times Mirror/Mosby, 1984.

Harper, D. *Online Etymology Dictionary,* 2013. Accessed September 16, 2013. http://etymonline.com/?term=health.

Health Canada. *Advisory Committee on Population Health Strategies for Population Health: Investing in the Health of Canadians.* Ottawa: Author, 1994.

Health Canada. *Towards a Healthy Future: Second Report on the Health of Canadians.* Ottawa: Federal, Provincial and Territorial Advisory Committee on Population Health, 1999.

Health Canada. *Economic Burden of Illness in Canada, 1998.* Ottawa: Author, 2000a.

Health Canada. *Population Health, 2002.* Ottawa: Author, 2000b. Accessed June 26, 2010. http://www.phac-aspc.gc.ca/ph-sp/phdd/determinants/index.html#determinants.

Health Canada. *SARS.* Ottawa: Author, 2008. Accessed September 13, 2013. http://www.hc-sc.gc.ca/hc-ps/dc-ma/sars-sras-eng.php.

Haque, A. "Psychology from Islamic Perspective: Contributions of Early Muslim Scholars and Challenges to Contemporary Muslim Psychologists." *Journal of Religion and Health* 43, no. 4 (2004): 357–77.

Hodge, R., R. Anthony, and J. M. J. Longo. "International Monitoring for Environmental Health Surveillance." *Canadian Journal of Public Health* 93, no. 1 (2002): S16–S23.

Holmes, D., A. Perron, and G. Michaud. "Nursing in Corrections: Lessons from France." *Journal of Forensic Nursing* 3, no. 3–4 (2007), 126–51.

Horstmanshoff, H. F. J., M. Stol, and C. Tilburg. *Magic and Rationality in Ancient Near Eastern and Graeco-Roman medicine.* London: Brill Publishers, 2004.

Howard, J. *An Account of the Principal Lazarettos in Europe.* London: Johnson, Dilly and Dadel, 1791.

Hudson, E. H. "Treponematosis and Man's Social Evolution. *American Anthropologist* 67 (1965): 885–901.

Hume, E. E. *Medical Works of the Knight Hospitallers of St. John of Jerusalem.* Baltimore: John Hopkins, 1940.

Hume, E. E. *Max von Pettenkofer.* New York: Hoeber, 1927.

Illich, I. *Medical Nemesis: The Expropriation of Health.* Toronto: McClelland and Stewart, 1975.

Institute of Population and Public Health (IPPH). *Health Equity Matters. IPPH strategic plan 2009–2014.* Ottawa: Canadian Institute of Health Research, 2009. Accessed September 13, 2013. http://www.cihr-irsc.gc.ca/e/40524.html.

Jackson, M. *The Oxford Handbook of the History of Medicine.* Oxford: Oxford University Press, 2011.

Kalisch, P. A., and J. B. Kalisch. *The Advance of American Nursing.* 2nd ed. Boston: Little, Brown and Company, 1986.

Katzmarzyk, P. T., N. Gledhill, and R. J. Shephard. The Economic Burden of Physical Inactivity in Canada. *Canadian Medical Association Journal* 163, no. 11 (2000): 1435–40.

Keating, D. P., and C. Hertzman. ed. *Developmental Health and the Wealth of Nations: Social, Biological, and Educational Dynamics.* New York: Guilford Press, 1999.

Kelly, L. *Dimensions of Professional Nursing.* 3rd ed. New York: MacMillan Publishing Company, 1975.

Kerr, M., D. Frost, and D. Bignell. *Don't We Count as people? Saskatchewan Social Welfare Policy and Women's Health.* Saskatchewan: Women's Health Centre of Excellence, 2004.

Klein-Frank, F. *Al-Kinda.* In *History of Islamic Philosophy,* edited by O. Leaman and H. Nasr, 172–85. London: Routledge, 2001.

Kordunsky, A. "Russia not Only Country With Anti-Gay Laws." *National Geographic Daily News,* 2013. Accessed August 15, 2013. http://news.nationalgeographic.com/news/2013/08/130814-russia-anti-gay-propaganda-law-world-olympics-africa-gay-rights/.

Lalonde, M. *A New Perspective on the Health of Canadians.* Ottawa: Health and Welfare Canada, 1974.

Loades, D. *Chronicles of the Tudor Kings.* Wayne: CLB International, 1990.

Lyons, A. S., and R. J. Petrucelli. *Medicine: An Illustrated History.* New York. Harry N. Abrams, Inc, 1978.

MacDonald, S., M. P. Joffres, S. J. Stachenko, L. Horlick, and G. Fodor. Multiple Cardiovascular Risk Factors in Canadian Adults. *Canadian Medical Association Journal* 11 (1992): 2021–29.

Marmot, M., G. Rose, M. J. Shipley, and P. J. Hamilton. "Employment Grade and Coronary Heart Disease in British Civil Servants." *Journal of Epidemiology and Community Health* 32 (1978): 244–49.

Masse, R., and B. Moloughney. "New Era for Schools and Programs of Public Health in Canada." *Public Health Reviews* 33, no. 1 (2011): 277–88.

McCommon, B. "Antipsychiatry and the Gay Rights Movement." *Psychiatric Services* 57 (2006): 1809–15. doi:10.1176/appi/ps.57.12.1809.

McDade, J., and D. Franz. "Bioterrorism as a Public Health Threat." *Emerging Infectious Diseases* 4, no. 3 (1998). Accessed June 27, 2010. http://www.cdc.gov.ncidod/eid/vol4no3/medade.htm.

McKeown, T. *The Role of Medicine: Dream, Mirage or Nemesis?* London: Nuffield Provincial Hospital, 1976.

McKeown, T. Determinants of Health. In *The nation's Health,* edited by P. Lee, N. Brown, and I. Red, 49–57. San Francisco: Boyd and Fraser, 1981.

Mikkonen, J., and D. Raphael. *Social Determinants of Health: The Canadian Facts.* Toronto: York University School of Health Policy and Management, 2010. Accessed August 15, 2013. http://www.thecanadianfacts.org/The_Canadian_Facts.pdf.

Muntaner, C., E. Ng, and H. Chung. *Better Health: An Analysis of Public Policy and Programming Focusing on the Determinants of Health and Health Outcomes that are Effective in Achieving the Healthiest Populations.* Ottawa: Canadian Health Services Research Foundation and Canadian Nurses Association, 2012.

Murray, N. D., B. J. Low, C. Hollis, A. Cross, and S. Davis. "Coordinated School Health Programs and Academic Achievement: A Systematic Review of the Literature." *Journal of School Health* 77, no. 9 (2007): 589–99.

Naidoo, J., and Wills, J. *Health Promotion: Foundations for Practice.* 2nd ed. Toronto: Bailliere Tindall/ Elsevier Limited, 2000.

National Expert Commission Canadian Nurses Association. *A Nursing Call to Action: The health of our Nation, the Future of our Health system.* Ottawa: Canadian Nurses Association, 2012. Accessed June 10, 2013. http://www.can-aiic.ca/expertcommission/.

National Forum of Health. *Canada Health Action: Building on the Legacy.* Final Report (Volume 1). Ottawa: Minister of Public Works and Government Services, 1997.

National Public Health Partnership (NPHP). *The Language of Prevention.* Melbourne: NPHP, 2006.

Naylor, D. *Learning from SARS: Renewal of Public Health in Canada: A Report of the National Advisory Committee on SARS and Public Health.* Ottawa: Her Majesty the Queen in Right of Canada, 2003.

Neuberger, M. *History of Medicine.* London: Oxford University Press, 1910.

Nunn, J. F. *Ancient Egyptian Medicine.* Norman: University of Oklahoma Press, 2002.

Nutting, M. A., and L. L. Dock. *A history of Nursing: The Evolution of Nursing Systems from Earliest Times to the Foundation of the First English and American Training schools for Nurses.* 4 vols. New York: Putnam's Sons, 1937.

O'Lynn, C. History of Men in Nursing: A Review. In *Men in Nursing: History, Challenges and Opportunities,* edited by C. E. O'lynn and R. Tranbarger, 5–42. New York: Springer Publishing Company, 2007.

ParticipACTION. *The ParticipACTION Archive Project.* Ottawa: Government of Canada, 1969. Accessed June 28, 2010. http://www.usask.ca:80/archieves/participaction/english/impact/index.html.

Pelley, T. Nursing: Its History, Trends, Philosophy, Ethics and Ethos. Philadelphia: W.B. Saunders, 1964.

Pierce, R. V. *The Peoples Common Sense Medical Adviser in Plain English; or Medicine Simplified.* 13th ed. Buffalo: Published at the World's Dispensary Printing Office and Binderly, 1886.

Polgar, S. Evolution and the Ills of Mankind. In *Horizons of Anthropology*, edited by S. Tax, 200–211. Chicago: Aldine, 1964.

Porta, M. *A Dictionary of Epidemiology*. 5th ed. Toronto: Oxford University Press, 2008.

Porter, R. *The Greatest Benefit to Mankind: A Medical History of Humanity from Antiquity to the Present*. New York: Harper Collins, 1997.

Porter, R. *The Cambridge Illustrated History of Medicine*. Cambridge: Cambridge University Press, 2011.

Public Health Agency of Canada (PHAC). *Ottawa Charter for Health Promotion: An International Conference on Health Promotion*. Ottawa: Government of Canada, 2001a. Accessed June 25, 2010. http://www.phac-aspc.gc.ca/ph-sp/docs/charter-chartre/pdf/charter.pdf.

Public Health Agency of Canada (PHAC). *Determinants of Health: What Makes Canadians Healthy or Unhealthy?* Ottawa: Author, 2001b. Accessed June 26, 2010. http://www.phac-aspc.gc.ca/ph-sp/determinants/index-eng.php#determinants.

Public Health Agency of Canada (PHAC). *Act to Establish Public Health Agency Outcomes into Force*. Ottawa: Author, 2006. Accessed September 13, 2013. http://www.phac-aspc-gc.ca/media/nr-rp?2006/2006_11_e.html.

Public Health Agency of Canada (PHAC) (September, 2007). *Core Competencies for Public Health in Canada: Release 1.1*. Ottawa: Author. http://www.phac-aspc.gc.ca/core_competencies or http://www.phac-aspc.gc.ca/php-psp/ccph-cesp/pdfs/cc-manual-eng090407.pdf.

Public Health Agency of Canada (PHAC). *The Chief Public Health Officer's report on the State of Public Health in Canada–2008—Chapter 2*. Ottawa: PHAC, 2008a. Accessed June 26, 2010. http://www.phac-aspc.gc.ca/publicat/2008/cphorsphc-respcacsp/cphorsphc-respcacsp)5B-2.

Public Health Agency of Canada (PHAC). *Minimizing the Risks of Cardiovascular Disease*. Ottawa: PHAC, 2008b. Accessed June 28, 2010. http://www.phac-aspc.gc.ca/cd-mc/cvd-mcv/risk-risques-eng.php.

Public Health Agency of Canada. *Master Programs in Public Health*. Ottawa: Author, 2012. Accessed September 13, 2013. http://www.phac-aspc.gc.ca/php-psp/master_of_php-eng.php.

Public Health Agency of Canada. *Government of Canada Invests in Project Promoting Walking to Prevent Chronic Disease*. Ottawa: PHAC, 2015. Accessed November 10, 2015. http://news.gc.ca/web/article-endo?nid=1013839&tp=1.

Public Health Action Support Team. *Epidemiological Basis for Preventive Strategies. Health Care Evaluation: Epidemiological Basis for Preventive Srategies*. Gerrards Cross: PHAST, 2011.

Quinlan, E., and H. D. Dickinson. The Emerging Public Health System in Canada. In *Health, Illness, and Health Care in Canada*, edited by B. Singh Bolaria and H. D. Dickinson, 42–55. Toronto: Nelson Education, 2009.

Rachlis, M., and C. Kushner. *Strong Medicine: How to Save Canada's Health*. Toronto: Harper Collins, 1994.

Raphael, D., ed. *Social Determinants of Health: Canadian Perspectives*. Toronto: Canadian Scholars Press, Inc, 2004.

Raphael, D. *Social Determinants of Health*. 2nd ed. Toronto: Canadian Scholars' Press International, 2009.

Raphael, D. *Health Promotion and Quality of Life in Canada: Essential Readings*. Toronto : Canadian Scholars' Press International, 2010.

Renouard, P. V. *History of Medicine: From its Origins to the Nineteenth century with an Appendix Containing a Philosophical and History Review of Medicine to the Present Time*. Charleston: Bibliolife, 2010.

Risse, G. B. *Mending Bodies, Saving Souls: A History of Hospitals*. London: Oxford University Press, 1990.

Romanow, R. J. *Building on Values: The Future of Health Care in Canada—Final Report. Commission on the Future of Health Care in Canada*. Ottawa: Government of Canada, 2002. www.hc-sc.gc.ca/english/care/romanow/hcc0023.html.

Rootman, I., S. Dupéré, A. Pederson, and M. O'Neil. *Health Promotion in Canada: Critical Perspectives on Practice*. 3rd ed. Toronto: Canadian Scholars' Press Inc, 2012.

Rosen, G. *History of Public Health*. New York: MD Publications, Inc, 1958.

Ross-Kerr, J. C. Nursing in Canada from 1760 to the Present: The Transition to Modern Nursing. In *Canadian Nursing: Issues and Perspectives*, edited by J. C. Ross-Kerr and M. J. Wood, 14–28. 4th ed. Toronto: Mosby, 2003.

Royce, M. *Eunice Dyke: Health Care Pioneer: From Pioneer Public Health Nurse to Advocate for the Aged*. Toronto: Dundurn Press, 1983.

Rutty, C., and S. C. Sullivan. *This is Public Health: A Canadian History*. Ottawa: Canadian Public Health Association, 2010. Accessed September 13, 2013. http://www.cpha.ca/uploads/history/book/History-book-print_ALL_e.pdf.

Saad, B., H. Azaizeh, and O. Said. "Tradition and Perspectives of Arab Herbal Medicine: A Review." *Evidence-based Complementary and Alternative Medicine* 2, no. 4 (2005): 475–79.

Saner, E. "Gay Rights Around the World: The Best and Worst Countries for Equality." 2013. *The Guardian,* Accessed July 16, 2013. http://www.theguardian.com/world/2013/jul/30/gay-rights-world-best-worst-countries.

Shah, C. P. *Public Health and Preventive Medicine in Canada.* 5th ed. Toronto: Elsevier Saunders, 2003.

Shaw Media. *Canadian Mine Safety in the Global context.* Toronto: Global Regional News, 2011. Accessed August 30, 2013. http://www.republicofmining.com/2011/06/10/canadian-mine-safety-in-a-global-context-global-regina-news-june-9-2011/.

Shryock, R. H. *The History of Nursing: An Interpretation of the Social and Medical Factors Involved.* Philadelphia: W.B. Saunders Company, 1959.

Singh Bolaria, B., and H. D. Dickinson. ed. *Health, Illness, and Health Care in Canada.* 4th ed. Toronto: Nelson Education, 2009.

Smith, S. *The Kingfisher Atlas of the Ancient World.* Boston: Kingfisher, 2006.

Sodipo, J. O., H. Gilly, and G. Pauser. "Endorphines: Mechanisms of Acupuncture Analgesia." *American Journal of Clinical Medicine* 9, no. 3 (1981): 249–58.

Soroka, S., and A. Mahon. *Analysis of the Impact of Current Health Care System Funding and Financing Models and the Value of Health and Health Care in Canada. Part III.* Ottawa: Health Services Research Foundation and Canadian Nurses Association, 2012.

Spitzer, R. L. "The Diagnostic Status of Homosexuality in DSM-III: A Reformulation of the Issues." *American Journal of Psychiatry* 138, no. 2 (1981): 210–15.

Standing Senate Committee on Social Affairs, Science and Technology, Subcommittee on Population Health. *A Healthy, Productive Canada: A Determinant of Health Approach.* Ottawa: Author, 2009. Accessed July 02, 2013. http://www.parl.gc.ca/Content/SEN/Committee/402/popu/rep/rephealth1jun09-e.pdf.

Starfield, B. "Politics, Primary Healthcare and Health: Was Virchow Rights?" *Journal of Epidemiology and Community Health* 65 (2011): 653–55.

Stewart-Brown, S. *What Is the Evidence on School Health Promotion in Improving Health or Preventing Disease and, Specifically, What Is the Effectiveness of the Health Promoting Schools Approach?* Copenhagen: WHO Regional Office for Europe Health Evidence Network report, 2006. Accessed August 15, 2013. www.euro.who.int/document/e88185.pdf.

St. John's Ambulance Foundation. (2018). *St. John Ambulance history: The most Vulnerable Order of the Hospital of St. John of Jersuleum.* Toronto, ON: Author. Retrieved March 3, 2018 from http://www.sja.ca/English/St-John-International/Pages/St-John-International-History.aspx?AcceptCookies=No&Branch=111.

Storch, J. Canadian Health Care System. In *Realities of Canadian Nursing: Professional, Practice, and Power Issues,* edited by M. McIntrye, E. Thomlinson, and C. McDonald, 29–53. Baltimore: Lippincott Williams Wilkins, 2006.

Sullivan, T., and P. Baranek. *First do no Harm: Making Sense of Canadian Health Reform.* Toronto: Malcolm Lester and Associates, 2002.

Swan, R. "The History of Medicine in Canada." A Paper Presented at the Symposium on the History of Medicine in the Commonwealth. Faculty of Medicine and Pharmacy, Royal College of Physicians of London: London, England, September 23, 1966, 42–51.

Swanson, J. M., and M. Albrecht. *Community Health Nursing: Promoting the Health of Aggregates.* Toronto: W.B. Saunders Company, 1993.

Syed, I. B. "Islamic Medicine: 1000 Years Ahead of its Times. *Journal of the Islamic Medical Association* 2 (2002): 2–9.

Taylor, M. G. "The Canadian Health Insurance Program." *Public Administration Review* 33 (1973) 31–39.

Taylor, M. G. *Health Insurance and Canadian Public Policy.* 2nd ed. Montréal: McGill University Press, 1987.

Thomas, V. D. *Health and Health Care Delivery in Canada.* Ottawa: Elsevier Canada, 2010.

Thompson, V. D. *Health and Health Care Delivery in Canada.* Toronto: Mosby/Elsevier, 2010.

UNAIDS. *Global Report: Overview of the Global AIDS Epidemic.* New York: Author, 2006. Accessed June 10, 2010. http://www.data.unaids.org/pub/GlobalReport/2006/2006_GRCH02_en.pdf.

Unschuld, P. U. *Huang Di Nei Jing Su Wen: Nature, Knowledge, Imagery in an Ancient Chinese Medical Text.* Berkeley and Los Angeles: University of California Press, 2003.

Van Loon, R. J., and M. S. Whittington. *The Canadian Political System: Environment, Structure and Process.* 2nd ed. Toronto: McGraw-Hill Ryerson, 1976.

Varia, M., S. Wilson, S. Sarwal, A. McGeer, E. Gournis, E. Galanis, and B. Henry. "Hospital Outbreak Investigation Team. Investigation of a Nosocomial Outbreak of Severe Acute Respiratory Syndrome (SARS) in Toronto, Canada." *Canadian Medical Association Journal* 169, no. 4 (2003): 285–92.

Vickers, A. J., A. M. Cronin, A. C. Maschino, G. Lewith, H. MacPherson, N. E. Foster, K. J. Sherman, C. M. Witt, K. Linde, and Acupuncture Trialists' Collaboration. "Acupuncture for Chronic Pain: Individual Client Data Meta-analysis." *Archives of Internal Medicine* 172, no. 19 (2012): 1444–53.

Walsh, J. J. *The Popes and Science: The History of the Papal Relations to science During the Middle Ages and Down to our own Time.* New York: Kessinger Publishing, 2003.

Watawaba, Y., I. Matsumoto, T. Kumazawa, and E. Ikezono. "Characteristics of Acupuncture Analgesia: Review of the Articles on Stimulation Produced Analgesic and Morphine-like Substance". *Masui* 27, no. 7 (1978): 667–75.

Watson, R. "Climate Change in Likely to Affect the Health of Millions, Report Warns." *British Medical Journal* 334, no. 7595 (2007): 768–78.

Weiner, M. A. *Weiner's Herbal: The Guide to Herb Medicine.* Briarcliff Manor: Stein and Day/Publishers/Scarborough House, 1980.

World Health Organization. "*Constitution of the World Health Organization as Adopted by the International Health Conference.*" Official records of the WHO, No. 2. Geneva: Author, 1948.

World Health Organization. "*Declaration of Alma Ata.*" *Geneva,* Switzerland: WHO, 1978. www.who.dk/About WHO/Policy/20010827_1.

World Health Organization. "New Players for a New Era: Leading Health Promotion into the 21st century." 4th International Conference on Health Promotion, Jakarta, Indonesia 21–25 July, 1997.

World Health Organization. "*NCD country profiles, 2011. Canada.*" Geneva. Author, 2011. Accessed August 16, 2013. http://www.who.int/nmh/countries/can_en.pdf.

World Health Organization. *Bangkok Charter for Health Promotion (11 August, 2005).* Geneva: Author, 2013. Accessed September 17, 2013. http://www.who.int/healthpromotion/conferences/6gchp/bangkok_charter/en.

World Health Organization Commission on the Social Determinants of Health. *Closing the Gap in a Generation: Health Equity Through Action on the Social Determinants of Health.* Final Report of the Commission on Social Determinants of Health. Geneva: WHO, 2008.

Wujastyk, D. *The Roots of Ayurveda.* New York: Penguin, 2003.

Zola, I. K. Medicine as an Institution of Social Control. *Sociological Review* 20 (1972): 487–504.

Zysk, K. G. *Asceticism and Healing in Ancient India: Medicine in the Buddhist Monastery.* London: Oxford University Press, 1998.

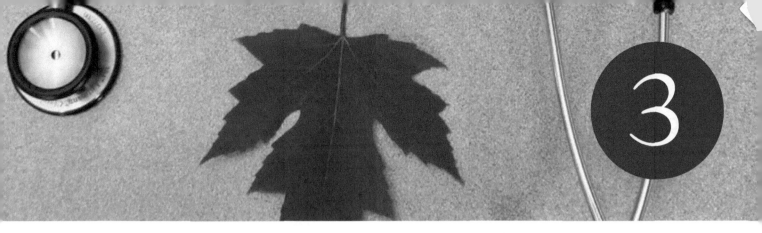

"Medicare" in Canada: History and Current Challenges

"The pessimist complains about the wind.
The optimist expects it to change.
The realist adjusts the sail."

(William Arthur Ward)

Learning Objectives

After completion of this chapter, the student will be able to:

- Describe the evolution of publicly insured health care (Medicare) in Canada and how it has been shaped and influenced by various social, political, and economic factors,
- List and differentiate between the roles and responsibilities of the federal, provincial and territories governments in delivering health care services to our residents,
- List and differentiate between the five criteria's of the Canada Health Act (1984),
- Describe how publicly insured health care is managed and delivered in Canada, and
- List and describe three current issues and challenges facing our publicly insured health care systems in Canada.

Core Competencies addressed in Chapter 3

Core Competencies	Competency Statements
1.0 Public Health Sciences	1.1, 1.2, 1.3, 1.4, 1.5
2.0 Assessment and Analysis	2.1, 2.4, 2.5, 2.6
3.0 Policy and Program Planning, Implementation, and Evaluation	3.1, 3.2, 3.6. 3.7
4.0 Partnerships, Collaboration, and Advocacy	4.1, 4.2, 4.3, 4.4
5.0 Diversity and Inclusiveness	5.1, 5.2
6.0 Communication	6.1, 6.2, 6.4
7.0 Leadership	7.1, 7.2, 7.3, 7.4

Note: Please see the following document or web-based link for a detailed description of these specific competencies. Public Health Agency of Canada (2007).

Introduction

In 2015, life expectancy for a male and female born in 2012 in Canada was 80 and 84, respectively (Canadian Broadcasting Corporation [CBC] 2014). By comparison, the top three countries for life expectancies for males born in 2012 for Iceland at 81.2 years, Switzerland at 80.7 years, and Australia at 80.5 years. For females born in 2012, the top three countries were Japan at 87.0 years, Spain at 85.1 years, and Switzerland at 85.1 years (CBC 2014). Statistics Canada (2010a, b, 2012a) predicts that Canada's population could exceed 40 million by 2036 with 1:4 expected to be foreign-born immigrants; and the third of us will belong to a visible minority; nearly 1:4 will be over at the age of 65 years, and the Indigenous population may reach 2.2 million. In fact, as of July 1, 2014, Canada's population was 35,540,400 and 15.7% (nearly 1:6) was aged 65 or older (Statistics Canada 2014). This was the first time that the proportion of older adults has exceeded those of younger adults. Specifically, 4.6 million Canadians were aged 15 to 24 years, compared to 4.7 million aged 55 to 64 (Statistics Canada 2014). This proportion has steadily increased since the mid-1960s as a result of lower fertility rates and increased life expectancies.

A country's commitment to public health care services is one of the indicators employed to measure its overall wealth, prosperity, success, and status from a global perspective (Butler-Jones 2012; National Expert Committee Canadian Nurses Association 2012; Suhrcke et al. 2005; World Health Organization 2000). The health care industry in one of the largest sectors of the Canadian economy, accounting for 10.9% of the gross domestic product (GDP) in 2015 or $219.1 billion ($6,105 per person) (Canadian Institute for Health Information [CIHI] 2015a,b).

Over the past five decades, Canada has secured significant gains in the health status of our citizens and residents across the lifespan through routine immunization and smoking cessation programs; reducing and managing the incidence of various communicable diseases (e.g., tuberculosis, measles, smallpox, and HIV/AIDS); investments in health infrastructures (e.g., hospitals, community clinics, laboratory, and diagnostic services, sewage, and water treatment facilities), and through legislation (e.g., mandatory seat-belt and infant/child-seat legislations) (Bartfay and Bartfay 2015). However, there are major areas in which significant improvements are required such as decreasing the rates of non-communicable diseases (e.g., heart disease, stroke, diabetes, and Alzheimer's disease) associated with a variety of social determinants of health (e.g., employment and working conditions, educational levels and literacy, poverty, homelessness); lifestyle choices (e.g., inactivity, smoking, diets high in saturated fats, sugar and salt); injuries, and disabilities.

In 2010, for example, 55% of Canadians aged 12 years and older reported living with at least one chronic non-communicable health condition (Butler-Jones 2012). Similarly, approximately 4.4 million Canadians (14.3% of the population) reported having a physical, mental/emotional or a combination type of disability (World Health Organization 2011). To put this in a global perspective, the World Economic Forum predicts that cancer, diabetes, mental illness, heart, and respiratory diseases could cost the global economy over $47 trillion (U.S.) over the next 20 years (Bloom et al. 2011).

The *fee-for-service model* that underpins current Medicare payment systems in Canada is based on the episodic acute care model of health care delivery, which suited most physicians and Canadians when Medicare programs were first introduced over five decades ago (Bartfay and Bartfay 2015). We shall explore the evolution of Medicare systems and associated funding models and payment schemes in greater detail in the following. In fact, disease and population health trends have significantly changed over time and this model is antiquated and ineffective to address current and emerging health issues and challenges facing Canadian residents and citizens across the lifespan. For example, when our Medicare systems were initially conceived, communicable diseases (e.g., tuberculosis, measles, smallpox) were still the dominant threat to the health of residents in Canada (Butler-Jones 2012; National Expert Commission Canadian Nurses Association 2011). Currently, non-communicable diseases are associated with approximately 89% of all avoidable or amendable mortalities in Canada, and chronic disease and illness have become the major drivers for increasing annually the associated publicly funded health care costs with concomitant lost economic productivity for our nation (World Health Organization 2011). In fact, it has been estimated that some 75% of "good health" is the result of factors beyond episodic care provided in acute care hospitals (National Expert Commission Canadian Nurses Association 2012; Standing Senate Committee on Social Affairs, Science and Technology, Subcommittee on Population Health 2009).

Avoidable or amendable mortalities are defined as untimely and premature deaths that should not have occurred with the presence of timely and effective primary health care services or other public health interventions, practices, programs, policy interventions, and/or health related legislations (Mackenbach et al. 1990; Manuel and Mao 2002; Nolte and McKee 2011; Treurniet et al. 2004). For example, in 2008 there were more than 238,600 mortalities in Canada, of which 39% of these were among individuals less than 75 years of age (Statistics Canada 2012). Of these total mortalities, it is estimated that approximately 72% were potentially avoidable; 65% were preventable health conditions (i.e., cardiovascular diseases, cancers, and injuries), and 35% of these were manageable and treatable health conditions (Statistics Canada 2012).

The concept of avoidable mortality dates back to 1976 and has been gaining interest over the past few decades because of its potential to link population-based health outcomes to the functioning of health care systems (Nolte and McKee 2008, 2011; Statistics Canada 2012). For example, preventing both communicable and non-communicable diseases from happening can be achieved via public health activities, interventions, programs, policies, and/or legislations that seek to maintain the health of individuals across the lifespan, and by addressing social, behavioural and environmental risk factors that make individuals susceptible to disease. Such public health prevention efforts can range from community-based immunization programs to national policy initiatives such as specific road safety designs (e.g., guard rails on bridges, and reflective paint on roads), car manufacturing safety standards (e.g., seat belts, air bags, and safety glass) and food safety legislation (e.g., pasteurization of milk) (Bartfay and Bartfay 2015).

These public health initiatives are also supported by the majority of Canadians. For example, based on a recent commissioned national poll conducted by Nanos Research, 6 out of 10 (60%) respondents surveyed reported that the federal government should have a greater role in helping Canadians live a healthy lifestyle by regulating things such as fat or salt content in processed foods (National Expert Commission Canadian Nurses Association 2012). Accordingly, the federal government has introduced legislation in 2006 governing the presence of harmful trans-fats in processed foods sold in Canada associated with the development of heart disease and stroke, which pushed food manufacturers and agencies to comply with total dietary recommendations based on published peer-reviewed scientific reports (2%–5% of total fat) (Health Canada and Heart and

Stroke Foundation of Canada 2006). Similarly, legislation in Ontario was introduced in 2008 entitled the "Healthy Food for Healthy Schools Act" which requires food items sold in the province's schools to meet these nutritional standards for trans-fats (Ontario Ministry of Education 2008).

Various provincial/territorial and national public health programs aimed at reducing the prevalence of smoking by Canadians have been initiated and, by extension, the illnesses and diseases (e.g., lung, throat, and mouth cancers, cardiovascular disease) associated with this lifestyle choice over the past four decades. These include public health education and promotion programs; increasing the legal age for obtaining tobacco-related products (e.g., cigarettes, cigars, chewing tobacco) to 19 years of age, and smoking bans in government offices, work places, libraries, malls, restaurants, and other enclosed spaces routinely accessed by individuals, and increased taxation (Bao et al. 2006; Health Canada 2003; Shields 2007). The prevalence of smoking has declined from approximately 50% in 1965 to less than 20% in 2008, with the rate of decline more pronounced in males

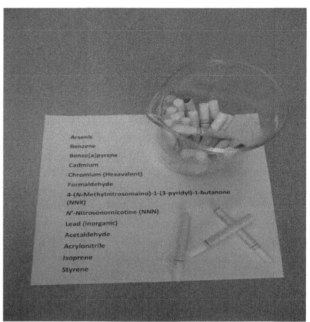

Source: Wally Bartfay

Photo 3.1 Tobacco smoke contains over 4,000 chemicals, of which more than 70% are known carcinogens, or substances that are reported to cause, initiate or promote cancer in humans (Health Canada 2011).

than females (Canadian Cancer Society and Statistics Canada 2011; Reid and Hammond 2011). According to the Canadian Tobacco, Alcohol and Drugs Survey (CTADS), 4.2 million Canadians aged 15 years or older were smokers in 2013, which represents approximately 15% of the total population (Government of Canada 2015a).

It is important to note that these public health efforts often take decades to manifest themselves in terms of actual declines in avoidable mortalities. The induction period between tobacco smoking and the development of lung cancer takes on average 21 years, so the direct impact of these collective public health efforts are not seen immediately at the population level per se (Canadian Cancer Society and Statistics Canada 2011; Reid and Hammond 2011).

In fact, it was not until the late 1980s that the rates of avoidable mortalities associated with tobacco use started to decline for males. For females, the reductions in the prevalence of smoking have not yet been translated into noted reductions in the incidence of lung cancer. Nonetheless, the rate of increase in the incidence of lung cancer for females has decelerated significantly in the past decade (Canadian Cancer Society and Statistics Canada 2011; Reid and Hammond 2011;

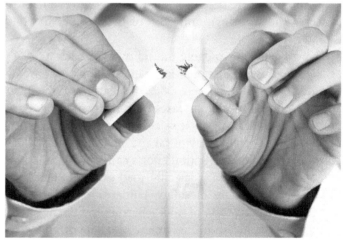

rangizz/Shutterstock.com

Photo 3.2 The prevalence of smoking has declined from approximately 50% in 1965 to less than 20% in 2008, with the rate of decline more pronounced in males than females (Canadian Cancer Society and Statistics Canada 2011; Reid and Hammond 2011). In 2012–2013, only 4% of Canadian students in grades 6 to 12 were current smokers (≈114,000 students) nationally (Health Canada 2014).

Statistics Canada 2012). In addition, the decreased prevalence of smoking over the past five decades has also resulted in significant reductions in the incidence of other forms of non-communicable diseases such as heart disease and stroke (Butler-Jones 2012; Public Health Agency of Canada 2009). These public health efforts related to the reduction of tobacco use by Canadian residents and citizens over the past five decades best exemplifies what can be achieved through interprofessional and sectorial collaborative public health efforts (Bartfay and Bartfay 2015).

If we consider and reflect about the present situation and context in Canada that involves individuals living with several chronic health conditions, illnesses, and disabilities, there is a growing need and recognition to fund collaborative primary care models of health delivered in communities and in individuals homes by teams of interdisciplinary public health professionals and workers (Browne et al. 2012; National Expert Commission Canadian Nurses Association 2012; Soroka and Mahon 2012;

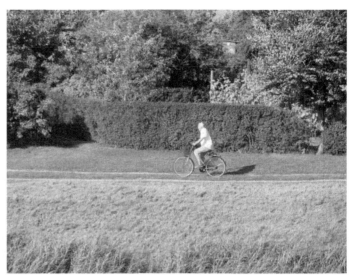

Source: Wally Bartfay

Photo 3.3 It is noteworthy that approximately 75% of good health that is maintained or achieved by an individual is the result of lifestyle factors and various social determinants of health (e.g., physical activity, eating a balanced diet, proper sanitation, and clean water supplies) which are beyond direct episodic acute care that is often delivered in hospitals (National Expert Commission Canadian Nurses Association 2012; Standing Senate Committee on Social Affairs, Science and Technology, Subcommittee on Population Health 2009).

Starfield 2012). The acute care physician-driven model which is largely provided in hospitals simply cannot meet the current and emerging needs of Canadians. We argue that one of the major challenges facing our publicly funded Medicare systems today is our continued reliance on an outdated and self-perpetuating funding model based on episodic hospital-based acute care administered and driven by physicians who act as gate keepers to a variety of specialized diagnostic and treatment procedures (Armstrong and Armstrong 2003; Browne et al. 2012; National Expert Commission Canadian Nurses Association 2011; Starfield 2011). Unfortunately, the status quo remains despite a growing body of evidence that show that this acute care physician-driven Medicare funding model is outdated, costly, and insufficient in meeting current and projected health care needs of Canadian residents; along with public support for the need to adopt and fund primary public health care models (Browne et al. 2012; Commission on the Future of Health Care in Canada 2002; National Expert Commission Canadian Nurses Association 2011; Soroka and Mahon 2012; Soroka 2007; Standing Senate Committee on Social Affairs, Science and Technology 2012; Starfield 2011). Hence, we argue there is a critical need to reform our Medicare systems and current funding models if we value health as an essential asset and right for all individuals, and for the continued growth and prosperity of our nation as a whole (Bartfay and Bartfay 2015).

In this chapter we shall explore the evolution of our publicly funded health insurance systems commonly referred to as *"Medicare"* by the mass and social media. We shall examine the role of the federal government and the provincial/territorial governments in providing health care services to our residents, and explore how various acts by Parliament and Royal Commissions on Health Services eventually led to the passage of the Canada Health Act (or Bill C-3) (Begin 2002; Mussalem 1992). Lastly we shall explore current challenges facing our Medicare systems in Canada including the rising costs of providing health care services; the growth of private clinics, and the implications of recent court challenges and rulings.

Medicare

Medicare (French: *assurance-maladie*) is the collective term that is widely employed by residents in Canada to refer to their publicly funded and administered universal health insurance systems (Bartfay 2010a; Bartfay and Bartfay 2015). It is publicly funded through taxes and administered on a provincial or territorial basis, within guidelines established by the federal government. The term **publicly funded** refers to a taxed based system to support health care services rendered in public hospitals, community clinics, or institutions in Canada. **Privately funded**, by contrast, refers to *out–of–pocket* health care services that are paid for by an individual or private insurance plan or benefit (e.g., employee health benefits) (Bartfay and Bartfay 2015).

Currently there is one federal, ten provincial and three territorial jurisdictions for the delivery of publicly funded health care services to our citizens and permanent residents. Medicare was conceived on the basis that health care in Canada be universally available to all permanent residents; comprehensive in terms of health care services covered; be portable across the ten provinces and three territories, and be operated on a non-profit basis (Armstrong and Armstrong 2003). Medicare was also created to foster national standards by establishing cost sharing health care programs providing these aforementioned criteria's were adhered to. Nonetheless, one of the major drawbacks of these funding schemes was the emphasis on hospital-based acute care services controlled and dominated by physicians and the medical model of health.

The terms "health care system" and "health systems" are often used interchangeable by the mass and social media's in Canada. However, they are in fact unique and distinctly different concepts. A **health care system** is a collective term employed to describe all the health care services (e.g., client education, consultations, conducting clinical assessments, and surgery) provided by health care professionals (e.g., physicians, nurses, dieticians, and dentists) in a variety of clinical and community-based settings (e.g., community clinics, school-based immunization programs, stroke rehabilitation units, emergency rooms, and surgical clinics) (Statistics Canada 2012b). Conversely, a **health system** encompasses a broader concept which is defined as all activities whose primary purpose is to promote, restore, and/or maintain the health of individuals across the lifespan (National Expert Commission Canadian Nurses Association 2012; World Health Organization 2000). Canada's health care systems consist of a group of publicly insured health care services, which have been conceived and developed with the objective of providing national health care and diagnostic services to all residents irrespective of their age, health condition, social status, or income level.

In our modern, technologically advanced and wealthy nation, it is easy to believe that access to health care services by Canadian citizens and residents have continued to improve overtime (Bartfay 2010a; Bartfay and Bartfay 2015). However, the current reality for a growing number of individuals including those who are disabled, live in rural and remote regions of Canada, are poor or marginalized (e.g., single mothers, Indigenous peoples, immigrants, elderly) is diminished publicly insured health care services with corresponding increases in out–of–pocket costs (CIHI 2013, 2009, 2007; National Expert Commission Canadian Nurses Association 2012; Romanow 2002; Villeneuve and MacDonald 2006). For example, a recent Canadian study found that out–of–pocket costs associated with the purchasing of required prescribed drugs to treat a variety of ailments kept 1:10 Canadians from obtaining needed medications (Law et al. 2012). Similar findings were reported by Human Resources and Skills Development Canada (2010) that found that out–of–pocket drug cost prevented approximately 13% of individuals with disabilities, and 25% of those with severe disabilities, from purchasing required medications. Over half (54%) of Canadians take one or more prescription medications on a regular basis, and more than one-third (36%) take two or more, which are often paid as an out–of–pocket expense (Commonwealth Fund 2015).

Historically, health care services were largely provided by charitable religious organizations to all those in need. The arrival of Medicare during the 1950s and 1960s also increased the demand for acute care hospital-based nursing services (Bartfay and Bartfay 2015). Not surprisingly, the number of health care professionals such as physicians and public health nurses practicing in home and community-based health care settings quickly diminished over time. Canada currently employs a mix of both public and private organizations to deliver health care services to residents. Table 3.1 provides a time line of major historical events, trends, and legislations in Canada that have led to the development of Medicare and our current health care systems in Canada. We shall explore these developments in greater details in the following.

Table 3.1 Time Line of Major Events, Trends and Legislations Related to Medicare in Canada

Time/Dates	Major Events, Trends, and Legislations
1867	BNA Act passed. Section 91 describes the federal government's role in establishing quarantine regulations and their responsibility for Native peoples. Section 92 states that the provinces/territories are responsible for establishing and maintaining hospitals and social services.
1910	The Flexner Report outlined the shortcomings of medical schools in the United States and Canada including their lack of standardized curriculums, graduation credentials, and inconsistent or inadequate education and training based on the medical model of health. Alternative schools of medicine were subsequently closed and the new scientific paradigm was installed as the dominate approach to medical education and training.
1919	Prime Minister King proposes a national tax based health care insurance plan for both hospitals and physicians, but his plan is rejected.
1930s	Coburn (1988) notes that only 25% of nurses work as salaried health care staff members in hospitals, while the majority are self-employed entrepreneurs who practice in private homes and/or community health settings.
1935	Prime Minister Bennett proposes the Employment and Social Insurance Act, where the federal government would collect taxes for certain social security benefits including health. His proposal is rejected by the premiers.
1937	British Privy Council rules in support of the provinces/territories that Bennett's proposal was *ultra vires* (meaning it is outside the mandate of the federal government).
1943	The Marsch and Heagerty Reports help to serve as a blueprint for the evolution and development of health and social programs in Canada.
1947–1948	The CCF party in Saskatchewan under the leadership of Tommy Douglas introduces the first universal and comprehensive hospital-based insurance plan in Canada. Subsequently, the National Health Grants Act is passed by Parliament with overwhelming public support.
1950s	The number of salaried nurses working in hospitals increases to approximately 65%.
1955	Armstrong and Armstrong (2003) report that by the year 1955, there are 1,216 hospitals in Canada and 90% of these are designated as non-profit. Although only 40% of the population has some form of private health care (hospital) insurance, these non-profit hospitals still charge for various health care services rendered.
1957	The Hospital Insurance and Diagnostic Services Act (HIDSA) is passed by Parliament.
1960	Justice Emmett Hall heads the Royal Commission on Health Services in Canada. His report supports the need for a national Medicare program in Canada. He also urges that private health insurance companies in Canada (N = 145), be replaced by publicly-funded provincial/territorial health insurance plans.
1961	Premier Woodrow Lloyd of Saskatchewan introduces the Medical Care Insurance Act, which enforces socialized medicine and fee schedules. This prompts outrage and a 23 day strike by physicians in the province, and the government agrees to amend the Act in an attempt to repair relationships.

(Continued)

Table 3.1 Time Line of Major Events, Trends and Legislations Related to Medicare in Canada (*Continued*)

Time/Dates	Major Events, Trends, and Legislations
1964–65	Justice Emmett Hall heads the first Royal Commission on Health Services in Canada, and recommends the establishment of a national Medicare program, in opposition to the intention of Prime Minister Diefenbaker and the Canadian Medical Association (CMA).
1966	Emmett Hall heads a second Royal Commission on Health Services in Canada to examine the effectiveness of the current system and his recommendations leads to the establishment of the Medical Care Act (MCA). The MCA effectively leads to the creation of the first publicly funded Medicare program in Canada.
1970s	Health care costs continue to escalate, and there is increased public concern regarding access to publicly insured health care services in Canada.
1972	The creation of a pan-Canadian Medicare program is realized when all provinces and territories finally enlist with the MCA, which is based on a 50/50 cost sharing model between the federal and provincial/territorial governments.
1975	Our national health care expenditure is estimated to be $12.2 billion (CIHI 2010a, b).
1977	The federal government decides to change the 50/50 cost sharing formula to a new per capita block grant funding model with the passage of the Federal-Provincial Fiscal Arrangement Fiscal Arrangement and Established Programs Financing Act (EPF).
1980	Our national health care expenditure is estimated to be $22.3 billion (CIHI 2010a, b).
1982	(May): The CMA is opposed to Monique Begin's Bill-C31 for fear it will create a socialized medical state in Canada. Despite intense opposition by the CMA, Parliament passes Bill C31 -the Canada Health Act (CHA) with the support of all political parties, and suggested amendments by the Canadian Nurses Association.
1984	(April): CHA is enacted and replaces HIDSA and MCA. The CHA is based on the following five founding criteria's: Public administration; comprehensiveness; universality; portability, and accessibility.
1985	(June/July): Jake Epp, the Federal Minister of Health, sends a letter to all his provincial and territorial health ministers to clarify the intent of the CHA and its five founding criteria's. Our national health care expenditure is estimated to be $39.8 billion (CIHI 2010a, b).
1986	(June): Physicians in Ontario take strike action to protest the government's position on extra-billing in the province, which they believe violates their right to contract directly with patients, and that it also undermines the quality of health care. Public opinion is opposed to the physician's position and the strike fails to stop the ban on extra billing (Brennan 1986; Kravitz et al. 1989).
1989	Approximately 85% of nurses in Canada are employed by hospitals, and only 15% choose to engage in private practice or community-based nursing (CIHI 2006a).
1990	Our national health care expenditure is estimated to be $61 billion (CIHI 2010a, b).
1995	-(January): Diane Marleau, the Federal Minister of Health, sends a follow-up letter to all provincial and territorial health ministers to express the growing public concerns over the expansion of private clinics in Canada, and the establishment of two-tied health care delivery systems. Our national health care expenditure is estimated to be $74.1 billion (CIHI 2010a, b).

(Continued)

Table 3.1 Time Line of Major Events, Trends and Legislations Related to Medicare in Canada (*Continued*)

Time/Dates	Major Events, Trends, and Legislations
1996	1995–1996 is the last year of EPF funding scheme, and the federal government transfers $22 billion to the provinces and territories of which 71% is allocated for health care. Canada Health and Social Transfer (CHST) funding scheme replaces the EPF. Health Canada (2000) reports that no federal penalties have been levied against the provinces and territories for extra-billing their residents since the end of the 1990s.
2000	Premier Ralph Klein of Alberta introduces Bill 11, which includes provisions for using public health care funds to subsidize various private acute care hospitals, imaging clinics and other private clinics. Our national health care expenditure is estimated to be $98.4 billion (CIHI 2010a, b).
2002	Auditor General of Canada (2002, p. 17) reports that Parliament *"cannot readily determine the extent to which each province and territory has satisfied the criteria and conditions of the Canada Health Act."*
2004	Private funds—including mostly private insurance and out–of–pocket payments—represents 30% of Canada's overall health care spending in 2004, compared to the Organization for Economic Cooperation and Development (OECD) average (27%) (CIHI 2010b). The federal government and the premiers agree to a $41-billion infusion into the publicly funded health care systems over 10 years. Among the key parts of the agreement: • Ensuring stable, predictable long-term funding; • Implementing a National Waiting Times Reduction; • Creating a National Home Care Program; • Developing a national strategy for prescription drug care, and • Respecting the Canada Health Act (CBC News Online, August 2006).
2005	(June): A landmark ruling by the Supreme Court of Québec overturns a previous law which prevented residents from purchasing their own private health care to pay for medical services available through publicly funded health care systems (Jacques Chaoulli et al. Versus the Attorney General of Québec). (November): The Provincial government of Québec declares that it will allow their residents to purchase private medical insurance to pay for publicly insured Medicare services. Our national health care expenditure is estimated to be $141 billion (CIHI 2010a, b). In 2005, the Federal government allocates $19 billion to the Canada Health Transfer for annual cash payments for health care and this transfer amount has increased by 6% per year, which the Federal government legislates as an annual increase through 2013/2014 (Government of Canada, Department of Finance 2006; Health Council of Canada 2011).
2006	Health care spending in Canada escalates to $148 billion annually in Canada, of which half of the total expenditures is related to physician services, hospitals, and retail sales of prescription and non-prescription drugs (CIHI 2007). CIHI (2006) reports that 62.5% of nurses work in hospital-based settings in Canada, while only 13.4% work in community settings, and 10.5% work in nursing homes and long-term care facilities.
2007	(March): Patient Wait Time Guarantee Trust Fund are established by the federal government, and requires each province and territory to specify their priority areas and implement a patient wait time guarantee.

(Continued)

Table 3.1 Time Line of Major Events, Trends and Legislations Related to Medicare in Canada (*Continued*)

Time/Dates	Major Events, Trends, and Legislations
2009	Our national health care expenditure is in excess of $183 billion (11.9% of GDP), compared with only $12.2 billion in 1975 (CIHI 2010a).
2010	Since the First Ministers Accords, the provincial and territorial governments have increased their annual health care spending by about $40 billion, from $85 billion to 2004 to a projected $125 billion in 2010, which represents an annual average increase of 6.7% (Canadian Institute for Health Information 2010; Health Council of Canada 2011).
2011	Approximately 10% of our gross domestic product (GDP) is tied up in health care costs which are estimated at $4,100 per person per year (Hall 2011).
2012	Health care costs continue to escalate and reach a record high of $207 billion or $5,948 per person (approximately 11.6% of GDP) (CIHI 2013).
2014–2015	Canada Health Transfer (CHT) payments move to a full equal per capital cash allocation, following the expiry of the *10-Year Plan to Strengthen Health Care*. This transaction affects provinces and territories differently, depending on their level of per capita CHT cash relative to the other provinces (Deraspe and Gauthier 2011; Gauthier 2011).
2015	Health care costs escalate to $219.1 billion or $6,105 per person. The following top three drivers makeup 60% of all expenditures: (a) Hospitals (29.5%); (b) drugs (15.7%); and (c) physician costs (15.5%) (CIHI 2015a).
2016	Total health expenditure was $228.1 billion (11.1% of GDP), a 2.7% increase from 2015 (CIHI 2016).
	Total health care spending per Canadian was $6,299, and acute care hospital spending accounted for the largest share of total health spending by the public sector at 37.7% (CIHI 2016).
2017	Canadians had more than 1 million potentially unnecessary medical tests and treatments performed each year (Choosing Wisely Canada and CIHI, 2017).
	Up to 30% of clients indicated in the 8 selected *Choosing Wisely Canada* recommendations had tests, treatments and procedures that are potentially unnecessary and/or harmful in nature.
	Unnecessary tests and care wastes health system resources, increases wait times for clients and can lead to harm.
	Approximately 1 in 3 low-risk clients with minor head trauma in Ontario and Alberta had an unnecessary head scan in an emergency department, despite a *Choosing Wisely Canada* recommendation.
	1 in 10 older Canadians aged 65+ were prescribed a benzodiazepine on a regular basis to treat insomnia, agitation or delirium.
	In Ontario, Saskatchewan and Alberta, 18% to 35% of clients undergoing low-risk surgery had an unnecessary preoperative test performed, such as a chest X-ray, ECG or cardiac stress test (Choosing Wisely Canada and CIHI, 2017).
	Total health expenditure in Canada was over $242 billion, (or $6,604 per person), which represented 11.5% of Canada's gross domestic product (GDP) (CIHI, 2018).
	Total health expenditure per person varied across the country from $7,378 in Newfoundland and Labrador and $7,329 in Alberta to $6,367 in Ontario and $6,321 in British Columbia (CIHI, 2018).

The Evolution of Health Services in Canada: A Brief History

This section provides the reader with a historical overview of key developments and how health care services were provided to residents in Canada since the time of colonization during the seventeenth century to present day. We shall explore the major social, political, economic influences, and forces that have led to the development of our current publicly funded Medicare systems in Canada, as well as current factors that are threatening its survival.

Pioneer Nurses

Free health services were initially provided by charitable religious organizations in Canada to all those in need. French Jesuit missionaries were, in fact, the first male nurses to tend to sick soldiers and Indigenous peoples in North America in 1629 at a French garrison in Port Royal Acadia (Kenton 1925; Parkman 1897). Two general charitable hospitals were founded in 1639: the Hospitalières nuns administered the one in present day Québec City and the Charon Brothers managed the one in Montréal.

Melle Jeanne Mance is credited as being the first female nurse and the founder of the Hôtel-Dieu Hospital in Montréal, Québec in 1644 (Bartfay 2010b; Donahue 1996; Gibbon and Mathewson 1947). The Hôtel-Dieu was the first charitable hospital built in Canada to provide a variety of health care services free of charge to soldiers, colonists, and Indigenous peoples. This tiny cottage hospital was built under the sponsorship of the wealthy female philanthropists Madame de Bullion of France (Bartfay 2010b). Donahue (1996) notes that this hospital consisted of a tiny cottage built inside the fort, surrounded by a palisade and protected by a moat because of the threat of attack by the Iroquois Indians. Jean Mance tended to soldiers with wounds from arrows, treated childblains and frostbite, practiced bloodletting and compounded her own medicines. By October 1644, a larger hospital was established in a building sixty-by twenty-four feet. For almost 15 years, she did all the nursing here with the help of a few assistants (Donahue 1966). The Hôtel-Dieu Hospitals were devoted to the care of the sick and wounded. By contrast, the general hospitals of the French regime attempted to resolve problems related to begging, poverty, and marginal living conditions. The main clientele of these general hospitals consisted of abandoned elderly people, vagabonds, the poor, the handicapped, and those labeled as being insane (Bartfay and Bartfay 2015).

The Grey Nuns

In 1738, the first female visiting home [public health] nurses in Canada were the French Catholic Grey Nuns (or "Les Soeurs Grises"). This charitable nursing order was founded under the direction of Marguerite d'Youville who was the niece of the French explorer La Vérendrye (Gibbon and Mathewson 1947). English forces eventually defeated the French at the Plains of Abraham in Québec City and established British rule of the new territory under the Treaty of Paris in 1763 (Morton 1983). Despite the takeover by the British, this had little impact on charitable home nursing services provided by the French Catholic Grey Nuns (Gibbon and Mathewson 1947). The Grey Nuns also extended their charitable services to other regions of Canada including present day St. Boniface in Manitoba, Lac Ste. Anne in Alberta, and Île à La Crosse in Saskatchewan (Ross-Kerr 2003).

These pioneer public health nurses in Canada had to face a series of epidemics which first began in 1846. The following account by Sister Laurent describes some of the health care challenges faced by the Grey Nuns:

> "Some of us went into the houses where sick people were. They used to have measles and dysentery and inflammatory rheumatism, and smallpox sometimes. We had medicines from Montréal, but we also learned the use of herbs that grew in the country, and how to help the sick so as to ease the pain and aid them to get better."
>
> (Cited in Gibbon and Mathewson 1947, p. 89).

This account helps to exemplify the resourcefulness of these early pioneer nurses who provided a variety of home based nursing services to those in need. Home nursing remains an important component of public health nursing in Canada today (Bartfay and Bartfay 2015). The Mack Training School was established in 1874 at St. Catherine's, Ontario, and was one of the earliest formal schools of nursing in Canada, but only admitted qualified female candidates (Bartfay 2008). The first major hospital-based training school for nursing in Canada was established at the Montréal General Hospital in 1890 by Nora Bertrude Livingston, a graduate of the New York Hospital.

By 1909, over 70 hospital-based training schools for nursing had been established across Canada. Approximately 60% of all trained nurses in Canada were self-employed in private duty home settings prior to World War II, as opposed to hospital-based practice. Visiting district and public health nurses, including the Victorian Order of Nurses, also provided nursing services in small towns and country districts.

Pioneer Surgeons and Physicians

Swan (1966) notes that conditions during early colonization were challenging due to the harsh climate and geography of Canada, and physicians were often required to be pioneers in other fields including exploration, legislation, and politics. The first recorded physician–surgeon in "New France" was Jehan de Broet who sailed up the St. Lawrence to Tadoussac in 1600 A.D. as surgeon of Chauvin's fleet (Abbott 1931). In 1608, Bonnerme accompanied Champlain to Québec City and thus became its first surgeon, but died the following year from either scurvy or dysentery.

Dr. Michel Sarazin was appointed in 1689 by King Louis XIV to be the Royal Physician at the French garrison in Québec (Swan 1966). Later he became the official physician of the Hotel-Dieu Hospital in present day Québec City. He was also a member of the Académie des sciences de Paris and sent back hundreds of plants and bulbs that he collected around the Gulf of St. Lawrence near Montréal and Québec City. In fact, Sarazin is recognized as one of Canada's premier botanists, and by the time he died in 1734 he had compiled close to 175 works, including the popular "Catalogue et histoire des plantes du Canada."

The earliest example of an insurance-based health care service in Canada can be traced backed to the seventeenth century in Ville-Marie, Québec (Bartfay and Bartfay 2015). A master surgeon, Dr. Bouchard offered his patients a health care agreement that could be renewed on an annual basis, and which he could withdraw if he cured his patients' ailments. Indeed, this would be regarded as a form of health care *"utopia"* for any health care provider today. According to Swan (1966), Bouchard was a master surgeon who undertook to provide full medical care services to a number of families in Ville-Marie (i.e., Montréal) for the sum of $1.00 per family per annum in 1655. It is interesting to note that his contract exempted him from providing his patients with medicines and also from treating certain conditions and diseases including the plague, smallpox, epilepsy, and kidney stones.

Early Outbreaks and Epidemics

The early European settlers exposed Indigenous people to infectious diseases which had not been known to them previously, including smallpox, typhoid, measles, diphtheria, and tuberculosis (Library and Archives Canada 2007a). In the year 1710, an outbreak of yellow fever called *"Mal de Siam"* struck Canada as a consequence of the *stegomyia* mosquitoe migrating north from New Orleans (Swan 1966). By 1720, Canada had established its first quarantine laws due to an outbreak of bubonic plague carried to our Canadian shores by rat-infested ships sailing from the Mediterranean.

During the eighteenth century, there was a curious epidemic amongst Scottish troops in Nova Scotia called *"la mal de la Baie St. Paul,"* which was in fact extragenital syphilis (Swan 1966). It was deemed a highly contagious disease that was treated aggressively with corrosive sublimate mercury, and later it was believed that some of the symptoms experienced were due to the treatment rather than to the infection itself. Upper Canada (Ontario) and Lower Canada (Québec) established boards of health between 1832 and 1833, respectively. These boards of health were mandated with enforcing quarantine and sanitation laws; stopping the sale of spoiled and rancid foods, and imposing restrictions on immigration to help prevent the spread of disease (Thompson 2010). During the nineteenth century, tuberculosis (TB) became a national health care issue, and it was especially prominent amongst Indigenous peoples (Swan 1966). In 1896, the Prince of Wales wrote to Lord Minto, the Governor General in Canada, to express his concern for the health of Canadians. This epidemic subsequently resulted in the formation of the Canadian Tuberculosis Society.

During the early 1900s, the provinces began to establish their first formally organized public health bureaus. For example, bureaus of public health were established in Saskatchewan in 1909; Alberta in 1918; Manitoba in 1928; and Nova Scotia in 1931 (Thompson 2010). These public health bureaus were responsible for overseeing a variety of public health activities including the pasteurization of milk, testing cattle for TB, managing TB sanatoriums, and controlling the spread of sexually transmitted infections (STIs) through various public health education efforts and venereal disease (VD) clinics (Bartfay and Bartfay 2015). Physicians and nurses also provided immunization clinics and maternal health education to those in need.

British North America Act (1867)

With the passage of the British North America (BNA) Act (renamed the Constitution Act in 1982), Confederation became a reality with Sir John A MacDonald as the first prime minister of the "*Dominion of Canada*" (Thompson 2010). The BNA Act was first drafted at the Québec Conference in 1864 and passed without amendments by the British Parliament in 1867. It was subsequently signed by Queen Victoria in England on March 29, 1867 and came into effect on July 1, 1867. The BNA Act united the three colonies of the time, which consisted of the British province of Canada comprised of Ontario (Upper Canada) and Québec (Lower Canada) in 1841; Nova Scotia, and New Brunswick (Bartfay 2010a; Government of Canada 2007a). Manitoba joined Confederation in 1870, followed by British Columbia in 1871, and Prince Edward Island in 1873. Alberta and Saskatchewan were given provincial status in 1905, and formally independent Newfoundland joined Confederation as Canada's tenth province in 1949 (Bartfay 2010a). Canada currently consists of ten provinces and the three territories of Yukon, Northwest Territory and Nunavut. In 1982, Canada moved to formally patriot its Constitution and become a sovereign nation with a royal proclamation from her Majesty Queen Elizabeth II.

When Sir John A. MacDonald and our other Fathers of Confederation set out the terms of the BNA Act (1867), they had no idea how industrialization, urbanization, global warming or the environment, might affect the health and well-being of our

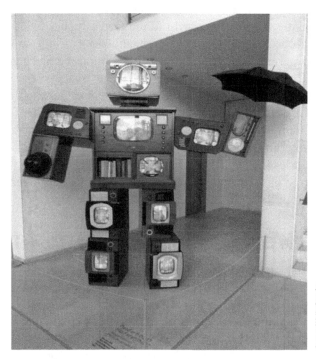

Source: Wally Bartfay.

Photo 3.4 The medical model of health comprehends the human body as a contraption or apparatus similar to a robot, in which all components or parts are interconnected but are capable of being replaced or treated separately and therefore in isolation by various specialists (e.g., cardiologists treats the malfunctioning heart; nephrologists treats the malfunctioning kidney, and the hepatologists treats the malfunctioning liver). Health is achieved when all the biological components or parts of the body function properly.

residents across the lifespan (Storch 2006; Wallace 1950). Although the BNA Act of 1867 did not mandate health care responsibility to either federal or provincial/ territorial jurisdictions per se, historically both levels of government in Canada have been involved and continue to be entwined in health care matters. The only reference to a health care theme in the BNA Act of 1867 are found in Sections 91 and 92, which defines the jurisdictions and responsibilities of the federal and provincial governments, respectively (Shah 2003).

Specifically, Section 91 of the Act describes the role of the federal government in economic matters including taxation, regulation of trade, external affairs, defense, criminal law, powers of reservations and disallowance, immigration, and quarantine. Section 92 of the Act describes the responsibilities of provincial governments, which include inter alia education, civil law, agriculture, and social welfare. Subsequent interpretations of Section 91 gave the provinces and territories in Canada jurisdiction over most health services. The federal government maintained jurisdiction for health related matters for Indigenous peoples, members of the Royal Canadian Mounted Police, veterans, military personnel, and inmates in federal prisons.

The first census in the new Dominion of Canada took take place in 1871, which showed a total population of 3,689,257 a population large enough to warrant growing concerns for delivering public health care services (Thompson 2010). From 1867 to 1919, Chenier (1999) reports that the Department of Agriculture covered all federal related health matters and concerns. The Department of Health was created in 1919 by the federal government largely in response to the increase in sexually transmitted infections (STIs) and the growing recognition for the importance of keeping children healthy and safe (Thompson 2010). In 1928, the Department of Health became known as National Health, and in 1944 the name was changed again to the Department of National Health and Welfare (Bartfay 2010a). The mandate of the federal government expanded to include food and drug control, the development of public health programs, the operation of the Laboratory of Hygiene and health care for members of the civil service (Thompson 2010).

During the 1990s, the Department of National Health and Welfare was renamed to Health Canada. Currently, the federal government is responsible for providing health care to members of the Canadian Armed Forces, Federal inmates in prisons, members of the Royal Canadian Mounted Police (RCMP), veterans and they also provide temporary health insurance for refugee claimants and their dependents under the Interim Federal Health (IFH) program (Bartfay 2010a; Thompson 2010). We shall explore the role of the federal and provincial/territorial governments in providing primary health care services in more detail in the following sections below.

The Emergence of the Medical Model of Health

This section highlights the evolution of the laboratory-based medical model of health for establishing disease causation and how it has shaped medical education, training and clinical practice during the past century. We shall also explore how physicians have subsequently emerged as gatekeepers to access diagnostic, laboratory, and other episodic health care services largely provided in acute care hospitals in Canada. A fundamental understanding of this model is critical to comprehend how it has served as the basis for subsequent publically funded models of health care in Canada and associated legislations.

Early eighteenth century is characterized as a period where medical quackery often flourished due to a lack of standardized education and training by those who employed the title of "*doctor of medicine*" (Library and Archives Canada 2007a). To help improve medical standards, an ordinance was passed in 1750 that declared that all medical practitioners where required to undertake an exam in the presence of the King's Physician in England (Swan 1966). Many physicians arrived in Canada as immigrants from the United Kingdom and the United States during the late eighteenth and early nineteenth centuries. In 1823, the first medical school was established at McGill University in Montréal, to help further standardize medical education and training in Canada. In 1853, Dr. Rolfe subsequently found the medical school at the University of Toronto, and by the end of the nineteenth century there were an additional nine medical schools established in Canada (Swan 1966).

Although public health efforts (e.g., sanitation, food inspections, and clean water supplies) were bringing about remarkable changes to the health of populations, the increased use of anesthetics and the increasing awareness of disease causing microorganisms led to the establishment of medical schools which emphasized a *one-to-one* practice mandate in North America and abroad (Swanson and Albrecht 1993). Many of these medical schools were funded by wealthy patrons or philanthropic organizations such as the Rockefeller and Carnegie Foundations.

During the 1850s, students enrolled in medical schools in Canada attended formal lectures, but received very little instruction in laboratory settings (Library and Archives Canada 2007a, b). It wasn't until the mid-1870s when Sir Dr. William Osler, the chair of the medical school at McGill University, revolutionized scientific medical education worldwide by introducing the use of microscopes and dissection into his anatomy classes and bedside teaching. Dr. Osler also helped to introduce a system of postgraduate medical training and education, which still remains a standard in North America and abroad today (Library and Archives Canada 2007b). In 1892, Dr. Osler wrote the landmark textbook in scientific medicine entitled "*The Criteria's and Practice of Medicine: Designed for the Use of Practitioners and Students of Medicine*." This textbook became the standard textbook for over 40 years and was subsequently translated into French, German, Spanish, and Chinese (Library and Archives Canada 2007b).

The Flexner Report (1910)

During the late nineteenth century, there were over 400 privately owned medical schools founded in the United States, which lacked standardized training requirements and curriculums (Greifinger and Sidel 1981). In 1910, the Flexner Report was commissioned by the Carnegie Foundation, which outlined the shortcomings of medical schools in the United States and Canada including their lack of standardized curriculums, graduation credentials, and inconsistent or inadequate education and training (Swanson and Albrecht 1993). It is interesting to note that this report was written by Abraham Flexner who was a school master by occupation, and had no formal medical training or education (Armstrong and Armstrong 2004; Moskop 1981). Despite this noted shortcoming, Flexner visited a total of 155 medical colleges in the United States and Canada and claimed that he could assess in a matter of hours whether the school met "*scientific standards*" or not. As a consequence of his report, alternative schools of medicine were closed and the new scientific paradigm became the established universal standard and benchmark for medicine to follow.

The Flexner Report (1920) resulted in the withdrawal of funding by philanthropic organizations such as the Rockefeller and Carnegie Foundations, which triggered the closure of scientifically inadequate or substandard medical schools in North America (Swanson and Albrecht 1993). The report was also instrumental in subsequently establishing medicine as a recognized profession in Canada and the United States, which required formal education, training and a license to practice. A new breed of physicians was promulgated, which closely adhered to the single agent germ theory of disease causation. Hence, the curriculum and training focus was dominated by the laboratory-based disease causation model of health; as opposed to the prevention of disability, caring for the whole person (holistic model), or on rehabilitative therapies (Greinfinger and Sidel 1981).

Medical Breakthroughs by Canadians

Despite the noted shortcomings of the medical model of health and education, it is also important to acknowledge that this approach or paradigm did result in significant advances in medicine during the twentieth and twenty-first centuries (Bartfay and Bartfay 2015). In fact, there are numerous contributions and medical breakthroughs made by Canadians and other physician scientists, which are beyond the scope and purpose of this chapter (e.g., x-rays, internal pacemaker, antibiotics, and anaesthesia). Nonetheless, two important breakthroughs are provided which exemplify how the pioneering work of Canadians has benefited individuals on a global scale.

The first is the discovery of insulin by Sir Dr. Frederick Banting, who is regarded as the principal discoverer of insulin through his laboratory-based research on the pancreas of beagles (Library and Archives Canada 2007a, d; Swan 1966). In 1923, Dr. Banting and his fellow researcher J. J. R. Macleod were awarded the Novel Prize in physiology, which he chose to share with his partner Charles Best (Swan, 1966). In 1934, Dr. Banting was amongst the last group of Canadians to be knighted by King George V for his discovery of insulin that has saved countless lives for individuals afflicted with diabetes worldwide (Library and Archives Canada 2007a, d).

The second example is the discovery of a revolutionary surgical intervention for the treatment of severe epilepsy by Dr. Wilder Penfield, known as the *"Montréal Procedure"* (Library and Archives Canada 2007c). Penfield would first administer a local anaesthetic and subsequently remove the skull cap to expose the brain while his patients were still awake and conscious. Penfield would probe the brain and ask his patients to describe their feelings and sensations to identify the exact location in the brain where the seizure was believed to originate. He would then surgically remove the affected tissue. Remarkably during this period, the Montréal Procedure was reported to be apparently successful in more than half of the patients he operated on. This technique also allowed Penfield to create the first detailed anatomical maps of the sensory and motor portions of the human brain.

In 1934, with a generous grant from the Rockefeller Foundation, Penfield founded the world renowned Montréal Neurological Institute. The institute today continues to provide state of the art treatments for various patients with neurological disorders and cutting edge scientific research (Library and Archives Canada 2007a, c). Penfield's pioneering work earned him many honours including the *"Companion of the Order of Canada"* in 1967, and induction into the Canadian Medical Hall of Fame in 1994 (Library and Archives Canada 2007c).

Shift from Home and Community to Hospital-Based Health Services

This section explores how the adoption and the increased reliance on the medical model of health have resulted in a shift of health care practice settings from the home and community to acute care hospitals. We shall explore the major driving forces, including the increased costs of associated laboratory and diagnostic technologies, and the increased demand for other health care professionals such as nurses to provide health care services in acute care hospital settings. Lastly, we shall explore the implications for public health and discuss why there is a growing need and recognition to provide primary health services in the home and community settings.

The growth of the laboratory-based medical model of health during the nineteeth and twentieth centuries with its increased reliance on technology (e.g., x-rays, electrocardiograms, and laboratory blood tests) to make clinical diagnosis resulted in a shift of practice settings from private homes and community settings to hospitals (Bartfay and Bartfay 2015). Storch (2006) reports that during the early 1920s, medical and surgical procedures that were previously performed at private medical offices or the patient's home were increasingly being performed in hospitals, and this amplified the demand for hospital-based physicians and nurses. Following World Wars I and II, many of the new medical technologies (e.g., x-ray machines and blood tests) were introduced in North America. The average physician could not afford these new diagnostic test equipment and technologies in their private practice (Storch 2006). Accordingly, hospitals became the logical plate for physicians to access these new tools of the trade, and this also increased the need and demand for nurses in this newly centralized practice setting.

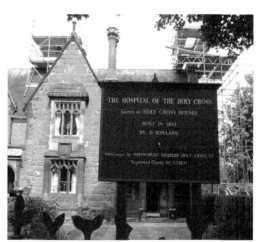

Source: Wally Bartfay.

Photo 3.5 The nineteenth century marks a turning point for the function of hospitals as places to house and care for the sick and feeble to training centres for nursing and medical students and centres of innovation, research, and discovery.

Stinson (1969) argues that the private duty nurse of the 1920s was a "near paragon of solo practice" (p. 333), in comparison to the hospital-based nurse of the 1960s. Indeed, public health and private duty nurses during the 1920s were rarely supervised by physicians or other nurses, and were quite autonomous in terms of their practice and interventions performed (Bartfay 2010b Bartfay and Bartfay 2015). Historically in Canada, nurses were hired by individuals and families to provide nursing services in their home environments.

Visiting district or public health nurses also provided nursing services in town or country districts that were organized at both the national and local levels (Gibbon 1947; Gibbon and Mathewson 1947). The Victorian Order of Nurses (VON) is perhaps the best known of these, and was founded in 1897 (Gibbon 1947; Gibbon and Mathewson 1947). Nurses in Canada also practiced in a variety of district or public health settings. Coburn (1988) notes that by 1948, approximately 65% of nurses were working in hospitals, in comparison to only 35% in 1930. Similarly, it has been estimated that up to 60% of all nurses in Canada were self-employed in private duty settings prior to World War II (Baumgart and Wheeler 1992; Canadian Nurses Association 1996).

The arrival of Medicare in Canada during the 1950s and 1960s also increased the demand for acute care hospital-based nursing services. By 1955, there were 1,216 publicly subsidized hospitals across Canada, which further amplified public demand for physician driven hospital-based health care services based on the medical model of health. Armstrong and Armstrong (2003) argue that there was little public critique of the methods employed by physicians and by guaranteeing payment for hospital-based health care services, governments at various levels were consolidating and reinforcing the power and monopoly of physicians in Canada at the time.

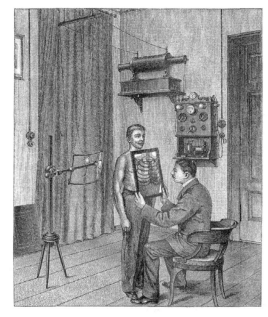

Photo 3.6 Diagnostic (e.g., X-rays, ECGs) and laboratory-based (e.g., CBC's, cell cultures for bacteria) tests became too expensive for the average physician to afford in their private practice, so physicians and subsequently nurses relocated to hospitals were these health care services were becoming increasingly centralized during the 19th and 20th centuries.

© Hein Nouwens/Shutterstock.com

Not surprisingly, the proportion of nurses working in community-based settings or as private home nurses, quickly diminished. By the early 1950s, these subsidized hospital-based health care reforms initiated by the federal government quickly increased the number of salaried nurses in acute care hospitals to approximately 65% (Coburn 1988). Stinson (1969) reports that the nurse of the 1960s had far more responsibility but less autonomy in the technology-laced hospital settings, and had many "*masters*" including physicians, hospital administrators (who were typically physicians themselves), and nursing supervisors (i.e., head nurses). By 1989, approximately 85% of all nurses were employed by acute care hospitals, and only 15% chose to engage in private practice or public health nursing (CIHI 2006b; Richardson 1997). There are presently over 268,500 registered nurses across Canada (National Expert Commission Canadian Nurses Association 2012), and the majority (>85%) of these continue to work in acute care hospital settings, as opposed to community-based or home settings. Currently, there is an increased desire to reintroduce the emphasis of home and community-based primary health care services in Canada (Bartfay and Bartfay 2015). We shall explore the effects of the various federal transfer payment schemes to the provinces and territories for publicly insured health care services based on the medical model of health in greater detail in the following sections below.

It has been argued that physicians still dominate our health care systems in Canada and exercise tremendous power and influence over how provincial and territorial governments fund "*medically necessary*" publicly insured health services (Armstrong and Armstrong 2003; Armstrong, Armstrong, and Coburn, 2001; Bartfay and Bartfay 2015). They also exercise a great deal of control, power and influence on how other public health care professionals practice. According to Whittaker (1984), nurses in Ontario were the first who attempted to gain control over the practice domains of physicians through certification and registration in 1905, but were blocked by provincial and federal medical associations in Canada until the 1950s. More recently, the Ontario Medical Association successfully lobbied the provincial government to eliminate payment for services performed by rehabilitation therapists and audiologists unless they work under the supervision of and in the same premises as physicians (Boyle 2001).

Moreover, the province of Ontario's pilot program entitled "Family Health Networks" have failed to hire significant numbers of nurse practitioners (NPs), who are trained to perform many of the tasks traditionally performed by family physicians (a.k.a, general practitioners), despite the shortage of physicians in many parts of the province. It is noteworthy that although 160 physicians were hired in Ontario to service these Family Health Networks, only seven NPs were hired according to a PricewaterhouseCoopers report commissioned by the provincial government (Mackie 2001). In 2010, there was renewed interested by the Minister of Health in Ontario to promote such primary care models of health, including NP-led clinics in underserviced regions of the province. Indeed, NP-led clinics offer a team-based approach to frontline health care services by collaborating with physicians and other health care professionals.

In fact, it can be argued that despite the need and growth of NP's, family physicians remain the major "*gatekeepers*" for accessing health care services (e.g., diagnostic imaging, blood tests) and other specialists (e.g., cardiologists, dermatologists, and neurosurgeons) in Canada (Bartfay and Bartfay 2015; Browne et al. 2012; Health Council of Canada 2010, 2011; National Expert Commission Canadian Nurses Association 2012; Starfield 2011). According to the September 27, 2010, news release by John G. Abbott, CEO of the Health Council of Canada, family physicians continue to act as the primary gatekeepers for diagnostic and health care services in Canada because of the way that our Medicare systems have evolved overtime (Abbott 2010). For examples, they act as gatekeepers in terms of obtaining prescription medications by clients, referrals to other medical specialists (e.g., cardiologists, orthopedic surgeon, neurologists, and psychiatrists), and to a variety of imaging and diagnostic procedures (e.g., ultrasounds, CT scans, mammograms, and blood tests) (Abbott 2010). The current fee–for–service payment systems set up by the various provincial and territorial governments also helps to reinforce this gatekeeper model for accessing publicly insured diagnostic and health care services in Canada.

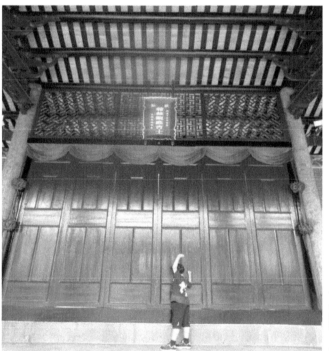

Source: Wally Bartfay.

Photo 3.7 A huge closed door used to symbolize the inability, powerlessness, and frustration of clients to access various publicly funded health care and/or diagnostic and imaging services without being first cleared by a physician who acts as "gatekeepers" to these vital amenities.

Redefining the Federal Governments Role in Health

A shift from the home and community to hospital-based health care from the 1920s and onwards, has created a growing public need for a more standardized and universal approach to access and receive health services in Canada (Bartfay 2010a; Bartfay and Bartfay 2015). A growing number of social and political movements have advanced this agenda over time. A number of grassroots movements have argued that a more equitable and stable funding mechanism would exist if the federal government spearheaded this social agenda related to access and affordable health care for all residents despite their social standing or income levels (Bartfay 2010a; Thompson 2010). As a consequence of these grassroots movements, Prime Minister Mackenzie King was the first to historically include a national health care insurance plan as part of his federal governments' platform in the year 1919 (Rachlis and Kushner 1994; Thompson 2010). Nonetheless, King's attempt to conceive a national health care insurance plan to cover both hospital and physician services was initially not successful due to vocal opposition by provincial and territorial governments.

Employment and Social Insurance Act (1935)

In 1935, Prime Minister R. B. Bennett pledged to address a variety of social issues such as minimum wage, unemployment, and public health insurance as part of his government's agenda (Thompson 2010). On the advice of the Royal Commission on Industrial Relations, Bennet's Conservative government presented the *Employment and Social Insurance Act*. Under this proposed Act, the federal government would gain the right to collect taxes to provide certain Canada wide social programs including unemployment insurance and health (Bartfay 2010b; Shah 2003). The provinces collectively revolted because they felt that it infringed on their provincial/territorial jurisdictions, and they subsequently took the matter to the British Privy Council for a constitutional ruling.

In 1937, the British Privy Council ruled that Bennett's proposal was *"ultra vires,"* meaning it was outside of the federal government's jurisdiction and mandate. This landmark ruling is important because it resulted in the first formal ruling that health was, in fact, a provincial/territorial responsibility (Bartfay 2010a). The Employment and Social Insurance Act was also deemed unconstitutional by the Supreme Court of Canada on the grounds that it violated provincial and territorial responsibility (Thompson 2010; Shah 2003). Nonetheless, the federal and provincial/territorial governments did subsequently agree to amend the BNA Act (1867) in 1940 to allow for the introduction of a national unemployment insurance program, which became fully operational in 1942 (Thompson 2010).

Marsh and Heagerty Reports (1943)

The Great Depression of the 1930s and World War II resulted in a shift in the growing public belief that governments should be responsible for providing their citizens and residents with a reasonable standard of living and acceptable access to basic services including health care, irrespective of their social standing or income levels (Thompson 2010). In 1939, the Minister for the Department of Pensions and National Health, Ian MacKenzie, wrote a letter to Prime Minister King "urging that unemployment and health insurance be introduced as war measures" and outlined the reasons why our nation required a national public health care system for our returning troops (Taylor 1987, p. 16). MacKenzie's arguments were persuasive and powerful because he carefully outlined in his report the fact that other countries were already developing such programs for their returning troops and citizens (Bartfay 2010a). MacKenzie commissioned Dr. J. J. Heagerty who was the Director of Public Health Sciences to develop a proposal for a national health insurance program. Dr. Heagerty established the Inter-Departmental Advisory Committee on Health Insurance that included representatives from all his provincial counterparts (Storch 2006; Taylor 1987).

Meanwhile, Leonard Marsh who was the Director of Social Research at McGill University in Montréal, was hired as an expert consultant by the federal government on post-war construction (1944–1945) (Storch 2006; Taylor 1987). Marsh's (1943) report entitled *"Report on Social Security for Canada"* is regarded by many authorities as the single most important document for the development of the postwar welfare state in Canada (Bliss 1975; Marsh 1975; Rice and Prince 2000; Taylor 1973). Marsh (1975) argued that the public social safety net in Canada embodied the collective pooling of risks for all involved.

Jointly, the 1943 reports by Heagerty and Marsh solidified postwar public sentiment in Canada and idealism including the right for freedom of citizens as detailed in the Atlantic Charter (March 1975; Taylor 1973). These reports also served as blueprints for the development of various national social insurance and health programs (Bartfay 2010a). For example, in 1944, the federal government introduced family allowances for each child under the age of 16, which was commonly referred to as the "*baby bonus*" by Canadians (Thompson 2010). Research Focus Box 3.1 describes a current investigation examining the social and health care challenges faced by women living on social assistance in the provinces of Saskatchewan and Manitoba employing a participatory research design. This investigation suggests that women who are dependent on provincial welfare programs for income are at higher risk for experiencing negative social and health effects including increased levels of stress and anxiety and housing and subsistence concerns, in comparison to similar individuals who are not social assistance.

Saskatchewan's Pioneering Health Care Reforms

Since the 1940s, Canadians have advanced the belief and public opinion that they do not want health care systems that are based on income versus need, or ones that are driven by the profit-driven corporate model of health (Armstrong and Armstrong 2003; Villeneuve and MacDonald 2006). The Ontario Coalition of Senior Citizens' Organizations has documented numerous testimonials and stories of suffering, pain, and death resulting from being poor and not being able to afford health care services prior to Medicare (Heeney 1995). For example, one Canadian woman described her experience of having her baby born at home as follows:

Research Focus Box 3.1

Saskatchewan Social Welfare Policy and Women's Health

Study Aim/Rationale
The aim of this study was to examine the effects of current social assistance policies on the health and well-being of women in the provinces of Saskatchewan and Manitoba.

Methodology/Design
The investigators employed a qualitative participatory action research approach to evaluate the impact of provincial social assistance policies and programs on the health of women. Data were collected from seven focus groups comprised of women from Indigenous, urban and rural communities in the provinces of Saskatchewan and Manitoba. All study participants were living on social assistance in their province of residence. Thematic analysis of the qualitative data collected from these seven focus group meeting were undertaken to identify the emerging themes and areas of concern.

Major Findings
Findings from this study suggest that women who are currently dependent on provincial social assistance experience high levels of stress and anxiety in meeting fundamental daily requirements for living. These stressors include basic nutritional needs (food); access to safe and affordable housing; affordable transportation; access to public health care services, and medications. Disruptions related to schooling on education that resulted from the need to move frequently due to high cost of living, were of particular concern to the respondents.

Implications for Public Health
The findings suggests that participatory research appears to be a valuable tool to qualitatively examine current health challenges faced by women living on social assistance from diverse backgrounds. The finding from the focus groups were subsequently summarized in an official report sent the provincial ministers responsible for welfare policies. The investigators challenged policymakers in their report to live on social assistance themselves in order to experience firsthand the many social and health challenges faced by women in these provinces. Lastly, the findings also suggest that women who live on social welfare are at significantly higher risk for experiencing negative alterations to their health and well-being, in comparison to those who are not on social assistance.

Source: Kerr, Frost, and Bignell (2004).

The doctor didn't come to the house when they called because they still hadn't paid the bill from the first child. The baby had trouble eating and the baby's health got worse. When the baby was almost two months old, the family finally had enough money to take the child to the hospital. The initial minor problem with the baby's digestive system was diagnosed, but the treatment was too late. The baby was starving to death and not even intravenous fluids could save her at this late stage.

(Heeney 1995, p. 78)

Similarly, when a young man required surgery to straighten his back and reduce his pain and suffering after being inflicted with polio, one third of his cattle had to be sold to pay for the operation and associated hospital costs (Heeney 1995).

The Saskatchewan government enacted the Municipal and Medical Hospital Services Act in 1939. This Act permitted municipalities in the province to charge either a land tax or a personal tax to help support acute care hospital-based medical services in the province. The late premier of Saskatchewan, Tommy Douglas, understood firsthand the importance of access to public health services as a boy whose family suffered as a consequence of disease and disability (Margoshes 1999). Douglas was premier of Saskatchewan from 1944 to 1961, and believed that all citizens and residents in his province should have access to public health care services based on their need, as opposed to their income levels. In fact, during one point in his political career, Douglas appointed himself Health Minister in Saskatchewan to help bring about his vision for health insurance to all his residents in his province despite their social class or income level (Bartfay 2010a; Bartfay and Bartfay 2015).

Douglas' governing party, the Cooperative Commonwealth Federation (CCF), was the first to introduce a universal hospital-based social insurance plan for all residents of Saskatchewan in 1947 (Bartfay 2010a). The Hospital Insurance Act (1947) guaranteed permanent residents of Saskatchewan hospital-based medical services in exchange for a modest insurance premium payment (Thompson 2010). The CCF party also introduced an insurance scheme for physician services provided in 1957. Consequently, Douglas is credited for providing the foundations for a national publicly funded Medicare program in Canada (Hales and Lauzon 2007; Rachlis and Kushner 1994; Wilson 2002). In 1961, Douglas left Saskatchewan to lead the federal National Democratic Party (NDP) in Ottawa.

Douglas' successor, Premier Woodrow Lloyd passed the Saskatchewan *Medical Care Insurance Act* in 1961, and it was enacted in July, 1962 (Thompson 2010). This Act proposed that physicians be salaried health care professionals of their province. The Act enforced socialized medicine and imposed fee schedules, which prompted outrage by physicians. The Act subsequently resulted in provincial strike action by physicians in Saskatchewan which lasted 23 days, but it left a legacy of discontent (Thompson 2010). In August of 1962, the Saskatchewan government revised the Medical Care Insurance Act in an attempt to appease the physicians in the province. Hence, the strike action by physicians was successful since the government agreed that a third-party billing system should remain in place to provide compensation for their health services rendered (Storch 2006; Villeneuve and MacDonald 2006). Bartfay (2010a) reports that this system of billing is still in existence today and physicians largely remain self-employed health care entrepreneurs. By contrast, the majority of health care professionals and workers in public health organizations (e.g., public health nurses, health promoters, and epidemiologists) remain as salaried employees.

The health care reforms introduced in Saskatchewan also stimulated other provinces to establish their own publicly administered hospital insurance plans, and they lobbied the federal government to share some of the associated costs (Gelber 1966; Margoshes 1999). British Columbia shortly followed Saskatchewan by introducing its own version of a universal hospital insurance program in 1949. Newfoundland and Labrador joined Confederation in 1949 with the stipulation that they uphold their "*Cottage Hospital Medical Care Plan*" (1934). This plan was developed taking into consideration the unique geography of the region, and provided outport care by having nurses and physicians regularly visit remote communities by the sea. In 1950, the province of Alberta implemented their own health care plan (Shah 2003).

National Health Grants Act (1948)

The federal government recognized that they could not move forward unilaterally with a national health insurance plan or system due to constitutional rulings, as noted earlier. Consequently, federal politicians decided to advance their agenda by offering cash incentives to the provinces and territories to subsidize health care services rendered (Shah 2003). With this strategy, the federal government could influence the health care system of delivery nationally by imposing certain conditions and restrictions. In return, the federal government agreed to share the associated health care costs with the provinces and territories.

The *"National Health Grants Act"* of 1948, marked the start of the federal government's role in partially subsiding provincial and territorial health care services largely rendered by physicians via tax-based funds (Shah 2003). Specifically, this Act provided grants-in-aid to provinces and territories for an assortment of health related services and projects, which included the construction of new hospitals, laboratory services, and training of health care professionals (e.g., physicians and nurses). These grants were gradually replaced with the introduction of the Medicare system in Canada. Armstrong and Armstrong (2003) note that by 1955, there were 1,216 hospitals and 90% of these were classified as non-profit in nature. Nonetheless, these so-called non-profit hospitals still charged for their services and only 40% of residents in Canada had hospital-based health insurance plans. Individuals without hospital insurance plans often risked enormous personal debts and were typically those with the lowest household incomes and the poor.

Hospital Insurance and Diagnostic Services Act (1957)

Prime Minister John Diefenbaker was reluctant to commit to the long promised public health Medicare program because of the growing popularity of private health insurance plans in Canada and the increased availability of acute care hospital-based health services (Storch 2006; Taylor 1987). As an alternative to a costly national Medicare program, Diefenbaker decided to consult with the Canadian Medical Association (CMA) and took their advice to establish a Royal Commission on Health Services to study the matter in greater detail. The federal government subsequently appointed Justice Emmett Hall to head a Royal Commission on Health Services in Canada, who carefully examined the health care needs of Canadians and public opinion. Ironically, neither the CMA nor Diefenbaker believed or contemplated the possibility that this Royal Commission would be in favor of recommending the establishment of a publicly funded national Medicare program (Bartfay 2010a; Bartfay and Bartfay 2015).

The Hall Commission had two major recommendations in 1964 (Taylor 1973, 1987). First, that a nationwide publicly funded (taxed-based) health insurance plan be established and modeled on the Saskatchewan system. Second, that public health care insurance plans should be extended to include physician services administered outside of hospital settings. Hall also urged that the 145 private health insurance companies across Canada be replaced by provincial/territorial publicly funded health insurance plans (Thompson 2010). Hall also encouraged that the various governments in Canada prepare for the predicted increases in the number of seniors in Canada by increasing enrollments in professional schools (e.g., nurses, physicians, and dentists). For example, Hall recommended that the estimated 19,000 physicians at the time be doubled by 1990, otherwise the health care systems in Canada might be seriously compromised (Thompson 2010). Hall also argued that a Medicare system did not equate a socialized welfare benefit per se, but should be seen as an economic investment in Canada since healthy citizens meant a healthy economy. Add to your knowledge of Supreme Court Justice Emmett Hall's position for the need for a national health care program on a radio broadcast by accessing the Web-Based Resource Box 3.1.

Public opinion and support for a comprehensive Medicare program as outlined by Hall was overwhelming (Bartfay 2010a; Bartfay and Bartfay 2015). Major corporations and businesses in Canada were also in favor of some sort of national Medicare program because unions were becoming increasingly powerful and successful in demanding that their contracts cover medical insurance costs (Armstrong and Armstrong 2003). Indeed,

Web-based Resource Box 3.1   Radio Broadcast of Justice Emmet Hall

Learning Resource	Website
This web link provides access to the National Farm Radio Forum broadcast with Justice Emmett Hall making a case for national health care in Canada, November 2, 1964.	http://archieves.cbc.ca/ health_care_system/clips/447/

employers were not interested in sharing the cost of providing health care benefits for their employees, but were highly motivated in maintaining a healthy workforce. Fortunately, by the time Hall had finished his final report and recommendations, a new federal government under the leadership of Prime Minister Lester B. Pearson was elected (Storch 2006). Pearson could now make good on the Liberal's campaign promise of a Medicare program for all residents in Canada. Accordingly, the federal government agreed to reimburse provinces and territories for a portion of the costs associated with providing health care insurance under the "*Hospital Insurance and Diagnostic Services Act*" (HIDSA). As its name implies, its main purpose was to establish and maintain services and facilities that would lead to better health and access to health care services for the population as a whole.

The Act was subsequently passed by Parliament in 1957 and officially enacted in 1958 (Health Canada 2001, 2003; Rachlis and Kushner 1994). Under this Act, the provinces and territories would continue to direct their own health insurance plans, but the federal government would agree to cover half of the associated costs of specified health care services in hospitals. Five provinces immediately agreed to the terms of the Act. By 1961, HIDSA was operating in all the provinces and territories and covered approximately 99% of the population of Canada (Shah 2003). HIDSA proposed that any province or territory willing to implement a comprehensive hospital-based publicly insured health plan would receive federal assistance in the form of 50 cents on every dollar spent on the plan (Thompson 2010). Included in the insured health care costs were accommodation and meals for patients admitted to hospitals, necessary nursing services, laboratory and diagnostic services, medications provided to patients, and facility costs such as operating room costs, surgical supplies, radiology and physiotherapy (Babson and Brackstone 1973; Soderstrom 1978).

Not surprisingly, the cash-strapped provinces were receptive to HIDSA and enthusiastic to receive federal transfer payments to help support hospital-based health care services because it literally cut their associated costs by half. It is notable that although health care services administered in hospitals was broadly defined, this definition did not cover homes for the aged, nursing homes, tuberculosis hospitals and sanatoriums, or hospitals or institutions for the mentally ill (Soderstrom 1978; Babson and Brackstone 1973).

Medical Care Act (1966)

In 1965, the federal government appointed Emmett M. Hall, a Justice of the Supreme Court of Canada, to chair another Royal Commission on Health Services in Canada. The Commission reported that nearly 60% of residents had some form of private health insurance against the costs of medical care; however, 30% of those insured had inadequate coverage (Shah 2003). The commission recommended the need for strong federal government leadership and financial support for medical care, and that it should be decentralized under the jurisdiction of provincial governments.

After a series of discussions between the federal, provincial and territorial governments, the *Medical Care Act* was passed by Parliament in December of 1966, and implemented on July 1, 1968. The Medical Care Act and HIDSA collectively established a formula for federal transfer payments to the provinces and territories to help cover the cost of public hospital-based health insurance plans that employed a formula of 50 cents to the dollar (CIHR 2001; Deber 2000; Government of Canada 2002a). Each province and territory was free to administer their own public health insurance plans as long as it conformed to the criteria of the Act which included: *universality, portability, comprehensive coverage, and public administration.* These criteria mirror those outlined in the Canada Health Act, which we shall explore in greater detail in the following. However, this funding scheme drastically reduced home and community-based public health services and health promotion strategies nationally because funding was limited to physician-driven hospital-based acute care services (e.g., diagnostic imaging and laboratory tests, and surgeries). Consequently, community based health promotion and primary prevention programs provided by a variety of health care professionals and workers (e.g., school nurses, health promoters and educators) took a back seat to acute care hospital-based health care services.

It is not surprising, therefore, that health care costs quickly escalated since transfer payments from the federal government were restricted to acute care models of health driven by physician services and diagnostic procedures performed in hospitals. Thompson (2010) argues that the Medical Care Act reinforced the dominate position of the physician as the primary health care professional within this practice domain and the provincial/territorial health care systems of delivery. Hence, the services of any other health care professional (e.g., nurse, physiotherapists, audiologists) would be subject to a fee. Accordingly, acute care hospitals that were controlled and dominated by physicians became the primary location for accessing health care services by individuals throughout the lifespan. Not only did acute care hospitals continue to grow in response to increased access and use by residents, their associated provincial and territorial health care expenses also grew exponentially. For example, the use of costly emergency room facilities to get access to a variety of non-emergency health care services (e.g., prescription renewals, common cold, dietary advice related to constipation, and lifestyle counseling) by residents became a commonplace.

Health care institutions and clinics in Canada are typically classified as either private (e.g., Copeman Health Care Centre in Vancouver); territorially/provincially (e.g., Québec's CLSC system), or as non-profit in nature (e.g., university hospitals). To be eligible for publicly insured health care services, the person in need must be a lawful resident of a province or territory in Canada. Table 3.2 shows the names of various health care plans for

Table 3.2 List of Provincial and Territorial Health Care Plans in Canada

Province or Territory	Name of Public Health Care Insurance Plan	Ministries Responsible for Public Health Care
Newfoundland and Labrador	Newfoundland and Labrador Medical Care Plan	Health and Community Services
Nova Scotia	Medical Service Insurance	Department of Health
New Brunswick	Medicare	Department of Health
Prince Edward Island	Medicare	Department of Health
Québec	Assurance maladie (Medicare)	Santé et Services Sociaux
Ontario	Ontario Health Insurance Plan	Ministry of Health and Long-Term Care
Manitoba	Manitoba Health	Manitoba Healthy Living
Saskatchewan	Saskatchewan Medical Care Insurance Plan	Saskatchewan Health
Alberta	Alberta Health Care Insurance Plan	Alberta Health and Wellness
British Columbia	Medical Services Plan	Ministry of Health Services
Yukon	Yukon Health Care Insurance Plan	Yukon Health and Social Services
Northwest Territories (NWT)	NWT Health Care Plan	Department of Health and Social Services

the ten provinces and three territories in Canada. Typically, every province and territory in Canada issues its residents with its own health care identification card and negotiates with the federal government for funds to cover associated health care costs. By comparison, as many as 33 million Americans lack health insurance and one in three young adults between the ages of 18 and 24 years have no health insurance (Hales and Lauzon 2007).

Although the provinces of Ontario and Québec objected to the Act based on the grounds that it would have an impact on their provincial priorities, both provinces had health insurance plans in place by 1969 and 1970, respectively (Thompson 2010). The last jurisdictions in Canada to create health insurance plans were New Brunswick (1971); the Northwest Territories (1971); and Yukon (1972); (Thompson,2010). The creation of a Canada-wide Medicare program for hospital and physician services was established in 1972, when all provinces and territories decided to join this plan (Bartfay 2010a).

Federal Health Care Funding Arrangements

During the 1970s, health care costs continued to escalate, and by 1976 the total health expenditures in Canada exceeded $13 billion annually (Shah 2003). One may argue that these elevated costs were associated, at least in part, with a decreased emphasis on home and community-based health care services and primary health promotion initiatives and programs nationally. The provincial and territorial governments became increasingly dissatisfied with the fiscal arrangements because innovative health care initiatives, such as community-based services instead of general hospital care, were not cost shared with the federal government. In December of 1976, a consensus with both levels of government was reached at the First Ministers Conference to include certain extended health care services.

In March of 1977, the federal government decided to alter the 50/50 cost sharing formula to per capita block grants by passing the *Federal-Provincial Fiscal Arrangements and Established Programs Financing* (EPF) Act (Bartfay 2010a). These block grants consisted of a formula comprised of both cash and tax points to the provinces and territories generated every two months, as was relative to the gross national product (GNP) and population growth trends (Thompson 2010). Tax points consists of a basic redistribution in the amount of taxes the federal government charged the provinces and territories (Department of Finance Canada 2008; Government of Canada 2002b). The provinces and territories could now increase their own tax base to pay for any funding shortcomings associated with their own health care services.

In essence, residents of the ten provinces and three territories in Canada pay the same amount of taxes for these health care services; however, the tax money is distributed differently. This EPF Act gave the provinces and territories increased freedom due to fewer restrictions by the federal government on how they spent the block grants (e.g., community-based services). The EPF Act also permitted the transfer of funds for the Extended Health Care Services Program, which covered services as such ambulatory health care, some components of home care, and residential care in nursing homes related directed to health issues (e.g., administration of prescription medications) (Thompson 2010).

Within a few years after the introduction of the EPF Act, health care spending in Canada continued to increase dramatically and, in fact, grew faster than that of our GDP. Since the funding for the EPF was based on the GDP, the provinces and territories ended up paying for progressively larger amounts of the costs associated with these health care services (Department of Finance Canada 2008; Government of Canada 2002b). Nonetheless, this basic funding formula remained in place until the year 1996. Armstrong and Armstrong (2003) maintain that this funding scheme encouraged provinces to move as many individuals as possible out of expensive acute care institutions into the less expensive residential care facilities and/or private homes. In the latter case, care is often performed by female caregivers and relatives without financial compensation.

Hence, rather than challenge the dominant medical model of health care, this move reinforced it by defining those who were curable versus those who were incurable (Bartfay and Bartfay 2015). Moreover, those who were now labeled as incurable in nature apparently required less-skilled care by trained health care professionals. Accordingly, during the 1980s and onwards, acute care hospitals began to cut back on the number and types of health care services provided, the number of staff (especially nursing services), and the number of available hospital beds (Thompson 2010). Hospitals have been also discharging patients earlier based on hospital care formulas developed for a variety of medical procedures and interventions. For example, whereas mothers of newborn children used to stay two weeks or more following a Cesarean delivery during the 1960s, it is now common practice to send these mothers home after a few days (Makeover 1998; Spitzer 2000). Moreover, data from Ontario hospitals show that approximately 12% of the babies born without complications who were sent home early were readmitted within a month (Abraham 1999).

It may be argued that although advances in surgical treatments and technology have helped reduce the length of hospital recovery times for patients, they have not eliminated the need for skilled care and support following discharge from an acute care hospital or facility (Bartfay and Bartfay 2015). For example, specific tasks such as bathing a bedridden patient with paralysis or giving an injection for insulin are far more complicated then they may appear on the surface to skilled health care professionals. Hence, when certain patients are discharged early based on hospital treatment formulas, they may increase costs in the long-term by risking the health of prematurely discharged patients and other household members (e.g., back injuries, caregiver strain, and depression) (Airo et al. 2001; Chou et al. 1999; Rombough et al. 2006). Indeed, an increasing number of patients are being sent home who may still need physical assistance, medical treatments and/or social psychological support and care (Canadian Home Care Association 1998; National Forum on Health 1977). New immigrants to Canada, for example, may be living alone or be far away from family caregivers (Brotman 1998; Cranswick 1999). Similarly, various Indigenous peoples who live in rural or remote areas of Canada and homeless individuals may not have access to skilled care providers (Buchignani and Armstrong-Esther 1999; Cloutier-Fisher and Joseph 2000). The problems with early discharge formulas for individuals with complicated conditions are illustrated by an example offered to the Ontario Minister of Health by an organization representing seniors:

A man of 70, his left side paralyzed as the result of a former stroke, is rushed to the hospital to be treated for congestive heart failure and pneumonia. In the course of the treatment that saves his life, he is given a powerful antibiotic. Recovering in hospital, the man is too weak to sit up assisted and finds himself incontinent. He also develops a severe case of diarrhea, a not uncommon reaction to the antibiotic. Still, he is sent home to his apartment, where he lives *alone*.

(Henderson 1994, H5)

In accordance with the acute care hospital standards, this elderly man had been "*fixed and repaired*" and therefore could be safely discharged home into the community in accordance with normal discharge formulas and treatment models based on the medical model of health (Leduc Browne 2000; Makeover 1998). Money is saved by these institutions because the care is transferred from the hospital to the home, despite the fact that some patients may not have family members or loved ones to care for them. In the aforementioned example, an elderly neighbour attempted to help this 70-year-old man with his recovery but his condition deteriorated quickly, and was subsequently readmitted to another acute care hospital. The elderly man was also prescribed medications upon discharge to his home that the pharmacists claimed should be administered in a hospital. Moreover, these medications would cost approximately $1,000 since they were not covered by Medicare because they were to be given outside of an acute care hospital setting (Henderson 1994). By ignoring the determinants of health and by not taking into account a holistic view of the health care needs of this elderly man, not only was his health and well-being compromised, but the associated health care costs were also significantly increased. This example highlights the negative ripple effects experienced by one elderly man that resulted from premature discharge and the lack of home and community-based health care services to support seniors with complex health care needs.

Furthermore, a shorter hospital stay is not always a true or suitable indicator for either improved quality of health care services delivered, improved efficiency, or an accurate quantitative measure related to the effectiveness of the medical treatments or interventions performed in a facility. Decreased readmission rates to hospitals may also simply masks the greater reliance of early discharged patients on family members, or other health care services not covered by Medicare insurance programs in Canada (e.g., private home nurses, personal care assistants, and physiotherapists) (Canadian Home Care Association 1998; Fuller 2001; Glazer 1990; Yelaja 2001).

In addition to the aforementioned strategies to reduce rising health care costs in Canada, certain previously covered medical services have been delisted from provincial and territorial coverage, while others have been eliminated altogether in certain jurisdictions. As a consequence of these provincial and territorial cuts, many physicians were outraged and began to bill their patients over and above what their province or territory paid them between 1977 and 1978. This practice, known as *"extra-billing,"* resulted in swift public outrage, disapproval and hostility (Thompson 2010; Toughill 1992). Furthermore, the practice of extra-billing contradicts the criteria's of the Canada Health Act. We shall explore this Act and the impact of extra-billing patients for health care services in greater detail in the following sections below. Add to your knowledge of federal block transfer payments to the provinces and territories and the tax point system by accessing the links in the Web-Based Resources Box 3.2.

During the mid-1980s, the *Territorial Formula Financing (TTF) Act* was introduced in an attempt to replace a system comprised of annual block grants provided by the federal government to the three territories. The TTF is similar to provincial transfer plans since it enables the territories to provide a wide range of health services. In 2001–2002, the Federal Government transferred $510 million to the Northwest Territories; $611 million to Nunavut, and $346 million to Yukon (Department of Finance Canada 2002). In the last year of the EPF (1995–1996), a total of $22 billion in EPF entitlements (cash and taxes) were dispensed, the majority (71.2%) of which was intended for health care and the remainder for post-secondary education (Shah 2003). This arrangement was replaced by the CHST in 1996, which had similar provisions for use and transfer.

The EPF and the Canada Assistance Plan (CAP) for welfare were collectively replaced by the *Canada Health and Social Transfer fund* (CHST) in 1996 (Bartfay 2010a). Specifically, the federal government

Web-based Resource Box 3.2 Federal Block Transfer Payments and Tax Point System

Learning Resource	Website
Department of Finance Canada (2008). Tax points transfer. Ottawa, ON: Author. This website highlights how the Federal government employs a point system for the transfer of funds to support provincial/territorial Medicare programs.	http://www.fin.gc.ca/transfers/taxpoint/taxpoint-eng.asp
Government of Canada (2002). The transfer of tax points to provinces under the Canada health and social transfer. Ottawa, ON: Author. This website details how transfer payments to the provinces and territories are derived under the Act.	http://dsp-psd.tpsgc.gc.ca/Collection-R/LoPBdp/BP/bp450-e.htm

announced in their February, 1995 budget for the CHST an additional cut of $7 billion for health and social spending for the 1996–1997 fiscal years and another $4.5 billion in 1997–1998 (Stewart 1995). The federal planned cuts for health and social spending were met with antagonism and outrage by the opposition parties in Parliament and horror and anger by the public. Consequently, the federal government later rescinded and promised modest increases in spending for health and social services. Nonetheless, the CHST remained in place and made it next to impossible for citizens and residents of Canada to hold either the federal or provincial/territorial governments accountable for their levels of spending (Armstrong and Armstrong 2003).

The CHST is simply a block transfer fund paid by the federal government which includes payments for health care, welfare, and post-secondary education in Canada (Sullivan and Baranek 2002). Hence, with the CHST cash transfers for health care services to the provinces and territories continues to be combined with postsecondary education and social assistance payments. Moreover, the federal government continues to justify its cash transfers based on the estimate of the value of the tax point transfer scheme it introduced back in 1977. Shah (2003) reports that in the fiscal year 1995–1996 to 1996–1997, total CHST entitlements to the provinces decreased by nearly $3 billion dollars (approximately 10%), and was reduced by an additional $1.1 billion (approximately 5%) the following fiscal year. Consequently, provincial and territorial governments had to incrementally increase their own financial contributions over the decades to sustain and maintain their own health care systems.

Due to growing budgetary deficits during the 1990s and onwards, the federal government has responded by reducing transfer payments for health services and postsecondary education in Canada (Deber 2000; CIHR 2001; Government of Canada 2002). Shah (2003) reports that Bills C-96, C-69 and C-20 were enacted to freeze the cash flow to the provinces and represented a diminished presence and willingness of the federal government to enforce health care policies and legislations. Although it may appear that Canada has a national Medicare program, this is, in fact, incorrect. In reality, Canada has ten provincial and three territorial health care systems that are structured on federal guidelines and provide mainly sickness care dominated by physicians and the medical model of health.

Since the 2003 "*First Ministers' Accord on Health Care Renewal*" and the 2004 "*10-Year Plan to Strengthen Health Care*" (a.k.a., the *Health Accords*), the provincial and territorial governments have increased their annual health care spending by approximately $40 billion, from $85 billion in 2004 to approximately $220 billion in 2015 (CIHI 2015a, b; Health Council of Canada 2011). This translates into an annual average increase of 6.7%, although the costs vary by province and territory. Unlike equalization payments which are unconditional in nature, the Canada Health Transfer (CHT) is a block transfer fund that must be used by the provinces and territories for "maintaining the national criteria" for publicly funded health care in Canada, as outlined in the Canada Health Act (detailed in the following). The federal government introduced legislation which permitted an annual transfer increase of 6% per year through 2013/2014. The *10-Year Plan to Strengthen Health Care* expires at the end of the 2013–2014 fiscal year (Deraspe and Gauthier 2011; Government of Canada 2015b). As announced in 2011, total CHT funds are set in legislation to increase at a rate of 6% until 2016–2017. In 2017–2018, total cash CHT will increase in line with a three-year moving average of nominal GDP, with funding guaranteed to increase by at least 3% yearly. This transition affects provinces differently, depending on their level of per capita CHT cash relative to other provinces. During the years 2015–2016, the provinces and territories received $68 billion through major transfers, which included $34,026 billion for CHT payments; $12,959 for Canada Social Transfer funds; $17,341 for equalization funds, and $3,561 billion for Equalization and Territorial Formula Financing (Government of Canada 2015b).

The Canada Health Act (1982)

During the 1970s, there was increased public concern related to the rising costs of Medicare in Canada and the growth of private for-profit clinics (Bartfay 2010a). In addition, there was increasing concern by physicians related to the growth of socialized medicine in Canada, which they argued interfered with their doctor–patient relationships and that government cutbacks were interfering with their professional mandates (Storch 2006). There was also a growing trend by physicians across Canada to engage in the controversial practice of extra-billing or "*balance billing*" for compensation of medical health care services rendered since current Medicare funds were inadequate in their opinion (Bartfay 2010a; Bartfay and Bartfay 2015).

Monique Bégin, the federal Minister of Health and Welfare, believed that extra-billing; user-fees, and the growth of private for profit clinics and institutions in Canada posed a serious threat to the survival of Medicare. Accordingly, Bégin introduced to Parliament Bill C-3 on December, 1983, which is commonly referred to as the "*Canada Health Act*" (CHA) (Begin 2002; Mussalem 1992). Passage of the CHA by Parliament occurred in May 1982 and was enacted in April, 1984. The CHA received Royal Assent in June 1985 and is still in place today. It is interesting to note that the introduction of the Medicare program was radically opposed by physicians and the Canadian Medical Association because they were understandable pleased with the hospital-based insurance plans which they dominated and controlled (Storch 2006). Consequently, physicians took strike action to protest what they regarded as a slip into so-called "*socialized medicine*." Add to your knowledge of Canada's publicly funded and administered health care systems and Acts by accessing the links shown in Web-Based Resources Box 3.3.

The CHA replaced HIDSA and the Medical Care Act, and had the support of all federal political parties at the time. The Act's primary objective was to provide equal, prepaid (tax-based) and accessible health care to eligible residents of Canada (Thompson 2010). The CHA defines an eligible resident as a person who makes Canada their permanent home and one who resides in a province or territory, but does not include individuals such as tourists or transients (Government of Canada 1984). The primary objective of the CHA was to promote and restore physical and mental well-being of residents of Canada and to facilitate reasonable access to health services without financial or other barriers such as age, sex, income level, or social status (Health Canada 2004).

Since the introduction of Medicare in Canada, physicians in private practice were regarded as entrepreneurs who would bill their provincial/territorial Medicare insurance system for their medical services rendered (Bartfay 2010a; Bartfay and Bartfay 2015). Not surprisingly, an earlier version of Bill C-31 only identified physicians as providers of insurable health care services in Canada. However, intense lobbying by the Canadian Nurses Association (CNA) was instrumental in getting Bill C-31 amended and when the Act was finally passed by Parliament, it also recognized other health care professionals as potential providers

Web-based Resource Box 3.3 Publicly Funded and Administered Health Care Systems and Acts

Learning Resource	Website
Canada Health Act (CHA) This website provides an overview of the CHA	http://www.laws.justice.gc.ca/en/C-6/index.html
Canada Health Act: Federal Transfers and Deductions This website details the mechanisms for federal transfer payments and deductions related to the CHA	http://www.hc-sc.gc.ca/hcs-sss/medi-auur/cha-1cs/transfer-eng.php
Canada Health Act: Frequently Asked Questions (FAQ) This website provides an user-friendly explanation of various FAQs related to what the CHA is, its criteria and its intent.	http://www.hc-sc.gc.ca/hcs-sss/medi-assur/res/faq-eng.php.
Health Canada (2004): What is the Canada Health Act? This website details the five criteria of the CHA, and discusses items such as extra-billing.	http://www.hc-sc.gc.ca/hcs.sss.medi-assur/cha-1cs.oveview-apercu-eng.php)

of insurable health care services (Begin 2002; Mussalem 1992). Nonetheless, no province or territory to date has enacted legislation permitting nurses or other health care professionals to directly bill provincial or territorial health insurance plans. The CHA also included two provisions that discouraged the practice of extra-billing (or balanced billing) and/or user charges for health care services rendered under provincial or territorial publicly insured health services (Bartfay 2010a). The CHA also served as a legislative vehicle for facilitating access to public health care services by residents of Canada without financial or other social barriers. The Act, in fact, helped to reaffirm national values and principles held dear by Canadians, including the right to health care for all regardless of their social status or ability to pay (Bartfay 2010a; Bartfay and Bartfay 2015).

The CHA established five founding criteria's for the delivery of health care services in Canada (see Figure 3.1), and two additional conditions related to information and recognition (Government of Canada 1984; Health Canada 2001, 2003; Library of Parliament 2005). The CHA clearly set out the five criteria's of health care in Canada, while bringing together hospital and medical insurances together into one comprehensive package. However, with the passage of the CHA the federal government had less and less control over health care issues and diminished power to ensure that the founding criteria's were indeed being respected. These new funding arrangements were not based on the scrutiny of provincial health care budgets, but were based on populations, economic trends and past performances. Consequently, the federal government could not assess whether or not services were being universally provided to all in need, accessible, comprehensive, portable in nature and administered by a non-profit organization (Armstrong and Armstrong 2003). We shall explore these five founding criteria's and conditions in greater detail in the following.

Federal and Provincial/Territorial Responsibilities Under the CHA

Health Canada (2003, 2001) reports that the federal government is responsible for administering the Canada Health Act, and ensuring that the five founding criteria's are respected and adhered to by all the provinces and territories (Section 22). The federal government is also responsible for providing direct health care services to Indigenous peoples in Canada, military personnel and veterans, the Royal Canadian Mounted Police, and inmates serving time in federal penitentiaries throughout Canada (Bartfay 2010a; Bartfay and Bartfay 2015).

Conversely, the 10 provincial and 3 territorial governments are responsible for the direct delivery of their health care systems, health care management including planning and financing, and the evaluation of health care services that they provide to their residents (Health Canada 2003, 2001). These provincial and territorial governments are also responsible for managing physician and health care services provided by other

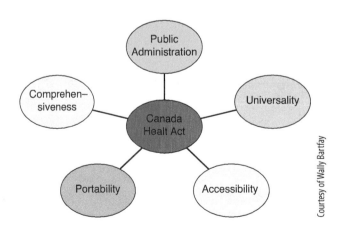

Figure 3.1 Conceptual diagram showing the five founding criteria's of the Canada Health Act

professionals (e.g., nurses, physiotherapists, rehabilitation and speech therapists), public and community health, and may also manage some components of prescription care available in their jurisdiction (Health Canada 2003, 2001; Government of Canada 1984).

The first condition of "*information*" in the CHA means that each province and territory must provide the federal government with information about their insured health care services rendered for the purposes identified in the Act. The second condition of "*recognition*" means that each province and territory must publicly recognize the federal contributions made to both insured and extended health care services (Thompson 2010). In addition, the 10 provinces and 3 territories must adhere to these criteria and conditions (in theory), if they are to receive transfer payments from the federal government for health care services rendered in their jurisdictions (Library of Parliament 2005). The Act also includes two provisions which discourage the practice of extra-billing and/or user charges for services covered under provincial and territorial health care insurance plans.

Public administration

The first criteria declares that health care is the responsibility of territorial and provincial governments, and therefore must be subject to regular public audits of how it is administered (Section 8). This criterion also states that health care services provided to residents and citizens in Canada must be administered and operated on a non-profit basis by a public authority (Health Canada 2001, 2003; Government of Canada 1984, 2007b). In other words, the provincial/territorial public health insurance plans must not be governed by a private enterprise or operated as a for-profit business. The public authority answers directly to the provincial/territorial government about its decisions to reimburse health care services rendered, and must also kept detailed records and accounts that are publicly audited (Thompson 2010). This criterion, however, gives each province and territory autonomy and flexibility in terms of determining its own administrative arrangements for its Medicare insurance plans and financing plans (e.g., sale taxes and other revenue mechanisms, premiums).

Comprehensiveness

The criteria of comprehensiveness states that residents of Canada should be allowed to access insured medical services provided by physicians and hospitals, and select services provided by dental surgeons (Thompson 2010). Moreover, these services should be made available to all residents of the province or territory and all insured individuals must be given equal opportunity to seek these insured health care services without barriers to access.

Section 2 of the Act provides a list of all health care services that the provinces and territories must insure. In accordance with their own laws, the territories and provinces could also insure additional public health care services deemed necessary or essential for the health of their residents (e.g., Pharmacare for individuals on social assistance) (Shah 2003). The criteria of comprehensiveness (Section 9) declares that the specific provincial and territorial health care insurance plans must cover all insured health services provided by hospitals, physicians, or dental surgeons performing "*necessary procedures*" in hospitals, as detailed in Section 2 of the Act (Health Canada 2001, 2003; Government of Canada 1984, 2007b). At a minimum, the intent was to cover all necessary medical services rendered by a medical practitioner, without exclusions or monetary limits.

Shimo (2006) reports that the differing levels of private care from province to province are part of a function of how open provincial and territorial governments are to private medicine and clinics. Indeed, private clinics are not illegal per se under the CHA, providing they do not charge patients for so–called "*medically necessary*" services rendered. However, what is considered medically necessary has changed overtime and become more difficult to clearly define. Indeed, why else would an individual need a hip replacement or a new knee if they were not necessary? However, a growing number of private clinics have started using this grey area of the law to muddle that distinction (Shimo 2006).

Universality

The previous Medical Care Act required that 95% of eligible residents be covered for insured health care services (Thompson 2010). Conversely, the CHA now requires that 100% of eligible residents be covered by their provincial or territorial Medicare insurance programs. Specifically, Section 10 of the CHA declares that all residents of the provinces and territories are entitled to insured health services provided for by their Medicare insurance plans.

It is up to each province and territory to determine whether its residents should be insured on a compulsory versus voluntary nature (Shah 2003). The federal government also allows the provinces and territories to charge their residents with insurance premiums based on personal income levels (e.g., Ontario) (Thompson 2010). However, if an individual could not pay these premiums (e.g., poor, homeless), it should not prevent them from seeking insured health care services in their province or territory.

Exceptions include those individuals who are under federal jurisdiction including members of the Canadian Armed Forces and veterans, the Royal Canadian Mounted Police (RCMP), Indigenous Peoples, prisoners in Federal institutions and transients. Transients include landed immigrants and returning expatriates. These individuals usually must often endure a waiting period before becoming eligible to be insured (Health Canada 2003, 2001; Government of Canada 1984, 2007b). Newcomers to Canada, which includes landed immigrants or Canadians returning from living

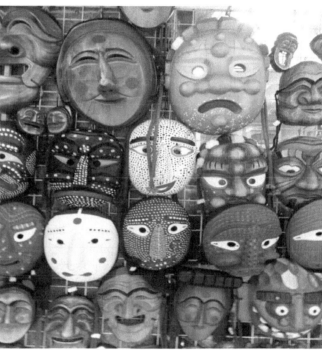

Source: Wally Bartfay

Photo 3.8 Canada is a multicultural and ethnically diverse country. Discrimination in terms of the previous health status of an individual, their age, race or non-membership in a group is not permitted under the CHA.

abroad, may be subject to a waiting period of up to three months before they may be entitled to receive insured health services by their province or territory (Government of Canada 2007b).

Portability

The criteria of portability declares that residents must continue to be covered who are temporarily out of their province or territory (Section 11). For example, Canadians moving from one province or territory to another are still eligible for health coverage which is paid for by their place of origin (Thompson 2010). This criterion also applies to individuals who are required to endure a waiting period in a new province or territory of residence. Most jurisdictions in Canada impose a three month waiting period before insured health insurance benefits in their new province or territory become active, because under the CHA this period cannot exceed three months. Individuals moving to Canada from abroad are therefore encouraged to purchase private health insurance plans during this waiting period.

Canadians who leave the country will continue to be eligible for publicly insured health insurance plans for a prescribed period of time, which is typically about 6 months (183 days) (Thompson 2010). Nova Scotia may permit a resident to be out of province for a period of up to 1 year; Newfoundland and Labrador offers out-of-province coverage for their residents for a period of 4 months; New Brunswick, Manitoba, Alberta and British Columbia state that a resident has to be present in their province for at least 6 months to retain coverage, and

Ontario states that a person may be out of province for a period of no more than 212 days in any given year (Thompson 2010).

The criteria also notes that regardless of the actual cost of delivery of health care services rendered out of their province or territory, payment is based on the amount that would have been paid by their home or formal province or territory for similar services rendered (Section 11.b.ii). Importantly, this criterion does not support residents in one province to actively seek out health care services or treatments outside of their home province or territory. In fact, most provinces require that individuals apply and obtain formal approval before having elective or non-emergency care provided to them outside of their home province (Shah 2003). This criteria, however, is intended to cover travelers abroad in case of emergency situations (Health Canada 2001, 2003; Government of Canada 1984, 2007b). The portability criterion, however, does not entitle a resident to seek out health care services in another province, territory, or country. It is intended to permit an individual to receive medically necessary services in relation to an urgent or emergent need when they are absent on a temporary basis from their home province or territory, such as being on a business trip or vacation (Government of Canada 2007b).

Accessibility

The criteria of accessibility declares that no individual can be discriminated against in terms of receiving health care services based on their age, lifestyle, or present health status or condition. Indeed, health care must be administered on uniform terms and conditions for insured individuals (Section 12.a) (Health Canada 2001, 2003; Government of Canada 1984, 2007b). According to the CHA, all eligible residents must have "*reasonable access*" to all insured health services on uniform terms and conditions. The interpretation of what constitutes reasonable access remains controversial. Indeed, an individual living in an isolated community in Nunavut will not have the same access to publicly insured health care services, in comparison to a person residing in an urban city such as Montréal, Toronto or Vancouver. Hence, accessibility under the CHA is generally interpreted as meaning access to health care services where and when it is available (Thompson 2010). For example, many Indigenous people in Canada grow up in overcrowded housing, especially in isolated northern communities, without adequate food, heating, or water supplies. As of March 31, 2012 there were 121 drinking water advisories issued for First Nations communities alone (Health Canada 2012). The availability and caliber of health care services remains problematic, especially in rural and less populated regions in Canada. Moreover, the health care services that are available even in large urban populated cities are not necessarily uniform in quality or accessibility across Canada.

Shimo (2006) reports that in December 1995 Barry Stein, a lawyer living in Montréal, was diagnosed with colorectal cancer. Mr. Stein was booked into the operating room on three separate occasions and each time the surgery was cancelled and had to be rescheduled. Stein believed that we would most likely die without the needed surgical intervention to treat his cancer and went to the United States to seek private treatment. Stein underwent months of vaccines, operations, and chemotherapies, and the associated medical costs rose to approximately $250,000 (U.S.). Mr. Stein strongly believed that the Government of Québec should pay for these "*medically necessary*" treatments which saved his life. He consequently sued the provincial government and received a full reimbursement for his medical expenses incurred (Shimo 2006).

In August 2007, an expectant mother in Calgary with quadruplets unexpectedly went into labour at 35.5 weeks gestation (Lang 2007). During this time, no available neonatal facilities were available in Alberta or the rest of Canada to adequately provide care to the quadruplets after birth. Hence, the expectant mother was flow to Montana in the United States, where the babies were safely delivered and then flow back to Alberta via air ambulance. This health care intervention costs $170,000 (CAN), which was subsequently paid for by Canadian taxpayers (Lang 2007).

Section 12.a also states that reasonable compensation for services rendered by physicians or dentists, and payments to hospitals to help cover the costs of health services rendered shall be provided. The intent of this criterion is to ensure that insured residents have reasonable access to insured hospital, medical and surgical dental services on uniform terms and conditions (Government of Canada 2007b). This access should not be precluded or impeded either directly or indirectly by charges (e.g., user fees or extra-billings); or other means such as discrimination on the basis of age, health, social status, or financial circumstances. Specific compensations for the provinces are established through negotiations between the provincial governments and organizations that represent physicians and dental surgical procedures that must be rendered in hospitals. Nonetheless, preventive dental care and routine dental surgical procedures (e.g., extraction of wisdom teeth) in Canada are currently not covered by any provincial or territorial insurance plan. Residents are therefore required to pay out of their own pockets for these dental services rendered, or may have private or employee-based insurance plans to help pay for some of these costs.

Moreover, the coverage of vision care varies greatly among provinces (Bartfay and Bartfay 2015). In general, specific vision care services for diabetic patients, individuals requiring surgery due to trauma or disease (including cataract surgery) are covered. The standard vision screening exam for adults, which is an example of primary prevention and health promotion, is not covered by all provincial and territorial plans and is often limited to children of a specific age range only. Cosmetic procedures and surgeries are typically not covered as well. Chiropractic treatments and procedures are covered by some provincial programs (e.g., Saskatchewan).

Chaoulli et al. Versus the Attorney General of Québec

The *Canadian Charter of Rights and Freedoms* was passed into law in 1982 (Makarenko 2005; Thompson 2010). The Charter does not specifically identify health care nor provides any guarantee in specific terms that Canadian citizens have a right to health care. Nonetheless, Section 7 of the Charter specifies that citizens have a right to life, liberty, and security and Section 15 Charter states that health care must be provided to all persons "*equally*" and "*fairly.*" Despite that fact that the 2003 First Ministers Accord created a separate $1.5 billion *Diagnostic and Medical Equipment Fund* aimed at decreasing patient wait times, long queues lines for diagnostic imaging (e.g., CT and MRI scans) persist in many jurisdictions across Canada (Health Council of Canada 2010, 2011). Several public challenges regarding the rights of Canadian citizens under the Charter have been prompted by long wait times and frustration over equal and fair access to needed medical diagnostic procedures and surgical treatments and interventions.

For example, Dr. Jacques Chaoulli and his patient, George Zeliotis challenged the Government of Québec's ban on private health insurance in court alleging that long wait times violated the Charter. Mr. Zeliotis was a 70-year-old salesman and resident of the province of Québec, and required a hip replacement. He was put on a lengthy provincial waiting list that he alleged resulted in decreased quality of life, immobility, loss of sleep, and unnecessary pain and suffering. Dr. Chaoulli decided to opt-out of Québec's publicly insured plan and was lobbying the government to establish a private hospital so that he could more effectively treat his orthopedic patients (Makarenko 2005).

In 1997, when this court case began, there were two main legislations governing health care services in the province of Québec: the *Hospital Insurance Act* (HOIA) and the *Health Insurance Act* (HEIA) (Makarenko 2005). HOIA regulated access to health care services in Québec, whereas HEIA regulated the provision of health care insurance in the province. These health care Acts in Québec effectively prevented any physician that choose to opt-out of the provincial Medicare health insurance plan from providing private medical care within a public hospital (Thompson 2010). Moreover, these Acts also prohibited residents from purchasing private medical insurance to cover so called "*medically necessary*" procedures, which are covered by the provincial health insurance plan (Chaoulli v. Québec Attorney General 2005; Lee-Arkazaki 2007; Monahan 2006). The key question in this landmark court case was whether restrictions on individuals to purchase private insurance for health care services covered by government plans violated the right to security of the person (Monahan 2006).

Three different courts heard this landmark case including two courts in Québec (Lower court and the Québec Supreme Court), followed by the Supreme Court of Canada (Makarenko 2005). The issue of legal challenge and debate in the courts centred on the question of whether or not there is an infringement of Charter rights that occurs when a provincial health care system is unable to provide timely access to needed services while simultaneously prohibiting an individual from buying these services using their own means and resources (Chodos and MacLeod 2004).

In June 2005, the Supreme Court of Canada overtuned a Québec law preventing a resident (*Jacques Chaoulli et al. versus Attorney General of Québec*) from purchasing their own private health insurance to pay for medical necessary health care services in hospitals available through the publicly funded health care system in that province (Chaoulli v. Québec Attorney General 2005; Lee-Arkazak 2007; Monahan 2006). In a four to three vote, the court ruled that such prohibitions in the province of Québec violated the Charter of Rights and Freedoms. Where the publicly insured health care system does not provide timely care, the Court ruled, forbidding individual purchase of care in unconscionable—"*access to a waiting list*," in a widely quoted declaration of judgment, "*is not access to health care*" (Monahan 2006, forward p. i). Essentially, the Supreme Court of Canada removed previous prohibitions placed on residents of Québec from using their own private health insurance plans to pay for medically necessary services rendered in the provincial hospital-based health care model (Makarenko 2005).

Subsequently, in November 2005, the provincial government of Québec declared that it would allow their residents to purchase private medical insurance in accordance with the Supreme Court's ruling. This ruling will undoubtedly have far-reaching implications for the future of publicly insured versus private health care in Canada, and how it is administered and delivered. Shimo (2006) argues that in the wake of this landmark court decision, there may be no more need for creative ways to stay within the law. In fact, many private health care providers are anticipating that many medical services can now be provided on a for-profit basis, and are quickly expanding their services and outlets across the country.

The Chaoulli court decision also has the potential to evoke major changes in the role that courts play in determining future health care policies in Canada. Indeed, now that the right to "*timely access*" to insured provincial/territorial health care services has been established by the Supreme Court of Canada, the role of the courts in making decisions related to a variety of health care issues will also likely be employed for rulings in the future. The courts will now be responsible, as in the case of the Chaoulli court decision, for determining what timely access means and whether it exists or not in various provincial and territorial insured health care systems in Canada.

Indeed, if the courts rule that provincial and territorial publicly insured health care standards are not being met, they can force the governments to change their policies accordingly. For example, few would argue against the fact that the ability to effectively communicate with one's health care provider is essential to receiving safe and effective health care services in Canada. This includes the need for a proper diagnosis based on presenting clinical signs and symptoms; the patients' history and their family's medical history (e.g., breast cancer has a genetic link), which are critical to assess treatment outcomes. John Eldridge, Linda Warren, and John Warren were patients who were born deaf and relied on a non-profit organization in British Columbia to provide sign language translations during physician appointments, hospital procedures and for diagnostic tests (Thompson 2010). Sign language was their preferred method of communication. Unfortunately, due to financial constraints in 1990s, this non-profit organization could no longer provider sign language translations during medical visits for these three patients. The patients alleged that their ability to communicate with their health care providers jeopardized their health and safety and their ability to make informed decisions related to their treatment options. Requests by these patients to both provincial and federal governments were denied. The patients subsequently appealed to the Supreme Court of British Columbia in 1997 and argued that failure to provide sign language interpretations as an insured benefit under the Medical Services Plan violated Section 15(1) of the Charter of Rights and Freedoms in Canada (Eldrige v. British Columbia 1997).

The Provincial Supreme Court ruled in 1992 that the need for a sign language translator by these patients was a supplementary service that the provincial government did not have to provide, since it was deemed not "*medically necessary*." The patients subsequently appealed to the Supreme Court of Canada, which ruled that the *Hospital Services Act* and the *Medical and Health Care Services Act* of British Columbia contravened Section 15(1) of the Canadian Charter of Rights (Thompson 2010). Specifically, the Supreme Court of Canada ruled that the government of British Columbia violated the patient's right to equality by failing to address the need for services to ensure safety and to effectively communicate with health care professionals and make informed decisions. Furthermore, the Supreme Court ordered that these two aforementioned provincial Acts be changed to accommodate these rights (Eldrige v. British Columbia Attorney General 1997).

Divergent Interpretations of the CHA

What Is "Medically Necessary"?

The term "*medically necessary*" within the context of the CHA has been hotly debated and contested (Armstrong and Armstrong 2003; Bartfay 2010a; Bartfay and Bartfay 2015). Typically, a physician or surgeon makes a clinical judgment based on their physical examination and diagnosis for a needed procedure, and then bills their provincial or territorial Medicare plan for the health services rendered. Although the term medically necessary appears throughout the CHA, is very subjective in nature and open to a wide range of interpretations by governments and health care professionals. Indeed, publicly insured health care services not only vary between the various provinces and territories in Canada, they also vary within these jurisdictions as well. For example, a surgeon in Québec may clinically determine that a breast reduction is a medically necessary procedure for a 25-year-old female patient because of associated back and muscle strain, sleep disturbances, pain, and discomfort and unnecessary physical and psychological stress and suffering. Conversely, another surgeon in Québec may simply determine that the same patient should undergo an elective cosmetic procedure (i.e., breast reduction), since her condition does not warrant a medically necessary surgical intervention.

In reality, the Act was only conceived to limit its focus to all medically necessary physician and dental hospital-based services. According to Brain J. Cohen, a health lawyer based in Toronto, Ontario, individuals who pay out-of-pocket for so-called "*medically necessary*" care may be eligible for reimbursement by their governments (Shimo 2006). In fact, Cohen reports that he has won several precedent setting cases for patients seeking treatment funding, both within Canada and the United States. For example, Cohen persuaded the Ontario Health Insurance Plan to pay for expenses for a resident of Ontario who was treated with the colon cancer drug Erbitux at a hospital in Buffalo in 2005. During this time, the drug Erbitux had not yet been approved for use by Health Canada (Shimo 2006).

Section 3 of the CHA endorses the concept of health promotion, but it does not mandate the provinces and territories to actively engage in such programs or activities (Government of Canada 1984). In reality, the components of health promotion described including protective, promotive, and preventive services are not required to meet the five criteria's detailed earlier in the Act in order to qualify for federal transfer payments. Consequently, the extent to which provincial and territorial governments provide health promotion services to their residents vary considerable in quantity and quality from one region to another (Romanow 2002; Sullivan and Baranek 2002). In hindsight, it may be argued that this major omission by the authors of the CHA has had wide reaching negative health effects in Canada. For example, the growing endemic of obesity in children and adults and the growing adaptation of sedentary lifestyles by many have resulted in increased

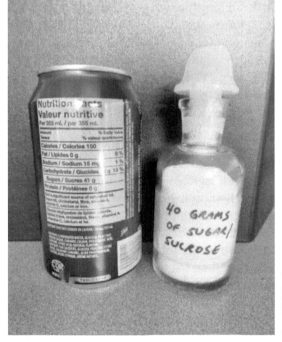

Source: Wally Bartfay

Photo 3.9 A carbonated beverage containing over 40 grams of sugar/sucrose. The consumption of soda and other sugary-rich drinks (e.g., fruit juices, energy drinks) has been linked to the development of obesity in children (Marchione 2012; Qi et al. 2011).

incidence of highly preventable chronic diseases (e.g., heart disease, stroke, hypertension, type two diabetes). In fact, between 1978/1979 and 2004, the combined prevalence of overweight and obese Canadians children and youth aged 2 to 17 years increased from 15% to 26% (Childhood Obesity Foundation 2015). Over 59% of Canadian adults are either overweight or obese and if the current trends continues, it is predicted that by 2040 up to 70% of adults aged 40 years or older will be overweight or obese (Childhood Obesity Foundation 2015).

Since the CHA does not specify or detail which medical and surgical interventions and diagnostic tests should be insured, the range of insured health care services may vary amongst the 10 provinces and 3 territories in Canada. Medical or surgical procedures or interventions should not be rendered simply for the convenience of the patient or physician (e.g., non-emergency elective Caesarian sections). Moreover, when more than one treatment option is available, the physician should first consider the less expensive or invasive option (Thompson 2010).

It is notably that the CHA does not guarantee health care per se (Thompson 2010). The Act simply states that permanent residents of a Canadian province or territory are eligible for publicly insured health care services for medically necessary services. However, which specific health care services are actually provided by the provinces and territories are open to interpretation and dependent on available resources, geography (e.g., rural and remote versus urban), expertise available, and finances.

Jake Epp's Letter

The growing concerns and limitations of the Canada Health Act were crystallized in a letter sent on June 18, 1985 to all provincial and territorial Ministers of Health by the Honourable Jake Epp, the federal Minister of Health and Welfare at the time (Government of Canada 2007b). The French equivalent of this letter was sent to Québec on July 15, 1985. In his letter, Epp attempted to clarify the intent and his government's interpretation of the Canada Health Act, and its five founding criteria's.

> "This letter strives to set out flexible, reasonable and clear ground rules to facilitate provincial, as much as federal, administration of the Canada Health Act. It encompasses many complex matters including criteria interpretations, federal policy concerning conditions and proposed regulations. I realize, of course, that a letter of this sort cannot cover every single matter of concern to every provincial Minister of Health. Continuing dialogue and communication are essential"
>
> (Government of Canada 2007b, p. 232- Annex A: Policy Interpretation Letters)

In addition to insured physician and hospital-based services, Section 2 of the Canada Health Act (1982) also provides transfer funds for so-called "*extended health services*," which includes ambulatory health care services; home care services; pharmaceuticals, and adult and nursing home services (Government of Canada 2004). The definition of extended health services can, therefore, be quite fluid in nature as opposed to a standardized national definition. Hence, provinces and territories can basically decide and define what these extended health care services are or are not accordingly to their perceived needs and their ability to fund these programs (e.g., *in vitro* fertilization procedures for couples in Québec). More importantly, funding for these extended health services are not contingent upon meeting the five criteria's of the Canada Health Act (Sullivan and Baranek 2002; National Forum of Health 1997).

Diane Marleau's Letter

A decade later, the Honourable Diane Marleau, who was the Federal Minister of Health at the time, sent a follow-up to Epp's letter dated January 6, 1995 to all her provincial and territorial ministers of health regarding the need to safeguard and protect the five founding criteria's of the Canada Health Act (Government of Canada 2007b). In her letter, Marleau described the mounting public concerns related the growth of a two tied health care system in Canada, and the growing fear that individuals without the ability to pay for private services or user facility fees will be most affected including those on fixed incomes, the poor, and elderly.

Marleau also highlighted the growing public fear related to the potential slow destruction of our publicly funded and administered health care systems due to the growth of private clinics (Bartfay 2010a; Bartfay and Bartfay 2015).

> "At a time when there is concern about the potential erosion of the publicly funded and publicly administered health care system, it is vital to safeguard these criteria's. As was evident and a concern to many of us at the recent Halifax meeting, a trend toward divergent interpretations of the Act is developing…I am convinced that the growth of a second tier of health care facilities providing medically necessary services that operate, totally or in large part, outside the publicly funded and publicly administered system, presents a serious threat to Canada's health care system"
>
> (Government of Canada 2007b, p. 233-Annex B: Policy Interpretation Letters).

Add to your knowledge of the debate surrounding public versus private for profit health care in Canada by assessing the link in Web-Based Resources Box 3.4.

When health care professionals have the option of working simultaneously in both the public and private sectors, waiting times for diagnostic services (e.g., MRI and CT scans, cardiac stress tests) and health care services (e.g., hip and cataract surgery) have been shown to actually increase. For example, waiting times in the provinces of Manitoba and Alberta for ophthalmological services were found to be significantly longer for physicians who provided health care services in both sectors (Alberta Consumers' Association 1994; Canadian Health Services Research Foundation 2001). Shimo (2006) reports that the national median wait time from seeing a general practitioner to actually having joint replacement surgery completed for hips, knees, ankles, or shoulders is 49.7 weeks, and is some provinces a two year wait time is not uncommon. By contrast, all surgeries can be performed within two weeks in private clinics (Shimo 2006).

To what extent do these wait times for publicly insured health care services affect users' satisfaction with the care they receive? CIHI (2007) reports that approximately 21% of Canadians surveyed who accessed publicly funded health care services within the 12 months prior to the 2005 Statistics Canada survey felt that their wait times for diagnostic tests were unacceptable. Almost three-quarters (71%) of those surveyed reported that wait times for diagnostic and health care services resulted in worry, anxiety, and stress. In addition, over one-third (38%) experienced pain and suffering while waiting to access health care services (CIHI 2007).

In February 1999, the federal government and the nine provincial governments (excluding Québec) signed the *Social Union Framework Agreement* (SUFA). The SUFA, along with other provisions, committed all provinces to support the five criteria's of the Canada Health Act. However, without effective sanctions for those who breech the Act, it is far from exactly clear how the provinces and territories are meeting these commitments. Instead of strengthening the federal governments' capacity to enforce the five criteria's of the CHA, improve care and prevent the growth of private health care in Canada, SUFA now requires that the federal government obtain agreement from the majority of provinces and territories before any new funding initiative can be introduced (Armstrong and Armstrong 2003). Hence, there may be no clear national legislative means to prevent the erosion of our publicly insured health care systems and the growth of private clinics across Canada.

Web-based Resource Box 3.4 Two-Tied Health Care

Learning Resource	Website
This web page provides an overview of two-tier health care services in Canada and provides a description of the various forms of private health care services in Canada	http://www.cbc.ca/news/background/health care/public_vs_private.html

Penalties and Deductions

Health Canada's current approach to the administration of the Canada Health Act is proclaimed to be one of transparency, consultation and dialogue with the 13 provincial and territorial health ministers. The "*Canada Health Act Dispute Avoidance and Resolution*" (DAR) process was formalized during the 2004 First Ministers Accord, in an attempt to help settle disputes related to penalties. The Government of Canada (2007b) reports that the application of financial penalties through deductions under the *Canada Health Transfer* agreement is considered only as a last resort. Although the DAR process includes dispute resolution provisions, the federal minister of health retains the final authority to interpret and enforce the Canada Health Act (Government of Canada 2007b).

The five criteria's described earlier set down the conditions that the provinces must abide by in order to receive transfer funds from the federal government to support a nationwide publicly insured Medicare system in Canada (Health Canada 2003, 2001; Government of Canada 2007b, 1984). The federal government has, in legislation at least, placed a restriction which allows them to withhold transfer payments to a province or territory that permit extra-billing (Section 18). For example, if a physician were to charge their patient for an office visit that is insured by their provincial or territorial health insurance plan, the amount charged would constitute extra-billing, and should be regarded as a violation of the CHA. Extra-billing of patients is seen as a barrier or impediment for individuals seeking medical care, and is therefore contrary to the accessibility criteria (Government of Canada 2007b).

The CHA also declares that user charges by physicians who charge for health care services rendered that are typically covered by their provincial or territorial health insurance plans is not permitted (Section 19) (Bartfay and Bartfay 2015). For example, if a patient were charged a facility fee for receiving an insured service at a hospital or clinic, that fee would be considered a user charge, which is not permitted under the Act (Government of Canada 2007b). Hence, if a province were to violate the prohibition on extra-billing or user charges, the federal government could deduct the corresponding amount from their transfer payment. The Group-Activity-Based Learning Box 3.1 seeks to promote classroom discussions and debate related to publicly funded health services and the growth of private clinics in Canada. Working in groups of three to five students, answer the following questions:

For examples, from November 1995 to June 1996, total reductions of $3.585 million were made to Alberta's cash contribution with respect to facility fees charged at clinics providing surgical, ophthalmological, and abortion services (Government of Canada 2007b). Similarly, due to facility fees allowed at an abortion clinic, a total of $284,430 was deducted from Newfoundland and Labrador's cash contribution. A deduction of $72,464 was

---

Group Activity-based Learning Box 3.1

Publicly Funded Health Services Versus the Growth of Private-For-Profit Clinics in Canada
Working in small groups of four to six individuals, critically discuss and debate the following questions:

1. What are some of the health challenges facing residents in your region, province or territory?

2. Are you in support of extra-billing, user fees and the growth of private clinics in your province or territory? Why or why not?

3. Should provincial and territorial governments in Canada allow permanent residents to purchase private health insurance plans to pay for medically necessary procedures offered by their publicly insured health care system? Why or why not?

4. How do these practices (i.e., extra-billing, user fees, growth of private clinics) negatively affect the health and well-being of marginalized individuals (e.g., the poor, homeless, elderly, and immigrants) in your province or territory?

made to British Columbia on the basis of charges reported by the province for extra-billing and patient charges at surgical clinics (Government of Canada 2007b). Shimo (2006) reports that there have been numerous documented occasions where clinics have charged both patients and their associated provincial or territorial governments for the same medically necessary services. Although this practice is known as double billings and violates the Canada Health Act, enforcement has been spotty at best. For example, in 2005 British Columbia kept track of private clinics charging for medically necessary services by searching through old newspaper clippings and clinic advertisements (Shimo 2006). Certainly this is not a very efficient means to monitor compliance by government officials and authorities or a means to boost public confidence in the system currently in place.

Passage of the CHA has only appeared to be successful in providing federal governments with a mechanism at the start to withhold transfer payments to the provinces and territories (Bartfay and Bartfay 2015). For example, the Auditor General of Canada (2002) reported that within the first three years (1984-1987), transfer penalties totaling $245 million dollars were levied against seven provinces. Initially, these penalties by the federal government have been successful in eliminating extra-billing and user fee charges to eligible residents in Canada. Nonetheless, the federal government has been increasingly reluctant to monitor and impose penalties in accordance with the five founding criteria's of the CHA over the subsequent decades. In fact, it appears that the federal government has been more eager to appease and pacify the provincial and territorial health ministers, as evidenced by the reimbursement of formal penalties levied (Bartfay 2010a). By June 1987, a total of $244.732 million in deductions were refunded to New Brunswick ($6.886 million), Québec ($14.032 million), Ontario ($106.656 million), Manitoba ($1.270 million), Saskatchewan ($2.107 million), Alberta ($29.032 million), and British Columbia ($84.749 million) (Government of Canada 2007b).

Consequently, there currently appears to be no fear, apprehension, or hesitation on the part of provincial and territorial governments to allow for the growth of private clinics, charge user fees and/or engage in the practice of extra-billing by physicians. This is not surprisingly since no recent federal government has levied any penalties for extra-billing since the end of the 1990s (Health Canada 2000). Similarly, the Auditor General of Canada (2002) reports that the federal government has never imposed financial penalties on five provinces identified for failing to put into force the criteria of portability detailed in the CHA. Federal governments have, instead, chosen to pursue a non-meddling and hands–off approach with the provincial and territorial governments in reference to publicly insured health care issues (Bartfay 2010a). Moreover, the Auditor General of Canada (2002, p. 17) has publicly criticized the federal government for failing to collect sufficient information required in accordance with the CHA to ensure compliance by the provinces and territories, and alarmingly reported that "Parliament cannot readily determine the extent to which each province and territory has satisfied the criteria and conditions of the Canada Health Act."

Rising Health Care Costs

It is not surprising that the cost of providing publicly insured health care services have grown steadily over the past five decades, and this trend is likely to continue with the current Medicare systems present in Canada (Bartfay and Bartfay 2015). We currently spend approximately 11% of our GDP on health care or an estimated $6,105 per person each year (CIHI 2015a, b). According to Hall (2011), Canada spends more per capita on health care than all but three of the world's most advanced nations, yet ranks tenth in the quality of medicine it delivers. For example, Japan with $2,729 per person spending on health care delivers the best health system, based on longevity and infant mortality. Italy has the second lowest costs and the third best life expectancies. By contrast, the United States spends substantially more (approximately $7,500 per person) and cannot match these outcome measures by far.

Based on 2013 data from twenty-nine countries with similar health care accounting systems in the *Organization for Economic Co-operation and Development* (OECD), per capita spending (US$) on health care remained highest in the United States ($9,086, 17.1% of GDP) followed by France ($4,361, 11.6% GDP), Germany ($4.920, 11.2% of GDP), Denmark ($4,847, 11.1% of GDP), Canada ($4,569, 10.7 GDP), Australia ($4,115, 9.4% of GDP), Japan ($3,713, 10.2% of GDP), Finland ($3,645, 9.1% of GDP), and the United Kingdom ($3,364, 8.8% of GDP) (CIHI 2015a).

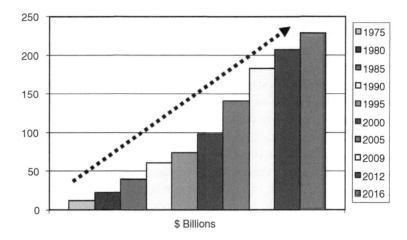

Figure 3.2 The rising costs of publicly funded health care in Canada—1975–2016

Source: Data adapted from the Canadian Institute for Health Information, (CIHI 2010). *National health expenditure trends, 1975 to 2010.* Ottawa, Ontario: Author, and Canadian Institutes for Health Information (CIHI 2013). *Canada's health care spending growth slows. Provincial and territorial government health expenditures expected to grow 3.1%, lowest since 1997.* Ottawa, ON: CIHI. Retrieved June 13, 2013 from http://www.cihi.ca/cihi-ext-portal/internet/en/document/spending+and+health+workforce/spending/release_30oct12. Canadian Institute for Health Information. (CIHI 2016). *National health expenditures: How much does Canada spend on health care?* Ottawa, Ontario: CIHI Retrieved April 14, 2017 from http://www.cihi.ca/en/nhex2016-topic1.

Note: Please note that figures have been rounded-off to the first decimal place and are in Canadian dollars.

Figure 3.2 shows the growing costs for providing our publicly insured health care systems in Canada from 1975 to 2015 (CIHI 2012, 2010a, b, 2015a, b). In 1975, the cost of providing our Medicare systems in Canada was $12.2 billion, which represented about 7% of our total GDP. By comparison, our national health care expenditure was in excess of $219.1 billion ($6,105 per person) in 2015 (10.9% of GDP) (CIHI 2015a). The costs ranged from $14,059 in Nunavut to $5,665 in Québec. The top three drivers for health care costs were: (a) Hospitals (29.5%); (b) drugs (15.7%) of which 13.3% were prescribed and 2.4% were non-prescribed, and (c) payments to physicians (15.5%) (CIHI 2015a, b). Notably, public health and all of its associated activities (e.g., health promotion and pre-vention campaigns and programs) accounted for only 5.5% of total health expenditures in 2015. Banswell (2015) reports that the public purse (taxes) comprises approximately 70% of the cost of health care in Canada, while the remaining 30% comes from out-of-pocket payments by individuals and/or insurance companies. Acute hospitals continue to make up the largest portion of health care spending accounting for approximately $63.5 billion in 2014. The average cost gross clinical payment per physician was $336,000, which represents an increase from the previous year by 6% reaching $24.1 billion in total payments (CIHI 2015b).

The number of seniors in Canada is expected to reach 6.7 million in 2020 and 9.2 million in 2041 (PHAC 2008, CIHI 2015a), and they account for a significant proportion of these health care costs, given that chronic disease (e.g., heart disease, diabetes, arthritis, and stroke) and disability increases with age.

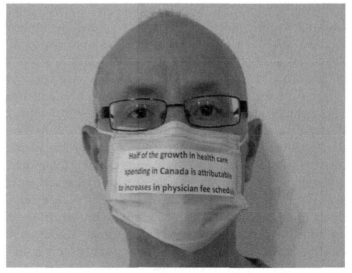

Source: Emma Bartfay.

Photo 3.10 Payments to physicians represents Canada's third largest share of health care expenditures.

Canadians aged 65 or older comprise approximately 15% of the total population, but consume more than 45% of all public sector health care costs (CIHI 2015a). Indeed, the average health care cost for a senior aged 65–69 years was $6,298; $8,384 for a senior aged 70–74; $11,578 for a senior aged 75–79 years, and $20,917 for a senior 80 years or more (CIHI 2015a).

One may argue that these elevated costs are associated, at least in part, with a decreased emphasis on home and community-based health care services and primary health promotion initiatives and programs nationally. In fact, acute care hospital-based health care services continue to account for the largest component accounting for 29.5% of health care expenditures in 2015 (CIHI 2015ab). In 2015, spending on drugs (including both prescription and non-prescription medications) made-up the second largest proportion of health care dollars, accounting for an estimated 15.7%, which represents a near doubling of the share of health care expenditures during the past three decades (CIHI 2010a, 2015a, b). Payments to physicians represent Canada's third largest share of health care expenditures, accounting for approximately 15.5% of health care expenditures in 2015.

Total health expenditures was $228.1 billion or 11.1% of GDP in 2016, which represents a 2.7% increase in comparison to 2015 figures. Total health care spending per Canadian was $6,299, and acute care hospital spending accounted for the largest share of total health spending by the public sector at 37.7% (CIHI 2016). Approximately 70% of total health expenditures came from the public sector and 30% from the private-sector. The private sector was comprised of 3 major spending categories; the largest of which was out-of-pocket spending (14.6%), followed by private health insurance (12.2%), and non-consumption (3.3%).

In 2017 a report released by Choosing Wisely Canada and the Canadian Institute of Health Information [CIHI] found that Canadians have more than 1 million potentially unnecessary medical tests and treatments performed each year (Choosing Wisely Canada and CIHI, 2017). Moreover, approximately 30% of clients indicated in the 8 selected *Choosing Wisely Canada* recommendations had diagnostic tests, treatments and/or procedures performed that were unnecessary and/or potentially harmful in nature. Indeed, unnecessary diagnostic tests and care wastes health system resources, increases wait times for clients and can potentially lead to harm (e.g., exposure to X-rays). Not surprisingly, total health expenditure in 2017 rose to $242 billion, (or $6,604 per person), which represented 11.5% of Canada's gross domestic product (GDP) (CIHI, 2018). Total health expenditure per person also varied across the country from $7,378 in Newfoundland and Labrador and $7,329 in Alberta to $6,367 in Ontario and $6,321 in British Columbia (CIHI, 2018).

Future Directions and Challenges

Improving the health of our nation will require large scale transformations and paradigm changes that focus on promoting health through the social determinants of health and supporting individuals, families, groups, and entire communities to take greater responsibility for health (Bartfay and Bartfay 2015). Groups and communities at risk for poorer health must be a priority for this major transformational challenge. Central to this transformation process is the way that public health professionals and workers are educated, so outdated curricula need to revised and updated based on the best available evidence.

There are several challenges facing our publicly funded health systems in Canada that must be addressed. We currently have had a physician-led and dominated funding model of health and health care services for the past five decades that has emphasized episodic acute care largely provided in hospital settings (Bartfay and Bartfay 2015). Our continued reliance on the fee-for-service medical model underpins this current system of funding and our reliance on costly acute care physician-driven diagnostic and laboratory health care services. For example, a study examining time usage in an acute care hospital revealed that emergency department physicians spent more time entering data into electronic medical records (44%) than any other activity including direct client care (28%) (Hill, Sears, and Melanson 2013). There is a growing need to nurture, fund, and support the delivery of evidence-informed primary health services delivered by interdisciplinary teams of public health professionals and workers in community settings and individual homes (Butler-Jones 2012; Browne et al. 2012; National Expert Commission Canadian Nurses Association 2012; Soroka and Mahon 2012; Standing Senate Committee on Social Affairs, Science and Technology 2012).

Our publicly insured health care systems are currently at a defining moment in our history as a nation with regards to its delivery and sustainability, and what we value as residents and citizens of Canada (Armstrong et al. 2001; Bartfay 2010a; Bartfay and Bartfay 2015). It may be argued that passage of the CHA in 1982 has been instrumental in perpetuating the dominant biomedical model since the turn of the century, which is characterized by physician and hospital-based services to address diverse public health care needs in Canada (Bartfay 2010a; Bartfay and Bartfay 2015). Conversely, the determinants of health and holistic definitions of health care have not been adequately incorporated into the current publicly insured health care models in Canada.

In 1994, the federal government established an eight-member-committee to examine and make recommendations about our "*national crisis*" in health care (National Forum on Health Care 1997). However, most of the committee's recommendations have yet to be implemented as regional and federal political agenda's change periodically with their mandated terms and election priorities. Health care costs continue to shore, waiting lists remain a significant barrier to timely care resulting in unnecessary stress, suffering or pain, and there is a growing shortage of health care professionals including family physicians and registered nurses.

There are several viable suggestions and successful pilot programs that could be implemented to curve current health care costs. Research reveals, for example, that community-based health centres in Ontario are better than acute care hospitals for providing a variety of primary health models and programs that are geared towards the needs and realities of the communities they serve in comparison to other models; provide superior management of chronic diseases, and result in lower rates of costly emergency department visits to manage these conditions (Glazier et al. 2012; Muldoon et al. 2010; Russell et al. 2010). Providing increased home care services could also result in significant health cost savings. Every day in Canada, approximately 14% or 5,200 of all costly acute care hospital beds in Canada are occupied by clients who could be cared for safely in some other setting, and 20% of these individuals stay more than a month in hospital after the point when they are not required to be there awaiting placement (e.g., nursing home) (National Expert Committee Canadian Nurses Association 2012). For example, moving only 25% of the 6,000+ clients who require palliative care in Ontario from costly acute care hospital facilities (costing $19,900 per client annually) to home care settings (costing only $4,700 per client annually), would mean a saving of more than $15,000 per palliative client alone (National Expert Committee Canadian Nurses Association 2012; Ontario Association of Community Care Access Centres, Ontario Federation of Community Mental Health and Addiction Programs, and Ontario Hospital Association 2010). Browne et al. (2012) estimate that if the home care daily maximum was doubled to $200/day in Ontario, this would result in a $250/day in hospital cost saving per client or $750,000 per day saving for 3,000 Ontarians resulting in a total annual associated hospital health care cost savings of $23,375,000. Hence, we argue that primary health models that emphasis home and community-based services by an interdisciplinary team of public health professionals and workers holds the promise to provide effective, affordable services as the mainstream of health care in Canada, in contrast to costly acute care hospital driven services which our current archaic funding models continue to perpetuate and support (Bartfay and Bartfay 2015).

In April 2001, the Prime Minister of Canada appointed Roy J. Romanow as head of the "*Commission on the Future of Health Care in Canada*" (Romanow 2002). The objective of this Royal Commission was to obtain a national perspective on the current challenges and barriers facing publicly insured Medicare systems, and to make recommendations related to its delivery and sustainability. Romanow sought to elicit this information by engaging in a Canada-wide forum with health care professionals, health care consumers and policy makers. Similar to the outcomes of previous Royal Commissions and numerous reports, political desire and movement to implement Romanow's 47 recommendations to improve and sustain our publicly-insured Medicare systems has been lethargic at best (Bartfay 2010a).

Despite these recommendations, our publicly insured health care systems remain physician dominated and controlled with the emphasis on acute health care services (Armstrong and Armstrong 2003; Villeneuve and MacDonald 2006). The current dominance of the medical model of health care, which has served as the foundation for our publicly insured Medicare systems in Canada since the 1960s, requires a dramatic shift focus to a more holistic one based on the primary health care approach to address the health care challenges facing Canadians in the new millennium (Bartfay 2010a; Bartfay and Bartfay 2015).

Hospitals in Canada and abroad originated as charitable non-profit institutions that offered a range of health care and social services despite the individuals' income level or social status. By contrast, hospitals today in Canada are, in fact, private corporations run by publicly funded hospital administers who report to an elected board of governors, and who are responsible for ensuring that the hospital remains profitable and therefore viable (Deber 2000). Falk-Rafael and Coffey (2005) note that hospital care in Canada in primarily delivered privately. Although hospitals are frequently referred to as "*public hospitals*" by residents, the reality is that they are run by private boards and their employees are not government employees or workers per se (Bartfay and Bartfay 2015).

Currently, our publicly insured health insurance systems in Canada are at a crossroads with mounting social and political pressures to loosen the restrictions based on the five founding criteria's of the CHA and create a parallel system of privately financed health care (Flood and Archibald 2001; Senate of Canada 2001). Opponents of a two-tiered health care system claim that it will further escalate health care costs; reduce access to health care services for the less affluent (e.g., seniors on fixed incomes, homeless); increase diagnostic and surgical wait times, and compromise equity and quality (Armstrong et al. 2001; Deber 2000). Conversely, advocates for a parallel privately financed health care system claim that it will improve health care services by offering more choices for health care consumers; improve overall access to publicly insured health care systems because of decreased waiting times, decrease stress, anxiety, pain and suffering, and improve quality of health care services provided because of the market driven for-profit health care model (Armstrong and Armstrong 2003; Danzon 1992).

Nonetheless, the fact remains that since the introduction of our publicly insured Medicare systems during the late 1960s, an increasing proportion of health care in Canada has, and continues to be financed through private sources (Armstrong and Armstrong 2003; Armstrong et al. 2001). There is an ever increasing and rapid growth of private for-profit health clinics in Canada, which directly challenges the validity of the CHA and the legislative powers of the federal government. In addition, the powerful and influential Canadian Medical Association (CMA) released a report in July 2007 which endorsed private health care in Canada as a means to improve our ailing health care systems. It is notable that Dr. Brian Day, who acted as President of the CMA in 2007–2008 when this report was released to the media and the provincial and territorial governments, is the owner of one of the largest private health care hospitals in Canada.

The Toronto based Medan Health Management, Ottawa-based La Vie Health Centre and Calgary-based Foothills Health Consultants are just a few of the growing number of private health care clinics in Canada (Thompson 2010). All the services offered by these private health clinics, including diagnostic tests and screening, receiving medical advice and consults, and health education (e.g., exercise or diet plans) are provided without long waiting lists for their clients.

For example, Shimo (2006) reports that the Copeman Health Care Centre operates a private clinic in Vancouver and has expanded its clinics to other major cities including Ottawa, Toronto, and London as part of its push to have centres in every major Canadian city. In Ontario, Don Copeman sees a huge potential market in the estimated 1.4 million individuals who don't have a family physicians or NP. Copeman claims that the current system will never be able to afford the provision of comprehensive, preventive health services that his facility offers. According to Shimo, (2006), governments don't have the funding to provide these services and politically it's unfathomable.

Similarly, the False Creek Surgical Centre is a private clinic in British Columbia which provides a wide range of health care services ranging from diagnostic ultrasounds to general surgery in its state of the art facility with three operating rooms, six recovery beds and five overnight stay rooms (False Creek Surgical Centre 2009). This private clinic provides health care services to individuals in need as well as services for the provinces Worker's Compensation Board.

Despite these current challenges facing enforcement of the CHA and our publicly insured health care systems, it can be argued that Medicare has, at least in part, come to define what it means to be "*Canadian*"

(Conference Board of Canada 2000; Lipset 1990). According to a 2012 national online survey of 2,207 individuals by Leger Marketing, 94% of respondents reported that they "loved our universal health care" and called it an "important source of collective pride," and 74% called it "very important" (Cheadle 2012, p. A6). Indeed, Medicare has come to define what we value as a free and autonomous democratic nation; our legislative rights to receive health care, and what is worth preserving through collective efforts at all levels of government, health care professionals and workers, and health care consumers (Bartfay 2010a; Bartfay and Bartfay 2015). After all, health is unquestionably a desired and positive asset desired by all individuals across the lifespan.

Even though significant funds have been allocated for reforming primary health care at all levels of government, the dominant policy remains acute illness care delivered predominately in acute care hospitals and a growing number of private clinics across Canada. Proponents for the importance of community-based care models, home care, long-term care and health promotion have not been able to attract sufficient funding to date to reform the present dominant medical models of health in place and reform health care funding systems and mechanisms. For example, we have not been effective enough in getting the message out that primary prevention will result in greater savings in the decades to come.

The terms *primary health* and *primary health care* are often used interchangeable and are poorly understood. Simply put, **primary care** is the care that an individual receives when they visit their health care provider for advice or treatment related to a disease or ailment (Bartfay and Bartfay 2015). By contrast, **primary health care** is a health-based model where its services take into account the social determinants of health and defined principles (i.e., essential accessible, equitable, collaborative, and the use of appropriate technologies) (Bartfay and Bartfay 2015). Adoption of the primary health care approach increases responsibility for health to include not just the provincial or territorial governments, but also includes individuals, groups, and entire communities. Currently, many government services are divided up into unique departments that function like silos. The primary health care approach, by contrast, requires contact at multiple levels and with a variety of government services including health, social development, public safety, justice, and education. One of the major challenges we face is how to do a better job in promoting the understanding and use of primary health care models in Canada.

Dykeman (2012) describes the experience at the Community Health Clinic (CHC) in Fredericton, New Brunswick, which has adopted such a primary health care model. The CHC is managed by the University of New Brunswick's faculty of nursing and the clinic provides a wide range of health and social services to their residents based on an interdisciplinary approach. The client is a respected member of the CHC health care team and programs are based on actual community input and needs assessments. The CHC serves a variety of residents in the community including the homeless, individuals with drug addictions, vulnerable populations, immigrants, and women without family physicians. In addition to these health care services, the CHC provides services that have positive "*ripple effects*" not just for individuals, but also groups and the community as a whole.

For example, nursing students provide CHC outreach services in shelters and a local soup kitchen. Clients who visit the CHC can also take a bath or shower; obtain necessary clothing at a clothing bank, and it offers hot or cold drinks depending on the weather. Staff members of the CHC sit on various governmental and

Group Review Exercise Box 3.1: "Sicko"

Overview of This Investigative Documentary
This 2007 investigative documentary by Michael Moore examines access to health care services and the pharmaceutical industry in the United States and compares and contrasts those with and without private health insurance. The film compares the for-profit, non-universal United States system with the non-profit universal health care systems of Canada, the United Kingdom, France, and Cuba. In Canada, Moore describes the case of Tommy Douglas, who was voted the greatest Canadian in 2004 for his contributions to the Canadian Medicare systems. According to Moore, almost fifty million Americans are uninsured while those who have medical insurance are often victims of insurance company fraud, confusing bureaucratic procedures and protocols,

and red tape. Interviews are conducted with people who thought they had adequate coverage but were denied care. Former employees of insurance companies are highlighted in the film that describe cost-cutting initiatives that give bonuses to insurance company physicians and others to find reasons for the company to avoid reimbursements payments for *"medically necessary"* treatments for policy holders, and thus increase the profit margins for the company. Various social determinants of health are examined along with the negative ripple effects for those who cannot afford private health care services.

Instructions

This assignment may be done alone, in pairs or in groups of up to five people (note: if you are doing this assignment in pairs or groups, please only submit one hard or electronic copy to your instructor. The assignment should be typewritten and 4 to 6 pages maximum in length (double-spaced please). View the documentary entitled *"Sicko,"* by Michael Moore and take detailed notes during the presentation See link: http:// topdocumentaryfilms.com/sicko/ view this documentary and take detailed noted during the presentation.

1. Provide a brief overview of the salient points in this investigative documentary.

2. List and describe three social determinants of health revealed in this film.

3. Compare and contrast the American system of health care with our Canadian system. What are the noted similarities and differences in terms of the Canada Health Act? How has "Obama Care" in the United States changed the American experience, if any?

4. Provide examples of what are deemed *"medically necessary"* procedures in the United States versus Canada according to this documentary film and those that are not medically necessary.

5. Describe some of the *"negative ripple effects"* experienced by those individuals who do not have access to private health insurance and those who have been denied reimbursements payments by their insurance companies for health care services rendered.

community-based committees to tackle current or emerging issues that affect their community (Dykeman 2012). As noted in this chapter, the costs of health care in Canada continue to escalate and we must find more effective means of providing health care services to our residents and citizens across the country. We believe that the adoption of more community-based primary health care models, such as the CHC described earlier, would result in the more efficient and effective use of our health care dollars with better outcomes uniquely tailored to the needs of the community in question.

The following Group Review Exercise Box 3.1 is based on an investigative documentary that compares the for-profit American health care system with publicly funded health care systems in Canada's, the United Kingdom, France, and Cuba. Various social determinants of health (e.g., poverty) and access to affordable health services are critically examined.

Summary

- Historically, health care services in the new colonies were largely provided by charitable religious organizations in Canada to all those in need.

- In 1738, the first female visiting home [public health] nurses were the Grey Nuns in Québec, who later extended their charitable nursing services to other regions of Canada including St. Boniface in Manitoba, Lac Ste. Anne in Alberta and Ile á la Crosse in Saskatchewan.
- Canada currently employs a mix of both public and private facilities to deliver health care services to residents.
- Medicare is the collective term widely employed to refer to our publicly funded and administered universal health insurance plans in Canada, and is publicly funded through taxes and administered on a provincial or territorial basis within guidelines established by the federal government.
- The British North American (BNA) Act (1867) was the first legislation to describe the jurisdictions and responsibilities of the federal and provincial governments for providing health care services (Sections 91 and 92).
- Subsequent interpretations of the BNA Act gave the provinces and territories jurisdiction over most health services.
- The growth of the medical model of health with its increased reliance on new technologies and laboratory-based diagnostic tests resulted in a shift from home and community-based practice settings to acute care hospitals following World Wars I and II.
- Similarly, the arrival of Medicare during the 1950s and 1960s in Canada also increased the demand for publicly subsidized hospital-based nursing services.
- Not surprisingly, home and community-based health care services quickly diminished over the subsequent five decades.
- Tommy Douglas, the late premier of Saskatchewan, was the first to introduce a universal hospital-based social insurance plan in 1948, and he is regarded as the *Father of Medicare* in Canada.
- The National Health Grants Act of 1948 marks the start of the federal government's role in partially subsiding provincial and territorial Medicare systems via tax-based funds.
- By 1961, HIDSA was operational in all provinces and territories in Canada and it covered approximately 99% of all permanent residents and citizens.
- In 1966, the Medical Care Act was passed and stated that each province and territory was free to administer their own public health insurance plans as long as it conformed to the following criteria detailed in the Act: Universality; portability; comprehensive coverage, and public administration.
- The Medical Care Act and HIDSA collectively established a formula for federal transfer payments to the provinces and territories to help cover the cost of hospital-based health insurance plans that employed a formula of 50 cents to the dollar.
- Consequently, home and community-based health promotion and primary prevention programs provided by a variety of public health care professionals and workers (e.g., school nurses, health promoters and educators) took a back seat to acute care hospital-based health care services controlled by physicians.
- This funding formula was subsequently replaced by the Federal-Provincial Fiscal Arrangements and Established Programs Financing (EPF) Act, which consisted of block transfer grants from the federal government to the various provinces and territories.
- The primary objective of the CHA (1982) was to promote and restore physical and mental well-being of residents of Canada and to facilitate reasonable access to health care services without financial or other barriers based on the following five criteria's: (a) Public administration; (b) universality; (c) accessibility; (d) portability, and (e) comprehensiveness.
- The term "*medically necessary*" within the context of the CHA has been open to wide interpretations, and is one that has been hotly debated.
- In 1975, national health care expenditures was approximately $12.2 billion (7% of GDP), and by 2012 the costs have increased significantly to $207 billion (11.6% of GDP) (CIHI 2010a, 2013) due largely to our continued reliance on antiquated health care funding models driven by episodic acute care hospital-based physician-driven health care services and diagnostic procedures.

- Currently, our publicly insured health systems are at a crossroad in Canada with mounting social and political pressures to loosen the restrictions based on the CHA and create a parallel system of privately funded health care models.
- We argued that the current dominance of the medical model of health care, which has served as the foundation for our publicly insured Medicare systems since the 1960s, requires a dramatic shift in focus which includes the need to embrace holistic definitions of health and the adoption of primary health care models that encourage interdisciplinary community-based collaborative health care services.
- There is an increased need to reexamine home and community-based models of care to properly address health challenges facing Canadians in the new millennium, such as an aging Canadian population and the growth in the incidence of non-communicable chronic disease (e.g., Alzheimer's disease, stroke, heart disease, type 2 diabetes) and disabilities.

Critical Thinking Questions

1. Review the five criteria of the Canada Health Act. Which of these criteria's/ criteria do you believe is most important in your community and why? How would you revise the Canada Health Act to make it relevant and enforceable nationally?
2. How would you define a "medically necessary" in your community? Do you feel additional health care interventions or procedures by other health care professionals and workers (e.g., public health nurses, health promoters, and rehab therapists) should be included in your definition? Why or why not?
3. List and identify for-profit clinics in your community or region. What health care services are being provided, and who is accessing them? Identify and contrast the current strengths and limitations of both private-for-profits clinics and your provincial/ territorial publicly funded health care system. How do you think the health of your residents in your community will be affected if health care services were based solely on the ability to pay rather than need?
4. If you had an opportunity to provide input into the creation of the ideal health care system designed to provide the best care to the most people in the most cost–efficient manner, how would you do it? Describe the principles of your health care system, priorities, how health care services would be allocated, mechanisms for delivery and financing.

References

Abbott, J. *New Report Shows Overuse of Diagnostic Imaging and Inappropriate Prescribing*, Health Council of Canada (news release), Ottawa, Ontario: Health Council of Canada, September 27, 2010. Retrieved August 25, 2011, http://www.newswire.ca/en/releases/archive/September2010/27/c5103.html.

Abbott, M. E. *History of Medicine in the Province of Québec.* Montréal: McGill University, 1931.

Abraham, C. "Early Release of Newborns Linked to Health Problems." *Globe and Mail*, 1999: A1–A2.

Alberta Consumers' Association. *Current Access to Cataract Surgery in Alberta.* Edmonton, Alberta: Author, 1994.

Armstrong, P., and H. Armstrong. *Wasting Away: The Undermining of Canadian Health Care,* 2nd ed. Don Mills, ON: Oxford University Press, 2003.

Armstrong, P., H. Armstrong, and D. Coburn. *Unhealthy Times: Political Economy Perspectives on Health and Care.* Don Mills, ON: Oxford University Press, 2001.

Auditor General of Canada. *1999 Report of the Auditor General of Canada to the House of Commons* (chapter 29). Ottawa, ON: Author, 2002. http://www.oag-bvg.gc.ca/domino/reports.nsf/html.9929ce.html/$file/9929ce-pdf].

Babson, J. H., and P. Brackstone. The Canadian Health Care System: Its History, Current Status and Similarities with the U.S. Health Care System. *Journal of Comparative Sociology* 1, no. 3 (1973): 24–30.

Bao, Y., N. Duan, and S. A. Fox. Is Some Provider Advice on Smoking Cessation Better than no Advice? An Instrumental Variable Analysis on the 2001 National Health Interview Survey. *Health Services Research* 41, no. 6 (2006): 2114–135.

Bartfay, W. J., and E. Bartfay. *Public Health in Canada.* Boston, MA: Pearson Learning Solutions, 2015 (ISBN:13:978-1-323-01471-4).

Bartfay, W. J. "Men in Nursing in Canada: Past, Present and Future Perspectives." In *Men in Nursing: History, Challenges and Opportunities,* edited by C. E. O'Lynn and R. E. Tranbarger, 205–18. New York, NY: Springer Publishing Company, 2008.

Bartfay, W. J. "Canada's Health Care System: History and Current Challenges." In *Community Health Nursing: Caring in Action,* edited by J. E. Hitchcock, P. E. Schubert, S. A. Thomas, and W. J. Bartfay, 23–41. Toronto, ON: Nelson Education, 2010a.

Bartfay, W. J. "A Brief History of Community Health Nursing in Canada." In *Community Health Nursing: Caring in Action,* edited by J. E. Hitchcock, P. E. Schubert, S. A. Thomas, and W. J. Bartfay, 11–22.Toronto, ON: Nelson Education, 2010b.

Baumgart, A. J., and M. M. Wheeler. "The Nursing Workforce in Canada." In *Canadian nurses Face the Future,* edited by A. J. Baumgart and J. Larsen, 45–69. Scarborough, ON: Mosby-Year Book, 1992.

Bliss, M. "A Preface." In *Report on Social Security for Canada,* edited by L. Marsh. Toronto, ON: University of Toronto, 1975.

Begin, M. *Revisiting the Canada Health Act (1984): What Are the Impediments to Change?* Paper presented at the Institute for Research on Public Policy, 30th Anniversary Conference, Ottawa, Ontario, 2002.

Bloom, D. E., E. Cafiero, E. Jane-Llopis, S. Abraham-Gessel, L. Bloom, S. Fathima, and A. B. Feigl. *The Global Economic Burden of Noncommunicable Diseases.* Geneva, Switzerland: World Economic Forum, 2011. Retrieved July 2, 2013, www.weforum.org.org/reports/global-economic-burden-noncommunicable-diseases.

Bothwell, R. *History of Canada Since 1867.* East Lansing, MI: Michigan State University Press, 1996.

Boyle, T. *New Rules Causes Chaos for Audiologists,* A27. Toronto, ON: Toronto Star, July 7, 2001.

Branswell, H. Canada's Health Spending Increase in 2014 Smallest in 17 Years. Toronto, ON: The Canadian Press, October 20, 2014. Retrieved November 15, 2015, https://www.questia.com/newspaper/1P3-3478376451/health-spending-increase-this-year-smallest-in-17.

Brennan, R. Doctor's Strike Memories Linger. *The Windsor Star.* Windsor, ON: A3, December 27, 1986.

Brotman, S. The Incidence of Poverty among Seniors in Canada: Exploring the Impact of Gender, Ethnicity and Race. *Canadian Journal of Aging/La Revue Canadienne du Viellissement* 17, no. 2 (1998): 166–85.

Brown, G., S. Birch, and L. Thabane. *Better Care: An Analysis of Nursing and Health Care System Outcomes.* Ottawa, ON: Canadian Health Services Research Foundation and Canadian Nurses Association, 2012.

Buchignani, N., and C. Armstrong-Esther. Informal Care and Older Native Canadians. *Ageing and Society* 19, no.1 (1999): 3–32.

Bullough, L. V., B. Bullough, and M. Stranton. *Florence Nightingale and Her Era: A Collection of New Scholarship.* New York: Garland Press, 1990.

Bumsted, J. *History of the Canadian Peoples.* Oxford, UK: Oxford University Press, 2004.

Butler-Jones, D. *The Chief Public Health Officer's Report on the Status of Public Health in Canada 2012.* Ottawa, ON: Her Majesty the Queen in Right of Canada, 2012. (ISSN: 1917-2656, Catalogue No. HP2-10/2012E).

Canadian Association of Schools of Nursing. *National Nursing Education Strategy Framework.* Ottawa, ON: Author, 2002.

Canadian Broadcasting Services. *Life Expectancy in Canada Hits 80 for Men and 84 for Women. For Both Sexes Life Expectancy is Up at Birth.* Toronto, ON: CBC, 2014. Retrieved November 10, 2015, http://www.cbc.ca/news/health/life-expectancy-in-canada-hits-80-for-men-84-for-women-1.2644355.

Canadian Health Services Research Foundation. *Myth Busters: A Parallel Private System Would Reduce Waiting Times in the Public System.* Ottawa, Ontario: Author, 2001.

Canadian Heritage. *Origin of the Name-Canada. Canadian Heritage.* Ottawa, ON: Government of Canada, 2004. http://www.canadianheritage.gc/progs/cpsc-ccsp/sc-o5_e.cfm.

Canadian Home Care Association [in collaboration with L' Association des CLSC et des CHSLD du Québec]. *Portrait of Canada: An Overview of Public Home Care Programs.* Ottawa, ON: Health Canada, 1998.

Canadian Institute for Health Information. *National Health Expenditure Database. National Health Expenditure Trends, 1975–2001.* Ottawa, ON: CIHR, 2001.

Canadian Institute for Health Information. *Health Care in Canada 2005.* Ottawa, ON: CIHR, 2005. https://secure.cihi.ca/cihiweb/disPage.jsp?cw_page=AR_43_E.

Canadian Institute for Health Information. Health Care in Canada, 2005. Ottawa, ON: CIHI, 2006a. www.secure.cihi.ca/cihiweb/dispPage.jsp?cw_page+AR_43_E.

Canadian Institute for Health Information. Workforce Trends of Registered Nurses in Canada. Ottawa, ON: Author, 2006b.

Canadian Institute for Health Information. *Health Care in Canada, 2006.* Ottawa, Ontario: CIHI, 2007. (ISBN 978-1-55465-049-1), www.cihi.ca.

Canadian Institute for Health Information. National Health Expenditure Trends 1975-2009. Ottawa, ON: Author, 2010a.

Canadian Institute for Health Information. *2010 Health Indicators Report.* Ottawa, ON: Author, 2010b.

Canadian Institute for Health Information. *National health expenditure trends, 1975 to 2010.* Ottawa, ON: Author, 2010c.

Canadian Institute for Health Information. *Canada's Health Care Spending Growth Slows. Provincial and Territorial Government Health Expenditures Expected to Grow 3.1%, Lowest Since 1997.* Ottawa, ON: CIHI, 2013. Retrieved June 13, 2013, www.cihi.ca/cihi-ext-portal/internet/en/document/spending+and+health+workforce/spending/release_30oct12.

Canadian Institute for Health Information. *Number of Doctors in Canada Continues to Increase.* Ottawa, ON: CIHI, 2014. Retrieved November 10, 2015, www.cihi.ca/sites/default/files/document/physicians2014_ps_final_en.pdf.

Canadian Institute for Health Information. *National Health Expenditure Trends, 1975 to 2015.* Ottawa, ON: CIHI, 2015a. ISBN 978-1-77-109-413-9 (PDF). Retrieved November 10, 2015, https://www.cihi.ca/en/spending-and-health-workforce/spending/canadas-slow-health-spending-growth-continues.

Canadian Institute for Health Information. (CIHI 2016). *National Health Expenditures: How Much Does Canada Spend on Health Care?* Ottawa, Ontario: CIHI. Retrieved April 14, 2017, http://www.cihi.ca/en/nhex2016-topic1.

Canadian Institute for Health Information. *More Doctors, Higher Spending: Data Sheds Light on Trends in the Physician Workforce.* Ottawa, ON: CIHI, 2015b.

Canadian Institute for Health Information (2018). *Health spending.* Ottawa, ON: Author. Retrieved March 3, 2018 from https://www.cihi.ca/en/health-spending.

Canadian Nurses Association. *On Your Own: The Nurse Entrepreneur. Nursing Now: Issues and Trends in Canadian Nursing, 1.* Ottawa, ON: Canadian Nurses Association, 1996. www.cna-nurses.ca/pages/issuestrends/nrgnow/On Your Own Entrepreneur September 1996.pdf).

Canadian Nurses Association. *Highlights of 2003 Nursing Statistics.* Ottawa, ON: Author, December, 2004. http://www.can-nurses.ca/CNA/nursing/statistics.

Chenier, N. *Health Policy in Canada. Library of Parliament, Research Branch, 1994, Revised 1999.* Ottawa, ON, 1999. http://www.dsp-psd.pwgsc.ca/Collection-R-LoPBdp/CIR/934-e.htm.

Chodos, H., and J. J. MacLeod. Romanow and Kirby on the Public/Private Divide in Health Care: Demystifying the Debate. *Health care Papers* 4, no. 4 (2004): 10–25.

Canadian Cancer Society and Statistics Canada. *Canadian Cancer Statistics 2011*. Toronto, ON: Canadian Cancer Society, 2011.

Chaoulli v. Québec Attorney General. *1 S.C.R. 791, 2005 SCC 35*. Montréal, QC: University of Montréal, 2005. Retrieved July 25, 2010, http://scc.lexum.umontreal.ca/en/2005/2005scc35.html

Cheadle, B. *What We're Proud of: Universal Health Care Give Us Glowing Hearts But Not the Queen, Poll Suggests*, A6. Toronto, ON: Toronto Star, November 26, 2012.

Childhood Obesity Foundation. *Statistics*. VGH Hospital Campus, Vancouver, BC, 2015. Retrieved November 10, 2015, http://childhoodobesityfoundation.ca/what-is-childhood-obesity/statistics/.

Choosing Wisely and Canadian Institute for Health Information. (April, 2017). *Uncessary care in Canada: Technical Report*. Ottawa, ON: Authors. ISBN: 978-1-771090583-9. Retrieved March 3, 2018 from https://www.cihi.ca/sites/default/files/document/choosing-wisely-technical-report-en-web.pdf.

Cloutier-Fisher, D., and Joseph, A. E. Long-Term Care Restructuring in Rural Ontario: Retrieving Community Service User and Provider Narratives. *Social Science and Medicine* 50, no. 7–8 (2000): 1043–47.

Coburn, D. The Development of Canadian Nursing: Professionalization and Proleterianization. *International Journal of Health Services* 18, no. 3 (1988): 437–56.

Cook, E. T. *The Life of Florence Nightingale*. Vols. I and II. London: The Macmillan Company, 1913.

Commission on the Future of Health Care in Canada. *Building on Values: The Future of Health Care in Canada-Final Report*. Ottawa, ON: Government of Canada, 2002. Retrieved July 02, 2013, http://publications.bc.ca/collections/Collection?CP32_85_2002E.pdf.

Commonwealth Fund. *Commonwealth Fund International Health Policy Survey of the General Public*. New York: Author, 2015. Retrieved December 03, 2015, www.commonwealthfund.org/interactives-and-data.

Conference Board of Canada. *Canadians Values and Attitudes on Canada's Health Care System: A Synthesis of Survey Results*. Ottawa, ON: Author, October 2000.

Cranswick, K. Help Close at Hand: Relocating to Give or Receive Care. *Canadian Social Trends* 12 (Winter 1999): 11–17.

Danzon, P. Hidden Overhead Costs: Is Canada's System Really Less Expensive?. *Health Affairs* XX (Spring, 1992): 21–34.

Deber, R. B. Getting What We Pay for: Myth and Realities About Financing Canada's Health Care System. *Health Law in Canada* 21, no. 2 (2000): 9–56.

Department of Finance Canada. *What Is Territorial Formula Financing?*. Ottawa, ON: Government of Canada, 2002. www.fin.gc.ca/FEDPROV/tffe.htm.

Department of Finance Canada. *Tax Points Transfer*. Ottawa, ON: Author, 2008. Retrieved July 08, 2010, www.fin.gc.ca/transfers/taxpoint-eng.asp.

Deraspe, R., and J. Gauthier. *Canada Health Transfer: Equal-Per-Capita Cash by 2014*. Ottawa, ON: Library of Parliament, 2011. Retrieved November 10, 2015, www.parl.gc.ca/Content/LOP/ResearchPublications/cei-14-e.htm.

Dickens, C. *Martin Chuzzlewit*. New York: The Macmillan Company, 1910.

Donahue, M. P. *Nursing the Finest Art: An Illustrated History*. 2nd ed. Toronto, ON: Mosby, 1996.

Dykeman, M. Primary Health Care Leads to Better Health. *The Canadian Nurse* 108, no. 7 (2012), 52.

Eldridge v. British Columbia Attorney General. *3 S.C. R. 624*. Ottawa, ON: Supreme Court of Canada, 2007.

Falk-Rafael, A., and S. Coffey. "Financing, Policy, and Politics of Health Care Delivery." In *Community Health Nursing: A Canadian Perspective*, edited by L. Lesseberg Stamler and L. Yiu, 17–34. Toronto, ON: Pearson Prentice Hall, 2005.

False Creek Surgical Centre. *Our Facility*. Vancouver, BC: Author, 2009. Retrieved July 25, 2010, http://www.nationalsurgery.com/facility.html.

Flood, M. C., and T. Archibald. The Illegality of Private Health Care in Canada. *Canadian Medical Association Journal* 164, no. 6 (2001): 825–30.

Fuller, C., ed. *Home Care: What We Know and What We Need*. Vol. ii. Ottawa, ON: Canada Health Coalition, 2001.

Gauthier, J. *The Canada Health Transfer: Changes to Provincial Allocations*. Ottawa, ON: Parliamentary Information and Research Service, Library of Parliament. Publication no. 2011-02-E, 2011.

Gelber, S. M. The Path to Health Insurance. *Canadian Public Administration* 9 (June 1966): 156–65.

Gibbon, J. W. *The Victorian Order of Nurses for Canada: 50th Anniversary, 1897–1947.* Montréal, QC: Southam Press, 1947.

Gibbon, J. W., and M. S. Mathewson. *Three Centuries of Canadian Nursing.* Toronto, ON: Macmillan Company of Canada Ltd., 1947.

Glazer, Y. N. The Home as Workshop: Women as Amateur Nurses and Medical Care Providers. *Gender and Society* 4, no. 4 (December 1990): 486–92.

Glazier, R., B. Zagorski, and J. Rayner. *Comparison of Primary Care Models in Ontario by Demographic, Case Mix and Emergency Department Use, 2008/09 to 2009/10. ICES Investigative Report.* Toronto, ON: Institute for Clinical and Evaluative Sciences, 2012. Retrieved July 04, 2013, http://www.ices.on.ca/file/ICES_Primary%20Care%20Models%20english.pdf.

Government of Canada. *Canada, House of Commons. An Act Relating to Cash Contributions by Canada in Respect of Insured Health Services Provided Under Provincial Health Care Insurance Plans and Amounts Under Provincial Health Care Insurance Plans and Amounts Payable by Canada in Respect to Extended Health Care Services and to Amend and Repeal Certain Acts in Consequence Thereof (The Canada Health Act).* Ottawa, ON: Author, 1984.

Government of Canada. *A Brief History of the Canada Health and Social Transfer (CHST).* Ottawa, ON: Department of Finance, 2002a. www.fin.gc.ca/FEDPROV/hise.html).

Government of Canada. *The Transfer of Tax Points to Provinces Under the Canada Health and Social Transfer.* Ottawa, ON: Author, 2002b. Retrieved July 9, 2010. dsp-psd.tpsgc.gc.ca/Collection-R/LoPbdP/BP/bp450-e.thm.

Government of Canada, Department of Finance. *The Budget Plan 2006: Focusing on Priorities.* Ottawa, ON: Author, 2006.

Government of Canada. Constitution *Acts 1867 to 1982.* Ottawa, ON: Department of Justice, 2007a. www.//laws.justice.gc.ca/en/const/index.html].

Government of Canada. *Canada Health Act Annual Report, 2005–2006.* Ottawa, ON: Author, 2007b.

Government of Canada. *Summary of Findings 2013. The Canadian Tobacco, Alcohol, and Drugs Survey (CTADS).* Ottawa, ON: Author, 2015a. Retrieved November 12, 2015, http://healthycanadians.gc.ca/science-research-sciences-recherches/data-donnees/ctads-ectad/summary-sommaire-2013-eng.php.

Government of Canada. *Federal Support to Provinces and Territories. Major Federal Transfers.* Ottawa, ON: Department of Finance, 2015b. Retrieved November 12, 2015, http://www.fin.gc.ca/access/fedprov-eng.asp.

Governor General of Canada. *Role and Responsibilities of the Governor General.* Ottawa, ON: Governor General of Canada, 2005. http://www.gg.cc/gg/rr/index_e.asp.

Greifinger, R. B., and V. W. Sidel. "American Medicine: Charity Begins at Home." In *The Nation's Health*, edited by P. Lee, N. Brown, and I. Red, 124–34. San Francisco: Boyd & Fraser, 1981.

Hales, D., and L. Lauzon. *An Invitation to Health*, 1st ed. Toronto, ON: Thomson/Nelson, 2007.

Hall, J. *Less Bang for Health Dollar in Canada*, A10. Toronto, ON: Toronto Star, May 13, 2011.

Health Canada. *Canada Health Act 1999–2000.* Ottawa, ON: Minister of Public Works and Government Services Canada, 2000, 14–15.

Health Canada. *Chapter C-6. Consolidated Statutes and Regulations (Canada Health Act).* Ottawa, ON: Government of Canada, 2001. www.hc-sc.gc.ca/medicare/Canada%0Health%20Act.htm.

Health Canada. *The National Strategy: Moving Forward. The 2003 Progress Report on Tobacco Control.* Ottawa, ON: Author, 2003a.

Health Canada. *Canada Health Act: Frequently Asked Questions.* Ottawa, ON: Government of Canada, 2003b. www.hc-sc.gc.ca/medicare/FAQ.htm.

Health Canada. *Canada Health Act Annual Report 2007–2009.* Ottawa, ON: Author, 2009. Retrieved June 23, 2010, www.hc-sc.gc.ca/hcs-sss/pubs/cha-1cs/2008-cha-1cs/2008-cha-ar-ra/page1-eng.php.

Health Canada. *Health Concerns. Carcinogens in Tobacco Smoke.* Ottawa, ON: Author, 2011. Retrieved November 12, 2015, www.hc-sc.g.ca-ps/pubs/tobac-tabc/carcinogens-carcerogenese/index-eng.php.

Health Canada. *First Nations, Inuit and Aboriginal Health. Drinking Water and Waste Water.* Ottawa, ON: Author, 2012. Retrieved July 03, 2013, www.hc-sc.gc.ca/fniah-spnia/promotion/public-publique/water-eau-eng.php#how_many.

Health Canada. *Summary of Results of the Youth Smokers Survey*. Ottawa, ON: Author, 2014. Retrieved December 03, 2015, http://www.hc-sc.gc.ca/hc-ps/tobac-tabac/research-recherche/stat/_survey-sondage_2012-2013/result-eng.php.

Health Canada and Heart and Stroke Foundation of Canada. *Transforming the Food Supply. Report of the Trans Fat Task Force*. Ottawa, ON: Minister of Health, 2006.

Health Council of Canada. *Decisions, Decisions: Family Doctors as Gatekeepers to Prescription Drugs and Diagnostic Imaging in Canada*. Toronto, ON: Author, 2010.

Health Council of Canada. *Progress Report 2011: Health Care Renewal in Canada*. Toronto, Ontario: Author, 2011. information@healthcouncilcanada.ca.

Henderson, H. *Group Wants to Do Something About Seniors Who Are Released From Hospital Too Early (Home Alone)*, H5. Toronto, ON: Toronto Star, July 16, 1994.

Heeney, H. *Life Before Medicare: Canadian Experiences*. Toronto, ON: Ontario Coalition of Senior Citizens' Organizations, 1995.

Heritage Canada. The Queen and Canada: 53 Years of Growing Together. Ottawa, ON: Heritage Canada, 2005. http://www.gg.ca/gg.ca/royalvisit2005/53_e.cfm.

Herstein, H. H., L. J. Hughes, and R. C. Kirbyson. *Challenge and Survival: The History of Canada*. Scarborough, ON: Prentice-Hall of Canada, 1970.

Hill R. G., Jr., L. M. Sears, and S. W. Melanson. 4000 Clicks: A Productivity Analysis of Electronic Medical Records in a Community Hospital ED. *The American Journal of Emergency Medicine* 31, no. 11 (November, 2013): 1591–94.

Hinshaw, A. S. A Continuing Challenge: The Shortage of Educationally Prepared Nursing Faculty. *Online Journal of Issues in Nursing*, 2001. http://www.nursingworld.org/ojin/topic14/tpc 14_3.htm.

Human Resources and Skills Development Canada. *Federal Disability Report*. Ottawa, ON: Author, 2010. Accessed July 03, 2013. www.hrsdc.gc.ca/eng/disability_issues/report/fdr/2010/fdr_1010.pdf.

Kenton, E. *The Jesuit Relations and Documents*. New York: The Vanguard Press, 1925.

Kerr, J. "Early Nursing in Canada, 1600 to 1760: A Legacy for the Future." In *Canadian Nursing: Issues and Perspectives*, edited by J. Kerr and J. MacPhail, 3–10. Toronto, ON: Mosby, 1996.

Kerr, M., Frost, D., and Bignell, D. *Don't We Count as People? Saskatchewan Social Welfare Policy and Women's Health*. Saskatchewan: SK. Women's Health Centre of Excellence, 2004.

Kravitz, R. L., M. F. Shapiro, L. S. Linn, and E. S. Froelicher. Risk Factors Associated With Participation in the Ontario Canada Doctor's Strike. *American Journal of Public Health* 79 (1989): 1233–77.

Lang, M. Calgary's Quads: Born in the U.S.A. *Calgary Herald*, August 17, 2007. Retrieved July 23, 2010, http://www.canada.com/topics/news/story/html?id=78b28230-d3ff-47d3-ab04-fff760931f1a.

Law, M., L. Cheng, I. Dhalla, D. Heard, and S. Morgan. The Effect of Cost on Adherence to Prescription Medications in Canada. *Canadian Medical Association Journal* 184, no. 3 (2012): 297–302.

Leduc Browne, P. *Unsafe Practices: Restructuring and Privatization in Ontario Health Care*. Ottawa, ON: Canadian Centre for Policy Alternatives, 2000.

Lee Akazaki, R. Unconscionable Delay of Civil Justice: Is It Also Unconstitutional? *Advocates Quarterly*, 32, no. 3, 2007. http://www.gilbertsondavis.com/publications/delay.htm.

Library and Archives Canada. *Introduction—Famous Canadian Physicians*. Ottawa, Ontario: Government of Canada, 2007a. http://www.collectionscanada.ca/physicians/index-e.html.

Library and Archives Canada. *Sir William Osler—Famous Canadian Physicians*. Ottawa, Ontario: Government of Canada, 2007b. http://www.collectionscanada.ca/physicians/002032-230-e.html

Library and Archives Canada. Dr. Wilder Penfield—Famous Canadian Physicians. Ottawa, ON: Government of Canada, 2007c.

Library and Archives Canada. *Sir Frederick Banting—Famous Canadian Physicians*. Ottawa, ON: Government of Canada, 2007d http://www.collectionscanada.ca/physicians/002032-200-e.html

Library and Archives Canada. *Dr. Emily Howard Stowe-Famous Canadian Physicians*. Ottawa, ON: Government of Canada, 2007e. http://www.collectionscanada.ca/physicians/002032-250-e.html]

Library of Parliament. *The Canada Health Act: Overview and Options*. Ottawa, ON: Author, 2005. Accessed July 13, 2010. http://www.parl.gc.ca/information/library/PRBpubs/944-e.pdf.

Lipset, S. M. *Continental Divide: The Values and Institutions of the United States and Canada*. New York: Routledge, 1990.

Loades, D. *Chronicles of the Tudor kings*. Wayne, NJ: CLB International, 1990.

Mackenbach, J. P., Bouvier-Colle, M. H., and Jougla, E. Avoidable Mortality and Health Services: A Review of Aggregate Data Studies. *Journal of Epidemiology and Community Health* 44 (1990): 106–11.

Mackie, R. Project Not Helping to Ease MD Shortage. *Globe and Mail,* A27. Toronto, ON, July 9, 2001.

Makarenko, J. *The Charter and Health Care in Canada*. Mapleleafweb, July 1, 2005. Accessed July 27, 2010. http://www.mapleweafweb.com/features/charter-health-care-canada.

Makeover, M. E. *Mismanaged Care: How Corporate Medicine Jeopardizes Your Health*. New York: Prometheus, 1998.

Manuel, D. G., and Y. Mao. Avoidable Mortality in the United States and Canada, 1980–1996. *American Journal of Public Health* 92, no. 9 (2002): 1481–84.

Miarchione, M. Soda, Other Sugary Drinks More Firmly Tied to Obesity in New Studies. *Huffington Post*, 2012. Accessed November 15, 2015. http://www.huffingtonpost.com/2012/09/21/obesity-soda-sugary-drinks_n_1904732.html.

Margoshes, D. *Tommy Douglas: Building the New Society*. Montréal, QC: XYZ Publishing, 1999.

Marsh, L. *Report on Social Security for Canada 1943*. Toronto, ON: University of Toronto Press, 1975.

Mobily, P. R., and A. M. Stineman. "Nursing Faculty: Opportunities and Challenges." In *Current Issues in Nursing*, 7th ed., edited by Slavik Cown, P., and S. Moorhead, 37–44. St. Louis, Missouri, Mosby/Elsevier, 2006.

Monahan, P. J. *Chaoulli v Québec and the Future of Canadian Health Care: Patient Accountability as the "Sixth Criteria" of the Canada Health Act. C.D. Howe Institute Benefactors Lecture*. Toronto, ON: i-30, 2006.

Moskop, J. C. "The Nature and Limits of Physician Authority." In *Doctors, Patients and Society*, edited by M. S. Straum and D. E. Larsen, 34–42. Waterloo, ON: Wildfrid Laurier University, 1981.

Muldoon, L., S. Dahrouge, W. Hogg, R. Geneau, G. Russell, and M. Shortt. Community Orientation in Primary Care Practices. Results from the Comparison of Models of Primary Health Care in Ontario study. *Canadian Family Physicians* 56, no. 7 (2010): 678–83.

Mussalem, H. K. "Professional Nurses' Associations." In *Canadian Nursing Faces the Future*, 2nd ed., edited by A. J. Baumgart and J. Larse, 495–18. Toronto, ON: Mosby, 1992.

National Expert Commission Canadian Nurses Association. *A Nursing Call to Action. The Health of Our Nation, the Future of Our Health System*. 50 Driveway, Ottawa, ON: Canadian Nurses Association, 2012 (ISBN: 978-1-55119-387-8). Accessed July 2, 2013. http://www.can-aiic.ca/expertcomission/

National Forum on Health, ed., *Canada Health Action: Building on the Legacy*. Vol. 2 of *Synthesis Reports and Issues Papers*. Ottawa, ON: Public Works and Government Services, 1997. http://www.hc.sc-gc.ca/english/care/health_forum/forum_e.htm.

Nolte, E., and M. McKee. Measuring the Health of Nations: Updating an Earlier Analysis. *Health Affairs* 27, no. 1 (2008): 58–71.

Nolte, E., and M. McKee. Variations in Amenable Mortality—Trends in 16 High Income Nations. *Health Policy* 103, no. 1 (2011): 47–52.

O'Brien-Pallas, L., C. Alksnis, and S. Wang. *Bringing the Future Into Focus: Projecting RN Retirement in Canada*. Ottawa, ON: Canadian Institute for Health Information, 2003 (ISBN 1-55392-263-8).

Ontario Association of Community Care Access Centres, Ontario Federation of Community Mental Health and Addiction Programs, and Ontario Hospital Association. *Ideas and Opportunities for Bending the Health Care Cost Curve*. Toronto, ON: Authors, 2010. Accessed July 03, 2013. http://www.oha.com?news?mediaCentre/Documents/Bending%20th%20Health%20Care%20Cost%20Curve%20(Final%20Report%20-%20April%2013%202010).pdf.

Ontario Ministry of Education. *Healthy Foods for Healthy Schools Act*. Toronto, ON: Author, 2008.

Pringle, D., L. Green, and S. Johnson. *Nursing Education in Canada: Historical Review and Current Capacity. The Nursing Sector Study Corporation*. Ottawa, ON: Government of Canada, 2004 (ISBN-0-9734932-9-1).

Parkman, F. *The Jesuits in North America in the Seventeenth Century*. Boston: Little, Brown, 1897.

Public Health Agency of Canada. *Core Competencies for Public Health in Canada: Release 1.1*. Ottawa, ON: Author, 2007. http://www.phac-aspc.gc.ca/core_competencies or http://www.phac-aspc.gc.ca/php-psp/ccph-cesp/pdfs/cc-manual-eng090407.pdf.

Public Health Agency of Canada. *Canada's Aging Population. Division of Aging Seniors*. Ottawa, ON: PHAC, 2008. Retrieved June 13, 2013, www.phac-aspc.gc.ca/seniors-aines/publications/public/various-varies/papier-fed-paper/index-eng.php.

Public Health Agency of Canada. *Tracking Heart Disease and Stroke in Canada*. Ottawa, ON: Author, 2009.

Public Health Agency of Canada. Government of Canada Invests in Project Promoting Walking to Prevent Chronic Disease. Ottawa, ON: Author, 2015. Retrieved November 9, 2015, http://www.newswire.ca/news-releases/government-of-canada-invests-in-project-promoting-walking-to-prevent-chronic-disease-520318011.html.

Qi, Q., A. Y. Chu, J. H. Kang, M. K. Jensen, C. C. Gary, R. P. Louis, and M. R. Paul. Sugar-Sweetened Beverages and Genetic Risk of Obesity. *New England Journal of Medicine* 367 (2011): 1387–96. doi:10.1056/NEJMoa1203039. Retrieved November 15, 2015, http://www.nejm.org/doi/full/10.1056/NEJMoa1203039.

Rachlis, M., and C. Kushner. *Strong Medicine: How to Save Canada's Health Care System*. Toronto, ON: Harper Perennial, 1994.

Rayburn, Al. *Naming Canada: Stories of Canadian Place Names* 2nd ed. Toronto, ON: University of Toronto Press, 2001.

Reid, J. L., and D. Hammond. *Tobacco Use in Canada: Patterns and Trends, 2011 Edition*. Waterloo, ON: Propel Centre for Population Health Impact, University of Waterloo, 2011. Retrieved July 2, 2013, http://www.tobaccoreport.ca/

Repplier, A. *Mere Marie of the Ursulines*. New York: Sheed and Ward, 1931.

Rice, J. J., and Prince, M. J. *Changing Politics of Canadian Social Policy*. Toronto, ON: University of Toronto Press, 2000.

Robinson Vollman, A., E. T. Anderson, and J. McFarlane. *Canadian Community as Partner: Theory and Practice*. New York: Lippincott, Williams & Wilkins, 2004.

Richardson, S. Lessons From the Past: Entrepreneurial Nursing Practice in Perspective. *AARN (Alberta Association of Registered Nurses) Newsletter* 53, no. 4 (1997): 19–29.

Romanow, R. J. *Building on Values: The Future of Health Care in Canada—Final Report*. Commission on the Future of Health Care in Canada (cat. No. CP32-85/2002E-IN), Ottawa, ON: Government of Canada, 2002. http://www.hc-sc.gc.ca/english/care/romanow/hcc0023.html.

Rombough, R., E. Howse, and W. J. Bartfay. Caregiver Stain and Caregiver Burden of Primary Caregivers of Stroke Survivors With and Without Aphasia: A Systematic Review. *Journal of Rehabilitation Nursing* 31, no. 5 (2006): 199–209.

Russell, G., S. Dahrouge, W. Hogg, R. Geneau, L. Muldoon, and M. Tuna. Managing Chronic Disease in Ontario Primary Care: The Impact of Organizational Factors. *Annals of Family Medicine* 7, no. 4 (2010): 309–18.

Senate of Canada. *The Health of Canadians—The Federal role. Interim Report of the Standing Committee on Social Affairs, Science and Technology*. Ottawa, ON: Government of Canada, 2001.

Shah, P. C. *Public Health and Preventive Medicine in Canada*. 5th ed. Toronto, ON: Elsevier Saunders, 2003.

Shields, M. Smoking Bans: Influence on Smoking Prevalence. *Health Reports* 18, no. 3 (2007): 9–24.

Shimo, A. Complete User's Guide to Private Medical Care in Canada. *MacLeans*, 119 (2006): 31–50.

Soderstrom, L. *The Canadian Health Care System*. London: Croom Helm, 1978.

Soroka, S., and A. Mahon. *Analysis of the Impact of Current Health Care System Funding and Financing Models and the Value of Health Care in Canada*. Ottawa, ON: Canadian Health Services Research Foundation and Canadian Nurses Association, 2012.

Soroka, N. S. *Canadian Perceptions of the Health Care System*. Toronto, ON: Health Council of Canada, 2007. Retrieved July 2, 2013, http://www.queensu.ca/cora/_files/PublicPerceptions.pdf.

Spitzer, D. L. "They Don't Listen to Your Body": Minority Women, Nurses and Childbirth Under Health Reform. In *Care and Consequences: The Impact of Health Care Reform*, edited by D. L. Gustafson, 85–106. Halifax: Fernwood, 2000.

Standing Senate Committee on Social Affairs, Science and Technology. *Time for Transformative Change. A Review of the 2004 Health Accord*. Ottawa, ON: Senate of Canada, 2012. Retrieved July 2, 2013, http://www.parl.gc.ca/Content/SEN/committee/411/soci/rep/rep07mar12-e.pdf.

Standing Senate Committee on Social Affairs, Science and Technology, Subcommittee on Population Health. *A Healthy, Productive Canada: A Determinant of Health Approach*. Ottawa, ON: Author, 2009. Retrieved July 2, 2013, http://www.parl.gc.ca/Content/SEN/Committee/402/popu/rep/rephealth1jun09-e.pdf.

Statistics Canada. *Population by Selected Ethnic Origins, by Provinces and Territories*. Ottawa, ON: Statistics Canada, 2005. http://www40.statcan.ca/101/cst01/demo26a.htm.

Statistics Canada. *Study: Projections of the Diversity of the Canadian Population*. Ottawa, ON: Author, 2010a. Retrieved July 2, 2013, www.statcan.gc.ca/daily-quotidien/100309/dq100526b-eng.htm.

Statistics Canada. Population Projections: Canada, the Provinces and Territories. *The Daily*. Ottawa, ON: Author, 2010b. Retrieved July 2, 2012, www.statcan.gc.ca/daily-quotidien/100526/dq100526b-eng.htm.

Statistics Canada. *2011 Census: Population and Dwelling Counts*. Ottawa, ON: Author, 2012a. Retrieved July 6, 2013, www.statcan.gc.ca/daily-quotidien/`20208a-eng.htm.

Statistics Canada. *Health Indicators 2012*. Ottawa, ON: Canadian Institute for Health Information, 2012b.

Statistics Canada. *Canada's Population Estimates; Age and Sex 2014*. Ottawa, ON: Author, 2014. Retrieved November 10, 2015, http://www.statcan.gc.ca/daily-quotidien/140926/dq140926b-eng.htm.

Stewart, E. *Ontario Health, Social Net Takes $1 Billion Cut*, A9, Toronto, ON: Toronto Star, February 28, 1995.

Stewart, G. T. *History of Canada before 1867*. East Lansing, MI: Michigan State University Press, 1996.

Storch, J. "Canadian Health Care System." In *Realities of Canadian Nursing: Professional, Practice, and Power Issues*, 2nd ed., edited by M. McIntyre, E. Thomlinson, and C. McDonald, 27–53. New York: Lippincott William & Wilkins, 2006.

Suhrcke, M., M. McKee, R. Arce, S. Tsolova, and J. Mortensen. *The Contribution of Health to the Economy in the European Union*. Luxembourg, EU: Office for the Publications of the European Communities, 2005. Retrieved July 02, 2013, http://ec.europa.eu/health/ph_overview/Documents/health_economy_en.pdf.

Sullivan, T., and P. Baranek. *First Do No Harm: Making Sense of Canadian Health Reform*. Toronto, ON: Malcolm Lester & Associates, 2002.

Swan, R. *The History of Medicine in Canada. A Paper Read at the Symposium on The History of Medicine in the Commonwealth, September 23, 1966. Faculty of the History of Medicine and Pharmacy, Royal College of Physicians of London*. London, 1966: 42–51.

Swanson, J. M., and M. Albrecht. Community Health Nursing: Promoting the Health of Aggregates. Toronto, ON: WB Saunders Company, 1993.

Taylor, M. G. *Health Insurance and Canadian Public Policy*. 2nd ed. Montréal, QC: McGill Queens University Press, 1987.

Taylor, M. G. The Canadian Health Insurance Program. *Public Administration Review* 33 (1973): 31–39.

Toughill, K. *Doctors Charging Extra Fees Up Front*, A2. Toronto, ON: Toronto Star, May 28, 1992.

Treurniet, H. F., H. C. Boshuizen, and P. P. M. Harteloh. Avoidable Mortality in Europe (1980-1997): A Comparison of Trends. *Journal of Epidemiology and Community Health* 58, no. 4 (2004): 290–95.

Trigger, B. G., and J. F. Pendergast. *Saint-Lawrence Iroquoians. Handbook of North American Indians*. Vol. 15-OCLS 58762737. Washington: Smithsonian Institution, 1978: 357–61.

Villeneuve, M., and J. MacDonald. *Toward 2020: Visions for Nursing*. Ottawa, ON, Canadian Nurses Association, 2006 (ISBN 1-55119-818-5).

Wallace, E. The Origins of the Social Welfare State in Canada, 1867–1900. *Canadian Journal of Economics and Political Science* 16 (1950): 383–93.

Whittaker, J. A. "The Search for Legitimacy: Nurses' Registration in British Columbia, 1813–1935." In *Not Just Pin Money*, edited by B. Latham and R. Pazdro, 315–20. Victoria, BC: Camosun College, 1984.

Wilson, R. *The Canadian Medicare System—An Overview*. Pulmonary Hypertension Central. 2002 www.phcentral.org. features/110102wilson.html.

Woodham-Smith, C. *Florence Nightingale 1820–1910*. London, UK: Constable, 1950.

World Health Organization. *The World Health Report 2000. HealthSystems: Improving Performance*. Geneva, Switzerland: Author, 2000.

World Health Organization. *Disability and Health: Fact Sheet No. 352*. Geneva, Switzerland: Author, 2011. Retrieved July 02, 2013, http:www.who.int/mediacentre/factsheets/fs352/en/index.html.

Yelaja, P. *Home Care Getting Worse, Report Says*, A3. Toronto, ON: Toronto Star, August 2, 2001.

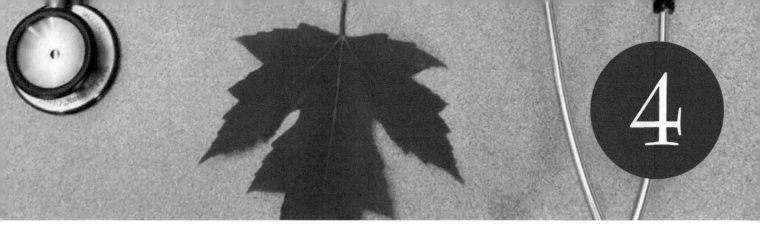

Indigenous Health in Canada

The significant problems we face cannot be solved at the same level of thinking we were at when we created them.

—Albert Einstein

Learning Objectives

After the completion of this chapter, the student will be able to:
- define and differentiate among the various types of Indigenous people in Canada,
- describe the historical, social and negative health impacts associated with contact with European colonizers and traders,
- describe the negative impacts of the Indian Act and treaty systems on Indigenous families and people,
- provide three examples of how the residential school system has negatively impacted Indigenous families and people,
- describe how health care is managed and delivered in Indigenous populations in Canada, and
- list and describe three major health challenges facing Indigenous populations in Canada currently.

Core Competencies addressed in Chapter 4

Core Competencies	Competency Statements
1.0 Public Health Sciences	1.1, 1.2, 1.3, 1.4
2.0 Assessment and Analysis	2.1, 2.2, 2.3, 2.4, 2.5, 2.6
3.0 Policy and Program Planning, Implementation, and Evaluation	3.1, 3.2, 3.3, 3.6
4.0 Partnerships, Collaboration, and Advocacy	4.1, 4.3, 4.4
5.0 Diversity and Inclusiveness	5.1, 5.2, 5.3
6.0 Communication	6.1, 6.2
7.0 Leadership	7.1, 7.2, 7.3, 7.6

Note: Please see the following document or web-based link for a detailed description of these specific competencies. Public Health Agency of Canada (2007).

Introduction

The term **"Indigenous"** is defined as people who are and remain the earliest or initial inhabitants of a place or land (Bartfay 2010; Bartfay and Bartfay 2015). According to Smith (2003), there are over 350 million indigenous people representing more than 5,000 unique cultures in over seventy countries globally. Indigenous peoples from various countries that include Canada, the United States, Africa, Australia and New Zealand unfortunately share in common a history of exploitation by the Caucasian Europeans colonizers. **Colonization** is defined as the process of establishing a colony or group of settlers in a new land or territory, whether previously inhabited or not, during which the settlers are both partially or fully subject to and accountable to their mother country of origin (Pearson and Trumble 1996). The historical evidence suggests that the social, spiritual, physical and mental health of Indigenous populations has been negatively impacted, and that colonization per se has resulted in their marginalization and disempowerment by white Europeans (Adelson 2005; Eckermann et al. 2006; Fleet 1997; McMurray 2007; WHO 1999, 2002a, 2002c).

This chapter explores the historical impact of European traders and colonizers on the health and well-being of Indigenous populations in Canada including First Nations, Inuit and Métis people. We will explore how Indigenous beliefs, concepts, health care practices and structures often conflict with western health care systems and definitions of health and well-being. We will

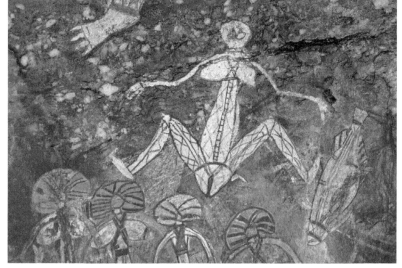

Photo 4.1 Example of Indigenous art from Australia. Indigenous peoples, also known as first peoples, aboriginals, or native peoples, are ethnic groups who are the original inhabitants of a given region or land, in contrast to groups that have settled, occupied or colonized the area more recently. There are currently an estimated 370 million Indigenous people globally.

examine the impact of various government policies that have been formulated to protect, civilize, and assimilate the First People into the Canadian society (Wasekeesikaw 2006). Similarly, we will explore the effects of Christian-based residential schools, which were first established during the late 1800s to assimilate First Nations children into the white-western-based society and culture of the colonizers. We will also explore some of the major current health issues and challenges facing Indigenous across the lifespan, including the growing incidence of sexually transmitted infections (STIs), tuberculosis, diabetes, depression, and suicide in youth.

Historical Perspectives

A fundamental understanding of the history of Indigenous peoples in Canada and the implications of contract with the Europeans colonizers provides health care professionals with a better understanding of the roots of various current social and political injustices and current public health challenges (Bartfay and Bartfay 2015). Table 4.1 provides the reader with a brief historical timeline of some of the major events affecting Indigenous in Canada. We will explore these in greater detail later.

Table 4.1 Historical Timeline of Major Events Affecting Indigenous people in Canada

Description of major historical event(s)	Time period
• Prior to contact with the European colonizers, it has been estimated that there were approximately eighteen million Indigenous inhabitants in North America and over 2,000 languages were spoken • Initial contact with the European traders and colonizers in 1535 • French Jesuit missionaries first attempt to convert First Nations people to Christianity • Introduction of previously unknown contagious diseases (e.g., smallpox, syphilis, tuberculosis) devastated the First Nations and Inuit populations	1600s
• Residential school system was first established by French Jesuit Missionaries • Primary objective was to convert the First Nations children to Christianity and to assimilate them into the European culture • Approximately 150,000 First Nations students are taken from their families and forced to attend residential schools until the closure of the last school in 1996	1800s
• Introduction of the "Indian Act" by the Federal government created a paternalistic wardship system with the creation of Indian reserves and the Treaty system • Indian Act was the first to legally define who was First Nation (Indian) versus those who were not • Royal Proclamation decreed that the British government had the right to negotiate treaties and purchase lands previously occupied by Indigenous people	1876
• Department of Indian Affairs transfers its health care portfolio over to Health Canada • This department is renamed the First Nations and Inuit Health Branch (FNIHB)	1945
• White Paper written • This policy document attempted to abolish the Indian Act of 1867 • Despite discussions and interest, the White paper is never implemented or passed by Parliament as a bill • Approximately 135 residential schools are in operation nationally	1969
• Indigenous communities across Canada express a desire to manage and control a greater proportion of their health care services • First Nations Environmental Network (FNEN) is formed to collectively deal with environmental challenges facing Indigenous communities across Canada	1980s

(Continued)

Table 4.1 Historical Timeline of Major Events Affecting Indigenous people in Canada (*Continued*)

Description of major historical event(s)	Time period
• Amendments to Section 35 of the Canadian Constitution formally recognize Indigenous peoples of Canada, including First Nations, Treaty Indians, Non-treaty Indians, Inuit and Métis • The Canadian Charter of Rights and Freedoms is passed into law • The Charter does not specifically identify health care or the right to health care, but it does demand that health care be provided to all persons "equally" and "fairly"	1982
• Bill C-31 passed by Parliament in response to complaints of discrimination and bias • Bill C-3l now permits a Status Indian women to marry a non-Indigenous man and permits their children to apply to be registered as well	1985
• The Government of Canada pledges $350 million to support the development of community-based healing initiatives for victims of the residential school system • Indigenous Healing Foundation established as an independent and non-profit organization to address healing needs of Indigenous peoples nationally	1998
• Federal government of Canada provides a formal apology to all First Nations' people as a gesture of reconciliation and accountability for past actions • Nunavut is given official territorial recognition and spans approximately one-fifth of Canada's land mass and has communities that spread across the three regions of Baffin, Bivilliq and Kitikmeot • Approximately 85% of the 30,000 people who inhabit Nunavut are Inuit • Government of Canada announces the Indigenous Diabetes Initiative program and allocates $58 million over next the five years to deal with this growing health challenge • Rates for diabetes are three to five times higher in Indigenous peoples than the national average	1999
• The Canadian Institute of Health Research (CIHR) announces the establishment of the "Institute of Indigenous Peoples' Health" (IAPH) • The IAPH provides funding to support research initiatives related to Indigenous health and well-being	2000
• Health Canada (2001b) reports that 244 of the 599 eligible (41%) rural Indigenous communities have signed the Health Services Transfer Agreement	2001
• Government of Canada—Department of Indian and Northern Affairs (DINA) attempts to clarify self-governance issues with proposed First Nations Governance Act (FNGA) • FNGA fails to be passed by Parliament due to intense lobbying and opposition by Indigenous groups	2002
• The Kelowna Accord—The first ministers met in Kelowna, British Columbia and the Federal government promises to spend $5 billion over the next five years to improve health, housing and education for Indigenous people • First ministers also establish the "Blueprint on Indigenous Health" that seeks to improve health outcomes for Indigenous peoples in comparison to those of the general population • Provinces and territories have yet to commit to the blueprint	2006
• Congress of Indigenous People (CAP) presents their report to the Senate's Subcommittee on Population Health • April, 2007, the first ever national food guide designed for First Nations, Inuit and Métis populations entitled "Eating Well with Canada's Food Guide—First Nations, Inuit and Métis" is launched in Yellowknife • This is the first food guide tailored to reflect the unique values, traditions and food choices of Indigenous populations • September, 2007, Federal government formalizes a $1.9 billion compensation plan for victims of the residential school system	2007

(Continued)

Table 4.1 Historical Timeline of Major Events Affecting Indigenous people in Canada (*Continued*)

Description of major historical event(s)	Time period
• June, 2008, Prime Minister Stephen Harper formally apologizes in the House of Commons for the treatment of Indigenous peoples in residential schools • June, 2008, Statistics Canada releases the first analysis of data on Indigenous people from the 2006 census, and reports that First Nations, Inuit and Métis collectively constitute a total population of approximately 1,172,790 • November 2008, in support of World Diabetes Day, the Government of Canada announces an additional $190 million to the Indigenous Diabetes Initiative	2008
• Pope Benedict XVI expresses "sorrow" to a delegation from Canada's First Nations over the abuse and "deplorable treatment" that Indigenous students suffered at the hands of the Catholic Church, but falls short of a formal apology for their wrong doings	April, 2009
• The Federal Court in Ottawa rules that Métis and non-status Indians have the same rights as Status Indians residing on First Nations reserves under the Canadian Charter of Rights and Freedoms	January, 2009
• The Indigenous population in Canada is more than one million (4% of the total Canadian population); more than half (54%) live in urban centres, and 8:10 live in Ontario and the four western provinces (Indigenous Affairs and Northern Development Canada 2010a, 2010b)	2010
• Between 1908 and 2013, 1,181 Indigenous women went missing, and of these 1,017 were murdered. On December 8, 2015, Prime Minister Justin Trudeau announced the launching of an investigation into the deaths and disappearances of Canada's Indigenous women (Wang 2015) • Justice Murray Sinclair, the chair of the "Truth and Reconciliation Commission" landmark report states that Canada's former Indigenous policy for the past 100 years can best be described as "cultural genocide" (CBC News 2015; Galloway and Curry 2015)	2015
• Report entitled "Honouring the Truth, Reconciling the Future: Summary of the Truth & Reconciliation Commission of Canada" released (See www.trc.ca, Cat No. IR4-71 2015E/PDF).	2016
• The Indigenous population is predicted to reach 2.2 million (Statistics Canada 2011c)	2031

From the late 1600s through the late 1800s, the new territory that we know as Canada today was increasingly populated by French and English colonizers, fur traders and military personnel (Bartfay 2010b). This period of time was characterized by very limited access to trained and formally educated health care professionals such as physicians, surgeons and nurses. Public health professionals and workers in Canada need to be aware of the negative historical effects of colonization and their continued impact on the health, well-being and health-seeking behaviours and beliefs of Indigenous peoples. First Nations, Métis and Inuit peoples face immense health challenges, and public health care professionals must work in collaboration with these populations to plan for effective health care access and delivery of primary health care services. It may be argued that Indigenous communities can be described as a unique society unto itself, and each community presents their own unique health care challenges (Bartfay 2010a).

The Venetian explorer John Cabot (circa 1450–1498) was commissioned by King Henry VII (Tudor) of England during the fifteenth century to find a safe trade passage to China, who was a valuable trading partner with Europe. Although Cabot was not successful in his efforts, he did discover a territory of land currently known as Newfoundland, Cape Breton and Nova Scotia. Cabot claimed the land for England, but King Henry VII was not eager to colonize these territories during his reign (Bartfay 2010a, 2010b).

In 1535, Cartier landed near the First Nations village of Stadocona near present-day Québec City. Cartier first utilized the word "Canada" to refer to the entire region lead by Chief Donnacona at Stadocona. It is interesting to note that the present name of our beloved country originates from the First Nations word "kanata," which means village or settlement (Canadian Heritage 2004; Rayburn 2001; Trigger and Pendergast 1978).

In 1547, maps referring to this new and unexplored region by European explorers began to refer to this area as Canada (Canadian Heritage 2004; Trigger and Pendergast 1978). Upon Confederation in 1867, the name Canada was officially referred to as the "Dominion of Canada" until the 1950s. In 1982, the Canada Act refers to our country as "Canada" solely in both official languages.

The first attempt to establish a permanent year-round colony in New France occurred in 1604 on Saint Croix Island in the territory named "La Cadie" or "l'Acadie" by the French nobleman Pierre Dugua Sieur Mons (Archives de Montréal 2010). The founding of Québec by Samuel de Champlain in 1608 and Montréal by Paul Comedey de Maisonneuve in 1642

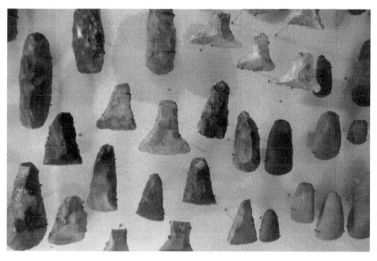

Source: Wally J. Bartfay

Photo 4.2 There is a growing body of archaeological evidence to confirm and establish that Indigenous people occupied various parts of North America for tens of thousands of years prior to the arrival of the European explorers and colonizers.

laid the groundwork for the major colonization of New France. During the sixteenth century, France was interested in expanding its economic and military power by discovering and colonizing new lands and territories (Bothwell 1996; Bumstead 2004; Trigger and Pendergast 1978). Canada was a land rich in natural resources including timber required for the construction of ships and houses and mineral resources. Animals including the beaver, fox and bear were also regarded as valuable trade commodities for the lucrative fashion industry in Europe. For example, beaver pelts were used for the fashionable top hats worn by gentlemen throughout Europe. The fur trade fuelled trans-Atlantic trade, and Europeans learned how to utilize the available national resources and adapt to the new land by First Nations peoples (Bartfay and Bartfay 2015).

Jacques Cartier's mission was to find new lands and territories and claim it the rightful property of France. Cartier landed on the east coast of Newfoundland in 1535 and dubbed the territory as "New France" (Fleet 1997). Cartier declared that the land was *"terra nullius,"* which implies that the land was considered uninhabited and empty, and therefore France had a legal claim to the land. This was despite the fact that there were approximately 500 distinct First Nations tribes in the early 1600s. Notably, Dickanson (2002a, 2002b) estimates that there were approximately eighteen million First Nations peoples who inhabited the North American continent prior to contact with the European colonizers. There is archaeological evidence for the presence of humans in northern Yukon dating 26,500 years ago. Furthermore, archaeological evidence reveals that southern Ontario was inhabited 9,500 years ago by First Nations peoples (Cinq-Mars 2001; Wright 2001). During the seventeenth century, the French empire expanded throughout North America as a result of various expeditions. During the eighteenth century conflicts between France and England, France eventually ceded Acadia, Newfoundland and the territory surrounding the Hudson Bay in 1713. Subsequently, France surrendered the entire colony of New France to England under the Treaty of Paris in 1763. British troops now occupied Québec and Montréal in 1759 and 1760, respectively (Archives de Montréal 2010).

Ensuring that the fur traders and colonizers were healthy was of prime importance for the economic and political interests of France and England (Abbott 1931). This was a noted challenge because of the harsh climate and geography of the land. One of the earliest recorded uses of Indigenous healers and herbal treatments was by Jacques Cartier. This is also the first documented account of widespread illness in the new colony. During one of Cartier's sailing expeditions up the St. Lawrence River in Québec, 127 of 130 of his men (97%) were struck with scurvy, and twenty-seven (21%) subsequently died as a result. Without the wisdom of First Nations' healers, significantly more of Cartier's sailors would have perished. Swan (1966) recounts that an observant officer noticed a native Indian, who suffered from similar symptoms, made a rapid recovery once he drank a decoction made from the sap and bark of a spruce tree. This brew saved Cartier and his remaining men.

These early fur traders and colonizers often had to provide for their own health care. They also relied on the wisdom of the traditional Indigenous healers or shamans who were often skilled in bloodletting, setting broken bones, the amputation of limbs, cauterizing wounds, and they also utilized a variety of herbal medicines to treat various ailments. The European colonizers and explorers were surprised and often astounded to learn about the extensive healing and medical practices known by First Nations people. In fact, many of the treatments and interventions employed, such as bloodletting, were regarded as state-of-the-art clinical practices in Europe at the time (Bartfay and Bartfay 2015). For examples, they knew about bloodletting and cupping, which were considered the contemporary treatments for fevers in Europe (Swan 1966). They also knew how to set fractures and perform amputations with great skill and to coagulate bleeding points with red-hot stones. First Nations' people also employed a variety of plants and herbs for a variety of ailments, and also practiced poulticing (Swan 1966).

Indigenous Status

Statistics Canada (2006b, 2008) reports that there were 1,172,790 people in Canada who identified themselves with an Indigenous identity, of which 572,090 were males and 600,695 were females according to the 2006 Census. The Indigenous population grew 45% between 1996 and 2006, in comparison to just 8% for non-Indigenous (Indigenous Affairs and Northern Development Canada 2010a, 2010b). More than half (54%) of all Indigenous people reside in urban centres, and 8:10 live in Ontario and the four western provinces. The largest population gain since 2006 was among the Métis for a total population of 389,785; First Nations populations–including status and non-status was reported at 698,025 (29% increase), and the Inuit population was 50,485 (26% increase) (Statistics Canada 2006). Between 1996 and 2001, the proportion of the Canadian population reporting an Indigenous identity increased by 22.2% (Villeneuve and MacDonald 2006). In 2011, the Canadian population was 33.5 million of which 1.4 million or approximately 4% of the total number of individuals who identified themselves as being Indigenous (Statistics Canada 2011a, 2011c). Of the total number of Indigenous, 62% identified themselves as First Nations, 31% as Métis and 4% of Inuit. Canada's population is predicted to exceed forty million by 2036, and the Indigenous population is expected to reach 2.2 million (Statistics Canada 2011c).

Although Indigenous seniors make up a relatively small proportion of Canada's Indigenous population, their numbers are predicted to significantly grow like the general Canadian population at large, and is predicted to triple between the years 1996 and 2016 (Health Canada 2002). The province of Ontario has the largest number of individuals who identify themselves as Indian, the territory of Nunavut has the largest number of Inuit and the province of Alberta has the largest number of Métis (Shah 2003). Eight out of every ten Indigenous people live in Ontario, Manitoba, Saskatchewan, Alberta or British Columbia. Approximately 108,000 live in northern parts of the province of Québec, and approximately 70% of all Métis reside in Western Canada with the largest population in the City of Winnipeg, Manitoba (Statistics Canada 2006).

According to Wasekeesikaw (2006), the term "Indian" originates from early French and English explorers to this continent who believed they had discovered India. The Indian Act of 1867 was the first to legally define who was Indian (First Nations), and it also provided a

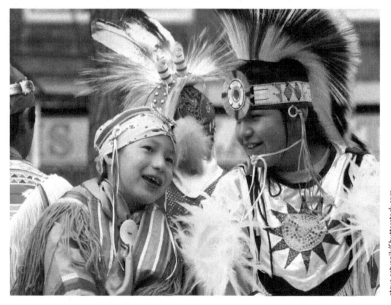

steve estvanik/Shutterstock.com

Photo 4.3 Having the designation and status as an "Indian" in Canada is acquired via a birth status and is also defined in the Canadian Indian Act of 1876.

vehicle for the European colonizers to legislate and rule over First Nations' peoples and the lands reserved for them (Bartfay 2010a; McMurray 2007).

First Nations/Indian

According to 2006 Census data, an estimated 698,025 people identified themselves as North American Indian or First Nations (Statistics Canada 2008). The First nation's population in Canada increased 29% between 1996 and 2006 and there are 615 First nations and ten distinct First Nations language families (Statistics Canada 2008). The Census recorded approximately sixty different Indigenous languages spoken by First Nations people in Canada including Algonquian, Athapaskan, Cree, Siouan, Salish, Tsimshian, Wakashan, Irogquoian, Haida, Kutenai, Ojibway and Tlingit. An estimated 87,285 could carry-on a conversation in Cree, followed by 30,255 in Ojibway.

Having the designation and status as an "**Indian**" in Canada is acquired via a birth status and is also defined by the Canadian Indian Act of 1876 (Bartfay, 2010a; Bartfay and Bartfay 2015; Waldram et al. 1995). A **treaty or registered Indian** (First Nations) is an individual who is recognized under the Canadian Indian Act of 1876, and also has obtained a unique registration number known as a "treaty number."

An Indian who is First Nations but does not have a registration number is still recognized as being "Indian" per se under the Canadian Indian Act of 1876 (Bartfay 2010a; Waldram et al. 1995). Conversely, **non-status Indians** are recognized as First Nations people in Canada, but the tribe or band to which they belong to did not wish to sign a treaty. Statistics Canada (2008) reports that the majority (n = 564,870 or 81%) of First Nations people are Status Indians, which means they are registered under the Indian Act, whereas an estimated 133,155 are not registered under the Indian Act. An estimated 40% lived on reserve, while the remaining 60% lived off reserve. The vast majority (98%) of the First Nations people living on reserve are Status Indian (Statistics Canada, 2008).

Inuit

The **Inuit** are believed to be descendants of the Thule culture that dates back to 1000 CE, and consists of a total of eight separate tribal groups (Bartfay and Bartfay 2015). Approximately 4% or 50,485 of the Indigenous persons in the 2006 Census identified themselves as Inuit, which represents a 26% increase in comparison from 1996 data (N = 40,220) (Statistics Canada, 2008). In 2006, the medium age of the Inuit population was twenty-two years, compared with forty years for those on non-Indigenous decent. Moreover, 12% of the Inuit population was four years old and under; 11% were in the five to nine years age group, compared with only 6% of non-Indigenous people surveyed. According to Statistics Canada (2008), just over three-quarters of Inuit in Canada (N = approximately 40,000 or 78%) live in one of the four regions within the Inuit Nunavut. This is the Inuktitut expression for "Inuit homeland," a region stretching from Labrador to the Northwest Territories. In 2006, 49% of all Inuit lived in Nunavut, 19% lived in Nunavik in northern Québec, 6% lived in the Inuvialuit region in the Northwest Territories and 4% lived in Nunatsiavut in Labrador. An estimated 17% lived in urban centres and 5% in rural areas outside Inuit Nunaat (Statistics Canada 2008).

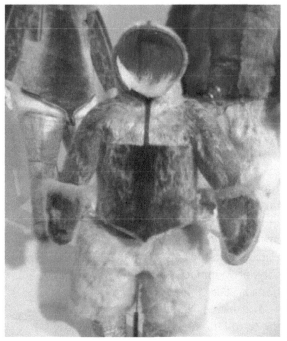

Source: Wally J. Bartfay

Photo 4.4 Traditional Inuit seal-skin outerwear. The Inuit people of Canada are renowned for their ability to adapt and survive in harsh environments and cold climates of Northern Canada and the Artic regions

Historically, the term "Eskimo" was used to describe indigenous people who occupied the cold Arctic regions of Canada, Newfoundland and Labrador (Bartfay 2010a). The word Eskimo, however, is regarded as offensive by some individuals because it has been utilized as a negative descriptor of people who eat raw flesh. Consequently, the designation and term has been replaced by the current term "Inuit." The Inuit peoples of Canada are renowned for their ability to adapt and survive in the often harsh environment and climate of Northern Canada and the Arctic regions (Bartfay 2010a; Bartfay and Bartfay 2015). There are absolutely no trees observed in the northern regions occupied by Inuit peoples, but there are some low stubby plants and berries. There are also a variety of alpine glaciers, icebergs as well as low-lying lakes and bays. The family remains the central economic unit of the Inuit, and everyone is assigned a particular job or task. Historically, the Inuit people lived semi-nomadic lives, in that they settled in accordance to their hunting needs. The women were responsible for transporting household's items and possessions; whereas the men fished and hunted for sea mammals such as seals, walrus and whales. In addition, the men also hunted caribou and polar bears and other game such as rabbits in the summer. Occasionally, the Inuit would also gather and store seasonal plants and berries.

According to Pearson and Trumble (1996, 479), Inuit languages tend to be polysynthetic and ergative in nature and are divided into the following two main types. First, the "Inupiag" or "Inuit" types that are spoken in Labrador, Northern Alaska and the Arctic Coast of Canada. Second, the "Yupik" types that are spoken in southern Alaska and Siberia. The Inuktitut language is strongest in the region of Nunavik and Nunavut where more than nine of ten Inuit can speak the language well enough to carry on a conversation. In contrast, the numbers are 27% in Nunatsiavut and 20% in the Inuvialuit region (Statistics Canada 2008). The Government of Canada regards Inuit peoples in the same manner as registered Indians, but they are classified in a separate category (Waldram et al. 1995).

Métis

The "**Métis**" are people formed between the union of Indigenous and non-Indigenous parents who were historically of European descent, and are legally considered the same as non-status Indians and Inuit in Canada (Bartfay 2010a; Bartfay and Bartfay 2015). The first records of Métis people are shown as early as 1600 on the East coast of Canada. The mothers were often Cree, Ojibwa, Algonquin, Saulteaux, Menominee, Mi'kmaq or Maliseet. Historically, there were distinctions between the French Métis born of francophone voyageur fathers, and the Anglo-Métis (A.K.A. Country-born) who descended from English or Scottish fathers. Today, these two cultures have coalesced into one Métis heritage and tradition. A majority of the Métis once spoke, and many still speak, either Métis French or a mixed language known as "Michif." The majority of Métis people today are not so much the direct result of First Nations and European intermixing, but are those who self-identify as being Métis due to intermarriages with others. The Supreme Court of Canada outlined three broad factors to identify Métis rights-holders in the Powley Ruling in 2003 as follows based on *section 35 of the Constitution Act, 1982*: (i) Self-identification as a Métis individual, (ii) ancestral connection to a historic Métis community and (iii) acceptance by a Métis community (Indigenous Affairs and Northern Development Canada 2012). The Powley Ruling dealt only with the Métis community in and around Sault Ste. Marie, although it did establish a legal precedent to determine the Indigenous rights of other Métis groups.

Data obtained from the 2006 Census suggest that the Métis population is on the rise in Canada, and this increase is outpacing other Indigenous groups in Canada as well as non-Indigenous populations

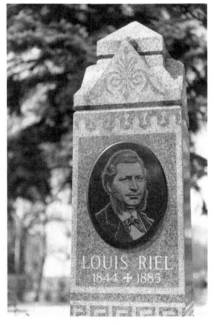

© Pierdelune/Shutterstock.com

Photo 4.5 Louis Riel was the founder of the province of Manitoba and leader of the Métis in St. Boniface. Riel led two popular Métis governments, was central in bringing Manitoba into Confederation, and was subsequently executed for high treason for his role in the 1885 resistance to Canadian encroachment on Métis lands by a all white male jury.

over the past decade (Statistics Canada 2008). Indeed, in 2006 an estimated 389,785 people reported that they were Métis and this figure has increased 91% in comparison to 1996 figures. Nonetheless, the Métis represent just 1% of the total population in Canada. Approximately nine of ten people (87%), who identified themselves as Métis, live in either the western provinces or Ontario. The census enumerated 85,500 (22%) in Alberta, 73,605 (19%) in Ontario, 71,805 (18%) in Manitoba, 59,445 (15%) in British Columbia and 48,115 (12%) in Saskatchewan (Statistics Canada 2008). In 2006, 25% of the Métis population in Canada was aged fourteen or younger, in comparison to 17% of non-Indigenous population, and seven of ten Métis lived in urban centres that represents a 67% increase in comparison to 1996 figures (Statistic Canada 2008).

Indigenous Languages

It is notable that the cultural and linguistic variations amongst First Nations, Inuit and Métis are reported to be greater than the sum total of all European nations combined (Kirmayer et al. 2000). Prior to contact with the European colonizers, it has been estimated that there were approximately eighteen million inhabitants in North America and over 2,000 distinct languages were spoken (Dickason 2002a, 2002b; Waldram et al. 1995). Health care professionals need to be culturally sensitive and informed about the various types of Indigenous peoples located across Canada and their traditions and beliefs. Traditionally, the Indigenous culture has been visual or oral in nature and therefore transmitted via works of art, story-telling or the spoken word, in contrast to written or electronic/digital mediums (Bartfay 2010a; Bartfay and Bartfay 2015; Beckman Murray et al. 2006). Language and art still serve as an important cultural vehicle for Indigenous peoples to connect with their rich history, traditions and culture (Smylie 2000). Nonetheless, many Indigenous languages currently spoken are threatened and endangered, and if lost will have profound negative consequences for the cultural survival and identify of Indigenous peoples in Canada (Kendall et al. 2001).

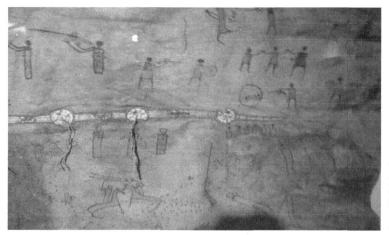

Source: Wally J. Bartfay

Photo 4.6 Traditionally, Indigenous culture has been visual and oral in nature and therefore transmitted via works of art, story-telling or the spoken word, in contrast to written or electronic / digital mediums.

Jesuit Missionaries and Residential Schools

Following the arrival of colonizers and fur traders to New France in the sixteenth and seventeenth centuries, Christian Jesuit missionaries arrived. Throughout the 1640s, Jesuit missionaries penetrated the Great Lakes and other inland regions and attempted to convert many of the Huron, Iroquois, Mohawk, Cree and other First Nations people to Christianity. This often created tensions and conflict between Europeans and First Nations Peoples. For example, Jesuit missionaries often came into conflict with the Iroquois, who frequently attacked Montréal. The primary objectives of these Jesuit missionaries were to befriend and convert the "savages" and "barbarians" to Christianity, which was the dominant religion in Europe during the time, and to civilize them according to their standards and beliefs. Early colonizers used canoes on the waterways, especially the St. Lawrence River and the Great Lakes, as their main form of transportation. During the winter when the lakes froze, individuals often travelled by sleds pulled by dogs or horses or on foot by snowshoes (an Indigenous invention). A land-based road transportation system was first developed during the 1830s.

The attempts of the Jesuits to convert First Nations people to a Christian-based faith were often regarded as hostile and unwelcomed attempts because they conflicted with their traditional values, beliefs and culture. Indeed, eight Jesuit missionaries and donnés who were killed between 1642 and 1649 were later canonized by the Catholic Church as the so-called "Canadian Martyrs" (Government of Ontario 2010). Detailed reports about their efforts to convert First Nations peoples to Christianity and the day-to-day lives of early colonizer's and fur traders in the region were regularly sent back to France via ships by the Jesuits. Collectively, these official reports were known as the "Jesuit Relations" documents and they span a period of more than seventy years (Kenton 1925; Kerr 1996; Parkman 1897). For example, Gariel Sagard (1636) described First Nations (Hurons) peoples as faithless savages who required enlightenment by teaching them about their Christian faith and beliefs.

Go into the entire world and preach the Gospel. It is for this last reason that of obedience to what is holy we took the trip to the Hurons and the Canadians . . . to come to the aid of our brothers in Canada, take the torch of the knowledge of the Son of God to them and chase away the darkness of barbarism and faithlessness.

Source: Sagard (1866).

During the 1800s, Jesuit missioners were even more aggressive in their attempt to convert Indigenous peoples to Christian-based faiths via the establishment of residential schools throughout Canada (Carney 1995; Miller 1996; Milloy 1999). The residential schools comprised a network of forced boarding schools for Indigenous children of Canada who were First Nations, Metis or Inuit. These residential schools were funded by the Canadian government's Department of Indian Affairs, and administered by Christian-based churches including the Catholic Church of Canada, Anglican Church of Canada and the Methodists (United Church) (Carney 1995; Miller 1996; Milloy 1999). The goal of these Christian-based residential schools was to better assimilate First Nations children into the dominant white-European culture, values systems and society (Indigenous Healing Foundation 1999). In fact, parents of First Nations children were legally required to send their children to these residential schools that taught them to be ashamed of their First Nations heritage, beliefs, value systems and society. This school system

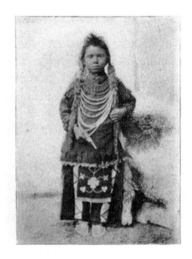
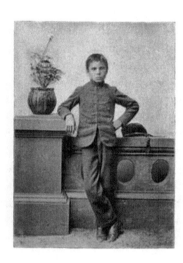

Source: Library and Archives Canada

Photo 4.7 The primary purpose of residential schools was to assimilate Indigenous children into the dominant white European culture, values and society.

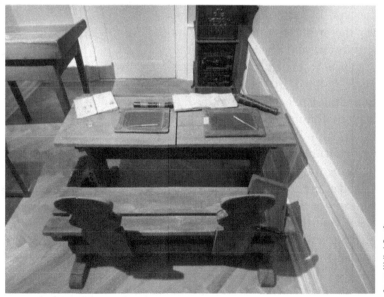

Source: Wally J. Bartfay

Photo 4.8 Residential schools were deemed compulsory for all Indigenous children from 1884 to 1948, but continued to exist in many parts of the country afterwards. The last residential school was closed in 1996 (Carney 1995; Miller 1996; Milloy 1999).

Web-based Resource Box 4.1 Truth and Reconciliation Commission Report

Resource	Web-Based Link
Truth and Reconciliation Commission of Canada: Calls to Action. (Winnipeg, MB). This report by Justice Murray Sinclair consists of ninety-four "calls to action" by various levels of government in Canada.	https://www.documentcloud.org/documents/2091412-trc-calls-to-action.html

had origins dating back to pre-Confederation times, but was primarily active following the passage of the Indian Act in 1876, until the mid-twentieth century.

There is currently a consensus in Canada from Indigenous groups, survivors and the Federal government that these residential schools did result in significant harm to children in attendance by forcibly removing them from their families, depriving them of their ancestral languages, cultures and traditions, and exposing many of them to physical, emotional, sexual and spiritual abuse at the hands of priests, nuns, vicars, clergy and other church officials and teachers. Evidence for this consensus includes the June 11, 2008 public apology offered, not only by Prime Minister Stephen Harper on behalf of the Government of Canada, but also by the leaders of all the other parties in the Canadian House of Commons.

Justice Murray Sinclair, the Chair of the "Truth and Reconciliation Commission" declared in his landmark report released in June, 2015 that Canada's former Indigenous policies could best be described as "cultural genocide" (CBC News 2015; Galloway and Curry 2015; The Truth and Reconciliation Commission of Canada 2015). This landmark report was based on over six years of testimonies from nearly 7,000 witnesses who were residential school survivors, and consisted of ninety-four specific recommendations. Add to your knowledge of the Truth and Reconciliation Commission's report by accessing the link shown in Web-Based Resource Box 4.1.

Treaties and Reserves

British colonizers introduced the concept of paternalistic wardship, via the creation of the reserve system in Canada. The creation of geographically defined "Indian reserves" often resulted in the forced isolation and/or relocation of entire First Nations' communities (Adelson 2005; Eckermann et al. 2006). England was instrumental in developing and implementing the "treaty system" in Canada. The **treaty system** provided a means for these colonizers to legally claim land that was originally occupied by First Nations people throughout North America (Dickason 2002a, 2002b). The British North America Act (BNA) of 1867 served as the impetus for Canada to become an independent nation. Despite the passage of the BNA Act of 1867, a Royal Proclamation stated that only

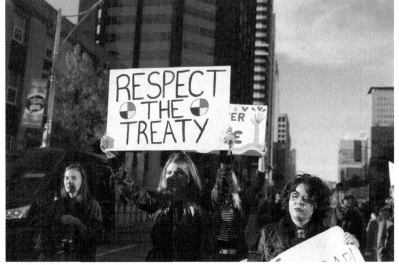

Photo 4.9 Colonization and the use of treaties by the British were not limited to Canada, but occurred in many regions of the world. A protest sign against the effects of colonization in Australia. Indigenous Australians and Torres Strait Islander people of Australia, descended from groups that existed in Australia and surrounding islands prior to British colonisation. Indigenous Australians are recognized to have arrived between 40,000 and 70,000 years ago.

England had the legal right to negotiate treaties or to purchase lands from First Nations peoples. In 1876, the **Indian Act** was passed to ensure that the terms and conditions of all signed existing treaties with Indigenous peoples were legally observed and enforced (Dickason 2002a, 2002b; Venne 2002).

Following Confederation, Indigenous peoples including First Nations, Inuit and Métis were often forced to be relocated and/or displaced from their traditional birth and hunting territories to make room for the ever-increasing numbers of Europeans (Wasekeesikaw 2006). For example, First Nations people were often forced to live on Indian reserves established for them by the Federal government, which often resulted in social or geographical isolation. These reserves were governed by the Federal government according to the terms and conditions of the Indian Act of 1867 (Department of Indian and Northern Affairs 1997; Dickason 2002a, 2002b; Venne 2002). The Federal government subsequently created the Department of Indian and Northern Affairs (DINA) whose specific mandate was to manage treaty Indians and the reserves. The DINA hired so-called "Indian agents" who were responsible for enforcing and carrying-out the specific terms of the treaties nationally (DINA 1997). First Nations people often felt that they were living in a police state, since they required special written permission from these agents to leave these established reserves. These required actions and behaviours often created conflicts since they were in marked contrast to their cultural and traditional beliefs related to autonomy and freedom. For example, individuals needed to obtain permission from an Indian agent to go hunting for food for their family off the reserve.

Indian Act and Bill C-31

The Indian Act (1876) was also discriminatory against status (treaty) First Nations (Indian) women who wished to marry a non-Indigenous person in Canada (Bartfay 2010b; Bartfay and Bartfay 2015). According to the Indian Act, this action would result in having her name stricken from the treaty list and her status would change from status Indian to a non-status Indian. Furthermore, any children born to the couple would be designated as non-status (non-treaty). Hence, the basic human right of choosing who you wished to be your husband had implications in terms of the status of First Nations women in Canada. In response to numerous complaints of bias and prejudice against these women, the Government of Canada responded by passing Bill C-31. In accordance with Bill C-31, a status Indian woman is now "permitted" to marry a non-Indigenous man, who can now also apply to become registered as well. In addition, the couple's children can also apply to be admitted into the band or tribe in accordance with their specific membership codes. The Canadian Constitution was amended in 1982, and now legally recognizes the status treaty rights of all First Nations peoples (Bartfay 2010a). Moreover, First Nations, Inuit and Métis peoples are now recognized under Section 35 of the Canadian Constitution (Waldram et al. 1995). In January 2013, the Federal Court in Ottawa ruled that Métis and non-status Indians have the same rights as status treaty Indians, in accordance with the Canadian Charter of Right and Freedoms.

A report entitled the "White Paper" was written in 1969 that strongly advocated for the abolishment of the treaty system and the Indian Act (1867), and DINA who were responsible for administering the reserve and treaty systems (DINA 1997; Schouls 2002). Despite support by Indigenous leaders and discussions with various politicians and policy makers, the White Paper never became official government policy or legislation in Canada. Nonetheless, it did serve as a critical catalyst for the resurgence of the Indigenous culture and their desire for self-governance in Canada (Schouls 2002).

Numerous ongoing treaty and land disputes remain to be settled (Johal 2006). McMurray (2007) reports that negotiations between Indigenous peoples and various levels of government are ongoing with the ultimate objective or aspiration of Indigenous self-government that will be grounded in the Constitution. For example, Nunavut was formally established and recognized as a separate territory from the Northwest Territories on April 1, 1999 by the *Nunavut Act* and the *Nunavut Land Claims Agreement Act*, although the actual boundaries had been established back in 1993. The creation of this new territory in Canada resulted in the first major change to Canada's political map since the incorporation of the new province of Newfoundland and Labrador in 1949. It is notable that Nunavut represents the largest expanse of land owned and governed by any Indigenous peoples (McMurray 2007).

Social and Health Consequences of Colonization

The result of European colonization often had devastating social and health consequences for Indigenous peoples in Canada and abroad (Bartfay 2010a; Bartfay and Bartfay 2015). For example, prior to contact with French and English colonizers in the new world, the Six Nations (Haudenosaunee) of Ontario cultivated and farmed approximately 80% of their subsistence requirements (Dickason 2002a, 2002b). By contrast, the vast majority of present-day subsistence nutritional requirements by Six Nations' people come from commercially available sources (e.g., supermarkets), and often consists of highly processed foods loaded with sugar, salt and fat. These alterations to their traditional subsistence means in the Six Nations has resulted in a growing incidence of obesity and associated cardiovascular disease (CVD) and Type 2 diabetes, which were not present fifty to sixty years ago (Bartfay 2010a; Hales and Lauzon 2007). According to the 2010 Canadian Community Health Survey, 66% of adults twenty years and older and 40% of children and youth not living on a reserve were overweight or obese, based on self-reported height and weight measures (Statistics Canada 2010b). For First Nations individuals who reside on reserves or northern communities, 62% of children (three to eleven years); 43% of youth (twelve to seventeen years) and 75% of adults eighteen years or older reported that they were overweight or obese (The First Nations Information Governance Centre 2011).

According to 2006 Census data, First Nations and Métis adults aged twenty or more were more likely to be diagnosed with one of several chronic conditions including heart disease, cancer, diabetes and arthritis (Statistics Canada 2007). According to Statistics Canada (2007), approximately 60% of non-Indigenous adults were reported having "excellent" or "very good health," a greater proportion than reported by First Nations peoples living off-reserves (51%), Métis (57%) or Inuit (49%) adults. It is also notable that approximately three-quarters of non-Indigenous adults reported no activity limitation, compared with 58% of First Nations living off-reserve, 59% of Métis and 64% of Inuit adults. In many cases, First Nations living off-reserve, Inuit and Métis adults reported poorer health than non-Indigenous adults even when the effects of differences in socio-economic characteristics, in health care access and in lifestyle risk factors were taken into consideration (Statistics Canada 2007).

French and English colonizers brought with them various diseases including STIs (e.g., syphilis, gonorrhoea), tuberculosis, measles and small pox, which devastated tens of thousands of First Nations' and Inuit people (Donahue 1996; Swan 1966).

> . . . a white trader who had suffered losses of equipment as the result of an Indian raid. His retribution was to invite the leaders of the Indian tribe concerned to smoke the pipe of peace. At the meeting he ceremoniously presented them with a keg of rum wrapped in a flag, with the instruction that they were not to unwrap the keg until they got back to their encampment. The flag had been impregnated with the smallpox virus, and many members of the tribe died as a consequence. This must be one of the earliest examples of germ warfare (Swan 1966, 44–45).

Inuit populations have a homicide rate that is ten times that of non-Indigenous populations in Canada, higher rates of crime and imprisonment, and alcohol and substance abuse (WHO 2002a). For example, Indigenous women make up 87% of prisoners in the province of Saskatchewan (Sapers and Zinger 2010), and are three times as likely as non-Indigenous women to be victims of violence (Statistics Canada 2011d). Indigenous women prisoners are twice as likely as their male counterparts to be diagnosed with mental health issues at time of admission, and are three times as likely to suffer from depression (Sapers and Zinger 2010). According to the 2006 Indigenous Peoples Survey, 78% of Indigenous aged fifteen years and older reported consuming alcohol in the past year, and 39% (48% of males and 32% of females) consumed alcohol at least once per week (Statistics Canada 2006a).

When European whalers and fur traders came to the Canadian Arctic, tens of thousands of Inuit lives were lost and their population was reduced by two-thirds in number (World Health Organization 2002a). These events had profound effects on Inuit health, culture and traditional ways of subsistence in the Arctic regions of Canada. Indeed, each of these groups added to the Inuit's sense of dispossession from their land and significantly destabilized their traditional ways of life (McMurray 2007). The Inuit's traditional ways of life, culture, health and environment are increasingly being threatened as a result of exploration and mining in the Arctic for resources such as diamonds, minerals, natural gas and oil (Bartfay 2010a; Bartfay and Bartfay 2015).

A growing number of Indigenous communities across Canada are being affected by alterations to their environments (Bartfay 2010a; Bartfay and Bartfay 2015). These include mining, forestry, the exploration of oil and natural gas, the polluting of rivers and lakes with various contaminates including pesticides, herbicides, mercury, lead and PCB's, and hydro-electric dam construction. All these activities negatively affect their environment and traditional ways of life including hunting, trapping and fishing. In response to this growing threat to their traditional ways of life, the FNEN was formed in the 1980s (FNEN 2004, 2002). The vision and mandate of the FNEN is to protect and restore the harmony of past, present and future life through traditional teachings by their ancestors and elders related to the mind, body and spirit (FNEN 2004, 2002). The mind consists of teachings and awareness related to the Mother Earth. The balance of body is achieved through grassroots activism by Indigenous peoples across Canada. To achieve balance with the spirit, various spiritual and cleansing ceremonies are often undertaken, such as healing circles. These ceremonies help to restore harmony and strengthen their unity with the powers of the *Mother Earth, Sky* and *All Relations*. The FNEN has been quite successful in preventing logging and clear cutting of forests in various provinces; bring to halt low-level flights by Canadian air force jets and aircraft over the traditional hunting grounds, and stopping the disposal of radioactive wastes on or near First Nations reserves (FNEN 2003). All Canadians, corporations, politicians and policy makers can certainly learn and benefit from the environmental planning and preservation efforts undertaken by the FNEN and other Indigenous groups (Burrows 1997; Duerden et al. 1996).

Government policies historically may be described as "assimilationist" in nature, implying the Indigenous people should be more like their European colonizers in terms of their culture, beliefs and ways of life (Bartfay 2010a, 2010b). Wasekeesikaw (2006) argues that the Federal government policies were specifically developed to civilize and assimilate First Peoples into their western-based society, values and belief systems. For example, First Nations' children were often placed into residential schools that were culturally inappropriate, insensitive and irrelative to their traditional belief systems and lifestyle (Chrisjohn et al. 1997). Consequently, First Nations' people were often blamed and wrongfully labeled by non-Indigenous as being lazy individuals waiting for government handouts, demoralized and living in squalor conditions (Adelson 2005; Eckermann et al. 2006).

The socially biased and unnatural geographical segregation of First Nations peoples onto reserves has often resulted in limited post-secondary educational, career and economic opportunities. Indigenous youth are more likely than non-Indigenous to drop out of school, and by leaving school without graduating increases the possibility of lifelong unemployment or jobs with low wages (Human Resources and Skills Development Canada 2010; Statistics Canada 2011e). In fact, the unemployment rate for Indigenous people aged twenty-five to sixty-four remains almost three times the rate for non-Indigenous (Indigenous Affairs and Northern Development Canada 2010a, 2010b). The medium income of First Nations families in 2005 was reported to be $11,224 for those living on reserves and $17,464 for those living off reserves, compared to the median income of $25,955 for non-Indigenous families (Statistics Canada 2009).

Indigenous people in Canada are six times more likely to be victims of homicide in 2014 (Grant 2015; Statistics Canada 2015). Although Indigenous people account for approximately 5% of the Canadian population, they account for approximately a quarter of all homicide victims reported by police. In 1991, Indigenous women accounted for 14% of all female victims of homicide in Canada, compared to 21% in 2014. Moreover, Indigenous women had a rate of 115 sexual assaults per 1,000 women in 2014, which was more than triple the rate of non-Indigenous women in Canada (Grant 2015; Statistics Canada 2015).

In 1999, the Canadian Federal government offered a public apology to all First Nations people as a gesture of reconciliation and accountability for the past actions of previous governments (McMurray 2007). In April,

Web-based Resources 4.2 Resources Related to Indigenous Healing and the Residential School System

Resource	Website
Indigenous Healing Foundation	http://www.ahf.ca
Documentary on impact of the residential school system by Kevin Annett and others.	http:video.goggle.com/videoplay?docid=-6637396204037343133
Truth and Reconciliation Commission	http://www.timescolonist.com/health/Residential+school+victims+share+horrific+stories/6293067/story.html.

2009, Pope Benedict XVI expressed "sorrow" to a delegation of First Nations representatives from Canada over the abuse and "deplorable treatment" that Indigenous students suffered at the hands of the Catholic Church in residential schools. Nonetheless, Pope Benedict XVI went short of providing a formal apology from the Catholic Church for its past wrongdoings. Add to your knowledge of Indigenous healing and the negative impacts associated with the forced residential school system by accessing the Web-Based Learning Resource Box 4.2.

It is also critical to report that the current depictions of Indigenous peoples in Canada are not all gloomy, negative or bleak in nature. Increasingly highly numbers of First Nations, Inuit and Métis peoples are pursuing higher education in community colleges and universities and/or seeking job or career training in various fields and disciplines (Bartfay 2010a). In fact, Indigenous are found in all of the trades in Canada (e.g., electrician, plumber, welder, carpenter, auto-mechanic), occupations and professions (e.g., lawyers, engineers, nurses, physicians). It is notable that the National Indigenous Achievement Awards are held and televised nationally by the Canadian Broadcasting Corporation (CBC). This annual award ceremony provides a vehicle to showcase the diverse talents and achievements of First Nations, Inuit and Métis peoples, and it also provides a critical vehicle for the promotion of positive role models for both Indigenous and non-Indigenous youth across Canada (Bartfay 2010a; Bartfay and Bartfay 2015).

Indigenous Perspectives of Health

First Nations, Inuit and Métis peoples are bound together by a rich tapestry comprising inherited cultural beliefs and values, customs, language, art and their spiritual bond with their surrounding environment (Bartfay 2010a; Bartfay and Bartfay 2015). According to McKenzie and Morrisette (2003), Indigenous perspectives on health and well-being emphasis a holistic and reciprocal relationship between the physical and spiritual world, the individual and their surrounding environment, and between the mind, body and spirit (see Figure 4.1). These holistic and reciprocal beliefs and values often contrast with the traditional western or European concepts of health and well-being related to the absence of disease and/or overt clinical signs and symptoms of illness or pathological processes (Lyons and Petrucelli 1978; Rosen 1958; WHO 1986, 1999, 2000c).

There are several versions of the origins of our world and the universe by the "Creator" told by Indigenous elders (Bartfay 2010a; Hales and Lauzon 2007). Nonetheless, they share in common their spiritual beliefs of holism and a strong bond or unity with the environment. These beliefs include a reciprocal and balanced relationship between individuals and the "Mother Earth," which will help to provide a path to good life or "Bimaadiziwin" (Kulchyski et al. 1999). An understanding of the relationship between the Mother Earth and Bimaadiziwin provides the individual with the sustenance necessary for high-quality spiritual and physical life (Bartfay 2010a; Bartfay and Bartfay 2015). Wasekeesikaw (2006) reports that the term "*miyupimaatis-siium*" means being alive well in First Nations culture and emphasize the relationship between the natural world and keeping one's spirit strong.

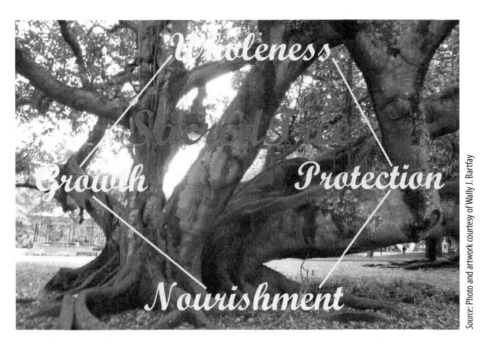

Source: Photo and artwork courtesy of Wally J. Bartfay

Figure 4.1 A Pictorial Representation of the "Sacred Tree"

"The Story of the Sacred Tree" exemplifies the common Indigenous belief that spiritual and physical life consists of a harmonious merger with all natural things (Bopp et al. 1985). This story begins with the great "Creator" who decides to plant a "Sacred Tree." The Sacred Tree is a spiritual place where all people can assemble and acquire or achieve required healing, strength and power, knowledge and wisdom, and a sense of security and sanctuary. The **Sacred Tree** is highly symbolic and is representative of the close connectedness to the "Mother Earth," since its roots are firmly and deeply embedded into her. Moreover, the branches of the Sacred Tree are also highly symbolic because they reach upwards towards "Father Sky." Figure 4.1 is a pictorial representation of this Sacred Tree, which displays the four great intended meanings of protection, nourishment, growth and wholeness.

The symbol of a circle is also significant spiritually and is often depicted or represented in the form of a Medicine Wheel (see Figure 4.2), which also helps to pictorially represent the teaching of Bimaadiziwin (Beckman Murray et al. 2006; Bopp et al. 1984). First Nations' Medicine Wheels are considered powerful and sacred symbols of the universe that depicts the circularity of life and the balance between the four required aspects of self: (a) Physical, (b) mental, (c) emotional and (d) spiritual (Bartfay 2010a; Bartfay and Bartfay 2015). The Northern component of the medicine wheel is often associated with the season winter, the colour white and a rock that represents strength and required action and the wolf (Bopp et al. 1985; Hales and Lauzon 2007; Beckman Murray et al. 2006). The Southern component of the medicine wheel is often associated with summer, the colour red and a tree that represents knowledge and honesty, and the bison or buffalo. The western aspect symbolizes the season fall, the colours black or blue, which represent sharing, reason and emotional responses and the bear. Lastly, the eastern component often symbolizes spring, the colour yellow and an eagle that represent the need for vision and kindness.

The totem pole, which dates back to the 1700s, also remains an important symbol of indigenous people in south-east Alaska, north-west Pacific coast and elsewhere (Halpin 2002; Huteson 2002; Jonaitis and Glass 2010). The word totem is derived from the Ojibway word "odoodem" that means "his kinship group" (Bartfay and Bartfay 2015). The carved symbols and figures represented on the totem poles are as varied as the cultures and clans that they originate from, but have never been employed as objects of worship per se. The lower the carved symbol or figure on the totem pole, the lower its importance. By contrast, the higher the symbol or figure, the more important it is. This is where the common phase "low man on the totem pole" comes from.

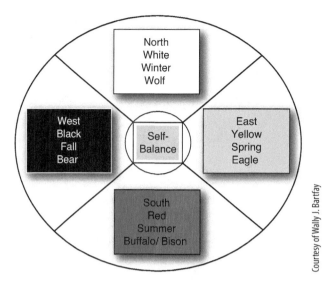

Courtesy of Wally J. Bartfay

Figure 4.2 First Nations Medicine Wheel

Totem poles are employed for a variety of reasons including purely artistic ventures; to illustrate stories that commemorate important historical events, accomplishments or persons; to represent shamanic powers; to recount familiar legends; to celebrate cultural beliefs and values; illustrate familiar lineages or prestige; serve as emblems for clans or families; symbolize unity; and illustrate links to spiritual ancestors (Halpin 2002; Huteson 2002; Jonaitis and Glass 2010).

Public health professionals and workers need to be cognizant of the fact that Indigenous beliefs, customs and values are often rooted in the context of their oral history and traditions. Decision making related to their way of life, including those surrounding the concept of health and well-being, are often situational in nature and dependent on the values and norms of their extended family unit and/or community (Daniel et al. 1999; Ellerby et al. 2000; Hernandez et al. 1999; Young 2003; Young et al. 2000). Indeed, the family and its children are recognized as the cornerstone of various Indigenous communities (Hammersmith and Sawatsky 2000). Indigenous values often emphasize holism, pluralism, autonomy, the importance of community- and family-based decision making and the maintenance of their overall *quality-of-life*, as opposed to the pursuit of a cure per se (Bartfay 2010a).

Delivery of Health Services

The role of the Federal government in providing delivery of health care services to Indigenous peoples dates back to 1945, when responsibility was transferred from the Department of Indian Affairs to the newly constituted Department of National Health and Welfare (Health Canada 2007c). Subsequently, a network of eighteen hospitals, thirty-three nursing stations, fifty-two

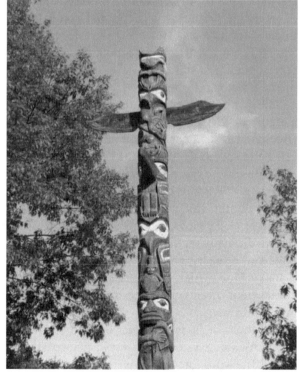

Source: Wally J. Bartfay

Photo 4.10 Originally, totem poles were the size of a walking cane, but slowly grew in grandeur and size over the centuries.

health centres with dispensaries and thirteen other health facilities with full-time physicians or nurses were established to serve the needs of Indigenous communities over the next ten years. In 1962, Health Canada was mandated with the responsibility for bestowing direct health service in Inuit communities in northern Canada and to First Nations people living on reserves (Bartfay 2010a, 2010b; Bartfay and Bartfay 2015).

During the mid-1980s, there was growing interest and movement by Inuit and First Nations communities to control and manage a greater proportion of their required health services (Health Canada 2007c). More recently, the *First Nations and Inuit Branch of Health Canada* (FNIHB 2008) has agreed to support the delivery of public health and health promotion services on reserves and in Inuit communities with this proposed model under the *Health Services Transfer Agreement* (HSTA). However, this transfer agreement of increased self-management and control of their health care services only applies to communities located south of the 60th parallel. According to Health Canada (2001b), since initiation of the transfer process of control and management of their health services more than a decade ago, 244 communities of the 599 eligible (or 41%, N = 388,712 total individuals) have agreed to sign the HSTA (Bartfay 2010a; FNIHB 2008).

Health care delivery approaches and systems vary in scope across provinces and territories in Canada, and between Indigenous communities and reserves. Larger and less-isolated communities, for example, often have designated health centres that provide their residents with more traditional public health and primary care services (Bartfay 2010a). Conversely, remote Indigenous communities will often have only nursing stations staffed by registered nurses (RNs) or nurse practitioners (NPs). NPs are licensed RNs who have advanced clinical and scientific knowledge and decision-making skills in assessment, diagnosis and health care management (Bartfay and Bartfay 2015; Stafanson and Bartfay 2010). Dalhousie University had the first educational program established for NPs in 1967 to deal with the critical shortage of physicians, and was targeted for RNs working in remote northern nursing stations in Nova Scotia (Stafanson and Bartfay 2010).

In 1998, the Ontario Minister of Health and Long-term Care (MOHLTC) passed Bill 127– the *Expanded Nursing Services for Patients Act*. This Act gives licensed NPs in the province of Ontario independent authority to prescribe a variety of medications, communicate a medical diagnosis (e.g., diabetes), and order a variety of blood tests, x-rays and diagnostic ultrasounds (College of Nurses of Ontario 2001, 2003). NPs in Ontario provide wellness screening activities (e.g., pap smears), monitor and assess infant growth and development, diagnose and treat minor illnesses (e.g., ear or urinary tract infections) and minor injuries (e.g., sprains and lacerations), provide screening and diagnostic evaluations for a variety of common clinical conditions (e.g., diabetes, heart disease) and clinically assess and monitor these patients. More recent legislation in Ontario has also expanded the role of NPs to include admitting and discharging patients from hospitals and prescription of various classes of medications. In 2004, representatives from all ten provinces and three territories meet and developed the first standardized national licensing exam for NPs in Canada. Despite these efforts, there remains of shortage of both RNs and NPs in Indigenous communities across Canada (Bartfay and Bartfay 2015; Stafanson and Bartfay 2010).

It is notable that approximately two-thirds of Indigenous peoples in Canada live in rural or remote areas (Shah 2003). There are few physicians and surgeons in rural and remote communities in Canada. Patients with serious illnesses in these communities must often wait eight to twelve hours for a flight to see a physician. In fact, only about 40% of the Inuit living in the Arctic get to see a physician throughout the year, in comparison to over 70% of other Canadians living in urban areas (World Health Organization 2007). There are also very few Indigenous physicians and surgeons. In 2002, Indigenous represented only 0.9% of all first-year medical students in Canada (Thompson 2010). The Indigenous Physicians Association of Canada, the National Indigenous Health Organization (NAHO) and the Association of Faculties of Medicine in Canada are currently collaborating on improving these stark numbers to better address the health care needs of Indigenous peoples across Canada.

Health care services, therefore, are often only provided by nurses. These nursing services are often delivered on need; or on an on-call basis 24-hours-a-day, seven-days-per-week (24/7) basis (Bartfay 2010a; Bartfay and Bartfay 2015). Nurses in these locations typically work in nursing stations (outposts) that are staffed alone by

Table 4.2 Classification of Community Types by FNIHB of Health Canada

FNIHB classification	Accessibility and community resources available	Types
Remote-isolated	There are no scheduled flights, no direct road access to physicians and minimal radio or telephone service	1
Isolated	Have regularly scheduled flights, lacks year-round road access to physicians and have good telephone and radio service	2
Semi-isolated	Have regularly scheduled flights, and road access to physician services is greater than 90 km, and may have paved or unpaved roads	3
Non-isolated	Have regularly scheduled flights, and often have paved or unpaved road year round access to physician services is less than 90 km	4

themselves or by a small group of nurses. Nurses in these isolated and remote communities provide a variety of essential public health services including physician and pharmacist replacement services, and advanced health assessments and referrals (Cradduck 1995; Tarlier et al. 2003). Nurses in these communities may be required to staff a small nursing station (outpost) and/or be flown in on a needs basis. Funding for these health care services depends on the size of the community, their accessibility and identified health care needs (Health Canada 2001a, 2001b). Table 4.2 shows the major types of communities by the FNIHB, which is based on their accessibility and community resources available (Health Canada 2001a, 2001b).

According to Health Canada (2007d), there are over 600 First Nations communities with 195 health centres and seventy-six nursing stations that provide primary health services in remote and/or isolated communities nationally. There are approximately 1,200 full-time RNs collectively employed either by the FNIHB and the transferred bands (Health Canada 2001a, 2001b). FNIHB nurses are employed by the Government of Canada (Federal), and they more than often serve as the only or main point of contact with our publicly funded health care systems. Nurses are also often employed by various Band Councils who have obtained responsibility for providing health care services in accordance with the HSTA (Health Canada 2007a, 2007b).

The Sioux Lookout Zone Hospital in Ontario had its control transferred to the province in 2002, as part of an amalgamation agreement reached with the local community hospital. In the province of Manitoba, the Percy E. Morre Hospital located in Hodgson, and the Norway House Hospital still operate under the jurisdiction of the FNIHB. In Alberta, The Blood Indian Hospital in Cardston also operates under FNIHB.

It is notable that although these hospitals were established to service the health care needs of Indigenous communities in these regions, the health care and diagnostic services provided by these hospitals are available to any non-Indigenous in need as well. In June of 2004, the non-profit All Nations' Healing Hospital was opened in Fort Qu'Appelle, Saskatchewan. This institution was built on First Nations land and integrates traditional Indigenous beliefs, values and health care practices with the conventional western-type of medical health care services employing a culturally sensitive approach (Bartfay 2010a; Hales and Lauzon 2007). Traditional healing practices and beliefs are integrated to meet the health care needs and challenges facing Indigenous peoples. These include the use of traditional herbal or folkloric remedies, shamanism and a variety of purification rituals including healing circles, smudging and sweat lodges (Donahue 1996; Mullin et al. 2001).

Cultural Safety and Public Health

The preservation and maintenance of the health and well-being of Indigenous peoples across Canada is a growing public health challenge. Indigenous beliefs surrounding the concept of health emphasis a holistic and reciprocal relationship between the physical and spiritual world, the individual and their environment, and their mind, body and spirit (Bartfay 2010a; Bartfay and Bartfay 2015). Indigenous beliefs are rooted in the context of oral history and culture, and decisions surrounding one's health and well-being are often situational and highly dependent on the values of the individual within the context of their family and community.

Public health care professionals and workers need to be aware of the history, beliefs, traditions and cultures of Indigenous communities they serve to effectively provide safe, effective and culturally appropriate primary health care services. The concept of **"cultural safety"** is based on a broad definition of culture care and on the public health care professional's interpretations and analyses of their own cultural selves and the impact of these on providing health care, and requires the mutual empowerment of both client and public health care professional or worker (De and Richardson 2008; Dion Stout and Downey 2008; Richardson and Williams 2007). With the concept of cultural safety, it is the client who ultimately judges whether the professional relationship is seen as beneficial, healing and/or therapeutic in nature. This concept first emerged during the 1980s in response to the poor treatment of the Maori who are indigenous New Zealanders. However, the concept of cultural safety has broadened to include a wide range of determinants of health.

It has been argued that public health care systems that are deemed culturally unsafe fail to acknowledge institutional discrimination and disregard the needs of Indigenous families and communities (Brown and Fiske 2001). The concept of cultural safety provides a mechanism for recognition of the indices of power inherent in any professional relationship or interaction, and the potential for disparity and inequality within any relationship (Bartfay 2010a; Bartfay and Bartfay 2015). An understanding of this concept is fundamental to providing safe, relevant and culturally appropriate public health care to Indigenous people. An understanding and acknowledgement by the public health professional or worker who imposes their own cultural beliefs and values may disadvantage the client is fundamental to the delivery of culturally safe primary health care services. Additional research by both Indigenous and non-Indigenous health care scientists and practitioners is needed to address the growing number and magnitude of health concerns and issues facing Indigenous populations in Canada. Accordingly, a proposal has been tabled for the need to create a unique research institute devoted solely to Indigenous health (Reading et al. 2002).

Group Activity-based Learning Box 4.1

Health Challenges Facing Indigenous People in Canada
This box provides the learner with opportunities to examine major health challenges and possible public health interventions to address these issues. Working in small groups of three to five students, discuss and answer the following questions:

1. What are some of the major health problems/challenges facing Indigenous peoples in your province or territory?

2. What is the role of Indigenous community leaders and elders in responding to these health problems/challenges?

3. What would you do as a public health care professional or worker to better address the health care needs of Indigenous people in your province/territory?

4. How can research findings be utilized to facilitate culturally sensitive evidence-based public health services in Indigenous communities across Canada?

Major Current Health Issues

The health of Indigenous peoples is one of the most pressing issues for public health in Canada. For example, arthritis is one of the most prevalent non-communicable chronic conditions among Indigenous populations in Canada (Butler-Jones 2012; Public Health Agency of Canada 2010a). According to the 2006 Indigenous Peoples Survey, 20% of respondents fifteen years and older reported being diagnosed with arthritis or rheumatism (Ng et al. 2010).

The life expectancy of Indigenous peoples is approximately ten years less in comparison to non-Indigenous Canadians (Bramley et al. 2005; Butler-Jones 2012; MacKinnon 2005; Statistics Canada 2004, 2008). For example, whereas the average life expectancy for non-Indigenous in Canada is seventy-six years for men and eighty-three years for women, First Nations men are expected to live 68.9 and 76.6 years (Health Canada 2005b; Health Council of Canada 2005). Statistics Canada (2004) reports that First Nations infants are more likely to be born pre-term, but have heavier birth weights than non-First Nations infants. Moreover, infant mortality rates are typically more than twice as high among First Nations, when compared to non-First Nations people. Post-neonatal mortality rates are 3.6 times as high and are independent of neighbourhood socio-economic status (Statistics Canada 2004). The birth rate among Indigenous women is higher than their non-Indigenous counterparts at 2.6 children per woman aged fifteen to forty-nine, 3.4 children per Inuit women, 2.9 children per First Nations women and 2.2 children per Métis women (Butler-Jones 2012; Statistics Canada 2010a, 2011b). In November 2010, a report based on a two-year study by the *House of Commons Standing Committee on Human Resources, Skills and Social Development and the Status of Persons with Disabilities* (HUMA) issued a comprehensive report that called for a Federal poverty-reduction plan (Canada 2010). Specifically, HUMA recommended that national initiatives be undertaken to:

> eliminate the gap in well-being between Indigenous and non-Indigenous children by granting as a first step adequate funding to social programs that provide early intervention to First Nations, Inuit and Métis children and their families including the Indigenous Head Start and the First Nations and Inuit Child Care Initiative (Canada 2010, Recommendation 4.3.2).

The Federal government responded by providing a list of current existing Indigenous programs in Canada. Add to your knowledge of current Indigenous health issues and resources by accessing the Web-Based Resource Box 4.3.

With each passing year, it appears that more and more Indigenous communities and groups are speaking out in protest at the imbalances and substandard levels of health care delivery received compared to non-Indigenous populations (Bartfay and Bartfay 2015). Deagle (1999) argues that the health care system in Canada is best categorized as a three-tier system, with Indigenous peoples on the last tier. The Assembly of First Nations has accused the Government of Canada for failing to appropriately invest in measures to improve the social and health conditions, and quality of life of First Nations peoples (Adelson 2005). For example, in November, 2005 an *Escherichia coli* outbreak in the water supply on the Kashechewan reserve near Timmons, Ontario resulted in

Web-based Resource Box 4.3 Indigenous Health Issues and Resources

Learning Resource	Website
Indigenous Nurses Association of Canada (ANAC)	http://www.anac.on.ca
Assembly of First Nations	http://www.afn.ca
First Nations and Inuit Health Branch	http://www.hc-sc.gc.ca/fnihb-dgspni
Indian and Northern Affairs Canada	http://www.ainc-inac.gc/pr//pub/ywtk/index_e.html
National Indigenous Health Organization (NAHO)	http://www.naho.ca

various health conditions including severe skin rashes and gastro-intestinal disorders (e.g., diarrhoea, vomiting) (Health Canada 2005c). Consequently, because their water supply was deemed not safe for human consumption, 946 residents of the Kashechewan reserve had to be evacuated and received treatment for their associated health conditions. The contamination of drinking water supplies in these First Nations' communities resulted from out-dated and/or poorly managed water treatment plants. In March, 2007 there were ninety-two First Nations' communities across Canada under a drinking water advisory due to unsafe or contaminated water supplies (Health Canada 2007a). Despite the passage of time, the situation appears to remain status quo given that 121 First Nations communities across Canada were under drinking water advisories as of March 31, 2012 (Health Canada 2012a; National Expert Commission Canadian Nurses Association 2012). The Council of Canadians (2015) reports that as of January 2015, there were 1,838 drinking water advisories issued across Canada, including 169 drinking water advisories issued on 126 First Nation communities.

Mental Health Issues, Injuries, and Drownings

Unemployment rates of 25% to 50% have been reported in certain Indigenous communities across Canada, with associated decreased life expectancies and negative physical and mental health outcomes (McMurray 2007). For example, the First Nations' and Inuit Health Branch of Manitoba reports that between 30% and 50% of all health related issues for which Indigenous were seeking assistance from nurses were of mental health origin (Migrone et al. 2003).

Self-inflicted injuries (e.g., cutting oneself) and the suicide rate are approximately six times higher in Indigenous youth aged fifteen to twenty-four, in comparison to the general population in Canada (Bolaria and Bolaria 2006, 2002; Crisis Intervention and Suicide Prevention Centre of British Columbia 2008). In fact, suicide and self-inflicted injuries in Indigenous youth and adults up to the age of forty-four years of age remain leading causes of death (Canadian Mental Health Association n.d.; National Expert Commission Canadian Nurses Association 2012). Moreover, the suicide rate among Inuit youth is among the highest in the world, and is eleven times the Canadian national average (Health Canada 2012b). The Canadian Institute for Health Information (CIHR 2004) reports that injury rates resulting in premature deaths among First Nations' people living on reserves are four times higher in comparison to the general Canadian population.

Mortality rates resulting from trauma and injuries (e.g., motor vehicle accidents, falls) in Indigenous children are significantly higher in comparison to non-Indigenous Canadian children (MacMillan et al. 1999). Every $1.00 invested toward road safety and prevention results in a $40.00 saving towards health care costs, or a return on investment (ROI) of 3,900%. Findings from the *First Nations and Inuit Regional Health Survey* show that injuries, trauma and drownings are major health concerns in school-aged and teenage Indigenous children (Canadian Institute of Child Health 2000). For examples, by the time Indigenous children reach the age of seventeen years, 13% of them will have broken a bone; 4% will receive a serious trauma to the cranium; 2% will report severe frostbite and 3% will have drowned. Similar findings were reported by Bristow et al. (2002) in their study that examined paediatric drownings in Manitoba.

Gasoline Sniffing

The sniffing of the toxic solvent gasoline is a growing problem in many Indigenous communities across Canada, and this disturbing health altering behaviour has been reported in teens and school-aged children (Schissel 2006; York 1992). Gasoline is a highly addictive neurotoxin that may result in permanent damage to the brain, nervous system, kidneys, liver and other vital organs (Schubert and Bartfay 2010c; Bartfay and Bartfay 2015).

On January 26, 1993, six Inuit youth from Davis Inlet, Labrador made national headlines in the news when they attempted to commit group suicide by sniffing gasoline (Schissel 2006). Luckily, their suicide attempt was thwarted by a counsellor who heard about their plans from fellow children. Alarmingly, twenty additional Inuit children attempted to end their lives in November, 2000 and were consequently air-lifted for medical treatment and counselling to Goose Bay. According to Schissel (2006), of the 169 children (aged 10–19) living in Davis Inlet at the end of 2000, 154 have attempted gas sniffing and seventy children were considered chronic gas sniffers.

Gasoline sniffing is not limited to Inuit populations in Canada, many Indigenous communities have been affected or are threatened due in part to the negative social, cultural and economic effects of colonization and/or the reserve system (Bartfay 2010a, 2010c). For example, during the 1940s the Shamattawa Crees of Northeastern Manitoba were relocated onto reserves created by the Federal government (York 1992). Gasoline has been referred to as their "lifeblood" of these reserves because residents are dependent on it for a variety of uses including heating their homes and fuelling their all-terrain vehicles and cycles (ATVs, ATCs), and snowmobiles so they can hunt and fish to feed their families (York 1992). Unfortunately, it is also a relatively inexpensive addictive substance of abuse that can easily be obtained by youths, and it is one of the most dangerous forms of addictions in the world.

> But gasoline is the deadliest poison at Shamattawa. Children and teenagers sniff to gain a quick escape, a cheap and immediate high–a few minutes of euphoria in the land of poverty and misery . . . At night, they break into snowmobile gas-tanks to steal more of the precious substance, until it finally dominates their existence . . . Medical experts have concluded that gasoline sniffing is one of the most dangerous addictions in the world . . . a single inhalation can hook a child . . . Once inhaled, gasoline harms the kidneys and liver, and inflicts permanent damage to the nervous system and the brain (York 1992, 8–9).

These highly publicized events above received both national and international coverage by various news media outlets. They have also brought with them a dramatic realization of the negative effects of colonization and the creation of reserves, which has often resulted in the social, economic and political marginalization of Indigenous peoples in Canada (Bartfay 2010c).

Health of Indigenous Families

Infant mortality rates are often employed as an indicator of the health of a nation or defined population because it is strongly associated with both adult mortality and overall life expectancy rates (Mandleco and Bartfay 2010). Over the past few decades, infant mortality rates have steadily declined in Canada. For example, in 1960 it was 27 per 1,000 live births, and by 2003 it had dropped to 5.3 deaths per 1,000 live births. Mortality rates amongst Indigenous infants remain two to three times higher in comparison to non-Indigenous Canadians (McMurray 2007). Infant mortality rates were highest in Nunavut (19.8 per 1,000 live births); among the provinces–Manitoba ranked the highest (8.0 per 1,000 live births), and New Brunswick and British Columbia had the lowest rates at 4.1 and 4.2 live births per 1,000, respectively (Statistics Canada 2006c).

The Research Focus Box 4.1 examines maternal psychosocial, situational and home-environments of Indigenous adolescent mothers residing on and off reserves, in comparison to non-Indigenous mothers in Canada. The findings suggest that teen First Nations and Métis mothers may be at increased risk for negative health and developmental outcomes as a result of their compromised socioeconomic living conditions and negative home environments.

The family unit as a collective whole is often faced with the challenge of providing adequate shelter. Based on findings from the 2006 Census, Indigenous children were almost nine times (26%) more likely to live in families with a crowded home, in comparison to non-Indigenous children (3%) (Statistics Canada 2009). Furthermore, remote and isolated communities are often confronted with the additional burden of having to secure affordable and nutritious food items for themselves and their children (Bartfay 2010a; Bartfay and Bartfay 2015). For example, the prevalence of iron-deficiency anemia and associated risk factors were found to be higher in one study that examined James Bay Cree infants in Northern Québec (Willows et al. 2000). The cost of food is also rising in many remote Indigenous communities and regions in Canada. Indigenous peoples are reported to be four times more likely than non-Indigenous people to experience hunger as a direct result of poverty (Food Banks of Canada 2011). For example, residents in Nunavut spend approximately 25% (or $14,815) of their total expenditures on food, compared to the national average of only 11%

Research Focus Box 4.1

Maternal Psychosocial, Situational, and Home-environmental Characteristics of Métis, First Nations and Caucasian Adolescent Mothers in Canada

Study Aim/Rationale

The aim of this study was to compare and contrast the maternal psychosocial, situational, and home-environmental characteristics of Métis, First Nations and Caucasian adolescent mothers in Canada. There are an increasing number of infants born to teenage adolescent mothers. Little is currently known about how their parenting environments may negative affect health and developmental outcomes.

Methodology/Design

A longitudinal exploratory study design was chosen by the researchers. A convenient sampling method was used to recruit seventy-one Métis, First Nations and Caucasian adolescent mother's subjects. The researchers assessed maternal psychosocial, situational and home-environmental characteristics at four weeks and twelve to eighteen months post-birth. The Human Development Index was employed to quantify these outcomes.

Major Findings

Caucasian mothers scored significantly higher on quality of home environment scores, in comparison to Indigenous mothers. Infants born to teen First Nations and Métis mothers have an increased risk for encountering negative parenting environments, health and developmental outcomes in comparison to those over nineteen years of age or older. Forty-nine percent of the variance was explained via a multiple regression model that contained the following variables: Infant-care emotionality, education level of the infant's maternal grandmother, ethnicity and enacted social support explained. The variables infant-care emotionality and grandmother's education level were found to be significant predictors of parenting environments, health and developmental outcomes. Scores obtained by Indigenous subjects on the Human Development Index showed that First Nations subjects who lived off reserves had similar scores to residents living in third world countries such as Trinidad and Tobago (ranked 35th globally). Furthermore, First Nations mothers living on reserves were only marginally better off than Brazilians (ranked 63rd globally).

Implications for Public Health

The findings suggests that teen First Nations and Métis mothers may be at increased risk for negative health and developmental outcomes as a result of their compromised socioeconomic living conditions and negative home environments, both on and off reserves. Public health workers and professionals can assist teenage First Nations and Métis mothers at risk by providing them with early intervention programs that focus on health promotion and coping strategies. In addition, culturally sensitive programs that train expectant Indigenous mothers in basic infant nutrition and care (e.g., bathing, feeding) would be beneficial.

Source: Secco and Moffatt (2004).

(or $7,626) of total expenditures (Statistics Canada 2011). Indeed, the cost for a litre of milk can be as high as $12, $17 per kilogram for green peppers and $29 for cheese spread (Food Banks of Canada 2012). The use of food banks has also grown in the territories over the past decade and food insecurity has become much more severe of late due to the high costs of delivering food items to these remote communities and the population boom. As of March 2008, the total number of individuals accessing food banks in the territories was 1,340, and by 2012 this number has grown to 2,420 (72.8% increase) (Food Banks of Canada 2012). Similarly, Statistics Canada (2009) reports that First Nations, Inuit and Métis people account for only 4% of the total Canadian population, yet make up 11% of individuals utilizing food banks nationally (Statistics Canada 2010c).

According to WHO (2000a, 2000b, 2000c), when treatment protocols for tuberculosis (TB) were first introduced in 1948, it was predicted that the respiratory disorder would be eradicated worldwide by the year 2000. A growing number of Indigenous families are forced to live in crowded houses. This over-crowding is an ideal breeding ground for respiratory infections such as TB. In addition to over-crowding, multidrug-resistant strains of TB have also emerged, and an estimated eight million people acquire TB worldwide each year. It is predicted that by 2020, nearly one billion people will be newly infected globally, 200 million will be severely ill, and thirty-five million will die if control measures are not further developed (WHO 2000a, 2000b, 2000c). The incidence of TB in 1999 in Indigenous in Canada was approximately seventy per 100,000, in comparison to only one per 100,000 in non-Indigenous (Fitzgerald et al. 2000; Long et al. 1999). Currently, the TB rate among Indigenous people is almost six times higher in comparison to non-Indigenous (Muntaner et al. 2012; National Expert Commission Canadian Nurses Association 2012). George (2012) reports that the incidence of TB among the Inuit is currently 284 times higher, in comparison to other Canadians, according to recent statistics released by the Government of Nunavut's Health Department. In 2010, the overall rate for TB among the Inuit was 198.6 per 100,000 people, compared to 0.7 per 100,000 for the Canadian-born, non-Indigenous members of the population. Moreover, the rate for Inuit in Nunavut was even higher at 434 times the national rate (George 2012). The WHO strategy for the detection and cure of TB consists of the following five elements: (i) Political commitment, (ii) microscopy services, (iii) drug supplies, (iv) surveillance and monitoring systems and (v) the use of efficacious regiments with direct observation of treatment (Bartfay and Bartfay 2015; Thomas and Bartfay 2010). This represents a significant public health challenge in various Indigenous communities across Canada.

Sexually Transmitted Infections

The incidence of STIs, including HIV/AIDS, chlamydia, gonorrhoea and syphilis has been increasing in recent years, especially among Indigenous teens and young women (Public Health Agency of Canada 2010c; Ship and Norton 2001; WHO 2000b). In 2005, for example, although Indigenous peoples comprised 3.3% of the entire population in Canada, 22.4% of new infections for HIV/AIDS were reported amongst Indigenous (National Indigenous Council on HIV/AIDS 2003; Public Health Agency of Canada [PHAC] 2006a, 2006b). Similarly, in 2013 Indigenous peoples comprised only 4.3% of the entire Canadian population (Statistics Canada 2013), yet 8.9% of all prevalent infections for HIV/AIDS reported were amongst Indigenous peoples (PHAC 2012). STIs are notifiable communicable diseases in Canada (PHAC 2003; 2005), and all provinces and territories have developed guidelines and recommendations for prenatal testing for these diseases (Canadian Paediatric Society 2006).

The Government of Canada has identified HIV/AIDS as an epidemic among Indigenous peoples (Jenkins et al. 2003; PHAC 2004). In May of 2001, the National Indigenous Council on HIV/AIDS (NACHA 2002) was established to address this epidemic. Furthermore, the council was also formed to advise Health Canada on STI prevention and treatment strategies that are culturally specific to Indigenous peoples (Figure 4.3).

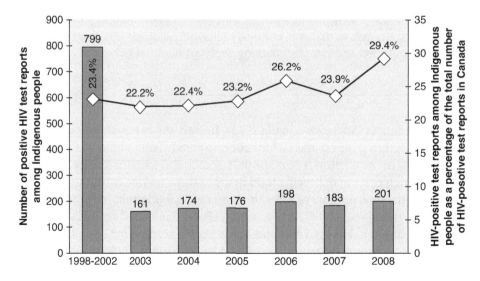

Figure 4.3 HIV-positive test reports among Indigenous people as a percentage of the total number of HIV-positive reports in Canada from 1998 to 2008.

Web-based Resource Box 4.4 HIV/AIDS Resources for Indigenous Populations

Learning Resource	Website
Indigenous AIDS Network	http://www.caan.ca
National Indigenous Council on HIV/AIDS: Canadian Strategy on HIV/AIDS (Health Canada 2000)	http://www.hc-sc.gc.ca/hppb/hiv_aids/can_strat/Indigenous/main/htm

Indigenous people remain disproportionately affected by HIV/AIDS and accounted for 13% of all new HIV infections in 2008, a rate estimated to be approximately 3.6 times higher than non-Indigenous (Butler-Jones 2012; PHAC 2010b, 2010d). Between the years 1998 and 2008, female Indigenous accounted for approximately 50% of all new reported HIV infections, compared with 21% among the non-Indigenous population (PHAC 2010b, 2010d). Add to your knowledge of STIs and current evidence-based public health programs and initiatives for Indigenous populations by accessing the Web-Based Resource Box 4.4.

Cardiovascular Disease and Diabetes

The Heart and Stroke Foundation's (HSF 2003) report entitled "The Growing Burden of Heart Disease and Stroke," notes that Indigenous are particularly vulnerable to the development of CVD, including heart disease and stroke. Findings from this report indicate that Indigenous peoples are more likely to have major risk factors associated with the development of CVD including a sedentary lifestyle, being overweight or obese, consuming large amounts of processed foods high in sugar, saturated and trans-fats and salt, smoking and diabetes. The *2002–2003 First Nations Regional Longitudinal Health Survey* found that women aged twenty to thirty-four were more likely to be obese or morbid obese, in comparison to non-Indigenous women (National Indigenous Health Organization [NAHO], 2006). The greater incidence of sedentary lifestyles can be attributed, in part, to a reduction in traditional fishing, trapping and hunting practices, and an increased reliance on motorized boats and vehicles such as ATCs and snowmobiles (Bartfay 2010a; Bartfay and Bartfay 2015). Furthermore, changes to the traditional fishing, trapping and hunting lifestyles by Indigenous peoples in Canada have resulted in an increased reliance on highly processed commercially available foods, an increased incidence of obesity in both children and adults, and Type 2 diabetes (Bartlett 2003; Bobet 1998; Ralph-Campbell et al. 2009; Young 2003; Young et al. 2000).

Obesity is a well-documented risk factor for the development of various chronic diseases including Type 2 diabetes, heart disease and stroke, metabolic syndrome, hypertension, hyperlipidemia and certain forms of cancer. Interestingly, although Inuit populations in Canada have also observed an increased incidence of obesity over the decades, they still have a relatively low incidence of Type 2 diabetes. The term "healthy obese" has thus been linked to Inuit peoples; where although individuals have increased levels of body fat present, this does not appear to predispose them to the development of Type 2 diabetes (Lemas et al. 2011; Reading 2010; Wildman 2009). It is speculated that a diet rich in polyunsaturated fatty acids (n-3 PUFA) by Inuit peoples may be a protector factor.

It is notable that diabetes was not known in Indigenous populations fifty to sixty years ago in Canada who engaged in traditional subsistence practices (e.g., hunting, fishing) without the use of motorized vehicles, ate traditional diets and had more active lifestyles (Bartfay 2010a). Further challenges to obtaining healthy and affordable food choices exist in northern and remote Indigenous communities (Butler-Jones 2012; Chan et al. 2006; Rosol 2009; Rosol, et al. 2011). For example, according to the 2007 to 2008 Inuit Health Survey, approximately 70% of households in Nunavut reported experiencing moderate-to-severe food insecurity over the past year (Egeland et al. 2011; Rosol 2009; Rosel 2011).

Tobacco has been employed by First Nations peoples as a sacred and purifying agent in their traditional ceremonies. However, the use of commercially available tobacco products such as cigarettes, cigars and chewing tobacco neither support nor is in concert with traditional sacred ceremonial uses of tobacco in First

Nations' cultures, as detailed in the First Nations and Inuit Tobacco Control Strategy (FNITC) (Health Canada 2005a). Indeed, there are significant differences between ceremonial uses of tobacco and smoking or chewing commercially available products, which have major health implications for Indigenous communities across Canada (Bartfay 2010a; Bartfay and Bartfay 2015).

The age-adjusted rate for adult onset Type 2 diabetes in Indigenous people is three to five times higher than the general non-Indigenous population (Bobet 1998; First Nations and Inuit Regional Health Survey 1999; Health Canada 2011; Macaulay et al. 2003; Statistics Canada 2007; Young 2003; Young et al. 2000). For example, Health Canada and the Public Health Agency of Canada (2011) report that 17.2% of on-reserve and 10.3% of off-reserve First Nations peoples in Canada were clinically diagnosed with Type 2 diabetes, compared to a national rate of 6.4% for non-Indigenous peoples. The *Indigenous Peoples Survey* conducted by Health Canada found that 6.5% of First Nations people over the age of fifteen years have already been diagnosed with Type 2 diabetes, and this number has been steadily increasing over the past decades (Hales and Lauzon 2007). Moreover, the survey found that 5.5% of Métis and 8.4% of First Nations people living on reserves have this disease. The *2002–2003 First Nations Regional Longitudinal Health Survey* found that women aged twenty to thirty-four years are now being diagnosed with diabetes earlier (HAHO 2006). Indigenous mothers are also at increased risk of having adult-onset Type 2 diabetes and/or developing gestational diabetes (Hegele et al. 2002; Young et al. 2000).

Discouragement and suppression of traditional lifestyles and diet, displacement of entire communities, the exploitation of natural resources for profit by multinational companies and increasing sedentary lifestyles are just a few of the associated factors associated with the higher incidence of diabetes in Indigenous communities in Canada. The Canadian Diabetes Association Clinical Practice Guidelines Expert Committee (2003) reports that public health professionals and workers now face major challenges in trying to provide Indigenous people with culturally appropriate health care programs and prevention strategies. For example, there has been increased attention by health care professionals and various levels of government to provide culturally appropriate food guides and educational toolkits (e.g., Health Canada 2007b, 2003; Northwest Territories Food Guide 2003). The National Indigenous Diabetes Association (NADA) was established to promote healthy lifestyles (e.g., dietary choices, exercise, stop smoking), and to provide educational materials and assistance for those affected by this potentially life-threatening disease and its associated health complications including heart disease, stroke, kidney disease, blindness and amputations of limbs (Bartfay 2010a; Bartfay and Bartfay 2015). For example, every $1.00 spent on a tobacco prevention campaign results in a $20.00 saving in health care costs, or a return on investment of 1,900%.

The Canadian Diabetes Association Clinical Practice Guidelines Expert Committee (2003, S111, Grade D, Consensus) have made the following recommendations for the prevention, treatment and management of diabetes in First Nations, Inuit and Métis peoples:

(a) Treatment of diabetes in Indigenous people should follow clinical practice guidelines.
(b) There must be recognition of, respect for and sensitivity regarding the unique language, culture and geographic issues as they relate to diabetes care and education in Indigenous communities across Canada.
(c) Culturally appropriate primary prevention programs should be initiated by Indigenous communities to increase awareness of diabetes, increase physical activity, improve eating habits and achieve healthy body weights, and to promote environments that are supportive of a healthy lifestyle.
(d) Community-based diabetes screening programs should be established in Indigenous communities. Urban people of Indigenous origin should be screened for diabetes in primary care settings.

Add to your knowledge of diabetes nutrition and current public health toolkits and programs that have been designed specifically for Indigenous populations by accessing the Web-Based Resources Box 4.5.

Web-based Resource Box 4.5 Indigenous Nutritional Guides and Toolkits

Resources	Website
Health Canada: Office of Nutrition Policy and Promotion. Nutrition Labeling Toolkit for Educators—First Nations and Inuit Focus (2003)	http://www.hc-sc.gc.ca/fn-an/label-etiquet/nutrition/fni-pni/nutri-kit-trouse/index-eng.php
Northwest Territories Food Guide (March, 2003)	http://www.hlthss.gov.nt.ca

Future Directions and Challenges

One of the major challenges involves educating public health professionals and workers about Indigenous definitions and meanings surrounding the concept of health. Public health care professionals need to be cognizant that western definitions of health and health care systems may often conflict with Indigenous culture, beliefs and health care practices (Bartfay 2010a; Bartfay and Bartfay 2015). Current curriculums and programs in public and community health need to include current (e.g., STIs, suicide in youth) and emerging health issues (e.g., growing rates of Type 2 diabetes, obesity trends) facing various Indigenous communities across Canada. Moreover, public health care professionals and workers also need to be educated and cognizant of the negative effects of colonization and its associated products (e.g., reserve system, residential schools) and how these have often marginalized and negatively impacted the health and well-being of First Nations, Inuit and Métis peoples. Indigenous families and communities face immense health challenges in the new millennium and public health care professionals, workers and policy makers must learn to work in collaboration with these populations to plan for effective access and delivery of primary health care services across the lifespan.

Collaborative public health initiatives and programs should be developed in consultation with Indigenous communities, elders and stakeholders and should be based on culturally appropriate and evidence-informed interventions. To better address these health care challenges, a delegation of Indigenous people and health care researchers have collectively lobbied the Government of Canada to consider funding research initiatives to more effectively deal with current Indigenous health issues based on evidence-informed initiatives. These recommendations were formally presented to the CIHR, and in the year 2000 the "IAPH was launched (Beckman Murray et al. 2006). The aim of the IAPH is to present the results from scientific investigations to Indigenous people and stakeholders in a manner that is culturally appropriate, accessible, and user friendly. National initiatives, such as the IAPH, are critical if we are to address current and emerging public health issues facing various Indigenous communities across Canada.

Group Review Exercise 4.1 "Sleeping Children Awake"

Overview of This Investigative Documentary
This short six-part documentary outlines the history of the residential school system and its negative ripple effects on First Nations' families and peoples in Canada. Sleeping Children Awake (SCA) was filmed in 1991 and televised in 1992 and was one of the earliest, feature documentaries to examine the impact of the residential school system. SCA won several awards including "Best Canadian Documentary 1993" (CanPro) and was screened at the Truth and Reconciliation Commission of Canada's national events held in Winnipeg, Manitoba 2010, and Saskatchewan 2012.

Residential schools operated in Canada from the 1800s until the year 1996 and their objective was to assimilate Indigenous people into the western culture and beliefs systems and to systematically destroy their native culture, traditions, language and belief systems. The former Grand Chief Phil Fontaine, a residential school survivor himself, stated "The first step in healing is disclosure," which this six-part documentary seeks to highlight through the voices and experiences of actual survivors including Elijah Harper (a former Member of Parliament) and the late Art Solomon (Elder and author). These recollections and experiences are bridged by dramatic excerpts from Shirley Cheechoo's autobiographical play entitled "Path with No Moccasins." In addition this documentary features songs by Maria Linklater and Indigenous art by various artists and painters. SCA is both a personal record of our nations' history and a tribute to the enduring strength of Indigenous peoples and culture.

Instructions

This assignment may be done alone, in pairs or in groups of up to five people (*Note:* if you are doing this assignment in pairs or groups, please only submit one hard or electronic copy to your instructor). The assignment should be type-written and no more than four to six pages maximum in length (double-spaced please). View the short six-part documentary entitled "Sleeping Children Awake (SCA)." See links: magicarrowproductions@gmail.com or http://www.youtube.com/watch?v=0zkUKbAaff0
View this documentary and take detailed notes during the presentation.

   i. Provide a brief overview of the salient points or outcomes highlighted in this short six-part documentary and comment on the aims of the residential school system.
   ii. Briefly discuss the "negative ripple effects" of the residential school system on Indigenous families, cultures and belief systems discussed in this documentary.
   iii. What are some of the current and future implications or challenges for public health addressed in this documentary in terms of healing?
   iv. Discuss the importance of "cultural safety" when providing primary health care interventions to Indigenous populations in your province or territory.

Summary

- European colonization often resulted in "negative ripple effects" that had devastating social and health consequences.
- For example, French and English colonizers brought with them various diseases that were previously unknown to Indigenous populations including various STIs, tuberculosis, measles and small pox that devastated tens of thousands of First Nations and Inuit peoples (Bartfay 2010a; Donahue 1996).
- Government policies such as the treaty and reserve systems, residential schools, and various legislations were developed to control and assimilate First Nations people into the western cultures and belief systems have negatively impacted on their health and well-being.
- For example, we learned that following Confederation, Indigenous peoples including First Nations, Inuit and Métis were often forced to be relocated and/or displaced from their traditional birth and hunting territories to make room for the ever-increasing numbers of European settlers.
- The First Nations' Medicine Wheel is considered a powerful and sacred symbol of the universe, which depicts the circularity of life and the balance between the four aspects of self: (i) Physical, (ii) mental; (iii) emotional, and (iv) spiritual.
- Indigenous beliefs, concepts, health care practices and structures often conflict with the western health care systems and definitions of health and well-being. Indeed, Indigenous perspectives on health and well-being emphasis a holistic and reciprocal relationship between the physical and spiritual world, the individual and their surrounding environment, and between the mind, body, and spirit.
- Larger and less-isolated Indigenous communities often have designated health centres that provide their residents with more traditional public health and primary health services.

- By contrast nurses and NPs are typically the major health care providers in remote communities, where two-thirds of Indigenous peoples live in Canada.
- Public health care professionals and workers need to be aware of the history, beliefs, traditions and cultures of Indigenous communities they serve to provide safe, effective, and culturally appropriate health care.
- Public health care professionals and workers also need to be cognizant of the concept of "cultural safety," which provides a mechanism for the recognition of the indices of power inherent in any professional relationship or interaction, and the potential for disparity and inequality within any relationship.
- Lastly, we examined some of the current major health issues and challenges facing Indigenous populations in Canada including mental health issues, tuberculosis, diabetes and heart disease.

Critical Thinking Questions

1. You are working as a public health manager in a remote First Nations' reserve in Canada. A routine water sample indicates significant growth of the bacteria *E. coli*. How would you deal with the major threat to the health and safety of the residents of the community? Who would you contact and what specific public health measures would you put into place. Justify your choices.
2. List and identify current public health issues facing Indigenous peoples in your community, province or territory. In your opinion, which are the top three issues and why? Identify public health strategies and interventions that could help decreasing the impact of these issues.
3. If you were a provincial/ territorial minister of health, what specific policies or legislations would you put in place to improve the health of Indigenous populations across the lifespan in your jurisdiction? Justify your choices.

References

Abbott, M. E. *History of Medicine in the Province of Québec*. Montréal: McGill University, 1931.

Aboriginal Affairs and Northern Development Canada. *Aboriginal Peoples and Communities*. Ottawa, ON: Author, 2010a. Retrieved July 4, 2013, http://www.aadnc-aande.gc.ca/eng/1100100013785.

———. *Fact Sheet: 2006 Census Aboriginal Demographics*. Ottawa, ON: Author, 2010b. Retrieved July 7, 2012, http://ainc-inac.gc.ca/eng/1100100016377.

———. *Powley Ruling*. Ottawa, ON: Author, 2012. Retrieved December 21, 2012, http://www.aadnc-aandc.gc.ca/eng/1100100014419/1100100014420.

Aboriginal Healing Foundation. *Annual Report 1999*. 1999. Retrieved April 24, 2010, http://www.ahf.ca/newsite/english/pdf/annual_report_1999.pdf.

Aboriginal and Torres Striat Islander Social Justice Commission. "Native Title Report 2005," 2005. http://www.humanrights.gov.au/social%5justice/ntreport05/ch1.html.

Adelson, N. "The Embodiment of Inequity: Health Disparities of Aboriginal Canada." *Canadian Journal of Public Health* 96, no. S2 (2005): S45–61.

Archives de Montréal. *Fonds Aegidius Fauteux. Canadian Historical Portrais*. Montréal, QC: Villes de Montréal, 2010. Retrieved April 28, 2010, http://www.2.ville.montreal.qc.ca/archieves/portraits/en/region/quebec/index.shtm.

Bartlett, J. G. "Involuntary Cultural Change, Stress Phenomenon and Aboriginal Health Status." *Canadian Journal of Public Health* 92 (2003): 165–67.

Bartfay, W. J. "Men in Nursing in Canada: Past, Present and Future Perspectives." In *Men in Nursing: History, Challenges and Opportunities*, edited by C. E. O'Lynn and R. E. Tranbarger, 205–18. New York: Springer Publishing Company, 2008.

———. "Aboriginal Health: Concepts and Current Challenges." In *Community Health Nursing: Caring in Action*, 1st Canadian ed., edited by J. E. Hitchcock, P. E. Schubert, S. A. Thomas, and W. J. Bartfay, 42–58. Toronto, ON: Nelson, 2010a.

———. "Canada's Health Care System: History and Current Challenges." In *Community Health Nursing: Caring in Action*, 1st Canadian ed., edited by J. E. Hitchcock, P. E. Schubert, S. A. Thomas, and W. J. Bartfay, 23–41. Toronto, ON: Nelson, 2010b.

———. "Environmental Perspectives on Health." In *Community Health Nursing: Caring in Action*, 1st Canadian ed., edited by J. E. Hitchcock, P. E. Schubert, S. A. Thomas, and W. J. Bartfay, 117–42. Toronto, ON: Nelson, 2010c.

Bartfay, W. J., and E. Bartfay. *Public Health in Canada*. Boston, MA: Pearson Learning Solutions, 2015. (ISBN:13: 978-1-323-01471-4).

Beckman Murray, R., J. Proctor Zentner, V. Pangman, and C. Pangman. *Health Promotion Strategies Through the Lifespan*, Canadian ed. Toronto, ON: Pearson/Prentice Hall, 2006.

Bobet, E. *Diabetes Among First Nations People: Information From the Statistics Canada 1991 Aboriginal people's Survey*. Ottawa, ON: Minister of Public Works and Government Services Canada; Publication H34-88/1998E, 1998.

Bolaria, B. S., and R. Bolaria. "Women's Lives, Women's Health." In *Health, Illness and Health Care in Canada*, 3rd ed., edited by B. S. Bolaria and H. D. Dickinson, 169–73. Toronto, ON: Nelson Thomson Learning, 2002.

Bopp, J., M. Bopp, L. Brown, and P. Lane. *The Sacred Tree*. Lethbridge: Four Worlds International Institute for Human and Community Development, 1984. www.4words.org.

———. *The Sacred Tree*. Lethbridge, AB: Four Worlds International Institute for Human and Community Development, 1985. http://www.4words.org.

Borrows, J. "Living between Water and Rocks. First Nations, Environmental Planning and Democracy." *University of Toronto Law Journal* XLVII, no. 4 (1997): 38. www.utpjournals.com/product/utlj/474/474_burrows.html.

Bothwell, R. *History of Canada Since 1867*. East Lansing, MI: Michigan State University Press, 1996.

Bramley, D., P. Hebert, L. Tuzzio, and M. Chassin. "Disparities in Indigenous Health: A Cross-Country Comparison Between New Zealand and the United States." *American Journal of Public Health* 95, no. 5 (2005): 844–50.

Bristow, K. M., J. B. Carson, L. Warda, and R. Wartman. "Childhood Drowning in Manitoba: A 10-year Review of Provincial Paediatric Death Review Committee Data." *Paediatric Child Health* 7, no. 9 (2002): 637–41.

Brown, A. J., and J. Fiske. "First Nations Women's Encounters With Mainstream Health Care Services." *Western Journal of Nursing Research* 23, no. 2 (2001): 126–47.

Bumstead, J. *History of Canadian Peoples*. Oxford: Oxford University Press, 2004.

Butler-Jones, D. *The Chief Public Health Officer's Report on the State of Public Health in Canada 2012*. Ottawa, ON: Her Majesty the Queen's in Right of Canada, 2012. ISSN:1917-2656. Cat. No. HP2-10/2012E.

Canada. *Federal Poverty Reduction Plan: Working in Partnership Towards Reducing Poverty in Canada*. Report of the Standing Committee on Human Resources, Skills and Social Development and the Status of Persons with Disabilities (HUMA). Ottawa, ON: Parliament of Canada, 2010. Retrieved October 15, 2015, http://www.parl.gc.ca/HousePublications/Publications.aspx?DocID=4770921.

Canadian Diabetes Association Clinical Practice Guidelines Expert Committee. "Type 2 Diabetes in Aboriginal Peoples." *Canadian Journal of Diabetes* 27, no. 4 (2003): S110–11.

Canadian Heritage. Origin *of the Name-Canada*. Ottawa, ON: Government of Canada, 2004. http://www.canadian heritage.gc.ca/progs/cpsc-ccsp/sc-o5_e.cfm.

Canadian Institute of Child Health. *The Health of Canada's Children: A CICH Profile*. 3rd ed. Ottawa, ON: CICH, 2000.

Canadian Institute for Health Information. *Canadian Population Health Initiative. Improving the Health of Canadians*. Ottawa, ON: CIHR, 2004.

Canadian Mental Health Association. *Aboriginal People/First Nations*. Toronto, ON: Author, n.d. Retrieved July 7, 2013, http://www.ontario.cmha.ca/about_mental_health.asp?cID=23053.

Canadian Paediatric Society. *Positive Statement: Recommendations for the Prevention of Neonatal Ophthalmia*. 2006. Retrieved May 14, 2010, http://www.cps.ca/English/statements/ID/ID02-03.htm.

Carney, R. "Aboriginal Residential Schools Before Confederation: The Early Experience." *Canadian Catholic Historical Association, Historical Studies* 61 (1995): 13–40.

CBC News. *Truth and Reconciliation Commission Urges Canada to Confront "Cultural Genocide" of Residential Schools*. Toronto, ON: Canadian Broadcasting Corporation, June 2, 2015. Retrieved December 16, 2015, http://www.cbc.ca/news/politics/truth-and-reconciliation-commission-urges-canada-to-confront-cultural-genocide-of-residential-schools-1.3096229.

Chan, H. M., K. Fediuk, S. Hamilton, L. Rotas, A. Caughey, H. Kuhnlein, G. Egeland, and E. Loring. "Food Security in Nunavut, Canada: Barriers and Recommendations." *International Journal of Circumpolar Health* 65, no. 5 (2006): 416–31.

Chrisjohn, R. D., S. L. Young, and M. Maraun. *The Circle Game: Shadows and Substance in the Residential School Experience in Canada. A Report to the Royal Commission on Aboriginal Peoples*. Penticton, BC: Theytus, 1997.

Cinq-Mars, J. On the Significance of Modified Mammoth Bones From Eastern Beringia. *The World of Elephants— International Congress, Rome*. 2001. http://www.cq.rm.cnr.it/elephants2001/pdf/424_428.pdf.

College of Nurses of Ontario. *A Primer on the Primary Health Care Nurse Practitioner*. Ottawa, ON: CNO, 2001. Retrieved May 9, 2010, http://www.cno.org/doc/standards/41030_rnecprimer.html#.

———. *The Nurse Practitioner*. Ottawa, ON: CNO, 2003. Retrieved May 9, 2010, http://www.cno.org.

Cradduck, G. R. "Primary Health Care." In *Community Nursing: Promoting Canadians' Health*, edited by M. J. Stewart, 451–71. Toronto, ON: Saunders, 1995.

Crisis Intervention and Suicide Prevention Centre of British Columbia. *Key Suicide Statistics*. BC: Author, 2008. Retrieved May 12, 2009, http://www.crisiscentre.bc.ca/learn/stats.php.

Daniel, M, K. O'Dea, K. G. Rowley, R. McDermott, and S. Kelly. "Social Environmental Stress in Indigenous Populations: Potential Biopsychosocial Mechanisms." *Annuals of the New York Academy of Science* 896 (1999): 420–23.

De, D., and J. Richardson. Cultural Safety: An Introduction. *Paediatric Nurse* 20, no. 2 (2008): 39–44.

Deagle, G. The Three-Tier System (Editorial). *Canadian Family Physician* 45 (1999): 247–49.

Department of Indian and Northern Affairs. *First Nations in Canada*. Ottawa, ON: Government of Canada, 1997.

Dickason, O. P. *Canada's First Nations: A History of Founding Peoples from Earliest Times*, 3rd ed. Don Mills, ON: Oxford, 2002a.

———. "Reclaiming Stolen Land." In *Nation to Nation: Aboriginal Sovereignty and the Future of Canada*, edited by J. Bird, L. Land, and M. Macadam, 34–42. Toronto, ON: Oxford, 2002b.

Dion Stout, M., and B. Downey. *Nursing, Indigenous People and Cultural Safety. So What? Now What?* Queensland, Australia: eContent Management Pty Ltd.,2008. Retrieved May 14, 2010, http://www.contemporynurse.com/22.2/2.2.22html.

Donahue, M. P. *Nursing the Finest Art: An Illustrated History*, 2nd ed. Toronto, ON: Mosby, 1996.

Duerden F., R. G. Kuhn, and S. Black. "An Evaluation of the Effectiveness of First Nations Participation in the Development of Land-Use Plans in the Yukon." *The Canadian Journal of Native Studies* 16, no. 1 (1996): 105–24.

Eckermann, A., T. Dowd, E. Chong, L. Nixon, R. Gray, and S. Johnson. *Binan Goonj: Cultures in Aboriginal Health.* Bridging First Nations Development Institute. 2006. http://www.firstnations.org/about.asp.

Egeland, G. M., L. Johnson-Down, Z. R. Cao, N. Sheikh, and H. Weiler. "Food Insecurity and Nutrition Transition Combine to Affect Nutrient Intakes in Canadian Arctic Communities." *The Journal of Nutrition* 141, no. 9 (2011): 1746–53.

Ellerby, J. H., J. McKenzie, S. McKay, G. J. Gariepy, and J. M. Kaufert. "Bioethics for Clinicians: 18. Aboriginal Cultures." *Canadian Medical Association Journal* 163, no. 7 (2000): 845–33.

First Nations and Inuit Regional Health Survey. *National Report 1999.* St. Regis, QC: First Nations and Inuit Regional Health Survey National Steering Committee, 1999.

First Nations Environmental Network. *Our Vision.* 2002. http://fnen.org.

———. *History and Profile.* 2003. http://fnen.org.

———. *Our Goals.* 2004. http://fnen.org.

FitzGerald, G., L. Wang, and R. Elwood. "Tuberculosis 13: Control of the Disease Among Aboriginal People in Canada." *Canadian Medical Association Journal* 162, no. 3 (2000): 351–55.

Fleet, C. *First Nations Firsthand: A History of Five Hundred Years of Encounter, War, and Peace Inspired by the Eyewitnesses.* Edison, NJ: Chartwell, 1997.

Food Banks of Canada. *Hungercount 2010. A Comprehensive Report on Hunger and Food Bank Use in Canada, and Recommendations for Change.* Toronto, ON: Author, 2011. Retrieved October 15, 2015, http://www.foodbankscanada._getmedia/12a3e485-4a4e-47d.

Food Banks of Canada. *Hungercount 2012. A Comprehensive Report on Hunger and Food Bank Use in Canada, and Recommendations for Change.* Toronto, ON: Author, 2012. ISBN: 978-0-9813632-8-8.

Galloway, G., and B. Curry. "Residential Schools Amounted to 'Cultural Genocide' Reports Says." *The Globe and Mail*, Ottawa, ON. June 2, 2015. Retrieved December 16, 2015, http://www.theglobeandmail.com/news/politics/residential-schools-amounted-to-cultural-genocide-says-report/article24740605/.

George, J. "TB among Inuit Needs 'Vigilant Action' Says National Inuit Org." *Nunatsiaq Online*, March 23, 2012, Nunavut. Retrieved December 30, 2012, http://www.nunatsiaqonline.ca/stories/article/65674tb_among_inuit_needs_vigilant_action_says_national_inuit_org/.

Government of Ontario. *Archives of Ontario French Ontario in the 17th and 18th Centuries—Making Contact.* Toronto, ON: Ministry of Government Services, 2010. Retrieved April 28, 2010, http://www.archives.gov.on.ca/english/on-line-exhibits/franco-ontario/contacts.aspx.

Grant, T. "Indigenous People Six Times More Likely to Be Murder Victims: Statscan." *The Globe and Mail.* November 25, 2015. Retrieved December 3, 2015, http://www.theglobeandmail.com/news/national/aboriginals-six-times-more-likely-to-be-homicide-victims-statscan/article27475106/.

Hales, D., and L. Lauzon. *An Invitation to Health*, 1st Canadian ed. Toronto: Thomson/Nelson, 2007.

Halpin, M. M. *Totem Poles: An Illustrated Guide.* Vancouver, BC: University of British Columbia (UBC) Press, UBC Museum of Archeology, 2002. (ISBN: 0-7748-0141-7).

Hammersmith, B., and L. Sawatsky. *The Beat of a Different Drum: An Aboriginal Cross-Cultural Handbook for Child-care Workers.* Sanichton, BC: Association of Aboriginal Friendship Centres, 2000.

Health Canada. *Indian Health Policy 1979. First Nations and Inuit Health Branch.* 2001a. www.hc-sc-gc-ca/fnihb-dgspni/fnihb/bpm/hfa/transfer_publications/indian_health_policy.htm.

———. "Ten Years of Health Transfer First Nations and Inuit control. First Nations and Inuit Health Branch." 2001b. www.hc-gc.ca/fnihb-dgspni/fnihb/bpm/hfa/ten_years_health_transfer/index.htm.

———. *Canada's Aging Population. Division of Aging and Seniors.* Ottawa, ON: Minister of Public Works and Government Services Canada, 2002. www.hc-sc-gc.ca/seniors-aines/.

———. *Office of Nutrition Policy and Promotion. Nutrition Labeling Toolkit for Educators—First Nations and Inuit Focus (2003)*. Ottawa, ON: Author, 2003. http:www.hc-sc.gc.ca/fn-an/label-etiquet/nutrition/fni-pni/nutria-kit-trousse/index-eng.php.

———. *First Nations and Inuit Health (2005, April). First Nations and Inuit Tobacco Control Strategy Program Framework*. Ottawa: Health Canada, 2005a. www.hc-sc.gc.ca/fnih-spni/pubs/tobac-tabac/2002_frame-cadre/intro_e.html.

———. *First Nations Comparable Health Indicators*. Ottawa, ON: Author, 2005b. Retrieved May 12, 2010, http://www.hc-sc.gc.ca/fniah-spnai/diseases-maladies/2005-01_health-sante_indicat-eng.php#life-expect.

———. *Progress on Kashechewan Action Plan*. 2005c. http://www.ainc-inac.gc.ca/nr/prs/s-d2005/2-02730_e/html.

———. *Drinking Water Advisories-First Nations and Inuit Health*. Ottawa, ON: Author, 2007a. http://www.hc-sc.gc.ca/fnih-spni/promotion/water-eau/advis-avis_concern_e.html.

———. *Eating Well With Canada's Food Guide. First Nations, Inuit and Métis*. Ottawa, ON: Minister of Public Works and Government Services Canada, 2007b.

———. *First Nations and Inuit Health*. Ottawa, ON: Author, 2007c. http://www.hc-sc.gc.ca/fnih-spni/index_ehtml.

———. *First Nations and Inuit Health: Nursing*. Ottawa, ON: Author, 2007d. http://www.hc-sc.gc.ca/fnih-spni/services/nurs-infirm/index_e.html.

———. *First Nations and Inuit Health Branch of Health Canada*. Ottawa, ON: Author, 2008. www.hc.sc.gc.ca/fnihb/.

———. *First Nations, Inuit and Aboriginal Health: Drinking Water and Waste Water*. Ottawa, ON: Author, 2012a. Retrieved July 7, 2013, http://www.hc-sc.gc/fniah-spnia/promotion/public-publique/water-eau-eng. Php#how_many.

———. *First Nations, Inuit and Aboriginal Health–Mental Health and Wellness*. Ottawa, ON: Author, 2012b. Retrieved July 7, 2013, http://www.hc-sc.gc.ca/fniah-spnia/promotion/mental/index-eng.php.

Health Council of Canada. *The Health Status of Canada's First Nations, Métis and Inuit Peoples*. Ottawa, ON: Author, 2005. Retrieved May 12, 2010, http://healthcouncilcanada.ca.c9.previewyour site.com/docs/papers/2005/BkgrdHealthyCdns.ENG.pdf.

Heart and Stroke Foundation of Canada. "The Growing Burden of Heart Disease and Stroke in Canada, 2003. Chapter 1-Risk Factors." 2003. www.cvdinfobase.ca/cvdbook/CVD_En03.pdf.

Hegele, R. A., H. Cao, A. J. G. Hanley, B. Zinman, S. B. Harris, and C. M. Anderson. "Clinical Utility of HNFIA Genotyping for Diabetes in Aboriginal Canadians." *Diabetes Care* 23, no. 2 (2002): 775–78.

Hernandez, C. A., I. Antone, and I. Cornelius. A Grounded Theory Study of the Experience of Type 2 Diabetes Mellitus in First Nations Adults in Canada. *Journal of Transcultural Nursing* 10, no. 3 (1999): 220–28.

Human Resources and Skills Development Canada. *Current Realities and Emerging Issues Facing Youth in Canada: An Analytical Framework for Public Policy Research, Development and Evaluation*. Ottawa, ON: Author, 2010. Retrieved July 7, 2013, http://www.horizons.gc.ca/2010-0017-eng.pdf.

Huteson, P. R. *Legends in Wood. Stories of the Totems*. Tigard, OR: Greatland Classic Sales, 2002 (ISBN: 1-886462-51-8).

Jenkins, A. L., T. W. Gyrokos, K. N. Culman, B. J. Ward, G. S. Pekeles, and E. L. Mills. "An Overview of Factors Influencing the Health of Canadian Inuit Infants." *International Journal of Circumpolar Health* 62, no. 1 (2003): 17–39.

Johal, A. *Canadian Court to Rule on Tribal Land Rights.*" 2006. www.worldpress.org/Americas/2272.cfm.

Jonaitis, A., and A. Glass. *The Totem Pole: An Intercultural History*. Washington, DC: University of Washington Press, 2010.

Kendall, D., R. Linden, and J. Lothian Murray. *Sociology in Our Times: The Essentials* 2nd Canadian ed. Scarborough, ON: Nelson Thomson Learning, 2001.

Kenton, E. *The Jesuit Relations and Documents*. New York: The Vanguard Press, 1925.

Kerr, J. "Early Nursing in Canada, 1600 to 1760: A Legacy for the Future." In *Canadian Nursing: Issues and Perspectives*, edited by J. Kerr and J. MacPhail, 3–10. Toronto, ON: Mosby, 1996.

Kirmayer, L. J., G. M. Brass, and C. L. Tait. "In Review: The Mental Health of Aboriginal Peoples: Transformations of Identify and Community." *Canadian Journal of Psychiatry* 45, no. 7 (2000): 607–16.

Kulchyski, P., D. McCaskill, and D. Newhouse. *In the Words of Elders: Aboriginal Cultures in Transition*. Toronto: University of Toronto Press, 1999.

Lemas, D. J., H. W. Wiener, D. M. O'Brien, S. Hopkins, K. L. Stanhope, P. J. Havel, and B. B. Boyer. "Genetic Polymorphisms in Carnitine Palmitoyltransferrase 1A Gene Are Associated With Variation in Body Composition and Fasting Lipid Traits in Yup-ok Eskimos." *Journal of Lipid Research* 53 (2011): 1–30.

Long, R., H. Njoo, and E. Hershfield. "Tuberculosis: 3. Epidemiology of the Disease in Canada." *Canadian Medical Association Journal* 160, no. 1 (1999): 1185–90.

Lyons, A. S., and R. J. Petrucelli. *Medicine: An Illustrated History.* New York: Harry N. Abrams, Inc., 1978.

MacKinnon, M. A. First Nations Voice in the Present Creates Healing in the Future. *Canadian Journal of Public Health* 96, no. S1 (2005): S13–S16.

MacMillan, H., C. Walsh, and E. Jamieson. *Children's Health.* Ottawa, ON: First Nations and Inuit Regional Health Survey National Steering Committee, 1999.

Mandleco, B., and W. J. Bartfay. "Care of Infants, Children and Adolescents." In *Community Health Nursing: Caring in Action,* 1st Canadian ed., edited by J. E. Hitchcock, P. E. Schubert, S. A. Thomas, and W. J. Bartfay, 325–73. Toronto, ON: Nelson, 2010.

McKenzie, B., and V. Morrisette. "Social Work Practice With Canadians of Aboriginal Background: Guidelines for Respectful Social Work." *Envision: The Manitoba Journal of Child Welfare* 2, no. 1 (2003): 13–19.

McMurray, A. *Community Health and Wellness: A Social-Ecological Approach,* 3rd ed. Toronto: Mosby/Elsevier, 2007.

Migrone, J., J. D. Neil, and C. Wilkie. "*Mental Health Services Review First Nations and Inuit Health Branch Manitoba Region.*" 2003. www.umanitoba.ca/cdentres/centre_aboriginal_health_research/researchreports/mental_health_review_fina_report.pdf.

Miller, J. R. *Shingwauk's Vision: A History of Canadian Residential Schools.* Toronto, ON: University of Toronto Press, 1996.

Milloy, John S. *A National Crime: The Canadian Government and the Residential School System 1879–1986.* Winnipeg, MB: University of Manitoba Press, 1999. ISBN 0-88755-646-9.

Mullin, J., L. Lee, S. Hertwig, and G. Silverthorn "Final Journey: A Native Smudging Ceremony." *Canadian Nurse* 97, no. 2 (2001): 20–22.

Muntaner, C., E. Ng, and H. Chung. *Better Health: An Analysis of Public Policy and Programming Focusing on the Determinants of Health and Health Outcomes That Are Effective in Achieving the Healthiest Populations.* Ottawa, ON: Canadian Health Services Research Foundation and Canadian Nurses Association, 2012.

National Aboriginal Council on HIV/AIDS. *Canadian Strategy on HIV/AIDS.* Ottawa, ON: Health Canada, 2003. http://www.hcsc.gc.ca/hppb/hiv_aids/can_strat/aboriginal/main/htm.

National Expert Commission Canadian Nurses Association. *A Nursing Call to Action. The Health of Our Nation, the Future of Our Health System.* Ottawa, ON: Canadian Nurses Association, 2012. Retrieved July 4, 2013, http://www.cna-aiic.ca/expertcommission/.

Ng., C., S. Chatwood, and T. K. Young. "Arthritis in the Canadian Aboriginal Population: North–South Differences in Prevalence and Correlates." *Chronic Diseases in Canada* 31, no. 1 (2010): 22–26.

Northwest Territories Food Guide. "Government of the Northwest Territories." 2003. http://www.hlthss.gov.nt.ca.

Parkman, F. *The Jesuits in North America in the Seventeenth Century.* Boston: Little, Brown, 1897.

Pearson, J., and B. Trumble, eds. *The Oxford English Reference Dictionary,* 2nd. ed. New York: Oxford University Press, 1996.

Public Health Agency of Canada. *National Notifiable Diseases.* Minister of Public Works and Government Services Canada. Ottawa, ON: Author, 2003. Retrieved May 14, 2010, http://dsol-smed.phac-aspc.gc.ca/dsol-smed/ndis/list_e.html.

———. *Canada's Report on HIV/AIDS 2004. The Federal Initiative to Address HIV/AIDS in Canada.* Ottawa, ON: Author, 2004. Retrieved May 14, 2010, http://www.phac-aspc.gc.ca/aids-sida/hiv_aids/report04/1_e.html.

———. *HIV/AIDS Epi Update, May 2005.* Ottawa, ON: Author, 2005.

———. *Canadian Sexually Transmitted Infections Surveillance Report, 2004: Pre-release.* Ottawa, ON: Author, 2006a. Retrieved May 12, 2010, http://www.phac-aspc.ca/std-mts/stddata_pre06_04/index.html.

———. *Focusing on Populations at Risk.* Ottawa, ON: Author, 2006b. Retrieved May 14, 2010, http://www.phac-aspc.ca/aids-sida/haic-vsac1205/index.html.

———. *Core competencies for public health in Canada: Release 1.1.* Ottawa, ON: Author, 2007. Web-based link: http://www.phac-aspc.gc.ca/core_competencies or http://www.phac-aspc.gc.ca/php-psp/ccph-cesp/pdfs/cc-manual-eng090407.pdf

———. *Arthritis Risk Factors.* Ottawa, ON: Author, 2010a. Retrieved July 7, 2013, http://www.phac-aspc.gc.ca/cd-mc/arthritis-arthrite/risk-risque-eng.php.

———. *HIV/AIDS Epi Updates, July 2010*. Prepared by Surveillance and Risk Assessment Division, Centre for Communicable Diseases and Infection Control. Ottawa, ON: Author, 2010b.

———. *HIV/AIDS: Populations at Risk*. Ottawa, ON: Author, 2010c. Retrieved July 7, 2013, http://www.phac-aspc.gc.ca/aids-sida/populations-eng.php.

———. *Report on Sexually Transmitted Infections in Canada: 2008*. Ottawa, ON: Author, 2010d.

———. *Population-Specific HIV/AIDS Status Report: Aboriginal People*. Ottawa, ON: Author, 2010e, http://www.phac-aspc.gc.ca/aids-sida/publication/ps-pd/aboriginal-autochtones/gfx/f6-eng.gif or http://www.phac-aspc.gc.ca/aids-sida/publication/ps-pd/aboriginal-autochtones/chapter-chapitre-3-eng.php

———. *Summary: Estimates of HIV Prevalence and Incidence 2011*. Ottawa, ON: Author, 2012. Retrieved October 15, 2015, http://www.phac-aspc.gc.ca/aids-sida/publications/survreport/estimat2011-eng.php.

Ralph-Campbell, K., R. T. Oster, T. Connor, M. Pick, S. Pohar, P. Thompson, and L. E. Toth. "Increasing Rates of Diabetes and Cardiovascular Risk in Métis Settlements in Northern Alberta." *International Journal of Circumpolar Health* 68 (2009): 433–42.

Rayburn, A. *Naming Canada: Stories of Canadian Place Names*, 2nd ed. Toronto, ON: University of Toronto Press, 2001.

Reading, J. *The Crisis of Chronic Disease among Aboriginal Peoples: A Challenge for Public Health, Population Health, and Social Policy*. Victoria, BC: Centre for Aboriginal Health Research, University of Victoria, 2010.

Reading, T., N. Jeff, and E. Nowgesic. Improving the Health of Future Generations: The Canadian Institutes of Health, Research Institute of Aboriginal Peoples' Health. *American Journal of Public Health* 92, no. 9 (2002): 1396–01.

Repplier, A. *Mere Marie of the Ursulines*. New York: Sheed & Ward, (1931).

Richardson, S., and T. Williams. "Why Is Cultural Safety Essential in Health?" *Medical Law* 26, no. 4 (2007): 699–07.

Robinson Vollman, A., E. T. Anderson, and J. McFarlane. *Canadian Community as Partner: Theory and Practice*. New York: Lippincott, Williams & Wilkins, 2004.

Rosen, G. *A History of Public Health*. New York: MD Publications, Inc., 1958.

Rosol, R. *Evaluating Food Security in Nunavut: Preliminary Results From the Inuit Health Survey*. Ottawa, ON: Statistics Canada, 2009.

Rosol, R., C. Huet, M. Wood, C. Lennie, G. Osborne, and G. M. Egeland. "Prevalence of Affirmative Responses to Questions of Food Insecurity: International Polar Year Inuit health Survey, 2007–2008." *International Journal of Circumpolar Health* 70, no. 5 (2011): 488–97.

Royal Commission on Aboriginal Peoples. *Report of the Royal Commission on Aboriginal Peoples*. Vol. 2—*Looking Forward, Looking Back*. Ottawa: Ministry of Supply and Services Canada, 1996.

Sagard, Gabriel. *Histoire du Canada et voyages que les frères Mineurs recollects y on faits pour la conversion des infidels depuis l'an 1615*. Vol. 1, p. 22. Nouvelle édition/Paris: Librairie Tross. 1866. Archives of Ontario Library, 971.01 SAG 1 (translation).

Sapers, H., and I. Zinger. *Presentation to the Canadian Human Rights Commission, April 7, 2010*. Ottawa, ON: Office of the Correctional Investigator of Canada, 2010. Retrieved July 7, 2013, http://www.oci-bec.gc.ca/comm/presentations/presentations20100407-eng.aspx#mentalHealth.

Secco, M. L., and M. E. K. Moffatt, "The Home Environment of Métis, First Nations, and Caucasian Adolescent Mothers: An Examination of Quality and Influence." *Canadian Journal of Nursing Research* 25, no. 2 (2004): 106–26.

Schissel, B. "The Pathology of Powerlessness. Adolescent Health in Canada." In *The Selling of Innocence: The Gestalt of Danger in the Lives of Youth Prostitutes*, edited by B. Schissel and K. Fedec. *Canadian Journal of Criminology* 41, no. 1 (2006): 33–56.

Schouls, T. The Basic Dilemma: Sovereignty or Assimilation. In *Nation to Nation: Aboriginal Sovereignty and the Future of Canada*, edited by J. Bird, L. Land, and M. Macadam, 34–42. Toronto: ON: Irwin, 2002.

Secco, M. L., and M. E. K Moffat. "The Home Environment of Métis, First Nations, and Caucasian Adolescent Mothers: An Examination of Quality and Influence." *Canadian Journal of Nursing Research* 35, no. 2 (2004): 106–26.

Shah, C. *Public Health and Preventive Medicine in Canada*, 5th ed. Toronto, ON: Elsevier Canada, 2003.

Ship, S., and L. Norton. HIV/AIDS and Aboriginal Women in Canada. *Canadian Woman Studies* 21, no. 2 (2001): 35–31.

Smith, R. "Learning from Indigenous People." Editorial. *British Medical Journal*, 327, no. 7412 (2003): 1.

Smylie, J. "Society of Obstetrician and Gynaecologists Policy Statement—A Guide for Health Professionals Working With Aboriginal Peoples: The Sociocultural Context of Aboriginal Peoples in Canada." *Journal for Society of Obstetricians and Gynaecologists* 100 (2000): 1070–81.

Stafanson, D., and W. J. Bartfay. "Varied Roles and Practice Specialties in Community Health Nursing." In *Community Health Nursing: Caring in Action*, 1st Canadian ed., 59–97. Toronto, ON: Nelson, 2010.

Statistics Canada. *2001 Census Release 5, January 21, 2003: Ethnocultural Portrait of Canada*. Ottawa: Government of Canada, 2003. http://www.12.statcan.ca/english/census01/release/release5.cfm

———. "Study: Infant Mortality Among First Nations and Non-First Nations People in British Columbia." *The Daily*, November 9, 2004. Ottawa, ON: Author. Retrieved July 23, 2011, http://www.statcan.gc.ca/daily-quoitidien/041109/dq041109c-eng.htm.

———. *Aboriginal Peoples Survey: Adults, 2006*, Public–Use Microdata File. Ottawa, ON: Statistics Canada, 2006a. Special Survey Division, Data Liberation Initiative.

———. *Census 2006*. Ottawa, ON: Government of Canada, 2006b. Retrieved April 29, 2010, http://www.12statcan.ca/english/Census06/data/topics.

———. *Infant Mortality Rates, by Province and Territory*. Ottawa, ON: Author, 2006c (CANSIM, Table 102-0504).

———. *Study: The Health of First Nations Living off-reserve, Inuit and Métis Adults*. Ottawa, ON: Author, 2007. Retrieved July 23, 2011, http://www.statcan.gc.ca/daily-quoitidien/100623/dq10062c-eng.htm.

———. "Aboriginal Peoples in Canada in 2006: Inuit, Métis and First Nations, 2006 Census." *The Daily*, January 15, 2008. Ottawa, ON: Author. Retrieved July 23, 2011, http://www.statcan.gc.ca/daily-quotidien/080115dq080115a-eng.htm.

———. *2006 Census: Aboriginal Peoples in Canada in 2006: Inuit, Métis and First Nations*. Ottawa, ON: Government of Canada, 2009a.

———. *Canadian Social Trends, First Nations People: Selected Findings of the 2006 Census*. Ottawa, ON: Author, 2009b. Retrieved October 15, 2015, http://www.statcan.gc.ca/pub/11-08-x/2009001/article/10864-eng-htm.

———. *Age-Specific Fertility Rate: Number of Live Births and Age-Specific Fertility Rate by Age of Mother and Number of Children Previously Born, 1961 to 1997*, data file. Ottawa, ON: Author, 2010a. Retrieved July 7, 2013, http://jeff-lab.queensu.ca/library/free/health-statistics/00060107.ivt.

———. *Canadian Community Health Survey, 2010: Annual*, Share Data File. Ottawa, ON: Author, 2010b.

———. *Spending Pattern in Canada. Table 4-1 (Canada) and Table 4-14 (Nunavut): Average Expenditure Per Household, Canada, Provinces and Territories, Recent Years*. Ottawa, ON: Government of Canada, 2010c.

———. *CANSIM Table 051-0001 Estimates of Population by Age Group and Sex for July 1, Canada, Provinces and Territories, Annual*, Custom data file. Ottawa, ON: Author, 2011a.

———. *CANSIM Table 102-4505 Crude Birth Rate, Age-specific and Total Fertility Rates (Live Births), Canada, Provinces and Territories, Annual*, data file. Ottawa, ON: Author, 2011b. Retrieved July 7, 2013, http://www5statcan.gc.ca/cansim/a05?lang=eng&id=10245505.

———. "Population Projections by Aboriginal Identity in Canada: 2006 to 2031." *The Daily*, 2011c. Ottawa, ON: Author. Retrieved July 4, 2013, http://www.statcan.gc.ca/daily-quotidien/111207/dq111207a-eng.htm.

———. *Violent Victimization of Aboriginal Women in Canadian Provinces, 2009*. Ottawa, ON: Author, 2011d. Retrieved July 7, 2013, http://www.statcan.gc.ca/pub/85-002x/2011001/article/11439-eng.htm.

———. *Women in Canada: A Gender-Based Statistical Report-First Nations, Métis and Inuit Women*. Ottawa, ON: Author, 2011e. Retrieved July 7, 2013, http://www.statcan.gc.ca/pub/89-503-x-2010001/article/11442-eng.pdf.

———. *2011 National Household Survey: Aboriginal Peoples in Canada: First Nations, Métis, and Inuit. The Daily*. Ottawa, ON: Author, 2013. http://www.statcan.gc.ca/daily-quotidien/130508a-eng.pdf.

———. *Homicide in Canada, 2014*. Ottawa, ON: Author, 2015. Retrieved December 3, 2015, http://www.statcan.gc.ca/daily-quotidien/151125/dq151125a-eng.htm?HPA.

——— Swan, R. *The History of Medicine in Canada. The History of Medicine in the Commonwealth Symposium, September 23, 1966*, 42–51. Faculty of Medicine and Pharmacy, Royal College of Physicians of London. London, UK, 1966.

Tarlier, D. S., J. L. Johnson, and N. B Whyte. Voices from the Wilderness: An Interpretive Study Describing the Role and Practice of Outpost Nurses. *Canadian Journal of Public Health*, 94 (2003): 180–84.

The Council of Canadians. *Report on Notice for Drinking Water Crisis in Canada*. Ottawa, ON: Author, 2015. Retrieved October 15, 2015, http://canadians.org/drinking-water.

The First Nations Information Governance Centre. *RHS Phase 2 (2008/10) Preliminary Results*. Ottawa, ON: Author, 2011.

Thomas, S. A., and W. J. Bartfay. Global Health Perspectives for Community Health Nurses. In *Community Health Nursing: Caring in Action*, 1st Canadian ed., edited by J. E. Hitchcock, P. E. Schubert, S. A. Thomas, and W. J. Bartfay, 143–72. Toronto, ON: Nelson, 2010.

Thompson, V. D. *Health and Health Care Delivery in Canada.* Toronto, ON: Mosby Elsevier, 2010.

Trigger, B. G., and J. F. Pendergast. *Saint-Lawrence Iroguoians. Handbook of North American Indians,* 357–361, Vol. 15— OCLC 58762737. Washington, DC: Smithsonian Institution, 1978.

Truth and Reconciliation Commission of Canada, 2015. *Honouring the Truth, Reconciling for the Future. Summary of the Final Report of the Truth and Reconciliation Commission of Canada.* Library and Archives Canada, Ottawa, Ontario. (ww.trc.ca). ISBN 978-0-660-02078-5. Cat no. IR4-7/2015E-PDF.

Venne, S. "Treaty-Making With the Crown." In *Nation to Nation: Aboriginal Sovereignty and the Future of Canada,* edited by J. Bird, L. Land, and M. Macadam, 45–52. Toronto, ON: Irwin, 2002.

Villeneuve, M., and J. MacDonald. *Toward 2020: Visions for Nursing.* Ottawa, ON: Canadian Nurses Association, 2006. (ISBN 1-55119-818-5).

Waldram, J. B., D. A. Herring, and T. K. Young. *Aboriginal Health in Canada: Historical, Cultural and Epidemiological Perspectives.* Toronto, ON: University of Toronto Press, 1995.

Wang, Y. "Trudeau Launches Investigation Into the Deaths and Disappearances of Canada's Indigenous Women." *The Washington Post,* December 9, 2015. Retrieved December 16, 2015, http://www.msn.com/en-ca/news/canada/ trudeau-launches-investigation-into-the-deaths-and-disappearances-of-canada%e2%80%99s-indigenous-women/ ar-AAgcKCX.

Wasekeesikaw, F. H. "Challenges for the New Millennium: Nursing in First Nations." In *Realities of Canadian Nursing: Professional, Practice and Power Issues,* 2nd ed., edited by M. McIntyre, E. Thomlinson, and C. McDonald, 414–33. New York, NY: Lippincott Williams & Wilkins, 2006.

Wildman, R. P. "Healthy Obesity." *Current Opinion in Clinical Nutrition & Metabolic Care* 12 (2009): 438–43.

Willows, N. D., Morel, J., and Gray-Donald, K. "Prevalence of Anemia Among James Bay Cree Infants of Northern Québec." *Canadian Medical Association Journal* 162, no. 3 (2000): 323–26.

World Health Organization. "Ottawa Charter for Health Promotion." *Canadian Journal of Public Health* 77, no. 12 (1986): 425–30.

———. *Indigenous and Tribal Peoples: Legal Frameworks and Indigenous Rights.* Geneva: WHO, 1999. http://www.who. int/hhr/activities/Indigenous/en/print.html.

———. *Communicable Diseases 2000: Highlights of Activities in 1999 and Major Challenges for the Future.* Geneva: WHO, 2000a. Retrieved May 12, 2010, http://www.who.int/infectious-disease-news/CDS2000/PDF/cd2000.pdf.

———. *Fact sheet. HIV, TB and Malaria. Three Major Infectious Disease Threats. Back 001.* Geneva: WHO, 2000b. Retrieved May 12, 2010, http://www.who.int.inf-fs/en/back001.

———. *Fact sheet. Tuberculosis F-S 104.* Geneva: WHO, 2000c. Retrieved May 12, 2010, http://www.who.int/inf-fsfact104.

———. *International Decade of the World's Indigenous People: Report by the Secretariat. Fifty-Fifth World Health Assembly Item 19.* Geneva: WHO, 2002a. http://www.who.int/hhr/activities/Indigenous/en/print.html.

———. *World Report on Violence and Health.* Geneva: WHO, 2002b. http://www.who.int/hhr/activities/Indigenous/en/ print.html.

———. *Health of Indigenous Peoples. Fact Sheet No. 326.* Geneva: WHO, 2007. Retrieved May 12, 2010, http: www.who. int/mediacentre/factsheets/fs326/en/index.html.

Wright, J. V. "A History of Native People in Canada: Early and Middle Archaic Complexes." Canadian Museum of Civilization Corporation. 2001. http://www/civilization.ca/archeo/hnpc/npvol04e.html.

York, G. *The Disposed. Life and Death in Native Canada.* Toronto, ON: Little Brown and Company, 1992.

Young, T. "Review of Research on Aboriginal Populations in Canada: Relevance to Their Needs." *British Medical Journal* 327 (2003): 419–22.

Young, T., J. Reading, B. Elias, and J. D. O'Neil. Type 2 Diabetes Mellitus in Canada's First Nations: Status of an Epidemic in Progress. *Canadian Medical Association Journal* 163, no. 5 (2000): 127–29.

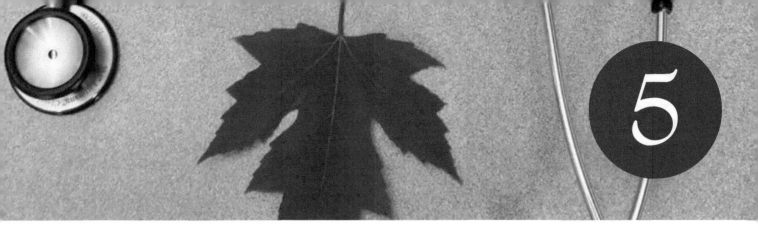

Essential Research Methods for the Practice of Public Health

A scientist is not a person who gives the right answers; he is the one who asks the right question.
—Claude Lévi-Strauss, 1908–2009

Learning Objectives

After completion of this chapter, the student will be able to:
- Describe how research has been employed by health care professionals and workers to advance public health in Canada and globally;
- Define and differentiate between the terms research and evidence-informed public health (EIPH);
- Define and differentiate between the terms basic and applied research;
- List and describe the nine steps of the research process utilized by public health researchers;
- Define and differentiate between qualitative, quantitative and mixed method design (hybrid) research methodologies employed by public health researchers and provide examples of each; and
- List and describe how quantitative, qualitative and mixed-design studies can be utilized by health care scientists to advance public health education, theory and practice in Canada.

Core Competencies addressed in Chapter 5

Core Competencies	Competency Statements
1.0 Public Health Sciences	1.3, 1.4, 1.5
2.0 Assessment and Analysis	2.1, 2.2, 2.3, 2.4, 2.5, 2.6
3.0 Policy and Program Planning, Implementation, and Evaluation	3.1, 3.2, 3.6, 3.7
4.0 Partnerships, Collaboration, and Advocacy	4.1, 4.4
5.0 Diversity and Inclusiveness	5.2
6.0 Communication	6.1, 6.2, 6.4
7.0 Leadership	7.3, 7.4, 7.6

Note: Please see the following document or web-based link for a detailed description of these specific competencies (Public Health Agency of Canada 2007).

Introduction

Research is defined as a systematic and purposeful method of scientific inquiry into the nature of phenomena of interests to public health care professionals and scientists in an attempt to develop new knowledge and practice standards, test existing hypotheses and to develop conceptual models and theories (Bartfay and Bartfay 2015). The ultimate goal of research is the development of a sound body of knowledge to guide and improve the practice of public health in Canada and globally. Public health research includes, but is not limited to, health promotion policies and strategies; socio-economic, political, cultural, and environmental determinants of health; disease, injury, and disability prevention strategies; public and community health issues (e.g., safe water); workplace and occupational health research; methods and practice; health policy formation and evaluation; toxicology and environmental health; identification of health advantages and risk factors related to the interaction of environments including cultural, social, psychological, behavioural, physical, and genetic; basic methodology development (e.g., risk evaluation and surveillance tools, epidemiological, and biostatistical procedures); development, implementation, and evaluation of health technologies and tools; risk factors associated with the development of chronic disease and their modification; ethical issues (e.g., poverty), and public health systems and services research (Alwan 2011; Bowling and Ebrahim 2007; Canadian Institutes of Health Research-Institute of Population and Public Health [CIHR-IPPH] 2013; United States Department of Health and Human Services, Centres for Disease Control and Prevention 2006).

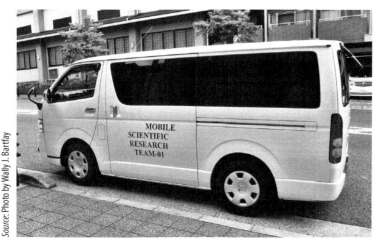

Source: Photo by Wally J. Bartfay

Photo 5.1 A mobile community-based research van in Japan. Research can be conducted in a variety of settings including the laboratory and in various community settings, schools, community centres, and workplaces to name but a few locations.

In addition, public health professionals and workers utilize research from a variety of disciples including the social sciences (e.g., sociology, psychology, anthropology, political science), urban planning and design, engineering, pharmacology, medicine, and nursing to name but a few. As public health care professionals and workers, you will be required to integrate data and research findings into your practice on a daily basis.

Group Activity-based Learning Box 5.1

How is research being used to influence public health services?

This Group Activity-Based Learning Box 5.1 highlights the central importance of employing published peer-reviewed scientific investigations in the public and allied health sciences for planning, implementing and evaluation public health initiatives and programs in your region or community. Working in small groups of three to five students, discuss and answer the following questions:

1. Provide an example of how published peer-reviewed research findings can be utilized to influence current public health care practices and standards of care in your province or territory?

2. How can research be utilized to assess the quality and effectiveness of primary health care services provided in your community?

3. How can published peer-reviewed research findings be employed to better facilitate culturally sensitive evidence-informed primary health care interventions in your community?

You will be required to critical appraise research reports, identify and implement safe and effective primary health care interventions for public health practice, and evaluate the impact and cost-effectiveness of primary health care services rendered across the lifespan. All public health care professionals and workers are accountable to society for providing safe, high-quality and cost-effective health care services, and the care provided must be constantly evaluated and improved upon via research. In the years ahead, you are likely to engage in individual, group and/or institutional efforts to utilized research as a basis for making clinical decisions and for planning primary health care interventions.

Research is also needed to generate knowledge about public health education, administration and the cost-effectiveness of health care services provided and health care delivery systems (Bowling and Ebrahim 2007; Polgar and Thomas 2008). You will be encouraged to ask questions such as: "Why is this primary health care intervention currently being used in our community?" "Would another intervention be more effective to promote the health of our residents in the community?" "Has any previous research been conducted on this topic or area?" "Do the findings from the investigations conducted provide sound evidence for use in public health practice?" "How can I use the evidence published in the scientific literature to improve my practice as a public health care professional or worker?"

This chapter provides an introduction to basic research methodologies employed by public health researchers in Canada and abroad. Although a discussion of all qualitative, quantitative and mixed-method design research and approaches is beyond the scope and purpose of this chapter, a survey of the most common ones employed will be highlighted.

The primary aim of public health is to empower residents and citizens to make informed decisions and partake in interventions that seek to preserve, promote and/or restore their health, and these interventions are often based on the best available evidence in the empirical literature (Public Health Agency of Canada (PHAC) 2007). Researchers seek to discover, investigate, understand, explain, and predict phenomena of relevance and interest to public health. Public health care professionals and workers may participate in the research process at multiple levels including the identification of problem areas; collecting, analyzing and interpreting data; applying findings to practice; and evaluating, designing and conducting research (Bartfay 2010a). At a minimum, all public health professionals and workers are expected to read current research investigations and apply the findings to practice as an ongoing component of their public health practice and services they provide (PHAC 2007).

Basic and Applied Research

A distinction between basic and applied research is often made in the empirical literature to distinguish between the nature of the investigations undertaken. **Basic (pure) research** is defined as activities undertaken to extend the knowledge base in public health or to formulate or refine an existing conceptual model or theory (Bartfay and Bartfay 2015). Basic investigations are conducted for the "pursuit of knowledge for knowledge's sake" or for the pleasure of learning and finding truth in nature (Burns and Grove 2007; Bryman, Bell, and Teevan 2012; Miller 1991; Polit and Tatano Beck 2012; Wysocki 1983). The purpose of basic research is to solve problems, make decisions related to health care delivery or services, and to predict or control outcomes in practice situations. For example, Cadena (2006) investigated the needs and functioning of individuals diagnosed with schizophrenia who were living in an assisted living facility in the community in relation to the residents' characteristics. Although the findings from this study had implications for public health practice, the research itself was not conducted to solve a particular problem per se.

Applied (practical) research is defined as public health investigations that focus on finding solutions to existing problems and to generate knowledge that will directly influence practice (Bartfay and Bartfay 2015). Findings from applied investigations can be employed by policymakers for making changes that address current or predicted health problems or concerns; to test existing conceptual models or theories and to validate their usefulness in practice (Burns and Grove 2007; Miller 1991; Polit and Tatano Beck 2012; Wysocki 1983). Hence, applied research tends to be of greater utility for evidence-informed public health (EIPH) by public health care professionals and workers. For example, Shaughnessy, Resnick, and Macko (2006) conducted a study to test a conceptual model to explain physical activity among older adults who had survived a stroke. The validity of the conceptual model to explain exercise behaviour was based on relevant concepts such as self-efficacy and outcome expectations by the stroke survivors.

Evidence-Informed Public Health and Research

Public health is a holistic and evidence-informed discipline that seeks to promote; maintain and/or restore the health and quality of life of individuals, families, communities and/or entire populations over the lifespan through health promotion and prevention and various primary health care initiatives, activities, policies and/or legislations (Bartfay and Bartfay 2015). **EIPH** is defined as a process for "distilling and disseminating the best available evidence from research, practice and experience and using that evidence to inform and improve public health policy and practice" (National Collaborating Centres for Public Health [NCCPH] 2011, 1). During the past decade, there has been a growing consensus for the need to employ *evidence* to direct practice and policy directives in public health (e.g., Bowen and Zwi 2005; Oxman, Lavis, and Fretheim 2007; Pach 2008; Rycroft-Malone 2008). The adoption of EIPH involves the utilization of the best available evidence for providing safe and effective primary health care interventions and services, which is often derived through research investigations (Gerrish and Clayton 2004; Melnyk and Fineout-Overholt 2005; Thurston and King 2004; Thomas et al. 2000).

For example, in 2005 the Registered Nurses Association of Ontario (RNAO) released a best practice guideline document entitled *Women Abuse: Screening, identification and initial response* for registered nurses in Ontario (see http://www.rnao.org/bestpractices or http://rnao.ca/bpg/guidelines/woman-abuse-screening-identification-and-initial-response). This document was developed by an interdisciplinary panel and the guidelines seek to facilitate the routine and universal screening for the abuse of women by nurses in all clinical practice settings. Moreover, this document provides a large selection of evidence-informed strategies along with information about the strength of the evidence in the scientific literature supporting each of these noted strategies. Refer Chapter 1 for a detailed description of EIPH and the types of evidence employed by public health professionals and workers. Add to your knowledge of EIPH by accessing the Web-Based Resource Box 5.1.

There is currently no consensus in the literature about what constitutes usable research-derived evidence for EIPH by health care professionals (DiCenso, Guyatt, and Ciliska 2005; Goode 2000; Guyatt and Rennie 2002; Sackett et al. 2000). Nonetheless, there is a general agreement that findings should be based on clearly described and rigorous investigations. Figure 5.1 provides a typical strength-ranking hierarchy for published investigations or reports (Bartfay and Bartfay 2015). Level I investigations typically consists of systematic reviews of randomized clinical trials (RCTs) or non-randomized trails. The strongest evidence according to this hierarchy comes from systematic reviews that compare and integrate consistent findings from multiple trails that employ rigorous and methodological procedures. Level II studies, in general, consist of a single RCT

Web-Based Resource Box 5.1   Evidence-Informed Public Health

Learning Resources	Website
Canadian Best Practices Portal (PHAC) Created and managed by the PHAC, this portal contains a searchable database of community-based interventions that have been evaluated and shown to be effective. This portal also provides public health care professionals and workers with several helpful links and evidence-informed resources.	http://cbpp-pcpe.phac-aspc.gc.ca/ or http://cbpp- pcpe.phac-aspc.gc.ca/interventions/
National Collaborating Centres for Public Health (November 2011). What is EIPH? This website provides a definition of EIPH, describes why it should be implemented for public health practice and policy making, and outlines a seven-step-model of EIPH.	http://www.nccmt.ca/eiph/
Middlesex-London Health Unit (2013). EIPH. This resource describes the types of evidence to be considered for public health practice and policy making and lists various helpful resources and databases	https:www.healthunit.com/evidence-informed-public-health
TRIP Database TRIP is a clinical search engine designed to allow users to quickly and easily find and use high-quality research evidence to support their practice and/or care, which has been online since 1997.	http://www.tripdatabase.com/
World Health Organization (WHO)/Europe Database Portal This portal provides the user with access to various health statistics and to detailed monitoring and assessment tools for key areas of health policy. These links also provide access to a broad range of information systems: from international comparisons of aggregate indicators to the results of detailed disease surveillance and the monitoring of specialized areas of health policy.	http://www.euro.who.int/en/data-and-evidence/databases

or a non-randomized trial. Level III hierarchical studies usually consist of a systematic review of observational and/or correlational investigations. Level IV investigations consist of a single observational or correlational study. Level V hierarchical studies typically consist of a systematic review of some laboratory-based physiological study, a descriptive study or a qualitative investigation. Level VI studies are usually comprised of a single laboratory-based physiological study, a descriptive study or a qualitative investigation. Lastly, level VII studies consist of opinions by single individuals in their noted field of expertise and/or expert panels or committees.

Over the past three decades, the widely accepted view that the health practitioner and/or researcher could act as the sole rationale agent who is capable of effectively identifying, retrieving, appraising and translating published research data for the purposes of designing new investigations or translating it into practice has served as the core of evidence-informed practice in the allied health sciences (e.g., Atkins et al. 2004, 2013; DiCenso, Ciliska, and Guyatt 2005; Sackett et al. 1996). Obviously, the ability of a public health professional or worker to identify, retrieve, appraise and apply published peer-reviewed publications for practice or research applications depends on a multitude of factors including their level of education and training related to research methods,

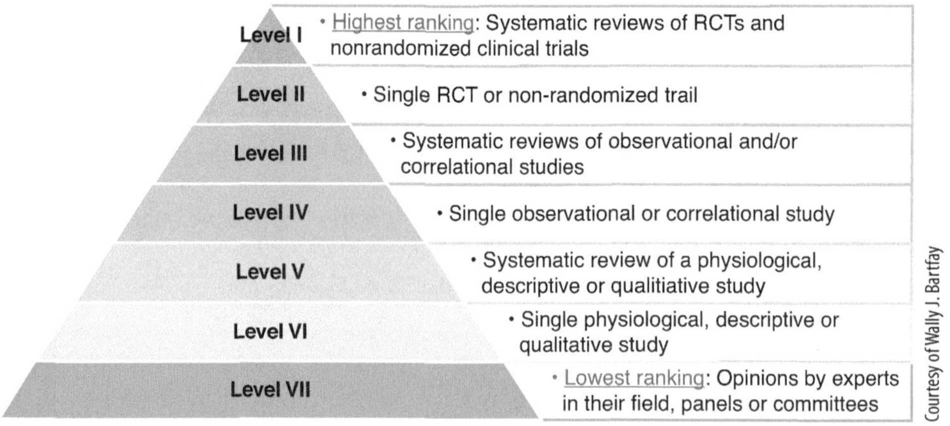

Level I	• Highest ranking: Systematic reviews of RCTs and nonrandomized clinical trials
Level II	• Single RCT or non-randomized trail
Level III	• Systematic reviews of observational and/or correlational studies
Level IV	• Single observational or correlational study
Level V	• Systematic review of a physiological, descriptive or qualitiative study
Level VI	• Single physiological, descriptive or qualitative study
Level VII	• Lowest ranking: Opinions by experts in their field, panels or committees

Courtesy of Wally J. Bartfay

Figure 5.1 Conventional evidence-based medicine (EBM) and evidence-based practice (EBP) strength-ranking hierarchy employed for published research articles

experience and personal comfort levels to name but a few variables. An additional major criticism and limitation of EBM and EBP is that they often assume that RCTs, meta-analyses and systematic reviews provide the highest level of credible and reliable evidence (Figure 5.1) (Bartfay and Bartfay 2015). Conversely, descriptive studies, observational studies, case reports, expert opinions and especially those that employ qualitative methodologies or approaches are the weakest and least credible and reliable sources of evidence (Ciliska, Thomas, and Buffet 2008; Cullins et al. 2005; Oxman, Lavis, and Fretheim 2007; Sawatzky-Dickson 2010).

During the past decade, however, there is a growing consensus that we have to collectively consider and appraise published evidence within the unique context it is to be appraised and employed by both researchers and stakeholders or the intended target population (Bowen and Zwi 2005; Rycroft-Malone 2008; Pach 2008). Furthermore, we also argue that for evidence to be adequate and meaningful in the public health context then it must also be suitable as a basis for theory, since public health research, practice and policies ought to be directed and guided by social and scientific theories (Bartfay and Bartfay 2015). Hence, unlike the traditional EBM and EBP approaches, EIPH involves a collaborative effort where public health professionals, workers and affected stakeholders partake in a transparent process of determining what sorts of evidence are required; and how it should be collected, appraised, synthesized, applied and formally evaluated based on their unique aims, needs, context, settings and environments (Bowen and Zwi 2005; Ciliska, Thomas, and Buffett 2008; McCormack et al. 2013; Pach 2008). Refer Chapter 1 for a further discussion on the use and rationale for EIPH in the new millennium.

Systematic Reviews

A **systematic review** is a narrowly focused synthesis of research investigations on a select topic, field of inquiry, practice intervention and/or related research problem (Bartfay and Bartfay 2015). Systematic reviews are often considered the cornerstone of evidence-informed practice (Craig and Smyth 2002; Forrest and Miller 2004; Jennings 2000; Neutens and Rubinson 2002; Sackett et al. 2000; Stevens 2001). Systematic reviews are scholarly reviews of the research literature that follow a rigorous and detailed format for analysis and are held to high standards of clarity, precision, accuracy and replication standards as primary research investigations. In addition, they provide state-of-the-art summaries of what the best published evidence is at the time of the review for a given time period (e.g., past 5-10 years). For example, Rombough, Howse, and Bartfay (2006) conducted a systematic review of the literature related to the concepts of caregiver strain and caregiver burden of primary caregivers looking after a stroke survivor with and without aphasia at home in their community. Comprehensive reviews of three electronic databases were undertaken by the authors: (a) Cumulative Index to Nursing and Health Literature (CINAHL 1982–2004), (b) Medical Literature Online (MEDLINE 1966–2004), and (c) Psychological Information (PsycINFO-1967 to 2004). Fourteen articles met the inclusion

Web-Based Resource Box 5.2   Systematic Reviews

Learning Resources	Website
Agency for Health Care Research and Quality This website provides reviews of research from a multidisciplinary perspective.	**http://www.ahrq.gov**
Cochrane Database of Systematic Reviews (CDSR) This database employs a standardized template and format for conducting systematic reviews on various health related areas of research and specialized fields of practice.	http://www.vichealth.vic.gov.au/cochrane
Database of Abstracts of Reviews of Effects (DARE) A user-friendly website that provides individuals with reviews on the effects of various peer-reviewed publications.	http://www.york.ac.uk/inst/crd/index.htm
Ontario Ministry of Health and Long-term Care-effective Public Health Practice Project (EPHPP) This website provides public health care professionals and workers with access to various websites and reviews related to public health practice in Canada and internationally.	http://www.hamilton.ca/phcs/ephpp

criteria for this systematic review. The reviewer's concluded that there was a lack of research in this noted area and that several key initiatives were required, including the development of an instrument with psychometric properties for assessing burden and strain for caregivers of stroke survivors in the community.

Fortunately, systematic reviews on a wide variety of topics relevant to public health and the health sciences in general are increasingly becoming available both in published forms and on the Internet. For example, the *Cochrane Data of Systematic Reviews* (CDSR) provides thousands of systematic reviews related to various health care interventions by health care professionals (Jabad et al. 1998). In Canada, the Ontario Ministry of Health and Long-term Care (MOLTC) has sponsored the *Effective Public Health Practice Project (EPHPP)* that provides systematic reviews on a wide range of health topics of relevance to the practice of public health in Canada. Refer Web-Based Resource Box 5.2 for these noted websites and additional agencies that provide systematic reviews on a variety of topics and practice interventions in the health sciences.

Meta-analysis

The translation of published research into public health practice remains an ongoing challenge in Canada and globally. **Meta-analysis** is a statistical technique for integrating and pooling completed and published numerical (quantitative) research findings on a select topic or area of inquiry, and treats the findings as a single summary piece of information (Bartfay and Bartfay 2015). In brief, the findings from a variety of quantitative research investigations on a single topic are combined and statistically analyzed. Here the person performing the meta-analysis assumes that the individual studies are the unit of analysis, in contrast to individual subjects in the original published studies.

This statistical method provides health care professionals and workers with an objective and convenient method for interpreting a large body of research into a single coherent outcome finding and/or pattern that might have otherwise gone undetected (Conn and Rantz 2003; Stetler et al. 1998; Whittemore 2005). The statistical approach allows for the application of various criteria including sample size considerations, the level of statistical significance obtained and the noted variable examined. Hence, meta-analysis permits health care professionals and workers to make objective, as opposed to subjective, interpretations of the best available evidence used to influence public health practice. For example, Snethen, Broome, and Cashin (2006) performed a meta-analysis to determine the effectiveness of seven completed intervention-based studies that targeted overweight children. The pooled resulted from these investigations suggest that these interventions have positive health effects on children in terms of influencing weight loss in this target population.

Meta-summaries and Meta-syntheses

Qualitative research investigations conducted by health care professionals and scientists generate important evidence and conceptual models and theories related to a variety of public health issues or concerns. Although these studies provide important insights and understandings of public health and practice situations, it is often difficult to generalize from the samples of the general population, which is an important criterion when developing EIPH guidelines and policies (Barbour 2000; Burns and Grove 2007). To address this limitation, meta-summaries and meta-syntheses of qualitative research are being conducted to provide a stronger rationale and basis for the generalizations of these findings for practice. **Meta-summaries** are interpretative summaries of primary qualitative research investigations that provide a synthesis of these studies to produce a narrative about selected phenomenon or a specific topic (Bartfay and Bartfay 2015). These interpretative summaries provide valuable knowledge for understanding various components and aspects related to practice by public health care professionals and workers (Beck 1999; Dixon-Woods, Fitzpatrick, and Roberts 2001; Sandelowski and Barroso 2003, 2006; Whittemore 2005).

Well-designed and well-conducted qualitative investigations in the health sciences provide important information for clinical practice, health-related concepts, and for the development of policies, conceptual models and theories related to public health care and practice (Beck 2002; Dixon-Woods, Fitzpatrick, and Roberts 2001; Sandelowski and Barroso 2003, 2006; Streubert Speziale and Rinaldi Carpenter 2007). A **meta-synthesis** is a scholarly synthesis of primary qualitative research studies and is conducted to provide a critical analysis and synthesis of the collective findings into a new conceptual model, framework or theory on a select topic or problem of interest. For example, Goodman (2005) performed a meta-synthesis of qualitative studies that examined the lived experiences of fathers during the early months following the birth of their child. Seven qualitative studies were critically examined, and a total of 134 fathers were represented. Based on a meta-synthesis of these seven primary qualitative investigations, Goodman (2005) identified the following four major phases of becoming a new father: (a) Entering with expectations and intentions, (b) confronting reality, (c) working to develop a role as an involved parent, and (d) reaping the benefits of fatherhood.

The Research Process in Public Health

Research in the public health sciences is needed in order to reduce the uncertainty associated with diagnosis, expected treatment outcomes and delivery of health care services to individuals across the lifespan (Bartfay and Bartfay 2015). There is a wide variety of research currently being conducted in the health sciences that range from strictly controlled laboratory investigations conducted on the molecular level to observations on complex health-related behaviour and concepts at the group or population level, or at the systems level for evaluating public health care delivery and services provides. However, all forms of research in the health sciences follow a standardize method or approach known as the "research process."

The **research process** is defined as a series of nine steps and techniques used to structure a study and to gather, analyze, interpret, disseminate and apply data and information in a systematic and formularized fashion (Bartfay and Bartfay 2015). Figure 5.2 provides a schematic summary of the fundamental steps of research process employed by health care researchers in Canada and globally. Each of the nine steps of the research process is logically linked to each other, as well as to the conceptual or theoretical foundations of the investigation (Burns and Grove 2007; Bryman, Bell, and Teevan 2012; Polit and Tatano Beck 2008). We will explore each step of the research process in greater detail below.

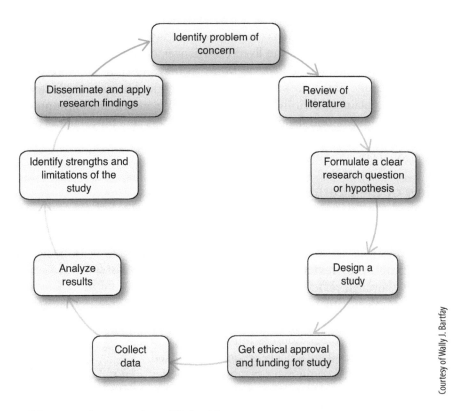

Courtesy of Wally J. Bartfay

Figure 5.2 Major steps of the research process in public health

Step I: Identification of a Problem (Conceptualization Phase)

The purpose of research is to ultimately solve or minimize the impact of a public health concern, issue or problem, and to contribute to its solution through the accumulation of relevant empirical information (Bowling and Ebrahim 2007; Loiselle and Profetto-McGrath 2004; Neutens and Rubinson 2002; Polgar and Thomas 2008). Hence, the first step of the research process involves the identification of an actual or potential public health concern, issue or problem. This step is also referred to as the "conceptualization phase," and personal interest or curiosity often serves as the impetus for this step. The **research problem** is a clear articulation of an actual or potential health concern, issue or problem to be investigated (Bartfay and Bartfay 2015). The research problem is often reflected in the title of the investigation and in the first line of the study abstract.

Depending on the specific research problem to be investigated, the researcher may choose to conduct a qualitative, quantitative or mixed-methods design study (detailed below). **Quantitative research** is defined as a formal, precise, systematic and objective process in which numerical data are used to obtain information on a variety of health-related phenomenon of interest or concern (Bartfay and Bartfay 2015). Quantitative investigations typically involve the study of concepts that are well-defined and well-developed. Moreover, there are usually reliable measurement techniques (e.g., scales, questionnaires, laboratory blood tests, clinical diagnostic measures or tests) that have been developed to measure and quantify the concept of interest to the researcher. For example, Olney (2005) utilized a quasi-experimental study to assess the effects of back massage taught by public health nurses to family members of hypertensive patients and its effects on blood pressure readings (a quantitative measure). Olney (2005) reported that ten minutes of back massage daily significantly decreased both systolic and diastolic blood pressure readings in these hypertensive subjects.

By contrast, qualitative investigators usually focus on a problem or concept that is poorly defined or there is little known about it (e.g., home care needs of elderly widows). **Qualitative research** is defined as a holistic and subjective process used to describe and to promote a better understanding of human experiences and phenomena via the collection of narrative data, and to develop conceptual models and theories that seek to describe these experiences and phenomena (Bartfay and Bartfay 2015). For example, Porter (2005) conducted a phenomenological study to evaluate the lived experiences of home care for elderly widows living alone in their communities. This qualitative investigation provides public health care professionals and workers with important insights into homecare services for the elderly and helps to facilitate an understanding of the growing problem of maintaining their independence in their homes and communities. Porter (2005) reports that home care must be understood as more than what providers actually do in the homes of service recipient clients. For example, an elderly woman who lives alone should be viewed as one who experiences home care and intends to negotiate reliance upon her standby helpers.

Step II: Review of the Literature

The second step of the research process is determining what, if anything, is already known about your research problem. Here the researcher assesses what is already known about the health concern, issue or problem by reviewing the best available scientific literature. A thorough review of the empirical literature also provides the researcher with a foundation on which to base new evidence and formulate new research questions and/or hypotheses. Print-based literature resources must be searched by the investigator manually and are quickly becoming outdated and replaced by Internet-based commercial vendors (e.g., Aries Knowledge Finder, Ovid, EbscoHost, ProQuest) that provide access to a variety of electronic databases in the health and social sciences. However, print remains an important source of information in many developing regions and countries where access to the Internet or even a steady supply of electricity remains a major challenge.

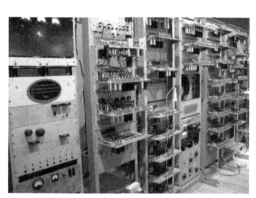

Source: Wally J. Bartfay

Photo 5.2 Freddie Williams and Tom Kilburn built the first computer nicknamed "Baby" in 1974 that could run a stored program at the University of Manchester, England (shown above). Today, a variety of Internet-based electronic databases that store millions of health-related abstracts and links to peer-reviewed journals are available to researchers globally.

In most cases, universities, hospitals and/or public libraries in Canada already subscribe to one of these commercial vendors, which offer user-friendly menu-driven programs with on-screen support so that retrieval of peer-reviewed articles can easily be achieved even by novice researchers or students.

For example, the *Cumulative Index to Nursing and Health Literature* (aka, CINAHL) database includes peer-reviewed published articles from 1982 to present; contains over one million records, and can be accessed online or by CD-ROM either directly (http://www.cinahl.com) or through a commercial vendor. The CINAHL database provides students, practitioners and researchers in the health sciences with bibliographic information for locating peer-reviewed articles including the author(s) name(s), title of the article, name of the journal, year of publication with volume and page numbers provided, and an actual published abstract of the article when available for over 300 journals. Supplementary information, such as the specific names of database instruments or scales employed (e.g., McGill Pain Scale, Becks Depression Inventory, Denver Developmental Scale, SF-36 Health Related Quality of Life Scale) is also available for several of the records in the database. Peer-reviewed articles of interest can typically be ordered electronically through an Internet provider. Table 5.1 provides a list of some of the available electronic databases in the public and health sciences.

Similarly, the *Medical Literature On-Line* (aka, MEDLINE) database was developed by the US National Library of Medicine (NLM) and is considered one of the foremost sources for bibliographic literature in the public and allied health sciences. This electronic database now dates back to 1966 to present and includes over 5,000 health-related journals published in approximately seventy countries, and contains over fifteen million records. Abstracts of systematic reviews from the Cochrane Collaboration also became available through MEDLINE in 1999.

Table 5.1 Electronic Databases in the Public and Allied Health Sciences

Name of Electronic Database	Abbreviation Utilized for Search
AIDS Information On-Line	AIDSLINE
Alcohol and Alcohol Problems Sciences Database	ETOH
Cancer Literature	CancerLit
Combined Health Information Database	CHID
Cumulative Index to Nursing and Health Literature	CINAHL
Education Resources Information Center database	ERIC
Excerpta Medica Database	EMBASE
Health and Psychosocial Instruments Database	HAPI
Health Services, Technology, Administration, and Research	HealthSTAR
Medical Literature On-Line	MEDLINE
Psychology Information	PsychINFO

The *Institute for Scientific Information* (ISI) also maintains an interdisciplinary resource known as the "Web of Knowledge," which provides access to a host of bibliographic databases in a variety of disciplines and fields including medicine, nursing and the social, pure and applied sciences. Individuals can conduct a general search by author or their topic of interest from 1992 to present. Available databases for screening in the Web of Knowledge resource include the *Current Contents Connect, Science Citation Index*, and the *Social Sciences Citation Index*.

In addition, many of the noted database search programs have an enormously helpful feature that allows individuals to find references to other similar studies. For example, after the researcher locates a study of relevance and interest in PubMed, they can click on the "Related Articles" icon on the right-hand side of the screen to search for similar peer-reviewed articles. Similarly, if the researcher is accessing the CINAHL database via OVID, they can click on the "Find Similar" icon.

There is some debate among qualitative researchers about the value of doing a literature review upfront prior to collecting and analyzing the data since certain researchers argue that prior knowledge of studies may influence their conceptualization of the phenomena under investigation (Creswell 2003; Polit and Tatano Beck 2012; Streubert Speziale and Rinaldi Carpenter 2007). Nonetheless, we argue that this is often not desirable and/or feasible since public health care professionals and workers are often expected to read scientific journals and attend research symposiums and conferences as part of their professional or job mandates. Furthermore, as part of the research culture and norms in Canada and globally, research ethics boards (REBs) and granting agencies will be hesitant to approve or fund a research proposal without a properly conducted review of the available published scientific literature. This also provides important context for the proposed study. Lastly, we argue that it is imperative to conduct a literature review for a proper analysis and comparison of the new data that are to be generated. Indeed, researchers are required to determine and describe what is new about their findings; how do these findings compare and contrast with other published findings, and how do the new findings advance public health practice and/or our understanding of the problem investigated?

Step III: Formulate Research Questions or Hypotheses

Advances in public health depend on the identification of researchable questions and/or hypotheses by health care practitioners and researchers. A **research question** is a clear statement of scientific inquiry that the investigator wants to answer through a specific study (Bartfay and Bartfay 2015). The formulation of a research question is a creative process that draws upon consideration of previous relevant work in the area or field of inquiry, clinical practice, emerging public health issues or concerns (e.g., obesity and immobility trends in Canada, aging population), socioeconomic issues (e.g., 2009 global economic recession resulting in increased unemployment and increased reliance on food banks by Canadians) and/or theory development (Burns and Grove 2007; Neutens and Rubinson 2002; Polgar and Thomas 2008; Polit and Tatnao Beck 2012; Streubert Speziale and Rinaldi Carpenter 2007). Moreover, inconsistencies or noted discrepancies in published research findings sometimes generate ideas for new research questions. A researcher may wonder, for example, whether a study conducted on a different age cohort (e.g., elderly Canadians vs. young adults) or target population (e.g., urban vs. rural Indigenous adolescents) would yield different findings.

Research questions need to be relevant to current or emerging public health problems and issues, and phrased in ways that direct the evidence searched to be relevant, applicable and precise in nature and context. One approach that may help researchers formulate quantitative research questions is the "PICOT" method, which is an acronym for *Population, Intervention, Comparison, Outcome and Timeframe* (Bassil and Zabkiewicz 2014; Haynes et al. 2006; Thabane et al. 2009). For example, a researcher may be interested in determining if menopausal women aged fifty-five to sixty-five (i.e., population) who receive a prescribed Mediterranean diet and mall-walking exercise programme (i.e., intervention), fare better, worse or the same in comparison to similar women who do not eat a prescribed Mediterranean diet or engage in a mall-walking exercise programme (i.e., comparison group); in regards to weight and abdominal circumference loss (i.e., outcome), over a twelve-week trail (i.e., timeframe).

However, it is important to note that not all research is interventional or quantitative in nature. Accordingly, Mantzoukas (2008) suggests employing the elements of *content*, *coherence*, and *structure*, when formulating research questions. For example, in terms of content a qualitative researcher may be interested in examining the "impact of having a diagnosis of terminal cancer relied to a young mother on her family." The coherence element often incorporates the methodology that will be employed by the qualitative researcher (e.g., ethnographic or phenomenological inquiry). The structure element of the research question incorporates who, what, where, when, why and/or how factors.

Research questions may be employed by both qualitative and quantitative researchers. For example, Draucker (2005) conducted a qualitative grounded theory study to explore the use of mental health services by adolescents who were diagnosed with depression and their families. The following three research questions were formulated by the investigator: (a) How do depressed adolescents and their families decide whether to use mental health services? (b) What are common processes of mental health service use by adolescent with depression and their families? and (c) Do service use processes differ for African American and Caucasian adolescents who are depressed and their families (Draucker 2005, 156)?

In qualitative studies, it is important to note that research questions often evolve over the course of the study. This is appropriate with qualitative investigations since boundaries are typically not cast in stone and can be altered and, in the typical naturalistic inquiry, will be (Lincoln and Guba 1985, 228). With qualitative studies and approaches, the research typically begins with a research question or set of questions that provides a general starting point for inquiry and discovery. The research questions are therefore regarded as being more fluid or flexible in nature, and often evolve or are modified through discovery of new information (Burns and Grove 2007; Bryman, Bell, and Teevan 2012; Neutens and Rubinson 2002; Polgar and Thomas 2008; Polit and Tatnao Beck 2012; Streubert Speziale and Rinaldi Carpenter 2007). We will explore qualitative research investigations in greater detail below.

An example of research questions posed by quantitative researchers is provided by Bottorff et al. (2005) who explored couple dynamics and interactions related to tobacco use before pregnancy. The investigators formulated the following two research questions: (a) What are the couple's routines that accommodate tobacco use by one or both individuals in intimate relationships and (b) How do couple interpersonal dynamics influence tobacco use- and how are these dynamics are influenced by tobacco use (Bottorff et al. 2005)?

A **hypothesis** is defined as a prediction statement made by the researcher regarding the expected relationships between two or more variables (Bartfay and Bartfay 2015). A variable is a defined attribute of a person or object that varies and/or takes on different values (e.g., age, heart rate, income). A hypothesis basically translates a quantitative research question into a precise prediction of expected outcomes that can be tested and verified mathematically. A research hypothesis, therefore, states the expected relationship between an independent variable X (presumed cause or antecedent variable) and the dependent variable Y (presumed effect or outcome variable) (Burns and Grove 2007; Neutens and Rubinson 2002; Polgar and Thomas 2008; Polit and Tatnao Beck 2012). Hypotheses are formally tested through a variety of statistical tests and procedures (e.g., T-tests, ANOVA, Chi-square) where the researcher seeks to determine the probability of having a correct hypothesis. Nonetheless, hypotheses are never proven per se through these statistical tests and procedures; rather, they are either accepted (supported) or rejected (not supported) based on specific mathematical perimeters.

An example of a simple hypothesis is provided by McFarlane et al. (2005) who predicted that children whose mothers partake in a nurse case management intervention for women exposed to intimate partner violence (X) will have fewer behavioural problems (Y) than children whose mothers receive routine screening and information only.

An example of a complex hypothesis with multiple independent variables is provided by Clingerman, Stuifbergen, and Becker (2004) who predicted that among women with multiple sclerosis, functional limitations (Y) are influenced by the women's external resources, such as their education (X_1), marital status (X_2), social support (X_3), employment status (X_4) and perceived economic adequacy (X_5).

An example of a hypothesis with multiple dependent variables is provided by a laboratory-based randomized experiment by Bartfay and Bartfay (2000) who predicted that chronically iron-loaded mice versus those in the placebo group (independent variables) would have dose-dependent increases in total heart iron concentrations, decreased antioxidant reserves as quantified by glutathione peroxidase activity, increases in oxygen free radical production in the heart as quantified by cytotoxic aldehydes, and decreases in cardiac function (dependent variables).

Given that qualitative researchers are not interested in determining cause-and-effect relationships or making predictions that can be mathematically validated per se, hypotheses are not utilized in qualitative research designs or approaches. Indeed, qualitative researchers are concerned with developing an understanding of the personal meanings, experiences and interpretations of individuals. Hence, words and thematic concepts serve as the core of data sets for qualitative studies; whereas numbers and statistics serve as the core of data sets for quantitative studies. We will explore the differences between qualitative and quantitative investigations in greater detail below.

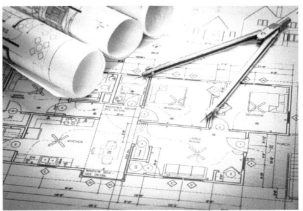

Source: Gargantiopa/Shutterstock.com

Photo 5.3 A research design is a detailed plan of action or "blueprint," which describes the various research methods and strategies that will be utilized by the researcher to answer specific research questions or hypotheses.

Step IV: Design a Study

A **research design** is a detailed plan or blueprint for the research methods and strategies that will be employed by the researcher in order to answer the research question or hypothesis (Bartfay and Bartfay 2015). The research design includes detailed information on how the study will be conducted and by whom; how subjects will be recruited; ethical considerations (e.g., informed consent); how the data will be collected (e.g., surveys, questionnaires, in-depth interviews, fasting blood samples) and stored (e.g., coded data in a locked metal safe); use of any instruments (e.g., scales, diagnostic tests); how the data will be analyzed (e.g., thematic analysis for qualitative study, descriptive and inferential statistics for quantitative data), and how the findings will be disseminated (e.g., publications, conference proceedings, mass and social medias) (Burns and Grove 2007; Neutens and Rubinson 2002; Polgar and Thomas 2008; Polit and Tatnao Beck 2012).

The research methods and study designs undertaken by health care scientists are diverse. Although a discussion of all the research designs and approaches that may be employed by health researchers is beyond the scope and purpose of this chapter, an overview of the most common published quantitative and qualitative approaches will be highlighted. Table 5.2 provides a comparison of qualitative and quantitative research methodologies and approaches.

Qualitative research methods

Qualitative research is grounded in the social sciences tradition and is interested in answering questions related to the study of human phenomena and experiences. Qualitative researchers embrace the idea of subjectively and holism in their quest to understand and describe human phenomena and experiences under study, and are committed to discovery through the use of multiple ways of knowing (Burns and Grove 2007;

Table 5.2 Comparison Between Qualitative and Quantitative Research Methodologies

Qualitative	Quantitative
Subjective in nature	Objective in nature (measureable, tangible)
The researcher is the instrument and builds close personal relationships with the subjects for data collection	The researcher is typically at arms-length, separate or detached from subjects during data collection
Multiple realities (fluid in nature)	One reality (fixed in nature)
Organismic	Mechanistic (machine model of the human body)
Whole is greater than the parts	Parts equal the whole
Seeks understanding, discovery, and descriptions	Seeks control, reduction, replication, and prediction
Data consists of words and phrases (narrative descriptions)	Data consists of numbers/statistics
Context dependent data	Context free data
Seeks to determine understanding of associations or links between concepts/variables being investigated	Seeks to determine relationships (e.g., cause-and-effect, functional) between concepts or variables (independent, dependent) being investigated
Sample size is typically small and non-random in nature, and no control groups are employed for making comparisons	Seeks large number of subjects to increase power of the study, randomization to increase generalizability of findings, and control groups are typically employed for comparison purposes for concepts or variables investigated
Data analysis is typically inductive, constant, and/or ongoing in nature	Data analysis is typically deductive in nature and done at the end of data collection
Primarily seeks to build theories or conceptual models based on where the researcher attempts to match interpretations with those of the subjects or other observers	Primarily seeks to test theories, conceptual models, and/or hypotheses

Neutens and Rubinson 2002; Polit and Tatano Beck 2012; Streubert Speziale and Rinaldi Carpenter 2007). The **holistic care paradigm** encompasses the belief that human being are more than the sum of their mind and body parts, but consist of dynamic and interrelated wholes that include the mind, body, soul, spirit, culture, and socio-political environments (Bartfay and Bartfay 2015). Refer Chapter 1 for a detailed description of the holistic care paradigm. It may be noted that the descriptive and subjective nature of qualitative research approaches may sit uneasily with those favouring objective and structured quantitative research methodologies in the public health sciences. Nonetheless, the acceptance of qualitative investigations as legitimate and valuable approaches continues to grow as a growing number of public and allied health researchers become educated and knowledgeable about these methodologies and publish their findings.

The reader should be aware that some published qualitative research reports do not identify a specific research approach per se (e.g., grounded theory, phenomenology, ethnography, historical), but simply identify the study as qualitative in nature. Hence, the research approach or tradition may have to be inferred by the types of research questions posed and the methods employed to collect and analyze the data. Moreover, a qualitative research study may sometimes report more than one research approach or tradition utilized. For example, Gibson and Kenrick (1998) described their investigation as a phenomenological study that utilized grounded theory methods to investigate the lived experiences of nine patients who had undergone vascular bypass surgery due to peripheral vascular disease. Baker, Wuest, and Stem (1992) have referred to this as "method slurring" and have criticized such research practices because each qualitative research approach or tradition has different intellectual assumptions, views, aims and methodological prescriptions.

Table 5.3 provides an overview of some of the ten major qualitative research traditions and their domains of origins, definitions, area of research inquiry, and an example of each research tradition is provided. Each of the ten qualitative research traditions highlighted in Table 5.3 is based on a philosophical orientation that influences the interpretation of data by the researcher. Nonetheless, each tradition is based on a worldview that is holistic in nature and that there may be multiple constructed realities or phenomenon of interests to public

Table 5.3 Ten Major Qualitative Research Traditions

Research Tradition and Domain	Definition	Area of Research Inquiry and Example
1. Action (aka, participative, cooperative) research or inquiry Social sciences, democratic principles/empowerment and participatory approaches	A qualitative research method characterized by the systematic study of the reported needs of individuals, groups or entire communities and the empowerment and implementation of a planned change to mutually and cooperatively solves real-life problems	Seeks to empower those who are part of the process to act on their own behalf to solve so-called "real-life problems" (e.g., To advance an understanding of the health reported needs of victims of the 2010 earthquake in Haiti and how to meet them)
2. Discourse analysis Human communication/ sociolinguistics	A qualitative research method that seeks to develop an understanding of the rules, mechanisms, and structure of human communication and conversations	Rules, patterns, and forms of conversation (e.g., physician to patient communication of a clinical diagnosis)
3. Ecological psychology Human behaviour and associated events	A qualitative research method that seeks to develop an understanding of the environment's influence on human behaviour and attempts to identify principles that explain the interdependence of humans and their environmental context	How the environment influences human behaviour (e.g., road rage due to vehicle traffic accidents)

(Continued)

Table 5.3 Ten Major Qualitative Research Traditions (*Continued*)

Research Tradition and Domain	Definition	Area of Research Inquiry and Example
4. Ethnographic research Culture/anthropology	A qualitative anthropological research method that seeks to study the evolution, meanings, patterns and experiences of a defined cultural group in a holistic fashion, and which seeks to develop conceptual models and theories of cultural behaviour	Seeks holistic understanding of a culture or a culture's shared meaning or value (e.g., Indigenous definitions of health)
5. Ethnomethodology Social settings/social group norms and assumptions	A qualitative research method that seeks to develop a better understanding of how individuals make sense of everyday activities, their social group's norms and assumptions, and how they interpret their social world to behave in socially acceptable ways.	Manner by which a mutual agreement is achieved in social settings and how people make sense of everyday activities and behave in socially acceptable ways (e.g., a host at a party orders a taxi for an intoxicated quest)
6. Ethology Psychology of human behaviour and events	Is a qualitative research method that seeks to develop a better understanding of human behaviour as it evolves in its natural setting or contexts	Human behaviour is observed overtime in their natural context (e.g., how fathers bond with their newborn infants overtime)
7. Grounded theory Social settings/sociology Symbolic interactionism/social symbols (e.g., language)	An inductive qualitative research approach based on symbolic interaction theory that seeks to discover the meaning of problems that exist in a real-life social context and the process that individuals employ to handle them, and it also involves the formulation and redevelopment of propositions until a theory is developed.	Socio-psychological and structural processes that occur within a social setting (e.g., A male obstetrician might view childbirth in quite a different way from a female midwife, and in turn their views may be quite different than those of the woman giving birth)
8. Hermeneutics Lived experiences	A qualitative research approach that utilizes interpretive phenomenology to develop a better understanding of the lived experiences of humans and how they interpret those experiences in the social, cultural, political and/or historical context	Interpretations and meanings of individuals' experience (e.g., a victim of torture who survived a brutal war or civil conflict)
9. Historical research Past events, trends, and effects	Is a qualitative research approach that seeks to systematically discover and critically analyze remote or recent past events, causes or trends and to shed light on present behaviour, practices or phenomenon	Systematic collection and critical evaluation of data (i.e., diaries, reports, photo's, film) related to past occurrences (e.g., Examining diaries related to the stress of living through the Great Depression of the 1930s in Canada)
10. Phenomenology Lived experiences	An inductive and descriptive qualitative research approach that seeks to describe and develop a better understanding of the lived experiences of humans	Experiences of individuals within their life-world (e.g., lived experience of being a primary caregiver looking after a family member post-stroke at home)

and allied health care researchers. Hence, the reasoning process for these approaches involves systematically placing pieces of narrative data together to make perceptual wholes (Burns and Grove 2007; Bryman, Bell, and Teevan 2012; Neutens and Rubinson 2002; Polit and Tatano Beck 2012; Streubert Speziale and Rinaldi Carpenter 2007).

The findings from qualitative investigations lead to a better understanding of a particular phenomenon in a defined situation or context, and are therefore not generalized in the same way as quantitative investigations. Hence, there are often no operational definitions provided for the study variables as one would expect to see in quantitative investigations, but rather the health-related experiences being studied are perceived and described as a whole in their specific contexts.

For example, a phenomenological investigation was undertaken to examine the effects of the 2008–2009 global economic recession on the health of unemployed blue-collar autoworkers in the Durham Region of Ontario, Canada (Bartfay, Bartfay, and Wu 2013). The researchers concluded that unemployed autoworkers in this region of Canada experienced negative health effects including high levels of stress, anxiety and depression; increased physical pain and discomfort; changes in weight and sexual function; and financial hardships including the inability to purchase prescribed medications. In sum, qualitative studies provide public health professionals and workers with a better understanding of individuals or groups as human beings. Indeed, qualitative research methodologies provide us with a better understanding of how disease, illness, disability and public health care services affect health consumer's lives as interpreted from their unique perspectives. The Research Focus Box 5.1 provides an example of a qualitative research study that employed a participatory action research framework to examine women's health and healing in the Canadian north.

Quantitative Research Methods

As noted in Table 5.2, quantitative research methods involve formal, precise and systematic processes for generating quantitative (numerical or statistical) information related to a variety of health care issues and concerns. For example, a researcher may be interested in describing the spread of the Avian (bird) H5N1 flu virus and its influence on morbidity and mortality rates globally for those infected. Another researcher may be interested in examining the influence of the diet, immobility and the time spent in front of a video display terminal on childhood obesity in Canada. Or a researcher may want to conduct a laboratory-based study with animals to examine the effect of a diet supplemented with conjugated linoleic acid (CLA) on muscle mass in mice with cancer cachexia, and extrapolate the findings for potential human applications.

A description of all the quantitative research methodologies that are utilized in the health sciences is beyond the scope and purpose of this chapter. Nonetheless, Table 5.4 provides an overview of some of the most common types of research approaches employed; their definitions, and an example of each. We will also examine some additional epidemiological methodologies and approaches in greater detail in the chapter entitled *Epidemiology: Essential Concepts for Public Health*, and we will also discuss health services and outcomes research in the chapter entitled *Program Planning and Evaluation in public health*.

Several of the studies summarized in Table 5.4 attempt to maximize the researcher's control over the research situation. **Research control** seeks to eliminate the effects of possible extraneous influences on the dependent variable so that the true relationship between the independent and dependent variables can be understood. A number of the approaches detailed in Table 5.4 also employ the process of randomization. The primary function of randomization is to secure comparable groups and to equalize the groups with respect to possible extraneous variables. When randomization is not possible or feasible, the researcher can employ other methods including homogeneity, matching or statistical controls. **Homogeneity** refers to the degree to which subjects in the study are similar, equivalent or consistent in nature with respect to the extraneous variables included in the study. For example, Zauszniewski and Chung (2001) utilized homogeneity in their study that examined the effects of symptoms of depression and learned resourcefulness on the health practices of individuals with diabetes. The researchers restricted their sample to adult women with type 2 diabetes without a prior known history of a mental disorder.

Research Focus Box 5.1

Example of a Qualitative Study

An Examination of the Social Determinants of Health as Factors Related to Health, Healing and Prevention of Foetal Alcohol Spectrum Disorder in a Northern Context—the Brightening Our Home Fires Project, Northwest Territories, Canada.

Study Aim/Rationale

Social determinants of health (SDH) including gender, culture and income levels are increasingly being investigated as key variables for various health outcomes in diverse populations in Canada and internationally. Foetal alcohol spectrum disorder (FASD) is a complex issue that requires an understanding of broad based SDH, not just the abstention from alcohol consumption during pregnancy by women. This includes an understanding related to location, economics and the unique social and cultural views of health according to Dene and Inuit peoples of northern Canada. The Brightening Our Home Fires (BOHF) project was conceptualized as an exploratory project to examine the issue of the prevention of FASD from a women's health perspective in the Northwest Territories (NT) of Canada. This qualitative research project was prevention focused via an SDH perspective.

Methodology/Design

The BOHF project employed a participatory action research framework to examine women's health and healing in the NT of Canada. The specific methodology utilized was "Photovoice"; where female participants ($N = 30$) were provided training in digital photography and given cameras to use and keep. The primary research question utilized was: What does health and healing look like for you in your community? Women described their photos, individually or in small focus groups around this central topic. Participants were recruited from Yellowknife, Lutsel 'ke, Behchokö and Ulukhaktok. These four different communities across the NT represented the Dene and Inuit cultures.

Major Findings

The qualitative data analysis offered seven major themes of importance to women's health in the north which included: (a) land and tradition; (b) housing; (c) poverty; (d) food; (e) family; (f) health, mental health, and trauma; and (g) travel. This research was FASD informed, and women participants were aware this was an FASD prevention funded project whose approach focused on a broader context of health and their lived experiences surrounding this public health issue in the NT.

Implications for Public Health

These findings suggest that Photovoice provides a non-threatening way to engage in dialogue on complex public health and social issues for Dene and Inuit women in the NT of Canada. Public health professionals and workers need to be cognizant of various SDH associated with FASD from the unique perspective of the stakeholders involved and their unique definitions of health and well-being. Participatory action frameworks appear to be an effective vehicle for engaging key stakeholders in the research process, and for engaging in targeted FASD public health prevention programs in the NT of Canada.

Source: Badry and Felske (2013)

Matching involves the deliberate pairing of subjects in one group with those in another comparison group based on their similarity on one or more diagnosis, characteristic, trait or dimension in order to enhance the comparability of groups (Bartfay and Bartfay 2015). For example, Talashek, Alba, and Patel (2006) conducted a study to compare inner city teenagers who were either pregnant or never pregnant to determine factors that might predict pregnancy status. The researchers controlled for participants' area of residence (i.e., inner city) and employed matching to control for the teenagers' age and ethnicity.

Statistical control involves the use of various statistical procedures to control for extraneous or possible confounding influences on the dependent (outcome) variable under investigation. Some readers who have not taken a class in biostatistics may be unfamiliar with these statistics procedures and analysis techniques, such

Table 5.4 Major Quantitative Research Approaches

Types	Definition	Examples
1. Case-control studies	A non-experimental quantitative research design that seeks to compare and contrast a "case" (i.e., a person or patient with a specific diagnosis or condition under investigation) with a matched control (i.e., a person without the condition or diagnosis)	A comparison of diet and body mass index (BMI) between Indigenous cases with Type 2 diabetes and healthy controls (i.e., Indigenous without Type 2 diabetes) in Québec
2. Case study	An in-depth description and analysis of a single individual, patient or group presenting with a specific health-related condition or phenomenon of interest	A group of Inuit stroke patients who had a stroke three years earlier and were experiencing eating difficulties
3. Clinical trials	A clinical study designed to assess the safety, efficacy and effectiveness of a new pharmaceutical agent, therapy or clinical intervention that involves four main phases: (a) Phase I: Occurs after the initial development of the medication or therapy and seeks to determine issues surrounding safety and tolerance; (b) Phase II: Seeks preliminary evidence related to the effectiveness and desirable clinical outcomes of the medication, therapy or clinical intervention; (c) Phase III: Involves a full experimental test that seeks to determine efficacy and includes randomization of subjects and a control group and is often referred to as "RCT." The RCT is utilized to establish approval of the experimental medication, therapy or clinical intervention for use by Health Canada, and (d) Phase IV involves long-term monitoring for unknown side effects and possible hazards related to the medication, therapy or intervention in general populations. This phase also seeks to determine the cost-effectiveness and clinical utility post approval	An RCT to determine the effectiveness of a work-based smoking cessation program for factory workers where 50% of the workers are assigned to a three-month experimental condition and the remaining 50% to the control group
4. Cohort studies	A quantitative trend or time-dimensional study that focuses on a specific subpopulation that is often an age-related subgroup from which different samples are selected at different points in time	A cohort of university students in Nova Scotia who graduated between 1970 and 1975 and their incidence of coronary artery disease in 2010
5. Correlational studies	A non-experimental quantitative study that seeks to examine the nature of relationships between two or more variables in a single clearly defined group or population	A study that seeks to determine the nature of the relationships between home-based chelation therapy with Deferral and the prevention of heart and liver failure in transfusion dependent patients with beta-thalassemia major
6. Cross-sectional studies	Are quantitative studies that involve the collection of data at one point in time to examine and describe the status of specific phenomena or relationships among phenomena from different age or developmental groups at a fixed point in time	A cross-section of individuals residing in Winnipeg, Manitoba aged twenty to sixty-five years of age is employed to determine the relationship between BMI and cholesterol profiles

(Continued)

Table 5.4 Major Quantitative Research Approaches (*Continued*)

Types	Definition	Examples
7. Descriptive studies	Studies that have as their main objectives the accurate portrayal and/or account of characteristics of persons; events, or groups in real-life situations in order to develop a better understanding of these as well as the frequency with which these phenomena occur	A study to examine quantitatively the concepts of caregiver burden in lay primary caregivers (i.e., parents and guardians) looking after a paraplegic school-aged child in their home following a traumatic motor vehicle accident (MVA)
8. Experimental studies	A study in which the investigator intentionally manipulates the independent variable; randomly assigns subjects to either experimental (treatment or intervention) group and to control groups (do not receive the treatment or intervention), and controls for experimental conditions in an attempt to decrease the possibility of error and increase the probability that the study's findings are an accurate reflection of reality. Hence, all true or classical experiments must have the following three conditions present: (a) random assignment; (b) manipulation, and (c) control	An experimental study to examine the effectiveness of an Internet-based learning and information resource site related to sexually transmitted infections (STIs) for highs school teens aged fifteen to seventeen years in Vancouver, BC. Teens in the experimental group receive six sessions of thirty minutes each on the STI Internet site; whereas controls receive six sessions of thirty minutes each on a site related to diet and exercise. Following the treatment sessions, knowledge related to STI is compared for the two groups via a paper and pencil knowledge test
9. Follow-up studies	A quantitative study undertaken to determine the outcomes of individuals or groups with a specified condition, diagnosis or who have received a specified treatment, therapy or intervention	A study to determine the health-related quality of life (HQOL) of patients in Calgary, Alberta who have undergone coronary bypass surgery
10. Outcomes research studies	Research designed to critically and objectively examine and document the effectiveness of health care policies and services and the end results of patient care	A study to evaluate the telephone callers ratings of perceived accessibility and satisfaction with health services received and the quality and usability of the information provided by nurses for a province-wide public health-based telehealth (telephone-based) program in Ontario
11. Panel studies	Are similar to follow-up studies, however the same individuals, patients or group of people (i.e., the panel) are employed to examine changes in data, clinical outcomes and/or phenomenon at two or more points in time	A study where data from 1990 and 2010 were compared to explore the antecedent characteristics of heavy smokers, defined as those who smoked twenty-five or more cigarettes per day in Newfoundland, who were later successful in quitting the habit
12. Prospective studies	A quantitative study design that commences with an examination of presumed causes or independent variables (e.g., inactivity, obesity, high levels of low-density lipoproteins (LDLs) and then goes forward in time to observe the presumed effects of these on the dependent variable that may include clinical outcomes, diagnosis or conditions (e.g., cardiovascular disease)	A study that begins with a sample of obese and inactive adults and non-obese active adults and that follows them over time and compares the two groups in terms of the development of heart disease and stroke

Table 5.4 Major Quantitative Research Approaches (*Continued*)

Types	Definition	Examples
13. Retrospective studies	A quantitative study design that begins with the manifestation of the dependent (outcome) variable, characteristic or phenomenon in the present (e.g., lung cancer), and then attempts to ascertain the antecedent factors or predictive independent variables that have caused it (e.g., smoking habits) before the study was initiated	A retrospective study to examine and compare infants who died of sudden infant death syndrome (SIDS—the cases) with infants who did not (controls) matched by date of birth on a number of suspected antecedent factors including birth weight, maternal characteristics, fetal heart rate variability, and sleep-wake cycles before birth
14. Surveys, self-reports, and questionnaires	Non-experimental research that seeks to obtain quantitative information about people's actions, behaviour, knowledge, intentions, opinions or attitudes and helps to provide knowledge related to the prevalence, distribution, and interrelationships of variables within a population	A survey to determine the health care needs of new immigrant single teenage mothers with low-birth infants in Toronto, Ontario
15. Time series studies	A type of quasi-experimental study that seeks to establish patterns and involves the collection of quantitative data over an extended time period and one with multiple data collection points both prior to and after an intervention, therapy or treatment to examine changes in a variable or variables across time	A time series study to assess the effect of a combination of antiretroviral medications on the frequency, severity and distress related to nausea among HIV-infected patients in New Brunswick. Measurements are taken prior to the start of treatment (the intervention) and then subsequently once a week for fifteen consecutive weeks once the treatment commences
16. Trend studies	Are studies in which samples from a general population are studied over time with respect to some characteristic or phenomenon; and where different samples are selected at specified repeated intervals, but the samples are always drawn from the same population. These studies permit researchers to examine patterns and rates of change and allow them to make predictions about future directions or needs	A trend study to examine the number of medical and nursing students enrolling in Canadian university programs where trend data are employed to make forecasts or predictions about future supplies of health care personnel in Canada
17. Quasi-experimental studies	An intervention-based study with a control group, however the subjects or comparative groups (e.g., schools, communities, regions) are not randomly assigned to treatment conditions	A community-based study to evaluate the effectiveness of a violence-prevention intervention program for staff working in long-term facilities in a community. The intervention program is implicated in five nursing homes, and five other nursing homes that do not receive the intervention serve as the control (comparison) group. Data on violence-prevention and recognition skills are assessed before and after the program for both experimental and control groups

as analysis of covariance or multiple step-wise regression techniques. Hence, a detailed description of powerful statistical control mechanisms is beyond the purpose and scope of this chapter and will not be discussed here. Nonetheless, the reader should recognize that an increasing number of researchers in the public and allied health sciences are utilizing a variety of powerful statistical procedures and techniques to control for extraneous variables. For example, Wishart et al. (2000) evaluated a community-based visiting/walking program designed to help decrease caregiver burden and stress for primary caregivers looking after a relative who was cognitively impaired. The researchers predicted in advance that the primary caregivers' level of formal education may influence their reported level of caregiver burden. Consequently, the researchers employed statistical control measures to make meaningful comparisons between the intervention and control groups so that the observed differences in reported caregiver burden levels could not be attributed to possible group differences in their level of education.

The Research Focus Box 5.2 provides an example of a quantitative study that examined the effects of sedentary versus active lifestyles on anthropometric measures (e.g., body mass index) and various biochemical measures (e.g., body iron stores, oxidative stress levels) believed to be associated with an increased risk for developing cardiovascular disease (CVD) in post-menopausal women in Ontario, Canada.

Mixed-methods Design Research

Given the increasing interest in collaboration by a variety of practitioners and researchers in the public health sciences, there has been significant growth in the utilization of mixed methods approaches in the past decades (Brewer and Hunter 2006; Creswell 2003; Green and Caracelli 1997; Happ et al. 2006; Moffatt et al. 2006; Tashakkori and Teddlie 2003). **Mixed-methods design** (i.e., hybrid design) research consists of a blending of both qualitative and quantitative approaches and methods (Bartfay and Bartfay 2015). Mixed-methods research design strategies and approaches for collecting and analyzing health related data are continually evolving and can be employed to gather a variety of information in the public and allied health sciences.

For example, Polit, London, and Martinez (2001) utilized a mixed-methods research design study to assess the health of poor urban women and their families. Quantitative data were collected longitudinally for nearly 4,000 women in four major cities in the United States. The researchers reported that findings from the quantitative data found that food insecurity and hunger were experienced by more than 50% of the families surveyed. Longitudinal qualitative ethnographic data were also collected from a small number of women in the same cities by different investigators. Qualitative data were utilized to explain how food insecurity was actually managed and experienced. For example, one respondent noted:

> It was hard, especially when you got kids at home saying
> 'I'm hungry.'…I was doing very odd jobs that most people
> would not dare to do. I was making deliveries of pizza in
> bad neighborhoods where most people wouldn't go. I mean,
> I literally took my life in my own hands.

—Polit, London, and Martinez 2001, p. 58

In sum, the dichotomy between qualitative and quantitative forms of data represents the key methodological distinction in the social and allied health care sciences, and the types of investigations vary according to their purpose as well as their research design or tradition. For example, if the aim of the proposed study is descriptive or exploratory in nature, then an experimental design study would be inappropriate. The major consideration in evaluating a research design is whether or not it enables the researcher to answer their research question or hypothesis. This is critical to determine for qualitative, quantitative or mixed-methods research design studies. Moreover, the specific research design or methodological approach utilized should be in concert with the noted aims of the investigation.

Research Focus Box 5.2

Example of a Quantitative Study

A Case-control Study Examining the Effects of Active Versus Sedentary Lifestyles on Measures of Body Iron Burden and Oxidative Stress in Post-menopausal Women

Study Aim/Rationale

One in eight women between the ages of forty-five and sixty-four lives with CVD, and they are ten times more likely to die from CVD than from any other disease including cancer. In activity and the adoption of sedentary lifestyles increase the risk for the development of CVD and all-cause mortality in post-menopausal women. There is preliminary evidence to suggest that excess body iron stores may catalyze the production of harmful oxygen free radical species including DNA, cellular membranes and proteins. Body iron stores increases two-to threefold following the onset of menopause in women. Preliminary evidence suggests that regular aerobic forms of exercise (e.g., walking, cycling, swimming, jogging, dancing, mowing the lawn, skating) may decrease body iron stores and increase protective antioxidant defenses. The aim of the present study was to compare different measures of body iron burden and their relationship to oxidative stress measures in active versus sedentary women in Ontario, Canada.

Methodology/Design

An age-matched case—control study was employed to examine the effects of active ($N = 25$) versus sedentary ($N = 25$) lifestyles on various measures of oxidative stress (e.g., malondialdehyde [MDA], hexanal); measures of body iron burden (e.g., serum ferritin, transferrin saturation); protective antioxidant enzymes (e.g., red cell glutathione peroxidase activity [GPx]), and BMI. Participants were from both urban and rural (farming) communities that were recruited from the greater Kingston, Ontario area. Women who self-reported that they engaged in thirty minutes or more of moderate-intensity forms of aerobic physical activity as active post-menopausal women, resulting in mild perspiration and increased respiratory rates three or more times per week. Conversely, women who self-reported that they engaged in ≤ 15 minutes total of moderate forms of aerobic physical activity per week were classified as sedentary. Exercise intensity was assessed via a brief self-reported questionnaire comprised of ten short questions that we developed in accordance with the Canadian Society of Exercise Physiology guidelines.

Major Findings

Measures of body iron burden and oxidative stress were significantly elevated in sedentary women in comparison to active women ($p < 0.001$). Red cell GPx activity was higher in active women compared to sedentary women ($p < 0.001$). BMI was also found to be significantly higher in sedentary women, in comparison to active post-menopausal women ($p < 0.001$).

Implications for Public Health

These findings suggest that sedentary post-menopausal women may be at increased risk of developing CVD due to increased body iron stores, increased oxidative stress levels, decreased protective RBC GPx activity and increased BMI in comparison to active post-menopausal women. In October 2005, the Secretariat for Intersectoral Healthy Living Network announced the Integrated Pan-Canadian Living Strategy. The goal of this national strategy is to recruit public health nurses and other public health professionals and workers in an effort to achieve a 20% increase in the number of Canadians who report that they are physically active on a regular basis. Given that menopause significantly increases the risk of developing CVD, public health professionals and workers need to target this group, especially given that the findings from this investigation suggest that aerobic forms of exercise may mitigate the risk of developing CVD in post-menopausal women.

Source: Bartfay and Bartfay (2013).

Step V: Ethical Approval

In the public health sciences, as in any discipline that involves research with humans or animals, investigators must address a wide range of ethical issues before the study can be formally approved by their institution (e.g., hospital, community clinic, university). However, this was not always the case. For example, from 1933 to 1945 the Nazi regime in Germany performed a variety of medical experiments on prisoners of war and persons that the Third Reich in Europe considered racially inferior such as mentally handicapped children and Jews in concentration camps (Berger 1990; Levine 1986; McNeill 1993; Steinfels and Levine 1976). The Nazi medical experiments violated numerous basic human rights because individuals were exposed to permanent physical or psychological harm and even death; no informed consent was obtained regarding the potential risks, and subjects could not refuse to participate. Wartime experiments that raised ethical concerns were also present in other countries including Australia, North Korea and Japan.

Another well-known example in public health involves the 1932 to 1972 Tuskegee, Alabama syphilis study by the US Public Health Service (Brandt 1978; Levine 1986; Rothman 1982; Vessey and Gennarao 1994). The study investigated the effects of the STI syphilis among 399 poor and disadvantaged rural African-American men over a period of forty years and 201 healthy controls without syphilis. This region had the highest rate of syphilis in the United States. Many of the men who consented to partake in the study were not informed about the purpose and procedures of the research investigation, and some weren't even aware that they were subjects in the study. The study was regarded as a "study in nature" as opposed to an experiment because its aim was to prospectively follow the natural course of the disease. The subjects were examined periodically and although a medically known cure for syphilis was available since the 1940s (i.e., penicillin), this treatment was knowingly withheld from those with this STI. Moreover, no effort was made by the US Public Health Service to stop the study until a 1972 account of the study was published in the *Washington Star* newspaper, which sparked public outrage nationally. Subsequently, the Department of Health, Education, and Welfare (DHEW) stopped the study, an investigation was undertaken and it was found to be ethically unjustified. From the Canadian context, research involving First Nations, Inuit and Métis people has been particularly subject to several noted unethical cases of conduct by university and government-sponsored investigators. Several Indigenous people have reported that they often felt over-researched with little or no real noted benefits for their respected communities (Bassil and Zabkiewicz 2014; Kovach 2010; Schnarch 2004). One of the major ethical issues has focused on the inability to obtain true informed consent of all the risks and benefits from the study participants. Schnarch (2004) reports that Indigenous people have often been persuaded to partake in various investigations without truly understanding actual or potential risks to their health and safety, the inappropriate use by government officials and policy makers and/or the misapplication of research outcomes that were not always culturally fitting.

For example, the Nuu-chah-nulth are a group of First Nations people who reside along the northwestern coast of British Columbia, have elevated rates of rheumatoid arthritis. In 1986, they agreed to partake in a study conducted by Ryk Ward, a university-based researcher from the University of British Columbia (UBC) (Kovach 2009; Wiwchar 2004). Approximately 900 First Nations people agreed to donate a blood samples for the study looking into the causes of rheumatoid arthritis. Nonetheless, the results for this noted investigation were determined to be inconclusive in nature. Shortly afterwards, Ward decided to leave UBC and took the blood samples with him without the prior knowledge or consent by the Nuu-chah-nulth First Nations community. Ward subsequently used these samples to publish various research reports related to migration and HIV/AIDS in Indigenous peoples, which first came to the attention of this First Nations community in 2000. Several members of the community felt betrayed, deceived, used, and hoodwinked by the researcher. The community subsequently decided to establish their own REB in response to this case and to critically review and evaluate all research being conducted in their community. Similarly, in response to this and other similar related grievances, Canadian Indigenous communities have responded by establishing a research-based political movement to create an ethical framework for knowledge generation known as the "Ownership, Control, Access, and Possession (OCAP)" principles (Bassil and Zabkiewicz 2014; Kovach 2009). The ownership principle means that the community in which the research will take place now collectively owns the information or data collected. The control principle means that the community or group will control all aspects of data management that may impact them directly or indirectly. This includes things like formulating actual research questions or hypotheses, how data will be collected and stored, to the dissemination and application of findings. The access principle means that Indigenous communities should have the right to manage and make decisions in reference to how the data collected regarding them will be utilized. Lastly, the possession principle refers to the mechanisms by which ownership will be asserted by Indigenous peoples.

In response to human rights violations, various codes of ethics have been developed. One of the first global efforts to protect human rights and establish ethical standards for researchers was the *Nuremberg Code* of 1949, which resulted from the Nuremberg Tribunals of Nazi physicians and surgeons (Fromer 1981; Levine 1986). Several other international standards have been subsequently developed including the *Declaration of Helsinki*, which was adopted in 1964 by the World Medical Association and revised most recently in October 2000 (see http://www.wma.net/e/policy/b3.htm). This document was based on the Nuremberg Code of 1949, but now differentiated between therapeutic and non-therapeutic research. **Therapeutic research** provides subjects/patients with an opportunity to receive an experimental treatment that may have beneficial results. Conversely, **non-therapeutic research** is conducted to generate new knowledge about an intervention, therapy or treatment. However, it will unlikely benefit the subject/patient partaking in the investigation, but may benefit future subjects or patients. These codes of ethics involve a variety of ethical standards that need protection including the respect for human dignity, right to privacy and anonymity, self-determination, full disclosure of the potential risks and benefits of the study, informed consent, and the right to withdrawal from the study anytime without penalty.

In addition to the above, most disciplines and professions have their own code of ethics. For example, Health Canada adopted the *Good Clinical Practice: Consolidated Guidelines* (1997) as their ethical standards for all clinical research involving human subjects. The first *Tri-Council Policy Statement: Ethical Conduct for Research Involving Humans* (aka, TCPS see http://www.pre.ethics.gc.ca/eng/policy-politique/initiatives/tcps2-eptc2/Default/) guidelines to protect human subjects in all types of research came into effect in the year 1998 (Minister of Supply and Services Canada 1998). The Tri-Council consists of the three major federal research funding agencies in Canada: (a) The Canadian Institutes of Health Research (CIHR), (b) Natural Sciences and Engineering Council of Canada (NSERC), and (c) the Social Sciences and Humanities Research Council of Canada (SSHRCC) (CIHR, NSERC, and SSHRC 1998, 2010). The original TCPS guidelines were based largely on the mechanistic medical model of health dominated by quantitative research approaches (Bryman, Bell, and Teevan 2011).

One of the major complaints of the original TCPS guidelines by qualitative researchers was that the standard research protocols, signed consent forms and other elements are often not compatible with certain qualitative research methodologies and approaches (e.g., ethnographic studies or natural observational studies) (van den Hoonaard and Connolly 2006). Moreover, research questions, topics investigated and even methodologies often emerge out of the research process itself, so standardized consent forms detailing the potential risks and benefits of participation and other features may not be feasible or appropriate. For example, imagine how an inner city gang involved with drug trafficking and prostitution may respond to an ethnographic researcher when they are handed a standardized information sheet and consent form to sign. Indeed, the original TCPS (1998) contained 476 paragraphs, of which only four pertain to "natural observation research" (Byrman, Bell, and Teevan 2012; van den Hoonaard and Connolly 2006).

The most recent Tri-Council Policy Statement (TCP2) came into effect in December 2010 and was created with input from both quantitative and qualitative researchers alike (see http://www.pre.ethics.gc.ca/eng/policy-politque/initiatives/tcps2-eptc2/Default/). In fact, there is now an entire chapter devoted to qualitative research approaches, and the new guidelines recognize that requiring formal written informed consent and other traditional elements of the biomedical model of research may not be appropriate and feasible in all research situations.

Both the original TCPS and updated TCPS2 identify three core principles, which are complementary and mutually reinforcing in nature: (a) Respect for persons, (b) concern for welfare, and (c) justice (CIHR, NSERC, and SSHRC 1998, 2010). **Respect for persons** stipulates that an individual's autonomy and their freedom to choose what will happen to them must be ensured. This principle also means that consent must be ongoing in nature. Hence, participants must be allowed to withdraw from the study at any time if they so choose to. **Concern for welfare** addresses all aspects of an individual's life as well as the welfare of groups and communities, which requires a favourable balance between the actual or potential risks and benefits of the research investigation. The principle of **justice** requires that individuals be treated fairly and equitably, so that no specific group, community or segment of the population bears an undue burden of risk associated with the study, and no part of society at large is excluded from the potential benefits that the research study may bestow.

Each of these principles provides valuable guidance for researchers and can also be employed to identify research practices and activities that should be potentially avoided for a variety of moral and ethical reasons (CIHR, NSERC, and SSHRC 1998, 2010). Several institutions (e.g., universities, hospitals) and agencies have now adopted the TCPS2 statement as their principle source for evaluating and determining ethical standards related to human investigations in Canada. Research in Canada is also subject to the Canadian law, in particular the *Charter of Rights and Freedoms* (see http://laws.justice.gc.ca/en/charter/1.html).

Another aspect of concern related to research in Canada involves the concept of sponsored research investigations by for-profit driven organizations or companies. For example, ethical issues may arise if the sponsor places restrictions on the ability of researchers to publish negative or detrimental results, places restrictions on the methodologies that can be employed and/or has certain expectations regarding the expected outcomes or findings (Bartfay and Bartfay 2015). Perhaps the most famous Canadian example involves Dr. Nancy Olivieri, a haematologists at the Hospital for Sick Children in Toronto who investigated a novel oral chelator (deferiprone or L1) for the clinical management of clients with thalassemia, a rare blood disorder resulting in severe anemia (Baylis 2004; Hoffbrand 2005; Naimark, Knoppers, and Lowy 1998; Thompson, Baird, and Downie 2001). This case made national and international headlines related to bioethics and the involvement of drug companies such as Apotex in RCTs. In 1998 Olivieri reported, in a publication that was not prior approved by the sponsor Apotex, that a substantial proportion of patients in the oral chelator deferiprone trial she was heading was ineffective at removing sufficient iron levels (Olivieri, Brittenham, and McLaren 1998). Moreover, deferiprone was found to be a significant cause of liver fibrosis—a previously unreported clinically serious side-effect.

Apotex subsequently sued Olivieri for breach of contract; which resulted in a long and very publicly debated court case, and an extensive ethical inquiry by the Ontario College of Physicians and Surgeons. Dr. Olivieri was eventually cleared of all wrong doings, and she also won substantial legal settlements from the Sick Kids Hospital and the University of Toronto. This case highlights important ethical considerations when accepting funding from for-profit corporations including the right to protect subjects from harm, remaining at "arms-length" and the right to publish and disseminate research outcomes or findings be they negative or positive in nature (Baylis 2004; Hoffbrand 2005; Naimark, Knoppers, and Lowy 1998; Thompson, Baird, and Downie 2001).

Research standards involving animals in Canada are governed by the Canadian Council of Animal Care (CCAC), and are articulated in the two-volume Guide to the *Care and Use of Experimental Animals* (see http://www.ccac.ca/en_/standards/guidelines or http://www.ccac.ca/en_/). The CCAC is an autonomous and independent body, created in 1968 to oversee the ethical use of animals in science in Canada. The *Three Rs tenet* for using and conducting research involving animals is comprised of the terms "Replacement," "Reduction" and "Refinement" (CCAC 2013). The term replacement refers to methods that avoid or replace the use of animals in an area where animals would otherwise have been used. **Reduction** refers to any strategy that will result in fewer animals being used for scientific investigations. Refinement refers to the modification of husbandry (i.e., care and housing of animals) and/or experimental procedures to minimize pain and distress (e.g., administration of analgesics) (CCAC 2013). Ethical considerations for animals are clearly different for those of human subjects. For example, the concept of informed consent is not appropriate or relevant. Nonetheless, all researchers employing animal models must attempt to minimize physical and emotional distress, discomfort, and harm, as with human subjects also.

Group Activity-Based Learning Box 5.2

Protecting Human Rights in Research Studies

This Group Activity-Based Learning Box 5.2 highlights the importance of protecting basic human rights when conducting research in the health sciences. Working in small groups of three to five students, discuss and answer the following questions:

1. What are some basic human rights requiring protection when conducting a study related to public health?

2. How does your institution REB ensure that the ethical research mandates of the Tri-Council (TCPS2) are being met by all researchers?

3. What is the process of submitting a research proposal for ethical approval by your institutions REB?

The external review of a human-based study and its ethical considerations is typically required by either the agency funding the investigation and the organization or agency from which participants may be recruited. This is often done by a so-called REB or "institutional review board" (IRB) for human studies, and animal care committees (ACC) for research involving animals. Researchers need to be cognizant of ethical requirements throughout the study's planning and implementation phases and ask themselves continually whether safeguards for protecting their subjects are sufficient.

Step VI: Collect Data (Empirical Phase)

Qualitative data collection

A major aim of qualitative research investigations is to place the researcher as close as possible to the subjects in an attempt to gain access to and describe and interpret their personal experiences (Burns and Grove 2007; Bryman, Bell, and Teevan 2012; Neutens and Rubinson 2002; Polgar and Thomas 2008; Polit and Tatnao Beck 2012; Streubert Speziale and Rinaldi Carpenter 2007). Moreover, data collection in qualitative research studies is regarded as more fluid in nature, in comparison to quantitative approaches. It is critical for the qualitative researcher to develop and maintain a high degree of trust with their subjects, which is often labour intensive and time consuming in nature. However, researchers who utilize qualitative research approaches need to be cognizant about maintaining their professionalism and guard against becoming too emotionally involved with their research subjects.

Qualitative researchers employ a variety of methods to record data, including the use of detailed field notes, digital tape recordings, video recordings or personal computers using a USB interface to record what the study participants stated. Written notes may be incomplete by themselves, they may be distracting to the participants and they may be biased by the interviewer's memory or personal recollections. Hence, researchers typically record and subscribe the statements verbatim. Tape-recorded interviews should be checked for audibility and completeness soon after the interview is completed to check for completeness, critique their own interviewing styles so that improvements can be achieved with future interviews, and also for possible follow-up questions that may require further probing or clarification.

There are a variety of approaches employed for the collection of self-reported verbal or narrative data forms, which can be broadly classified into the following three main types: (a) Unstructured, (b) structured, and (c) or semi-structured interviews (Burns and Grove 2007; Mann and Stewart 2001; Neutens and Rubinson 2002; Polgar and Thomas 2008; Polit and Tatnao Beck 2012; Streubert Speziale and Rinaldi Carpenter 2007). **Unstructured interviews** are informal in nature and consist of general or broad questions posed by the researcher that are not predetermined or planned in nature regarding their content or specific nature of the data sought to be collected. Unstructured interviews should be conducted by experienced and well-seasoned researchers, as opposed to those with limited qualitative research experiences. Although interviews are typically conducted face-to-face with subjects, a growing number of researchers are utilizing the Internet to collect unstructured data (Fitzpatrick and Montgomery 2004; Mann and Stewart 2001; Robinson 2001).

For example, Beck (2009) utilized the Internet to examine the lived experiences of mothers caring for children with obstetrical brachial plexus injuries in their homes. The researcher posted the following broad unstructured and open-type of question on the United Brachial Plexus Network, an Internet-based support group: "*Please describe in as much detail as you wish to share your experience of caring for your child with a brachial plexus injury.*" Mothers provided their written responses describing their personal lived experiences to the researcher via e-mail attachments.

Semi-structured interviews consist of a list of predetermined probing topics or questions that are fluid in nature and therefore can be elaborated on by the researcher to seek additional information or clarification as so desired. The probing topics or questions provide the researcher with a interview guide, which serves as a platform to gain additional insights into topics or phenomenon of interests based on the responses obtained. For example, Wu et al. (2010) investigated the experiences of cancer-associated fatigue among fourteen Chinese children diagnosed with leukemia in focus groups held in a clinical setting. A total of nine probing questions were asked by the researchers. "*Could you describe what it feels like to be tired and lacking in energy,*" is an example one of the probing questions asked to the children (Wu et al. 2010)?

Structured interviews consist of predetermined and fixed questions or categories of information (e.g., fixed response options) that are specified in advance by the researcher and which cannot be deviated from. Structured interview questions are regarded as closed-ended or fixed in nature, from which the researcher does not deviate (e.g., a health history questionnaire). For example, Berger, Treat Marunda, and Agrawal (2009) examined the effects of menopausal status and hot flashes throughout breast adjuvant chemotherapy on various predetermined sleep outcomes employing a structured personal diary format. The predetermined and fixed sleep outcomes included the number of awakenings, total sleep time in minutes per day and the minutes awake after sleep onset.

Quantitative data collection

Quantitative researchers collect data employing highly structured and predetermined data collection plans and protocols. There are a variety of methodologies that may be employed to gather quantitative data by public and allied health scientists including scales (e.g., McGill Pain Scale, Denver Developmental Scale), questionnaires (e.g., SF-12 Medical Outcome Study Short Form), clinical inventories and assessment tools (e.g., Beck's Depression Inventory; Functional Independence Measure [FIM]); laboratory tests (e.g., lipid profiles, white blood cells counts), diagnostic tests (e.g., CT-scans, electrocardiograms), bio-physiological measures (e.g., pulse, blood pressure, oxygen saturation, temperature), surveys and other self-reports to name but a few. Multiple measures of some variable may be needed if the concept under investigation is complex in nature. For example, the presence of anemia can typically be determined by routine haemoglobin and hematocrit levels. However, this may be insufficient for research purposes involving the metabolism of iron and factors that may affect it. Hence, the researcher may also seek to illicit additional laboratory-derived data related to iron metabolism such as serum ferritin levels, total iron-binding capacity, and transferring saturation. In addition, the researcher may also seek to evaluate detailed dietary records and their use of iron supplements and multivitamins, clinical history for genetic disorders of iron metabolism (e.g., hemochromatosis, beta-thalassemia major, Sickle Cell anemia), blood donation history, and menstrual status.

The quantification of objective measures should be clearly defined and established rather than haphazard in nature prior to data collection by the researchers. Indeed, with quantitative data (i.e., numbers) the language of communication should be precise in nature, as opposed to words as with qualitative data. For example, if a researcher reported that the average oral temperature of a cohort of subjects was "somewhat high," different readers may have very different interpretations about this physiological measure. Conversely, if the researcher reported an average oral temperature of 37.8°C, there is no uncertainty.

An early step in developing a data-collection plan is the identification and prioritization of data needs by the researchers. The list of possible data needs may appear daunting, but categories and data sources often overlap. Quantitative researchers often collect detailed demographic information (e.g., age, sex, level of education, social and economic status, time of diagnosis) that may also be possible confounding variables that can be controlled for during the data analysis phase. All researchers should be familiar with the procedures, instruments and/or tools used to collect quantitative data. Similarly, all research assistants should be given a formal training manual and partake in a training session that provides them with a mock data-collection scenario.

Lastly, there should be some discussion about the reliability and validity of the instruments, tools or measures utilized by the researchers in the research report so that the reader can judge the overall quality of the data collected. For example, Irvine et al. (2000) conducted a study to evaluate the reliability and validity of two different psychometric health outcome measures: the Medical Outcome Study Short Form (SF-36) and the Quality of Life Profile, Senior Version (QOLPSV). The study was designed to assess the health status of fifty patients as quantified by these forms at admission (Time 1) and discharge (Time 2) from home health care services provided by nurses. The researchers determined internal consistency using Cronbach's alpha for the eight subscales of the SF-36 which ranged from 0.76 to 0.94, and for the nine subscales of the QOLPSV which ranged from 0.47 to 0.82. Moreover, construct validation for both scales was undertaken through the testing of a series of hypotheses (e.g., the number of nursing diagnosis reflected the patient's need for nursing resources). The researchers concluded that the SF-36 may be a better measure of health outcomes following nursing care than the brief version of the QOLPSV (Irvine et al. 2000).

Step VII: Data Analysis (Analytical Phase)

Qualitative data analysis

The main objective of data analysis, regardless of the type of data collected, is to formally organize and structure the data so that the researcher can extrapolate the meaning of the data in terms of the research questions posed and/or the hypotheses. The analysis of qualitative data is a dynamic, intuitive, cerebral and creative process that is more fluid in nature due to its holistic nature, in comparison to the more linear and formulaic nature of quantitative data analysis (detailed below). There are no clearly defined rules for the analysis of

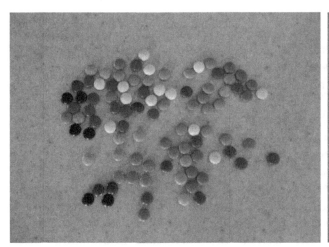 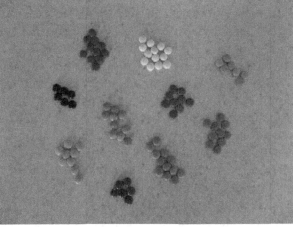

Source: Wally J. Bartfay

Photo 5.4A and B A pictorial representation of how qualitative data are analyzed using assorted coloured candies. The first step involves transcribing and coding the data, represented by various colours for the candy (Photo 5.3A). The process of data analysis then often takes the form of data clusters, which are comprised of specific data sets with similar themes represented by the sorting of candies by specific colour codes (Photo 5.3B).

qualitative data such as field notes taken or verbatim transcription of audiotapes. Nonetheless, the first challenge faced by qualitative researchers is to organize and reduce the vast amounts of raw data that can best be characterized as an editing style.

There are four main prototypical editing styles that are utilized by qualitative researchers: (a) Editing analysis style, (b) immersion/crystallization analysis style, (c) template analysis style, and (d) quasi-statistical/manifest content style (Burns and Grove 2007; Neutens and Rubinson 2002; Polgar and Thomas 2008; Polit and Tatnao Beck 2012; Streubert Speziale and Rinaldi Carpenter 2007). The **immersion or crystallization style** is a subjective and interpretive style that requires the total immersion and reflection of the text materials, which eventually leads to an intuitive crystallization of the data. Insights and theories derived from the qualitative data cannot crystallize unless the qualitative researcher is completely familiar with the data and therefore reads their narrative data over-and-over numerous times in their search for a deeper meaning and understanding of the phenomenon or concepts under investigation.

With the **editing analysis style,** the qualitative researcher acts as an interpreter who critically reads and examines the subjective data in an attempt to discover meaningful segments or categorization schemes that can be subsequently employed to sort and organize the data. The researcher then searches for emerging patterns and structures. This method is typically employed by grounded-theory researchers; however, researchers whose tradition is ethnomethodology, hermeneutics or phenomenology may also employ data analysis procedures that fall within the editing analysis style.

With the **template analysis style,** the qualitative researcher develops a rudimentary analysis guide or template to which narrative data units are applied (e.g., behaviour, events, linguistic expressions), and these templates undergo constant revision as more subjective data are gathered and interpreted. This style is often adopted by researchers who's research tradition is discourse analysis, ethnography, ethno-science or ethological in nature.

Quasi-statistical or manifest content analysis style consists of an accounting-type of frequency inventory or system used to determine the number of times an underlying word, phrase, insight, phenomenon, construct or theme appears in a qualitative data set. This results in the determination of frequency counts of qualitative data that can be subsequently analyzed statistically. Sandelowski (2001) argues that numbers are underutilized by qualitative researchers because of two myths. The first myth is that true or real qualitative investigators *do not count* and second, they *cannot* count. Nonetheless, a growing number of qualitative researchers are employing quasi-statistical techniques to better describe phenomenon, events, experiences and behaviour across the lifespan.

For example, Hawkins et al. (2009) employed this technique to better describe data derived from in-depth interviews of partners related to their sexuality and intimacy patterns who looked after loved ones who were diagnosed and underwent treatment for cancer. The researchers used quasi-statistical methods to tabulate a variety of patterns of change derived from their qualitative data set. The researchers reported that cessation or severely decreased frequency of sex was noted in 59% of the women and 79% of the men, and renegotiation of intimacy and sex was reported by 19% of women and 14% of men.

In addition to the four prototypical editing styles described above, a variety of methods based on different philosophical traditions have been published to help guide qualitative researchers through the data analysis phase. For example, Glaser and Strauss (1967) describe a grounded-theory approach for generating theories from qualitative data sets utilizing a constant comparative method of analysis. With this method, the researcher simultaneously collects, codes and analyzes the data. Throughout this process, the researcher documents their ideas about the data, categories and emerging conceptual schemes in the form of memos, which encourage the researcher to critically reflect on and describe patterns and relationships in the data and their emergent conceptualizations. Similarly, phenomenological researchers have developed a variety of approaches for data analysis based on Husserl's philosophical tradition (e.g., Colaizzi 1978; Giorgi 1985; Van Kaam 1966). Regardless of the analytical approach utilized, the reader can have more confidence in the interpretations derived from the data set if the report indicates that two or more individuals were involved in the coding, clustering and interpretations of the data, and this also helps to ensure inter-coder reliability.

Once the data have been transcribed and coded, the process of data analysis takes the form of data clusters, which are comprised of data sets with similar themes. Desantis and Ugarriza (2000) define a theme as an abstract entity that brings meaning and identity to a current experience and its variant manifestations. Hence, a theme captures and unifies the nature or basis of the experience into a meaningful whole for the researcher. Once the researcher has identified and exhausted all relevant themes for the study, they report them in a manner that is meaningful to the intended audience and often in concert with the philosophic tradition used (e.g., Grounded theory, phenomenology).

Themes are never universal in qualitative studies and thematic analysis involves the process of not only discovering commonalities among study participants, but also seeking natural variations that may be present and how they are patterned. The identification of themes from qualitative data clusters and categories is not a linear process. In fact, the researcher typically derives a theme from the narrative clusters, then revisits the materials with the themes in mind to ascertain if the data really do fit, and then refines or abandons the theme as necessary.

For example, Strang et al. (2006) investigated the experiences of family caregivers looking after family members with dementia and their transition to long-term care facilities in the community. The researchers noted that they were required to abandon an earlier dance metaphor theme that emerged from their data set as they continually re-examined and refined their themes in light of the material. They subsequently coded data categories in stages with each stage representing a higher level of conceptual complexity, and the interplay within the caregiver dyad reminded them of a dancing metaphor. As the analysis progressed, the dance metaphor failed to fully represent the increasingly complex nature of the interactions between the caregiver and their family member with dementia, so it was consequently abandoned by the researchers (Strang et al. 2006).

The traditional manual methods (e.g., coloured file cards, post-it notes to code narrative content, conceptual files with cut-up narrative material) for organizing qualitative data have a rich history, but are slowly being replaced by a variety of software programs that can perform various labour-intensive indexing functions. Currently, more than a dozen computer assisted qualitative data analysis software (aka, CAQWAS) packages are available that function as text retrievers, code and retrieve data, build theory, do data conversion/collection, help develop concepts maps and diagrams, and voice recognition software that converts voice to text (Bryman, Bell, and Teevan 2012; Fogg and Wightman 2000; Lewins and Silver 2007; Novak and Canas 2006; Taylor 2005). Examples of some of these commercially available qualitative software packages include ATLAS/TI, HyperRESEARCH, MaxQDA, NVivo 8, NUD*IST 6 and Qualitative Solutions and Research (QSR). For example, CmapTools (www.ihmc) was developed at the Institute for Human and Machine Cognition for concept mapping that helps qualitative researchers to illustrate concepts (enclosed in circles or boxes) and the proposed relationships between them (indicated by connecting lines or dots), and is available free for educational and not-for-profit organizations (Novak and Canas 2006).

In the final stages of data analysis, qualitative researchers strive to weave thematic concepts or pieces together into an integrated whole of the experience. Ultimately, qualitative researchers should seek to provide structure to the meaning of the data as a whole in the form of a conceptual model or theory by interrelating and weaving together the various themes that emerged from their data set. The integrity of quality research findings will be judged on the ability of the investigators to successfully tell the story of their subjects with truthfulness and attention to context and power (Streubert Speziale and Rinaldi Carpenter 2007). Lastly, qualitative researchers require a certain degree of creativity in uncovering the meaning of their data. As noted by Hunter et al. (2002), strategies for creativity often take great amounts of time and patience, and require incubation periods for new ideas to percolate fully. Insight into the incubation of data is critical to the final theoretical revelations.

Quantitative data analysis

During quantitative data analysis, the researcher utilizes statistical procedures to organize, interpret and communicate numerical data. The findings are typically summarized in the form of tables, graphs or other pictorial representations (e.g., pie charts). Quantitative measurement of data makes it possible to obtain reasonably precise and objective information based on explicit rules and conditions for performing a variety of descriptive and inferential statistical procedures according to the classification or level of numerical measurement. A variety of user-friendly software packages with pull-down menus are available to quantitative researchers, such as the Minitab Statistical Package (http://www.minitab.com/), Mathematica (http://www.wri.com/). S-Plus for Exploratory Data Analysis (http://www.splus.mathsoft.com/), Statistical Analysis System (SAS) (http://www.sas.com/), and the Statistical Package for the Social Sciences (SPSS) (http://www.spss.com/) to name but a few.

Descriptive statistics are used to describe and synthesize data. Examples include means, medium, mode, ranges, frequency distributions and percentages. **Inferential statistics** are based on the laws of probability and provide a means for drawing conclusions about a population based on quantitative data derived from a sample. Statistical inference consists of two major techniques: (a) Estimation of parameters and (b) statistical hypothesis testing. The current emphasis on evidence-informed practice in the public and allied health sciences has heightened awareness for not only determining whether a hypothesis was supported or not by traditional hypothesis tests, but also the need to estimate the value of a population parameter and the level of accuracy of the estimate via a parameter estimate. Hence, this information is richer in nature because it provides information about both the clinical and statistical significance of the published findings (Braitman 1991; Sackett et al. 2000).

Parameter estimates are used to estimate a given parameter, such as a mean, proportion or a mean difference between the experimental and control groups in a study. With interval estimation, for example, the researcher may report their calculated confidence interval (CI) around the estimate. For example, suppose a researcher wanted to answer the following research question: "*What is the percentage of adult Canadians exposed to asbestos in the workplace who will develop lung cancer?*" To answer this research question, the researcher will be required to estimate the proportion (e.g., absolute risk index) of individuals affected. The UBC provides a fast and user-friendly method for calculating CI known as the *Clinical Significance Calculator*, which is available to researchers and students on the Internet (http://spph.ubc.ca/sites/health-care/files/calc/clinsig.html).

Statistical hypothesis testing provides an objective means for determining whether or not the stated hypotheses were supported by the data collected, and permits researchers to make decisions about whether the results likely reflect chance sample differences or true population differences (Bartfay and Bartfay 2015). In sum, statistical hypothesis testing is basically a process for rejecting the null hypothesis, which states that there is no relationship among the variables investigated. When a researcher calculates a test statistic (e.g., chi-square test, paired Student's t-test, one-way analysis of variance [ANOVA]) that is beyond the stated critical limit (e.g., 0.05 level of significance), the study results are referred to as being "statistically significant" in the report. It is important that the reader keeps in mind that the word "significant" does not imply that the research findings are clinically or socially important per se, it simply means that the results obtained from a statistical point of view are not likely to have resulted from chance at a specified level of probability. By contrast, a non-significant result implies that an observed result may reflect chance fluctuations.

For example, Badger, McNiece, and Gagan (2000) conducted a study to examine depression, service needs, and service use in vulnerable populations. The researchers were interested in comparing enabling characteristics that assist or inhibit health seeking care in these individuals. During the analysis stage, study participants were assigned to one of two groups: (a) depressed and (b) non-depressed. The chi-square test was employed and the level of significance was set at 0.05 for this investigation. The researchers reported that significant differences between the two groups for work status (x^2 [4] = 18.10, p = 0.001) were detected. Moreover, depressed participants (70%) were disabled compared to non-depressed participants (43%), and fewer retirees were noted among depressed subjects in the study (Badger, McNiece, and Gagan 2000). Table 5.5 provides a description of the four major levels of measurement for quantitative types of data.

A quantitative researcher may often utilize multiple levels of measurement in their study. For example, Bozak, Yates, and Pozehl (2010) investigated the effects of an Internet-based physical activity intervention

Table 5.5 The 4 Major Levels of Measurement

	Classification	Definition	Examples
I	Nominal/Categorical data	The lowest level of measurement that involves the assignment of characteristics into mutually exclusive and collectively exhaustive categories. Numbers in this category cannot be meaningfully treated in the mathematical sense	Sex (male or female), blood type, and marital status (i.e., married = 1, separated or divorced = 2, widowed = 3 not married = 4)
II	Ordinal/Ranked data	Attributes are ordered according to a defined criterion that captures information about equivalence and its relative rank. However, they do not inform us about how much greater one rank or category is in comparison to the other	Frequency of visits of a family caregiver to a long-term care facility in the community ranked as 1 = daily; 2 = several times a week; 3 = several times a month and 4 = rarely
III	Interval data/Continuous	Interval data: There is a specified rank ordering on a defined attribute and the distance between those objects are assumed to be equivalent in nature along a continuum, but there is no true zero	Temperature, various psychometric scales (e.g., Duke Activity Status Index, Denver Developmental Scale)
IV	Ratio data	Is the highest level of measurement that provides information about the ordering and exact magnitude between the levels of the critical attribute due to a clearly defined true zero	Weight, height, lipid biomarkers, physical activity duration, total daily calorie consumption

targeted for adults diagnosed with metabolic syndrome. The researchers reported nominal-level data including race and sex of the study participants, the consumption of alcohol was measured on an ordinal-level scale, the subjects self-efficacy was measured on an interval-level scale using the Cardiac Exercise Self-Efficacy Instrument, and a variety of dependent (outcome) variables were assessed employing ratio-level data such as energy expenditure, physical activity duration and lipid profiles.

Step VIII: Determine Strengths and Limitations of the Findings

The reader should critique all published research studies and reports for their overall quality, completeness and significance for EIPH. This requires that the reader carefully examine the research problem, its stated aim or purpose, the stated research questions or hypotheses, design and methods employed, the results obtained, and the possible implications for practice. High-quality research investigations typically focus on a single significant problem; demonstrate sound research design and methodologies, produce credible research findings that can be easily replicated by other investigators, and which provide a sound scientific basis for additional investigations in the field of inquiry.

Performing a critique of a published research report is a cerebral process that requires practice and knowledge of the research process. Systematic reviews of the literature often provide the reader with insightful critiques of published peer-reviewed articles, their noted strengths and limitations and directions for further research or clarification. Moreover, letters to the editor also provide rich sources of critiques of research investigations. Table 5.6 provides a template/checklist that can help guide the reader for critiquing research reports in the health sciences.

Table 5.6 Template/Checklist for Critiquing Research Reports

Critiquing Guidelines	Yes	No	Additional Comments
1. Is the problem and rationale for the study clear to the reader?			
2. Is a review of relevant literature provided?			
3. Are the research questions and/or hypotheses clearly stated?			
4. Is the study design and sampling method employed clearly described?			
5. Did the researchers clearly provide their rationale and justify why they choose this research design or sampling technique over others?			
6. Did the researchers seek ethical approval for their investigation and is this clearly described in the report?			
7. Did the researchers clearly detail their data collection procedures, including the validity and reliability of instruments or techniques employed so that there is sufficient information to replicate the study by other researchers?			
8. Is the method for data analysis appropriate for the type of data collected (qualitative, quantitative, mixed-methods design research) and clearly explained to the reader (e.g., coding methods, statistical methods employed)?			
9. Do the researchers describe the strengths and limitations of their findings?			
10. Were possible sources of error, bias and/or confounding variables considered by the researchers?			
11. Did the researchers appropriately discuss the generalizability of their research findings based on the findings obtained for their specific target sample?			
12. Do the researchers compare and contrast their findings in light of other relevant published research reports?			
13. Were possible alternative explanations for the study findings considered by the researchers?			
14. Are the implications for practice in the public or allied health sciences highlighted?			
15. Are directions for future research or additional questions/hypotheses arising out of the findings that require further investigation discussed by the researchers?			

Step IX: Dissemination and Application of Research Findings

The final step of the research process involves the dissemination and application of the research findings. Researchers who want to communicate their research findings to others can do so using a variety of methods including: peer-reviewed journals; oral or poster presentations at local, national or international conferences; public lectures; workshops, the mass media (e.g., television, radio, newspaper) and social media (e.g., Facebook, YouTube, Twitter). The lead author on the report is typically the first listed author, and has overall responsibility for the research report. The coauthors are listed by convention according to their noted contribution and intellectual input provided in the report.

Although each peer-reviewed journal provides potential contributors with detailed formatting instructions for the submission of manuscripts, they typically follow the IMRAD format. The IMRAD format is an acronym for dividing the manuscript into the following four main sections: (a) [I]ntroduction, (b) [M]ethods, (c) [R]esults, and (d) [D]iscussion. Each peer-reviewed report resulting from the study should make a significant and independent contribution to the scientific literature. It is both inappropriate and unethical to write several reports when one-single report would suffice, a practice that has been termed "salami slicing" publications (Baggs 2008).

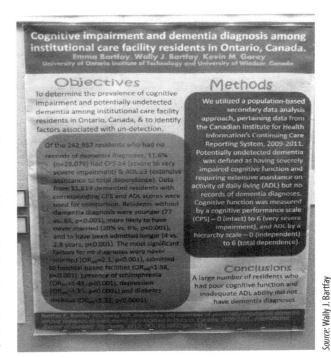

Source: Wally J. Bartfay

Photo 5.5 A collaborative research poster presented at an international conference on gerontology and geriatrics. Dissemination and application of research findings are the last steps of the research process. Research poster by Bartfay, Bartfay, and Gorey (2013).

Knowledge Utilization in Public Health

Researchers often have to keep in mind multiple target audiences for the dissemination of their research findings. Although it is generally important to speak and write for a broad target audience, it is also critical to consider the primary intended audience. Indeed, will the consumers of the oral or written report be primarily researchers, public health professionals and workers, or the general lay public? The research report, be it written, oral or both, should provide a clear and concise overview of the research problem, how it was studied and analyzed, and what the findings mean. Findings from a given study often generate new research questions and/or hypotheses and the cycle of research continues on and repeats itself (see Figure 5.2).

Research is conducted to generate knowledge for use in clinical practice. The term **knowledge utilization** relates to the process for formally applying and utilizing research findings to guide EIPH, including its practice, the development and evaluation of programs and public health policies (Bartfay and Bartfay 2015). Hence, reading, critiquing and synthesizing finding from the empirical literature are essential for generating research evidence for use by public health care professionals and workers.

Using the best-available-evidence enables us to provide high-quality care, improve client and population outcomes, develop new programs and policies and decrease associated health care costs. Nonetheless, there is often a time lag between the generation and application of new findings. For example, the time lag between the discovery of citrus juice by James Lind as a preventive measure against scurvy and its use on British naval ships was 264 years (Glaser, Abelson, and Garrison 1983). Similarly, it took over two decades of research that documented the benefits of so-called "baby aspirin" (81 mg) in protecting individuals against stroke and heart disease before it became formally approved as a prophylactic intervention (Marwick 1997).

Various models for knowledge utilization and the incorporation of research into practice have been developed and evaluated over time. For example, the *Stetler Model* (2001, 1994) was designed with the premise that research could be undertaken and applied not only by large organizations, but also by individual managers and clinicians. Similarly, the *Iowa Model of Evidence-based Practice to Promote Quality Care* (Titler et al. 2001) was developed to promote the utilizing of EIPH, and outlines a series of activities and critical decision paths. The *Ottawa Model of Research Use* (OMRU) is a Canadian model developed by Logan and Graham (1998), which consists of six key components that are interrelated through the process of evaluation. These components deal specifically with the practice environment (e.g., home-based nursing care; community clinics), the potential research adopter (administrators and staff), the evidence-informed innovation (the research intended for use in practice), strategies for transferring the innovation into practice (e.g., training of staff), adoption/use of the evidence in practice settings, health outcomes achieved and other measures (e.g., cost-effectives of services) (Logan et al. 1999). For example, Logan et al. (1999) employed their model at four sites in Ontario, Canada as part of a province-wide nursing project related to pressure-ulcer treatment and practices. Since the initiation of this project, the investigators reported significant change in the attitudes and organizational culture to support the use of evidence at both the practitioner and organizational levels (Logan et al. 1999).

Future Directions and Challenges

While only a few public health professionals and workers will direct programs of research, all will need to participate in research, critical read and review research findings and apply the best available evidence to their practice of public health. EIPH involves the conscientious integration, conduct and synthesis of numerous high-quality investigations in a defined field or specific area of research inquiry. The ultimate goals of research are to improve public health practice and education, improve delivery of these health care services, evaluate the effectiveness of various health care delivery models and decrease the associated costs. Most individuals believe that "a good idea will sell itself." Unfortunately, this is seldom the case in the public and allied health sciences and we have to do a better job in effectively communicating our research findings to a variety of professional and lay audiences.

Traditionally, the strategies for communicating research findings were limited to studies published in professional journals and scientific conference proceedings. Currently, a growing variety of communication strategies are being employed by researchers to communicate their research findings to fellow researchers, practitioners and to the lay public including the mass media (e.g., television, newspapers, radio shows) and social media (e.g., Facebook, Twitter, YouTube). The use of evidence-informed guidelines is increasingly becoming the standard for providing primary health care services in Canada and other nations globally (Commission on the Social Determinants of Health 2008; Bowen and Zwi 2005; NCCPH 2011; Pach 2008; Rycroft-Malone 2008).

A variety of organizational, social-political, professional and/or economic barriers impede the implication of sound and high-quality research findings. For example, in many public health practice settings, administrators and managers have established procedures to reward competence in practice. However, few practice settings have established a formal system to reward public health professionals and workers in Canada for critiquing research, utilizing research in their practice and/or discussing research findings with their clients.

Phillips (1986) notes that another historical barrier to bridging the research-practice gap was the shortage of role models who could be emulated for their success in using or promoting the use of research to guide EIPH. Fortunately, much progress has been made over the past few decades in Canada and internationally in highlighting the importance of research to guide practice in the public health sciences. Lastly, educators in the public health sciences must continue their efforts to teach the importance of research and EIPH to their students. Indeed, the valuing of research as the *sine qua no* on which practice is based must be conveyed throughout undergraduate and graduate degree programs in public health. This is not teaching of the conduct of research per se, but rather the valuing of it as a way of knowing and as the foundation on which practice is based (Funk et al. 1991). Hence, a fundamental knowledge of the research process is critical for all students and practitioners in the public and allied health sciences.

Group Review Exercise

"Spinning a Pill"

Overview of this investigative documentary

Before medical products (e.g., new knee prosthesis, medications), equipment or assistive devices (e.g., pace-makers) or medications can be sold, clinically employed or prescribed in Canada, they have to undergo a special form of experiment termed a RCT. Although a product may be approved by governmental officials for use in Canada following the required RCTs, the long-term health consequences or negative outcomes and ripple effects are often not revealed during these clinical trials. A controversial oral contraceptive called "Yasmin" and its sister drug "Yaz" have become one of the country's top-selling birth control pills for women of child-bearing age. In this investigative television documentary by Marketplace which aired on the Canadian Broadcasting Corporation (CBC-TV), co-host Erica Johnson interviews young women who have taken Yasmin or Yaz believing that they were tested and proven safe for use. Nonetheless, these women consequently experienced serious negative health side effects and problems. Johnson asks why so many young women are unaware of the potential health risks associated with taking these noted birth control pills. In the United States more than 4,000 women have taken legal action against the pharmaceutical manufacturer of this product, and more than 800 women in Canada have joined a major class-action lawsuit against Bayer.

Instructions

This assignment may be done alone, in pairs or in groups of up to five people (note: if you are doing this assignment in pairs or groups, please submit only one hard or electronic copy to the instructor). The assignment should be type-written and no more than four to six pages maximum in length (double-spaced please). View the documentary entitled "Spinning a pill," which aired on CBC-TV investigative programme *Marketplace*. See link: http://www.cbc.ca/marketplace/2011/spinningapill/. View this documentary and take detailed notes during the presentation.

Provide a brief overview of the salient points in this investigative documentary.

1. What clinical and/or scientific evidence is presented in the investigative documentary to highlight actual and/or potential negative health effects associated with taking the drugs Yasmin or Yaz?

2. In order for the drug to be approved for human use, it had to undergo which phase of a clinical trial? Briefly describe this phase and its intended objectives.

3. Describe which phase of a clinical trial monitors the long-term health outcomes and consequences of drugs approved for use by humans?

4. Is there currently sufficient evidence to issue public health warnings related to actual and/or potential negative side effects or health outcomes associated with these drugs? Why or why not?

Summary

- Research is defined as a systematic and purposeful method of scientific inquiry into the nature of phenomena in an attempt to develop new knowledge and practice standards, test existing hypotheses and for the development of conceptual models and theories.
- Basic (pure) research entails activities undertaken to extend the knowledge base in public health or to formulate or refine an existing conceptual model or theory.
- Applied (practical) research is defined as public health interventions that focus on finding solutions to existing problems and to generate knowledge that will directly influence practice.

- Research is an essential pillar of public health because it is critical for evidence-informed practice, for the critical appraisal and utilization of current and sound scientific research and data to develop health policies and procedures, determine health outcomes and trends in diverse populations across the lifespan and to evaluate the effectiveness of public health care services and interventions.
- Qualitative research is defined as a holistic and subjective process used to describe and promote a better understanding of human experiences and phenomena via the collection of narrative data, and to develop conceptual models and theories that seek to describe these experiences and phenomena.
- Quantitative research is defined as a formal, precise, systematic and objective process in which numerical data are used to obtain information on a variety of health-related phenomenon of interest or concern.
- Mixed-methods design (aka, hybrid) research consists of a blending of both qualitative and quantitative approaches and methods.
- The research process consists of a series of nine steps and techniques used to structure a study and to gather, analyze, interpret, disseminate and apply data and information in a systematic and formularized fashion.
- High-quality research studies typically focus on a single problem; demonstrate sound research design and methodologies; produce credible research findings that can be easily replicated by others, and provide a sound scientific basis for additional investigations in the area of inquiry.
- The term knowledge utilization relates to the process of formally applying and utilizing research findings to guide EIPH.

Critical Thinking Questions

1. Select a peer-reviewed article that evaluated a specific intervention relevant to a current or emerging public health issue or problem in your community (e.g., growing rates of obesity in school-aged children; caregiver burden and stress for family members looking after a family member in their home; elder abuse, environmental hazard). Use the criteria detailed in Table 5.6 to appraise this article and come to a decision about the merits of employing this intervention in your own practice as a public health care professional or worker.

2. Review current standards of evidence-informed practice for public health care professionals and workers in your province/territory or community. How was published scientific reports employed to develop these standards? What factors limit our ability to effectively process and employ the vast amounts of information that is available, and how can we overcome these obstacles?

3. Research and articulate your own evidence-informed standard of practice for public health that you feel is important. Why is this standard important to you and why did you choose it? What sources did you consult to develop and justify this standard of practice?

References

Alwan, M. S. *A Prioritized Research Agenda for Prevention and Control of Noncommunicable Diseases.* Geneva, Switzerland: World Health Organization, 2011. ISBN 978 924 1564205. Accessed December 02, 2013. http://whqlibdoc.who.int/publications/2011/9789241564205_eng.pdf.

Atkins, D., D. Best, P. A. Briss, M. Eccles, Y. Falck-Ytter, S. Flottorp, G. H. Guyatt, R. T. Harbour, M. C. Haugh, D. Henry, S. Hill, R. Jaeschke, G. Leng, A. Liberati, N. Magrini, J. Mason, P. Middleton, J. Mrukowicz, D. O'Connell, A. D. Oxman, B. Phillips, H. J. Schünemann, T. Edejer, H. Varonen, G. E. Vist, J. W. Williams Jr, S. Zaza. "Grading Quality of Evidence and Strength of Recommendations." *British Medical Journal* 328, no. 7454 (2004): 1490–5002.

Atkins, L., J. A. Smith, M. P. Kelly, and S. Michie. "The Process of Developing Evidence-based Guidance in Medicine and Public Health: A Qualitative Study of Views from the Inside." *Implementation Science* 4, no. 8 (2013): 101–08. PMID: 24006933.

Badger, T. A., C. McNiece, and M. J. Gagan. "Depression, Service Needs, and Use in Vulnerable Populations." *Archieves of Psychiatric Nursing* 14, no. 4 (2000): 173–82.

Badry, D., and A. W. Felske. "An Examination of the Social Determinants of Health as Factors Related to Health, Healing and Prevention of Foetal Alcohol Spectrum Disorder in a Northern Context—The Brightening Our Home Fires Project, Northwest Territories, Canada." *International Journal of Circumpolar Health* 72 (2013). doi:10.3402/ijch.v72i0.21140.

Baggs, J. G. "Issues and Rules for Authors Concerning Authorship Versus Acknowledgements, Dual Publication, Self-plagiarism, and Salami Publishing." *Research in Nursing & Health* 31 (2008): 295–97.

Baker, C., J. Wuest, and P. N. Stern. "Method Slurring: The Grounded Theory/Phenomenology Example." *Journal of Advanced Nursing* 17 (2008): 1355–60.

Barbour, R. S. "The Role of Qualitative Research in Broadening the 'Evidence Base' for Clinical Practice." *Journal of Evaluation in Clinical Practice* 6, no. 2 (2000): 155–63.

Bartfay, W. J. "Introduction to Community Health Nursing in Canada." In *Community Health Nursing: Caring in Action.* 1st Canadian ed., edited by J. E. Hitchcock, P. E. Schubert, S. A. Thomas, and W. J. Bartfay, 1–10. Toronto, ON: Nelson Education, 2010a.

———. "Perspectives on Health and its Promotion and Preservation." In *Community Health Nursing: Caring in Action.* 1st Canadian ed., edited by J. E. Hitchcock, P. E. Schubert, S. A. Thomas, and W. J. Bartfay, 98–116. Toronto, ON: Nelson Education, 2010b.

Bartfay, W. J., and E. Bartfay. "A Case-Control Study Examining the Effects of Active Versus Sedentary Lifestyles on Measures of Body Iron Burden and Oxidative Stress in Postmenopausal Women." *Biological Research for Nursing* (September 19, 2013): 1–8. [EPUB PMID 24057220]. doi:10.1177/109980041350171.

———. Iron-Overload Cardiomyopathy: Evidence for Free Radical-mediated Mechanisms of Injury and Dysfunction in a Murine Model. *Biological Research for Nursing* 2 (2000): 1–11.

———. *Public Health in Canada.* Boston, MA: Pearson Learning Solutions, 2015. ISBN:13:978-1-323-01471-4.

Bartfay E., W. J. Bartfay, and K. M. Gorey. "Cognitive Impairment and Dementia Diagnosis Among Institutional Care Facility Residents in Ontario, Canada." The 20th IAGG World Congress of Gerontology and Geriatrics, Seoul, South Korea, July 2013 (Poster Presentation).

Bartfay, W. J., E. Bartfay, and T. Wu. Impact of the Global Economic Crisis on the Health of Unemployed Autoworkers." *Canadian Journal of Nursing Research* 45, no. 3 (September 2013): 66–79.

Bassil, K., and D. Zabkiewicz. *Health Research Methods: A Canadian Perspective.* Toronto, ON: Oxford University Press, 2014.

Baylis, F. "The Olivieri Debacle: Where were the Heroes of Bioethics?" *Journal of Medical Ethics* 30 (2004): 44–49. doi:10.1136/jme.2003.005330.

Beck, C. T. "Focus on Research Methods: Facilitating the Work of a Meta-analyst. *Research in Nursing & Health* 22, no. 6 (1999): 523–30.

———. "Mothering Multiples: A Meta-synthesis of Qualitative Research. *American Journal of Maternal Child Nursing* 27, no. 4 (2002): 214–21.

———. "The Arm: There is No Escaping the Reality of Mothers of Children with Obstetric Brachial Plexus Injuries. *Nursing Research* 58 (2009): 237–45.

Berger, R. L. "Nazi Science: The Dachau Hypothermia Experiments." *The New England Journal of Medicine* 322, no. 20 (1990): 1435–40.

Berger, A. M., H. A. Treat Marunda, and S. Agrawal. "Influence of Menopausal Status on Sleep and Hot Flashes Throughout Breast Adjuvant Chemotherapy. *Journal of Obstetric, Gynecologic, & Neonatal Nursing* 38 (2009): 353–66.

Bottorff, J. L., C. Kalaw, J. L. Johnson, N. Chambers, M. Stewart, L. Greaves, and M. Kelly. "Unraveling Smoking Ties: How Tobacco Use is Embedded in Couple Interactions." *Research in Nursing & Health* 28 (2005): 316–28.

Bowen, S., and A. B. Zwi. "Pathways to "Evidence-informed" Policy and Practice: A Framework for Action. *PLoS Medicine* 2, no. 7 (May 31, 2005): 1–6. doi:10.1371/journal.pmed.0020166.

Bowling, A., and S. Ebrahim. *Handbook of Health Research Methods: Investigation, Measurement and Analysis.* Berkshire, England: Open University Press/McGraw-Hill Education, 2007.

Bozak, K., B. Yates, and B. Pozehl. "Effects of an Internet Physical Activity Intervention in Adults with Metabolic Syndrome. *Western Journal of Nursing Research* 32 (2010): 5–22.

Brandt, A. M. "Racism and Research: The Case of the Tuskegee Syphilis Study. *Hastings Center Report* 8, no. 6 (1978): 21–29.

Braitman, L. "Confidence Intervals Assess both Clinical Significance and Statistical Significance. *Annals of Internal Medicine* 114 (1991): 515–17.

Brewer, J., and A. Hunter. *Foundations of Multi-methods Research: Synthesizing Styles.* Thousand Oaks, CA: Sage Publications, 2006.

Bryman, A., E. Bell, and J. J. Teevan. *Social Research Methods.* 3rd Canadian ed. Don Mills, ON: Oxford University Press, 2012. ISBN 978-0-19-544296-0.

Burns, N., and S. K. Grove. *Understanding Nursing Research: Building an Evidence-based Practice.* 4th ed. Philadelphia, PA: Saunders/Elsevier, 2007.

Cadena, S. V. "Living Among Strangers: The Needs and Functioning of Persons with Schizophrenia Residing in an Assisted Living Facility." *Issues in Mental Health Nursing* 27, no. 1 (2006): 25–41.

Canadian Council on Animal Care (CCAC). *Three Rs alternatives.* Albert St., Ottawa, ON: CCAC, 2013. Accessed December 01, 2013. http://www.ccac.ca/en_/three.

Canadian Institute of Health Research–Institute of Population and Public Health (CIHR-IPPH). *Institute of Population and Public Health.* Ottawa, ON: CIHR-IPPH, June 27, 2013. Accessed December 02, 2013. http://www.cihr-irsc.gc.ca/e/13777.html.

Canadian Institutes of Health Research, Natural Sciences and Engineering Council of Canada, and Social Sciences and Humanities Research Council of Canada. *Tri-Council Policy Statement: Ethical Conduct for Research Involving Humans.* Ottawa, ON: Public Works and Government Services Canada, 1998, with 2000, 2002, 2005 amendments.

———. *Tri-Council Policy Statement: Ethical Conduct for Research Involving Humans.* Ottawa, ON: Her Majesty the Queen in Right of Canada, 2010.

Ciliska, C., H. Thomas, and C. Buffet. "*An Introduction to Evidence-informed Public Health and a Compendium of Critical Appraisal Tools for Public Health Practice.*" 2008. Accessed November 23, 2013. http://www.nccmt.ca/pubs/eiph_backgrounder.pdf.

Clingerman, E., A. Stuifbergen, and H. Becker. "The Influence of Resources on Perceived Functional Limitations Among Women with Multiple Sclerosis. *Journal of Neuroscience Nursing* 36, no. 6 (2004): 312–21.

Colaizzi, P. "Psychological Research as the Phenomenologist Reviews it." In *Existential Phenomenological Alternatives for Psychology*, edited by R. Valle and M. King. New York: Oxford University Press, 1978.

Commission on the Social Determinants of Health. *Closing the Gap in a Generation. Health Equity Through Action on the Social Determinants of Health.* Geneva, Switzerland: World Health Organization, 2008. ISBN 978 92 4 156370 3.

Community Health Nurses Association of Canada (CHNAC). *Canadian Community Health Nursing Standards of Practice.* CHNAC, May 2003. Accessed March 23, 2008. www.communityhealthnursescanada.org.

Conn, V. S., and M. J. Rantz. "Research Methods: Managing Primary Study Quality in Meta-analyses. *Research in Nursing & Health* 26, no. 4 (2003): 322–33.

Craig, J. V., and R. L. Smyth. *The Evidence-based Practice Manual for Nurses.* Edinburgh, UK: Churchill Livingstone, 2002.

Creswell, J. W. *Research Design: Qualitative, Quantitative, and Mixed Methods Approaches.* 2nd ed. Thousand Oaks, CA: Sage, 2003.

Cullins, S., T. Voth, A. DiCenso, and G. Guyatt. "Finding the Evidence." In *Evidence-based Nursing: A Guide to Clinical Practice*, edited by A. Dicenso, G. Guyatt, and D. K. Ciliska, 20–43. St. Louis, MO: Elsevier/Mosby, 2005.

DeSantis, L., and D. N. Ugarriza. "The Concept of Theme as Used in Qualitative Research. *Western Journal of Nursing Research* 22, no. 3, (2000): 351–77.

DiCenso, A., G. Guyatt, and D. Ciliska. *Evidence-based Nursing: A Guide to Clinical Practice*. St. Louis, MO: Elsevier Mosby, 2005.

Dixon-Woods, M., R. Fitzpatrick, and K. Roberts. "Including Qualitative Research in Systematic Reviews: Opportunities and Problems." *Journal of Evaluation in Clinical Practice* 7, no. 2 (2001): 125–33.

Draucker, C. B. "Processes of Mental Health Service Use by Adolescents with Depression." *Image-The Journal of Nursing Scholarship* 37, no. 2 (2005): 155–62.

Fitzpatrick, J. J., and K. S. Montgomery. *Internet for Nursing Research: A Guide to Strategies, Skills and Resources*. New York: Springer, 2004.

Fogg, T., and C. W. Wightman. "Improving Transcription of Qualitative Research Interviews with Speech Recognition Technology." Paper presented at the Annual Meeting of American Educational Research Association, New Orleans, April 2000.

Forrest, J. L., and S. A. Miller. "The Anatomy of Evidence-based Publications: Article Summaries and Systematic Reviews. *Part I. Journal of Dental Hygiene* 78, no. 2 (2004): 343–48.

Fromer, M. J. *Ethical Issues in Health Care*. St. Louis, MO: C. V. Mosby, 1981.

Funk, S. G., M T. Champagne, R. A. Wiese, and E. M. Tornquist. "Barriers to Using Research Findings in Practice: The Clinician's Perspective." *Applied Nursing Research* 4 (1991): 90–95.

Gerrish, K., and J. Clayton. "Promoting Evidence-based Practice: An Organizational Approach. *Journal of Nursing Management* 12 (2004): 114–23.

Gibson, J. M. E., and M. Kenrick. "Pain and Powerlessness: The Experience of Living with Peripheral Vascular Disease." *Journal of Advanced Nursing* 27 (1998): 737–45.

Giorgi, A. *Phenomenology and Psychological Research*. Pittsburg, PA: Duquesne University Press, 1985.

Glaser, B. G., and A. Strauss. *The Discovery of Grounded Theory: Strategies for Qualitative Research*. New York: Aldine de Gruyter, 1967.

Glaser, E. M., H. H. Abelson, and K. N. Garrison. *Putting Knowledge to Use*. San Francisco, CA: Jossey-Bass, 1983.

Goode, C. J. "What Constitutes "Evidence" in Evidence-based Practice?" *Applied Nursing Research* 13 (2000): 222–25.

Goodman, J. H. "Becoming an Involved Father of an Infant. *Journal of Obstetric, Gynecologic, & Neonatal Nursing* 34, no. 2 (2005): 190–200.

Green, J. C., and V. J. Caracelli, eds., *Advances in Mixed Method Evaluation: The Challenges and Benefits of Integrating Diverse Paradigms*. San Francisco, CA: Jossey-Bass, 1997.

Guyatt, G., and D. Rennie. *Users' Guide to the Medical Literature: Essentials of Evidence-based Clinical Practice*. Chicago: American Medical Association, 2002.

Happ, M., A. Dabbs, J. Tate, A. Hricik, and J. Erlen. "Exemplars of Mixed Methods Data Combination and Analysis. *Nursing Research* 55, no. 2S (2006): S43–S49.

Hawkins, Y., J. Ussher, E. Gilbert, J. Perz, M. Sandoval, and K. Sundquist. "Changes in Sexuality and Intimacy After the Diagnosis and Treatment of Cancer. *Cancer Nursing* 32 (2009): 271–80.

Haynes, R. B., D. L. Sackette, G. J. Guyatt, and P. S. Tugwell. *Clinical Epidemiology: How to do Clinical Practice Research*. 3rd ed. Philadelphia, PA: Lippincott Williams and Wilkens, 2006.

Hoffbrand, A. V. "Research Conduct and the Case of Nancy Olivieri." *The Lancet* 366, no. 9495 (October 2005): 1432–33.

Hunter, A., P. Lusardi, D. Zucker, C. Jacelon, and G. Chandler. "Making Meaning: The Creative Component in Qualitative Research. *Qualitative Health Research* 12 (2002): 388–98.

Irvine, D., L. L. O'Brien-Pallas, M. Murray, R. Cockerill, S. Sidani, B. Laurie-Shaw, and J. Lochhaas-Gerlach. "The Reliability and Validity of Two Health Status Measures for Evaluating Outcomes of Home Care Nursing." *Research in Nursing & Health* 23 (2000): 43–54.

Jabad, A. R., D. L. Cook, A. Jones, T. P. Klassen, P. Tugwell, M. Moher, and D. Moher. "Methodological and Reports on Systematic Reviews and Meta-analyses: A Comparison of Cochrane Reviews with Articles Published in Paper-based Journals." *Journal of the American Medical Association* 280 (1998): 278–80.

Jennings, B. M. "Evidence-based Practice: The Road Best Traveled. *Research in Nursing & Health* 23 (2000): 343–45.

Kovach, M. E. *Indigenous Methodologies: Characteristics, Conversations, and Contexts.* Toronto, ON: University of Toronto Press, Scholarly Publishing Division, 2010.

Levine, R. J. *Ethics and Regulation of Clinical Research.* 2nd ed. Baltimore and Munich: Urban & Schwarzenberg, 1986.

Lewins, A., and C. Silver. *Using Software in Qualitative Research.* Thousand Oaks, CA: Sage, 2007.

Lincoln, Y. S., and E. G. Guba. *Naturalistic Inquiry.* Newbury Park, CA: Sage Publications, 1985.

Logan, J., and I. Graham. "Toward a Comprehensive Interdisciplinary Model of Health Care Research Use. *Science Communication* 20 (1998): 227–46.

Logan, J., M. B. Harrison, I. D. Graham, K. Dunn, and J. Bissonnette. "Evidence-based Pressure-ulcer Practice: The Ottawa Model of Research Use." *Canadian Journal of Nursing Research* 31 (1999): 37–52.

Loiselle, C., and J. Profetto-McGrath. *Canadian Essentials of Nursing Research.* New York: Lippincott Williams & Wilkins, 2004.

Mann, C., and F. Stewart. "Internet Interviewing." In *Handbook of Interview Research: Context and Method,* edited by J. F. Gubrium and J. A. Holstein, 603–27. Thousand Oaks, CA: Sage, 2001.

Mantzoukas, S. "Facilitating Research Students in Formulating Qualitative Research Questions." *Nurse Educator Today* 28 (2008): 371–77.

Marwick, C. "Aspirin's Role in Prevention Now Official." *The Journal of the American Medical Association* 277, no. 9 (1997): 701–02.

McCormack, B., J. Rycroft-Malone, K. Decorby, A. M. Hutchinson, T. Bucknall, B. Kent, A. Schultz, E. Snelgrove-Clarke, C. Stetler, M. Titler, L. Wallin, and V. Wilson. "A Realist Review of Interventions and Strategies to Promote Evidence-informed Healthcare: A Focus on Change Agency." *Implementation Science* 8, no. 8 (September 2013): 107–14. PMID: 24010732.

McFarlane, J. M., J. Y. Groff, J. O'Brien, and K. Watson. "Behaviors of Children Exposed to Intimate Partner Violence Before and 1 Year After a Treatment Program for Their Mother. *Applied Nursing Research* 18, no. 1 (2005): 7–12.

McNeill, P. *The Ethics and Politics of Human Experimentation.* Cambridge, UK: Cambridge University Press, 1993.

Melnyk, B. M., and E. Fineout-Overholt. *Evidence-based Practice in Nursing and Healthcare: A Guide to Best Practice.* Philadelphia, PA: Lippincott Williams & Wilkins, 2005.

Miller, D. C. *Handbook of Research Design & Social Measurement.* 5th ed. Newbury Park, CA: Sage, 1991.

Minister of Supply and Services Canada. Medical Research Council of Canada, Natural Sciences and Engineering Research Council of Canada, and Social Sciences and Humanities Research Council of Canada. *Tri-council Policy Statement: Ethical Conduct for Research Involving Humans.* Ottawa, ON: Author, 1998.

Moffatt, S., M. White, J. Mackintosh, and D. Howel. "Using Quantitative and Qualitative Data in Health Services Research—What Happens When Mixed Method Findings Conflict?" *BMC Health Services Research* 6 (2006): 28.

Naimark, A., B. M. Knoppers, and F. H. Lowy. *Clinical Trials of L1 (deferiprone) at the Hospital for Sick Children: A Review of Facts and Circumstances,* 89–90. Toronto, ON, 1998. Accessed November 30, 2013. http://www.sickkids.on.ca/L1trials/revcontents.asp.

Neutens, J. J., and L. Rubinson. *Research Techniques for the Health Sciences.* 3rd ed. Toronto, ON: Benjamin Cummings, 2002.

Novak, J., and A. Canas. "The Theory Underlying Concept Maps and How to Construct Them." *IHMC CmapTools Technical Report 2006-01.* Pensacola, FL: Institute for Human and Machine Cognition, 2006.

Olivieri, N. F., G. M. Brittenham, C. E. McLaren, D. M. Templeton, R. G. Cameron, R. A. McClelland, A. D. Burt, K. A. Fleming. "Long-term Safety and Effectiveness of Iron-chelation Therapy with Deferiprone for Thalassemia Major." *New England Journal of Medicine* 339 (1998): 417–23.

Oxman, A. D., J. N. Lavis, and A. Fretheim. "Use of Evidence in WHO Recommendations." *The Lancet* 369, no. 9576–9578 (June 2007): 1883–89.

Pach, B. *What Is the "Evidence" in Evidence-based Public Health? Pathways to Evidence Informed Public Health Policy and Practice.* Toronto, ON: Ontario Public Health Libraries Association (OPHL) Foundation Standard Workshop, November 14, 2008.

Phillips, L. R. F. *A Clinician's Guide to the Critique and Utilization of Nursing Research.* Norwalk, CT: Appleton-Century-Crofts, 1986.

Polgar, S., and S. A. Thomas. *Introduction to Research in the Health Sciences.* 5th ed. Toronto, ON: Churchill Livingstone Elsevier, 2008.

Polit, D. F., A. S. London, and J. M. Martinez. *The Health of Poor Urban Women.* New York: MDRC, 2001. http://www.mdrc.org.

Polit, D. F., and C. Tatano Beck. *Nursing Research: Generating and Assessing Evidence for Nursing Practice.* New York: Wolters Kluwe/Lippincott Williams & Wilkins, 2012.

Porter, E. J. "Older Widows' Experiences of Home Care. *Nursing Research* 54, no. 5 (2005): 296–303.

Public Health Agency of Canada. *Core Competencies for Public Health in Canada: Release 1.1.* Ottawa, ON: Author, September 2007.

Robinson, K. M. "Unsolicited Narratives from the Internet: A Rich Source of Qualitative Data." *Qualitative Health Research* 11 (2001): 706–14.

Rombough, R. E., E. L. Howse, and W. J. Bartfay. "Caregiver Strain and Caregiver Burden of Primary Caregivers of Stroke Survivors with and without Aphasia. *Rehabilitation Nursing* 31, no. 5 (2006): 199–209.

Rothman, D. J. "Were Tuskegee and Willowbrook 'studies in nature'?" *Hastings Center Report* 12, no. 2 (1982): 5–7.

Rycroft-Malone, J. "Evidence-informed Practice: From Individual to Context. *Journal of Nursing Management* 16, no. 4 (May 2008): 404–08. doi:10.111/j.1365-2834.2008.00859.x.

Sackett, D. L., S. E. Straus, W. S. Richardson, W. Rosenberg, and R. B. Haynes. *Evidence-based Medicine: How to Practice and Teach EBM.* 2nd ed. Edinburgh, UK: Churchill Livingstone, 2000.

Sandelowski, M. "Combining Qualitative and Quantitative Sampling, Data Collection, and Analysis Techniques in Mixed-methods Studies." *Research in Nursing & Health* 23 (2000): 246–55.

———. "Real Qualitative Researchers Do Not Count: The Use of Numbers in Qualitative Research." *Research in Nursing & Health* 24 (2001): 230–40.

Sandelowski, M., and J. Barroso. "Creating Meta-summaries of Qualitative Findings. *Nursing Research* 52 (2003): 226–33.

———. *Synthesizing Qualitative Research.* New York: Springer Publishing Company, 2006.

Sawatzky-Dickson, D. *Evidence-informed Practice Resource Package.* Winnipeg, MB: Winnipeg Regional Health Authority, November 2010.

Schnarch, B. "Ownership, Control, Access, and Possession (OCAP) or Self-determination Applied to Research: A Critical Analysis of Contemporary First Nations Research and Some Options for First Nations Communities. *Journal of Aboriginal Health* 1 (2004): 80–95.

Schumacher, K. I., B. J. Stewart, P. G. Archbold, M. J. Dodd, and S. L. Dibble. "Family Caregiving Skill: Development of the Concept." *Research in Nursing and Health* 23 (2000): 191–203.

Shaughnessy, M., B. M. Resnick, and R. F. Macko. "Testing a Model of Post-stroke Exercise Behavior." *Rehabilitation Nursing* 31, no. 1 (2006): 15–21.

Snethen, J. A., M. E. Broome, and S. E. Cashin. "Effective Weight Loss for Overweight Children: A Meta-analysis of Intervention Studies." *Journal of Pediatric Nursing* 21, no. 1 (2006): 45–56.

Skinner, H., S. Biscope, and E. Goldberg. "How Adolescents Use Technology for Health Information: Implications for Health Professionals from Focus Group Studies." *Journal of Medical Internet Research* 5 (2003): 32.

Strang, V., P. Koop, S. Dupuis-Blanchard, M. Nordstrom, and B. Thompson. "Family Caregivers and Transition to Long-term Care." *Clinical Nursing Research* 15 (2006): 27–45.

Stetler, C. B. "Refinement of the Stetler/Marram Model for Application of Research Findings to Practice. *Nursing Outlook* 42 (1994): 15–25.

———. "Updating the Stetler Model of Research Utilization to Facilitate Evidence-based Practice. *Nursing Outlook* 49 (2001): 272–79.

Stetler, C. B., M. Brunell, K. K. Giuliano, D. Morsi, L. Prince, and V. Newell-Stokes. "Evidence-based Practice and the Role of Nursing Leadership." *Journal of Nursing Administration* 28, no. 7/8 (1998): 45–53.

Stevens, K. R. "Systematic Reviews: The Heart of Evidence-based Practice." *AACN Clinical Issues* 12 (2001): 529–38.

Steinfels, P., and C. Levine. "Biomedical Ethics and the Shadow of Nazism. *Hastings Center Report.* 6, no. 4 (1976): 1–20.

Streubert Speziale, H. J., and D. Rinaldi Carpenter. *Qualitative Research in Nursing: Advancing the Humanistic Imperative.* New York: Lippincott Williams & Wilkins, 2007.

Tashakkori, A., and C. Teddlie. *Handbook of Mixed Methods in Social and Behavioral Research.* 2nd ed. Thousand Oaks, CA: Sage Publications, 2003.

Talashek, M. L., M. L. Alba, and A. Patel. "Untangling Health Disparities of Teen Pregnancy." *Journal for Specialists in Pediatric Nursing* 11, no. 1 (2006): 14–27.

Taylor, C. "What Packages Are Available?" 2005. Accessed February 15, 2011. http://caqdas.soc.surrey.ac.uk/.

Thabane, I., T. Thomas, C. Ye, and J. Paul. "Posing the Research Question: Not So Simple." *Canadian Journal of Anaesthesiology* 56 (2009): 71–79.

Thomas, L., M. Cullum, E. McColl, N. Rousseau, J. Soutter, and N. Steen. "Guidelines in Professions to Medicine." *Cochrane Database of Systematic Reviews* (2000) No. CD000349.

Thompson, J., P. Baird, and J. Downie. *Report of the Committee of Inquiry on the Case Involving Dr. Nancy Olivieri, the Hospital for Sick Children, the University of Toronto and Apotex Inc.* Toronto, ON: CAUT, 2001. Accessed November 30, 2013. www.dal.ca/committeeofinquiry.

Thurston, N. E., and K.M. King. "Implementing Evidence-based Practice: Walking the Talk." *Applied Nursing Research* 17 (2004): 239–47.

Titler, M. G., C. Kleiber, V. Steelman, B. Rakel, G. Budreau, L. Everett, K. Buckwalter, Tripp-Reimer, T., and C. Goode. "The Iowa Model of Evidence-based Practice to Promote Quality Care." *Critical Care Nursing Clinics of North America* 13 (2001): 497–509.

United States Department of Health and Human Services, Centres for Disease Control and Prevention. *Advancing the Nation's Health: A Guide to Public Health Research Needs, 2006–2015.* Washington, DC: Author, December 2006. Accessed December 02, 2013. http://www.cdc.gov/od/science/quality/docs/AdvancingTheNationsHealth.pdf.

van den Hoonaard, W. C., and A. Connolly. "Anthropological Research in Light of Research-ethics Review: Canadian Master's Theses, 1995–2004. *Journal of Empirical Research on Human Research Ethics* 1 (2006): 59–69.

Van Kaam, A. *Existential Foundations of Psychology.* Pittsburg, PA: Duquesne University Press, 1966.

Vessey, J., and S. Gennarao. "The Ghost of Tuskegee." *Nursing Research* 43, no. 2 (1994): 67–68.

Wiwchar, D. "Nuu-chach-nulth Blood Returns to West Coast." *Ha-Shilth-Sa* 31, no. 25 (2004): 1–4.

Whittemore, R. "Combining Evidence in Nursing Research: Methods and Implications." *Nursing Research* 54, no. 1 (2005): 56–63.

Wishart, L., J. Macerollo, P. Loney, A. King, L. Beaumont, G. Browne, and J. Roberts. "'Special Steps': An Effective Visiting/Walking Program for Persons with Cognitive Impairment." *Canadian Journal of Nursing Research* 31 (2000): 57–71.

Wu, M., L. Hsu, B. Zhang, N. Shen, H. Lu, and S. Li. "The Experiences of Cancer-related Fatigue Among Chinese Children With Leukaemia." *International Journal of Nursing Studies* 47 (2010): 49–59.

Wysocki, A. B. "Basic Versus Applied Research: Intrinsic and Extrinsic Considerations." *Western Journal of Nursing Research* 5, no. 3 (1983): 217–24.

Zauszniewski, J. A., and C. W. Chung. "Resourcefulness and Health Practices of Diabetic Women." *Research in Nursing & Health* 24 (2001): 113–21.242   Chapter 5: Essential Research Methods for the Practice of Public Health

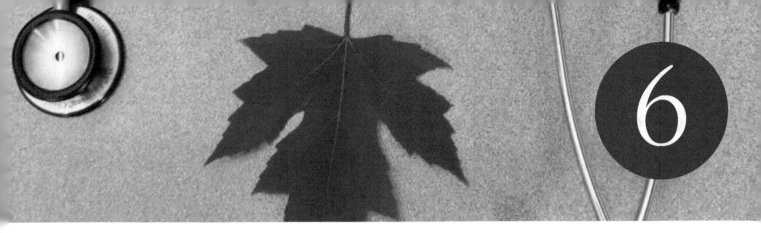

Epidemiology: Essential Concepts for Public Health

To predict the future, you have to create it.

—*Thomas J. Peters*

Learning Objectives

After completion of this chapter, the student will be able to:

- define and differentiate between the terms epidemiology, descriptive epidemiology, and analytical epidemiology,
- identify activities performed by epidemiologists and their relevance to the practice of public health in Canada and globally,
- define and differentiate between the terms endemic, epidemic, and pandemic,
- Define the term surveillance in the context of public health and describe its importance for the tracking of disease or health events in Canada and abroad,
- List and describe the four common stages for the natural history of disease,
- Describe and compare the components of the traditional epidemiological triangle for communicable disease, with the updated and revised epidemiological triangle for noncommunicable disease,
- Define and differentiate between the following measures of disease frequency: prevalence, incidence attack rates, mortality rates, and
- Define and differentiate between the following common measures of association: the relative risk or risk ratio; attributable risk or risk difference; attributable risk percentage; population-attributable risk (PAR); odd ratios.

Core Competencies addressed in Chapter 6

Core Competencies	Competency Statements
1.0 Public Health Sciences	1.2, 1.3, 1.4, 1.5
2.0 Assessment and Analysis	2.2, 2.3, 2.4, 2.5, 2.6
3.0 Policy and Program Planning, Implementation and Evaluation	3.1, 3.6
4.0 Partnerships, Collaboration and Advocacy	4.1
5.0 Diversity and Inclusiveness	5.1, 5.2, 5.3
6.0 Communication	6.1, 6.2
7.0 Leadership	7.2, 7.3

Note: Please see the following document or Web-based link for a detailed description of these specific competencies. Public Health Agency of Canada (2007).

Introduction

A fundamental understanding of the core principles and approaches utilized by epidemiologists are critical to the study and practice of public health in Canada and internationally (Health Canada 2002; Public Health Agency of Canada [PHAC] 2007). Epidemiologists employ a variety of descriptive and analytical epidemiological methods and approaches to provide information to public health professionals and workers that will help them to determine the appropriate primary health care interventions to control, prevent, or manage various identified health problems and concerns affecting diverse populations of Canadians (Bartfay and Bartfay 2015; Schubert and Bartfay 2010).

Epidemiology is defined as the scientific study of the distribution and determinants of health-related states or events in human populations across the lifespan, and the application of this study to maintain, control, and prevent alterations to health and well-being (Bartfay and Bartfay 2015). The term *epidemiology* is derived from the Greek words *epi* meaning upon, on or befall; *demos* meaning the people; and *logos,* a suffix meaning the study of (Merrill 2010). Epidemiology encompasses two basic approaches: (a) *Descriptive epidemiology* and (b) *analytical epidemiology.*

Descriptive epidemiology involves the identification, description, observation, measurement, interpretation, and dissemination of health-related states (e.g., disease present or not), events (e.g., chemical spill), patterns (e.g., how disease may cluster in certain occupations), trends (e.g., aging population in Canada) and/or injury (e.g., work-related, motor vehicle accidents) described by *person, place,* and *time* (Bartfay and Bartfay 2015). Describing epidemiological information by *person* (e.g., age, sex, occupation, ethnicity, race, illicit drug use) allows for the identification of the frequency of disease or other health-related events and helps to identify which individuals are at greatest risk in a defined population or community. High-risk individuals, groups, or populations can be identified by studying their inherent characteristics (e.g., age, sex, race), acquired characteristics (e.g., education level, social and economic status, immunity status), activities (e.g., occupation, exercise, and dietary habits), and access to public primary health care services in their community (e.g., walk-in clinics, availability of public health nurses in a rural community). Describing health information by *place* (e.g., place of employment, residence, province, or town) provides important geographical clues to the presence of causal agents in communities, and how disease or infectious agents may multiple, spread, and be transmitted.

Lastly, providing descriptive epidemiological information by *time* provides valuable information to public health professionals and workers in relation to when the health problem or event began and whether the presence of a disease is predictable. The time aspects may range from a few hours to weeks, years, and decades.

Moreover, when we examine health-related information in terms of *person, place*, and *time*, it often provides important insights into the nature of a disease and other health-related events.

Analytical epidemiology seeks to identify risk factors and/or social determinants of health that help to explain the causation or aetiology of a health-related state, event, or condition (Bartfay and Bartfay 2015). **Aetiology** is the scientific study of all known and suspected risk factors, causes, and/or social determinants of health that may be involved with the development of a health-related state, event, or condition and includes the susceptibility of the individual and the nature of disease agents. The primary purpose of an analytical investigation is to test hypothesized cause-and-effect relationships between a suspected risk factor (e.g., immobility, high fat diet) or social determinant of health (e.g., education, income) and a health-related state, injury, event, or disease outcome (e.g., development of heart disease or stroke). For example, in February 2011, the federal government, in partnership with Genome Canada and the Canadian Institutes of Health Research announced a $4.5 million investment in two national research initiatives aimed at identifying specific genes that cause paediatric cancers and rare genetic diseases (Canadian Institutes of Health Research 2011; Health Council of Canada 2011).

Epidemiologists seek to describe, quantify, and propose causal associations and mechanisms related to health and wellness in diverse populations and communities (Aschengrau and Seage III 2008; Friis and Sellers 2009; Merrill 2010; Neutens and Rubinson 2002; Valanis 1999). The discipline of epidemiology has a population focus since epidemiological investigations are concerned with the collective health and well-being of individuals in a defined population or community. The science of epidemiology is critical to the practice of public health because its methods and approaches provide for a means to assess and understand health-related states or events, noncommunicable and communicable disease processes, injury, morbidity, and mortality. Some of the activities performed by epidemiologists and their importance to the public health include (Bartfay and Bartfay 2015):

- The identification of risk factors related to disease events, injury, morbidity, and death,
- monitoring and describing their natural history,
- identifying which individuals, groups, or populations are at greatest risk, and
- evaluating the efficacy and effectiveness of various primary health care programs and interventions.

This chapter provides an introduction to core epidemiological concepts, approaches, methodologies, and measures that are critical to the education and practice of public health in Canada and globally.

Group Activity-based Learning Box 6.1

How Is Epidemiology Important to the Practice of Public Health in Your Community?
This group activity seeks to highlight the importance of epidemiological resources, methods, and approaches employed by various public health care professionals and workers in diverse communities across Canada. Working in small groups of three to five students, discuss, and answer the following questions:

1. As a public health professional or worker, what epidemiology resources would you utilize to find information about the leading causes of morbidity and mortality in your community?

2. Are there specific diseases, types of injuries, or health concerns that affect your community?

3. How have epidemiological methods or approaches been utilized to describe the characteristics of these affected individuals, groups, or populations?

4. How can epidemiological investigations and findings be utilized to promote the health and well-being of residents in your community?

Historical Developments in Epidemiology: A Brief Overview

Although a detailed review of all the historical developments related to the discipline of epidemiology is beyond the scope and purpose of this chapter, we shall highlight major developments that have impacted the scope and practice of public health in Canada and internationally in this section. An understanding of these historical developments are critical to understanding communicable and noncommunicable diseases and associated measures of disease frequency, morbidity, and mortality rates and trends.

Hippocrates of Cos (460–377 BC)

The use of epidemiological approaches can be traced back to the fifth century BC. The Greek physician and father of modern medicine Hippocrates of Cos (460–377 BC) was the first individual who attempted to explain disease causation from a non-secular or divine perspective. That is to say, Hippocrates was the first to formally dismiss the common belief that disease or states of ill health resulted from angry spirits, demons, or deities, but resulted as a consequence of a break in the laws of nature.

His theory of disease causation was based on an imbalance in the four essential body humours identified as (a) phlegm, (b) yellow bile, (c) black bile, and (d) blood (Adams 1886; Aschengrau and Seage III 2003; Garrison 1963; Lyons and Petrucelli 1978). For example, he believed that fever was caused by too much blood in the body and its treatment, therefore, consisted of returning the body to its natural balance via phlebotomy or the application of leeches. Remarkably, Hippocrates' theory of disease causation was taught to medical students for over 2,000 years following its conception until it was replaced by the germ theory of disease causation in the nineteenth century. Hippocrates suggested that the development of disease or states of ill health might be related to the external as well as the personal environment and lifestyle of individuals (Galin and Ognibene 2007; Hennekens, Buring and Mayrent 1987). The idea of an imbalance (e.g., excess stress levels, high-cholesterol profiles) or deficiencies (e.g., specific vitamins or minerals, lack of exercise) remain key concepts in epidemiology and public health today.

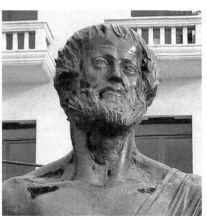

Source: Photo by Wally J. Bartfay

Photo 6.1 Statue of Hippocrates in Thessaloniki, Greece. Hippocrates' theory of disease causation revolutionized medicine in ancient Greece by establishing medicine as a discipline and profession distinct from other fields with which it had traditionally been associated (theurgy and philosophy).

Hippocrates was the first to formally coin the terms *epidemic* and *endemic* in his books entitled *Airs, Waters and Places, Epidemics I* and *Epidemics II*. In his writings, he attempted to explain the occurrence of disease on a rational basis, as opposed to a supernatural one. For example, he argued that disease is, in fact, a mass phenomenon that can affect individuals, groups, or entire populations. **Endemics** are defined as those diseases or illnesses which tend to always be present at low levels in a population in a defined geographical area or region (e.g., chicken pox, seasonal influenza). **Epidemics** are defined as the occurrence of a given disease or illness in clear excess of the normal frequency in a defined geographical area or region (e.g., cholera, West Nile Virus). A **pandemic** is defined as a massive epidemic that involves populations in widespread geographic areas or regions of the world (e.g., HIV/AIDS, SARS). These terms coined by Hippocrates remain in use today in Canada and internationally.

Hippocrates was also the first to describe communicable (aka infectious) diseases such as tetanus and mumps based on the collection of data and careful observations (Garrison 1963; Schubert and Bartfay 2010; Bartfay and Bartfay 2015). His emphasis on the art of clinical inspection, observation and meticulous documentation of findings is evidenced in forty-two preserved case records that are, in fact, the first known documents of clinical assessments (Adams 1886; Galin and Ognibene 2007). These case records describe and detail a variety of ailments and clinical conditions such as dysentery, diarrhoea, pulmonary oedema, malarial fevers, melancholia. and mania. For example, his clinical observations on pulmonary oedema were as follows:

"Water accumulates; the patient has fever and cough; the respiration is fast, the feet become edematous; the nails appear curved and the patient suffers as if he has pus inside, only less severe and more protracted. One can recognize that it is not pus but water … if you put your ear against the chest you hear it seethe inside like sour wine."

(cited in Lyons and Petrucelli 1987, p. 216)"

It is interesting to note that even before the work of Semmelweis (detailed below) and the discovery of germ theory in the nineteenth century, Hippocrates recognized the importance of using clean water for irrigating wounds and the importance of clean hands and nails. For example, he wrote, "*If water is used for irrigation, it had been very pure or boiled, and the hands and nails of the operator* [physician] *were to be cleansed*" (cited in Garrison 1963, p. 98).

Hippocrates also identified diseases as being hot or cold in nature with corresponding treatments that sought to bring the client's condition back to a balanced state (Buck et al. 1988; Cumston 1974). For example, Hippocrates classified diarrhea as a hot disease and believed it could be clinically managed with cold treatments such as eating fruit. Hence, cures for sickness and protection against various diseases and states of ill health were achieved by maintaining a balance and avoiding imbalance in the constitution of individuals. His contributions are still relevant today in reference to the importance of having detailed clinical information for making clinical diagnosis and his observations on how diseases may spread and affect populations.

John Graunt (1620–1674)

The systematic recording of births and deaths in London was initiated in 1603 and was referred to as the *Bills of Mortality* (Garrison 1963; Merrill 2010; Rosen 1958). This was the first official recording of population-based vital statistics in the world. When John Graunt overtook this record keeping task during the mid-seventeenth century, he systematically recorded information related to the person's age, sex, and when the deaths occurred. These demographic characteristics would be examples of descriptive epidemiology employed today in regards to *person, place, and time*. Graunt also employed analytical epidemiological approaches since he sought to determine what killed them (if known), and calculated how many people died each year based on their cause or aetiology. Hence, through his careful analysis of the Bills of Mortality in London, he was able to develop a more comprehensive understanding of a variety of diseases, their sources, and causes of mortality employing both descriptive and analytical epidemiological techniques. The Bills of Mortality were collected in the following manner as described by Graunt:

"When any dies, then, either by tolling, or ringing a Bell, or by bespeaking of a Grave of the Sexton, the same is known to the Searchers … repair to the place, where the dead Corps lies, and by view of the same, and by other enquiries, they examine by what Disease, or Casualty the Corps did die. Hereupon they make their Report to the Parish-Clerk, and he, every Thursday night, carries in an Accompt of all the Burial, and Christning, hapning that Week, to the Clerk of the Hall. On Wednesday the general Accompt is made up, and Printed, and on Thursdays published and dispersed to the several Families, who will pay four shillings per Annum for them.

(Graunt 1939, pp. 25–26)

In 1662, Graunt published his landmark book entitled the *Natural and Political Observations Made Upon the Bills of Mortality*, in which he carefully analyzed the weekly reports of births and death in London, England (Graunt 1662, 1939). Through careful recordings and analysis of the data, Graunt identified variations in mortality rates according to sex, residence in London, age and season of the year (Garrison 1963; Merrill 2010; Rosen 1958). As any good scientist and epidemiologist does today, Graunt kept meticulous records to provide evidence for his findings and conclusions and to establish patterns of disease occurrence. It is interesting to note how many causes of death were attributed to poverty and infectious diseases which were the leading causes of death in Europe before the turn of the present century.

For example, Graunt (1662) reported that there were 5 deaths attributed to gangrene; 8 to plague; 10 deaths related to cancer and wolves; 12 to French pox; 34 deaths in the street attributed to starvation; 38 related to

Table 6.1 Number of Births and Deaths by Sex in England as Reported by Gaunt (1662)

Christened	Buried
Males 4,994	Males 4, 932
Females 4,590	Female 4,603
In All 9,584	In All 9,535

Note: Increase in the burials in the 122 parishes and at the penthouse this year —993. Decrease of the plagues in the 122 parishes and at the penthouse this year—266.

King's Evil; 80 to measles; 445 abortive and stillborn-related deaths; 531 related to flox and smallpox; and 1,108 deaths related to fever. Gaunt utilized a variety of tables to summarize his findings. Table 6.1 is based on data reported by Graunt (1662) related to the number of births (as measured by Christened children) and deaths (as measured by burials) by sex. For example, Graunt reported that only 25:100 children born lived to the age of 26 years. Although mortality rates of adults were found to be lower in comparison, it is noteworthy that only 3:100 adults in London survived to the age of 66 years.

Graunt was the first to classify or divide death (aka mortality) into two major causes: (a) *acute* (sudden in nature) or (b) *chronic* (those which lasted over long periods of time). Graunt was also the first to develop and calculate life expectancy tables or actuarial tables as they are also known today. Walter Wilcox, a noted statistician, recognized the importance of Graunt's pioneering work on births, mortality, and causes of disease in England. For example, Graunt (1939) discovered the numerical regularity of deaths and births, the ratios of males and females at birth and death and the proportion of deaths from certain causes to all causes in successive years and in different areas. Hence, it may be argued that Graunt pioneered and lead the way both for the later discovery of uniformities in many social and volitional phenomena like marriage, suicide, and crime and for a study of these uniformities, their nature, and their limits.

Thomas Sydenham (1624–1689)

Thomas Sydenham (1624–1689) was a graduate of the Oxford Medical School in England. While at Souls College in Oxford, he became acquainted with Robert Boyle who first sparked his interest in epidemics and diseases. Like Hippocrates, Sydenham believed in the importance of detailed clinical observation, and his clinical interpretations resulted in his 1676 book entitled *Observationes Medicae* (Garrison 1963).

Sydenham described and distinguished a variety of diseases, including some psychological disorders and advanced the importance of fresh air, exercise, and eating a healthy diet, which other physicians rejected at the time as relative. These variables remain relevant today in terms of health promotion and prevention and for the management of various noncommunicable chronic diseases (e.g., cardiovascular disease, diabetes). One of the major contributions was his classification of fevers based on three levels that were plaguing London, England, during the 1660s and 1670s: (a) continued fevers, (b) intermittent fevers, and (c) smallpox (Garrison 1963; Merrill 2010). Sydenham gained an excellent reputation with the public and some of his younger open-minded colleagues. Nonetheless, he was also criticized because his ideas and theories sometimes conflicted with traditional Hippocratic approaches that still dominated medical practice during this time.

James Lind (1716–1794)

During the 1700s, it was often stated that "*more armies lost men to disease than to the sword.*" James Lind was a native of Scotland and a Royal Navy surgeon during the eighteenth century who noticed that sailors often developed scurvy in as little time as four to six weeks at sea (Gallin and Ognibene 2007; Merrill 2010; Valanis 1999). Scurvy is a potentially fatal clinical condition marked by extreme weakness, bruising, bleeding of the gums and elsewhere. Lind was influenced by Hippocrates and first looked to the water supply, provisions, and air and weather conditions as possible sources for scurvy. He observed that although the water supply and provisions were of good quality, British seamen still became sick with scurvy. He noted that the incidence of scurvy was most prevalent during ocean voyages for the months April, May, and June, and that thick fog, rainy weather, cold, and dampness were often present.

Lind later examined the eating habits of sailors and noted that their diet was extremely stout and consistent in nature comprising of biscuits, water gruel sweetened with sugar, sago, puddings, barley, mutton broth, and dried meats that were hard on the digestion. While serving upon the HMS Salisbury in 1747, Lind decided to set up an experiment to see if he could treat scurvy via a dietary intervention in twelve sailors affected with the disease. He assigned two sailors each to the following six dietary intervention groups: (a) A quart of cider a day on an empty stomach; (b) two spoonsful of vinegar three times daily on an empty stomach; (c) surgeons elixir; (d) a combination of garlic, mustard seed, and horseradish; (e) a half-pint of sea water daily; or (f) citrus fruit (e.g., limes, oranges, lemons) daily. In addition to these dietary interventions, all sailors with scurvy were given their traditional diet (Lind 1753). In only six days, the groups receiving the dietary intervention of citrus fruits daily were fit to report back to active duty. Conversely, those receiving the other noted dietary interventions remained ill. Lind concluded the following from his experiment at sea:

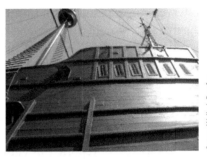

Photo 6.2 Prior to the 19th century, sailors often suffered from scurvy on long ocean voyages, which is a potentially life-threatening condition that we now know is attributed to low levels of ascorbic acid (vitamin C).

Source: Wally J. Bartfay

> I shall here only observe, that the result of my experiments was, that oranges and lemons were the most effective remedies for this distemper at sea. I am apt to think oranges preferable to lemons though perhaps both given together will be found most serviceable.

> (Cited in Stewart and Guthrie, 1953, p. 148)

Although Lind's sample size was relatively small ($N = 12$), he employed the important experimental principle of ensuring that the subjects in his study were similar in nature for comparison purposes (e.g., standard diet also received and all had scurvy). Moreover, he did not base his final conclusions about the beneficial effects of citrus fruit against scurvy from a single experiment, but made his conclusions from replicated studies and data obtained during other voyages at sea. As a consequence of Lind's epidemiological investigations into the nature, causes and observed cure for scurvy, the Royal British Navy has required all sailors to include a daily ration of limes or lime juice in their diet since 1895. This is why British sailors are still affectionately referred to as "Limeys" today.

This example of using scientific evidence to guide dietary practices upon British sailing vessels remains relevant today in regards to evidence-informed practice for public health in Canada and globally. It is also noteworthy that Lind employed scientific approaches to carefully document and assesses the effects of dietary interventions on a specific disease, considered a variety of possible sources and causes for scurvy, and considered sources of disease in reference to *person, place,* and *time.* Hence, Lind employed both descriptive and analytical epidemiological methods to examine how various dietary interventions could be employed to treat scurvy in British sailors. His findings remain relevant today because we have identified various nutritive agents (e.g., vitamins, minerals) that are critical for the promotion and maintenance of health for individuals across the lifespan.

Edward Jenner (1749–1823)

During the mid-1700s, a dairy farmer named Benjamin Jesty observed that although his female dairymaids often contracted cowpox, they never contracted the more deadly smallpox (Buck et al. 1988; Cumston 1926; Gallin and Ognibene 2007; Garrison 1963; Merrill 2010). Jesty believed there was a direct link between this noted observation and the prevention of smallpox. Hence, in 1774 he deliberately inoculated his uninfected wife and children with material taken from an infected dairy maid with a cowpox blister. Although this intervention was successful in providing protection against smallpox, little was publicized about this link.

The Chinese had also made similar observations about so-called "weaker" and "stronger" strains of smallpox, and reported that it was wise to be exposed to a weaker strain so that the client would not get the full-blown and more severe form of the disease. This intervention was known as *variolation*, and similar experiences were reported in Hungary, Turkey, and in the Orient. **Variolation** is defined as a prophylactic intervention that was widely practiced prior to the development of vaccines that involved the intentional and planned inoculation of an uninfected individual with content consisting of pustule matter (containing the virus) derived from an infected person to protect against the more severe form of smallpox.

For example, in 1721, Cotton Mather employed variolation to protect individuals in Massachusetts. Similarly, George Washington ordered the first massive immunization campaign in 1777 to inoculate his Army against smallpox (Fenn 2001; Harper 2000). Sir Hans Sloane had also conducted small studies using variolation, that is, inoculating healthy individuals with pus obtained from blisters of individuals infected with smallpox (Gallin and Ognibene 2007; Garrison 1963).

James Jurin published a series of articles between 1723 and 1727 on mortality rates resulting from smallpox in non-inoculated individuals versus those who had been inoculated (Lilienfeld 1982; Miller 1957).

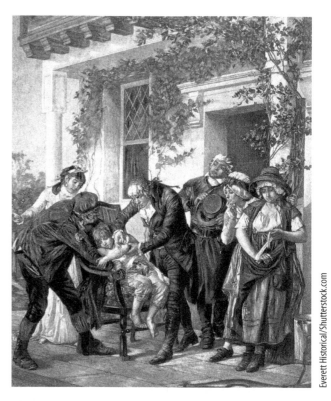

Everett Historical/Shutterstock.com

Photo 6.3 Edward Jenner vaccinating 8-year-old James Phipps with cowpox to provide immunity against the more serious and deadly smallpox in 1796. Immunization remains the most cost-effective public health intervention for controlling and managing vaccine-preventable diseases in Canada and internationally.

For example, Jurin reported that mortality occurred in five of six patients that were not inoculated, in comparison to one in sixty in those inoculated (Lilienfeld 1982; Miller 1957). These reports provide one of the earliest examples in the scientific literature that employed mortality rates as the critical endpoint. In 1734, Voltaire reported that "The Cirassians [a Middle Eastern people] perceived that of a thousand persons hardly one was attacked twice by full blown smallpox … that in a word one never truly has that illness twice in life" (cited in Plotkin 2005).

Edward Jenner was an English rural physician who was aware of these studies and reports, and is credited for developing the first known vaccine against smallpox. Like Jesty, Jenner also personally observed that dairymaids in the English countryside where he practiced contracted cowpox, but did not contract smallpox which was often more fatal by comparison. He noticed that dairymaids, who were servants, were also often required to tend to the sores on the heels of horses affected with cowpox, and the infected pus and fluids discharged from these sores were referred to as *the grease* of cowpox. The dairymaids often would not clean their hands affected with this grease, and would consequently spread the incidence of cowpox on the farm they worked at. In turn, the infected cows would transmit the cowpox to the dairymaids. Jenner convinced a dairymaid to permit him to rub a small amount of "infectious grease" into a small wound (incision) on her arm that he made. The dairymaid did not become ill and Jenner subsequently utilized this knowledge to invent a vaccine against smallpox.

It is notable that the Worldwide Global Smallpox Eradication Campaign began in the late 1960s. On October 26, 1977, World Health Organization workers reported that they tracked down the last known case of naturally occurring smallpox in the world. The patient was Ali Maow Maalin, a hospital cook residing in Merka, Somalia. Vaccination remains a prominent public health primary prevention intervention in Canada and globally against a variety of communicable (infectious) diseases.

William Farr (1807–1883)

When Graunt died, little was done to advance or continue on with his work related to the Bills of Mortality (described earlier) until almost 200 years later when William Farr (1807–1883) was appointed registrar general of London in 1839 (Garrison 1963; Hennekens, Buring, and Mayrent 1987; Humphreys 1885; Merrill 2010; Rosen 1958). Farr was a trained physician and self-taught mathematician. Farr embraced and built upon the ideas and work of Graunt. One of his most important contributions involved calculations that combined registration data on births, deaths, and marriages (as the numerator) with census data on the population size (as the denominator).

He recognized that data collection from human populations could be employed to learn about disease and illness. He replaced Graunt's concept of *political arithmetic* with the contemporary term *statistics*. Farr extended the use of vital statistics as measures of public health and developed a modern population-based vital statistics system, which serves as the basis for recording vital health statistics in Canada and internationally today. He established a system for the routine compilation of vital statistics such as mortality rates and published his findings during the next forty years in his *Annual Reports of the Registrar General*.

Farr invented the standardized mortality rate, which is a method for making fair comparisons between groups with different age structures. For example, Table 6.2 shows the annual mortality rate per hundred males and females in England and Wales for the years 1838 to 1871 by specific age groups. Standardized mortality rates for various age groups are still routinely reported and employed to identify demographic trends and at risk groups in public health. In his first annual report in 1839, Farr noted the "superior precision of numerical expressions" over literary expressions (Farr 1975, p. 214). He also reported that mortality rates decreased following improvements in sanitation; individuals who lived in densely populated areas had higher mortality rates due to cholera than those who lived in less crowed areas, and individuals who lived at higher elevations had lower death rates than those residing in lower elevations (Farr 1975).

Farr made several insightful observations based on meticulous comparisons between various cohorts of individuals such as mortality patterns for single versus married individuals; workers in different occupations such as metal mines, and those in the earthenware industry. He investigated the effects of imprisonment on mortality rates, and reported associations between the elevation of sea level and deaths from cholera. He also advanced

Table 6.2 Annual Mortality per Hundred Males and Females in England and Wales 1838–1871

Age (years)	Males	Females
0–4	7.26	6.27
5–9	0.87	0.85
10–14	0.49	0.50
15–24	0.78	0.80
25–34	0.99	1.01
35–44	1.30	1.23
45–54	1.85	1.56
55–64	3.20	2.80
65–74	6.71	5.89
75–84	14.71	13.43
85–94	30.55	27.95
95+	44.11	43.04

Source: Data adapted from William Farr (1975).

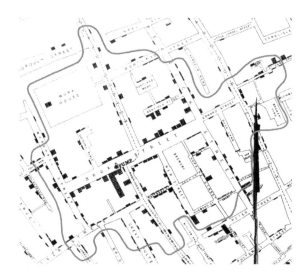

Figure 6.1 John Snow's map showing deaths attributed to cholera by location in London.

John Snow found that cholera deaths in London were clustered near the Broad Street water pump. Each black block represents a death and can be interpreted as a primitive bar graph.

Source: Snow (1855).

the notion that certain diseases, especially those which are chronic in nature, may have multifactorial aetiology (causes). Farr also devised a categorization system for the causes of death in England, which was an antecedent for the modern *World Health Organization's International Statistical Classification of Diseases & Related Health Problems (ICD-10)* classification system that is utilized around the world. Hence, Farr established a methodological tradition in epidemiology and public health which remains relevant today including the importance of defining your target population at risk, choosing an appropriate comparison (control) group, and ascertaining how other contributing factors (e.g., age, duration of exposure) may affect mortality outcomes (Figure 6.1).

John Snow (1813–1858)

John Snow was a highly respected physician of the royal family in England during the 1850s. He was also a noted researcher of anaesthetic gases, and administered chloroform to Queen Victoria during the birth of her children (Aschengrau and Seage III 2008; Friis and Sellers 2009; Gallin and Ognibene 2007; Merrill 2010). Snow became interested to determine the cause of cholera in London, and reasoned that the epidemic was linked to water supplies contaminated with fecal material. Cholera is a sudden potentially life-threatening enteric disease characterized by watery diarrhea, vomiting, severe fluid and electrolyte loss, rapid dehydration, weakness, and circulatory collapse. On the basis of descriptive data and careful observation, Snow hypothesized that cholera was transmitted by sewage-contaminated water. Snow reported:

> Within two-hundred and fifty yards of the spot where Cambridge Street joins Broad Street, there were upwards of five hundred fatal attacks of cholera in ten days. The mortality in this limited area probably equals any that was ever caused in this country, even by the plague; and it was much more sudden, as the greater number of cases terminated in a few hours …. As soon as I became acquitted with the situation and extent of this irruption of cholera, I suspected some contamination of the water of the much-frequented street-pump in Broad Street…. (Snow 1965, pp. 38–39)

Snow conducted two major descriptive epidemiological investigations on cholera in London. The first involved a cholera outbreak in the Soho district of London in the Broad Street area. The second entailed an analytic epidemiological investigation of the cholera epidemic in which he compared mortality rates based on the source of the water supply drunk, namely the Lambeth Water Company or the Southwark and Vauxhall Water Company (Snow 1855, 1965).

Consequently, Snow was finally able to provide statistical evidence in support of his water-borne hypothesis for cholera. Snow skilfully utilized observational methods, conducted neighbourhood interviews, and analyzed mortality records according to geographical locations and the specific water supply company source from August 1853 to January 1854. He carefully researched and mapped his data where deaths were occurring in London by households. Snow personally walked from house to house and for every dwelling in London in which a cholera death was reported to assess which water company supplied the household.

The data shown in Table 6.3 provides numerical evidence that water supplied by the Southwark and Vauxhall Company were responsible for the cholera outbreaks. Snow noted that residents who obtained their water supplies from this company had more fecal contamination present because it was obtained from a downstream source on the Thames River ($N = 1263$). Conversely, upstream sources of water obtained from the Lambeth company had less fecal contamination and therefore less associated incidences of cholera ($N = 98$). To make comparisons more meaningful between the two water supply companies, Snow also standardized the deaths rates per 10,000 houses for the Southward and Vauxhall company ($N = 315$) versus the Lambeth company ($N = 37$).

Today, we know that cholera is caused by the bacterial agent *Vibrio cholerate*, which flourishes in contaminated water supplies. Although Snow did not identify the specific bacterial agent responsible for the cholera epidemics in London, his work on the importance of having safe and clean water supplies still has significance today in public health. At present, ensuring a clean and safe water supply for a community (i.e., the environment) continues to play a key role in controlling water-borne diseases such as cholera and dysentery in humans. In fact, we argue that maintaining a safe water supply remains one of the most basic yet all-important public health measures in Canada and globally. During the summer of 2000, the water supply in Walkerton, Ontario, became contaminated with *Escherichia coli* 0157:57 (Ali 2004; O'Conner 2002). Consequently, more than 2,300 residents of Walkerton became severely ill, 7 died and the economic impact was estimated to be in excess of $64.5 million (Canadian) (Sullivan 2004).

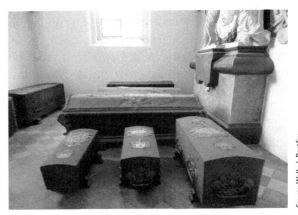

Source: Wally J. Bartfay

Ignaz Philipp Semmelweis (1818–1865)

Ignaz Semmelweis (1818–1865) was a Hungarian-born physician who performed the most sophisticated preventive clinical trial of the nineteenth century and confirmed the importance of proper handwashing by health care professionals to prevent the spread of clinical infections (Gallin and Ognibene 2007; Friis and Sellers 2009; Merrill 2010). During the mid-1800s, one of the greatest fears of

Photo 6.4 Childbed fever claimed the lives of many mothers and their children (small coffins) in Europe prior to Semmelweis' handwashing intervention. It is important to acknowledge that his scientific insights predate those of the germ theory for infectious diseases by Louis Pasteur (1822–1895) and Robert Koch (1843–1910). Today handwashing remains a critical primary preventive component for infection control in both clinical and community-based settings.

Table 6.3 Death Rates From Cholera in London, England 1853–1854 According to Water Supply Company

Water supply company	Number of houses	Deaths from cholera	Deaths per 10,000 houses
Southwark and Vauxhall	40,046	1,263	315
Lambeth	26,107	98	37
Rest of London	256,423	1,422	59

Source: Adapted from John Snow (1855).

expectant mothers was dying of childbed fever (aka puerperal sepsis). Childbed fever, as the name suggests, is a potentially life-threatening streptococcal uterine infection characterized by high fever, which is usually of the placental site and occurs shortly after delivery. Often the child would also become infected and die.

Semmelweis became an assistant in the first obstetric ward of the Allgemerines Krankenhaus in Vienna in 1846. Semmelweis observed that when the medical education system changed in 1840, he found a much higher mortality rate among the women on the teaching wards (i.e., First Maternity Division) where medical students and physicians were present, in comparison to the midwife-run ward (i.e., Second Maternity Division). From 1841 to 1846, the maternal mortality rate was approximately 10%–50% for the First Division of the Vienna General Hospital, in comparison to 2%–3% for the Second Division. The general public knew of this marked disparity and feared being assigned to the First Maternity Division to have their babies delivered by medical students and physicians.

Semmelweis and his fellow physician Jakob Kollestschka became frustrated by this mystery and began to dissect victims of childbed fever in the hope of shedding more light onto the nature or cause of the disease. Kollestschka received a small cut on his finger during one of these autopsies and later died of a high fever that was similar in characteristics with childbed fever. Semmelweis hypothesized that medical students and physicians on the First Maternity Ward had somehow contaminated their hands while performing autopsies on cadavers, and that childbed fever was "caused by conveyance to the pregnant women of putrid particles derived from living organisms, through the agency of the examining fingers" (Gallin and Ognibene 2007, p. 7). In fact, medical students and physicians would often come directly from the death house after performing autopsies on decaying bodies and then conduct internal pelvic exams on expectant mothers without washing their hands. Consequently, medical students and physicians transmitted infections while attending to women in the First Maternity Ward. By contrast, midwives did not perform autopsies on cadavers and therefore did not pass along these putrid particles derived from living organisms to the women they attended on the Second Maternity Ward of the hospital (Semmelweis 1861; Semmelweis and Murphy 1941; Iffy et al. 1979).

In 1847, Semmelweis conducted a preventive clinical trial that required all medical students, physicians, and midwives to scrub their hands with chlorinated lime before entering any maternity ward in the hospital and administering care to women. The percentage of deaths in 1848 after this intervention was 1.3%, compared with 12.1% in 1842 (Semmelweis 1861; Semmelweis and Murphy 1941). Despite the convincing evidence, Semmelweis' discovery was discounted by most of his colleagues who accused him of insubordination. The dominant thinking of the time was that the high mortality was due to women being impoverished. Nonetheless, he decided to publish his findings which showed the remarkable effects of his handwashing intervention with chlorinated lime (intervention group) on decreasing mortality, in comparison to the non-chlorinated lime handwashing group (i.e., pre-1847 control group comprised of medical students and physicians) (Semmelweis 1861; Semmelweis and Murphy 1941). It is important to note that the scientific insights of Semmelweis predated those of the germ theory for infectious disease by Louis Pasteur (1822–1895) and Robert Koch (1843–1910). Today, handwashing remains a critical primary preventative component for infection control in both clinical and community-based practice settings.

Twentieth-Century Developments in Epidemiology and Public Health

The twentieth century marks the beginning of major developments in our understanding of modifiable (e.g., smoking, diet) and nonmodifiable (e.g., sex, genetic predisposition) risk factors and various social determinants of health (e.g., poverty, level of education, unemployment) associated with the development of noncommunicable

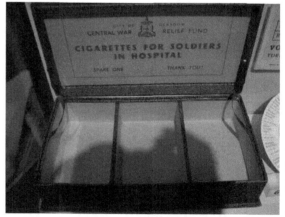

Source: Wally J. Bartfay

Photo 6.5 A war-time cigarette donation box for hospitalized soldiers in Scotland. Cigarette smoking was widely promoted as a social pleasure and norm during and after WWII by large tobacco companies and was glamorized by the film industry in Hollywood.

chronic diseases such as heart disease and cancer. Although a discussion of all epidemiological contributions made to our understanding of noncommunicable diseases is beyond the scope and purpose of this chapter, we shall highlight two major studies that remain as gold standards in the field of population-based epidemiology.

Doll and Hill's Landmark Studies on Smoking and Lung Cancer

Most scholars in the public and allied health sciences consider Richard Doll and A. Bradford Hill's study on the relationship between smoking by British physicians, and the development of lung cancer and mortality to be one of the major milestones of epidemiology during the twentieth century (Doll and Hill 1950, 1954; Doll et al. 2004). These researchers were disturbed by the striking increase in mortality related to lung cancer in males and females in England and Wales following World War II. It was thought by some that this increase was simply attributed to better diagnosis through technological innovations such as X-ray machines. However, Doll and Hill reasoned that improved diagnosis could not be entirely responsible, especially in light of the fact the lung cancer mortality rates had increased in geographical areas that did not have these modern diagnostic X-ray facilities. Like the Framingham Heart Study (described below), this study was emblematic of a shift in public health from infectious to chronic diseases following World War II. Indeed, the shift was fuelled by the belief that chronic diseases were not merely attributed to degenerative disorders of aging, but may have preventative environmental and lifestyle origins (Aschengrau and Seage III 2008; Susser 1985).

Doll and Hill's first study consisted of a case–control study which included 709 subjects (British physicians) who had lung cancer (the cases) and 709 subjects (also British physicians) who had diseases other than cancer (the controls). Controls were chosen based on the same sex, had to have practiced in the same hospital at approximately the same time as cases and were within a five-year age group (Doll and Hill 1950). The researchers found that 99.7% of male lung cancer subjects and 95.8% of male noncancerous subjects smoked; 68.3% of female lung cancer subjects and only 46.7% of female noncancerous subjects were smokers. Moreover, a higher proportion of subjects who self-identified themselves as heavy smokers, defined as twenty-five or more cigarettes smoked per day, had lung cancer (26% of male cancer subjects and 13.5% of male noncancerous subjects). Although the researchers did not identify any potential carcinogens in tobacco that may account for these findings, they did conclude that smoking is an important lifestyle factor in the cause of lung cancer.

In 1951, Doll and Hill (1954) conducted a prospective study comprised of a short smoking questionnaire covering 59,600 male and female registered members of the British Medical Association. The investigators divided the respondents into the following four main groups based on the responses obtained on their questionnaire: (a) nonsmokers, (b) light smokers, (c) moderate smokers, and (d) heavy smokers. After a period of 29 months following completion of their smoking questionnaire, the researchers reported 789 deaths among the 24,389 male physicians aged 35 years or older. After adjusting for age differences between the four smoking groups, Doll and Hill (1954) found that mortality rates attributed to lung cancer were 0.0 per 1,000 among the nonsmokers, 0.48 per 1,000 among light smokers, 0.67 per 1,000 among moderate smokers, and 1.14 per 1,000 among heavy smokers.

The researchers subsequently followed this cohort of British physicians for the next five decades (Doll et al. 2004). During this study period, the researchers reported that of the 34,439 male subjects studied, 25,346 died between the period of 1951 and 2001. Notably, mortality rates were found to be two to three times higher in lifelong smokers, in comparison to nonsmokers. The associated causes of deaths not only included lung cancer but also heart disease, a variety of vascular diseases and stroke, and chronic obstructive lung diseases. The researchers also found that the risk of mortality attributed to smoking steadily declined among ex-smokers in terms of the number of years they had stopped smoking.

This investigation was important for a number of reasons. First, it identified that lung cancer may have important lifestyle risk factors in terms of smoking history, intensity, and duration. Second, the prospective nature of the study was critical in determining the development of various chronic diseases (e.g., lung cancer, heart disease) that often take decades to clinically manifest. Third, the researchers incorporated changes in smoking habits over time in their analysis of the data, and therefore were able to objectively examine the health benefits of smoking cessation. Fourth, the researchers employed epidemiological approaches to help bring about a shift in public health after World War II from infectious to chronic noninfectious diseases.

Framingham Heart Study

The pioneering Framingham Heart Study, which began in 1948 in Framingham, Massachusetts, is an ongoing prospective cohort study which has identified a number of modifiable lifestyle (e.g., diet, exercise, smoking) and non-modifiable (e.g., sex, age, genetic predisposition) risk factors and social determinants of health (e.g., poverty, socioeconomic status, education level) for the development of heart disease (Dawber 1980; Dawber, Kannel and Lyell 1963; Dawber, Meadors, and Moore 1951; Kannell 2000; Kannell and Abbott 1984). Framingham is a small town located approximately 18 miles west of Boston. This location was chosen because it was implied that it represented a cross section of the American population; it was a fairly stable population; residents could easily access the two major hospitals in the community; local physicians were eager to help recruit subjects for the study; an annual updated population list was kept, and a broad range of occupations, industries, and incomes were represented. Framingham had a population of 28,000 residents when the investigation first began. The study design consisted of a random sample of 6,500 subjects from the targeted age range of 30–59 years for this large-scale epidemiological investigation. It is important to note that subjects in this prospective cohort study were not heterogeneous in terms of their exposures nor were they selected because of a particular exposure level or risk factor per se for disease. Hence, the frequency of the exposures within this study was expected to be representative of the target population.

The subjects were subsequently followed for a period of almost seven decades now, and were given physical examinations (e.g., blood pressure, pulse, height and weight); laboratory tests (e.g., cholesterol levels, glucose levels, bone mineral density, genetic characteristics), questionnaires and a variety of other health-related end points were examined every two years. The quantitative data was assessed to track changes in the incidence of disease and changes in identified risk factors. Several clinical categories of heart disease were distinguished in this cohort study, including myocardial infarction, angina pectoris, coronary insufficiency, and death from coronary heart disease. This study is notable because it has brought about a global shift in the focus for public health from noninfectious diseases post World War II to noncommunicable chronic diseases (e.g., cardiovascular disease, diabetes, Alzheimer's disease) (Aschengrau and Seage III 2008; Susser 1985). Susser (1985) maintains that the Framingham study has become the epitome of successful epidemiological research and is undisputedly the foundation keystone for current ideas about risk factors in general, and the prevention of ischemic heart disease in particular.

Current Developments in Epidemiology and Public Health

The use of epidemiological approaches to investigate various health and disease outcomes in diverse populations across the lifespan has exploded during the past few decades. For example, in a widely quoted editorial in the *New England Journal of Medicine,* Angell (1990) argued for the need and growth of epidemiological investigations, especially those which examine the associations between chronic degenerative diseases and modifiable lifestyle risk factors such as exercise and diet in our modern society. Indeed, it would be difficult to investigate specific lifestyle risk factors or the impacts of various social determinants of health through experimental studies. In addition, in certain cases it would be deemed impractical or unethical in nature.

For example, it would be unethical for researchers to expose half of a group of children to lead for ten years to compare their IQ scores twenty years later with those of the unexposed children (controls). Consequently, we must therefore rely on epidemiological (or observational) studies to arrive at these conclusions (Angell 1990). Almost every day, Canadians encounter media reports of epidemiological research into such diverse public health concerns such as the H1N1 pandemic, colon cancer screening, the health effects of second-hand smoke, chemical spills into our environment, growth of obesity in children and adults, increases in the incidence of type 2 diabetes in First Nation's peoples, and the increasing incidence of Alzheimer's disease in our aging population, for example.

Health Surveillance

The Public Health Agency of Canada (2007) reports that surveillance is a critical feature of public health and consists of the systematic collection and analysis of health-related data and timely communication of these associated health reports to health professionals, workers, and the general public when action is required. The Kirby Commission (2003, p. 26) defines health **surveillance** in Canada as:

> the tracking and forecasting of any health event or health determinant through the continuous collection of high-quality data, the integration, analysis and interpretation of those data into reports, advisories, alerts, and warnings, and the dissemination to those who need to know.

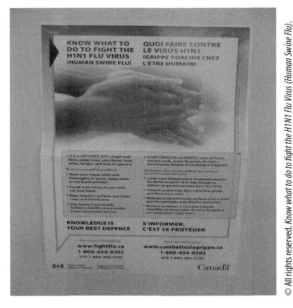

Photo 6.6 A public health primary prevention poster by the PHAC encouraging individuals to wash their hands to help combat the H1N1 flu virus.

The information gathered can be utilized to estimate the magnitude of disease or health conditions in various geographical regions in Canada, better understand the natural history of a disease and/or detect potential emerging epidemics (Teutsch, Churchill, and Elliot 1994).

Both national and provincial/territorial legislation decrees which diseases will be reported and which public health agency is responsible for reporting them. In addition, certain communicable diseases are also tracked globally and reported to the International Health Regulations (IHR) Branch of the World Health Organization (WHO 2006a, 2006b). At present, the only communicable diseases that require international notification are the plague, yellow fever, and cholera (Heymann 2004). Nonetheless, a number of communicable diseases (e.g., Avian flu, influenza, HIV/AIDS, tuberculosis) are regarded as diseases under surveillance and require reporting at varied frequencies to the IHR Branch of WHO. The emergence of Avian flu, Severe Acute Respiratory Syndrome (SARS) and West Nile virus has highlighted the critical public health need for tracking and surveying diseases in Canada and globally. Refer Chapter 9 for a detailed discussion of reportable diseases in Canada and internationally, along with emerging communicable and noncommunicable diseases under surveillance.

For example, Quinlan and Dickinson (2009) report that the West Nile virus first appeared in Canada in 2001. Public health officials responded by including the surveillance of infected humans, mosquitoes, horses, and birds (e.g., crows, blue jays). By 2002, public health officials in Canada documented the presence of this virus in Nova Scotia, Quebec, Ontario, Manitoba and Saskatchewan. The Public Health Agency of Canada (2006) reported that 1,300 human cases were identified in 2003, 29 in 2004, and 224 in 2005. In 2012, ten species of mosquitoes were identified that could transmit the West Nile virus to humans (PHAC 2012). Figure 6.2 shows the number of clinical cases and asymptomatic infections of West Nile virus in Canada in 2012.

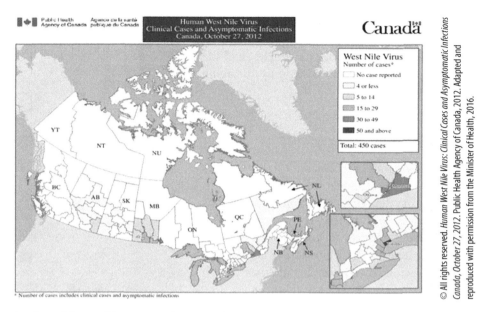

Figure 6.2 A map by the Public Health Agency of Canada showing the distribution of the West Nile Virus in Canada in 2012 (number of clinical cases and asymptomatic infections).

West Nile Virus first appeared in Windsor, Ontario on August 8, 2001, and has quickly spread to other regions. As of October 27, 2012, there have been a total of 450 West Nile Virus human clinical cases and asymptomatic infections reported in Canada.

Basic Concepts in the Epidemiological Approach

The Epidemiological Triangle of Communicable Disease

One of the major functions in epidemiological investigations for public health entails the study of altered states of health and communicable (i.e., infectious) disease in relation to their cause or aetiology (Schubert and Bartfay 2010). In order to ascertain the root cause of a communicable disease or altered states of health, the epidemiologist must first carefully consider the following four multifactorial elements (see Figure 6.3): (a) host, (b) agent, (c) environment, and (d) time.

The interactions between the host, agent, environment, and time are critical for tracing the aetiology (i.e., cause) of a communicable disease or other altered health condition. One of the primary aims of epidemiology is to provide information to public health professionals and workers that results in the disruption or breaking of one or more of the components of this triangle (Figure 6.3). A communicable disease, therefore, can potentially be stopped when one or more of the components of the triangle are intersected with a primary health care intervention. For example, primary prevention public immunization campaigns against a variety of known communicable diseases (e.g., tuberculosis, measles, rubella, chicken pox) help to prevent both the development and spread of disease by boosting the active immunity status of the host which develops antibodies (i.e., immunity) against the disease. Similarly, the importance of public health handwashing education campaigns can help break the chain of infection from person to person in a defined community. The reader is referred to Chapter 5 for a detailed description of the five levels of prevention.

Host

The **host** refers to the animal and/or human on which the agent acts to create disease or altered states of health and well-being. The host offers subsistence or a home for the pathogen to become established, although the host may or may not always develop the particular disease (see the following Typhoid Mary). Indeed, the level of immunity, genetic makeup, level of exposure and/or overall level of health and well-being can determine the extent of the effects of the pathogen on the host (Aschengrau and Seage III 2008; Friis and Sellers 2009; Merrill 2010). Similarly, the existences of preexisting disease or immune-competence are also key factors

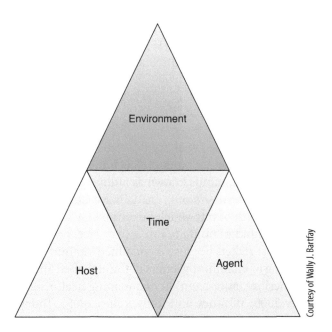

Figure 6.3 Epidemiological triangle of communicable disease.

known to affect the host's susceptibility and resistance to disease. For example, the development of opportunistic infections such as toxoplasmosis or tuberculosis in hosts already infected with HIV/AIDS is an example of a poor host resistance. Hence, all of these factors need to be considered when examining the role of the host in the epidemiological triangle.

During the early 1900s, approximately 350,000 cases of typhoid fever were reported annually in the United States alone (Health News 1968; Merrill 2010; Nester et al. 1973). **Typhoid fever** is a highly infectious disease clinically characterized by a high fever, rose-coloured spots on the chest or abdomen, electrolyte imbalance due to diarrhea, mental depression, physical weakness, and occasional intestinal haemorrhage and perforation of the bowel. Mary Mallon (aka *Typhoid Mary*) was responsible for transmitting typhoid fever to several hundred of individuals during a fifteen-year time period. Mallon was an Irish cook who worked in several people's home and in hospitals in New York and New Jersey. Bacteriological examination of Mallon's stool revealed that she was a chronic carrier of the disease, but like 20% of all carriers she exhibited no overt signs or symptoms. From 1907 to 1910, Mallon was placed under quarantine by public health officials in New York. As a consequence of legal actions she initiated, Mallon was released in 1910 and then disappeared.

Two years later, public health officials discovered that 200 individuals became infected in two hospitals in New York and New Jersey where Mallon worked as a cook under a different alias. This incident taught public health officials about the importance of keeping track of known carriers, and that carriers of typhoid should never be permitted to handle food or drink intended for consumption by others. In her later years, Mallon accepted voluntary quarantine to help public health officials break the chain of infection, and she later died at the age of 70 years in isolation (Health News 1968; Merrill 2010; Nester et al. 1973). Today, antibiotic therapy is used in the treatment of typhoid fever and the surgical removal of the gallbladder provides cure in approximately 60% of confirmed carriers (Mauser and Bahn 1974; Shindell, Salloway, and Oberembi 1976).

Agent

The **agent** is defined as "a toxic substance, microorganism, or environmental factor, such as radiation or a lifestyle, which must be present (or absent) for the problem to occur" (Schubert and Bartfay 2010, p. 176). Analytical epidemiology seeks to define and establish the link between the agent and the communicable disease or altered state of health in order to determine causality. An example is the link between exposure to asbestos (i.e., the agent) and mortality in building trade insulation workers and miners due to cancer of the lung, stomach and colon (Enterline 1965; Friis and Sellers 2009; Hales and Lauzon 2007; Selikoff, Hammond, and Churg 1968). According to Lillienfeld and Stolley (1994), disease agents or aetiological factors can be classified into the following four categories: (a) nutritive agents/elements, (b) chemical agents/elements, (c) physical agents, and (d) infectious agents.

Nutritive Agents

Nutritive agents consist of nutritional substances that are deficient or excessive within a host (Bartfay and Bartfay 2015). In 1911, the Polish chemist Casimir Funk (1884–1967) isolated a chemical substance that he believed belonged to a class of chemical compounds known as amines. He later added the Latin term for life (*vita*) to these compounds and coined the term *vitamin*. In 1916, McCollum subsequently showed that two factors were required for the normal growth of rats which he termed fat-soluble "A" factor (present in butter and fats) and water-soluble "B" factor found in nonfatty foods (e.g., rice, grains). It was later discovered that cod liver oil was an effective cure against rickets because it contained vitamin D.

These discoveries lead to the labeling of vitamins by letters of the alphabet, and also the importance of other trace elements (e.g., zinc, iron, magnesium, potassium) in maintaining health across the lifespan (Krause and Hunscher 1975; Sizer and Whitney 2000; Whitney and Rady Rolfes 2005). Today, dietary interventions are critical for both the preservation and maintenance of health for individuals across the lifespan. Public health care professions and workers seek to educate targeted groups which have been shown to be a high risk of having a deficit of a critical nutritive agent.

For example, infants who are exclusively breast-fed may be at risk for developing a vitamin D deficiency. Hence, public health professionals (e.g., physicians, public health nurses, dieticians) recommend that these infants receive a daily supplement of 400 international units (IU) of vitamin D per day in accordance with Canadian national nutritional guidelines (Health Canada 2000, 1999). On the other hand, public health care professionals and workers must also educate individuals about the risk of taking nutritive agents in excess. For example, although nutritive deficiencies of vitamin C (ascorbic acid) have been associated with the development of scurvy, excess consumption of this water-soluble vitamin can lead to the development of renal calculi (kidney stones) (Sizer and Whitney 2000; Whitney and Rady Rolfes 2005).

Chemical Agents

Chemical agents consist of a variety of chemicals, solvents and compounds (e.g., pharmaceuticals, acids, alkali compounds, heavy metals, poisons, and some enzymes) that can result in the development of disease or alterations to health (Bartfay and Bartfay 2015). For example, lead exposure either through ingestion (e.g., lead-based paint chips, drinking water from lead pipes) or inhalation (e.g., industrial emissions, stained-glass making) remains an environmental threat to the health and safety of Canadians. Lead may continue to leach into drinking water supplies in homes built in Canada prior to the 1930s (Donatelle et al. 2006). Similarly, homes built prior to the 1960s remain a treat due to lead-based paints that were widely utilized (Hales and Lauzon 2007).

Figure 6.4 shows possible environmental sources of toxic lead in Canada. Shah (2002) reports that automotive emissions were a significant source of environmental lead exposure until 1975, when unleaded gasoline was finally introduced into Canada. Lead poisoning, or plumbism, occurs in both urban and rural settings and is characterized by lethargy, anorexia, sporadic vomiting, intermittent abdominal pain, constipation, hyperactivity, and alterations to behaviours, damage to the nervous system, encephalopathy, seizures, and coma (Mandleco and Bartfay 2010; Sanborn et al. 2002; Shah 2003). There is a growing body of evidence which indicates that even small amounts of lead *in utero* or during infancy and early childhood can have profound effects on the child in reference to impaired intellectual development, behavioural difficulties, problems concentrating, neurological impairments, decreased intellectual and physical growth and hearing loss (Mandleco and Bartfay 2010; Sanborn et al. 2002). In fact, lead is easily and rapidly absorbed

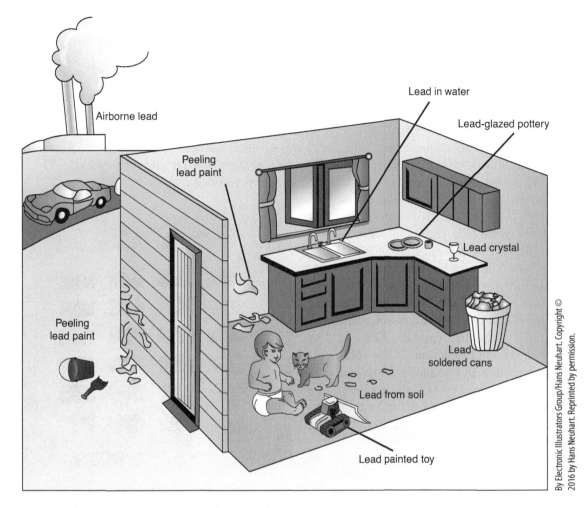

Figure 6.4 Possible environmental sources of toxic lead.

Lead in the environment remains a significant public health challenge, especially in homes built prior to the 1960s in Canada.

into the bloodstream and is often deposited in soft tissues and bone, and children absorb a higher proportion of ingested lead than adults (50% compared to 10% in adults) (Shah 2003).

Physical Agents

Physical agents include natural forces, forms of energy or mechanical agents that may negatively affect the health and well-being of humans (e.g., radiation, excessive exposure to ultraviolet waves, vibrations, excessive heat, or noise) (Bartfay and Bartfay 2015). For example, when jet aircrafts were in their infancy for commercial uses, many pilots being trained to fly these new aircraft were exposed to excessive levels of noise (>75 decibels) (Schubert and Bartfay 2010). It was determined that high-pitched sounds emitted by these jet aircrafts

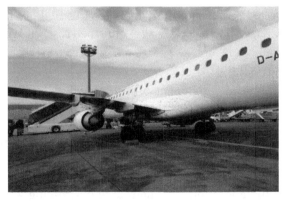

Source: Wally J. Bartfay

Photo 6.7 Noise from modern jet aircrafts is an example of a physical agent that can result in alterations to health including hearing loss, stress, anxiety, headaches, and sleep disturbances.

damaged the hearing of these pilots. Currently, pilots and ground-crew personnel working around these aircrafts are required to wear protective ear muffs to help minimize exposure to excessive levels of noise emitted by jets and other aircraft.

Infectious Agents

Infectious agents are defined as pathogens that can lead to the development of a disease and include bacteria, fungi, viruses (e.g., West Nile virus), metazoan (e.g., hookworm) and protozoa (e.g., malaria). A **pathogen** is defined as any microorganism (e.g., virus, bacteria) or other matter (e.g., prion) that can cause disease in humans or animals and/or result in a morbid process or state (Bartfay and Bartfay 2015). The reader is referred to Chapter 7 for a detailed discussion of these aforementioned pathogens.

For example, the first reported human case of West Nile virus was isolated in a woman living in the West Nile region of Uganda, Africa in 1937. As a consequence of global warming, West Nile virus has spread from the continent of Africa to colder countries such as Canada (PHAC 2012). West Nile virus has been reported in various provinces in Canada including Nova Scotia, Quebec, Ontario, Manitoba, and Saskatchewan. West Nile virus first appeared in Canada in 2001, and the Public Health Agency of Canada (2006) reports that 1,300 confirmed human cases of West Nile virus were identified in 2003, 29 in 2004, and 224 in 2005. This infectious agent has been associated with the development of severe swelling of the brain, coma, and death (Quinlan and Dickinson 2009). Public health officials in Canada have responded by monitoring mosquitoes (i.e., the vector) levels in ponds, creeks and other bodies of stationary water sources; reports of dead birds especially crows and blue jays, and infected humans. As

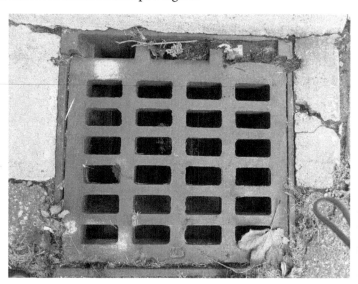

Source: Wally J. Bartfay.

Photo 6.8 A sewer basin spray-painted fluorescent green (upper right corner), which indicates that it has been treated by a public health worker for the West Nile mosquitoe larvae. Preventative public health actions, such as this one, often go unnoticed by the general public but are critical to ensure the health and well-being of all citizens in communities throughout Canada.

of October 2004, for example, public health officials reported that of 416 dead birds tested for the virus, 6,232 tested positive for the West Nile virus (Public Health Agency of Canada 2006). During the summer of 2012, Canada had 249 clinically confirmed cases of West Nile virus (PHAC 2012).

Environment

The third component of the epidemiological triangle is the **environment,** which comprises those factors outside of the host that are associated with the development of a disease, disorder or injury (Bartfay and Bartfay 2015). For example, epidemiologists must consider the physical environment in which the agent and host reside because certain diseases are more prevalent in particular climates or geographical locations (e.g., malaria, dengue fever). Similarly, individuals living in crowded and highly populated urban centres in Canada may be more susceptible to the influenza virus than those residing in less populated and congested rural or remote locations. A safe source of drinking water and efficient sewage treatment infrastructure system to manage raw sewage in communities are also essential components of all public health systems (Quinlan and Dickinson 2009; Schubert and Bartfay 2010). The Council of Canadians (2015) reports that as of January 2015, there were 1,838 drinking water advisories issued across Canada, including 169 drinking water advisories issued on 126 First Nation communities.

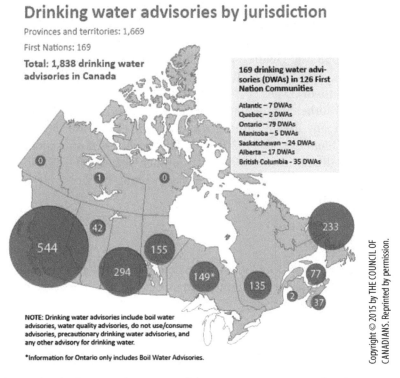

Figure 6.5 A snapshot of Canadian boil water advisories and do not consume water orders in 2015.

Approximately 25% of all Canadians utilize private wells, cisterns, or other water supply sources as their drinking water and have to assume responsibility for the monitoring of their own drinking water (Canadian Water and Wastewater Association, n.d.). Health Canada (2004) has developed specific guidelines for all public and private drinking water supplies. Depending on the province or territory, bacterial testing of the water supply for contaminates (e.g., *E. coli*, coliform bacteria) is done by either provincial health labs and/or certified private labs (Health Canada 2008). The presence of coliform bacteria in the drinking water may result from surface water infiltration or seepage from a nearby septic system. The presence of *E. coli* bacteria indicates that the water supply has been contaminated with fecal material. These contaminates can cause serious alterations to the health and well-being or even mortality of humans (e.g., 2000 *E. coli* outbreak in Walkerton, Ontario).

Time

The time or temporal component is also critical in determining the natural evolution or course of a disease. The **time component** helps to establish the required incubation periods for communicable agents, the life expectancy of the host or pathogen, and the duration and course of the disease or altered health condition. The epidemiologists may ask questions such as *Is there a sudden increase in the incidence of sexually transmitted infections (STIs) in a community*; *Is the influenza problem greater in winter or the summer months*, or *When did the Swine Flu pandemic first appear?* Variations in the patterns of disease associated with the time or temporal component provide important insights into the pathogenesis of disease; for determining seasonal or cyclic variations in the rate of disease, and for the recognition of emerging epidemics (Aschengrau and Seage III 2008; Friis and Sellers 2009; Merrill 2010; Neutens and Rubinson 2002; Valanis 1999). The time component may vary from a few hours, to a few weeks or months to several decades. For example, exposure to the agent diethylstilbestrol (DES) *in utero* is regarded as a possible cause of adenocarcinoma of the vagina because this exposure occurs on average twenty years before the diagnosis is made among affected women (Aschengrau and Seage III 2008; Herbst, Ulfelder, and Poskanzer 1971).

Time clustering of health reports also provides important insights into the aetiology of diseases and/or altered health conditions. For example, time clustering of health reports related to *toxic shock syndrome* (TSS) between January 1977 and October 1981 in the United States led to the formation of an aetiological hypothesis related to tampon use (Hennekens and Burings (Friis and Sellers 2008; Hennekens, Buring, and Mayrent 1987). TSS is a severe and acute disease associated with *staphylococci* of Phage Group 1 that produces a unique epidermal toxin (Davis et al. 1980; Todd et al. 1978). The striking increase in TSS appeared to be linked to the superabsorbent tampon Rely, which was introduced to the market in August 1978 by the Proctor and Gamble Company. The hypothesis was confirmed in various analytic studies (e.g., Davis et al. 1980; Latham et al. 1982; Shands et al. 1982, 1980). The product was subsequently removed in September 1980, which resulted in a dramatic decrease in the number of cases of TSS. Nonetheless, improper use of tampons including leaving them in the vaginal canal too long or forgetting to remove them, remains a potential cause for TSS today.

Natural History of Disease

The natural history of a disease can be viewed as a time-dependent process from its inception to its final resolution. Figure 6.6 depicts the four common stages associated with the development of most diseases. The **natural history of a disease** is defined as:

> the unaltered course that a disease would take without any intervention such as therapy or lifestyle changes … [and] can be understood by viewing the concept as a continuum, with exposure to the agent suspected of causing the disease or condition at one end, through the development of signs and symptoms of illness in a progression of severity, to the ultimate outcome of the disease, whether that be disability or death, at the other end.

(Schubert and Bartfay 2010, p. 178)

The stage of susceptibility is the first stage of the disease process and defines the likelihood a host has of developing the disease or altered health condition due to exposure to a specific external agent. For communicable diseases (e.g., measles, mumps, polio, syphilis, tuberculosis) this period is also referred to as the **incubation period** that begins with exposure to an infectious agent and subsequent pathological changes that occur in the host before the onset of overt clinical signs or symptoms.

For example, the incubation period for malaria is approximately 15 days (range 10–35 days) from the time the victim was bitten by an infected female mosquitoe to the time the victim exhibits overt clinical signs and symptoms (e.g., fever, chills, sweating, malaise, headaches). This lasts for approximately 24 hours and then reoccurs every 48 hours. Some diseases are also transmissible in the last 2 or 3 days

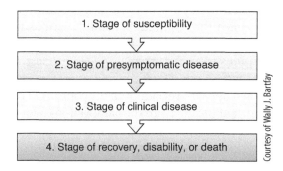

Figure 6.6 The four common stages for the natural history of disease.

of their incubation period (e.g., measles, chicken pox). For noncommunicable diseases (e.g., tetanus, Legionnaire's disease, anthrax), the time from exposure to clinical symptoms may also be referred to as the **latency period.** The host is unaware that they have a disease during the early stages of the disease process.

The stage of clinical disease begins when clinical signs and symptoms manifest themselves. The host typically seeks attention by a health care professional when signs and symptoms appear. However, the actual time of obtaining a confirmed diagnosis may be a function of available health care personnel and/or laboratory and diagnostic facilities. Once the diagnosis is made, treatment can begin (e.g., antibiotics, antiviral medications). The final stage reflects the clinical prognosis of the host recovering from the disease, their likelihood to recover fully, be disabled as a consequence of exposure to the agent, or die. A variety of factors can affect the natural history of the disease process including early detection and effective treatments. The central goal of public health is to preserve, protect, and promote the health and well-being of individuals, groups, and populations via primary health interventions for each stage of the disease process. Add to your knowledge of the disease process and disease trends for both communicable and noncommunicable diseases in Canada and abroad by accessing Web-Based Resource Box 6.1.

Revised and Updated Epidemiological Triangle

The epidemiological triangle (see Figure 6.3) was originally developed for understanding and managing infectious/communicable diseases, which were the leading causes of mortality during the second half of the twentieth century (Aschengrau and Seage III 2008; Friis and Sellers 2009; Merrill 2010; Neutens and Rubinson 2002; Valanis 1999). During its infancy, epidemiology, and public health focused on a single disease, pathogen, or cause for a disease with the objective of identifying and isolating the causal agent, and decreasing the susceptibility of the potential host (i.e., through immunization programs, quarantining of infected hosts). Although infectious diseases are still present and can affect the health and well-being of Canadians across the lifespan (e.g., influenza, tuberculosis, West Nile virus, HIV/AIDS), they are no longer the leading causes of mortality and morbidity in Canada and other developed and industrialized nations in

Web-Based Resource Box 6.1 Communicable and Non-communicable Diseases and Current Disease Trends

Learning resources	Website
Centers for Disease Control and Prevention Epidemiology Program Office. This website provides Information on current outbreaks, statistical data related to disease trends, and public health information and educational resources.	http://www.cdc.gov/epo
Public Health Agency of Canada—Notifiable Diseases Monthly Report. These monthly reports provide detailed information related to communicable disease alerts and trends for a variety of notifiable diseases (e.g., HIV/AIDS, TB, hepatitis B).	http://www.phac-aspc. gc.ca/bid-bmi/dsd-dsm/ ndmr-rmmdo/index.html.
World Health Organization (WHO) Weekly Epidemiological Record. This website provides weekly reports related to a variety of communicable and noncommunicable diseases from a global health perspective, and also provides links to various associated public health resources.	http://www.who.int/wer.

the world (Canadian Institute for Health Information 2007; Public Health Agency of Canada 2008b; World Health Organization 2010).

In fact, infectious diseases as leading causes of mortality and morbidity have been replaced by the so-called *chronic noncommunicable diseases* such as cardiovascular disease (e.g., heart disease, stroke), cancer, diabetes, and mental health issues (e.g., depression, dementia) (Alzheimer Society of Canada 2010; Canadian Cancer Society 2005; Canadian Institute for Health Information 2007; Donatelle et al. 2008; Hales and Lauzon 2007; Public Health Agency of Canada 2008a, 2008b; Statistics Canada 2002). Heart disease, for example, remains the second eading cause of mortality in adult Canadians, which claims the lives of approximately 50,000 adults annually and costs our public health care systems an estimated $7.3 billion (Canadian) in direct health care costs alone (Foot, Curnew, and Pearson 2005; Statistics Canada 2010, 2014).

Similarly, the Alzheimer Society of Canada (2010) reports that in 2008, 103,700 new dementia cases per year (or one new case every 5 minutes) were made, and this is projected to increase to 257,800 new cases in 2038 (one new case every 2 minutes) with an associated cumulative economic burden of $872 billion (Canadian) and the total informal caregiver opportunity costs are projected to exceed $301 billion annually (see Table 6.4). The current life expectancy in Canada is more than 80 years (Canadian Institute for Health Information 2007), and the number of seniors is expected to reach 6.7 million in 2020 and 9.2 million in 2041 (Public Health Agency of Canada 2008a). Given that age is a primary and unchangeable risk factor for developing dementia, the incidence of dementia will quickly increase as our population continues to age and the first baby boomers enter their senior years (65+) in the year 2011 and beyond (see Table 6.4).

The Research Focus Box 6.1 provides an example of a recent community-based study which sought to determine how adult day programs and caregiver support groups may positively affect the quality of life (QOL) of primary caregivers looking after loved ones with Alzheimer's disease in Ontario, Canada. The researchers conducted a pilot study to compare self-reports of QOL for primary caregivers with controls who were subjects not looking after family members with Alzheimer's disease or dementia. The investigators predicted that primary caregivers who accessed adult day programs in the community would have similar QOL scores in comparison to control subjects. This study provides an example of how adult day programs are having positive ripple effects for both clients with Alzheimer's disease and their primary caregivers in the community.

Table 6.4 Annual Total Economic Burden Attributed to Dementia Future Values, 2008–2038

Year	Total direct costs (e.g., include costs of prescription medications, hospital and physician costs and long-term care staff costs) (i)	Total unpaid caregivers opportunity costs (i.e., lost wages that could have been earned by informal caregivers in the labour force) (ii)	Total indirect costs (e.g., lost wages and corporate profits) (iii)	Total economic burden (i+ii+iii)
2008	$8,063,733,967	$4,995,340,836	$1,864,955,665	$14,924,030,467
2018	$19,573,547,540	$12,303,233,856	$4,845,163,396	$36,721,944,792
2028	$43,842,755,134	$26,921,613,083	$4,380,174,051	$75,144,542,267
2038	$92,832,808,780	$55,708,854,294	$4,097,831,931	$152,639,495,005

Source: Adapted from the Alzheimer Society of Canada (2010).

Research Focus Box 6.1

Quality-of-Life Outcomes Among Alzheimer's Disease Family Caregivers Following Community-Based Interventions

Study Aim/Rationale
This pilot study sought to determine how community-based interventions such as adult day programs and caregiver support groups affect the quality of life (QOL) of caregivers looking after family members with Alzheimer's disease in the Durham Region of Ontario, Canada.

Methodology/Design
The investigators used a cross-sectional comparative design to examine how adult day programs for family members were benefiting the QOL of sixty-two self-identified primary caregivers. The study was comparative because a control group consisting of individuals without Alzheimer's disease or dementia was used to evaluate QOL levels against primary caregivers looking after loved ones with Alzheimer's disease. All primary caregivers identified were female (i.e., spouse or partner). The authors hypothesized that using and accessing community-based interventions comprised of adult day programs would increase the QOL of caregivers of Alzheimer's disease clients. Individuals were recruited at five adult day programs and at six caregiver support groups in the Durham Region of Ontario. Primary data collection consisted of a self-report questionnaire administered to both primary caregivers and controls along with a thirteen-item QOL scale.

Major Findings
All Alzheimer clients who were accessing adult day programs were seniors. The mean age for caregivers of Alzheimer's disease adult day programs was 71 years (SD = 6.9; range = 60–86 years) and for Alzheimer's disease-free (controls) adults was 61.3 years (SD = 11.8; range = 37–83 years). The mean length of time in the caregiver role for caregivers of adult day programs was 65.5 months (SD = 38; range = 18–156 months) and for controls was 67.5 months (SD = 54.9; range = 12.184 months). The findings reveal that caregivers of Alzheimer's disease clients who utilize community-based interventions enjoyed similar levels of QOL (QOL rating = 2.76, SD = 0.5), in comparison to controls (QOL rating = 2.75, SD = 0.37).

Implications for Public Health
Maintaining one's QOL is also critical for the health and well-being of primary caregivers looking after loved ones with chronic noncommunicable diseases such as Alzheimer's disease and dementia. Findings from this pilot study suggest that community-based interventions such as adult day programs and caregiver support groups may be beneficial in maintaining or promoting the QOL of primary caregivers of Alzheimer's clients. Community-based programs should also target the multiple needs of primary caregivers, including their knowledge of available community resources and coping strategies.

Source: Bartfay and Bartfay (2013).

Although epidemiological investigations of causal associations in disease had historically began with communicable disease, one cannot, for example, single-out a single pathogen or microbe as the cause in noncommunicable chronic diseases associated with one's lifestyle, occupation, environment, and/or social determinant of health per se. It is notable that to date, we have been unable to identify any single "cause" resulting in the development of various noncommunicable chronic diseases including diabetes, heart disease, stroke, COPD, rheumatic arthritis, multiple sclerosis, ALS, Alzheimer's disease, bi-polar disorder or schizophrenia, to name but a few examples. This is because their causes, or associated risk factors and social determinants of health are currently deemed to be multifactorial in nature. Hence, this updated epidemiological triangle is more comprehensive in nature and recognizes that alterations to health and well-being are often fluid in nature and more complex in reference to the environment, determinants of health, and/or associated risk factors which can be both modifiable (e.g., physical inactivity, smoking, diet high in saturated fats) and non-modifiable (e.g., genetic predisposition, sex) in nature (Aschengrau and Seage III 2008; Friis and Sellers 2009; Merrill 2010; Neutens and Rubinson 2002; Valanis 1999). For example, currently only 7% of children and youth in Canada are meeting the recommended guideline of 60 minutes of moderate to vigorous intensity activity per day (Active Healthy Kids Canada 2014; Statistics Canada 2013). Moreover, between 1978/79 and 2004, the combined prevalence of being overweight or obese in Canadian children and youth aged 2–17 years increased from 15% to 26%, respectively (Childhood Obesity Foundation 2015). Currently, over 59% of adults in Canada are obese or overweight, and it is predicted that by 2040 up to 70% of adults aged 40 years of older will be either overweight or obese (Childhood Obesity Foundation 2015). Hence, it is well documented that physical inactivity and obesity in children can lead to a host of noncommunicable diseases including type 2 diabetes, hypertension, certain forms of cancer, heart disease and stroke during adulthood.

Time

Figure 6.7 provides an updated and expanded epidemiological triangle which takes into consideration all facets of the original epidemiological triangle developed for communicable disease (see Figure 6.3), but it also takes into account the chronic nature of noncommunicable diseases, conditions, disorders, defects, injuries, and associated morbidities and mortalities (Bartfay and Bartfay 2015). The time component remains a critical component, but the updated model also recognizes the nature of both acute and chronic communicable and noncommunicable diseases and altered states of health and well-being. Hence, the *time* component of the updated epidemiological triangle recognizes that noncommunicable diseases often take several years or even decades to manifest themselves (e.g., heart disease, stroke, type 2 diabetes, arthritis, Alzheimer's disease).

Determinants of Health

The term *agent* in the original epidemiological triangle (Figure 6.3) has been replaced and updated by the social determinants of health. Accordingly, this updated model (Figure 6.7) implies the need to consider multiple associated risk factors, causes, or aetiological factors associated with altered states of health and well-being, disability, injury, morbidity and/or mortality. We contend that the art and science of public health embodies and consists of the following five essential pillars: (a) evidence-informed public health, (b) health promotion and prevention, (c) primary health care, (d) social determinants of health, and (e) the holistic care paradigm (Bartfay and Bartfay 2015). These pillars are in concert with the updated epidemiological triangle. The reader is referred to Chapter 1 for a detailed discussion of the five essential pillars of public health.

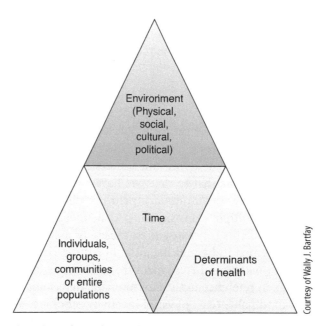

Figure 6.7 Revised and updated epidemiological triangle.

Evidence-informed public health (EIPH) "is the process of distilling and disseminating the best available evidence from research, practice and experience and using that evidence to inform and improve public health policy and practice" (National Collaborating Centres for Public Health 2011, p. 1). Health promotion and prevention activities enhance and/or reinforce the ability of an individual, family, group, community, or entire population to take control and maintain, improve, or restore their health and quality of life.

The **primary health care approach** is defined as a model of health care that emphasizes equity, accessibility, full participation by individuals and communities, the use of universally acceptable and affordable technologies and methods, intersectoral collaboration, and is based on practical scientifically sound and socially acceptable health care approaches and interventions which embrace the following five types of health care: (a) promotive, (b) preventive, (c) curative, (d) rehabilitative, and (e) supportive/palliative.

The **social determinants of health (SDH)** are defined as:

the structural determinants and conditions of daily life responsible for a major part of health inequities between and within countries. They include the distribution of power, income, goods and services, and the circumstances of people's lives, such as their access to health care, schools and education; their conditions of work and leisure; and the state of their housing and environment. The term "social determinants" is thus shorthand for the social, political, economic, environmental and cultural factors that greatly affect health status.

(Commission on the Social Determinants of Health 2008, p. 1)

The updated epidemiological triangle recognizes that the determinants of health are broad based and holistic in nature and include individual biology and genetic endowment, health behaviours, lifestyles, social and economic factors including income, education, food security, social exclusion, housing shortages, social support networks, employment and working conditions, social and physical environments, personal health practices and coping skills, access to health care services, sex and culture (Health Canada 2002; PHAC 2002; Raphael 2010, 2003). For example, employment status (e.g., working vs. unemployed) may also be a powerful predictor (i.e., a determinant of health) for developing a particular disease or altered health condition (e.g., depression, heart disease).

Lastly, the **holistic health care paradigm** incorporates the belief that human beings are more than the sum of their mind and body parts, but are dynamic and interrelated wholes that include their mind, body, spirit, culture, and environments (Bartfay and Bartfay 2015). In the Canadian context of public health practice, providing holistic care to individuals, families, groups, communities, or entire populations is based on the principle of social justice, in which the public health professional or worker brings an awareness of equity and the fundamental rights of all residents to accessible, competent practice, and the essential SDH. The reader is referred to Chapter 1 for a detailed description of these five noted essential pillars of public health.

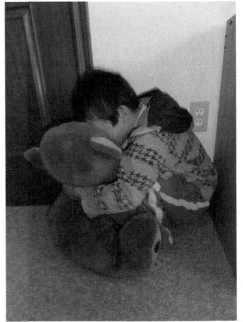

Source: Wally J. Bartfay

Photo 6.9 All health care professionals are legally required to report all suspected cases of child abuse in Canada.

Political, Social, and Cultural Environments

The term *environment* in the original epidemiological triangle (see Figure 6.3) was limited to the physical conditions and surroundings that were external to humans or animals that cause or allow for the transmission of infectious disease (e.g., contaminated water supplies). The updated epidemiological triangle expands on this condition and recognizes the impact of political, social, and cultural environments on states of health and well-being.

For example, all public health agencies and institutions in Canada have specific procedures and guidelines for identifying and reporting suspected cases of child abuse and neglect (Mandleco and Bartfay 2010). In fact, public health professionals (e.g., public health nurses, physicians, social workers) and workers are legally required to report all suspected cases of child abuse, including those which are physical, sexual, or emotional in nature. Child neglect often entails both physical and emotional harm to a child in terms of depriving them of their basic human needs for growth and development and needs for survival including a safe home environment, adequate nutrition, clothing, shelter, and/or health care (McAllister 2000). In 2003, the number of children living in poverty was 1.2 million or 17.6% (National Council of Welfare 2006). Because it is often underreported, we do not know the true extent of child abuse and neglect in Canada. Health Canada (2002) reported that in 1998 alone, child welfare agencies nationally investigated more than 130,000 child mistreatment cases, 31% for physical abuse, 19% for emotional maltreatment, 10% for sexual abuse, and 10% for neglect. Moreover, it is well documented that one's socioeconomic situation can play a significant role in morbidity and mortality patterns in the development of various chronic noncommunicable diseases (e.g., cardiovascular disease, diabetes) (e.g., Auger et al. 2004; Marmot and Theorell 1988; Ross et al. 2000; Wilkins, Berthelot, and Ng 2000).

The updated epidemiological triangle recognizes the impact of various social and political determinants of health on our public health systems. For example, the rapid growth of private for-profit health clinics in Canada is directly challenging the validity of the Canada Health Act and the legislative powers of the federal government to enforce the Act nationally (Armstrong and Armstrong 2003; Monahan 2006; Romano 2002). These sociopolitical influences all have significant impact on how public primary health care services are funded and delivered in Canada. The reader is referred Chapter 3 for a detailed discussion of these sociopolitical influences.

Group Activity-Based Learning Box 6.2

Understanding and Employing the Epidemiological Triangle

This group activity seeks to reinforce key concepts in this section by further examining and applying the updated and revised epidemiological triangle to examine current noncommunicable health conditions or altered states of health and wellness in your community. Working in small groups of three to five students, discuss, and answer the following questions:

1. What are the current major noncommunicable health conditions or altered states of health and wellness (e.g., chronic diseases, conditions, disorders, or injuries) in your community?

2. How can the updated epidemiological triangle be utilized to better understand these health conditions or altered states of health and wellness in your community?

3. What types of epidemiological data are still missing or lacking?

4. What forms of epidemiological research is still needed to fill these gaps in knowledge or practice?

5. Based on the best available scientific literature, how would you plan for primary health care interventions in your community to address these noncommunicable health conditions or altered states of health and wellness?

Individuals, Groups, Communities, and Entire Populations

Lastly, the individual host shown in Figure 6.3 has been expanded to include aggregates such as groups, communities, or entire populations (see Figure 6.7), which is in concert with the primary health care approach in Canada (Public Health Agency of Canada 2007). The primary goal of primary health care in Canada is to build community capacity to achieve sustainable health through health promotion efforts, as first detailed in the Ottawa Charter for Health Promotion (Frank and Smith 1999; WHO, Health and Welfare Canada and CPHA 1986). Hence, the process of public health promotion in Canada embraces actions directed at strengthening the skills and capabilities of both individuals and aggregates across the lifespan (Public Health Agency of Canada 2007). Although the host is, technically, always an individual, or animal, epidemiology is a science that examines the presence of disease and risk factors in populations over time. Hence, epidemiologists examine a group or population of hosts in which a particular agent or risk factor is present. To draw conclusions about a particular disease, injury, or health condition in a population without closely examining individual host characteristics for common factors can lead to misinterpretation of data and in turn, false conclusions (Schubert and Bartfay 2010).

When epidemiologists currently examine the individual host, group, community, or entire population affected, they often examine a multitude of demographic characteristics (e.g., age, sex, ethnicity), socioeconomic status, (e.g., employment history, occupation, income), nutritional and immune status, and the presence of preexisting diseases or conditions (e.g., respiratory disorders, diabetes) and lifestyles. Each of these noted characteristics or factors can have an impact on the development of a noncommunicable disease or health condition. Sex, for example, plays a prominent role in the development of certain disorders. Indeed, breast cancer typically affects women (approximately 99% of cases), whereas only a small proportion of cases (approximately 1%) are men (Canadian Cancer Society 2005; Ries et al. 2006). Ethnicity also plays a critical role. For example, the presence of type 2 diabetes in Indigenous people is three to five times higher in comparison to the general non-Indigenous population in Canada (First Nations and Inuit Regional Health Survey 1999; National Indigenous Health Organization [NAHO] 2006). Sickle cell anaemia, haemophilia, and beta-thalassemia major are examples of clinical blood disorders that have a strong genetic link.

Common Epidemiological Measures

Epidemiological measures and analysis of quantitative data permits epidemiologists, public health professionals and workers, and researchers to measure the health status of our nation and the occurrence of disease and other altered states of health in diverse populations across the lifespan. A variety of health status indicators are employed to provide a snapshot of the major diseases, conditions, altered states of health, disabilities and injuries in a defined population or community. This information is critical for establishing public health priorities (e.g., immunization against H1N1), planning for primary health care initiatives in targeted groups or populations (e.g., school-aged children, elderly, Indigenous groups) and for evaluating the effectiveness of public health programs (Schubert and Bartfay 2010). The Canadian Institute for Health Information (CIHI), the Canadian Public Health Agency (CPHA), Statistics Canada and the various provincial and territorial ministries of health routinely collect health-related data (Schubert and Bartfay 2010). In additional to these governmental agencies, various charitable foundations and organizations also collect and tabulate health-related data such as the Canadian Cancer Society, Canadian Diabetes Association and the Heart and Stroke Foundation of Canada to name but a few. Health-related data is routinely collected from a variety of sources including population-based surveys, cause-of-death reports, cancer registries, laboratory reports, and hospital admission records (Public Health Agency of Canada 2007).

Although a discussion of all the health indicators, statistical measures and research methodologies employed by epidemiologists and public health professionals and workers is beyond the purpose and scope of this chapter, an overview of some of the most common measures and health indicators shall be highlighted. The reader is referred to Chapter 5 for a detailed discussion of various research methodologies and approaches. The reader is referred to Chapter 9 for a detailed discussion of common global burden of disease measures (e.g., disability adjusted life years, quality adjusted life years).

Disease Frequency

The most basic measure of a disease frequency consists of a simple count of individuals or cases that have the disease, health condition, or altered state of health. However, this provides limited information in reference to its distribution in a given population and the time component when the count was obtained. Knowing the size of the population and the time period for which the data was obtained permits epidemiologists to make comparisons between disease frequencies among two or more groups or populations.

To illustrate this concept, consider the following hypothetical scenario. City A reports fifty-two cases of tuberculosis (TB) to provincial health officials and City B reports only thirty-seven cases of TB. Based on this limited information, public health officials may conclude that City A has a greater outbreak of TB in comparison to City B, and therefore may require more public health resources (e.g., public health nurses, physicians) to combat its spread. However, City A has a population of 1,000,500 residents, whereas City B has a population of only 8,700 residents. Therefore, City B actually has a more severe public health problem confronting them in terms of their total population. Moreover, if the epidemiologists also considered the time factor or temporal component for the TB outbreaks in Cities A and B, the public health problem becomes more crystallized and clear. Especially given that the reported cases for TB in City A was covered over a one-year period, whereas those for City B were reported during a four-month period.

The measures of disease frequency that are employed most often by epidemiologists and public health professionals and workers fall into two broad categories: (a) prevalence and (b) incidence (Bartfay and Bartfay 2015). Table 6.5 depicts a typical two-by-two table that is often used to organize data by epidemiologists and other health care researchers to compare proportions such as the cumulative incidence or prevalence data. The light-shaded boxes directly under the headings Disease or health condition (YES) or (NO) (i.e., a, b, c, d) are called the *cells* and the boxes located under the Total column in orange are called the *margins* (e.g., a + b and c + d). The data are cross-tabulated by two categories of exposure (i.e., yes or no) and by two categories of a disease or health condition (i.e., yes or no).

Table 6.5 The Typical Two-by-Two Table for the Organization of Cumulative Incidence or Prevalence Data

	Disease or health condition (YES)	Disease or health condition (NO)	Total
Exposure (YES)	a	b	a + b
Exposure (NO)	c	d	c + d
Total	a + c	b + d	a + b + c + d

Note:
Total number exposed = a + b
Total number unexposed = c + d
Total number in the study = a + b + c + d
Number exposed and diseased = a
Number exposed but not diseased = b
Number not exposed but diseased = c
Number neither exposed nor diseased = d
Total number diseased = a + c
Total number not diseased = b + d

Prevalence

Prevalence is defined as the proportion (percentage) of individuals in a given population who have the disease or altered states of health at a given point in time, and provides an estimate of the probability (or risk) that an individual will be ill at a stated point in time (Bartfay and Bartfay 2015). This point in time can be denoted by a specific fixed calendar time, or can also be a fixed point in the course of events that may vary in real time from person to person. For example, Tu et al. (2008) reported that the age-and-sex-adjusted prevalence for hypertension in Ontario, Canada increased from 153.1 per 1,000 adults in 1995 to 244.8 per 1,000 in 2005, which represents a significant increase of 60.0% ($p < 0.001$).

The term *prevalence rate* is often used interchangeably with "prevalence" in published reports; although by strict definition the latter is a proportion and not a rate per se. The formula for calculating the prevalence (P) is shown in the following

$$P = \frac{\text{Number of existing cases}}{\text{Total population}} \text{At a given point in time}$$

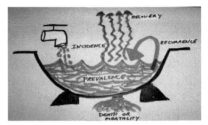

Source: Drawing and photo by Wally J. Bartfay

Photo 6.10 The "*bath tub analogy*" in epidemiology. Incidence consists of new cases represented by the addition of new water to the bath tub via the tap. Prevalence is represented by existing cases in the main body of water in the tub. Death or mortality is represented by water that is leaving or leaking-out of the bath tub. Recurrence (e.g., reinfection) is represented by the red arrow that effects prevalence, and recovery is represented by green arrows that symbolize water this is evaporating from the bath tub.

Prevalence Rate Calculation Example

During the month of July, a total of 14 workers in a steel mill in Hamilton, Ontario were found to have diabetes mellitus (DM), and the steel mill had a total of 2300 workers. What is the prevalence rate of DM for the month of April per 1000 workers?

$$P = \frac{14}{2300} \times 1000 = 6.09 \text{ per } 1000 \text{ workers}$$

Incidence

Incidence quantifies the number of new events or cases of a disease or condition that develop in a population of individuals at risk during a specified time period (Bartfay and Bartfay 2015). The incidence provides a measure which determines the rate of change from a non-diseased state to a diseased state among persons at risk and also reflects new cases of the disease or condition for a specified time period. There are two major types of incidence measures reported in the epidemiological literature: *Cumulative incidence* (CI)

Incidence Rate Calculation Example

During the month of January, a total of 4 clients were diagnosed with mumps in a small rural community of 2400 in northern Manitoba. What was the incidence rate for mumps for the month of January per 1000 residents?

$$ID = \frac{4}{2400} \times 1000 = 1.67 \text{ per } 1000 \text{ residents}$$

and the *incidence rate* or *incidence density* (ID). The **CI** is defined as the proportion of people who become diseased during a specified time period, and provides an estimate of the probability or risk that an individual will develop a disease or condition during this specified time period. The relevant time period must be clearly specified when reporting the CI. When calculating the CI, the epidemiologists assume that the entire population at risk at the commencement of the investigative period has been followed for the specified time period for the development of the disease, health condition, or outcome under study. However, the length of follow-up for the subjects or the time during which the outcome could be observed may not be uniform for all subjects.

The **incidence rate** or **incidence density (ID)** determines the impact of exposure in a defined population and is a measure of the instantaneous rate of development of a disease or condition in a population (Bartfay and Bartfay 2015). For example, Tu et al. (2008) reported that the age-and-sex-adjusted incidence of hypertension in Ontario, Canada, increased from 25.5 per 1,000 adults in 1997 to 32.1 per 1000 in 2004, which represents a significant relative increase of 25.7% ($p < 0.001$). The formula for calculating the ID is shown in the following:

$$ID = \frac{\textit{Number of new cases of a disease or condition during a specified time period}}{\textit{Total person} - \textit{Time of observation}}$$

The numerator of the ID is the number of new cases in the population, whereas the denominator is the sum of each person's time at risk or the sum of time that each individual remained under study and was free from disease or an altered state of health. It is important to note that the ID as a measure of incidence should in theory include only those subjects who are regarded at risk of developing the disease or condition. Hence, individuals who already have the disease or condition or cannot develop the disease (e.g., age, removal of the target organ, immunization against the disease) should be excluded. When presenting the ID, it is critical that the epidemiologist or public health professional or worker specify the relevant time units (e.g., number of cases per person-day, -month, -year, or -decade).

Attack Rate

When new cases of a disease or condition occur rapidly over a relatively short period of time in a well-defined population, the incidence rate is referred to as an **attack rate**. For example, on April 19, 1940, an outbreak of acute gastrointestinal illness following a church picnic was reported to the District Health Officer in Syracuse, New York (Gross 1976). Attack rates were calculated for each of the food items consumed by individuals at this church picnic.

The highest attack rate was found for those eating vanilla ice cream, where forty-three who ate the dessert became ill and ill did not, producing an attack rate of 80%. Of those who did not consume ice cream at the

---

Attack Rate Calculation Examples

During the month of November, a primary measles outbreak in an elementary school in Prince George, BC resulted in the absence of 100 of its 400 students enrolled. During the subsequent month of December, a secondary outbreak of measles resulted in an additional 100 students being diagnosed with measles, as were 150 of the 200 siblings (i.e., brothers and sisters) for the first 100 students. What was the primary attack rate for students during the month of December?

$$\text{Attack rate (AR)} = \frac{\text{Number of new cases during a specific period}}{\text{Number of people at risk during the same period}} \times 100\%$$

$$\text{Primary (AR)} = \frac{100}{400-100} \times 100\% = 33\%$$

What was the secondary attack rate? (Note: Always remember to reduce the number of people at risk by the number of people who are no longer at risk during the specified time period).

$$\text{Secondary (AR)} = \frac{150}{200} \times 100\% = 75\%$$

picnic, three became ill and eighteen did not, producing an attack rate of 14%. The ratio of these two attack rates is 5.7; which means that those who ate ice cream at the church picnic were 5.7 times more likely to suffer from gastrointestinal illness, in comparison to those who did not consume this dessert.

Morbidity and Mortality Rates

Other common measurements of disease frequency that all public health professionals and workers should be familiar with are *morbidity* and *mortality rates*. The **morbidity rate** is defined as the incidence of nonfatal cases of a disease or health condition in the total population at risk during a specified point in time. The formula for calculating the morbidity rate is shown in the following:

$$Morbidity\ rate = \frac{new\ nonfatal\ cases\ of\ a\ disease\ or\ condition}{total\ population\ at\ risk}$$

Infant Mortality Rate Calculation Example

A First Nations community in northern Labrador reported a total of 12 infant deaths per 10,000 live births in 2017. What was the infant mortality rate for this community per 1000 live births?

$$\text{Infant mortality rate} = \frac{\text{Number of infant deaths less than one year of age}}{\text{Total number of live births during the same year}} \times 1000$$

$$\text{Infant mortality rate} = \frac{12}{10,000} \times 1000 = 1.2\ \text{per 1000 live births per year}$$

Case-Specific Mortality or Fatality Rate Calculation Example

In a community located in Sub-Saharan, Africa, there were 500 individuals diagnosed with HIV/AIDS in 2017 of whom 17 died within one year of their initial diagnosis. What was the cause-specific mortality rate for this community?

$$\text{Case-specific mortality rate} = \frac{\text{Number of deaths due to a disease}}{\text{Number of people with the same disease}} \times 100\%$$

$$\text{Case-specific mortality rate} = \frac{17}{500} \times 100\% = 3.4\%$$

The **mortality rate** is defined as the incidence of death in a defined population during a specified period of time and is calculated by dividing the total number of fatalities (deaths) during that period by the total population (Bartfay and Bartfay 2015). Table 6.6 shows the ten leading causes of mortality in Canada in 2007 for both sexes (Statistics Canada 2010). The top three causes of mortality for Canadians were cancer, heart disease and stroke in 2007. In 2014, the top three leading causes of mortality for Canadians (both sexes) have remained status quo: (a) cancer 29.9%, $N = 72,476$ cases); (b) heart disease (19.7%, $N = 47,627$ cases), and (c) stroke (5.5%, $N = 13,283$ cases) (Statistics Canada 2014b).

Mortality rates can be expressed in a variety of ways including the crude mortality rate for all causes of death, age-specific mortality rate, cause-specific mortality rate (e.g., liver cancer, tuberculosis), maternal mortality rate (deaths of mothers giving birth or shortly after) or infant mortality rate.

Based on a 2008 report, David Stewart-Patterson, vice president of the Conference Broad of Canada, notes that with 10% of our gross domestic product tied up in health care costs, we spend approximately $4,100 per person each year on health care (Hall 2011). Yet in terms of longevity and infant mortality, two common points of comparison when ranking health care systems internationally, Canada is well down on the list of the seventeen nation's surveys. In fact, Canada was placed seventh on the list in terms of longevity and second from the bottom in terms of infant mortality statistics (Hall 2011).

Historically, it is notable that the health of a nation was assessed by the health indicators of maternal and infant mortality rates. For example, the infant mortality rate per 1,000 live births in Canada was 18.8 in 1970, 5.3 in 2000 and 5.1 in 2008 (Organization for Economic Cooperation and Development [OECD] 2010). However, these statistics are often not collected in developing nations. Nonetheless, it is estimated that 1,400 women die during labour or shortly after and approximately 28,000 children under the age of 5 die every day in developing nations (United Nations Children's Fund [UNICEF] 2005). What is most tragic is that many of these deaths are often easily treatable or preventable (e.g., proper handwashing, nutrition) (Heiby 1998; Thomas and Bartfay 2010).

Table 6.6 The Ten Leading Causes of Mortality in Canada, 2007

Causes of mortality	Rank	Number	%
Malignant neoplasms (cancer)	1	69,595	29.6
Diseases of the heart (heart disease)	2	50,499	21.5
Cerebrovascular diseases (stroke)	3	13,981	5.9
Chronic lower respiratory diseases	4	10,659	4.5
Accidents (unintentional injuries)	5	9,951	4.2
Diabetes mellitus (diabetes)	6	7,394	3.1
Alzheimer's disease	7	5,903	2.5
Influenza and pneumonia	8	5,452	2.3
Nephritis, nephritic syndrome and nephrosis (kidney disease)	9	3,803	1.6
Intentional self-harm (suicide)	10	3,611	1.5
Total (All ten causes combined)		**252,217**	**100**

Source: Adapted from Statistics Canada (2010).

Survival Rate

A measure used to express an individual's prognosis after being clinically diagnosed for a specific disease (e.g., breast cancer, liver cancer, prostate cancer, lung cancer) is the survival rate. The **survival rate** is defined as the percentage of individuals who are alive five years after being diagnosed or after commencement of a treatment regime, or the number of living cases per number of cases of the disease. Although the five-year survival of these clients is referred to a "rate" by convention, it is actually a *proportion*. Despite the widespread use of this measure in Canada and internationally, it is critical to point out that there is nothing "magical" about this five-year time period in terms of the natural history of specific diseases to justify this endpoint. Nonetheless, most deaths for cancer occur after this noted time period after diagnosis, so it has become an index or milestone measure for the success of cancer treatment and management.

One of the major challenges of employing this measure of survival has become more evident in recent decades with the advent of screening programs. Let us consider the following hypothetical example. Suppose a woman had the biological onset of breast cancer occur in the year 2005. Given the natural history of breast cancer which often takes several years to develop and manifest itself, the disease was considered subclinical and therefore no overt presenting clinical signs or symptoms were present (e.g., palpable lump or mass, dimpling of the breast, abnormal discharge from the nipple). Now suppose the woman first felt an abnormal mass/lump in 2008, which subsequently prompted a visit to her physician and an oncologist to do various clinical assessments and diagnostic procedures. Subsequently, a diagnosis of breast cancer was made following an abnormal mammogram and a biopsy of the mass/lump, which resulted in the diagnosis of Stage II breast cancer (see Figure 6.8). The woman subsequently underwent a mastectomy of the affected breast. Unfortunately, despite having the mastectomy and receiving follow-up treatments (e.g., tamoxifen), she died in 2012. As measured by the five-year survival rate, which is often employed by oncologists as a measure for the success of treatment following diagnosis, this woman was not a "successful" case because she survived for only four years after diagnosis. Another major limitation of employing the five-year survival rate occurs when we want to examine the survival experience of a group of clients who were diagnosed less than five years ago. In fact, we cannot employ this criterion because five years of observation post diagnosis is required to calculate the five-year survival rate. Hence, if we want to critically examine the effectiveness of a new therapy or drug that was introduced less than five years ago, for example, this measure would not be an appropriate or fitting measure.

Measures of Association

Measures of association are defined as statistical measures used to investigate the degree of dependence between two or more events or variables. Events are regarded as statistically associated when they occur more frequently together than they could be accounted for by chance alone (Schubert and Bartfay 2010). However, it is important to note that the presence of a statistical association does not alone imply causality.

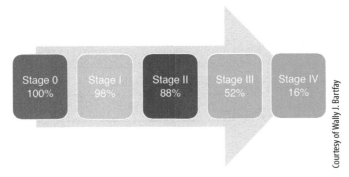

Figure 6.8 Predicted five-year survival rates for breast cancer based on stage diagnosed.

Note: Stage 0—carcinoma in situ (early form); Stage I—localized; Stage II—early locally advanced; Stage III—late locally advance; and Stage IV—metastasized.

For example, suppose you find an association between having yellow-coloured stains on the thumbs, index and ring fingers and lung cancer in a population of chronic smokers. We can be reasonably confident in stating that the presence of these yellow stains does not cause lung cancer per se. Rather, the presence of these yellow stains is due to holding cigarettes (which contain tar and nicotine) by individuals who smoke. The *cause* of lung cancer is, in fact, associated with the lifestyle behaviour (i.e., determinant of health) of chronic smoking. Hence, the observed association between having yellow stains on one's fingers and lung cancer would be considered *noncausal* in nature.

Two of the most commonly reported measures of association in epidemiological and public health reports are the *relative risk* and *attributable risk*. These measures indicate the degree of increased risk and/or frequency that one group will develop a disease or health condition in comparison to another group.

Relative Risk

The **relative risk** or **risk ratio** is defined as the ratio between the rates in the exposed and unexposed groups (Bartfay and Bartfay 2015). The relative risk comparison provides information about the strength of the relationship between the exposure and the disease or health condition, and is most often employed in aetiological investigations. Most epidemiologist and health care researchers prefer to use the relative risk measure for comparisons in aetiological investigations because it is anchored by a baseline value. That is to say, it provides researchers with an indication of how many times higher or lower the disease risk or health condition is among the exposed, when compared to the baseline risk among unexposed subjects. The relative risk (RR) is expressed mathematically in the following, where I_e represents the incidence rate among the exposed, and I_u represents the incidence rate among the unexposed:

$$RR = (I_e \, / \, I_u)$$

If there is no relationship between the exposed and disease or health condition, the numeric value for the relative risk will be 1.0. If there is a positive association observed between the exposure and disease or health condition (i.e., the exposure increases the risk of having the disease or health condition), then the numeric value will be greater than 1.0. Conversely, if the exposure prevents the development of the disease or health condition, the numeric value will be less than 1.0, which also indicates the presence of an inverse association. For example, a RR of 0.5 means that the exposed group has one half the risk of the unexposed group, or a 50%

Calculation of Relative Risk Example

A prospective cohort study examined the relationship between exposure to the fire retardant asbestos as an occupational risk in firefighters and the subsequent development of mesothelioma, a form of lung cancer. A cohort of 1000 firefighters were followed and the distribution was mesothelioma was as follows:

		Mesothelioma		
Asbestos	+	A 225	B 75	A + B = 300
	−	C 75	D 625	C + D = 700
		A + C = 300	B + D = 700	

The incidence rate among firefighters exposed to asbestos $= \dfrac{A}{A+B} = \dfrac{225}{300}$

The incidence rate among firefighters not exposed to asbestos $= \dfrac{C}{C+D} = \dfrac{75}{700}$

Hence, as noted in the 2 × 2 table above, 225 out of 300 firefighters exposed to asbestos were eventually diagnosed with mesothelioma, in comparison to 75 of the 700 firefighters who were not exposed to asbestos at work. What was the relative risk among firefighters exposed to the occupational hazard of asbestos for this cohort study?

$$\text{Relative risk} = \frac{\text{Incidence rate among risk group or } A/(A+B)}{\text{Incidence rate among non-risk group or } C/(C+D)}$$

$$\text{Relative risk} = \frac{225/(225+75)}{75/(75+625)} = \frac{0.750}{0.107} = 7$$

Hence, in comparison to firefighters who were not exposed to asbestos, exposed firefighters were 7 times more likely to develop mesothelioma based upon this prospective cohort study.

decreased risk of developing the disease or health condition. Similarly, a RR of 0.33 means that the exposed group has one-third the risk or a 67% reduction in risk, and so on.

Attributable Risk

The **attributable risk** or **risk difference** is defined as a measure of association that provides information about the effect of the absolute effect of the exposure or the excess risk of disease or health condition in those exposed compared to those unexposed (Bartfay and Bartfay 2015). This measure expresses the number of cases of disease or health condition attributable to the exposure of interest. In other words, the attributable risk (AR) provides information about the difference between the incidence rates in the exposed and unexposed groups, as can be mathematically calculated as shown in the following:

$$AR = (I_e / I_u)$$

The attributable risk is used by epidemiologists and public health researchers to quantify the risk of having the disease or health condition in the exposed group that is considered directly attributable to the exposure by removing the risk of the disease or health condition that would have occurred anyway due to other causes (i.e., risk of unexposed). The interpretation of attributable risk measures is dependent on the assumption that a *cause-and-effect* relationship exists between exposure and the development of the disease or health condition. Hence, the attributable risk is considered a very useful measure for the public health impact of a particular exposure in a defined population.

For example, if the attributable risk measure is 0, this means that there is no *causal* association observed between the noted exposure and the development of the disease or health condition. However, if the calculated value is greater than 0, this value indicates the number of cases of the disease or health condition among the exposed that can be directly attributed to the exposure itself. The **attributable risk percentage** is defined as the proportion of the disease or health condition of interest in the population being investigated that could be prevented by eliminating the exposure. The formula for calculating the attributable risk (AR%) is shown in the following:

$$AR\% = \frac{(I_e / I_u)}{I_e} \times 100\%$$

A similar measure that is also often employed by epidemiologists and public health care professionals and workers is the *attributable risk percentage*. Hence, this measure is also based on the assumption of a *cause-and-effect* association and provides a measure of the impact of the exposure on public health. In addition to these measures, the **population-attributable risk (PAR)** provides a measure of a disease or health condition in a population attributed to the exposure, and is typically expressed per 10^n. Moreover, the **population-attributable risk percentage (PAR%)** also appears in epidemiological and public health reports and provides a measure of the percentage of the disease or health condition in the population that can be attributed to the exposure.

Odds Ratio

The last relative measure of association that will be highlighted is the exposure *odds ratio* or *relative odds*, which is calculated by epidemiologists and health care researchers when incidence rates are not readily available. The **odds ratio** is typically calculated for case–control studies and provides a measure of the strength of the association between exposure and the disease or health condition under investigation. A case–control study often precedes a cohort study as an important initial attempt to identify the risk factor for a particular disease, health condition or event (Schubert and Bartfay 2010). The reader is referred to Chapter 5 for a discussion of case–control and cohort studies. The odds ratio (OfR) is mathematically expressed as follows:

$$OR = \frac{a/c}{b/d} = \frac{ad}{bc}$$

Calculation of Odds Ratio Example

The following table shows the association between smoking and stroke:

	Stroke	No Stroke
Smoker	A = 90	B = 60
Non-smoker	C = 60	D = 90

$$\text{Odds ratio} = \frac{A \times D}{B \times C} = \frac{90 \times 90}{60 \times 60} = \frac{8100}{3600} = 2.25$$

A two-by-two table can be utilized to derive this measure and can range from 0 to infinity in theory. If the odds ratio calculated equals 1, this is interpreted as no association between exposure and the disease or health condition. If the odd ration is greater than 1, this indicates a positive association between exposure and disease, whereas an odds ratio less than 1 would be indicative of an inverse or negative association between exposure and the disease or health condition.

Future Directions and Challenges

The historical roots of epidemiology illustrate the necessity of investigating a disease, health condition or event even before anything is often known about its aetiology per se. For example, prior to the discovery of the pathogen responsible for cholera, John Snow successfully employed epidemiological methods to show that a contaminated water supply on the Thames River in London, England, was associated with the cholera outbreaks. This finding had huge public health benefits in preventing and controlling cholera outbreaks long before the actual discovery of the pathogen responsible. The safety of our water supplies remains a major public health challenge in Canada and abroad. For example, contaminated water supplies in the past decade in Walkerton Ontario, North Battleford Saskatchewan, and the Kashechewan First Nation's reserve in Ontario have reminded us about how a contaminated water supply can threaten the health and safety of entire communities (O'Conner 2002; Quinlan and Dickinson 2009; Schubert and Bartfay 2010).

Our public health systems are also facing challenges related to combating infectious diseases due to multi-drug-resistant pathogens in a variety of clinical and community settings. Indeed, the indiscriminate, inappropriate, and widespread use of antibiotics in clinical (e.g., hospitals) and community health care settings (e.g., nursing homes, community walk-in clinics) and by the agricultural industry (e.g., poultry and dairy farmers) are increasingly producing strains of bacteria that are resistant to the current and limited number of available antibiotics on market (Baggett et al. 2003; Bax, Mullan, and Verhoef 2000; Boucher et al. 2009). There is also growing concern regarding potential acts of bioterrorism. For example, in 2001 bioterrorists deployed anthrax spores via the United States postal system which resulted in twenty-two confirmed infections and five deaths (Centers for Disease Control and Prevention 2008).

Marchant-Short and Whitney (2012) suggest that strategies that have helped public health care professionals and officials deal with infectious outbreaks such as SARS in Toronto should be considered and reflected upon in preparation for potential bioterrorist events. Hence, an understanding of the classic epidemiological triangle remains relevant today in terms of understanding communicable disease processes and how the spread of communicable diseases may be prevented (e.g., infection control measures, handwashing).

Although epidemiology and public health has historically focused on the detection and prevention of communicable disease, their mandate and foci has been expanded to include noncommunicable chronic diseases (e.g., cancer, heart disease, diabetes, stroke, Alzheimer's disease), which are currently the leading causes of morbidity and mortality in Canada (Statistics Canada 2010a, 2010b).

The life expectancy is more than 80 years in Canada, and the number of seniors is expected to reach 6.7 million in 2020 and 9.2 million in 2041 (PHAC 2008a). As of July 1, 2014, 15.7% (nearly 1:6) of Canada's population ($N = 35,540,400$) was aged 65 years or older (Statistics Canada 2014a). This was the first time that the total number of young Canadians aged 15–24 years ($N = 4.6$ million) was lower compared to the total number of older Canadians aged 55–64 years ($N = 4.7$ million) (Statistics Canada 2014a). Given that the likelihood of developing chronic noncommunicable disease increase with age, their incidence is predicted to dramatically increase over the next few decades also. This will continue to place increased burden and stress on our already strained publicly funded health care systems in Canada. In 2015 alone, the average health care cost for a senior aged 65–69 years was $6,298; $8,384 for a senior aged 70–74; $11,578 for a senior aged 75–79 years; and $20,917 for a senior 80 years or more (CIHI 2015a).

Accordingly, we have presented a revised and updated epidemiological triangle to address these health care issues and trends in Canada in light of our current understanding of the determinants of health; the holistic care paradigm of public health in Canada; and our expanded focus from individuals to groups, communities or entire populations (Health Canada 2002; Public Health Agency of Canada 2007).

Among the current challenges facing the science of epidemiology and public health in Canada and globally is an undue and continued emphasis on reductionist thinking that seeks answers and explanations on the molecular and laboratory level for complex social-psychological, political, cultural, and environmental phenomena. Consider, for example, the health links between poverty and health with a disproportionate burden of poverty falling on children, the unemployed or underemployed, one parent families and immigrants. For example, the National Population Health Survey found that new immigrants to Canada are generally in better overall health in comparison to the general Canadian population at large, but overtime they become twice as likely as Canadian-born individuals to report deterioration in their health status and income (Statistics Canada 2005). A reductionist and mechanistic approach to solving this complex issue based on the molecular- or laboratory-based level is simply not appropriate here. Hence, we argue that future gains in our understanding of health and disease processes may be less related to gains achieved based on mechanistic laboratory-based investigations, but will be attributed to more holistic interpretations which include a better understanding of the social determinants of health and multiple lifestyle risk factors. It is clear that much remains to be done from the new holistic public health perspective in this new millennium. Epidemiological and population health research provides the essential knowledge base that enables public health professionals and workers in Canada and abroad to meet current and anticipated future public health care needs and challenges facing Canadians across the lifespan.

Another challenge related to epidemiology and public health's scientific heritage is the fondness for dichotomous forms of reasoning related to health phenomena and the reluctance to view health as a continuous and complex state (Bartfay and Bartfay 2015). For example, let us consider the development of coronary heart disease (CHD). Traditional dichotomous forms of reasoning and thinking often draw attention to individual risk factors (e.g., smoking, diet high in saturated fat) and pathophysiological processes (e.g., atherosclerosis). By contrast, if we view CHD as a complex and continuous state, this encourages a population or community-wide perspective and the development of public health interventions and policies that will reduce overall incidence and prevalence rates by influencing frequency distributions in communities or entire populations.

For example, public health legislation banning smoking in public environments (e.g., workplace settings, shopping malls, restaurants) will help decrease unwanted exposure to second-hand smoke and therefore decrease the likelihood of developing CHD. Similarly, designing urban environments (e.g., wide sidewalks, parks, designated bicycle lanes in cities) that encourage individuals to be more active and adopt healthy lifestyles will also have positive ripple effects in terms of reducing the incidence and prevalence of CHD in communities and entire populations.

Another challenge surrounding the use of epidemiological approaches to understand and address public health challenges in the new millennium is not, however, purely scientific in nature. We need to consider the impact of collective actions and values which are at the heart of public health interventions and policies, and ascertain whether or not issues affecting individuals are more important than issues affecting entire communities or populations at large. Should public health inventions and policies emphasize the health of individuals, communities or entire populations? Which public health interventions and policies will result in the greater social good and have the greatest impact factor in terms of health outcomes achieved? The reader is referred to Chapter 10 for a more detailed discussion of these ethical issues related to the practice of public health in Canada.

We argue that when we concentrate on the individual level, this places emphasis on a biomechanistic view of health which views health largely as the absence of disease and the need to cure those individuals affected (Bartfay and Bartfay 2015). Conversely, when we adopt a community- or population-based perspective, a more holistic view of health will embody health promotion and prevention. This holistic view believes that individuals are more than their sum of functioning biological components or systems, and sees health as a complex blend of various socio-psychological, cultural, political, biological, environmental, and spiritual determinants of health along a continuum of health (Bartfay and Bartfay 2015).

An understanding of epidemiological approaches is particularly useful in public health because its focus is population based and it provides the necessary tools to monitor, collect, describe, analyze and interpret public health-related data that is collected (Aschengrau and Seage III 2008; Friis and Sellers 2009; Merrill 2010; Neutens and Rubinson 2002; Valanis 1999). The use of epidemiological techniques also helps to alert public health professionals and workers to the possible aetiology of diseases, health conditions, or events in populations and communities. Hence, current epidemiological approaches not only provides a vehicle to understanding disease processes at various levels but also provides a means to assess, monitor, and influence entire communities or populations.

Lastly, despite remarkable achievements related to the field of epidemiology and our understanding of both infectious (communicable) and noncommunicable disease processes during the nineteenth century and onwards, continued progress is by no means assured because of a new constellation of emerging threats (e.g., SARS, West Nile Virus, H1N1, growing rates of obesity and immobility in children and adults, bioterrorism) to human health and well-being in the new millennium. Accordingly, we argue that a basic understanding of epidemiological methodologies, principles, and measures are critical to provide safe and effective evidence-informed practice by all public health professionals and workers in Canada and globally (Canadian Nurses Association 2001, 1998; Public Health Agency of Canada 2007; Shah 2003). Public health care professionals and workers must receive education and training in epidemiology in order to address persisting, reemerging and emerging threats; to monitor health care and population trends; and to appropriately address health care challenges across the lifespan in Canada and abroad. For example, the Community Health Nurses Association of Canada (2003) notes that all public health nurses are required to identify and seek to address the root cause of illness and disease and to actively apply "epidemiological principles in using strategies such as screening, surveillance, immunization, communicable disease response and out-break management and education" (p. 12).

Group Review Exercise Box 6.1   Severe Acute Respiratory Syndrome (SARS) Crisis in Toronto

About this Canadian film

In 2003, a new virus emerged in Asia and quickly spread around the world. The condition known as *Severe Acute Respiratory Syndrome* (SARS) was spread by airborne droplets and resulted in severe congestion of the lungs, respiratory failure, and death in those infected. Over a period of just five months since entering the City of Toronto 375 residents fell ill and a total of 44 residents of Ontario died as a consequence of this global pandemic. The impact of this pandemic on the public health care system was enormous in Canada. By comparison, there were a total of 774 deaths reported worldwide. SARS resulted in a public health crisis in Toronto and other Canadian cities. This film documents the 2003 SARS crisis in Toronto and how organizations such as the World Health Organization (WHO) in Geneva, Switzerland, the provincial Ministry of Health and Long-term Care (MOHLTC), Toronto Public Health and other health care officials and organizations responded to this pandemic. The film is based on real events and is supplemented with actual news footage and press releases issued during this crisis in Canada and abroad. As a consequence of the SARS pandemic, we realized there was a national need to build and strengthen our public health care systems in Canada, and this included the establishment of the Public Health Agency of Canada.

Instructions:

This assignment may be done alone, in pairs or in groups of up to five people (note: if you are doing this assignment in pairs or groups, please only submit one hard or electronic copy to your instructor). The assignment should be typewritten and no more than four to six pages maximum in length (double-spaced please). View the film entitled "Plague city: SARS in Toronto." *Source*: Anchor Bay Entertainment, Inc. (2005). Plague city: SARS in Toronto, Toronto, ON: SWE Plague City Productions, Inc. (DV14938). Take notes during the viewing of this Canadian film.

  i. Provide a brief overview of how the SARS virus entered into Canada from abroad and how it quickly spread in the environment.
 ii. Describe the role of public health professionals in monitoring, tracking, and treating this previously unknown virus in Toronto, Ontario.
iii. Describe the interventions and actions taken by the World Health Organization (WHO), the Ministry of Health and Long-Term Care (MOHLTC), Toronto Public Health and other public health officials to limit the spread and impact of the SARS virus.
 iv. What did public health professionals and officials learn from the global SARS pandemic, and how can we better prepare to manage future events in Canada?

Summary

- Epidemiology is the scientific study of the distribution and determinants of health-related states or events in human populations across the lifespan and the application of this study to maintain control and prevent alterations to health and well-being (Schubert and Bartfay 2010).
- Activities of epidemiologists involve a host of undertakings including the identification of risk factors or determinants of health related to disease events, injury, disability, and deaths; monitoring and describing their natural history; monitoring and tracking diseases and outbreaks in communities; identifying which individuals or populations are at greatest risk; and evaluating the efficacy and effectiveness of various community-based primary health care services, interventions, or programs.
- Hippocrates (466–377 B.C.) coined the terms *epidemiology*, *endemics* and *pandemics* and was the first to establish a scientifically based model of disease causation based on the body humours which challenged traditional beliefs of his time associated with supernatural causes of disease states.
- John Graunt's (1620–1674) statistical analysis of the *Bills of Mortality* in London lead to the development of a more comprehensive understanding of a variety of diseases, their distributions in populations, and the causes of mortality.

- Richard Doll and Bradford Hill were the first to examine the association between smoking history (i.e., lifestyle choice), intensity, and duration with the development of the noncommunicable chronic disease lung cancer in England following World War II employing epidemiological methods.
- The Framingham Heart Study began in 1948 and was the first prospective cohort study to identify a number of modifiable lifestyle (e.g., diet, exercise) and non-modifiable (e.g., sex, age, genetic predisposition) risk factors associated and social determinants of health (e.g., poverty, level of education) with the development of heart disease and stroke.
- We examined the importance of collecting accurate and high-quality data for disease surveillance and tracking so that public health professionals can integrate, analyze and interpret the data to ensure the health and safety of Canadian residents through the dissemination of health reports, advisories, alerts, and warnings.
- The epidemiological triad, comprised of the (a) host; (b) agent, (c) environment, and (d) time, was developed to examine communicable diseases (e.g., TB, plague, smallpox) in relation to their cause and aetiology, which were the leading causes of disease before the turn of the present century.
- Currently, noncommunicable forms of disease (e.g., heart disease, stroke, certain cancers, diabetes), which have been linked to lifestyle risk factors (e.g., diet, smoking, immobility) and various social determinants of health (socioeconomic status, environmental factors), are the major causes of morbidity and mortality in Canada.
- Consequently, an updated version of the epidemiological triangle was presented that consists of the (a) environment which has been expanded to include physical, social, cultural, and political aspects; (b) individuals, groups, communities, and entire populations as the focus; (c) the social determinants of health; and (d) time.
- The four stages for the natural history of a disease consist of the (a) stage of susceptibility; (b) stage of presymptomatic disease; (c) stage of clinical disease; and (d) the stage of recovery, disability, or death.
- The central goal of public health is to preserve, protect, and promote the health and well-being of individuals, groups, and populations via primary health care interventions for each stage of the disease process.
- Lastly, we examined various measures of disease frequency (e.g., prevalence, incidence, attack rates) and associations (e.g., relative risk, attributable risks, odds ratio) that are critical for reading and understanding governmental reports, public health alerts and warning, and peer-reviewed articles in the public and allied health sciences.

Critical Thinking Questions

1. A producer at a local television station has asked you to provide input into the development of a short video highlighting the current and historical improvements epidemiology has made to public health in Canada and abroad. What themes, content, or public health messages would you suggest for this video and justify why you have chosen these?
2. What are the pros and cons of having reportable national and international disease registries for a select communicable disease (e.g., TB, HIV/ AIDS, hepatitis B, SARS, H1N1)?
3. What does it mean when the prevalence and incidence rates for a given health problem (e.g., type 2 diabetes, cardiovascular disease, breast cancer) are similar, and what does it mean when they are very different in nature?
4. How might public health care professionals and workers employ epidemiological data (e.g., prevalence, incidence, morbidity, and mortality rates) to influence their practice for a defined population (e.g., school-aged children, elderly, Indigenous peoples, homeless)?
5. Why are infant and child mortality rates widely employed by public health officials as a proxy measure of health of population health?
6. What epidemiology data would you employ to determine the current top three leading causes of mortality and morbidity in your province or territory, and how have these data changed over the past decade?

References

Active Healthy Kids Canada. *2014 Report Card on the Physical Activity of Children and Youth: Is Canada in the Running?*. Toronto, ON: Author, 2014. Retrieved November 15, 20125, http://dvqdas9jty7g6.cloudfront.net/reportcard2014/AHKC_2014_ReportCard_ENG.pdf.

Adams, F. *The Genuine Works of Hippocrates.* New York: William Wood, 1886.

Ali, S. H. "A Socio-Ecological Autopsy for the *E. coli* 0157:H7 Outbreak in Walkerton, Ontario, Canada." *Social Science and Medicine* 58 (2004): 2601–12.

Alzheimer Society of Canada. *Rising Tide: The Impact of Dementia on Canadian Society.*(A Study Commissioned by the Alzheimer Society). Executive Summary. Toronto, ON: Author, 2010 (ISBN: 978-0-9733522-2-1).

Angell, M. "The Interpretation of Epidemiologic Studies." Editorial. *New England Journal of Medicine* 323 (1990): 823–25.

Armstrong, P., and H. Armstrong. *Wasting Away: The Undermining of Canadian Health Care,* 2nd ed.. Don Mills, ON: Oxford University Press, 2003.

Aschengrau, A., and G. R. Seage III. *Essentials of Epidemiology in Public Health.* 2nd ed. Toronto, ON: Jones and Bartlett Publishers, 2008.

Auger, N., M. F. Raynalut, R. Lessard, and R. Choiniere. "Income and Health in Canada." In *Social Determinants of Health: Canadian Perspectives,* edited by D. Raphael, 39–52. Toronto, ON: Canadian Scholars' Press, 2004.

Baggett, H. C., T. W. Henessy, R. Leman, C. Hamlin, D. Bruden, A. Reasonover, P. Martinez, and J. C. Butler. "An Outbreak of Community-Onset Methicillin Resistant *Staphylococcus aureus* Skin Infections in Southwestern Alaska." *Infection Control & Hospital Epidemiology* 24, no. 6 (2003): 397–402.

Bartfay, E., and W. J. Bartfay. "Quality-of-Life Outcomes Among Alzheimer's Disease Family Caregivers Following Community-Based Interventions." *Western Journal of Nursing Research* 35 no. 1 (January 2013): 98–116. doi:10.1177/0193945911400763.

Bartfay, W. J., and E. Bartfay. *Public Health in Canada.* Boston, MA: Pearson Learning Solutions, 2015.

Bartfay, W. J. "Introduction to Community Health Nursing in Canada." In *Community Health Nursing: Caring in Action,* edited by J. E. Hitchcock, P. E. Schubert, S. A. Thomas, and W. J. Bartfay, 1–10. Toronto, ON: Nelson Education, 2010.

Bax, R., N. Mullan, and J. Verhoef. The Millennium Bugs—The Need for a Development of New Antibacterials. *International Journal of Antimicrobial Agents* 16 (2000): 51–9.

Boucher, H. W., G. H. Talbot, J. S. Bradley, J. E. Edwards, D. Gilbert, L. B. Rice, and J. Bartlet. "Bad Bugs, No Drugs: No ESKAPE! An Update From the Infectious Diseases Society of America." *Clinical Infectious Diseases* 48 (2009): 1–12.

Buck, C., A. Llopis, E. Najera, and M. Terris, eds. *The Challenge of Epidemiology: Issues and Select Readings.* Washington, DC: World Health Organization, 1998.

Canadian Cancer Society. *Media Backgrounder: Canadian Cancer Statistics 2005. Fast Facts. Media Release.* Retrieved May, 26, 2010, http://www.cancer.ca/ccs/internet/mediareleaselist/0,,3172_343093094_399060511_landld-en.html.

———. *Canadian Cancer Statistics 2012.* Retrieved January 02, 2013, http://www.cancer.ca/canada-wide/about%20cancer/cancer%20statistics/stats%20at%20a%20glance/breast%20cancer.aspx.

Canadian Institute of Health Information (CIHI). *Health Care in Canada.* Ottawa, ON: Canada. Author, 2007.

Canadian Institute of Health Research. *Government of Canada Boosts Efforts to Find Treatments for Pediatric Cancers and Rare Genetic Diseases (News Release).* Ottawa, ON: Author, February 22, 2011. www.cihr-irsc.gc.ca/e/43211.html.

Canadian Nurses Association. *Evidence-based Decision-Making and Nursing Practice.* Ottawa, ON: Author, 1998. Retrieved April 12, 2013, http://www.can-nurses.ca.

———. *Why Is Nursing Education Changing? To Meet the Changing Needs of the Health Care System.* Ottawa, ON: Author, 2001. Retrieved April 12, 2012, http://www.can-nurses.ca/pages/careers/why_is_nrsg_edu.changing.htm.

Canadian Water and Wastewater Association. (n.d.). *Private Water Supplies: Frequently Asked Questions.* Retrieved March 10, 2011, http://www.cwwa.ca/faqprivate_e.asp.

Centers for Disease Control. *Questions and Answers about Anthrax.* Washington, DC: Author, 2008. Retrieved June 05, 2013, http://emergency.cdc.gov/agent/anthrax/faq.

Childhood Obesity Foundation. *Statistics.* VGH Hospital Campus, Vancouver, BC: Author, 2015. Retrieved November 10, 2015, http://childhoodobesityfoundation.ca/what-is-childhood-obesity/statistics/.

Community Health Nurses Association of Canada (CHNAC). *Canadian Community Health Nursing Standards of Practice*. Retrieved April 14, 2013, http://www.communityhealth-nursing-canada.org.

Commission on the Social Determinants of Health. *Closing the Gap in a Generation. Health Equity through Action on the Social Determinants of Health*. Geneva, Switzerland: World Health Organization, 2008.

Cumston, C. G. *An Introduction to the History of Medicine*. New York: Alfred A. Knopf, 1926.

Davis, J. P., P. J. Chesney, P. J. Wand, M. LaVenture, and the Investigation and Laboratory Team. "Toxic-Shock Syndrome: Epidemiologic Features, Recurrence, Risk Factors, and Prevention." *New England Journal of Medicine* 303 (1980): 1429–1435.

Dawber, T. R. *The Framingham Study: The Epidemiology of Atherosclerotic Disease*. Cambridge, MA: Harvard University Press, 1980.

Dawber, T. R., W. B. Kannel, and L. P. Lyell. "An Approach to Longitudinal Studies in a Community: The Framingham Study." *Annuals of the New York Academy of Science* 107 (1963): 539–556.

Dawber, T. R., G. F. Meadors, and F. E. Moore. "Epidemiological Approaches to Heart Disease: The Framingham Study." *American Journal of Public Health* 41 (1951): 279–286.

Doll, R., and A. B. Hill. "Smoking and Carcinoma of the Lung." *British Medical Journal* 2 (1950): 739–748.

———. "The Mortality of Doctors in Relation to Their Smoking Habits." *British Medical Journal* 1 (1954): 1451–1455.

Doll, R., R. Peto, J. Boreham, and I. Sutherland. Mortality in Relation to Smoking: 50 Years' Observations on Male British Doctors. *British Medical Journal* 328, no. 7455 (2004): 1519.

Donatelle, R. J., L. G. Davis, A. J. Munroe, A. Munroe, and M. Casselman. *Health: The Basics*. 3rd Canadian ed. Toronto, ON: Pearson Benjamin Cummings, 2006.

Enterline, P. E. Mortality Among Asbestos Products Workers in the United States. *Annuals of the New York Academy of Science* 132 (1965):156–164.

Farr, W. *Vital Statistics: A Memorial Volume of Sections From the Reports and Writings of William Far*. New York: Academy of Medicine, 1975.

Fenn, E. A. *Pox Americana. The Great Small Pox Epidemic of 1775–82*. New York: Hill and Wang, 2001.

First Nations and Inuit Regional Health Survey. *National Report 1999*. St. Regis, QC: First Nations and Inuit Regional Health Survey National Steering Committee, 1999.

Foot, D., G. Curnew, and L. Pearson. *The Shape of Things to Come: A National Report on Heart Disease and the Challenges Ahead*. Toronto, ON: Commissioned by Becel, 2005. Retrieved March 30, 2013, http://www.becel.ca/pdf. shapeothings_en.pdf.

Frank, F., and A. Smith. *The Community Development Handbook: A Tool to Build Community Capacity*. Ottawa, ON: Human Resources Development Canada, 1999.

Friis, R. H., and T. A. Sellers. *Epidemiology for Public Health Practice*. 4th ed. Toronto, ON: Jones and Bartlett Publishers, 2009.

Gallin, J. I., and F. P. Ognibene. *Principles and Practice of Clinical Research*. 2nd ed. Burlington, MA: Academic Press—Elsevier, 2007.

Garrison, F. H. *History of Medicine*. Philadelphia: Saunders, 1963.

Graunt, J. *Natural and Political Observations Made Upon the Bills of Mortality*. London: John Hopkins Press, 1662/1939.

Gross, M. "Oswego Country Revisited." *Public Health Reports* 91 (1976): 168–170.

Hales, D., and L. Lauzon. *An Invitation to Health*. 1st Canadian ed. Toronto, ON: Nelson Education, 2009.

Hall, J. *Less Bang for Health Dollar in Canada*, A10. Toronto, ON: Toronto Star, 2011.

Harper, D. P. "Angelical Conjunction: Religion, Reason, and Inoculation in Boston, 1721–1722." *The Pharos*, (2000): Winter, 1–5.

Health Canada. *Nutrition for Healthy Pregnancy: National Guidelines for the Childbearing Years*. Ottawa, ON: Minister of Public Works and Government Services, 1999.

———. *Nutrition for a Healthy Pregnancy: National Guidelines for the Childbearing Years*. Ottawa, ON: Minister of Public Works and Government Services, 2000.

———. *Population Health, 2002*. Ottawa, ON: Minister of Public Works and Government Services, 2002. Retrieved March 2, 2012, http://www.phac-aspc.gc.ca/ph-sp/phdd/determinants/index.html#determinants.

──────. *Guidelines for Canadian Drinking Water Quality. Supporting Documents*. Ottawa, ON: Author, 2004. Retrieved March 10, 2013, http://www.hc.sc.gc.ca/ewh-semt/pubs/water-eau/doc_sup-appui/index_e.html.

──────. *What's in your Well? A Guide to Well Water Treatment and Maintenance*. Ottawa, ON: Author, 2008. Retrieved March 10, 2012, http://www.hc-sc.gc.ca/ewh-semt/pubs/water-eau/well-puits_e.html.

Health Council of Canada. *Progress Report 2011: Health Care Renewal in Canada*. Toronto, ON: Author, 2011, information@healthcouncilcanada.ca.

Health News. *Medical Milestone: Mary Mallon, Typhoid Mary, November 1968*. New York: New York Department of Health, 1968.

Heiby, J. R. "Quality Improvement and the Integrated Management of Childhood Illnesses: Lessons from Developed Countries." *Quality Improvement* 24, no. 5 (1998): 264–68.

Hennekens, C. H., J. E. Buring, and S. L. Mayrent. *Epidemiology in Medicine*. Toronto, ON: Little, Brown and Company, 1987.

Herbst, A. L., H. Ulfelder, and D. C. Poskanzer. "Adenocarcinoma of the Vagina: Association of Maternal Stilbestrol Therapy with Tumor Appearance in Young Women." *New England Journal of Medicine (NEJM)* 284 (1971): 878–81.

Heymann, D. L. *Control of Communicable Diseases Manual: An Official Report of the American Public Health Association*. 18th ed. Washington, DC: American Public Health Association, 2004.

Hippocrates. "On Airs, Waters, and Places." *Medical Classics* 3 (1938): 19–42.

Humphreys, N. A., ed. *Vital Statistics: A Memorial Volume of Selections From the Reports and Writings of William Farr, 1807–1883*. London: Sanitary Institute of Great Britain, 1885.

Iffy, L., H. A. Kaminetzky, J. E. Maidman, J. Lindsey, and W. S. Arrata. "Control of Perinatal Infection by Traditional Preventive Measures." *Obstetrics and Gynecology* 54 (1979): 403–11.

Kannel, W. B. "The Framingham Study: Its 50-Year Legacy and Future Promise." *Journal of Atherosclerosis and Thrombosis* 6 (2000): 60–66.

Kannel, W. B., and R. D. Abbott. "Incidence and Prognosis of Unrecognized Myocardial Infarction: An Update on the Framingham Study." *New England Journal of Medicine (NEJM)* 311 (1984): 1144–47.

Kirby, M. *Reforming Health Protection and Promotion in Canada: Time to Act. 14th Report on the Standing Senate Committee on Social Affairs, Science and Technology*. Ottawa, ON: Government of Canada, 2003.

Krause, M. V., and M. A. Hunscher. *Food, Nutrition, anSSd Diet Therapy*. 5th ed. Philadelphia, PA: Saunders, 1972.

Latham, R. H., M. W. Kehrberg, J. A. Jacobson, and C. B. Smith. " Toxic Shock Syndrome in Utah: A Review of a Case-Control Study and Surveillance." *Annuals of Internal Medicine* 96 (1982): 906–18.

Lilienfeld, A. M. "Centers Paribus: The Evolution of the Clinical Trial." *Bulletin of History and Medicine* 56 (1982): 1–18.

Lind, J. *A Treatise of the Scurvy*. Edinburgh, Scotland: Kincaird and Donaldson, 1753.

Lyons, A. S., and R. J. Petrucelli. *Medicine: An Illustrated History*. New York: Harry N. Abrams, Inc., 1978.

Mandleco, B., and W. J. Bartfay. "Care in Infants, Children, and Adolescents." In *Community Health Nursing: Caring in Action*. 1st Canadian ed., edited by J. E. Hitchcock, P. E. Schubert, S. A. Thomas, and W. J. Bartfay, 325–73. Toronto, ON: Nelson Education, 2010.

Marchant-Short, S., and L. Whitney, Leeann, L. "Communicable Diseases." In *Community Health Nursing: A Canadian Perspective*. 3r ed., edited by L. Leeseberg Stamler and L. Yiu, 189–212. Toronto, ON: Pearson Canada, 2012.

Marmot, M., and T Thorell. "Social Class and Cardiovascular Disease: The Contribution of Work." *International Journal of Health Services* 18, no. 4 (1988): 659–74.

Mausner, J., and A. K. Bahn. *Epidemiology: An Introductory Text*. Philadelphia, PA: WB Saunders, 1974.

McAllister, M. "Domestic Violence: A Life-span Approach to Assessment and Intervention [Electronic Version]." *Lippincott's Primary Care Practice* 4, no. 2 (2000): 174–89.

Merrill, R. M. *Introduction to Epidemiology*. 5th ed. Toronto, ON: Jones and Bartlett Publishers, 2010.

Miller, G. *The Adoption of Inoculation for Smallpox in England and France*. Philadelphia, PA: University of Pennsylvania Press, 1957.

Monahan, P. J. *Chaoulli v Québec and the Future of Canadian Healthcare: Patient Accountability as the "Sixth Principle" of the Canada Health Act. C.D. Howe Institute Benefactors Lecture, November 29, 2006*, Toronto, ON: i-30, 2006.

National Aboriginal Health Organization (NAHO) First Nations Centre. *First Nations Longitudinal Health Survey 2002/2003: Report on Selected Indicators by Sex.* Retrieved April 10, 2013, http:rhs-ers.ca/English/pdf/rhs2002-03reports_on_selected_indicators_by_sex.pdf.

National Collaborating Centres for Public Health (NCCPH). *What Is Evidence-Informed Public Health? Fact Sheet.* Retrieved October 12, 2013, http://www.nccmt.ca/eiph/

National Council of Welfare. *Poverty Facts 2003.* Ottawa, ON: Author, 2006.

Nester, E. W., B. J. McCarthy, C. E. Roberts, and N. N. Pearsall. *Microbiology, Molecules, Microbes and Man.* New York: Holt, Rinehart and Winston, 1973.

Neutens, J. J. and L. Rubinson. *Research Techniques for the Health Sciences.* 3rd ed. Toronto, ON: Benjamin Cummings, 2002.

O'Conner, D. B. *Part One: A Summary of the Walkerton Inquiry: The Events of May 2000 and Related Issues. Ontario Ministry of the Attorney General.* Toronto, ON: Publications Ontario, 2002.

Organization for Economic Co-operation and Development (OECD). *OECD Health Data 2010: Statistics and Indicators for 30 Countries.* Retrieved April 12, 2012, http://www.ecosante.org/index2.php?base=OCDE&langs=ENG&langh=ENG.

Pamuk, E., D. Makuc, K. Heck, C. Reuben, and K. Lochner. *Socioeconomic Status and Health Chartbook. Health, United States.* Hyattsvill, MD: National Centre for Health Statistics, 1998, http://www.cdc.gov/nchs/hus/htm.

Plotkin, S. A. "Vaccines: Past, Present and Future." *Nature and Medicine,* 11 (2005): S5–11.

Public Health Agency of Canada. *The Social Determinants of Health: An Overview of the Implications for Policy and the Role of the Health Sector,* 2002. Retrieved March 30, 2011, http://www.phac-aspc.gc.ca/ph-sp/phdd/pdf/overview_implications/01_overview_e.pdf.

———. *West Nile Virus MONITOR: Human Surveillance (2003–2005),* 2006. Retrieved May 2012, http://www.phac-aspc.gc.ca/wnv-vwn.monhumunsurv-archieve_e.html.

———. *Core Competencies for Public Health in Canada: Release 1.1.* Ottawa, ON: Author, 2007.

———. *Canada's Aging Population. Division of Aging Seniors.* Ottawa, ON: PHAC, 2008a. Retrieved April 02, 2012, http://www.phac-aspc.gc.ca/seniors-aines/publications/public/various-varies/papier-fed-paper/index-eng.php.

———. *Minimizing the Risks of Cardiovascular Disease.* Ottawa, ON: Author, 2008b. Retrieved March 30, 2012, http://www.phac-aspc.gc.ca/cd-mc/cvd-mcv/risk0risques-eng.php.

Quinlan, E., and H. D. Dickinson. "The Emerging Public Health System in Canada." In *Health, Illness, and Health Care in Canada.* 4th ed., edited by B. Singh Bolaria and H. D. Dickinson (eds.), 42–55. Toronto, ON: Nelson Education, 2009.

Raphael, D. *Health Promotion and Quality of Life in Canada: Essential Readings.* Toronto, ON: Canadian Scholars' Press Inc., 2010.

——— (ed.). *Social Determinants of Health: Canadian Perspectives.* Toronto, ON: Canadian Scholars Press, Inc., 2004.

Ries, L. A. G., D. Harkins, M. Krapcho, A. Mariotto, B. A. Miller, E. J. Feuer, L. Clegg L, et al. *SEER Cancer Statistics Review, 1975–2003.* Bethesda, MD: National Cancer Institute, 2006.

Romanow, R. J. *Building on Values: The Future of Health Care in Canada-Final Report. Commission on the Future of Health Care in Canada* (cat. No. CP32-85/2002E-IN), Ottawa, ON: Government of Canada, 2002, http://www.hc-sc.gc.ca/english/care/romanow/hcc0023.html.

Rosen, G. A. *History of Public Health.* New York: MD Publications, 1958.

Ross, N., M. Wolfson, J. Dunn, J. M. Berthelot, G. Kaplan, and J. Lynch. "Relations between Income Inequality and Mortality in Canada and in the United States: Cross Sectional Assessment Using Census Data and Vital Statistics." *British Medical Journal* 320 (2000): 898–902.

Sanborn, M. D., A. Abelsohn, M. Campbell, E. Weir. "Identifying and Managing Adverse Environmental Effects: 3. Lead Exposure." *Canadian Medical Association Journal* 166, no. 1 (2002): 287–92.

Schubert, P. E., and W. J. Bartfay. "Introduction to Community Health Nursing in Canada." In *Community Health Nursing: Caring in Action,* 1st Canadian ed., edited by J. E. Hitchcock, P. E. Schubert, S. A. Thomas, and W. J. Bartfay. 173–90. Toronto, ON: Nelson Education, 2010.

Scotto, C. J. "A New View of Caring." *Journal of Nursing Education* 42, no. 7 (2003): 289–91.

Selikoff, I. J., E. C. Hammond, and J. Churg. "Asbestos Exposures, Smoking and Neoplasia." *Journal of the American Medical Association* 204 (1968): 104–10.

Semmelweis, I. P. *Die aetiologie der Begriff und die prophylaxis des kindbettfiebers*. Budapest: C.A. Hartleben and Vienna, 1861.

Semmelweis, I. P., and F. B. Murphy (translation). "The Etiology, the Concept and Prophylaxis of Childbed Fever." *Medical Classics* 5 (1941): 350–773.

Shah, C. P. *Public Health and Preventative Medicine in Canada*. 5th ed. Toronto, ON: Elsevier Canada, 2003.

Shands, K. N., W. F. Schleck III, N. T. Hargrett, B. B. Dan, G. P. Schmid, and J. V. Bennett. "Toxic Shock Syndrome: Case-Control Studies at the Centers for Disease Control." *Annuals of Internal Medicine* 96 (1982): 895–992.

Shands, K. N., G. P. Schmid, B. B. Dan, D. Blum, R. J. Guidotti, N. T. Hargrett, R. L. Anderson, et al. "Toxic Shock Syndrome in Menstruating Women: Association With Tampon Use and Staphylococcus Aureus and the Clinical Features of 52 Cases." *New England Journal of Medicine* 303 (1980): 1436–48.

Shindell, S., J. C. Salloway, and C. M. Oberembi. *A Coursebook in Health Care Delivery*. New York: Appleton-Century-Crofts, 1976.

Sizer, F., and E. Whitney, E. *Nutrition: Concepts and Controversies*. 8th ed. Belmont, CA: Wadsworth, 2000.

Snow, J. *On the Mode of Communication of Cholera*. 2nd ed. London, UK: Churchill, 1855.

———. *Snow on Cholera*. Cambridge, MA: Harvard University Press, 1855.

Statistics Canada. *Mental Health and Well-Being. Canadian Community Health Survey*. Ottawa, ON: Author, 2002. Accessed April 02, 2011, http://www.statcan.ca/bsolc/English/bsolc?catmp=82-617-X&CHROPG=1.

———. Dynamics of Immigrants Health in Canada. Evidence From the National Population Health Survey. *The Daily*. Ottawa, ON: Author, February 23, 2005. Accessed June 05, 2013, http://www.statcan.ca/Daily/English/050233/d/5050223c.htm.

———. *Age-Standardized Mortality Rates by Selected Causes, by Sex (Both Sexes)*. Ottawa, ON: Author, 2010a (CANSIM Table 102-0552 and Catalogue No. 84F0209X). Accessed April 14, 2011, http://www40.statcan.gc.ca/cbin/fl/cstsaveas-flg2.cgi?filename=health30a-eng-htm&lan=eng.

———. *Leading Causes of Death by Sex (Both Sexes)*. Ottawa, ON: Author, 2010b. (CANSIM table 102-0561 and Catalogue No. 84-215-X). Accessed April 14, 2011, http://www40.statcan.gc.ca/cbin/fl/cstsaveasflg2.cgi?filename=hlth36a-eng.htm&lan=eng.

———. *Physical Activity Levels of Canadian Children and Youth, 2007 to 2009*. Ottawa, ON: Author, 2013. (Report 82-625-X). Accessed November 10, 2015, http://www.statcan.gc.ca/pub/82-625-x/2011001/article/11553-eng.htm.

———. *Canada's Population Estimates; Age and Sex 2014*. Ottawa, ON: Author, 2014a. Retrieved November 10, 2015, http://www.statcan.gc.ca/daily-quotidien/140926/dq140926b-eng.htm.

———. *Leading Causes of Death by Sex (Both Sexes). CANSIM table 102-0561*. Ottawa, ON: Author, 2014b. Retrieved July 02, 2014, http://www5.statcan.gc.ca/cansim/a26?lang=eng&retrLang=eng&id=1020561&paSer=&pattern=&stByVal=1&p1=1&p2=37&tabMode=dataTable&csid=

Stewart, C. P., and D. Guthrie, eds. *Lind's Treatise on Scurvy. A Bicentenary Volume Containing a Reprint of the First Edition of a Treatise of the Scurvy by James Lind, MD, with Additional Notes*. Edinburgh, Scotland: Edinburgh University Press, 1953.

Sullivan, P. *Safety of Drinking Water Remains a Crucial Health Issue: CMA President Says. Canadian Medical Association*. Retrieved March 2, 2012, http://www.cma.ca/index.cfm/ci_id/10013192/la_id/1.html.

Susser, M. "Epidemiology in the United States After World War II: The Evolution of Technique." *Epidemiological Review* 7 (1985): 147–77.

Swanson, K. M. "What Is Known About Caring in Nursing Science: A Literary Meta-Analysis." In *Handbook of Clinical Nursing Research*, edited by A. S. Hinshaw, S. L. Feetham, and J. L. F. Shaver, 31–60. Thousand Oaks, CA: Sage Publications, 1999.

Teutsch, S., R. Churchill, and R. Elliot. *Principles and Practice of Public Health Surveillance*. New York: Oxford University Press, 1994.

The Council of Canadians. *Report on Notice for Drinking Water Crisis in Canada*. Ottawa, ON: Author, 2015. Retrieved October 15, 2015, http://canadians.org/drinking-water or https://www.google.ca/search?q=boil+water+advisory+-canada&biw=1280&bih=631&source=lnms&tbm=isch&sa=X&ved=0CAgQ_AUoA2oVChMIsYmbsO3EyAIVwpoeCh3G4gBG#imgrc=UqPAKvcqi5zvPM%3A.

Thomas, S. A., and W. J. Bartfay. "Global Health Perspectives for Community Health Nurses." In *Community Health Nursing: Caring in Action.* 1st Canadian ed., edited by J. E. Hitchcock, P. E. Schubert, S. A. Thomas, and W. J. Bartfay, 1–10. Toronto, ON: Nelson Education, 2010.

Thompson, V. D. *Health and Health Care Delivery in Canada.* Toronto, ON: Mosby Elsevier, 2010.

Todd, J., M. Fishaut, E. Kapral, and T. Welch. "Toxic-Shock Syndrome Associated With Phage-Group-I *Staphylococci.*" *Lancet* 2 (1978): 1116–18.

Tu, K., Z. Chen, L. L. Lipscombe, and The Canadian Hypertension Education Program Outcomes Research Taskforce. "Prevalence and Incidence of Hypertension From 1995 to 2005: A Population-Based Study." *Canadian Medical Association Journal* 178, no. 11 (May 20, 2008): 1429–35.

United Nations Children's Fund (UNICEF). *The State of the World's Children 2006.* New York: Author, 2005. Retrieved April 12, 2013, http://www.esa.un.org.unpp.

Valanis, B. *Epidemiology in Health Care.* 3rd ed. Stamford, CT: Appleton and Lange, 1999.

Whitney, E., and S. Rady Rolfes. *Understanding Nutrition.* 10th ed. Toronto, ON: Thompson Wadsworth, 2005.

Wilkins, R., J. M. Berthelot, and E. Ng. "Trends in Mortality by Neighbourhood Income in Urban Canada From 1970–1996." *Health Reports* 13 (2000): 1–28.

World Health Organization (WHO). *International Health Regulations.* Geneva, Switzerland: Author, 2006a. Retrieved April 14, 2011. http://www.who.int.csr/ish/en.

———. *Working for Health: An Introduction to the World Health Organization.* Geneva, Switzerland: Author, 2006b. Retrieved April 14, 2011. http://www.who.int/about/brochure_en.pdf.

———. *WHO Mortality Data.* Geneva, Switzerland: Author, 2010. Retrieved http://www.who.int/who.sis.mort.en.

World Health Organization and Health and Welfare Canada and the Canadian Public Health Agency. "Ottawa. Charter for Health Promotion." *Canadian Journal of Public Health* 77, no. 12 (1986): 425–30.

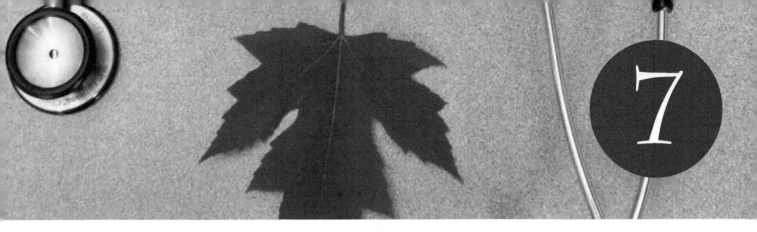

Human Responses to Disease, Illness, and Sickness

The History of Medicine:

- 2000 BC—Here, eat this root.
- 1000 AD—That root is heathen. Here, say this prayer.
- 1850 AD—That prayer is superstition. Here, drink this potion.
- 1920 AD—That potion is snake oil. Here, swallow this pill.
- 1945 AD—That pill is ineffective. Here, take this penicillin.
- 1955 AD—Oops…bugs mutated. Here, take this tetracycline.
- 1960–1990 AD—39 more "opps"…. Here, take this more powerful antibiotic.
- 2000 AD—The bugs have won! Here, eat this root.

—Anonymous

Learning Objectives

After completion of this chapter, the student will be able to:
- define and differentiate among the terms disease, illness, and sickness;
- describe why the classification of diseases is essential to public health practice in Canada and globally;
- list and define the five general categories for classifying diseases and provide examples of each;
- list and describe the five stages of the illness process;
- define and differentiate between the terms acute and chronic disease and provide examples of each;
- define the terms communicable and non-communicable disease and provides examples of both;
- list and describe common modes of disease transmission;

(Continued)

(*Continued*)

- describe the importance for the surveillance, control, and management of diseases by public health professionals and workers;
- define and differentiate among acquired, natural, active, and herd forms of immunity and provide examples of each;
- describe the role of public health professionals and workers for planning and implementation immunization programs in Canada and globally;
- identify and describe current barriers and challenges for controlling and managing communicable and non-communicable diseases in Canada and globally;
- define and differentiate between the terms injury and disability and provide examples of each; and
- define bioterrorism and discuss the growing implications for public health and safety.

Core Competencies Addressed in Chapter 7

Core Competencies	Competency Statements
1.0 Public Health Sciences	1.1, 1.2, 1.3, 1.4
2.0 Assessment and Analysis	2.1, 2.2, 2.4, 2.5, 2.6
3.0 Policy and Program Planning, Implementation, and Evaluation	3.1, 3.2, 3.6
4.0 Partnerships, Collaboration, and Advocacy	4.1, 4.2, 4.3, 4.4
5.0 Diversity and Inclusiveness	5.1, 5.3
6.0 Communication	6.1, 6.2
7.0 Leadership	7.1, 7.2, 7.4, 7.5

Notes: Please see the following document or web-based link for a detailed description of these specific competencies (Public Health Agency of Canada 2007a).

Introduction

The words disease, illness, and sickness are often used interchangeably in published health reports, the mass medias (e.g., newspapers, television, radio), and by Internet-based social medias (e.g., Facebook, Twitter, YouTube), but the terms are not synonymous in nature (Bartfay and Bartfay 2015). In this chapter, we shall explore human responses to disease, illness, and sickness. We shall also examine the various common classifications and nomenclatures employed to describe disease, common modes of disease transmission, and the stages of the illness process, and examine sickness and health from a social–cultural perspective. We shall also explore how an individual's interpretation of an altered state of health, condition, or disability may have different meanings based on the individual's dominant social and cultural context. Lastly, we shall examine the threat of bioterrorism and how it may affect the health and safety of residents in Canada and globally.

The responsibility for the preservation and promotion of health in Canada is multi-sectorial and shared among our residents, communities and healthcare regions, public health professionals and workers, healthcare services agencies, institutions and organizations, and all levels of government (Advisory Committee on

Population Health 2001; Bartfay and Bartfay 2015; Bartfay 2011; Canadian Public Health Association 2001; Public Health Agency of Canada 2007; Romanow 2002). This responsibility includes the implementation of national and provincial/territorial primary healthcare initiatives which seek to empower individuals, families, groups, or entire communities to make informed decisions about their health and well-being.

For example, public health primary prevention immunization campaigns have been shown to be the most efficient and cost effective means to prevent the occurrence of a variety of vaccine preventable diseases and illnesses (e.g., Chicken pox, measles, mumps, polio, rubella, tuberculosis [TB]) (Plotkin 2005; Plotkin and Orenstein 2008, Public Health Agency of Canada 2006b).

Nonetheless, one of the current challenges facing public healthcare professionals and workers in Canada and globally is the fear that vaccines cause autism by some misguided and misinformed individuals. This is largely due to fraudulent research first published in the medical journal *Lancet* by Dr. Andrew Wakefield, a gastroenterologists in the United Kingdom, who claimed a link between the measles, mumps, and rubella (MMR) vaccine and autism in a small study of only 12 children (Wakefield et al. 1998). Due to international social and mass media exposure of this report, parents and guardians of children began to fear that the MMR vaccine and others containing thimerosal (a mercury-based preservative) caused autism (Associated Press 2007; Anekwe 2009; Deer 1998; Konner 2011; Ross 2011).

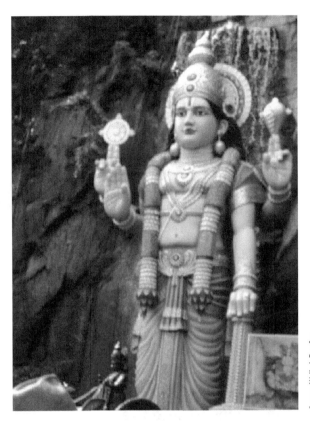

Source: Wally J. Bartfay

Photo 7.1 Statue of Dhanvantari, (Batu Caves, Malaysia) is one of the Hindu gods of healing and the father of Ayurvedic medicine. Beliefs about the origins and meanings of disease, illness and sickness often have great cultural, spiritual and social variations globally. Canada consists of a multicultural and ethnically diverse society in which public health care professionals and workers need to be cognizant and respectful of these noted beliefs.

Immunization rates in the United Kingdom and globally declined significantly as a result of Wakefield's article and widespread media exposure. For example, vaccination rates dropped by almost half in London and it was estimated that over 125,000 children born in the late 1990s did not receive the MMR vaccine because of fear by parents and guardians that they may develop autism (Associated Press 2011). Subsequent follow-up studies done by a variety of investigators refuted the claims made by Wakefield (e.g., Chai 2015; Demicheli et al. 2005; Honda, Shimizu, and Rutter 2005; Kemp 2010; Madsen et al. 2002; Price et al. 2010).

It was later discovered that the data reported in the original article by Wakefield (1998) was, in fact, fictitious and invalid in nature and the article was subsequently retracted. Despite the official retraction of Wakefield's (1998) article and the discrediting of the science behind the claims made including those by the co-authors of the original article, the claim that *vaccines cause autism in children* is still being perpetuated by radical anti-vaccine groups and certain social media sites (e.g., Twitter, Facebook, YouTube).

Hence, public health professionals and workers are faced with the challenge of educating misinformed individuals due to corrupt or fraudulent claims made by Wakefield. This example illustrates how misleading and incorrect information related to the MMR vaccine can be perpetuated via the mass media, Internet, and social media sites, and may have negative ripple effects in terms of potentially increasing the incidence and spread of vaccine-preventable diseases in Canada and globally (Bartfay and Bartfay 2015).

In this chapter, we shall examine the nomenclature of diseases and how they are broadly classified in Canada and globally. We shall highlight the importance of surveillance and tracking of these diseases by Canadian and global public health organizations and agencies. We shall also examine the role of public healthcare professionals and workers in their prevention, surveillance, control, and management, and highlight current challenges facing Canadians across the lifespan.

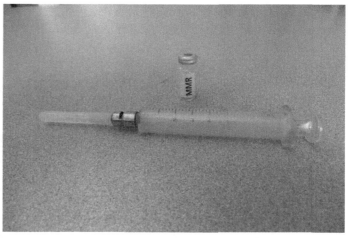

Source: Wally J. Bartfay

Photo 7.2 A small British study involving only 12 children linking the MMR vaccine to autism was found to be totally bogus and fraudulent, and subsequent large-scale studies conducted in various countries involving hundreds and thousands of children found no evidence for this. However, the belief that vaccines cause autism remains a major public health challenge in Canada and globally due to this false claim still being reported and spread by radical anti-vaccination special interests groups and certain misguided celebrities. In fact, every $1.00 spent on immunization results in a $16.00 saving for associated healthcare costs or a return on investment (ROI) of 1500%.

Nomenclature and the Common Classifications of Disease

All public health professionals and workers need to have at their disposal a standardized nomenclature and system for the classification of disease, its surveillance in groups and populations across the lifespan, communication of research findings, health trends and outcomes, and for the standardization of evidence-informed practice standards (American Psychiatric Association [APA] 2000; Friis and Sellers 2009; MacMahon and Pugh 1970; World Health Organization [WHO] 2004). A *nomenclature* is defined as a set of highly detailed and precise collection or a set of terms that are utilized by public health professionals and workers for both recording and describing clinical diagnoses for the purposes of classifying ill persons into defined groups (Bartfay and Bartfay 2015). A nomenclature system, therefore, must be extensive enough so that all possible clinical conditions encountered in public health practice can be effectively recorded, tracked, and communicated.

The *classification of disease* consists of a standardized system and terminology used for the purposes of categorizing diseases by their clinical nature, and permits the statistical compilation of a group of cases of disease by arranging disease entities into categories that share similar clinical manifestations (Bartfay and Bartfay 2015). Each category of a disease classification system must refer to diseases that are sufficiently frequent in nature in defined populations so that cases of the disease fall into a single category (APA 2000; Friis and Sellers 2009; MacMahon and Pugh 1970; WHO 2004). Otherwise, the disease classification system would contain an unmanageable list of disease categories. For example, it is possible to classify cases of disease according to a known causal agent (e.g., hepatitis B, TB, syphilis), or according to a known clinical manifestation such as the affected anatomical location (e.g., breast or prostate cancer). Finally, a well-defined disease classification system permits public health professionals and researchers to employ a standardized approach and scheme which can then be utilized across regional or provincial/territorial health jurisdictions in Canada or even other countries so that comparisons in morbidity and mortality outcomes from disease can be examined and compared.

ICD-10

For example, one of the most widely used disease classification systems in Canada and globally is the *International Statistical Classification of Diseases and Related Health Problems* (aka ICD-10) by the WHO Collaborative Centers for Classification of Diseases (WHO 2009), which helps to provide a wide-angled picture of the general health situation of countries, various regions of the world and populations. Currently, the ICD-10 is the world's standardized tool to capture mortality and morbidity data related to a variety of diseases. The ICD-10 also serves as a vehicle to organize and code health information that is used for biostatistics and epidemiology, monitoring and evaluation, prevention, treatment, and for research purposes. Hence, the ICD-10 has been designed for various purposes in mind including clinical and public health practice, healthcare management, allocation of primary healthcare resources, general epidemiological and public health purposes, and for the evaluation of healthcare programs and policies. The ICD-10 is in its 10th revision and currently spans three volumes. Volume I, for example, provides healthcare professionals and workers with the classification of diseases into three- and four-character levels. This new alphanumeric coding scheme replaces the numeric ones employed in previous editions. The reader is referred to Chapter 6 for a discussion of the *Bills of Mortality* by John Graunt (1620–1672) in England, which eventually evolved overtime into the present ICD-10. The revised and updated ICD-11 is scheduled for release in the year 2018 by WHO (see http://www.who.int/classifications/icd/revision/en/ and http://www.who.int/classifications/icd/revision/icd11faq/en/).

DSM-V

The *Diagnostic and Statistical Manual of Mental Disorders* (aka DSM-IV-TR and DSM-V) by the APA (2013, 2000, 1994) is widely employed worldwide and provides a standardized means for the classification and diagnosis of psychiatric disorders. The DSM-V was released on May 18, 2013, and is similar to the DSM-IV-TR with the following major changes: Asperger syndrome was dropped as a distinct classification, the various subtype classifications for variant forms of schizophrenia was deleted (e.g., formally paranoid, disorganized, catatonic, undifferentiated, and residual), the bereavement exclusion for depressive disorders was dropped, gender identity disorder was renamed "gender dysphoria," gambling disorder and tobacco use disorders are new, and the A2 criterion for post-traumatic stress disorder was removed and is included in the new section entitled *Trauma and Stressor-Related Disorders* (APA 2013; Friedman et al. 2011a, 2011b).

The previous DSM-IV-TR manual employed a 5-axis evaluation system, which was based on a holistic diagnostic approach. Axes I and II included all the mental disorders, which were broadly classified as clinical syndromes and personality disorders. Axes III contained physical disorders and conditions and Axes IV and V provided the user with a coded outline of supplemental information (e.g., psychosocial stressors and adaptive functions), which could assist mental health professionals and workers in planning treatment regimes and their associated predicted outcomes. Each of the mental disorder classifications also contained a link code to the ICD-10, and provided the user with useful information such as diagnostic criteria and associated clinical manifestations of the disorders (e.g., sex ratios, age of onset, complications, predisposing factors, prevalence, familial patterns). It is notable that the revised and updated DSM-V has discarded this multi-axial system of diagnosis (formerly Axis I, Axis II, and Axis III), and now lists all disorders in Section II. Moreover, it has replaced Axis IV with significant psychosocial and contextual features and dropped Axis V, which was formerly referred to as the *Global Assessment of Functioning* (aka GAF) (APA 2013).

The updated DSM-V has been criticized by various authorities and mental health organizations and associations due to a lack of empirical support for several of the revisions or additions made, a low inter-relater reliability for many disorders listed, confusing and/or contradictory information provided, and corporate influences by the psychiatric drug industry to name but a few (de Leon 2013; Kowa and Giordano 2012; Nemeroff et al. 2013).

For example, it has been reported that approximately 70% of task force members for the DSM-V had ties to the pharmaceutical industry, which represents an increase of 57% in comparison to DSM-IV task force membership (Cosgrove and Drimsky 2012; Cosgrove, et al. 2006). Criticism of the DSM-V resulted in a formal petition signed by approximately 13,000 individuals and mental health professionals and several mental health organizations and associations (Coalition for DSM-5 Reform 2013). Nonetheless, the DSM-V remains the most widely employed manual globally for the diagnosis and classification of mental disorders.

In Canada, both the delivery and planning for mental health services falls under the jurisdiction of the provincial and territorial governments (Public Health Agency of Canada [PHAC], 2013d). The federal government, primarily through *Health Canada*, collaborates with the provinces and territories to develop responsive, coordinated, and efficient mental health service systems. The PHAC also contributes to these efforts via surveillance activities by their Centre for Chronic Disease Prevention and Control. The Government of Canada announced the creation of the *Mental Health Commission of Canada* in its March, 2007, budget in Parliament (PHAC 2013d). The Commission was created to focus national attention on various mental health issues and challenges facing Canadians and to work to improve the health and social outcomes of individuals living with mental illness. Following this announcement, a board of directors and eight advisory committee members have been established to assist the work of the Commission.

What Is a Disease?

A *disease* is defined as an interruption, cessation, or disorder either mental or physical in nature that may arise from a single or combination of factors such as an infectious agent or determinant of health (e.g., genetic predisposition, biochemical imbalance, lifestyle, environment) that is characterized by a recognizable set of clinical signs and symptoms (Bartfay and Bartfay 2015). The identification of the etiology and natural history of disease remains an important component of public health in Canada and globally. Diseases processes and associated alterations to health and well-being are often complex in nature and require a holistic understanding of various measures, features, and aspects including one's physiology and biochemistry, microbiology, epidemiology, and various socio-political and environmental factors.

Health indicators are measures of health and factors that can affect health and are employed to measure, monitor, and compare important factors that influence the health of Canadians across the lifespan and healthcare systems (Health Council of Canada 2011). For example, the report entitled *Health Indicators 2010* provides more than 40 measures and aspects of health and health system performance in Canada for larger health regions, and the 10 provinces and 3 territories (Canadian Institutes for Health Information 2010). This report highlights the importance of various social determinants of health (SDH) across the lifespan (Commission on Social Determinants of Health 2008; Raphael 2009). The reader is referred to Chapter 1 for a detailed discussion on the SDH.

Similarly, Muntaner, Ng, and Chung (2012) reported that income is a significant determinant of health for Canadians. Low-income Canadians and families have the highest rates of mortality, illness, and healthcare use, while middle-income individuals and families have worse health outcomes in comparison to highest income groups. This finding was found to be consistent for this determinant of

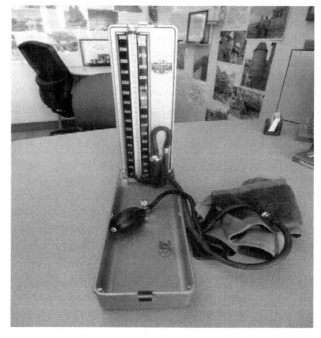

Source: Wally J. Bartfay

Photo 7.3 The Health Indicators 2010 report found that Canadians who lived in the least-affluent neighbourhoods were 37% more likely (255 per 100,000 population) to have an acute myocardial infarction (i.e., heart attack) than those in more-affluent areas (186 per 100,000 population) (Canadian Institutes for Health Information 2010). Moreover, Canadians who lived in low-income neighbourhoods had higher rates of hypertension, diabetes, smoking, and other known cardiac risk factors.

health regardless of whether the income was measured at the individual, household, or neighbourhood levels (Muntaner, Ng, and Chung 2012). Poverty in Canada affects over 3 million Canadians including 600,000 children (Ontario Association of Food Banks 2008; UNICEF 2012), and over 150,000 Canadians live on the street and have no permanent home or residence (Salvation Army 2011). Hence, poverty and income levels remain significant SDH in Canada and globally (Commission on Social Determinants of Health 2008; Raphael 2009).

What Is Illness and the Stages of the Illness Experience

Illness is defined as a subjective or psychological state experienced by an individual who feels aware of not being well or their experience with a disease, and it is a social construct fashioned out of transactions between healthcare professionals and affected individuals in the context of their common culture (Porter 2008). The individual's acceptance of their clinical diagnosis and treatment regime or plan follows a relatively predictable and typical path through the illness process (Anderson and Anderson 1998; Thompson 2010).

The Public Health Agency of Canada (PHAC 2009e) reports that the most recent *Economic Burden of Illness in Canada (EBIC)* study shows that the total costs of illness were estimated to be over $202 billion (Canadian) in 2000 alone. In a recent analysis, the total economic burden of illness associated with obesity has been estimated to be $4.3 billion (in 2005 dollars), $1.8 billion in direct healthcare costs, and $2.5 billion in indirect costs (PHAC 2009e).

Stage I

During stage I, illness begins when the individual notes that something is wrong, as evidenced by abnormal signs or symptoms. *Signs* are defined as manifestations of an illness that an individual can see (e.g., rash on extremities, edema of the feet, and blood in the urine or stool) (Bartfay and Bartfay 2015). *Symptoms* are defined as those aspects of the illness that an individual experiences, feels, or perceives (e.g., shortness of breath, fatigue, headaches, abdominal pain) (Bartfay and Bartfay 2015). This stage ends with the person's acceptance of the reality of their condition and that they may be becoming ill. Some individuals may take additional time and effort to engage in the process of self-analyzing these abnormal signs and symptoms via available health literature and/or other resources (e.g., Internet). Some individuals may also engage in the process of self-diagnosis and treatment (e.g., antacids to treat acid reflux, acetaminophen to relieve a migraine or pain in the joints).

Each of the five stages depicted in Figure 7.1 is characterized by certain decisions, socially or culturally expected behaviours and endpoints.

Public health professionals and workers should be cognizant that concepts related to states of ill health and their associated signs and symptoms are often derived from the dominant social and cultural norms, traditions and expectations they subscribe too. Swanson and Albreacht (1993) note that for individuals, symptom labeling and diagnosis depend on the degree of differences between their behaviour and those of their reference group. These are defined as normal beliefs about the causation of illness, level of stigma attached to a particular set of symptoms, prevalence of the pathology, and meaning of the illness to the individual and family.

For example, in a study conducted on Italian women, Ragucci (1981) reported that being healthy or not ill meant the ability to continue to interact socially and perform routine household chores and tasks such as cleaning and cooking. By contrast, some individuals of Hispanic origin believe that coughing,

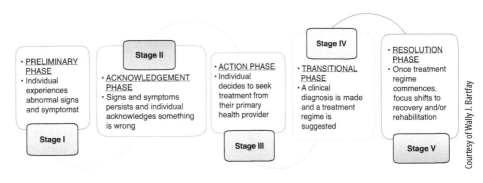

Figure 7.1 The five main stages of the illness experience.

sweating, and diarrhea are normal part of living rather than symptoms of ill health—perhaps because of their high frequency in their country of origin (Swanson and Albrecht 1993).

Indeed, an individual's interpretation of an altered state of health, condition, or disability may have different meanings based on the individual's dominant social and cultural context. For example, Tripp-Reimer (1984) notes that epilepsy is viewed by Ugandans as untreatable and contagious in nature, as a cause of family shame for Greek families, as a reflection of a physical imbalance among Mexican-Americans, or as a divine sign of having gained favor to endure a trail by a God according to the Hutterities. Hence, there may be wide social-cultural variation in the manner in which individuals from different cultures perceive signs and symptoms and associated diagnosis (Davitz and Davitz 1977; Hartog and Hartog 1983; Kobayashi 2009; Waxler-Morrison et al. 2005).

These altering perspectives are important to keep in mind from the Canadian perspective also, especially given that we are a country of immigrants. In fact, according to the 2001 Census, 13.4% (4,000,000) of the population reported that they were visible minorities and two-thirds (70%) indicated that they were foreign born, which represents a significant increase from 1991 (Statistics Canada 2005c). According to recent census data, the total population of Canada in the year 2006 was 31,241,030, and 5,068,090 (16.2%) individuals identified themselves as a visible minority, which represents a further increase of 13.4% in comparison to 2001 Census data (Statistics Canada 2006). These visible minorities included 1,262,865 South Asians, 1,216,570 Chinese, 783,795 blacks, 410,695 Filipinos, 304,245 Latin Americans, and 239,935 Southeast Asians (Statistics Canada 2006). Moreover, more than 200 different ethnic origins were reported. Indeed, as immigrants and their families attempt to adjust to Canadian culture and lifestyles and formulate a new cultural identity, they often experience cultural and generational conflicts and various healthcare challenges (Bartfay and Bartfay 2015; Klaas and Bartfay 2010).

According to the *National Population Health Survey*, immigrants who arrive in Canada are generally in better overall health in comparison to the general Canadian population, but overtime they become twice as likely as Canadian born to report deterioration in their health status (Statistics Canada 2005a). In addition, in comparison to Canadian born residents, new immigrants to Canada have been found to have a 10% increase on average in their body mass index (BMI) over a period of only 8 years, and this weight gain may compromise their health or increase their risk for disease (e.g., heart disease, diabetes) (Statistics Canada 2005a). Therefore, acculturation to a Canadian lifestyle may also have detrimental health consequences for new immigrants.

Hyman and Dussault (2000) compared the experiences of newly landed non-English- and non-French-speaking pregnant Southeast Asian women in Montréal, Québec. The aim of this investigation was to compare these newly arrived Southeast Asian women with their so-called more acculturated counter parts. That is to say, Southeast Asian pregnant women who have resided in Montréal for longer periods of time. The findings revealed that the more acculturated women were less likely to give birth to low-birth-weight-infants, had lower levels of stress, and better social support systems, in comparison to their less acculturated Southeast Asian counterparts (Hyman and Dussault 2000). Public health professionals and workers need to be cognizant of these challenges. Providing culturally competent care is seen as an essential component of public health that can help reduce health disparities and enhance positive health outcomes in ethnically diverse populations across the lifespan (Brach and Fraser 2000; Fraas and Bartfay 2010; Public Health Agency of Canada 2007). For example, the Canadian Nurses Association (CNA 2000a) notes that in order to achieve optimum health outcomes, nurses must provide care that is culturally competent by demonstrating consideration for client diversity, providing culturally sensitive care (e.g., openness, sensitivity, and recognizing culturally based practices and values), and incorporating cultural practices into health promotion activities.

Stage II

During stage II, the signs and symptoms persist and do not diminish in severity over time even with self-treatment (e.g., rest, over-the-counter medications). Consequently, the individual decides that the illness is serious and real and that they now require validation, advice, and/or guidance by others (Anderson and Anderson 1998; Thompson 2010). Some individuals may discuss the problem or condition with a friend or family member, while others may make an appointment to see their primary healthcare provider. Hence, this stage gives the individual permission to act and to become overtly sick according to cultural and social norms (e.g., be excused from normal obligations such as work or school). It may be argued that a person's illness can also influence the behaviour of those they associate with, in large part because these individuals often have a burden placed on them. For example, they may be required to provide extra support for the ill person or to assume their tasks and responsibilities. This often results in an undesired change in their daily routine and increased stress. Individuals who are ill are relieved from the roles and responsibilities they have in society, which specific ones to be exempted from, and to what extent depend on the nature and severity of their illness (Thompson 2010).

Stage III

During stage III, the individual formally seeks professional advice and assistance for dealing with the illness, and to further legitimize the sick role (Bartfay and Bartfay 2015). During this stage, they visit their primary healthcare provider to be formally assessed (e.g., physical exam, blood work, diagnostic tests). The primary healthcare provider will assess the results obtained to derive at a clinical diagnosis or professional opinion regarding the individual's state of overall health.

Stage IV

During stage IV, the individual considers the clinical diagnosis and the professional advice or treatment regime suggested to manage their illness by their primary healthcare provider (Anderson and Anderson 1998; Thompson 2010). Each individual responds differently to a clinical diagnosis. For example, if the problem is relatively simply in nature, non-life threatening, and easily treated (e.g., common cold), the individual typically accepts the diagnosis and suggested treatment plan or regime. On the other hand, if the problem is deemed complex, potentially life-threatening in nature (e.g., cancer) and requires more complicated treatments or interventions, the individual may initially deny the clinical diagnosis or seek a second opinion.

Moreover, there may be differences in opinion between the individual and their healthcare provider in terms of desired treatment plans or regimes. For example, an individual who is diagnosed with a terminal illness may request aggressive treatments or interventions (e.g., chemotherapy, radiation therapy, surgery) although their healthcare provider feels that these treatments or interventions would be futile in nature. Conversely, the individual with a potentially life-threatening illness may refuse the available treatment options or interventions, opting for a better quality of life instead of having to endure undesirable side effects. It is also important to keep in mind that family members and their significant others will also need to go through the process of acceptance when confronted with a diagnosis of a terminal illness (Bartfay and Bartfay 2015).

Stage V

During stage V, the individual eventually relinquishes the sick role, and works toward recovery or rehabilitation (Anderson and Anderson 1998; Thompson 2010). The shift in focus now is toward restoring the health of the individual, making them feel more comfortable, and/or preventing further deterioration. If the illness is deemed short term or acute in nature, the individual will quickly recovery and resume their normal activities of daily living. Conversely, if the illness is deemed long term or chronic in nature, the individual will ideally focus on achieving maximum recovery or preventing further deterioration through the interventions or treatment regimens agreed upon. Compliance with the treatment regime and/or interventions may waver during this stage, and it is imperative that follow-up routine assessments be made by the healthcare provider. A detailed discussion of acute and chronic forms of disease is provided below.

What Is Sickness and the Sick Role?

Sickness is defined as a state of social dysfunction of an individual with a disease or the result of being defined by others in one's culture as unhealthy, and the expected role that the individual should assume when ill (Porta 2008). The *sick role* is defined as a behavioural pattern in which an individual accepts and readily adopts the signs and symptoms of a physical or mental disorder in order to receive care, seek sympathy, and/or be protected from the demands and stresses of life in their defined culture (Bartfay and Bartfay 2015). It is widely accepted that when an individual is sick, their behaviours, roles, attitudes, and expectations toward others change as a consequence.

Sickness and the sick role adopted by an individual are often defined by social and cultural norms, expectations, and traditions (Kleinman 1988; Kleinman, Eisenberg and Good 1978; Twaddle 1981). For example, the image of an ideal weight has changed over the centuries due to social and cultural expectations, which has been reflected in works of art (i.e., painting, drawings, sculptures). Indeed, during the Baroque art period (17th and 18th centuries) in Europe, being a women of heavy set (i.e., overweight or obese) was regarded as healthy and as the ideal body image. Conversely, according to current social and cultural standards in North America, being "thin-is-in" and healthy, whereas being overweight or obese (BMI over 30) is associated with the potential for sickness (Findlay 1996; Groesz, Levine, and Murnen 2002; Schissel 2009). This new standard of the ideal body image has been shaped by a variety of social and cultural factors including a growing body of scientific literature on weight standards and morbidity, mortality rates for various health conditions, and the associated influence of the mass and social medias and the fashion industry.

In effect, a growing body of scientific literature has shown that excess body weight and obesity are major risk factors/indicators for the development of various diseases (e.g., heart disease, stroke, diabetes, cancer) in Canada and globally for several decades now (e.g., Chaput and Sharma 2011; International Obesity Task Force 2006; Sharma and Lau 2013; Statistics Canada 2003). Health Canada's standard weight scale, which displays acceptable weights based on the heights of adults and children, has become an acceptable clinical and social standard for assessing whether or not an individual is at risk for becoming sick and unhealthy (Schissel 2009; Statistics Canada 2005b). Research has shown that following tobacco, obesity is the second major contributor for premature death and disability worldwide (Worldwatch Institutes 2000). The WHO (2013b) reports that global obesity rates have doubled since 1980, and in 2008 more than 1.4 billion adults 20 years or older were classified as being overweight, and of these 200 million males and 300 females worldwide were classified as being obese. In addition, more than 40 million children under the age of 5 years were classified as being overweight (WHO 2013b).

Between 1985 and 2001, the number of obese Canadians has almost tripled from 5.6% to 14.9% (Hales and Lauzon 2007). According to the *Canadian Community Health Survey*, 23.1% of adult Canadians (22.9% of males and 23.2% of females) aged 18 years or older were classified as obese, and 36.1% were classified as overweight (42% of males and 30.2% of females) (Statistics Canada 2005b). Similarly, Shields (2006) reports that being overweight or obese in Canadian youth aged 12–17 years has more than doubled in the past 25 years, and is becoming a major public health concern. A report by the *Standing Committee of Health in Canada* has revealed that 26% of Canadian children aged 2–17 years are overweight or obese, and 55% of Indigenous youth living on reserves are either obese or overweight (Parliament of Canada 2007).

The *Canadian Community Health Survey* found that a child who has one parent that is obese has a 50% chance of being obese themselves by the age of 5 years, and this number increases to 80% if both parents are obese (Statistics Canada 2010). Leitch (2007) predicts that given the current prevalence of childhood obesity, and its link with many diseases, this could be the first generation that may not live as long as their parents. This trend is also affecting developing nations in the world. For

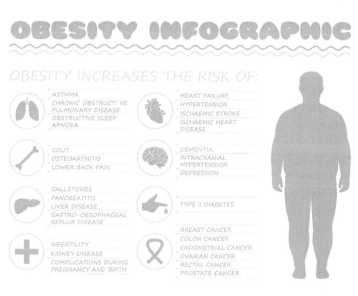

Photo 7.4 Complications associated with obesity. Obesity, unhealthy diets and physical inactivity are growing public health concerns in Canada. Currently, approximately 1:4 adult Canadians are obese.

example, it is estimated that 69.5% of all adults in Paraguay are either overweight or obese, with 37.9% being overweight and 31.6% being obese (Obesity HQ 2012–2013). Moreover, 64.5% of all males are either overweight or obese, with 41.6% of males being overweight and 22.9% obese. Data regarding females show that 71.8% are either overweight or obese. Specifically, 36.1% are overweight and 35.7% are obese (Obesity HQ 2012–2013).

In addition to the clinical height and weight standards and the growing health concerns associated with being overweight or obese described above, the socially constructed image of an acceptable body image and weight by the mass and social medias and fashion industry also plays a critical role in promoting cultural standards for beauty. Schissel (2009) notes that one has to look no further than advertisements for brand-name cosmetics or clothing which emphasize a thin and youthful body type. This socially constructed image of the ideal thin women propagated by the fashion and cosmetic industries results in a constant and never-ending struggle to avoid being labeled as weak, ugly, or potentially sick. Findlay (1996) argues that the social and mass media's along with the health and beauty industries promote their products by suggesting that *success and beauty* will belong to every woman if she diets properly or purchases the latest stay thin diets, supplements, or products. Healthcare professionals (e.g., physicians, nurses, registered dieticians), for their part, tend to advocate a thin build over a heavy one, thus reinforcing this dominant social norm in developed nations. Hence, it may be argued that the consistent exposure to impossible images of the ideal and beautiful body conveys a sense of perpetual deficiency in our society (Findlay 1996).

One's weight and body image in North America and the European continent has come to preoccupy the thoughts of many, especially young girls and women, to the point where weight control may lead to the development of self-injurious conditions such as anorexia and bulimia (e.g., Mosley 1997; Schissel 2009; Waller 1998; White 2000; Wolf 1990). Mandleco and Bartfay (2010) argue that because of the increasing social pressures to be slim propagated by the mass and social medias and the health and beauty industries, some adolescents severely limit their food intake to a level significantly below that required to meet the demands of normal growth. This phenomenon has been referred to as a "sickness of body image." For example, one investigation by the *Jacob Institutes for Women's Health* noted that "sickness of body image" was found in 40% of third-grade girls surveyed who reported that they were dieting to lose weight, and this figure rose to 75% in fifth graders (Mosley 1997). In fact, hospitalization rates for eating disorders in Canada for girls aged 15 or more increased 34% from 1987 to 1999 (Canadian Institutes of Health Information 2005). Schissel (2009) reports that the final irony is when governments proclaim eating disorders, especially obesity, as a national health problem or "epidemic," they paradoxically target and blame individuals who are often the most exploited and vulnerable ones in society, and ultimately they lay blame on the victim for taxing an already heavily burdened healthcare system in Canada.

The Five Disease Categories

Diseases are typically classified into five general categories by convention: (a) allergies and inflammatory disease, (b) cancer, (c) congenital and hereditary diseases, (d) degenerative diseases, and (e) metabolic diseases (Bartfay and Bartfay 2015). Table 7.1 provides the definition for each of these disease categories and examples of each. For example, the ragweed plant (*Ambrosia artemisifolia L.*) is a common invasive species of plant

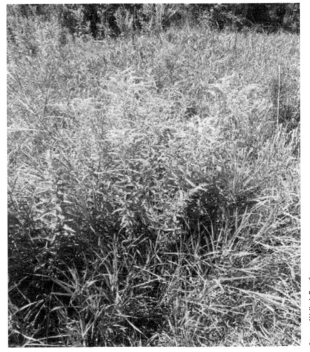

Photo 7.5 Ragweed (*Ambrosia artemisifolia L.*) is the most common cause of hay fever during the months of August to October in Canada, and pollen from these plants can be carried for distances up to 200 km away.

Source: Wally J. Bartfay

Table 7.1 Five Major Disease Classification Categories

Disease category	Definition	Examples
i. Allergies and inflammatory disease	Allergies are caused by the body's reaction to an invading foreign agent, substance or allergen, which results in the development of antibodies. Subsequent exposure causes the release of chemical mediators and a variety of signs and symptoms (e.g., anaphylaxis bronchospasm, dyspnea, eczema, laryngospasms, rhinitis, sinusitis, urticaria). Inflammations are protective responses by body tissues to an irritation or injury and may be acute or chronic in nature and histamine, kinins, and other various substances mediate the inflammatory process. Cardinal signs and symptoms of inflammation are redness (rubor), heat (calor), swelling, and pain (dolor), which may result in loss of function.	– Allergic rhinitis caused by localized reaction to animal dander, house dust or pollen – Allergy to penicillin or other antibiotics – Crohn's disease and inflammatory bowel disease – Egg allergies – Inflammatory scoliosis – Peanut allergies – Rheumatoid arthritis – Ulcerative colitis
ii. Cancer	Collective term used to describe a group of diseases characterized by uncontrolled cell growth and division or the loss of the cell to perform normal apoptosis. It is a neoplasm clinically characterized by uncontrolled cell growth of anaplastic cells which typically invades surrounding tissues and may also metastasize to other surrounding or distant tissues or organs in the body.	– Breast cancer – Colon cancer – Leukemia (cancer of the blood) – Lung cancer – Non-Hodgkin's lymphoma (NHL) – Testicular cancer
iii. Congenital and hereditary diseases	A group of diseases caused by familiar genetic tendencies by which particular traits or conditions are genetically transmitted from the parents to their offspring's. May also result due to injury to the fetus or embryo in-utero caused by environmental, biological or chemical agents.	– Cooley's anemia (beta-thalassemia major) – Congenital adrenal hyperplasia – Congenital heart defects (i.e., aortic stenosis, atrial septal defects, patent ductus arteriosus, tetralogy of Fallot and valvular stenosis) – Congenital non-spherocytic hemolytic anemia – Congenital rubella syndrome – Down syndrome – Familial cretinism – Familial histiocytic reticulosis – Hemophilia – Hereditary multiple exostoses – Morquio's disease – Sickle cell disease

(Continued)

Table 7.1 Five Major Disease Classification Categories (*Continued*)

Disease category	Definition	Examples
iv. Degenerative diseases	A disease or a group of diseases characterized by the progressive deterioration of the structure or function of tissue, organ or a body part over time which eventually results in mental or physical alterations to function.	– Alzheimer's disease – Arteriosclerosis – Arthritis – Degenerative joint disease – Osteoarthritis
v. Metabolic diseases	Are caused when glands or organs in the body fail to maintain or secrete adequate amounts of hormones or other biochemicals necessary to maintain homeostasis which result in dysfunction or malfunction of certain organs involving physiologic or metabolic processes that result in disease states.	– Addison's disease – Cretinism (hypothyroidism) – Diabetes mellitus – Gout – Hyperthyroidism

that is present throughout Canada, the United States, and many European countries (Canadian Biodiversity Information Facility 2013; Ministry of Agriculture, Food and Rural Affairs Ontario 2015; Wopfner, et al. 2005). This yellow weed grows in gardens, poorly kept lawns, roadsides, pastures, meadows, and open fields.

What Are Acute and Chronic Diseases?

Diseases are further classified by convention as first being either acute or chronic in nature. *Acute diseases* are defined as those disorders or conditions that are relatively severe in nature with a sudden onset, but have a short duration of clinical signs and symptoms (Bartfay and Bartfay 2015). For example, chickenpox is an acute and highly contagious viral disease caused by the herpes *varicella–zoster virus* (VSZ) (Baumgardner 1998; Guris, Marin, and Seward 2008). The virus can be spread by direct contact with skin lesions or by droplets from the respiratory tract of infected clients. Indirect transmission through uninfected persons or via objects in the environment is rare. The incubation period for chickenpox averages 2–3 weeks, followed by fever, mild headache, and general malaise, which occur typically 24–36 hours before the rash appears. The rash begins as macules and progresses in 24–48 hours to papules, and lastly to vesicles. The vesicles turn cloudy, are easily broken when scratched, and become encrusted within 24–48 hours.

By contrast, *chronic diseases* are defined as those disorders or conditions which tend to be relatively less severe in nature but are continuous in duration, and which can last for long periods of time including an entire lifetime (Bartfay and Bartfay 2015). For example, TB is a chronic granulomatous infection caused by the acid-fast bacillus *Mycobacterium tuberculosis*, which can be transmitted by the inhalation or ingestion of infected droplets (Hornick 2008; Rodnick and Gude 1998). Globally, respiratory TB was the single most dominant cause of mortality during the mid-ninteenth century, when it was first registered in England and Wales as a cause of mortality (McKeown 1994). During the twentieth century, the rates for TB declined steadily in most developed and industrialized nations in the world, but re-emerged during periods of social or economic stress (e.g., wars, high unemployment rates), especially in immigrant populations (Dubos and Dubos 1952).

The WHO (2009b, 2000a) reports that when treatment protocols for TB were first developed and implemented in 1948, it was predicted that the disease would be globally eradicated by the year 2000. Unfortunately, TB has re-emerged as a global threat due to increased international trade and travel, poverty, overcrowding, and increased multidrug resistance strains of TB (WHO 2000b, 2009a). In 1993, the WHO organization declared TB to be a global emergency, since approximately 8 million individuals were acquiring TB each year (WHO 2000b, 2000c). By the end of 1998, the WHO global strategy for TB detection and control was adopted by 22 of the high-burden countries, which had approximately 80% of the estimated cases of TB (WHO 2000c, 2009a).

Group Activity-Based Learning Box 7.1

How Does Public Health Manage Acute and Chronic Diseases In Your Community?
The Group Activity-Based Learning Box 7.1 explores the role of public health in managing acute and chronic diseases in your community. Working in small groups of three to five students, discuss and answer the following questions:

1. What are some of the major acute and chronic diseases in your community, province, or territory?

2. How have these acute and chronic diseases affected the residents of your community?

3. What public health efforts (e.g., support groups, public health campaigns) are currently in place to help individuals, families, or groups manage these acute and chronic diseases?

4. How can published epidemiological and public health research related to acute and chronic disease be better utilized to promote the health and well-being of citizens in your community?

Nonetheless, in 2006, 9.2 million new cases of TB and 1.7 million deaths worldwide were reported (The Lung Association 2009). In fact, it is estimated that between 2000 and 2020, there will be 1 billion newly infected individuals with TB, 200 million will become sick, and 35 million will die from TB if public health control measures are not further developed and implemented (WHO 2000c).

In Canada, TB remains a significant threat to the health and well-being of our residents, especially Indigenous populations, individuals, and families that are homeless, alcoholics, individuals infected with HIV/AIDS, and new immigrants and refugees from countries where TB is endemic (Thomas and Bartfay 2011). For example, while the 2006 Census reports that Indigenous peoples account for just under 4% of the Canadian population, 21% of all TB cases occurred in this population in 2008 (Health Canada 2012a, 2012b). In fact, from 2000 to 2008, the age-standardized active TB reported incidence rates for First Nations people living on-reserve were between 32 and 59 times higher than the Canadian-born non-Indigenous population, and between 2 and 3 times higher than the foreign-born Canadian population (Health Canada 2012a, 2012b). The WHO strategy for the detection and cure of TB is composed of

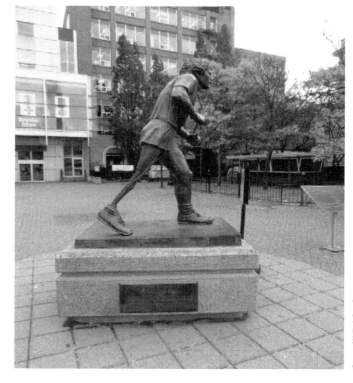

Photo 7.6 Bone cancer is an example of a non-communicable disease. In 1980, Terry Fox (1958–1981) after having one leg amputated due to bone cancer, embarked on a cross-Canada run to raise funds related to cancer research. Although the spread of his cancer eventually forced him to end his quest after 143 days and 5373 km and he subsequently lost his life, his efforts resulted in a lasting worldwide legacy and inspiration for clients and their families dealing with cancer.

Source: Wally J. Bartfay

five major elements: (a) political commitment by governments, (b) microscopy services, (c) available drug supplies, (d) the use of efficacious regiments with direct observation of treatments, and (e) surveillance and monitoring systems (WHO 2000c, 2000b, 2009a). We shall examine the importance of surveillance and monitoring systems in greater detail below.

What Are Communicable and Non-communicable Diseases?

Non-communicable diseases are defined as diseases that cannot be transmitted from one individual to another or from a group to a population (Bartfay and Bartfay 2015). Examples of these include heart disease, stroke, chronic obstructive pulmonary disease (COPD), diabetes, and melanoma. The WHO (2011a), for example, reports that ischemic heart disease is the leading cause of death in developed regions of the world and resulted in approximately 1.42 million deaths in 2008 alone. Non-communicable diseases result in 89% of all deaths in Canada, and are the major drivers of healthcare costs and lost productivity (WHO 2011). In fact, more than 40% of Canadian adults report having least one non-communicable disease, which includes cancer, heart disease, diabetes, arthritis, emphysema or COPD, and mood disorders (Canadian Academy of Health Sciences 2010; National Expert Commission Canadian Nurses Association 2012). Chad (2012) from the *Centre on Global Health Security* reports that modest public health investments to prevent and treat non-communicable diseases could result in major economic returns for countries around the world and literally save millions of lives. Moreover, it is predicted that every dollar spent on managing non-communicable diseases results in a saving of three dollars in return (Chad 2012).

The *communicability of the disease* is the ability of a disease to be transmitted from one individual to another or from one group or population to another (Bartfay and Bartfay 2015). The communicability of a disease is determined by how likely an agent or pathogen can be transmitted from an infected or diseased individual to another who is not immune and susceptible. Health Canada (2003) defines a *communicable disease* as an illness caused by a specific agent or its toxic products that arise through transmission of that agent or its products from an infected person, animal, or reservoir to a susceptible host, either directly or indirectly through an intermediate plant or animal host, vector, or the inanimate environment. A communicable disease may occur as an individual case or a group of cases, known as an outbreak, and this occurs when the number of new cases of a disease exceeds the normal occurrence during a given period of time. For example, invasive pneumococcal disease and TB are two common outbreaks present typically during the winter and spring seasons in Canada, especially in under-housed populations (Marchant-Short and Whitney 2012). According to Heymann (2008), communicable diseases kill more than 14 million people each year mainly in the developing world. In these countries, approximately 46% of all deaths are due to communicable diseases, and 90% of these deaths are attributed to acute diarrheal and respiratory infections of children, HIV/AIDS, TB, malaria, and measles.

New dimensions of communicable disease have recently come to the attention of public health officials in Canada and globally, which include a better understanding of the bacterium *Helicobacter pylori* in the development of gastric ulcers, appearance of extremely virulent viruses (e.g., H1N1 Swine flu, H5N1 Avian [Bird] flu, Ebola virus), and prions. A *prion* is defined as a self-replicating, protein-based pathogenic agent that can infect humans and animals (Bartfay and Bartfay 2015). Although cooking foods at sufficiently high temperatures will kill most bacteria and parasites, heat does not kill prions because the proteins have already been denatured or unraveled (Jacobsen 2008).

Certain Fore tribe people of Papua New Guinea suffered from a strange illness that caused shaking, paralysis, and death and its cause was not known for several years. It was eventually discovered that the disease Kuru was caused by eating the brains of dead relatives, as part of the Fore tribe people's burial ritual. Infections were apparently transmitted by the direct ingestion of the brain or nervous tissue from infected individuals or animals (Collinge et al. 2006; Jacobsen 2008). As Kuru disease is the only human epidemic caused by a prion in history, it has provided important insights into the variant Creutzfeldt–Jakob disease (vCJD).

An example of a current emerging disease caused by a prion is Mad Cow disease or bovine spongiform encephalopathy (BSE) in cattle and the new vCJD in humans (National Center for Infectious Diseases 2007; Public Health Agency of Canada 2009a). BSE is a fatal brain-wasting disease in cattle that first appeared in

England in 1986, and public health officials are concerned that it may be transmitted to humans in the form of vCJD. Indeed, since 1987, BSE has been confirmed in Canada, the United States, Japan, Israel, and 20 European countries, and BSE transmission to humans has led to more than 150 cases of invariably fatal vCJD; the vast majority occurring in Britain (Beisel and Morens 2004; Belay and Schonberger 2005; Donnelly 2004). Both the cattle variant and the human form result in a fatal brain disease with unusually long incubation periods measured in years or decades. BSE is thought to be transmitted when cows are fed leftovers from slaughterhouses from sheep or other cows as a protein source in their feed. The disease is believed to be transmitted to humans through the consumption of meat from these infected cattle. vCJD is characterized by a slow yet progressive damage to the neurological system in humans and eventual death (Beisel and Morens 2004; Belay and Schonberger 2005; Donatelle 2010; Donnelly 2004).

The first case of BSE diagnosed in Canada was a cow that had been imported from the United Kingdom in 1987 at the age of six months, and the diseased animal was promptly destroyed (Forge and Freclette 2005). The federal government subsequently attempted to trace every other head of cattle imported from the United Kingdom between 1982 and 1990. In July 2003, 15 farms were quarantined in Alberta and 25 other herds were examined. Investigations by the Canadian Food Inspection Agency led to the slaughter of more than 2700 heads of cattle (Forge and Frechette 2005).

These examples above illustrate the importance for all public health professionals and workers to understand modes of disease transmission and classifications, and the importance of thorough history taking during contract tracing. For example, it would be important to determine if instruments used in invasive procedures involving the brain or neural tissue on an individual diagnosed with NcCJD may have been contaminated. We will examine the importance of tracking and surveillance for public health in greater detail below.

As international travel and trade increases, with the potential of transporting pathogens from remote regions of the world to densely populated urban centres within hours or days, the likelihood of contracting and spreading a previously unknown communicable disease on Canadian soil increases. The WHO (2008) reports that as of September 2008, the Avian flu virus has resulted in 245 clinically confirmed human deaths worldwide. The Ebola virus, which is endemic is parts of Africa, is fatal in up to 75% of cases who contract it and there is no current immunization or clear understanding on how it is transmitted (Hahn et al. 2006; Jacobsen 2008). The reader is referred to Chapter 9 for a detailed discussion

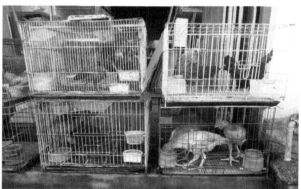

Photo 7.7 Chickens for sale in Hong Kong. The first outbreak of avian (AKA bird flu) influenza A (H5N1) virus in humans occurred in Hong Kong in 1997, and was confirmed in 18 individuals, 6 of whom died. Infections were acquired by humans directly from chickens, without the involvement of an intermediate host. The outbreak was halted by a nation-wide slaughter of more than 1.5 million chickens. Currently, H5N1 is an emerging avian influenza virus that is a global public health concern as a potential pandemic threat to humans. The mortality rate for humans with H5N1 is approximately 60%.

Source: Wally J. Bartfay

of international health issues and the spread of communicable diseases globally. There is also concern about the increasing resistance of bacteria such as *Staphylococcus aureus, Enterococcus,* and *Mycobacterium* (which causes TB) to current available antibiotics due to over and/or improper prescription, and the biochemical redesign of the organisms themselves (Larson 2007; Ritterman 2006; Weber 2006). Donatelle (2010) reports that diarrheal diseases cause almost 3 million deaths per year mostly in developing countries where resistance forms of *Campylobacter, Shigella, Escherichia coli, Vibrio cholera,* and *Salmonella* food poisoning have emerged. In certain regions, as much as 50% of the *Campylobacter* cases are resistant to Cipro, the most effective treatment currently available.

A potentially deadly *superbug* called *Salmonella enteric typhimurium* is resistant to most antibiotics and has now appeared in various parts of Europe, Canada, and the United States (Donatelle 2010). We shall explore the public health concerns related to the growing resistance of bacteria to antibiotics in institutional and community-based settings further below in the section entitled *Community and Hospital-acquired Nosocomial Infections.*

Table 7.2 Examples of Common Communicable and Non-communicable Diseases According to Acute or Chronic Classification

	Communicable (acute)	Communicable (chronic)	Non-communicable (acute)	Non-communicable (chronic)
Communicable (aka infectious)	– Chicken pox – German measles – Influenza – Lyme Disease – Mumps	– HIV/AIDS – Polio – Syphilis – Tuberculosis	– Anthrax – Legionnaire's disease – Tetanus	
Non-communicable (aka non-infectious)			– Cerebral vascular accident (stroke) – Motor vehicleaccidents (MVA) – Post-partum depression – Suicide	– Alcoholism – Arthritis – Diabetes mellitus – Heart disease – Renal disease – Rheumatoid arthritis – Schizophrenia

Communicable (infectious) and non-communicable (non-infectious) diseases are often further classified and clinically distinguished by convention as being either acute or chronic in nature. Table 7.2 provides examples of some common acute and chronic communicable and non-communicable diseases.

It is critical for all public health professionals and workers to develop effective partnerships with their community stakeholders and populations they serve in order to provide safe and cost-effective primary healthcare services and initiatives across the lifespan for the management of both communicable and non-communicable acute and chronic diseases (Public Health Agency of Canada 2007a, 2007b). For example, the Mantoux Tuberculin Skin Test (MST) compact disk (CD) was developed in partnership with the Regional Infection Control Network (RICN) of Ontario, Toronto Public Health and community stakeholders to address noted knowledge and information gaps. This included material required to administer the test, proper test site selection, and how to interpret and record usual test reactions for the MST (RICN 2009). This CD was distributed to various public health professionals and workers, regional public health units, community agencies, long-term care facilities and homes and hospitals, and has been endorsed by the Ontario Lung Association's Tuberculosis Committee.

The impact and dissemination of findings related to communicable diseases in a community or population has migrated over the past few decades from public health journals and conferences to greater access and use of the mass medias (e.g., television, radio, newspapers), social medias (e.g., Twitter, Facebook, YouTube), and the Internet (e.g., PUBMED, MEDLINE, governmental reports). For example, the 2003 Severe Acute Respiratory Syndrome (SARS) pandemic resulted in various headlines and articles which described public health efforts in Canada and globally related to surveillance; quarantine efforts, clinical signs and symptoms to be aware of, investigations into its origins and etiology, and primary prevention efforts (e.g., coughing into one's sleeve, proper hand-washing practicing). A total of 8098 people worldwide became sick during the 2003 SARS pandemic.

In addition to the above, misinformation or public health information that is contradictory in nature about a potential outbreak or pandemic may have negative ripple effects in a community, region or nation. According to Boyle (2010), the large amount of misinformation about vaccination safety that circulated during the 2009–2010 H1N1 pandemic may have accounted for the drop in the number of people who got vaccinated for seasonal flu in subsequent years. In addition, confusion about the vaccine, in general, as well as more specific concerns about the adjuvanted vaccine versus the non-adjuvanted vaccine in certain groups of

---

Group Activity-Based Learning Box 7.2

Examining the Impact of Non-communicable Disease and Associated Health Conditions and Altered States of Health and Wellness in Your Community?

The Group Activity-Based Learning Box 7.2 explores current major non-communicable diseases or associated health conditions and altered states of health and wellness in your community. Working in small groups of three to five students, discuss and answer the following questions:

1. What are the current major non-communicable disease or associated health conditions and altered states of health and wellness (e.g., health conditions, disorders, or injuries) in your community?

2. How can SDH be utilized to better understand these non-communicable diseases, health conditions or altered states of health and wellness in your community?

3. What forms of health research or data are still needed to fill these gaps in knowledge and/or practice?

4. Based on the best available evidence, how would you plan for primary healthcare interventions in your community to address these non-communicable diseases, health conditions, or altered states of health and wellness?

---

individuals (e.g., young children, expectant mothers) was commonplace. Indeed, complacency may have set in after the pandemic turned-out to be not as bad as predicted by public health officials.

Some 58.2% of long-term care workers got vaccinated for seasonal flu in 2010, compared to 51% who got the H1N1 shot in 2009. The average coverage for the previous 4 years was 80% (Boyle 2010). During the 2012–2013 flu seasons in Canada, public health officials reported an increase of approximately 30% more confirmed cases, in comparison to previous years. For example, Toronto Public Health reported 1180 confirmed cases of the flu between September 2012 and January 15, 2013, which represented a spike over a five-year average of 318 cases for the same time period (McDiarmid 2013). Moreover, there were 68 institutional (e.g., hospitals, nursing homes) outbreaks, compared to a five-year average of only 16 (McDiarmid 2013).

Types of Immunity

Immunity is defined as the specific amount of resistance to disease by an individual (Bartfay and Bartfay 2015). One of the public health means to control, manage, and prevent the spread of communicable disease is through mass vaccination campaigns and public health education detailing its many benefits for the individual and community at large. It is possible, at least in theory, to completely eradicate an

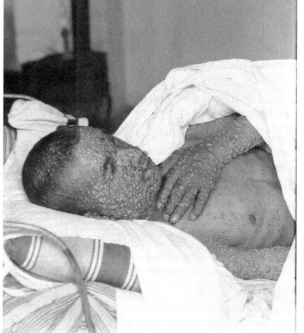

Photo 7.8 Although smallpox is considered eradicated by the WHO, it is still considered a public health concern because of the possible treat that terrorists may access government laboratories that still store the virus and deploy it as a biological weapon.

infectious disease globally (WHO 1998, 2000). *Eradication* is defined and achieved when there is no risk of infection or disease globally even in the absence of immunization and/or other public health disease control measures, and when the agent is no longer present in nature (Bartfay and Bartfay 2015). The disease is not extinct because it remains present in certain government laboratories worldwide.

The last recorded case of naturally acquired smallpox was reported in Somalia in 1977, and in 1980 the WHO declared that smallpox was completely eradicated through global public health immunization campaigns (Centers for Disease Control 1991; Swansom and Albrecht 1993). Although smallpox is considered eradicated by the WHO, it is still considered a public health concern because of the possible threat that terrorists may access government laboratories that still store smallpox and employ it as a biological form of terrorism (Heymann 2008). We shall examine the possible public health implications associated with the deployment of biological agents/weapons by terrorists in a community in the section below entitled *Bioterrorism*.

Research Focus Box 7.1

Immunization Services Offered in Québec (Canada) Pharmacies

Study Aim/Rationale

Access and a lack of education are factors associated with the success of vaccination campaigns that seek to promote herd immunity in communities. It may be argued that pharmacists are typically easier to access in both urban and rural community settings, in comparison to public health professionals such as nurses and physicians. Although Québec pharmacists are currently not permitted to administer vaccines themselves, they can (1) promote vaccinations in their communities, (2) counsel clients on vaccination, (3) sell vaccines, and (4) provide vaccine administration by a registered nurse in their pharmacy. The aim of this investigation was to describe immunization services given in Québec pharmacies and assess the relation between pharmacist and nurses.

Methodology/Design

In 2008–09, an anonymous questionnaire was mailed to all pharmacy owners ($N = 1663$) in the province of Québec, Canada. The questionnaire sought to illicit information about the characteristics of the pharmacy owners, their attitudes related to vaccine administration, their perceptions related to working with nurses in their pharmacy to administer the vaccines, and perceived challenges.

Major Findings

Among the 1102 (66%) respondents, 90% stated that vaccines were sold in their pharmacy in Québec, 27% reported that a registered nurse administered vaccines in their pharmacy, and 44% were planning to offer vaccine administration within the next five years. Three out of four respondents stated that they were currently engaged in vaccine health promotion, and 65% were involved with vaccine counseling. Recommendations for cold chain maintenance were followed in 23% of pharmacies selling vaccines. The presence of another health professional in the pharmacy, extended opening/operating hours, not being located in the same building as a medical clinic, and having an agreement to collaborate with a public health unit or a medical clinic for immunization were positively associated with vaccine administration in multivariate analysis. Higher perceived difficulties with lack of demand from clients were negatively associated with vaccine administration.

Implication for Public Health

Pharmacies are typically easier to access by the majority of Canadians residing in both urban and semi-rural communities where access to healthcare professionals such as public health nurses or physicians may be a challenge. This study suggests that pharmacists appear to be willing to increase their involvement in public health immunization campaigns. Half of respondents said that they would be willing to administer vaccines themselves if legislative modifications were made (e.g., similar to what is currently permitted in Ontario). Collaboration between public health professionals and pharmacists need to be further developed and fostered to encourage both access and vaccination coverage to promote herd immunity.

Source: Sauvageau C., E. Dubé, R. Bradet, M. Mondor, F. Lavoie, and J. Moisan. "Immunization Services Offered in Québec (Canada) Pharmacies." *Human Vaccination and Immunotherapies* 9, mo. 9 (September 1, 2013): 1943–49. doi:10.4161/hv.25186.

Antigenicity

Antigenicity refers to the ability of the antigen system to have the required strength, activity, and effectiveness to respond to a disease threat where the antigens stimulate the immune system to make the body think it has the disease, and the immune system responds appropriately by developing the necessary antibodies (Bartfay and Bartfay 2015). If the pathogen later enters the body, the immune system recognizes it and the individual is protected from the disease via a rapid response of the immune system. If the antigens and antibodies disappear over time, then a booster shot or vaccine will be required to strengthen or reactivate the immune response in the body (e.g., tetanus booster given every 10 years). When the individual cannot effectively elicit an effective immune response, or if it is not sufficient in nature or strength, then there is an increased probability that the individual will contract the disease. There are four ways an individual can acquire immunity or protection against a potentially infectious disease: (a) acquired immunity, (b) natural, (c) active immunity, and (d) herd immunity (Heymann 2008; Merrill 2010; Public Health Agency of Canada 2006b). We shall examine each in greater detail below. The Research Focus Box 7.1 describes a study which examined the perception and potential role of pharmacists in the promotion, distribution, and administration of vaccines in Québec, Canada. Currently, pharmacists in Québec are not permitted to administer vaccines themselves. The Canadian Pharmacist Association (2013) reports that pharmacists in the provinces of British Columbia, Alberta, Ontario, and New Brunswick can administer the seasonal flu vaccine to their clients, whereas Manitoba, Québec, and Nova Scotia should be able to provide vaccinations once regulations are finalized.

Acquired (Passive) Immunity

Acquired or *passive immunity* occurs when there is a transfer of antibodies from the mother to the infant or child via the placenta or through routine breast feeding, or may come from already-produced antibodies by another host (e.g., immune globulin) (Bartfay and Bartfay 2015). This form of immunity typically lasts for a few weeks or months in duration. This is an important reason for public health professionals such as family physicians and public health nurses to educate women about the many benefits associated with breast feeding their infants (Jo Damazo and Bartfay 2010). For example, colostrum, which is the milk produced in the first few days after giving birth, is especially beneficial since it contains large quantities of the antibody called "secretory immunoglobulin A" (IgA). The WHO reports that if every new born infant was exclusively breast-fed for the first 6 months of life, an estimated 1.5 million children could be saved each year (Jacobsen 2008).

Natural Immunity

Natural immunity is defined as an innate resistance to a specific antigen or toxin by the individual that results from the development of antibodies as a result of the host's having acquired the primary infection and which protects against acquiring subsequent infections by the same toxin or antigen (Bartfay and Bartfay 2015). Diseases such as diphtheria, measles, and pertussis are examples of diseases that produce lifelong immunity as a consequence of the individual developing antibodies. Nonetheless, not all pathogens produce natural immunity in the host (e.g., sexually transmitted HIV infections). Hence, without appropriate treatment, re-infection may occur (Jo Damazo and Bartfay 2010).

Active Immunity

Active immunity occurs through vaccination and is present when the body develops its own antibodies against a pathogen or antigenic substance (Bartfay and Bartfay 2015). The proper administration of vaccines can provide lifelong protection from a variety of diseases. The two primary objectives of public health immunization programs are: (a) disease prevention and (b) the global eradication of diseases. Indeed, it has been estimated that six children worldwide die from a vaccine-preventable disease each minute (WHO 1998, 2000). The *WHO Expanded Program on Immunization* began in 1974, and this global public health initiative has resulted in the vaccination of approximately 85% of children around the world against measles, mumps, rubella, tetanus, pertussis, diphtheria, poliomyelitis, and smallpox (WHO 1998, 2000).

The Public Health Agency of Canada (2006b) estimates that between 4000 and 8000 individuals die each year from influenza-related illnesses or associated complications. Human influenza viruses are typically spread by droplets in the air via sneezing or coughing (Jo Damazo and Bartfay 2010). Routine vaccination, which typically begins in the month of October in Canada, can provide up to six months of protection. The *Canadian Immunization Guide* (PHAC 2013a) consists of the following five parts: (a) key immunization information, (b) vaccine safety, (c) vaccination of specific populations (e.g., infants and children), (d) active vaccines, and (e) passive immunizing agents (see http://www.phac-aspc.gc.ca/publicat/cig-gci/p01-eng.php).

The National Advisory Committee on Immunization (NACI) has developed the *Canadian Immunization Guide* (7th ed.) to assist healthcare professionals (e.g., family physicians, public health nurses) to critically examine their standards of practice in regard to immunization. Specifically, the NACI has developed the following 17 practices related to immunization in Canada (Public Health Agency of Canada 2006b, 22):

1. Immunizations should be made available to all residents of Canada.
2. There should be no restrictions, barriers, unnecessary preconditions, or requirements for receiving vaccines (e.g., financial, language constraints).
3. Healthcare professionals such as physicians and nurses should screen all clients for required vaccines during all clinical opportunities that arise, and encourage vaccination when required or indicated.
4. Healthcare professionals should educate parents and guardians of children and adults about the benefits of immunization in general and easily understandable terms.
5. Healthcare professionals should update and inform parents and guardians of children and adult recipients about the potential risks (e.g., mild bruising and discomfort at injection site, mild fever) and benefits (e.g., individual and herd immunity against a variety of diseases) associated with vaccines.
6. Healthcare professionals should recommend, postpone, reschedule, and/or withhold the administration of vaccines for true contraindications only (e.g., client is severely immunocompromised, client is febrile).
7. Healthcare professionals should administer all required or indicated vaccine doses for which a client is eligible at the time of their visit and consultation.
8. Healthcare professionals should ensure that all vaccinations administered are accurately and completely recorded and documented (e.g., name of client, date, specific name or type of vaccine administered, dose, lot number of vaccine, route administered such as oral or intra-muscular).
9. Healthcare professionals should keep and maintain easily retrievable vaccination summary records for their clients to facilitate age-appropriate vaccination scheduling.
10. Healthcare professionals should report all clinically significant adverse events or side effects following vaccination in a prompt, accurate, and complete fashion (e.g., severe adverse allergic reactions, excessive bleeding, deafness, seizures, coma).
11. Healthcare professionals should report all cases of vaccine-preventable diseases as required under provincial and territorial legislation (e.g., measles, mumps, hepatitis A & B).
12. Healthcare professionals should observe and follow appropriate procedures and standards for vaccine management in their province or territory of practice.
13. Healthcare professionals should maintain current, up-to-date, and easily accessible protocols and standards at all locations where vaccines are dispensed.
14. Healthcare professionals should be properly trained and licensed to administer vaccines, and engage in ongoing education regarding current immunization recommendations and standards.
15. Immunization errors should be reported by healthcare professionals to their local health jurisdiction.
16. Healthcare professionals who administer vaccines should maintain and operate a tracking system for their clients.
17. Routine audits should be conducted at all immunization clinics or facilities to assess the overall quality of immunization records kept and immunization coverage achieved in their designated geographical region.

Immunization remains the most efficient and cost-effective public health intervention for controlling vaccine-preventative disease in Canada and globally. Vaccines are either live and inactivated (attenuated) or killed—meaning that the virulence has been removed, which leaves only the antigenic components necessary to stimulate the immune system to produce the necessary antibodies. Vaccines may also be viewed as a kind of public health infection control measure that limits the incidence of infection in a local community or region. Mild common illnesses such as otitis media, upper respiratory tract infections, colds, and diarrhea are not contraindications for immunization (Jo Damazo and Bartfay 2010). In communities with poor immunization rates, barriers to successful immunization should be assessed and, where possible, removed through various public health initiatives. Vaccination status should be assessed by public health professionals at all health visits in an effort to complete necessary immunizations. Lastly, community clinics and health departments should be proactive and flexible in scheduling appointments and should not penalize individuals who do not have transportation or adequate financial resources (Bartfay and Bartfay 2015; Jo Damazo and Bartfay 2010). The Research Focus Box 7.2 describes a study which examined the integration of a barcode scanning technology versus traditional

---

Research Focus Box 7.2

The Integration of Barcode Scanning Technology into Canadian Public Health Immunization Settings

Aim and Significance

Immunization is one of the most effective community-based primary prevention interventions to decrease the incidence of various preventable communicable diseases across the lifespan. As part of a series of feasibility studies following the development of Canadian vaccine barcode standards, the researchers compared a barcode scanning technology with traditional manual methods for entering vaccine data into electronic client immunization records in public health settings.

Methodology/Design

A comparative pilot study was undertaken to examine and compare the ease and quality of data entered into client electronic records using barcode technology versus traditional manually entered (i.e., drop-down menu) methods. Two software vendors incorporated barcode scanning functionality into their systems so that Algoma Public Health (APH) in Ontario and four First Nations (FN) communities in Alberta could participate in this feasibility pilot study. The researchers compared the recording of client immunization data (vaccine name, lot number, expiry date) using barcode scanning of vaccine vials versus pre-existing manual methods. In addition, time and motion methodology was employed to determine the actual amount of time required for data recording, record audits to assess data quality, and qualitative analysis of immunization staff interviews to gauge user perceptions. Data was collected between July and November 2012, with 628 (282 barcodes) vials processed for the APH investigation and 749 (408 barcoded) vials for the study in the FN component of the study. Seventeen immunization nurses were also interviewed afterwards to evaluate their perceptions of the barcode versus traditional methods for entering client immunization data.

Major Findings

The researchers found that barcode scanning technologies led to significantly fewer immunization record errors than using drop-down menus (APH study: 0% versus 1.7%; $p=.04$) or typing in vaccine data (FN study: 0% versus 5.6%; $p<.001$). Although no statistically significant difference in time to enter vaccine data between scanning and using drop-down menus (27.6s versus 26.3s; $p=.39$), scanning was found to be significantly faster than typing data into the record (30.3s versus 41.3s; $p<.001$). All 17 of the nurses interviewed noted improved record accuracy with scanning. In addition, the majority of nurses felt that a more sensitive scanner was required to reduce the occasional failures to read the 2D barcodes on some vaccine vials.

Implications for Public Health

Finding from this pilot study suggest that entering vaccine data into electronic immunization records through barcode scanning may led to improved data quality during public health immunization campaigns. The use and integration of barcode technologies was well received by public healthcare professionals. Further research and work is needed to formally evaluate and improve barcode readability, particularly for unit-dose vials.

Source: Pereira et al. (2013).

manually methods for entering data via electronic records during public health immunization campaigns in community-based settings. These findings suggest that barcode scanning technology can improve data quality and ease of entry when using electronic client records during primary prevention immunization campaigns.

Herd Immunity

Herd immunity is based on the notion that if a significant percentage (e.g., 95%) of a given population has been immunized against an infectious agent; this can protect the whole population including the non-immunized individuals, by severely limiting its ability to spread. Immunization or past experience with a disease (e.g., chickenpox) reduces the number of those individuals who are susceptible in a defined herd (i.e., a population or group) (Bartfay and Bartfay 2015). Herd immunity is achieved or realized in the herd when the total number of susceptibles is reduced and the total numbers of protected individual's or non-susceptibles dominate the herd. That is to say, the lack of susceptible individuals in the herd halts the spread of the disease (see Figure 7.2).

For example, assume that each infected individual in a community has contact with 10 other individuals in that community. In a completely susceptible community, there is a high probability that all of the 10 contacts might become infected also. In addition, these 10 newly infected individuals could infect another 10 individuals each, and so on. If 80% of the total population in this community were immunized against the agent, only 2 of the 10 contacts are now likely to become infected. Hence, those two infected individuals will not be able to spread the infection to large numbers of non-immunized individuals in their community and therefore prevent the development of an outbreak or epidemic. The estimated herd-immunity thresholds needed to effectively stop the transmission of a specific communicable disease depends on its transmissibility.

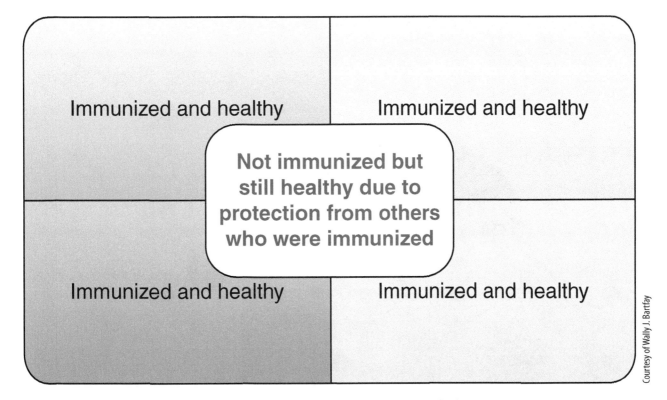

Courtesy of Wally J. Bartfay

Figure 7.2 Conceptual representation of how herd immunity halts the spread of infections in a community.

Infections can easily spread when individuals lack immunization against the agent. Herd immunity is based on the notion that if a significant percentage of a given population has been immunized against an infectious agent; this can protect the whole population, including those who are non-immunized against the infectious agent present in a defined population or community.

For example, the herd immunity threshold for pertussis is 92–94%, 83% for diphtheria, 83–94% for measles, 83–85% for rubella, and 75–86% for mumps (Merrill 2010).

Common Modes of Disease Transmission

Vertical and Horizontal Modes

The *mode of disease transmission* is defined as the mechanism or means by which an infectious agent or pathogen is transferred from an infected or diseased host to an uninfected and susceptible non-immunized host (Bartfay and Bartfay 2015). Public health professionals and workers must be cognizant and aware of the different modes of transmission to be able to understand and utilize the most efficient, safe, and cost-effective public health interventions to interrupt disease prevalence and to prevent its transmission in communities or entire regions. Disease transmission can take place either horizontally or vertically (Gordis 1996; Jo Damzo and Bartfay 2010; Bartfay and Bartfay 2015).

Vertical transmission occurs when an infectious disease is transmitted between a parent and child or off-spring via sperm, placenta, breast milk, or contact with the vaginal canal at birth (e.g., sexually transmitted infections such as HIV/AIDS, herpes, syphilis). Transmission may also occur through open sores or lesions on the infected individual. *Horizontal transmission* involves the direct transport of an infectious agent or pathogen from person-to-person. This can occur through direct or indirect modes of transmission, fecal or oral transmission or by airborne means (detailed below).

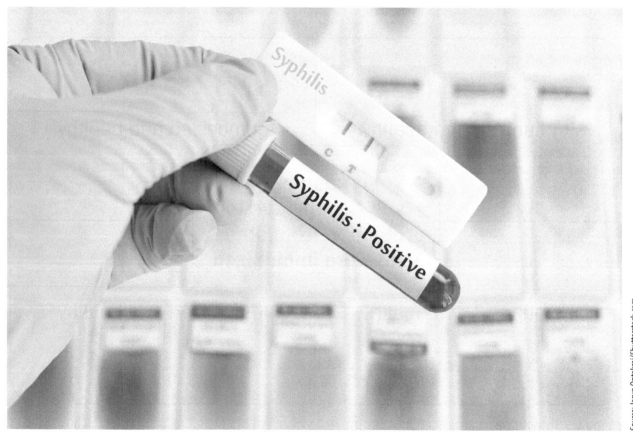

Photo 7.9 Syphillis is an example of a common STI. STI's such as syphilis can occur via vertical modes of transmission and remain a major global public health concern.

Airborne or Respiratory Mode of Transmission

Airborne or *respiratory mode of transmission* occurs when microorganisms or pathogens become suspended in droplet nuclei or aerosols in the air (e.g., via coughing, sneezing) and enter a susceptible host through a port of entry (e.g., nose or mouth) (Jo Damazo and Bartfay 2010). An example of a microorganism that can be transmitted via airborne means is the measles virus of an infected individual to another via sneezing or coughing. Contaminated droplets with the measles virus can enter a susceptible host through a number of ports of entries including the mucous membranes or conjunctiva of the eyes (Chin 2000).

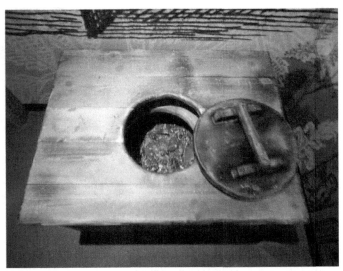

Photo 7.10 The fecal/oral model of transmission of an infectious microorganism or pathogen can occur via direct contact with hands or other contaminated objects (e.g., latrines, toilet seats, water taps on sinks or wash-basins) with organisms from human and/or animal feces and then placed in the mouth.

Fecal/Oral Mode of Transmission

Fecal/oral mode of transmission of an infectious microorganism or pathogen can occur directly by physical contact with hands or other contaminated objects with organisms from human or animal feces and then placed in the mouth (Jo Damazo and Bartfay 2010). This can occur, for example, when a cook in a restaurant fails to properly wash their hands after defecation and returns to cook for customers. Indeed, proper hand-washing and cooking of foods helps to significantly decrease the potential spread of disease in the environment. Examples of diseases spread via this mechanism include hepatitis A and hemolytic uremic syndrome, which is caused by the bacterium *E. coli* 0157:H7. The *Food and Drug Act (FDA)* in Canada is the federal legislation which helps Health Canada to monitor and ensure the safety of all food items, drugs, cosmetics, and therapeutic devices used nationally (see http://laws.justice.gc.ca/eng/acts/F-27/). Despite this legislation, Canadian's are still vulnerable to foodborne illnesses.

In June of 2011, an unusually lethal strain of *E. coli* 0104:H4 bacteria infected more than 1500 individuals in the Hamburg region of Germany and killed 15 Germans and 1 Swede who visited the country (Cowell and Neuman 2011). The potential source of the outbreak was believed to be contaminated raw vegetables such as lettuce, cucumbers, and tomatoes. On June 6, 2011, the media reported that a male from Peel, Ontario, who recently visited family in the Hamburg region of Germany and ate raw salad had developed a mild case of this *E. coli* infection. There are many types of *E. coli* and most are harmless, but a small number can produce a poison known as "shiga toxin," which has the ability to attach to an individual's intestinal wall, allowing them to release the poison in large amounts in the infected victim. According to Cowell and Neuman (2011), public health officials are alarmed because a startling high proportion of those infected suffer from a potentially lethal complication attacking the kidneys, called hemolytic uremic syndrome. This syndrome can provoke comas, seizures, and stroke.

Among the confirmed cases reported by the Robert Koch Institutes, Germany's disease control agency, 470 people had been diagnosed with this noted kidney syndrome. Scientists are currently at loss to explain why this little known organism identified as *E. coli* 0104:H4 has proven so virulent. European authorities have reported several differences from previous outbreaks including that women make up more than two-thirds of those affected and that young and middle-aged adult's account for a high percentage of the most severe cases (Cowell and Neuman 2011).

In September 2012, the Canadian Food Inspection Agency issued a recall of all beef products processed at the XL meat processing plant located in Brooks, Alberta due to *E. coli* contamination. This recall affected all provinces and territories in Canada, the United States, and Hong Kong (see http://www.inspection.gc.ca/food/information-for-consumers/food-safety-investigations/xl-foods/eng/1347937722467/1347937818275).

Marchant-Short and Whitney (2012) report that foodborne diseases and illnesses can be prevented and controlled by avoiding food contamination, destroying contaminants (e.g., via meat irradiation), and eliminating the spread or multiplication of possible contaminates. Ultimately, the prevention of foodborne disease rests on the handlers and preparers of food, which include proper hand washing and hygiene of food preparation items (e.g., knives, cutting boards), cooking methods, and storage.

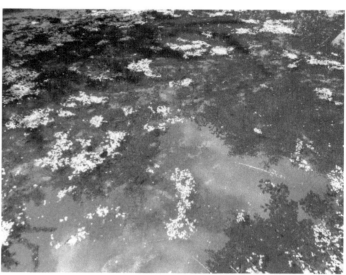

Source: Wally J. Bartfay

Photo 7.11 A safe and clean water supply is critical to the health of individuals, families and entire communities. Examples of common waterborne diseases and complications include cholera, dysentery, typhoid fever, shigellosis, coliform bacteria including *E. coli* 0157:H7 and vibrio.

The WHO (2009b) notes that the prevention of foodborne diseases includes five key elements: (a) keeping clean (hygiene), (b) separating raw and cooked food, (c) cooking the food properly and thoroughly, (d) keeping food items at safe temperatures (e.g., refrigeration), and (e) using safe water supplies and raw materials.

Waterborne Mode of Transmission

Waterborne mode of transmission occurs via contract or consumption of contaminated water supplies, and includes contamination of water supplies from fecal contamination from humans or animals which result in enteric illness or disease (Bartfay and Bartfay 2015). Recent outbreaks of cryptosporidium in North Battleford, Saskatchewan, and *E. coli* in Walkerton, Ontario, have raised national public awareness related to the importance of monitoring and maintaining safe municipal water supplies in Canada (Ali 2004; O'Conner 2002; Public Health Agency of Canada 2001, 2000; Sullivan 2004).

Community- and Hospital-Acquired Nosocomial Infections

Although the immune systems of healthy individuals are remarkably adept to respond to challenges posed by communicable diseases and microbial agents, pathogens have been slowly gaining ground over the past five decades globally. Added to the growing public health impact and challenges posed by these emerging or re-emerging infectious agents in hospitals and community settings is the growing resistance of these pathogens to currently available anti-microbial drugs (Levy and Marshall 2004; Rybak and LaPlante 2005; Weinstein 2001). In fact, not only are antimicrobial-resistant pathogens increasing in number, they are also expanding their geographical ranges, increasing the breadth of their resistance and impact, and spreading from institutional healthcare settings (e.g., hospitals, nursing homes) into the general community (Bartfay and Bartfay 2015). The PHAC (2013f) reports that over 200,000 individuals in Canada get infections every year while receiving healthcare services in hospitals, and more than 8000 die as a result annually.

For example, *S. aureus* is one of the most common causes of both hospital- and community-acquired infections. Methicillin-resistant *S. aureus* (MRSA) was first recognized as a nosocomial pathogen in 1961, shortly after methicillin was approved for market. By 2000, approximately half of all nosocomial *S. aureus* isolates in North America were methicillin resistant (Rybak and LaPlante 2005; Weinstein 2001). Donatelle (2010) reports that antibiotic strains of *S. aureus* are often endemic in many hospitals in North America. In some cities, 31% of *staph* infections are resistant to antibiotics, and in nursing homes as many as 71% of *staph* infections defy traditional antibiotic regimens.

In recent years, MRS infections have started to spread from healthcare settings into the community, where outbreaks are occurring among individuals with no prior hospital exposure. Indeed, outbreaks have been reported in day-care centres, among First Nation's individuals on reserves, inmates in correctional facilities, military personnel, and competitive athletes such as football players and wrestlers (e.g., Baggett et al. 2003; Centers for Disease Control 2003; Kazakova et al. 2005; LaMar et al. 2003; Pan et al. 2003). Alarmingly, an increasing proportion of MRSA also show low-level resistance to vancomycin, which is currently considered the last resort treatment options available (Hiramatsu et al. 2001; Weigel et al. 2003).

Similarly, the failure to properly treat individuals with TB is leading to the emergence of *M. tuberculosis* strains that are becoming increasingly drug resistance and undermining disease elimination efforts (Espinal et al. 2001; WHO 2003). In fact, of the estimated 300,000 new cases of drug-resistant TB occurring globally each year, 79% are resistant to three of the four first-line drugs (WHO 2013b, 2003). For example, *M. tuberculosis* strains resistant to isoniazid and rifampin (MDR-TB) are currently 10 times more frequent in Europe and central Asia than other parts of the world (WHO 2013b). Figure 7.3 shows a map with the estimated number of TB cases per 100,000 individuals by specific regions of the world for the year 2010. Hence, TB remains a growing public health concern and challenge in the new millennium (WHO 2013a).

Although NDM-1 is not transmitted through the air, it can be passed from one individual to another through improper hand-washing (Bartfay and Bartfay 2015). Of the 19 cases that have tested positive for NDM-1 to date, 17 had recently returned from India. However, one of two confirmed cases in Toronto (i.e., an 86-year-old man) has not been out of the country for years, which suggests that this superbug is now being transmitted within the province of Ontario (Hall 2011). Hall (2011) reports that it is a sliver of DNA that turns ordinary bacteria into superbugs and could become a new scourge in Ontario hospitals, long-term care facilities, and

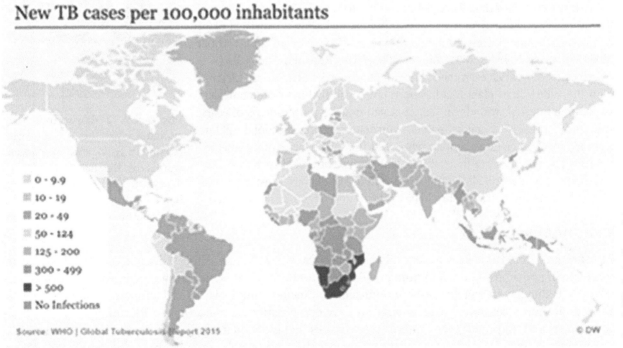

Figure 7.3 The estimated number of tuberculosis cases (all types) per 100,000 individuals by regions of the world

nursing homes. These tiny genetic packages originated in India and Pakistan and can worm their way into the normal bacteria that colonize our bodies by the billions and produce an enzyme that makes them immune to most major antibiotics currently available. In hospital or nursing home settings, where weakened clients are more susceptible to infections or face disease spreading procedures, it could join the list of ailments such as methicillin-resistant *S. aureus* (MRSA) that perpetually threatens these facilities and their residents (Hall 2011).

This growing public health concern to antibiotic resistance of pathogens has been linked to inappropriate prophylactic prescriptions and/or use by healthcare professionals. Indeed, Weber (2006) estimates that approximately 50% of antibiotics in Canada and the United States are prescribed incorrectly or inappropriately (e.g., to treat viral infections). The other public health challenge entails the uneven supply and availability of new classes of antibiotics to combat drug-resistant bacteria, and the reduced number of pharmaceutical companies investing in research to produce new classes of antibiotics (Talbot et al. 2006; Vergidis and Falagas 2008; Weber 2006). In the early part of the last century, antibiotic research and development was at an all-time high. Indeed, four classes of antibiotics were developed during the 1930s and 1940s (sulfonamides, beta-lactams, aminoglycosides, and chloramphenicol) and six classes during the 1950 and 1960s (tetracycline, macrolides, glycopeptides, rifamycins, quinolones, and trimethoprim) (Bartfay, Bartfay, and Green-Johnson 2010).

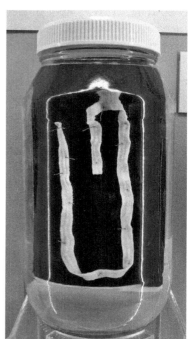

Since the 1970s to present, only two additional new classes of antibiotics have been researched and developed for commercial use (oxazolidinones and cyclic lipopeptides) (Boucher et al. 2009; Wenzel 2004). A major factor the precludes pharmaceutical companies from investing in the development of new antibiotics is the poor financial return, especially in light of the fact that antibiotics are typically prescribed for short durations (e.g., 2 weeks) as opposed to drugs that have to be taken for long durations or even decades (e.g., blood pressure or cholesterol-lowering drugs) (Amyes 2000; Overbye and Barrett 2005). For example, Wenzel (2004) reports that antibiotics are estimated to have a $100 million risk-adjusted net present value compared to musculoskeletal medications that have an estimated net value of $1,150 million to pharmaceutical companies.

With the current lack of financial incentives to research and develop new antibiotics, new alternatives need to be explored, including a variety of plant species which may possess antibiotic properties (Bax, Mullan' and Verhoef 2000; Projan and Shales 2004; Zinner 2005). The Research Focus Box 7.3 describes a study which examined antioxidant properties of an extract derived from the willow herd plant that has been employed by First Nation's healers for treating infected wounds on the Canadian prairies for hundreds of years. This study provides laboratory-based confirmation of the anecdotal folklore accounts by First Nation's peoples who used this plant for treating infected wounds. The authors argue that natural plant-derived products, such as Willow herb, may be a practical alternative to current drugs that are resistant to various pathogens and therefore should be explored and scientifically validated.

Photo 7.12 Tapewormes are common parasites. Tapeworms (Cestoda) is a class of parasitic worms of the flatworm phylum. Tapeworm eggs normally enter the human host from animals via food, especially raw or undercooked meat.

Source: Photo By Wally J. Bartfay

Parasitic Mode

Parasites are defined as eukaryotic organisms that are capable of causing illness, disease, or disability and survive by living off a host (animal or human) (Bartfay and Bartfay 2015). Eukaryote organisms have a complex cell or cells that have a membrane-bound nucleus and include fungi, plants, and animals. Although parasitic illnesses are more commonly encountered in developing nations around the world, immigration, international travel and trade and recent outbreaks remind us that individuals in Canada are not immune to these.

For example, over 7.4 million Canadians travelled globally for business or holidays, including 300,000 (4%) of children which accounted for a disproportionate number of travel-related hospitalizations in Canada (Crockett

Research Focus Box 7.3

Gram-negative and Gram-positive Antibacterial Properties of the Whole Plant Extract of Willow Herb (*Epilobium augustifolium*).

Study Aim/Rationale
The emergence of new pathogens and the increase in the number of multidrug-resistant strains in a variety of well-established pathogens during the past decade represents a growing public health concern globally. With the current lack of research and development for new antibiotics by large pharmaceutical companies due to poor financial returns, new alternatives need to be explored including natural herbal or plant-based extracts with reported antibacterial properties. Anecdotal evidence notes that extracts from the plant Willow herb (*Epilobium augustifolium*) have been used for centuries by First Nation's peoples in Canada and in folk medicine preparations externally to treat infected wounds. Willow herb is an invasive species in Canada, the United States, and parts of Europe that often inhabits riverbeds and areas following natural disasters such as forest fires and avalanches. It is argued that natural products, such as Willow herb, may be a practical alternative to current drugs that are resistant to these pathogens and therefore should be explored and validated. Accordingly, the aim of this investigation was to validate anecdotal reports in the laboratory by first determining if a crude extract of this plant possessed any antimicrobial properties against gram-positive and negative bacteria.

Methodology/Design
A laboratory-based experiment was undertaken to test the antibacterial properties of a whole plant extract of Willow herb grown on the Canadian prairies. It was hypothesized that the whole plant extract of willow herb would exhibit antimicrobial properties against a variety of common gram-positive (e.g., *S. aureus, Micrococcus luteus*) and negative (e.g., *Escherichia coli, Pseudomonas aeruginosa*) bacteria. The antibiotics vancomycin and tetracycline were employed as commercial positive controls. The negative control consisted of sterile water.

Major Findings
In comparison to growth controls, the whole plant extract of Willow herb significantly inhibited the growth of *Micrococcus luteus* ($p < .01$); *S. aureus* ($p < .05$), *Escherichia coli* ($p < .001$), and *Pseudomonas aeruginosa* ($p < .05$). Moreover, Willow herb extract was found to inhibit the growth of bacteria in culture more effectively than positive commercially available controls vancomycin ($p < 0.05$) or tetracycline ($p < 0.004$).

Implications for Public Health
These findings provide preliminary laboratory-based support for the anecdotal traditional folkloric claims that a whole plant extract of Willow herb possesses antibacterial properties against a variety of Gram-positive and negative bacteria. Given that whole plant extract was employed for this investigation, further studies are warranted to determine which specific part of the plant (e.g., leaves, stem, roots, flowers) possesses the desired properties. Further dose–response studies are also required as well as the need to isolate and identify the beneficial biochemical compounds present in the active part(s) of the plant via high-pressure liquid chromatography and/or gas chromatography mass spectrometry. Although it may take decades to isolate and purify these compounds present before animal and human clinical trials can take place, the effort appears warranted and critical in nature given the growing public health concern of multidrug-resistant strains of bacteria in Canada and globally.

Source: Bartfay, Bartfay, and Johnson (2012).

et al. 2009, 2011). In order to determine clinical manifestations and risk factors associated with travel-related diseases and illnesses in Canada, the *Canadian Paediatric Surveillance Program* routinely surveys over 2500 pediatricians and pediatric subspecialists across Canada. The acquisition of this data is utilized by public health professionals and workers to help monitor disease and illness outbreaks in this vulnerable population and also helps to develop public health promotion strategies, health education and advocacy (Crockett et al. 2009, 2011). An accurate diagnosis is dependent on obtaining a complete travel history, clinical manifestations, and recognition of associated signs and symptoms, and appropriate specimen and laboratory confirmation of the parasite.

Helminthes are endoparasitic worms that live inside the body of a host human or animal (Bartfay and Bartfay 2015). Jacobsen (2008) reports that it has been estimated that approximately one-third of all people in the world have a worm or nematode living in their body at any given time. These endoparasitic worms may take up residence in the individual's blood stream, brain, liver, lungs, intestines, or other body organs. For example, hookworms often latch onto the intestinal lining and cause bleeding and increase the risk of developing anemia and malnutrition (Bethony et al. 2006; de Silva et al. 2003; Hotez et al. 2004).

Guinea worm disease (dracunculiasis) is an extremely painful condition caused by ingestion of drinking water that contains fleas infected with the guinea worm larva. According to Jacobsen (2008), a mature Guinea worm may grow to up to 3 feet in length. Once the worm achieves maturity, it often crawls down the inside of an infected individual's leg and emerges from a painful blister near the foot. In fact, it often takes weeks for the worm to leave the host's body. The worm cannot simply be pulled out of the body because if it breaks it can cause massive infection. Instead, the worm is often tied to a stick that is used to coil the guinea worm as it slowly makes its way out of the human body.

Evidence for this disease has even been found in a 3000-year-old female mummy (Hopkins 2008). Over 3.5 million people were infected in 1986 in parts of India, Pakistan, Yemen, and 17 sub-Saharan countries in Africa. This number dropped to approximately 16,000 cases globally in 2006,

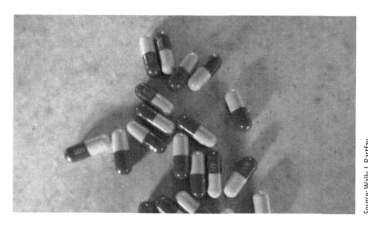

Photo 7.13 Photo of amoxicillin, a widely prescribed broad-spectrum antibiotic used against both aerobic gram-positive and gram-negative bacteria. Antibiotic resistance to various strains of bacteria is a growing public health concern in Canada and globally.

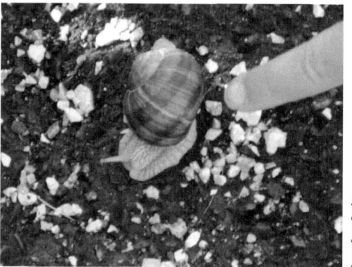

Photo 7.14 Schistosomiasis, also known as "Snail fever" and "Katayama fever," is an example of a helminth infection caused by fresh water parasitic worms of the schistoma type which infect the urinary tract and/or intestines. The parasites can damage the liver, lead to kidney failure, infertility, and bladder cancer and affects more than 240 million people worldwide annually (WHO 2014).

and over 98% of the cases were from Ghana and Sudan (Hopkins 2008). There is no known drug or cure for Guinea worm disease, although the prevalence can be decreased through the use of clean filtered water supplies. This includes teaching villagers in developing nations of the world to filter their drinking water through a finely woven cloth to remove copepods (Bartfay and Bartfay 2015).

Although boiling the water will often kill copepods and Guinea worm larvae, most villagers are often too poor to afford the fuel to boil their drinking water supplies regularly. Moreover, the application of temephos (Abate larvicide at 1 part per million) to ponds, wells, and other drinking water supplies at four-week intervals during the transmission season is a safe and effective public health means of vector control, which does not harm humans, fish, plants, or other aquatic species. These collective public health efforts are making a major contribution to decreasing the incidence of this disease, and the *World Health Organization International Commission for the Certification of Dracunculiasis Eradication* has already certified 180 countries as free of Guinea worm (Hopkins 2008).

Personal hygiene practices including effective hand washing, effective sanitation, and safe sexual practices are all paramount in the control of parasitic disease. Table 7.3 shows some of the common infections caused by tapeworms found in uncooked fish (e.g., sushi), pork or beef, flatworms which include liver, lung or blood intestinal

Table 7.3 Common Diseases and Illnesses Caused by Worms Globally

Agent	Disease or Illness	Common Location and Mode of Transmission
Ascaris lumbricoides (roundworm)	Ascariasis	– Worldwide – Eating food that is contaminated with fecal material or soil
Clonorchis sinensis (flatworm)	Clonorchiasis	– Southeast China and Asia – Eating raw or undercooked fish from freshwater sources (e.g., rivers, lakes)
Dracunculus medinensis (Guinea worm)	Guinea worm disease (Drancunculiasis)	– Parts of Asia and Africa – Drinking contaminated and unfiltered water sources
Echinococcus granulosus (tapeworm)	Hydatid cyst disease (Echinococcosis)	– Domesticated dogs worldwide – Contact with infected dogs or food
Enterobius vermicularis (pinworm)	Enterobiasis	– Worldwide – Fecal to hand to mouth spread
Fasciola hepatica (liver fluke)	Fascioliasis	– Cattle and sheep farms – Eating uncooked or undercooked aquatic plants (e.g., watercress) which grows in focally contaminated water supplies
Necator americanus and Ancylostoma duodenale (hookworm)	Hookworm disease	– Common in subtropical and tropical regions of the world – Typically enters through skin between toes or bare feet
Hymenolepsis nana (tapeworm)	Hymenolepiasis	– India, Middle-East, Australia and South America – Fecal to hand to mouth spread
Paragonimus (lung fluke)	Paragonimiasis	– China and Asia, Africa and South America – Eating raw or undercooked shellfish (e.g., crabs or crayfish)
Schistosoma (blood fluke)	Bilharzia (Schistosomiasis)	– Asia, Middle East, Africa, South America, Caribbean Islands
Stronglyloides stercoralis (nematode)	Strongyloidiasis	– Tropical and subtropical regions of the world – Enters through skin

(Continued)

Table 7.3 Common Diseases and Illnesses Caused by Worms Globally (*Continued*)

Agent	Disease or Illness	Common Location and Mode of Transmission
Taenia solium and Taenia saginata (tapeworm)	Taeniasis	– Worldwide – Eating uncooked or undercooked pork or beef
Trichinella spiralis (threadworm)	Trichinosis (Trichinellosis)	– Worldwide – Eating uncooked or undercooked pork or beef
Trichuris trichiura (whipworm)	Trichuriasis	– Worldwide – Eating focally-contaminated foods or soils

flukes, roundworms, pinworms, and hookworms. Pinworms are common in young children and often appear in crowded locations in the world and institutional settings.

Vector-borne Mode

Vector-borne diseases are caused by infectious agents that are transmitted via a vector or carrier, such as an insect (e.g., fly, tick, mosquitoe) (Bartfay and Bartfay 2015). Common vector-borne diseases in Canada include Lyme disease, West Nile virus and Eastern equine encephalitis (Marchant-Short and Whitney 2011). *Arthropod-borne viruses* or *arboviruses* are viruses that are spread by arthropods which include insects and arachnids (e.g., ticks, mites, spiders), and include yellow fever, dengue fever, and Venezuelan equine encephalitis (Bartfay and Bartfay 2015).

For example, Lyme disease is a tick-borne disease caused by the spirochete *Borrelia burgdorferi* that may result in multisystem, multistage, inflammatory disease principally affecting the skin, joints, nervous system, and the heart (Brouqui et al. 2004; Piesman and Gern 2004; Reed 2002). The portal of entry into humans is the dermis where the tiny infected tick attaches itself. After an incubation period that is typically 7–10 days (range

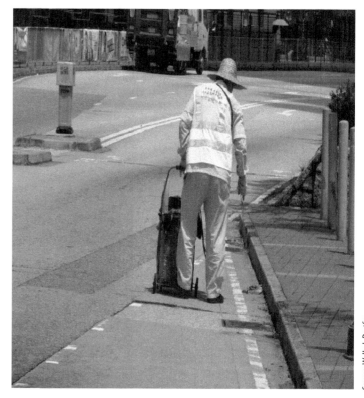

Source: Wally J. Bartfay

Photo 7.15 A public health worker in Hong Kong spraying a sewer basin to treat it for the *Aedes* mosquitoe, which can spread several diseases including Yellow Fever, Zika virus, Dengue fever, Mayaro and Chikungunya in tropical and subtropical regions of the world.

3–32 days), the infected individual often develops the hallmark erythema migrans rash for Lyme disease that resembles a red "bulls-eye," which occurs in approximately 70–80% of victims during the first stage of the disease (i.e., 3 days to 1 month) (Public Health Agency of Canada 2010c). This rash is often accompanied by symptoms of fever, headache, myalgia, arthlagiam, muscle and joint pain, and swollen lymph nodes. If not treated, the second stage of the disease can last up to several months in duration and include central and peripheral nervous system disorders, multiple skin rashes, arthritis and arthritic symptoms, heart palpitations and extreme fatigue and general weakness. If the disease remains untreated, the third stage can last several months or even years in duration with symptoms that can include recurring arthritis and neurological problems, although fatalities are relatively rare.

Lyme disease is present throughout North America and Europe and is transmitted by deer ticks or black-legged ticks that are often transported by small animals (e.g., rodents, squirrels, mice, birds) and/or deer that can carry the bacterium (Bartfay and Bartfay 2015). Although family pets such as dogs and cats can contact Lyme disease, there is currently no evidence to indicate that they can spread to humans, nor is there any evidence that it can be contracted from eating infected deer. Areas of high concern include the southern regions of British Columbia especially in the Fraser Valley and Vancouver Island, Lunenburg County in Nova Scotia, the southern regions of Ontario, southern Québec, and the southeastern corner of Manitoba (PHAC 2009d, 2010c, 2011). Most cases of Lyme disease can be cured with a 2–4-week treatment of doxycycline, amoxicillin, or ceftriaxone. Individuals can also protect themselves when walking in tick-infected areas by wearing clothing that will keep ticks aware from bare skin such as long sleeve shirts and pants, wearing closed shoes and tucking your socks into the pants or boots, and through the application of insect repellents containing DEET. In 2010, Lyme disease became a nationally reportable disease in Canada (Public Health Agency of Canada 2010c).

Malaria is perhaps the best known example of a vector-borne disease present in temperate regions of the world (e.g., sub-Saharan Africa, Caribbean island of Hispaniola, Middle East, Indian continent, Southeast Asia, Oceania, and South America), and affects between 300 and 500 million individuals each year worldwide (WHO and UNICEF 2005). The WHO and UNICEF (2005) report that 107 countries and territories are known to have the disease and that 36% of the global population live in these areas, 70% of the world's population reside in regions where malaria has never been under control, and 29% live in areas where malaria was once transmitted at low levels or not at all but where transmission has been significantly reestablished.

The suspected cause of malaria during the 1800s, also commonly known as "ague" was believed to be caused by "bad air" or "malaria" present near and around swamps, which was most likely methane gas (McManus 1998, 2011). Today, we know that malaria is caused by a microscopic parasite carried by mosquitoes. By the 1900s, malaria had disappeared from Eastern Ontario after learning that draining swamps could eliminate mosquitoe breeding grounds. Although no longer endemic to Canada, malaria was once wide-spread in Ontario (Upper Canada), along the shores of the St. Lawrence River, the Cataraqui River, the Rideau River, and the Great Lakes basin (McManus 1998, 2011). For example, during the construction of the 220-km Rideau Canal from Ottawa to Kingston from 1826 to 1832 by British Royal Engineers under the direction of Colonel John By, several individuals contracted malaria, especially near Jones Falls. McManus (1998) reports that during the construction of this canal, malaria ravaged the population of canal workers each summer. There are no accurate counts or mortality statistics related to those who died during the construction of the canal, but the numbers were certainly high. The only treatment at the time was quinine, derived from a tropical tree bark. Unfortunately, few laborers could afford this drug. Interestingly, workers were encouraged to drink "Gin and Tonics" during the summer. The tonic contains quinine, and was originally designed as a malaria treatment for British troops in India (McManus 1998).

In humans, malaria is caused by one or more of the following five species of intracellular protozoan parasites which differ in geographical distribution, clinical features (e.g., periodicity of infections, tendency for clinical relapses, potential for severe or complicated disease) and immunogenic potential: (a) *Plasmodium falciparum*, (b) *P. vivax*, (c) *P. ovale*, (d) *P. malariae*, and (e) *P. knowlesi* (see http://www.cdc.gov/malaria/about/biology/parasites.html). Although *P. vivax* infections are the most common type globally, *P. falciparum* malaria represents the most serious public health concern because of its tendency toward more severe and fatal infections (Centers for Disease Control and Prevention 2012; Kachur, de Oliveria, and Bloland 2008; WHO 2004; WHO and UNICEF 2005). Moreover, *P. knowlesi* is found throughout Southeast Asia as a natural pathogen of long-tailed and pig-tailed macaques. This species has recently been reported to be a significant cause of zoonotic malaria in that region, particularly in Malaysia (Centers for Disease Control and Prevention 2012). *P. knowlesi* has a 24-hour replication cycle, so it can rapidly progress from an uncomplicated to a severe infection in a relatively short period of time, and fatal cases have also been reported.

Malaria results from the bite of an infected female *Anopheles* mosquitoe and may be contacted by travelers from Canada to infected regions of the world (Jacobsen 2008; Snow, Korenromp, and Gouws 2004; WHO 2004). Anopheles mosquitoes breed near standing bodies of water (e.g., ponds, lakes, puddles) and require a blood meal to produce and lay eggs. Once a female mosquitoe acquires malaria by biting an infected host, the malaria parasite undergoes a reproductive stage in the gut of the mosquitoe, which can then spread malaria to humans through its saliva.

Malaria has been a reportable communicable disease in Canada since 1929, when a national surveillance system for communicable disease was first developed and implemented (MacLean et al. 2004). Although no longer considered an endemic disease in Canada, malaria has remained an important imported disease principally from immigrants and refugees to our country and travelers who visit affected countries and regions of the world, and rarely through blood transfusions (Kain et al. 2001; Slinger et al. 2001). Changes in the malaria attack rates in endemic countries of exposure for these individuals are also likely to influence the incidence of imported disease. Changes in Canadian immigration and refugee patterns from 1990 to 2002 are

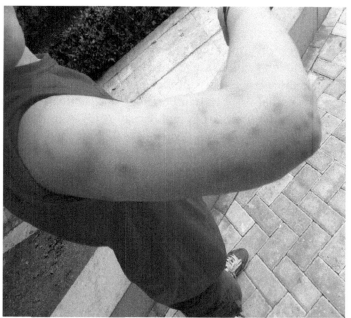

Photo 7.16 Severe mosquitoe bites due to not wearing insect repellent with DEET and a long sleeve shirt in LaBoca, Cuba. In 2014 Cuban health authorities confirmed the country's first 6 cases of chikungunya fever, a debilitating, mosquitoe-borne virus that is suspected of afflicting tens of thousands across the Caribbean since its arrival in the region in 2013. Chikungunya is not usually fatal, but causes high fever, severe joint pain, headaches and vomiting, and there is no known cure. According to a report by the Pan American Health Organization, there have been approximately 166,000 suspected and 4,600 laboratory confirmed cases of chikungunya in the Caribbean as of June, 2014 (Associated Press, 2014).

noteworthy because of a threefold increase in the annual immigrant numbers from the Indian subcontinent and relatively stable numbers from sub-Saharan Africa (MacLean et al. 2004). The Canadian infectious disease surveillance system has reported an average of 538 confirmed cases of malaria in Canada since 1990 (range 364–1029) with an average of 1 death per year (MacLean et al. 2004; Statistics Canada 2000). MacLean and coworkers (2004) note that in the past decade, fluctuations in numbers of imported malaria cases have been seen in Canada. In 1997 to 1998, malaria case numbers more than doubled before returning to normal. This increase was not seen in any other industrialized country.

Although a massive insecticide spraying campaign spear-headed by WHO during the 1950s and 1960s eliminated malaria from dozens of countries, it has slowly began to reemerge due to the development of insecticide resistance in mosquitoes. For various decades, the drug of choice for clinically treated malaria was chloroquine, but in most parts of the world the common strains of malaria are increasingly becoming resistant to this drug (WHO and UNICEF 2005; WHO 2004). This remains a growing global health concern because additional strains of malaria are also becoming resistant to other drug options including sulfadoxone/pyrimethamine (SP or Fansidar), mefloquine (Lariam), and artemisinin derivatives are also becoming less effective (Jacobsen 2008). Hence, although travelers from Canada and other non-endemic areas who visit known malaria regions or countries of the world are encouraged to take prophylactic (preventive) antimalarial drugs, they are becoming increasingly less effective. The only way to prevent malaria is to avoid being bitten by infected female mosquitoes through the use of insecticide-treated bed nets, wearing of clothes that cover the arms and legs during the times when mosquitoes are most active (e.g., evening, nights), use of mosquitoe repellents containing the chemical DEET, and the draining of stagnant water supplies (e.g., ponds, puddles, bird baths) and water-filled containers that encourage the breeding of mosquitoes.

Zoonotic Mode

Zoonotic mode infections are defined as diseases which are transmissible between animals and humans, and which do not necessarily require a human host to maintain their life cycles (Bartfay and Bartfay 2015). The term zoonosis is derived from the Greek words "zoon" (meaning animal) and "nosis" (meaning illness). The presence of the deadly Ebola-Reston virus in a quarantine population of primates located in a Texas holding station in the United States highlights the importance of understanding zoonotic modes of disease transmission by healthcare professionals and workers and the potential threat it poses to the health of humans (Jo Damazo and Bartfay 2010; Strausbaugh 1997). Moreover, it is also important to understand that family pets can be common sources of disease including worms from dogs, cat-scratch fever, rabbit fever (tularemia), and parrot fever (psittacosis).

Table 7.4 shows common carriers of infectious organisms that can be zoonotic in nature. Zoonotic disease may be classified according to their specific infectious agent including bacteria, fungi, parasites pria or viruses, or by the specific ability of the disease to be transmitted to humans. Common examples include listeriosis, Hantavirus pulmonary syndrome, salmonellosis, brucellosis, and rabies. More than 185 diseases have been reported to be transmitted to humans by animals (Acha and Szyfres 1989; Merrill 2010). It is important to note that although

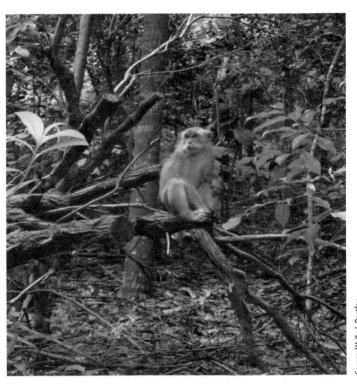

Source: Wally J. Bartfay

Photo 7.17 Primates in rainforests located near communities and villages can transmit a variety of communicable diseases to humans such as the monkey malaria parasite (*Plasmodium Knowlesi*).

Table 7.4 List of Common Carriers of Infectious Organisms that Can Be Zoonotic in Nature

Assassin bugs	Bats	Birds	Cats
Cattle	Chimpanzees	Coyotes	Dogs
Fish	Fleas	Flies	Foxes
Geese	Goats	Hamsters	Horses
Lice	Mice	Monkeys	Mosquitoes
Pigs	Possums	Rabbits	Raccoons
Rats	Rodents	Sloths	Skunks
Sheep	Snails	Ticks	

certain animals can be known carriers of a disease, they may not develop the disease themselves or show any signs or symptoms of the disease they carry. For example, coyotes can carry the plague and never become sick themselves (Merrill 2010). Nonetheless, coyotes can spread it to rodents and humans via a flea vector when humans are in wooden areas. A few days later, they may get ill and not connect their symptoms to the inoculation caused by the insect that bit them.

Rabies is a common global zoonotic viral infection of the central nervous system that affects warm-blooded vertebrates. The etiological agent is a rod-shaped RNA virus that belongs to the genus *Lyssavirus* in the *Rhabdoviridae*, a diverse family that includes a number of other agents that affects vertebrates, invertebrates, and plants (Jackson 2002; Warrel and Warrell 2004). All mammals are susceptible to the occurrence of rabies, but it tends to be skewed in certain major groups. For example, rabies manifests in two major epidemiological forms: (a) "Urban rabies," which is present in dogs and (b) "wildlife rabies," which is principally present in wild *Canidae* (i.e., foxes), *Herpestidae* (i.e., mongoose, meerkats), *Mephitidae* (i.e., skunks), *Procyonidae* (i.e., raccoons), and the *Chiroptera* (i.e., bats).

The occurrence of human rabies in Canada, the United States, and Europe has been dramatically reduced from the noted historical scores of deaths to only a few documented cases per year currently. Human cases are much higher in the developing parts of Asia, Africa, India, and Latin America (Coleman, Fevre, and Cleaveland 2004; Meslin 2003). Rabies has one of the highest case fatality rates of any known human infection, nearly 100%. It is estimated that more than 50,000 individuals and millions of animals die of rabies worldwide each year, and several million individuals receive prophylaxis rabies treatment after exposure (e.g., bite or scratch from a raccoon, dog, bat or skunk). The number of individuals vaccinated for potential rabies exposure in North America is estimated to be 20,000–40,000 per year (Meslin 2003). By comparison, prophylaxis treatment in India is estimated to be over a million exposures per year (Meslin 2003).

The major carriers of rabies in Canada are bats, foxes, raccoons, and skunks and the virus may be transmitted via a bit, scratch, or infection of a pre-existing open wound. The best protection against rabies is prevention through the administration of an oral vaccine for wildlife and pre-exposure vaccination of high-risk individuals including animal control workers, veterinarians and veterinary technicians and researchers who employ experimental animal models (e.g., rats, mice, monkeys) (Marchant-Short and Whitney 2012; Rupprecht, Hanlon, and Slate 2004). Rabies baiting for large areas (e.g., woodlands, forests) are typically carried-out by airplanes that drop vaccine baits. For smaller areas, which are typically less than 1000 km², animals may be trapped and manually injected with the rabies vaccine. This procedure is known as the "Trap-Vaccinate-Release" method (Ontario Ministry of Natural Resources 2013). While oral vaccines for immunizing raccoon and fox have been used since 1989, there has not been a similar vaccine to immunize skunks until recently. The Ontario Ministry of Natural Resources (2013) and partners have developed a new oral vaccine for skunks and, in 2006, began distributing this vaccine in southern Ontario.

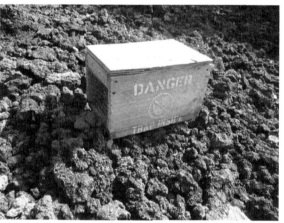

Source: Photo by Wally J. Bartfay

Photo 7.18 A trap set to catch small animals such as skunks and racoons known to carry the rabies virus. Rabies is spread to humans or animal animal when virus in the saliva of an infected animal enters through a bite, scratch, broken skin, the mucous membranes or the respiratory tract. The virus then gains access to the central nervous system through peripheral nerves.

Post-exposure prophylaxis (PEP) is recommended after the potential exposure of a rabid animal and is done in consultation with a public health professional. Determination of the need for follow-up care by a public health professional (e.g., public health nurse or physician) requires assessment of the endemic rates for animals in the region. For example, exposure in Eastern Ontario where raccoon rabies is still endemic requires follow-up treatment, whereas exposure in Newfoundland would require further investigation to assess the history of the animals habitation given that rabies in not usually present in this province. Nonetheless, the animal may have been brought into Newfoundland or migrated from an area that is considered endemic. For those who have been potentially exposed to the virus, it is often recommended that the individual receive rabies immune globulin with the calculated dose based on the individual's weight, and a series of follow-up rabies treatments.

If the animal can be located, they should be kept in a confined area for a period of 10 days in order to assess if the animal was infected with rabies at the time of exposure (Marchant-Short and Whitney 2012). Most infected animals will succumb to rabies within a five-day period, but 10 days is used to avoid any possible exceptions. If the animal exhibits signs and symptoms of rabies or dies during the isolation period, the exposed person is started on PEP as soon as possible. The Public Health Agency of Canada (2006b) notes that if the animal dies immediately following exposure, rabies validation of the animal's brain will take place at the national laboratory. The exposed individual may be offered PEP based on the findings of the laboratory. If the individual is started on PEP, but the laboratory testing of the animal's brain failed to detect the presence of any rabies virus, the PEP may be stopped prior to completion of the treatment regime.

Hantavirus have occurred in many parts of the world for long periods of time, but hantavirus pulmonary syndrome (HPS) was first recognized in 1993 when a cluster of fatal unexplained adult respiratory distress syndrome cases occurred among an otherwise group of healthy young adults in the Four Corners region of the southwest United States (Centers for Disease Control 2002; LeDuc 2008). Several young adults developed severe pneumonia via the inhalation of aerosolized rat urine and/or feces while cleaning homes, barns, or sheds in rural locations. *P. maniculatus* and other genetically and antigenically related viruses are capable of causing HPS. Approximately 400 cases of HPS have been documented in the United States with a mortality rate of 36% of which three-quarter of the cases are rural, and approximately 60% of the cases are male (LeDuc 2008). The disease is clinically characterized by fever, myalgia, headaches, cough, and gastrointestinal symptoms followed by abrupt onset of non-cardiogenic pulmonary edema and shock, which can quickly progress to death if not treated.

In Canada, Hantavirus can be carried by deer mice and it can be transmitted to humans through direct or indirect contact. The mice can shed the virus in their saliva, feces, and/or urine and humans may subsequently inhale the virus and develop HPS. The first case of HPS in Canada was reported in 1989 in Alberta (Marchant-Short and Whitney 2012; Public Health Agency of Canada 2009b). Since then, approximately 70 confirmed cases have occurred in Canada and most of cases were from the western provinces (Manitoba, Saskatchewan, Alberta and British Columbia), and two fatal cases were also contracted by Canadians outside the country from South America. HPS is a serious zoonotic public health concern and challenge because 30–40% of confirmed cases are fatal in nature (Public Health Agency of Canada 2009b). Individuals at risk include agricultural workers, workers in rural settings, and hikers and campers. Preventative strategies include keeping woodpiles away from dwellings, keeping items off the floor to prevent rodent nesting, trapping rodents, wet-mopping areas where droppings are located to prevent aeration of feces, and not camping or hiking near rodent-infected areas (Marchant-Short and Whitney 2012).

Health Surveillance

Health surveillance is a central component for public health efforts to track, control and manage communicable and non-communicable diseases in Canada and globally (Public Health Agency of Canada 2007b, 2010; WHO 2010a, 2010b, 2000c). Health surveillance entails the systematic collection and analysis of health-related data and timely communication of these health reports to health professionals and workers, and the public when action is required. The Kirby Commission (2003, 26) defines *health surveillance* in Canada as

the tracking and forecasting of any health event or health determinant through the continuous collection of high-quality data, the integration, analysis and interpretation of those data into reports, advisories, alerts, and warnings, and the dissemination to those who need to know.

Implicit in this definition is the formation of a continuous cycle that links health surveillance, data collection and analysis, prompt dissemination and communication of findings, public health practice (e.g., control, prevention), and public health policy and legislation when necessary. Health surveillance provides information for both urgent (e.g., 2003 SARS outbreak in Toronto, Ontario) and routine actions in public health (e.g., annual influenza vaccines) (Thompson 2010; Wallace 2008). Health surveillance is employed by public health professionals and governmental agencies to estimate the magnitude of disease or health conditions in various geographical regions in Canada, to better understand the natural history of a disease, and to detect potential emerging epidemics (Public Health Agency of Canada 2010; Teutsch, Churchill, and Elliot 1994). Public health surveillance utilizes established data collection procedures and sets, which are designed to detect changes in the occurrence of health conditions or events in time and to control and prevent alterations to health. Hence, health surveillance focuses on descriptive information that is analyzed with respect to time trends and the rates of occurrence are estimated. These findings are subsequently fed back to public health professionals and workers who originated the data. Communication of this information is essential for directing public health practice and policy initiatives.

We shall examine the two major types of public health surveillance, active and passive, in the following text. Health surveillance, be it active or passive in nature, does not seize with the notification of the disease case to public healthcare authorities. Rather, it initiates a critical process toward the control, containment, prevention, and/or management of the disease, health condition or event. The reader is referred to Chapter 6 for a discussion of the importance of surveillance and tracking for the practice of public health in Canada and globally.

Active Surveillance

Active surveillance is defined as the collection of health-related data via sentinel public health tracking systems, screening tools, and interviews in order to identify the occurrence of disease in a defined community or geographical region when individuals present with suggestive clinical signs and symptoms (Bartfay and Bartfay 2015). This often entails the creation of surveillance screening tools that help public health professionals to screen potential cases of disease and to also heighten their awareness.

For example, in 1937, the West Nile Virus was first isolated in an adult woman who lived in the West Nile district of Uganda, Africa (Public Safety Canada 2003). West Nile is spread by infected female mosquitoes, and most species breed on standing or stagnant water and require a blood diet to produce eggs. The virus can also be transmitted by organs/tissues during organ or tissue transplantation, blood transfusions, and possibly through breast milk during breastfeeding of infants. As a consequence of global warming, infected female mosquitoes were able to migrate to more northern and previously temperate regions such as Europe, the United States and Canada. West Nile virus was first recognized as a threat to individuals in North America in 1999 and first appeared in Canada in August, 2001, in birds (e.g., crows, blue jays) and mosquitoes (Public Health Agency of Canada 2006c; Public Safety Canada 2003; Quinlan and Dickinson 2009). In 2002, public health authorities documented the presence of West Nile virus in humans in the provinces of Nova Scotia, Québec, Ontario, Manitoba, and Saskatchewan. By 2007, more than 2200 human cases were identified in Canada (Public Health Agency of Canada 2009f). Public health authorities responded by developing a screening tool to assist with the active surveillance of this disease during the early periods in Canada. As of October 2012, the total number of West Nile cases and asymptomatic infections in Canada was 421 (Canadian Cooperative Wildlife Health Centre 2012; PHAC 2012). Add to your knowledge of West Nile virus by accessing the resources in the Web-Based Resource Box 7.1.

Similarly, a screening tool has been developed by the Ontario Ministry of Health and Long-Term Care (MOHLTC 2009) for the active screening of influenza-like-illnesses (ILI) (see below). The ILI screening tool is routinely utilized in acute care facilities in Ontario, urgent care clinics and emergency rooms, and provides a standardized and consistent tool for the early detection of respiratory ailments by healthcare professionals (e.g., physicians, nurses) such as SARS and influenza. This screening tool also provides a provincial-wide standard in terms of initiating standardized clinical assessments and control measures to help decrease the risk of transmission in public healthcare settings. The ILI screening tool can also be employed to help detect outbreak clusters and any new or virulent strains of microorganism-associated respiratory infections (MOHLTC 2009).

Web-Based Resource Box 7.1

Learning Resources	Website
Public Health Agency of Canada: West Nile Virus Monitor (2013) This website provides updates surveillance information and maps related to the West Nile virus in Canada	http://www.phac-aspc.gc.ca/wnv-vwn/
Public Health Agency of Canada (PHAC 2009). West Nile Virus-Protect Yourself! This website provides the general public with helpful information and tips on how they can protect themselves against the West Nile virus.	http://www.phac-aspc.gc.ca/wn-no/ index-eng.php
World Health Organization (July, 2011). West Nile Virus. Fact sheet No. 354 This website provides a fact sheet related to the West Nile virus and its current global health impact.	http://www.who.int/mediacentre/ factsheets/fs354/en/

Screening Tool for Influenza-Like Illness (ILI) in Healthcare Settings
1. Do you have new/worse cough or shortness of breath?   If "no," no further action is required. If "yes," ask patient to follow directions and continue with next question.   If the answer is "yes," patient should perform hand hygiene using alcohol-based hand rub and put on a mask covering their nose and mouth.   2. Are you feeling feverish,* or have you had shakes or chills in the last 24 hours?   If "no," no further questions. If "yes," nurse to take temperature as part of clinical assessment.

Note: Some people, such as the elderly and people who are immuno-compromised, may not develop fever.

If the answer is "yes," move patient to a separate area if possible.

Source: Ontario Ministry of Health and Long-Term Care (2009).

It is critical that public health professionals and workers remain current and updated regarding health surveillance and reporting practices in their province or territory. The *Canadian Network for Public Health Intelligence* (CNPHI) is a secure web-based collective of applications designed to facilitate national, integrated, real-time collection and processing of laboratory and epidemiological surveillance data, dissemination of strategic intelligence, and coordination of public health responses (PHAC 2013b). The CNPHI leverages the integration of disparate public health information resources and expertise for the direct benefit of local, regional, and national decision makers and authorities. The CNPHI is certainly scalable in nature and application, and therefore has the potential to expand beyond the biological community (see http://www.ncceh.ca/ sites/default/files/Surveillance_Workshop_Feb_2013-Beattie.pdf).

The *Integrated Public Health Information System* (iPHIS) is an electronic computer-based system of reporting that was developed by the Public Health Agency of Canada (2007a). The iPHIS allows various public health agencies and health jurisdictions within a province or territory to communicate disease patterns in an efficient and standardized way, and may also be employed as a mechanism for contacting other healthcare agencies (see http://www.phac-aspc.gc.ca/php-psp/surveillance-eng.php). Similarly, the *Canadian Integrated Outbreak Surveillance Centre* (CIOSC 2009) is an electronic computer-based system developed for public healthcare professionals and workers by Health Canada to communicate outbreak information related specifically to enteric or respiratory illness inter-provincially/territorially in Canada. CIOSC permits public healthcare professionals and authorities to make critical links in terms of person, place, and time data for infected individuals with similar clinical signs and symptoms across Canada. The reader is referred to the Web-Based Resource Box 7.2 for additional information related to CNPHI, iPHIS, CIOSC and surveillance for public health activities in Canada.

Web-Based Resource Box 7.2 CNPHI, iPHIS, CIOSC, and Public Health Surveillance

Learning Resource	Website
Canadian Integrated Outbreak Surveillance Centre (CIOSC 2013) (Health Canada) This website provides detailed information related to what CIOSC is, how it provides tracking and surveillance data related to various diseases and outbreaks, security surveillance and how public health alerts are issued.	http://www.acronymfinder.com/Canadian-Integrated-Outbreak-Surveillance-Centre-(internet_based-alerting-system)-(CIOSC).html
Canadian Integrated Public Health Surveillance (CIPHS 2007b) (Public Health Agency of Canada) This database is used to report and track human cases of reportable diseases to public health authorities and public health units and to the PHAC.	http://www.phac-aspc.gc.ca/php-psp/ciphs-eng.php#wiphis.
Canadian Network for Public Health Intelligence (CNPHI) Describes the web-based collection of applications and resources by the CNPHI designed to fill critical gaps in Canada's public health info-structure.	http://www.viu.ca/cch/aded/documents/CNPHIFeb2005.pdf

Passive Surveillance

Passive surveillance is defined as the notification of health authorities by public health professionals of individuals who have clinical signs and symptoms, and this relies on laboratory tests for confirmation of the diagnosis of the disease on the notifiable/reportable disease list for their respective province or territory in Canada (Bartfay and Bartfay 2015). The health report must be comprehensive in nature and include all the relevant demographic (e.g., age, sex, address, occupation), clinical information (e.g., presenting signs and symptoms, date of onset, travel history, sexual history), and prescribed treatment interventions. Collecting and communicating information by public healthcare professionals and workers is essential for health surveillance and for providing safe and effective public primary health services and programs. Indeed, the ability to effectively engage in health surveillance is a critical and ongoing component of public health in Canada. The list of over 50 diseases (see Table 7.7) that are currently under national surveillance is detailed below in the section entitled *Reportable/Notifiable Disease List* (see http://www.phac-aspc.gc.ca/surveillance-eng.php).

Contact tracing is the process of identifying relevant contacts of a person with an infectious disease and ensuring that they are aware of their exposure, and occurs in response to a communicable disease report made to a local health authority (Bartfay and Bartfay 2015). This process consists of interviewing the infected individual regarding their social, work or professional contacts of people they may have come into contact with during the known incubation period of the disease. Public healthcare professionals and workers gather a list of contacts from the first identified case and contact these individuals when deemed necessary based on the mode of transmission, incubation period, and infectious period of the particular communicable disease in order to determine what public health interventions are most appropriate for each case. Although contract tracing appears to be an infringement of the individual's right to privacy on the surface, it is critical to contain the spread of disease in populations (Bartfay and Bartfay 2015). It is also critical for ensuring public safety while providing ethically competent care by public health professionals and workers.

For example, during the SARS outbreak that occurred in Toronto, Ontario in 2003, quarantine acts of both the Ontario and federal Ministries of Health legislated and mandated public health professionals and authorized them to conduct contact tracing by naming those with SARS in the public media. The public health objective was to protect all individuals in the general public forum as well as to notify the contacts of first infected individuals and encourage them to self-identify and promptly come forward for health screening and clinical assessments. In fact, 44 individuals in Ontario died and 375 fell ill over a period of only 5 months (Campbell 2006; Health Canada n.d.; Naylor 2003). Infected clients and healthcare professionals (e.g., critical care nurses) with SARS or suspected carriers were quarantined. In addition, the WHO issued travel warnings to Toronto, Ontario, and cross-border travel to the United States was restricted to prevent the spread of SARS.

The SARS event in Toronto, Ontario, and how health public health professionals and workers did case findings and its associated health and social–political impacts is realistically depicted in a Canadian film entitled *Plague City: SARS in Toronto* (Anchor Bay Entertainment Inc. 2005). The reader is encouraged to view this film which realistically depicts how public healthcare professionals (e.g., physicians, clinical and public health nurses, epidemiologists, clinical microbiologists) and workers, various healthcare agencies and ministries of health worked cooperatively to deal with the SARS pandemic in Canada.

The reports of the National Advisory Committee on SARS and Public Health (Naylor 2003), the SARS Commission Reports in Ontario (Campbell 2004, 2005, 2006), and the Expert Panel on SARS and Infectious Disease Control (Walker 2004) all underscored the critical importance of public health in preventing the spread of disease in Canada. In response to the SARS pandemic and other public health concerns, the Public Health Agency of Canada was established in September, 2004, to further help coordinate and strengthen public health efforts in Canada. Subsequently, the Public Health Agency of Canada was given Royal Accent by Parliament in December, 2006, which formally recognized the agency and the Chief Public Health Officer (CPHO) (Public Health Agency of Canada 2006a). This Royal Accent by Parliament empowers the Public Health Agency of Canada and the CPHO to introduce legislation in the interest of public health and safety. The Public Health Agency of Canada also serves as a hub to gather and disseminate health-related information to public health professionals, government agencies, and institutions. Moreover, a variety of agencies, laboratories, and branches now directly report to the CPHO of the Public Health Agency of Canada. These public institutions and agencies include The Centre for Emergency Preparedness and Response (CEPR), Infectious Disease and Emergency Preparedness (IDEP), Laboratory for Foodborne Zoonoses, Office of Public Health Safety, National Microbiology Laboratory, and Pandemic Preparedness Secretariat (Public Health Agency of Canada 2006a). The Public Health Agency of Canada also collaborates closely and shares health-related information, findings and expertise with various international health agencies including the United States Centers for Disease Control and Prevention (CDC), European Centre for Disease Prevention and Control, and the WHO. It is critical to note that the list of contacts with the infected individual is only as accurate and reliable as the person relaying the information and the parameters required for reporting. For example, if the physician or nurse is not aware of the clinical signs and symptoms of the disease that requires reporting or the need for health surveillance, reporting and contract tracing will not be achieved or delayed.

The *basic Ro (transmissibility index or reproductive number)* of an infectious disease agent gives an indication of the transmissibility of the known agent, and can also be employed to estimate the vaccine coverage (if available) in an otherwise susceptible population to prevent person-to-person spread in a community or geographical area (Bartfay and Bartfay 2015). Table 7.5 shows the transmissibility indexes (basic Ro's) for select respiratory pathogens. For example, among the respiratory pathogens with higher transmissibility rates are measles, pertussis, mumps, and influenza, whereas the SARS coronavirus has relatively low case reproduction numbers (Dye and Gay 2003; Ena 2008; Garner 1996).

Table 7.6 shows a partial list of the incubation periods of select major communicable diseases. The *incubation period* is defined as the time that elapses between inoculation and infection by a pathogen in the host and the appearance of the first clinical signs or symptoms of the disease (Bartfay and Bartfay 2015). Incubation periods may vary between individuals with active immune systems that retard the growth of the pathogen, thus lengthening the incubation period. Conversely, those who are immune-compromised (e.g., HIV/AIDS, transplant patients) have chronic diseases (e.g., diabetes), are highly stressed, and/ or malnourished, for example, may have shorter incubation periods. In general, diseases with short incubation periods tend to produce more acute, intense, and severe illness, whereas those with long incubation periods are usually less severe in nature.

Therefore, contract tracing of potentially infected individuals is based on the possibility of transmission, and the window of risk will vary in accordance with the specific disease under investigation by the public

Table 7.5 Transmissibility Indexes (Basic Ro's) for Selected Respiratory Pathogens

Respiratory Pathogens	Basic Ro
Diphtheria	5–6
Influenza	1.68–20
Measles	15–17
Mumps	10–12
Pertussis	15–17
Rubella	7–8
SARS	2–3

Table 7.6 Incubation List of Select Communicable Diseases

Communicable Disease	Incubation Period	Communicability Period
Chickenpox	12–36 hours	From 5 days before the appearance of vesicles on the skin to 6 days after
Common cold	Typically 24 hours, but up to 72 hours	24 hours before the onset to 5 days after
Conjunctivitis (pink eye)	24–72 hours	For the entire duration of the infection, while still present and active
Diphtheria	48 hours to 5 days	Usually <2 weeks, but not more than 4 weeks total
Epstein-Barr virus	4–7 weeks	During the entire presence of clinical symptoms
Gonorrhea	48 hours to 5 days or more	Indefinite in nature unless clinically treated
Herpes simplex virus (e.g., common cold sores on lip)	Up to 2 weeks	As long as 7 weeks post disappearance of symptoms
Influenza	24–72 hours	Often 72 hours from clinical onset of signs and symptoms
Mumps	12–26 days, but usually around 18 days	From 6 days before the onset of signs and symptoms to 9 days after
Pediculosis (head lice)	Usually 2 weeks	As long as lice remain active and alive and continue to lay eggs
Rabies	2–8 weeks or longer	72 hours to 5 days before clinical signs and symptoms and during the course of the disease

(Continued)

Table 7.6 Incubation List of Select Communicable Diseases (*Continued*)

Communicable Disease	Incubation Period	Communicability Period
Ringworm	4–10 days	As long as lesions are present on the skin
Rubella (German measles)	8–10 days (usually 2 weeks)	1 week before and up to 4 days after the onset of a rash on the skin
Salmonella (food poisoning)	6–72 hours (usually 36 hours)	A wide variation from 72 hours to 3 weeks in duration
Scarlet fever	24–72 hours	24–72 hours if clinically treated, and 10–21 days if not treated
Smallpox	7–17 days (usually between 10 and 12 days)	Usually within 7–10 days of onset of skin rash
Syphilis	10 days to 10 weeks (usually 3 weeks)	Indefinite and variable in nature if not clinically treated
Tuberculosis	4–12 weeks (for primary stage of the disease)	Indefinite, as long as the *tubercle bacilli* are being discharged (e.g., via coughing) by the patient
Typhoid fever	1–3 weeks (usually 2 weeks)	Indefinite, as long as the *typhoid bacilli* appear in the feces of the patient
Whooping cough	7–21 days (usually 10 days)	Usually from 7 days post exposure to 3 weeks after onset of typical clinical paroxysms

health professional or worker. For example, when a public health nurse or physician investigates a case of rubella (German measles), they would list all individuals who were in contact with the infectious individual seven days prior to the onset of a rash. Conversely, while contract tracing for TB, the public health nurse or physician may identify recent contacts and those as far back as 12 weeks ago.

Reportable/Notifiable Disease Lists

In Canada, the list of communicable diseases which require notification at the federal level is agreed upon through a consensus of the provincial/ territorial and federal health agencies, experts, and authorities. The terms "reportable" and "notifiable" diseases are commonly used interchangeable by public health professionals and agencies. National and provincial/territorial legislation decree which diseases will be reported and which public health agency is responsible for reporting them. The list of reportable diseases is mandated by provincial/territorial legislation and therefore may differ slightly, but is based on the recommendations of the Public Health Agency of Canada (PHAC 2010, 2009). Hence, local public health personnel are mandated by their provinces and territories to report all notifiable diseases (e.g., hepatitis A, B or C, HIV/AIDS, TB, Lyme disease) to their respective ministries of health, and some diseases are also required to be reported to federal health authorities. How communicable diseases are tracked and reported varies according to each provincial or territorial health authority. For example, the Regional Infection Control Network (RICN 2010) for the province of Ontario consists of 14 regions served: (a) Erie St. Clair, (b) South Western Ontario,

(c) Waterloo Wellington, (d) Central South, (e) Central West, (f) Mississauga Halton, (g) Toronto Central, (h) Central Region, (i) Central East, (j) South Eastern Ontario, (k) Champlain, (l) North Simcoe Muskoka, (m) Northeastern Ontario, and (n) Northwestern Ontario. These boundaries are aligned with the Local Health Integration Networks. This network does not duplicate the work of public health professionals and workers, but serves as their partner and resource network across the province to develop the best evidence-informed practice standards for the management of communicable diseases in the province of Ontario (RICN 2010). The mandate of the RICN is to maximize the coordination and integration of activities related to the prevention, control and surveillance of infectious diseases in the province of Ontario across the healthcare spectrum on a regional basis.

This network does not duplicate the work of public health professionals and workers, but serves as their partner and resource network across the province to develop the best evidence-informed practice standards for the management of communicable diseases in the province of Ontario (RICN 2010).

Prior to 2009, Ontario's hospitals and healthcare institutions lacked a uniform surveillance system for the consistent tracking and reporting of significant organisms. The RICNs took on this challenge in 2009 by creating and implementing a uniform and standardized monitoring and surveillance electronic database tool for organisms of interests known as the *Infection Prevention and Control Surveillance and Education Tracking* (IPACSET), which is based on the Microsoft Access® platform. RICN (2010) reports that effective communication results in the successful gathering and circulation of information. The power of the RICNs is in the sharing of knowledge, expertise, and research with healthcare professionals, community leaders, and public health authorities. Through various communication strategies, RICNs ensure that critical information is in the hands of those who need it, when they need it (RICN 2010).

Currently, there are 52 notifiable diseases under national surveillance through a coordinated effort with federal, provincial, and territorial governments (PHAC 2013e, 2010; see http://www.phac-aspc.gc.ca/aids-sida/about/dis-eng.php). Table 7.7 provides a list of these notifiable/reportable diseases in Canada, which are constantly being monitored and updated. For example, Lyme disease became a nationally notifiable/reportable disease in Canada in 2010 (PHAC 2010c, 2013). This list helps to ensure uniformity among provincial/territorial and federal public health surveillance sources, and also helps to ensure conformity with international reporting and tracking efforts by public healthcare professionals and workers (PHAC 2009c, 2010, 2013e). In addition, certain communicable diseases are also tracked globally and reported to the *International Health Regulations* (IHR) Branch of the WHO (2010a, 2010b). The WHO routinely revises and updates the IHR to address the threat of new, emerging, or re-emerging infectious diseases and to accommodate new reporting sources. A growing number of diseases under surveillance (e.g., AIDS/HIV, H5N1) are also required to be reported at specified frequencies, depending on the disease and the geographic region of the world where it has occurred.

Heymann (2008) reports that although communicable diseases kill an estimated 14 million people annually in developing nations, at present the only three communicable diseases that require international notification, namely the plague, yellow fever, and cholera. However, a growing number of communicable diseases, such as Avian flu, influenza, and HIV/AIDS, are monitored and considered as diseases under surveillance and are actively tracked by the IHR Branch of WHO. Public health professionals and workers must be proactive in their efforts to be knowledgeable about various types of communicable and non-communicable diseases that threaten their communities in order to play a role in their effective surveillance, diagnosis, management, and prevention. In addition, they play a vital role in disease surveillance by investigating sources of disease outbreaks, collecting data regarding their nature, reporting cases found, and providing information to the public about primary healthcare interventions, disease morbidity and mortality within their geographical regions or communities of practice.

Non-reportable/Notifiable Diseases

Certain communicable diseases are regarded as non-reportable or non-notifiable in nature in Canada. These are typically regarded as communicable diseases that are common in populations and the public burden of the disease to the community is not considered large or great in nature per se. Examples include the common cold,

Table 7.7 Notifiable/Reportable Diseases Under National Surveillance in Canada

1. Acquired Immunodeficiency Syndrome (AIDS)
2. Acute Flaccid Paralysis
3. Anthrax
4. Botulism
5. Brucellosis
6. Campylobacteriosis
7. Chlamydia
8. Cholera
9. *Clostridium difficile* Associated Diarrhea Congenital Rubella Syndrome (CRS)
10. Creutzfeldt-Jakob Disease (CJD), Classic and New Variant
11. Cryptosporidiosis
12. Cyclosporiasis
13. Diphtheria
14. Giardiasis
15. Gonorrhea
16. Group B Streptococcal Disease of the Newborn
17. Hantavirus Pulmonary Syndrome (HPS)
18. Hepatitis A
19. Hepatitis B
20. Hepatitis C
21. Human Immunodeficiency Virus (HIV)
22. Influenza, laboratory-confirmed
23. Invasive *Haemophilus influenzae* type b (Hib) and non-b Disease Invasive Group A Streptococcal Disease
24. Invasive Listeriosis
25. Invasive Meningococcal Disease
26. Invasive Pneumococcal Disease
27. Legionellosis
28. Leprosy (Hansen's Disease)
29. Lyme Disease
30. Malaria
31. Measles
32. Mumps
33. Norovirus infection
34. Paralytic Shellfish Poisoning
35. Pertussis
36. Plague
37. Poliomyelitis
38. Rabies
39. Rubella
40. Salmonellosis
41. Severe Acute Respiratory Syndrome (SARS)
42. Shigellosis
43. Smallpox
44. Syphilis
45. Tetanus
46. Tuberculosis
47. Tularemia
48. Typhoid
49. Varicella (Chickenpox)
50. Verotoxigenic *Escherichia coli* Infection Viral Hemorrhagic Fevers
51. West Nile virus Infection
52. Yellow Fever

Source: Adapted from *Archived-National Notifiable Diseases* (Public Health Agency of Canada [PHAC] 2010). Ottawa, ON: Author. Accessed July 2, 2014. http://www.phac-aspc.gc.ca/bid-bmi/dsd-dsm/duns-eng.php.

bed bug infestations, conjunctivitis (pink-eye), pediculosis, and scabies. The role of public health professionals and workers in reference to these non-reportable communicable diseases is typically supportive and educational in nature. For example, public health nurses may be called upon to provide educational sessions and materials (e.g., brochures, website information) related to a recent outbreak of conjunctivitis (or pink-eye) to teachers, daycare staff, parents and guardians regarding its transmission, prevention and management.

Poisonings

Poisoning is a much larger public health issue than is generally recognized and there is currently no comprehensive poison prevention or control system in place nationally (Safe Kids Canada and Alberta Centre for Injury Control 2011). For example, in 2005 alone the Ontario Poison Centre (2007) reported that they responded to 46,047 actual poison exposures and 6139 poison information calls, and that 62% of all poisonings were managed at the site of the poisoning in the community, thus preventing costly emergency room visits located in acute care hospitals. In order to provide some cohesiveness and sense of "system" to a fragmented group of poison centres dispersed across the country, a voluntary association, the *Canadian Association of Poison Control Centres* (CAPCC) was formed at a meeting of Medical Directors in Toronto in 1982. The CAPCC provides a centralized forum for communication, information, and idea exchange among Canadian poison centres. While its members are primarily professionals (e.g., nurses and medical consultants) working in poison control centres, other members have included pharmacists, pharmaceutical companies, forensic toxicologists, and public health staff.

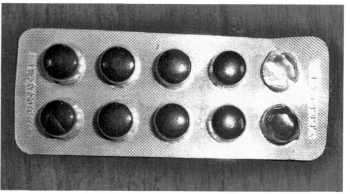

Source: Photo by Wally J. Bartfay

Photo 7.19 Activated Charcole Tables for Poisoning. Clients may be given activated charcoal to manage an acute poisoning event or overdose. When used along with other treatments, activated charcoal may be effective for an acute poisoning. But it is not useful in some cases, including poisoning from cyanide, lithium, alcohol and iron tablets, for examples. If you are in a rural or remote area and do not have access to activated charcoal, burnt toast may be given to the client while awaiting medical assistance.

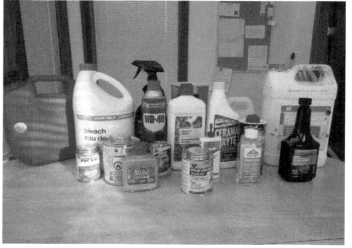

Source: Wally J. Bartfay

Photo 7.20 There are a variety of common household items that are poisonous to humans and pets. For Canadians of all ages, poisoning is the fourth leading cause of injury-associated deaths and permanent total disability; and the fifth leading cause of injury-associated hospitalizations, non-hospitalizations and permanent partial disabilities with an associated cost of $19.8 billion annually (Smartrisk 2009).

Poisoning was initially viewed as a problem of young children but now it is a concern across the entire lifespan. It is estimated that half of all *poison exposures* occur among children less than 5 years of age; however, only about 10% of the more severe poisonings occur among young children. More than two-thirds of severe poisonings happen to adults over 19 years (Safe Kids Canada and Alberta Centre for Injury Control 2011). Although a discussion on all forms of poisoning are beyond the scope and purpose of this chapter, we shall concentrate on the following two salient areas that are of growing concern to the health and safety of Canadians: (a) pesticide poisoning and (b) food safety and poisoning.

Poisonous Plants

There are a variety of poisonous plants which can be toxic to humans and other animals, which are generally caused by a variety of toxic chemical compounds that are produced by the plants themselves and/or absorbed from the soil (Canadian Biodiversity Information Facility 2013; Ministry of Agriculture, Food and Rural Affairs Ontario 2015; Scheider and Pautler 2010). For example, certain species of plants can absorb minerals such as selenium, lead, copper, molybdenum, and nitrates or nitrites for their surrounding environment in sufficient quantities to cause poisoning when ingested by gazing animals. These toxic reactions can range from mild discomfort and

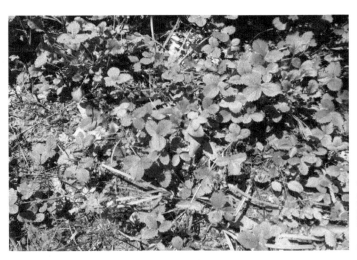

Source: Wally J. Bartfay

Photo 7.21 The allergen responsible in poison ivy (*Rhus radicans*) is urushiol, which is an oily mixture found in the sap throughout the plant that can stick to exposed skin, clothing, footwear, garden tools and even pet fur resulting in contact dermatitis. Remember the old adage for poison ivy: Leaves of three let them be.

localized swelling to organ damage, failure, and even death. Such poisons may be assimilated by being ingested, inhaled, or absorbed through the skin. The type of toxins include: (a) alkaloids, which are bitter tasting, that occur in the form of soluble organic acid salts, (b) polypeptides and amines, which or organic compounds containing nitrogen, (c) glycosides which are compounds that breakdown to form sugars and toxic aglycones, (d) oxalates, which occur as either soluble or insoluble salts, (e) calcium salts which are deposited in the kidneys, (f) resins or resinoids which can irritate muscle tissue, and (g) phytotoxins or toxalbumins which break down natural proteins resulting in the bioaccumulation of ammonia and protein deficiency.

A variety of poisonous plants in Canada have been identified (Canadian Biodiversity Information Facility 2013; Ministry of Agriculture, Food and Rural Affairs Ontario 2015; Scheider and Pautler 2010). Examples include bloodroot (*Sanguinaria canadensis*), climbing or bittersweet nightshade (*Solanum dulcamara*), may apple (*Popophyllum peltatum*), poison ivy (*Rhus radicans*), white baneberry (*Actaea pachypoda*), Jack-in-the-pulpit (*Arisaema triphyllum*), water-hemlock (*Cicuta maculata*), and white snakeroot (*Eupatorium rugosum*). For example, poison ivy is a common creeping plant that can cause mild skin irritation, itchiness, contact dermatitis, redness, and swelling to oozing painful blisters and high fevers resulting from contact with the plant. This plant is found throughout southern Canada except for the province of Newfoundland. This glossy perennial spreads easily in a variety of environments (e.g., sandy, stony, rocky shores, thickets, roadsides) by seed or by producing shoots from its extensive underground stems. Most individuals who come into contact with poison ivy develop symptoms within 24–48 hours post-contact. The inflamed areas often develop into blisters, which results in intense itchiness, swelling, and redness of areas exposed to the sap. Hence, a person has to come into contact with the sap as opposed to the plant per se. Moreover, if poison ivy is burned and the smoke in inhaled by an individual, a rash may also appear on the lining of the lungs resulting in extreme pain and possibly fatal breathing difficulties. Individuals are advised to wash all potential areas of their skin with cold water and soap. Cold water is advised because hot water may promote the opening of pores, which increases the chances that the resin may enter more deeply into the skin. Symptoms typically disappears 7–15 days after contact with the sap.

Pesticide Poisoning

Pesticides include various biochemical classes of agents and substances that are employed for killing or destroying insects or other organism harmful to plant species or animals and include insecticides, herbicides, fungicides, rodenticides, algaecides, and slimicides (Bartfay and Bartfay 2015). Experts generally agree that reducing exposure to pesticides reduces health risks (Bassil et al. 2007; Boyd 2007; Jerschow et al. 2012). There are approximately 1000 commercial pesticide products for sale in Canada that cannot be sold in other nations because of health and environmental concerns. All levels of government in Canada share the responsibility for protecting Canadians and the environment from the risks posed by pesticides. The federal government, pursuant to the *Pest Control Products Act* (see http://laws-lois.justice.gc.ca/eng/acts/P-9.01/), decides which pesticides are approved for use in Canada (Government of Canada 2013). Under the *Food and Drug Act* (see http://www.hc-sc.gc.ca/fn-an/legislation/acts-lois/act-loi_reg-eng.php), the federal government sets limits on the amount of pesticide residues that can remain on food sold in Canada, and conducts monitoring in an effort to ensure that these limits are not exceeded (Health Canada 2007). Canada passed a new and improved *Pest Control Products Act* (*PCPA*) in 2002. However, the new law did not come into force until June 2006.

In 2007, the first comprehensive national survey related to pesticide associated poisoning was released in a report entitled *Northern Exposure: Acute Pesticide Poisoning in Canada* by the David Suzuki Foundation (Boyd 2007). The survey found that more than 6000 individuals, including 2832 cases that were children less than 6 years of age, suffer from acute pesticide poisoning each year. The report tracked only victims with acute pesticide poisoning that resulted in immediate effects such as blistering of the skin, respiratory distress and breathing problems, heart palpitations, nausea, and vomiting (Boyd 2007). The chronic health effects of exposure to these agents were not assessed in this report (e.g., birth defects, organ dysfunction and damage, increased risk of certain cancers, neurological diseases such as Parkinson's disease). Québec had the highest number of reported pesticide poisonings with 2096 cases, followed by Ontario with 1,629, and Alberta with 1021 cases. The national average was 18 cases per 100,000. Moreover, the prairie provinces of Saskatchewan and Alberta which have a large number of farmers had the highest per-capita incidence rates of 33 per 100,000 and 30 per 100,000, respectively (Boyd 2007). The reader is referred to Chapter 8 for a detailed discussion on the science of toxicology, and various environmental hazards and poisons (e.g., DDT, mercury, lead, nuclear waste products, bisphenol A).

Food Safety and Poisonings

Food safety is a concern shared by consumers, industry and governments at all levels in Canada. Health Canada (2012) recognizes that a safe food supply is a major contributing factor to the health of Canadians across the lifespan. The *Canadian Food Inspection Agency* (CFIA) is responsible for enforcing the food safety legislations, policies, and standards that Health Canada sets. There are currently over 7200 employees with the CFIA (2013) who are stationed in field offices, laboratories, and food processing facilities across Canada. The CFIA also delivers inspection and quarantine programs related to foods, plants, and animals in 18 regions and 160 field offices across Canada. Products that may be subject to inspection certification by the CFIA range from agricultural inputs (e.g., seeds, feeds, and fertilizers), to fresh foods (e.g., meat, fish, eggs, grains, dairy products, fruit, and vegetables), and prepared and packaged foods (e.g., frozen dinners). The *Canadian Food Inspection Agency Act* was created in 1997 by Health Canada and requires that this agency report to the Minister of Agriculture and Agri-Food. The CFIA mandate is to verify industry compliance with federal acts and regulations through activities that include the registration and inspection of abattoirs and food processing plants, and the testing of food related products. The CFIA (2013)

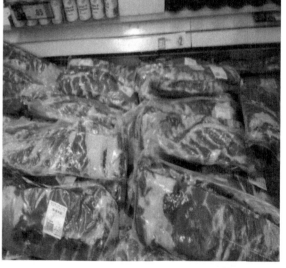

Source: Wally J. Bartfay

Photo 7.22 An example of a food item (i.e., meat) requiring refrigeration improperly stored above the so-called "safe load lines" which are clearly marked on all refrigerator units in grocery stores in Canada. Food safety is a concern shared by consumers, industry and governments at all levels in Canada. Public health inspectors help to monitor and enforce legislations to help protect against food poisoning in community settings.

encourages the food industry to adopt science-based risk management practices to minimize food safety risks.

Food-borne outbreaks are recognized when illness presents among individuals in a defined group or community who have consumed a common food source. This usually occurs within a variable but short time frame (i.e., a few hours) after consuming the contaminated food source with typical presenting clinical signs and symptoms (e.g., nausea, vomiting, abdominal cramps, diarrhea, fever, headache). Foodborne outbreaks are recognized when illness presents among individuals who have consumed contaminated food items or manufactured products (Piemann and Cliver 2006; WHO 2009c). For example, a community-wide foodborne outbreak of *E. coli* 0157:H7 was reported in the North Bay and Parry Sound District of Ontario for the time period of October to November, 2008 (North Bay Parry Sound District Health Unit 2009). During this outbreak, public health officials reported that 350 individuals became ill who all consumed contaminated food from a single restaurant, and 50 individuals had laboratory-confirmed disease. If a food safety emergency does occur (e.g., *E. coli* or *listeria* outbreak in meat products), the CFIA, in partnership with Health Canada, provincial agencies and the food industry, operates an emergency response system. The CFIA collaborates closely with public health author-

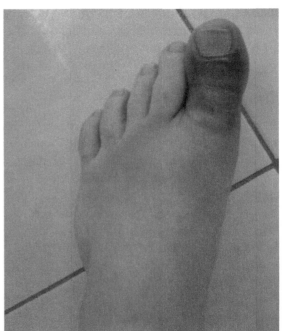

Source: Wally J. Bartfay

Photo 7.23 A badly bruised toe resulting from a construction-related injury. Safety equipment such as mandatory steel-toed boots, hard hats, safety glasses, and filtered breathing masks has significantly helped to decrease work-related injuries and disabilities in Canada.

ities at the federal, provincial, and municipal levels to monitor and analyze food-related outbreaks and potential hazards in the food supply. Based on health-risk assessments, the CFIA works with stakeholder partners such as industry associations and consumer protection groups to implement food safety measures that protect Canadians. The CFIA (2013) relies on the cooperation of stakeholders (i.e., producers, processors, distributors, and retailers) when public health actions such as disease control quarantines and food recalls become necessary. In cases where the product poses a serious health risk to Canadians, the CFIA will issue formal public health warnings via the mass and social medias. Canadians and public health professionals and workers can sign-up for the CFIA's *Allergy Alerts and Food Recalls* via an e-mail subscription service (see www.inspection.gc.ca).

In fact, food safety and contaminated food sources reported in the mass and social medias are a growing public health concern for Canadians. The CFIA manages approximately 350 food recalls each year in Canada, of which a third are related to undeclared ingredients that may cause severe allergic reactions (e.g., peanut products, soy products, eggs), and the remainder may pose a significant health risk to consumers (CFIA 2013). For example, on August 20, 2008, Maple Leaf Foods stopped production at its Toronto deli meat processing plant due to a national outbreak of *listerosis*, which resulted in several documented cases of associated illness and sickness and 20 deaths (Bouzane and Wylie 2000; Canadian Food Inspection Agency 2008). This outbreak resulted in the recall of 191 meat products sold across Canada over fears that they may be tainted and caused food poisoning by the CFIA and public health authorities. The outbreak was traced back to two contaminated deli-meat slicing machines with the gram-positive bacterium *Listeria monocytogens*.

This bacterium is widespread in the environment and may be present in soil, water, sewage, silage, and in the feces of humans and animals. *Listeria* is more likely to cause death than other bacteria that causes food poisoning, and it is estimated that up to 30% of infections occur in high-risk individuals (i.e., individuals with compromised immune systems such as HIV/AIDS and transplant clients, pregnant women and their fetuses, elderly) may be fatal (Canadian Food Inspection Agency 2008; Ramaswamy and Cresence 2007). The Canadian Food Inspection Agency has also issued public health warnings for possible contamination of mushrooms with the *listeria* bacterium from Ravine Mushroom Farms Inc., in Woodbridge, Ontario, and cheese from Ivanhoe Cheese Inc., based in Madoc, Ontario, in September, 2008 (Bouzane and Wylie 2008). These events described above highlight the critical need to strengthen and cultivate our public healthcare initiatives, agencies and systems of delivery in Canada (Advisory Committee on Population Health 2001; Joint Task Group on Public Health and Human Resources 2006).

Injuries and Disabilities

An *injury* is defined as an act, either intentional or unintentional, in nature that results in a wound, damage, and/or trauma to an individual (Bartfay and Bartfay 2015). According to findings from the *Canadian Community Health Survey* (CCHS), 4.27 million (15%) Canadians aged 12 years or older suffered an injury severe enough to limit their usual activities in 2009–2010, which represents an increase from 13% compared to 2001 results (Billette and Janz 2013).

Falls were a leading cause of injury and accounted for 63% of injuries in seniors; approximately 50% in adolescents and 35% in working age adults. Over half (55%) of injuries in seniors occurred while walking or doing household chores. Two out of three (66%) injuries among adolescents were linked to sports (e.g., hockey, skate-boarding, skiing, cycling). Among working adults aged 20–64 years, work and sports were associated with almost half (47%) of all injuries in this age group (Billette and Janz 2013). Similarly, the PHAC (2013c) reports that sports and recreation-related injuries make up a significant proportion of unintentional injuries among children and youth up to the age of 19 years, and account for approximately 40% of injuries treated in acute care hospitals with emergency departments.

According to the CCHS, an estimated 630,000 Canadian workers experienced at least one activity-limiting occupational injury based on cross-sectional estimates of the proportion of workers injured on the job by occupational category, and select work-related and socio-demographic characteristics (Wilkins and Mackenzie 2008). Nine percent of workers in trades (e.g., carpenter, plumber, carpenter, welder), transport (e.g., trucking, railway), and heavy equipment operators (e.g., bulldozers, diggers) in Canada sustained an on-the-job injury, compared with only 2% of workers in the "white-collar" sector (e.g., office workers, bankers, teachers) (Human Resources and Skills Development Canada 2013). In addition, men experienced a higher rate of injury (18.8 cases per 1000 employed men), compared to women (11.2 cases per 1000 employed females).

Mining remains one of the most dangerous jobs accounting for approximately 12,000 preventable deaths globally each year (Shaw Media 2011). For example, between the years 2006 and 2009, 80 miners died in Canada's mining, quarrying, and petroleum industries, compared to 34 deaths in the United States and a staggering 2631 deaths in China (Shaw Media 2011). In Ontario alone, there are over 38 mines in operation that generates approximately $22 million dollars annually toward our GDP (Ontario Ministry of Labour 2014).

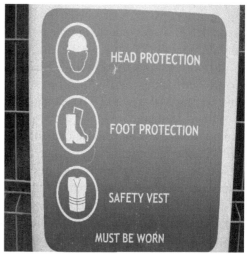

Source: Wally J. Bartfay

Photo 7.24 A safety warning notice on a construction site indicating which safety equipment must be worn by workers to minimize their chances of injury, disability or death.

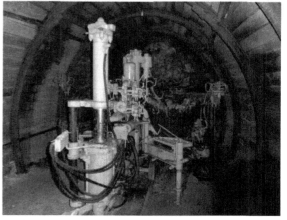

Source: Wally J. Bartfay

Photo 7.25 Heavy drilling equipment in an underground silver mine shaft. Mining remains one of the most dangerous occupations in Canada and abroad.

Each mine creates approximately 300 direct jobs and 2200 indirect jobs. Over the past 10 years, 337 critical injuries, 24 fatalities, and 193 occupational diseases resulting in fatality claims have been reported to the Ministry of Labour (Ontario Ministry of Labour 2014).

A *disability* is defined as any degree of physical infirmity, impairment, malformation, or disfigurement that is caused by a bodily injury, birth defect, illness, or disease that may be physical, cognitive, mental, sensory, emotional, developmental, or some combination of these (Bartfay and Bartfay 2015). Approximately 4.4 million (14.3%) of residents in Canada reported having a disability in the year 2006, and the percentage of individuals with disabilities increased with age ranging from 3.7% in children 14 years and younger to 56.3% in individuals 75 years or older (Human Resources and Skills Development Canada 2007, 2010; Statistics Canada 2007). The percentage of individuals with disabilities was lowest in Nunavut (6.4%) and highest in Nova Scotia (20%), which a national average of 14.3% reported (Human Resources and Skills Development Canada 2007; Statistics Canada 2007). A greater proportion of females (15.2%) reported having a disability, in comparison to 13.4% in males. There were 202,350 children (or 3.7%) between the ages of 0 and 14 years with a disability, and a greater proportion of boys (4.6%) were found to have a disability, in comparison to girls (2.7%). Among school-aged children (5–14 years) in Canada, learning disabilities were reported to be the most common disability for boys (72.7%), whereas chronic health conditions were the most common type for girls (65%). For adults aged 15 years or older, lack of mobility (11.5%), pain (11.7%), and reduced agility (11.1%) were the three most common types of disabilities reported (Human Resources and Skills Development Canada 2007; Statistics Canada 2007).

Individuals with disabilities are more likely to have lower incomes, live in substandard housing, live alone, and have considerably more difficulty in finding employment and gaining skills (Human Resources and Skills Development Canada 2010; Mikkonen and Raphael 2010). More than 40% of Canadians with disabilities are unemployed, and many are dependent on social assistance. For those who are employed, they earn approximately 22.5% less on average than adults without disabilities (Human Resources and Skills Development Canada 2010).

The WHO (2006) reports that a growing body of evidence suggests that public policy-makers and healthcare professionals may be unprepared to cope with the predicted rise of neurological and other chronic disorders, disabilities resulting from aging populations globally, and expanding life expectancies in developed nations. The *Global Burden of Disease* study conducted by the WHO, the World Bank, and the Harvard School of Public Health found that neurological and psychiatric conditions accounted for 38.2% of the Disability Adjusted Life Year Scores (DALYs) globally (Murray and Lopez 1996; WHO 2006). The reader is referred to Chapter 9 for a detailed discussion related to DALYs and other global measures of disability, and how they are calculated. Moreover, the WHO (2004a, 2004b) reports that 5 of the 10 leading causes of disability globally for individuals aged 15–44 years are psychiatric/ mental health conditions (e.g., depression, alcohol abuse, self-infected injuries, schizophrenia, bipolar disorder). In fact, mental and behavioral disorders account for approximately 12% of the global burden of disease and contribute to as many days of lost work as physical ailments and disease. The reader is referred to Chapter 9 for a detailed discussion on disability and global measures of morbidity (e.g., disability-adjusted life years, quality-adjusted life years) and mortality (e.g., infant mortality).

Bioterrorism

The Public Health Agency of Canada (2001) defines *bioterrorism* as the use of a microorganism with the deliberate intent of causing infection in order to achieve certain goals. This includes the release of infectious biological agents, toxic chemicals, and radioactive materials into the environment with the deliberate intent or objective or causing death, injury, disability, or harm to a defined group or population (Goodwin Veenema 2007; Rodriguez and Long 2006). Biological agents (e.g., anthrax, brucellosis, plague, smallpox, Q-fever, viral encephalitis, viral hemorrhagic fevers such as Ebola, Marburg, Lassa, and Machupo) are of special concern because they are relatively inexpensive to produce, can be rapidly produced in short periods of time if desired, can be distributed over large geographical areas, can have a simple mode of delivery (e.g., air, water, food supply), and may result in mass fatalities through exposure (Jacobsen 2008; McDade and Franz 1998).

Canada has not been immune to terrorist attacks and plots. For example, on October 22, 2014, the extremist Michael Zehaf-Bibeau fatally shot Corporal Nathan Cirillo, a Canadian reserve soldier who was on ceremonial sentry duty at the Canadian National War Memorial in Ottawa (Fantz and Schoichet 2014; Tuker 2014). Zehaf-Bibeau then stormed the centre block of the Parliament buildings where members of Parliament were attending caucus, where he was subsequently shot by security personnel. On June 2, 2006, counter-terrorism raids carried out in the Greater Toronto area resulted in the arrests of 14 adults and 4 youths, dubbed the "Toronto 18" (Loriggio 2014; Thompson 2016). The Toronto 18 consisted of extremist who were inspired by the terrorist group al-Qaeda, and planned to carry out various acts of terrorism in Canada including det-onating truck bombs, opening gun fire in crowed areas, storming the Canadian Broadcasting Corporation headquarters in downtown Toronto, and storming the Canadian Parliament buildings in Ottawa. On the evening of November 13, 2015, a series of carefully planned and coordinated terrorist attacks occurred in Paris, France (Durando 2015; Steafel 2015). The attacks consisted of suicide bombings in a soccer stadium, mass shootings in restaurants and cafés, and storming of a concert Hall in Paris which resulted in the murder of 130 individuals and 368 were wounded, including an estimated 80–99 who were seriously wounded with life-threatening injuries. These examples highlight the unfortunate fact that Canada and many of its allies are at risk for terrorist acts by extremists. Public health officials need to be prepared to deal with such emergencies which can result in vast causalities, deaths, and/or threats to public safety and security (e.g., contamination of water supplies) (Haddow, Bullock, and Coppola 2011; Landesman 2012).

The use of biological agents to infect humans, animals, or plants is not new in the history of mankind. For example, Jacobsen (2008) notes that during the Tartar siege of the city of Kaffa (now in the Ukraine) in the fourteenth century, the bodies of plague victims were launched over city walls with catapults to induce an epidemic. In 1763, during the French and Indian War, the British army sent smallpox-infected blankets to American Indians. During World War I, several European nations used biological agents against livestock and enemies. What is new today is that there are significantly more tools and means available for causing and spreading infectious diseases on a global scale (Jacobsen 2008).

All levels of government are involved in preparing for and responding to a potential biological threat in Canada (Public Health Agency of Canada [PHAC] 2005). In the event of a biological emergency that poses a risk to public health, the PHAC under the co-ordination of Public Safety (PS) and other government depart-ments (e.g., Health Canada, Department of National Defense) plays a critical role in protecting the health and safety of individuals in Canada. The PHAC helps to co-ordinate a national emergency system known as the *Emergency Operation Centers* (EOCs) that may be mobilized in response to calls for assistance from provin-cial, territorial, and/or other government agencies as well as from other international health organizations (e.g., WHO). The reader is referred to Chapter 8 for a detailed discussion of the *Emergencies Act*, which allows the federal government to grant the use of special powers to ensure public safety and security of Canadians

Table 7.8 Operation Levels of the Emergency Operation Centers (EOCs) in Canada

Level	Level of Alert/Activation	Description of Activities
1	Normal readiness	EOC staff carry-out day-to-day routine activities and the facil-ity is available for emergency training exercises, meetings and ongoing surveillance activities
2	Increased vigilance	Normal activities continue to be carried out, but EOC staff begins monitoring an evolving situation. Contingency plans are reviewed and personnel are put on stand-by status
3	Partial activation	Ongoing surveillance is increased and some partial staffing may occur
4	Full activation	The PHAC of Canada Emergency Response Plan is formally activated. The number of staff in the EOCs is expanded to pro-vide 24/7 support

Source: Adapted from the Public Health Agency of Canada (2005).

during a national emergency. Table 7.8 shows the four levels of operation for the EOCs in Canada. The EOC systems features so-called user friendly communication capacities including satellite, two-way radios, telephones with video displays and landline connections, smart boards, video display capabilities, media monitoring capabilities, emergency response software, and emergency back-up power supplies.

The PHAC's (2005) bioterrorism and emergency response include many duties and obligations which are highlighted below:

1. Developing and maintain national emergency response plans (e.g., National Smallpox Contingency Plan, H1N1 global pandemic in 2009).
2. Enforcing the *Quarantine Act* at Canadian border crossings and other ports of entry, developing laboratory protocols for testing for biologic terrorism agents and training the Canadian Public Health Laboratory Network in their use.
3. Developing protocols and rapid diagnostic tests for bioterrorists agents.
4. Maintaining a deployable laboratory capacity (e.g., mobile equipment) and *Microbiological Emergency Response Teams*.
5. Acting as the focal point for *Canada's National Emergency Response Assistant Plan* for the transportation of Human Risk Group IV agents (e.g., Ebola, Marburg, nipah, Crimean-Congo hemorrhagic fever).
6. Monitoring disease outbreaks and global disease events via the *Global Public Health Intelligence Network*.
7. Managing the *National Emergency Stockpile Systems*, which is a $330 million system that provides a stockpile of medical supplies and pharmaceuticals for quick deployment when needed (e.g., Tamifu, antibiotics, smallpox vaccines).
8. Working with provinces, territories, and local public health authorizes and officials to ensure that front-line healthcare workers have the necessary tools and knowledge to identify, diagnose, and manage an event requiring emergency medical supplies.
9. Establishing emergency medical response surge capacity in the form of *Health Emergency Response Teams*, to assist provinces, territories, or other health jurisdictions in relieving the effects of medical and health major disasters when requested.

Canada also plays an active role in the *Global Health Security Action Group* which seeks to improve public health preparedness and responses to possible attacks by bioterrorists. This group includes the countries from the G7, Mexico, the European Commission, and the WHO (PHAC 2005). Furthermore, the PHAC has worked with the WHO to develop and implement the *Global Public Health Intelligence Network*. This network is a secure Internet-based early warning system that actively gathers information about potential global public health issues, treats, and concerns, which include chemical, biological, radiological, and nuclear (CBRN) threats on a "real-time" 24/7 basis. This network is multilingual in nature and also monitors global media sources in seven languages including Arabic, traditional and simplified Chinese, English, French, Russian, and Spanish.

On October 18, 2001, the federal government pledged $11.6 million for national initiatives designed to improve the health security of Canadians which included $5.62 million to increase stockpiles of antibiotics on hand in the *National Emergency Stockpile System*, $2.24 million for sensors and detection equipment and to establish a database of information, $2.12 million to better equip a Canada-wide network of laboratories to quickly diagnose biological agents, and $1.61 to train front-line health emergency teams to enable them to better recognize, diagnose, and treat suspicious illnesses resulting from a terrorists incident (Canadian Broadcasting Corporation News 2004). Many of these initiatives have already been employed to deal with public health and safety issues. For example, in January 2013 the federal government announced that it would be releasing stockpiles of the Tamiflu to deal with the flu outbreaks in many parts of Canada. The number of flu cases in the City of Toronto was 30% higher than previous years, despite free provincial wide flu vaccines for residents of Ontario, and a similar number was reported in other major cities in Canada. In December 2001, the federal government further announced a $7.7 billion security package aimed at protecting Canadians from terrorists, which included $1.6 billion for public emergency preparedness which includes high-tech bio-suits for emergency response teams and stockpiles of antibiotics and supplies such as the smallpox vaccine and portable hospitals (Canadian Broadcasting Corporation News 2004).

In order to effectively respond to a biological threat or public emergency in a timely manner, healthcare professionals and workers require special training and expertise in disaster and emergency healthcare services and management (Goodwin and Veenema 2007; Public Health Agency of Canada 2001; Rodrigues and Long 2006). During an act of bioterrorism in Canada, the demand for both acute care and public health services would greatly increase, and the demand for active surveillance and contact tracing would also be in high need and demand. The particular biological agent used by the terrorists would determine the overall risk for person-to-person transmission and communicability in a defined community. A strong public health infrastructure is necessary to deal with rapid and effective detection and response mechanisms through emergency preparedness and funding activities.

Marchant-Short and Whitney (2011) note that strategies that have helped public health deal with infectious disease

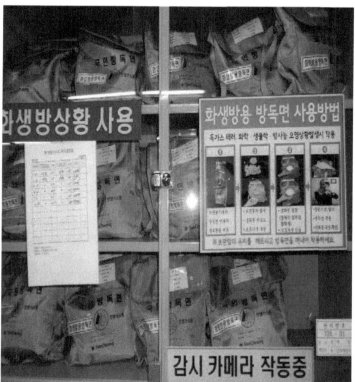

Source: Wally J. Bartfay

Photo 7.26 The treat of bioterrorism is a growing public health issue in Canada and globally. Stockpile of supplies including first aid kits, portable oxygen masks, gas masks and protective biological suits in an underground civilian emergency shelter in Seoul, Korea.

outbreaks such as SARS should be considered and reflected upon in preparation for potential bioterrorist events. Special training of personnel may include basic emergency management, how to communicate with the *Incident Management System*, infection control measures, dealing safely with specimens being collected in the field, and decontamination procedures (Marchant-Short and Whitney 2011). The best defense against a biological attack is early detection so that the outbreak can be properly confined and exposed individuals can be properly assessed and rapidly treated as required. Treatment may include, when deemed appropriate, PEP or immunization.

For example, in 2001 bioterrorists deployed anthrax spores via the US postal system, which caused 22 confirmed infections and 5 deaths (Centers for Disease Control and Prevention 2008). Moreover, more than 32,000 individuals who may have come into contract with anthrax-contaminated mail envelopes were provided with antibiotics by public health officials. In addition, public health education and the dispersion of updated information by public health authorities via the mass and social medias, Internet, or other means is critical to prevent the possibility of mass hysteria and panic regionally and/or nationally. The reader is referred to Chapter 8 for a detailed discussion of natural (e.g., tornado, tsunami, floods) and man-made disasters (e.g., nuclear accidents), the *Emergency Preparedness Act of Canada*, and the *Incident Command System* (ICS) that allows public officials to rapidly assess and respond in a coordinated manner to public health emergencies and disasters, including acts of bioterrorism. Add to your knowledge of bioterrorism and emergency preparedness by accessing the resources shown in the Web-Based Resource Box 7.3.

Web-Based Resource Box 7.3 Bioterrorism and Emergency Preparedness

Learning Resource	Website
Canadian Emergency Department Triage and Acuity Scale This website provides detailed information for health-care professionals and the general public related to how emergencies are graded based on an acuity scale.	http://www.srpc.ca/librarydocs/stasjoint statement.html
Department of Justice Canada (2007) Emergencies Preparedness Act, R. S. 1985 This website details Canadian Federal legislation dealing with national emergencies.	http://www.laws.justice.gc.ca/en/showtdm/cs?E-4.6
Public Health Agency of Canada's Centre for Emergency Preparedness and Response This federal website provides several useful links and information related to emergency preparedness.	http://www.phac-aspc.gc.ca/cepr-cmiu/index.html

Future Directions and Challenges

Life expectancy during the Roman Empire (27 BC to 476 AD) was approximately 29 years. During the 1900s, life expectancy had only been extended by 9 years (Preston 1975, 1995; Shine 2002). Infectious diseases were the leading cause of mortality that resulted from exposure to pathogens that produced diseases such as diphtheria, influenza, pertussis (whooping cough), TB, tetanus, and typhoid. However, by the mid-century, improvements in public sanitation including clean and safe water supplies, the widespread use of vaccinations as a primary public health intervention against infectious diseases and the development of antibiotic drugs have considerably reduced the mortality rates from infectious diseases. During the 1990s, the global life expectancy rose to 65 years (Preston 1975, 1995; Shine 2002). The major burden for industrialized nations has shifted from communicable diseases (e.g., TB, smallpox) to chronic and non-communicable diseases (e.g., heart disease, diabetes) during the twenty-first century. Marks and McQueen (2002) note that it is not simply that communicable disease has declined over the past century, but also that the success of public health has allowed populations to survive, age, and alas, acquire the diseases of privilege, including the privilege of age in the new millennium.

In fact, the current life expectancy in our industrialized nation of Canada is more than 80 years (Canadian Institutes for Health Information 2007), and the number of seniors is expected to reach 6.7 million in 2020 and 9.2 million in 2041 (Public Health Agency of Canada 2008). Statistics Canada (2010b) predicts that Canada's population could exceed 40 million by the year 2036, with approximately 1:4 over the age of 65 years. As of July 1, 2014, 15.7% (nearly 1:6) of Canada's population ($N = 35,540,400$) was aged 65 or older (Statistics Canada 2014). This proportion has steadily increased since the mid-1960s as a result of lower fertility rates and increased life expectancies in Canada. Given that the likelihood of developing chronic non-communicable disease increases with age, their incidence is also predicted to dramatically increase over the next few decades as the Canadian population continues to age and the first baby boomers enter their senior years (65+) in the year 2011 and beyond. This will continue to place increased demands on our already strained publicly funded healthcare systems in Canada. Indeed, in 2015 alone the average healthcare cost for a senior aged 65–69 years was $6298, $8384 for a senior aged 70–74, $11,578 for a senior aged 75–79 years, and $20,917 for a senior 80 years or more (CIHI 2015a).

Harlem Brundtland (2002) argues that the available interventions against these diseases, which includes preventive ones, yield less decisive results than we have achieved for most vaccine preventable diseases (i.e., via immunization campaigns), and that their associated costs can be very high. The PHAC (2011a) estimates that chronic diseases (e.g., heart disease, stroke, diabetes, depression) cost Canadians at least $190 billion annually in direct and indirect healthcare costs. The Ontario framework for *Preventing and Managing Chronic Disease* estimates that every 10% reduction in expenditures for chronic disease management could save the province $1.2 billion in return annually (Ontario Association of Community Care Access Centres Ontario Federation of Community Mental Health and Addiction Programs and Ontario Hospital Association 2010).

All public health professionals and workers must arm themselves with knowledge and the information about current and emerging acute and chronic diseases in Canada. They must also be armed with the necessary knowledge, skills (e.g., infection control measures, surveillance, contract tracing), and protocols for reporting and effectively responding when they encounter new disease entities (e.g., SARS pandemic of 2003) that have not yet been identified or adequately described.

An example of how quickly the health and well-being of individuals across the lifespan can be compromised and our public healthcare systems challenged is illustrated by the contamination of water supply sources during the past decade in several communities in Canada including Walkerton, Ontario, the Kashechewan Reserve in Ontario, and North Battleford, Saskatchewan. For example, in May 2000, more than 2300 residents becoming seriously ill and 7 died in Walkerton, Ontario, due to contamination of the town's water supply with *E. coli* 0157:57 bacteria, and the economic impact was estimated to be in excess of $64.5 million (Ali 2004; O'Conner 2002; Sullivan 2004).

In 1935, the Canadian Public Health Association established qualifications for the awarding of a *Certificate in Sanitary Inspection* (Canadian Institute of Public Health Inspectors [CIPHI] 2013). In 1963, there was a change in designation from *Sanitary Inspector* to *Public Health Inspector*. Currently, the CIPHI represents and unites environmental public health professionals and inspectors across Canada (see http://www.ciphi.ca/boc). At present, there are six Canadian schools which offer degree programs that can lead to CIPHI certification: Ryerson University (Toronto, ON), British Columbia Institute of Technology (Burnaby, BC), Concordia University College of Alberta (Edmonton, AB), Cape Breton University (Sydney, NS), New Brunswick Community College (Bathurst, NB), and First Nations University of Canada (Regina, SK).

A report written by representatives from both the federal and provincial/territorial health ministry's entitled *Building the Public Health Workforce for the 21st Century* was the first to formally propose a pan-Canadian framework to strengthen public health capacity (Joint Task Group on Public Health Human Resources 2006). The Joint Task Group on Public Health Human Resources (2006) were also the first to identify interdisciplinary core competencies deemed essential for all public health professionals and workers in Canada as one of the essential building blocks for their framework (see http://www.phac-aspc.gc.ca/core_competencies). These interdisciplinary core competencies provide the fundamental building blocks for providing safe, effective, and cost-efficient public primary healthcare services and programs. The reader is referred to Chapter 1 for a detailed discussion of the 36 essential competencies for public health.

The major challenge, however, remains to implement these recommendations on a Canada-wide basis to ensure consistency and standards of practice and education for public health. Indeed, universities that have the formal educational and professional mandates for training future healthcare professionals (e.g., schools of nursing, medicine) must ensure that their educational curriculums address all of the 36 core competencies for public health in Canada (Bartfay 2010; Bartfay and Bartfay 2015; Public Health Agency of Canada 2007). Work is already underway to expand on these core competencies for public health by developing discipline specific competencies.

For example, these 36 core competencies already complement the scope, standards of practice and essential entry-to-practice competencies for community health nurses in Canada in several areas including the need for evidence-informed practice, knowledge of research methods and epidemiology, population health assessment, surveillance, disease and injury prevention, and health promotion and protection for diverse populations across the lifespan (e.g., Alberta Association of Registered Nurses 2000; Canadian Association of Schools of Nursing n.d.; Canadian Nurses Association 1998, 2000b; Community Health Nurses Association of Canada 2003). The Community Health Nurses Association of Canada (CHNAC 2003, p. 3) standards of practice states that community health nurses "are registered nurses whose practice specialty promotes the health of individuals, families, communities and populations, and an environment that supports health." This practice requires that community nurses build collaborative partnerships with community stakeholders and other public healthcare professionals and workers to conduct holistic assessments of the assets and needs of individuals, families, groups or entire communities they serve to identify, prevent, and/or address states of illness, sickness, or disease (CHNAC 2003).

We argue that public health prevention is critical to averting many diseases, injuries, and disabilities in Canada. The reader is referred to Chapter 1 for a detailed discussion on the five levels of prevention. Primordial prevention involves actions and measures that seek to eradicate, eliminate, and/or minimize the impact of disease, injury, or disability and includes health policies and legislations (B.C. Minister of Health 2013; Kindig 2011). The Emergency Preparedness Act of Canada is a salient example of this level of prevention designed to protect Canadians on a national basis.

Informing individuals of disease risk and ways to prevent disease occurrence is a valuable component of primary prevention (Jo Damzo and Bartfay 2010). For example, immunizations are by far the most efficient and cost-effective public health intervention to prevent the occurrence of many communicable diseases (e.g., Chicken pox, measles, mumps, polio, rubella, TB) (Plotkin 2005; Plotkin and Orenstein 2008, Public Health Agency of Canada 2006b). The impact that vaccination has had on decreasing mortality on a global scale is hard to exaggerate. Plotkin and Orenstein (2008) note that with the exception of safe drinking water supplies, no other modality, not even antibiotics, had such a major effect on mortality reduction and population growth to date.

The goal of primary prevention immunization programs and campaigns in Canada is the elimination of vaccine-preventable diseases (Public Health Agency of Canada 2006b). For example, poliomyelitis has been eradicated in developed countries such as Canada, the United States, and Great Britain due to successful immunization programs. Similarly, MMR have been significantly reduced as a result of public health education and immunization campaigns.

Secondary prevention efforts, or disease treatments, should focus on minimizing possible negative health consequences for the affected individual. The effective clinical management of adult-onset type 2 diabetes is an example of how early interventions and treatment (e.g., weight management, diet, exercise) can change the natural history of this disease and increase the individual's health and quality of life. For example, changes in traditional lifestyles (i.e., hunting, fishing, trapping) resulting in increases in sedentary lifestyles and increased reliance on commercially prepared foods high in salt, sugar, and fat content have led to a higher incidence of diabetes in Indigenous communities across Canada (Bartlett 2003; National Indigenous Health Organization 2006; Young 2003; Young et al. 2000). It is notable that diabetes was virtually non-existent in Indigenous communities 6 decades ago. According to the Canadian Diabetes Expert Committee (2003), public healthcare professionals and workers and policymakers face major challenges to provide Indigenous people with culturally appropriate primary prevention programs and initiatives. In response to the growing incidence of obesity and diabetes, agencies such as the National Indigenous Diabetes Association (NADA) have been established to help facilitate the promotion of active and healthy lifestyles and eating habits in these target populations.

In reference to tertiary prevention initiatives, effective case management can help to eliminate the debilitating effects of disease (Jo Damzo and Bartfay 2010). For example, public health professionals and workers should be aware of community resources and agencies that can assist individuals and families with chronic disease (e.g., Alzheimer's disease support groups and adult day care programs). Healthcare professionals and workers should also be proactive in the development of public health policy at the local, regional, provincial/territorial, and national levels. The awareness of community or regional public health needs or issues will help to ensure that accurate information is collected for public health policy strategies and policy development that will help to maintain the public health infrastructure.

Quaternary prevention seeks to protect vulnerable groups (e.g., elderly, uneducated, homeless) from over diagnosis, being excessively medicated or other iatrogenic health interventions that may result in injury, harm, disability, illness, or death (Jamoulle and Roland 1995; Kuehlein et al. 2010). For example, Mitty (2010) found that 65% of older residents in nursing homes are at risk for iatrogenesis resulting from adverse drug interactions, especially if they are also physically frail and have one or more geriatric syndromes.

Lastly, public health professionals and workers must also be involved in research and investigations examining disease processes and formally document the clinical- and cost-effectiveness of their public health programs and interventions. For example, in 2009 through a partnership between the Public Health Agency of Canada and the Canadian Institutes of Health Research, the federal government committed $10.8 million over a three-year period to support a national influenza research network to strengthen Canada's capacity to prepare and respond to a global influenza pandemic (Canadian Institutes of Health Research 2009; Health Council of Canada 2011). This will help to ensure that financial resources and the appropriate healthcare personnel are available to address current and emerging diseases in Canada across the lifespan.

Group Review Exercise "The Vaccine Wars"

Overview of this investigative documentary
Vaccines, as primary public health interventions, have been shown to be effective in the eradication of various diseases worldwide including smallpox, polio and diphtheria since the turn of the century. Nonetheless, a growing number of parents are fearful of vaccines due to misinformation being propagated by certain politicians, celebrities, the Internet and social media sites (e.g., Twitter, YouTube and Facebook). This Public Broadcasting Station (PBS) documentary by Frontline critically examines the history, scientific effectiveness and growing movement fueled by certain celebrities, parents and the social media that are fearful of this potentially lifesaving intervention. In some communities, significant numbers of parents are rejecting vaccines altogether due to pseudo-scientific claims or anecdotal testimonials by parents regarding the safety of these vaccines. These negative campaigns and social media movements raise a number of public health concerns include the potential return of a variety of vaccine -preventable diseases such as measles, mumps, rubella and whooping cough. This Frontline documentary examines the science of vaccine safety and the increasingly bitter debate between public health professionals and a formidable populist coalition of parents, celebrities, politicians and activists who are armed with the latest social media tools. Despite the overwhelming consensus in the scientific and public health community, fear of vaccines are being propagated by testimonials by parents and disputed scientific investigations such as Dr. Andrew Wakefield vaccine and autism study ($N = 12$). This study was in fact retracted by the peer-reviewed journal Lancet where it first appeared in because it was proven to be bogus and totally false in nature. This discredited study claimed that the mercury-based preservative thimerosal which is present in the measles, mumps, and rubella (MMR) vaccine is associated with the development of autism in children. Despite the fact that this controversial study was shown to be bogus in nature, and numerous large-scale credible epidemiological investigations conducted in a variety of countries that have shown no link between autism and either the MMR vaccine or thimerosal, parents remain fearful.

Instructions
This assignment may be done alone, in pairs or in groups of up to 5 people (note: if you are doing this assignment in pairs or groups, please only submit one hard or electronic copy to your instructor).The assignment should be type-written and no more than 4–6 pages maximum in length (double-spaced please). View the PBS Frontline documentary entitled "The Vaccine War." Source: http://www.pbs.org/wgbh/pages/frontline/vaccines/ Take notes during the viewing of this investigative documentary.

1. Provide a brief overview of how the history and scientific evidence presented regarding the effectiveness of vaccines as a primary public health intervention.

2. Discuss why certain community leaders, celebrities or parent groups are lobbying against vaccines, and the negative role played by social media.

3. Discuss some of the "negative ripple effects" these fear campaigns and social media movements are having on public health and safety.

4. What do you believe are some of the challenges faced by public health professionals in promoting vaccination against various diseases in your province or territory in Canada?

5. Discuss how the Internet and social media (e.g., Twitter, Facebook, YouTube) may be employed by public healthcare professionals in Canada or globally to educate the public about the "positive ripple effects" of vaccines.

Summary

- The classification of disease consists of a standardized system and terminology used for the purposes of categorizing diseases by their clinical nature, and permits the statistical compilation of a group of cases for a disease by arranging disease entities into categories that share similar clinical manifestations.
- A disease is as an interruption, cessation, or disorder either mental or physical in nature that may arise from a single or combination of factors such as an infectious agent that is characterized by a recognizable set of clinical signs and symptoms.
- An illness is a subjective or psychological state felt by the individual who feels aware of not being well; and it is their experience with disease and a social construct fashioned out of transactions between healthcare providers and themselves in the context of their common culture.
- The individual's acceptance of their clinical diagnosis and treatment regime or plan typically follows a predictable path through the following five stages of the illness process: (a) Preliminary, (b) acknowledgement phase, (c) action phase, (d) transitional phase, and (e) resolution phase.
- Both sickness and the associated sick roles adopted are often defined by social and cultural norms, expectations, and traditions.
- Diseases are typically classified into five general categories by convention: (a) allergies and inflammatory disease, (b) cancer, (c) congenital and hereditary diseases, (d) degenerative diseases, and (e) metabolic diseases.
- Acute diseases are those disorders or conditions that are relatively severe in nature with a sudden onset, but have a short duration of clinical signs and symptoms (e.g., chickenpox caused by VSZ).
- Chronic diseases tend to be relatively less severe in nature but are continuous in duration, and which can last for long periods of time including an entire lifetime (e.g., TB).
- Communicable disease is defined as an illness caused by a specific agent or its toxic products that arise through transmission of the agent or product from an infected individual, animal, or reservoir to a susceptible host either directly or indirectly through an intermediate plant, animal host, vector, or inanimate environment.
- Non-communicable diseases are those that are non-transferrable or contagious in nature (e.g., heart disease, diabetes).
- Immunity is defined as the specific amount of resistance to a disease by an individual.
- Eradication of a disease is achieved when there is no risk of infection or disease globally even in the absence of immunization and/or other public health disease control measures, and when the agent is no longer present in the environment (e.g., smallpox).

- There are four ways an individual can acquire immunity or protection against a potentially infectious disease: (a) acquired (passive) immunity, (b) natural, (c) active immunity, and (d) herd immunity.
- Surveillance and tracking of diseases are critical components of public health practice in Canada and globally and provide information on both urgent (e.g., 2003 SARS outbreak in Toronto) as well as routine actions in public health (e.g., tracking of annual influenza strains).
- Active surveillance is defined as the collection of health-related data via sentinel public health tracking systems, screening tools, and interviews in order to identify the occurrence of disease in a defined community or geographical region when individuals present with suggestive clinical signs and symptoms.
- Passive surveillance involves the notification of health authorities by public health professionals of individuals who have clinical signs and symptoms, and this relies on laboratory tests for confirmation of diagnosis of the disease on the reportable disease list for their respected province or territory.
- For Canadians of all ages, poisoning is the fourth leading cause of injury deaths and permanent total disability, and the fifth leading cause of injury hospitalization, non-hospitalization, and permanent partial disability in Canada with an associated cost of $19.8 billion annually.
- An injury is as an act, either intentional or unintentional in nature, that results in hurt, damage and/ or trauma to an individual.
- A disability is as any degree of physical infirmity, impairment, malformation, or disfigurement that is caused by bodily injury, a birth defect, illness, or disease that may be physical, cognitive, mental, sensory, emotional, developmental, or some combination of these.
- Approximately 4.4 million (14.3%) of residents in Canada reported having a disability in the year 2006.
- Bioterrorism is the use of microorganisms with the deliberate intent of causing infection in order to achieve certain goals.
- Biological agents (e.g., anthrax, plague, Q-fever, Ebola) are of growing concern in Canada and globally because they are relatively inexpensive to produce, can be produced in short-periods of time and distributed over large geographical areas, often have simply modes of transmission (e.g., air, water, food supplies), and have the potential to result in mass fatalities through exposure.

Critical Thinking Questions

1. Population trends and projections in Canada suggest that life expectancy will continue to increase during the first half of the twenty-first century. What effect will this increased life expectancy have on both communicable and non-communicable diseases? What effect will this increased life expectancy have on public health needs, resources, and costs for managing both communicable and non-communicable diseases?

2. How should public health professionals and workers involved with health promotion and prevention deal with voluntary health risk-takers (e.g., smokers, heavy drinkers, intra-venous drug users), and with corresponding public health policies that seek to allocate scarce resources in your community (e.g., access to public health services)?

3. If you were designing a cardiovascular health promotion program for adults in your community, which specific stakeholders would you consider and seek their input on when developing your program and why? If you were designing a similar program for school-aged children in your community, which specific stakeholders would you consider and seek their input on when developing your program and why? What are the similarities and differences between the two programs and stakeholders?

References

Alberta Association of Registered Nurses. *Entry-to-Practice Competencies*. Calgary, AB: Author, 2000. Accessed May 17, 2011. http://www.nurses.ab.ca/publications/papers.html.

Ali, S. H. "A Socio-ecological Autopsy for the *E. Coli* 0157:H7 Outbreak in Walkerton, Ontario, Canada." *Social Science and Medicine* 58 (2004): 2601–12.

Allen, U. A. "Public Health Implications of MRSA in Canada." *Canadian Medical Association Journal* 175, no. 2 (2006): 161–62.

American Psychiatric Association (APA). *Diagnostic and Statistical Manual of Mental Disorders*. 4th ed. *Text Revisions: DSM-IV*. Washington, DC: Author, 1994.

———. *Diagnostic and Statistical Manual of Mental Disorders*. 4th ed. *Text Revisions: DSM-IV-TR*. Washington, DC: Author, 2000.

———. *Diagnostic and Statistical Manual of Mental Disorders*. 5th ed. Washington, DC: Author, 2013. ISBN 978-0-889042-555-8.

Amyes, S. G. "The Rise of Bacterial Resistance is Partly Because There Have Been No New Classes of Antibiotics since the 1960s." *British Medical Journal* 320 (2000): 199–200.

Anchor Bay Entertainment Inc. *Plague City: SARS in Toronto*. Toronto, ON: SWE Plague City Productions, Inc. (DV14938), 2005.

Anderson, K. N., and L. E. Anderson, eds. *Mosby's Medical, Nursing, and Health Dictionary*. 5th ed. Toronto, ON: Mosby, 1998.

Acha, P. N., and B. Szyfres. *Zoonese and Communicable Diseases Common to Man and Animals*. 2nd ed. Washington, DC: Pan American Health Organization, 1989.

Associated Press. *Will Autism Fraud Report Be a Vaccine Booster?* 2007. Accessed May 26, 2011. http://www.msnbc.msn.com/id/40955417/ns/health-kids_and_parenting/.

Associated Press (June 18, 2014). *Chikungunya Virus in Cuba Confirmed in 6 Travelers*. Associated Press and CBC News, Toronto, ON. Retrieved April 15, 2017, http://www.cbc.ca/news/health/chikungunya-virus-in-cuba-confirmed-in-6-travellers-1.2679905.

Anekwe, L. "UK MMR Uptake One of the Worst in Europe." *Pulse*, January 7, 2009. Accessed May 26, 2011. http://www.pulsetoday.co.uk/story.asp?storycode+4121589.

Baggett, H. C., T. W. Henessy, R. Leman, C. Hamlin, D. Bruden, A. Reasonover, P. Martinez, and J. C. Butler. "An Outbreak of Community-onset Methicillin-resistant *Staphylococcus aureus* Skin Infections in Southwestern Alaska." *Infection Control and Hospital Epidemiology* 24, no. 6 (2003): 397–402.

Bartfay, W. J. "Introduction to Community Health Nursing in Canada." In *Community Health Nursing: Caring in Action*. 1st Canadian ed., edited by J. E. Hitchcock, P. E. Schubert, S. A. Thomas, and W. J. Bartfay, 1–10. Toronto, ON: Nelson Education, 2010.

Bartfay, W. J., E. Bartfay, and J. Green Johnson. "Gram-negative and Gram-positive Antibacterial Properties of the Whole Plant Extract of Willow Herb (*Epilobium augustifolium*)." *Biological Research for Nursing* 14, no. 1 (January 2012): 85–89. doi:10.1177.1099800410393947. http://brn.sagepub.com.

Bartfay, W. J., and E. Bartfay, E. *Public Health in Canada*. Boston, MA: Pearson Learning Solutions, 2015. ISBN:13:978-1-323-01471-4.

Bartlett, J. G. "Involuntary Cultural Change, Stress Phenomenon and Aboriginal Health Status." *Canadian Journal of Public Health* 92 (2003): 165–67.

Bassil, K. L., C. Vakil, M. Sanborn, D. C. Cole, J. S. Kaur, and K. J. Kerr. "Cancer Health Effects of Pesticides: Systematic Review." *Canadian Family Physician* 53, no. 10 (October 2007): 1704–11.

Baumgardner, D. J. "Communicable Diseases of Children." In *Family Medicine: Principles and Practice*. 5th ed., edited by 163–72. New York: Springer Publishing, 1998.

Bax, R., N. Mullan, and J. Verhoef. "The Millennium Bugs. The Need for and Development of New Antibacterials." *International Journal of Antimicrobial Agents* 16 (2000): 51–59.

B.C. Ministry of Health. *Prevention Interventions*. Vancouver, BC: Author, 2013. Accessed December 17, 2013. http://www.health.gov.bc.ca/public-health/strategies/preventive-interventions/.

Bethony, J., S. Brooker, M. Albonico, S. M. Geiger, A. Loukas, D. Diemert, and P. J. Hotez. "Soil-transmitted Helminth Infections: Ascariasis, Trichuriasis, and Hookworm." *Lancet* 367, no. 9521 (2006): 1521–32.

Beisel, C. E., and D. M. Morens. "Variant-Creutzfeldt-Jakob Disease and the Acquired and Transmissible Spongiform Encephalopathies." *Clinical and Infectious Diseases* 38, no. 5 (2004): 697–704.

Belay, E. D., and L. B. Schonberger. "The Public Health Impact of Prion Diseases." *Annual Review of Public Health* 26 (2005): 191–212.

Billette, J. M., and T. Janz. *Injuries in Canada: Insights from the Canadian Community Health Survey.* Ottawa, ON: Statistics Canada, 2013.

Boucher, H. W., G. H. Talbot, J. S. Bradley, J. E. Edwards, D. Gilbert, L. B. Rice, and J. Bartlett. "Bad Bugs, No Drugs: No ESKAPE! An Update from the Infectious Diseases Society of America." *Clinical Infectious Diseases* 48 (2009): 1–12.

Bouzane, B., and D. Wylie. "Slicing Machines Likely *listeria* Source. Maple Leaf." *CanWest News Services*, 2008. Accessed May 17, 2011. http://www.canada.com/windsorstar/news/story.html?id=d542f8eb-aaa2-4b3a-af40-c67.

Boyd, D. R. *Northern Exposure: Acute Pesticide Poisoning in Canada. Health Environments, Healthy Canadian Series.* Vancouver, BC: David Suzuki Foundation, June, 2007. ISBN 1-897375-06-9. Accessed December 12, 2013. http://www.davidsuzuki.org/publications/downloads/2007/DSF-pesticide-poisoning.pdf.

Boyle, T. "Health Workers Get Fewer Flu Shots." *Toronto Star*, October 14, 2011. Toronto, Ontario: A3.

Brach, C., and I. Fraser. "Can Cultural Competence Reduce Racial and Ethnic Health Disparities? A Review and Conceptual Model." *Medical Care Research and Review* 57, Suppl no. 1 (2000): 181–217.

Brigham, M., and M. Hoefer. "Comparing Benefits and Risks of Immunization." *Canadian Journal of Public Health* 92, no. 3 (2001): 173–77.

Brouqui, P., F. Bacellar, G. Baranton, R. J. Birtles, A. Bjoërsdorff, J. R. Blanco, G. Caruso, M. Cinco, P. E. Fournier, E. Francavilla, M. Jensenius, J. Kazar, H. Laferl, A. Lakos, S. Lotric Furlan, M. Maurin, J. A. Oteo, P. Parola, C. Perez-Eid, O. Peter, D. Postic, D. Raoult, A. Tellez, Y. Tselentis, and B. Wilske. "Guidelines for the Diagnosis of Tick-borne Bacteria Diseases in Europe." *Clinical Microbiology and Infectious Diseases* 10, no. 12 (2004): 1108–32.

Campbell, A. *SARS Commission. Interim Report: SARS and Public Health in Ontario.* Toronto, ON: Ministry of Health and Long-Term Care, 2004. Accessed April 16, 2011. http://www.health.gov.on.ca/english/public/pub/ministry_reports/campbell04/campbell04.html.

———. *SARS Commission. Second Interim Report: SARS and Public Health Legislation.* Toronto, ON: Ministry of Health and Long-Term Care, 2005. Accessed April 16, 2011. http://www.health.gov.on.ca/english/public/pub/ministry_reports/campbell05/campbell05.pdf.

———. *The SARS Commission. Spring of Fear: Final Report.* Toronto, ON: Ontario Ministry of Health and Long Term Care, December, 2006. Accessed April 17, 2011. http://www.health.gov.ca/english/public/pub/ministry_reports/campbell06/online_rep.index.html.

Canadian Academy of Health Sciences. *Transferring Care for Canadians with Chronic Health Conditions.* Ottawa, ON: Author, 2010. Accessed December 17, 2013. http://www.dfcm.utoronto.ca/Assets/DFCM+Digital+Assets+CAHS+Transforming+Care+for+Canadians+with+Chronic+Health+Conditions.pdf.

Canadian Association of Schools of Nursing. *CASN Research Mandate and Goals Discussion Paper.* Ottawa, ON: Author, n.d. Accessed May 17, 2011. http://www.causn.org/research/casn_research_mandate.htm.

Canadian Biodiversity Information Facility. *Canadian Poisonous Plants Information System.* Ottawa, ON: Government of Canada, 2013. Accessed October 16, 2015. http://www.cbif.gc.ca/eng/species-bank/canadian-poisonous-plants-information-system/.

Canadian Broadcasting Corporation (CBC) News. *In Depth: Biological Weapons—Bioterrorism Spending in Canada.* Toronto, ON: CBC, February 18, 2004. Accessed June 2, 2011. http://www.cbc.ca/news/background/bioweapons/canada_spending.html.

Canadian Cooperative Wildlife Health Centre. "West Nile Virus." 2012. Accessed September 12, 2012. http://www.ciwhc.ca/wnv-report_2012.php?/language=en.

Canadian Diabetes Association Clinical Practice Guidelines Expert Committee. "Type 2 Diabetes in Aboriginal Peoples." *Canadian Journal of Diabetes* 27, no. 4 (2003): S110–S111.

Canadian Food Inspection Agency. *CFIA at a Glance.* Ottawa, ON: Author, December, 2013. Accessed December 12, 2013. http://www.inspection.gc.ca/about-the-cfia/organizational-information/at-a-glance/eng/1358708199729/1358708306386.

———. *Food Safety Facts on Listeria: Listeria Investigation and Recall-2008*. Ottawa, ON: Government of Canada, 2008. Accessed May 17, 2011. http://www.inspection.gc.ca/english/fssa/concen/cause/listeriae.shtml.

Canadian Institutes for Health Information (CIHI). *Government of Canada Announces Funding for Research to Further Protect Canadians from the H1N1 Flu Virus (News Release)*. Ottawa, ON: Author, June 5, 2009. www.cihr-irsc.gc. ca/e/39485.html.

———. *Health Care in Canada*. Ottawa, ON: Author, 2007.

———. *Health Indicators 2010*. Ottawa, ON: CIHI, May, 2010 (Figure 2 in report).

———. *Improving the Health of Canadians: Canadian Population Health Initiative*. Ottawa, ON: CIHI, 2005.

Canadian Institute of Public Health Inspectors (CIPHI). *Our Mission*. Toronto, ON: Author, 2013. Accessed December 12, 2013. http://www.ciphi.ca/boc.

Canadian Integrated Outbreak Surveillance Centre: Enteric Alerts (CIOSC). *Enteric Alerts*. Ottawa, ON: Health Canada, 2009. Accessed April 16, 2011. http://www.hc-sc.gc.ca/hc-ps/ed-ud/respond/food-aliment/fiorppriti_11-eng.php.

Canadian Nurses Association. "Cultural Diversity: Changes and Challenges." *Nursing Now: Issues and Trends in Canadian Nursing* 7 (February 2000a): 1–6.

———. *Evidence-based Decision Making and Nursing Practice*. Ottawa, ON: Author, 1998.

———. *Fact Sheet. The Primary Health Care Approach*. Ottawa, ON: Author, 2000b.

Community Health Nurses Association of Canada. *Canadian Community Health Nursing Standards of Practice*. Ottawa, ON: May, 2003. Accessed April 5, 2011. http://www.communityhealth-nursescanada.org.

Canadian Pharmacist Association. *Pharmacist`s Role in Flu Vaccination*. Ottawa, ON: Author, 2013. Accessed December 14, 2013. http://www.pharmacists.ca/index.cfm/education-practice-resources/patient-care/influenza-resources/ pharmacists-role-in-flu-vaccination/.

Canadian Public Health Association. *The Future of Public Health in Canada*. Ottawa, ON: Author, 2001.

Centers for Disease Control and Prevention (CDC). "Hantavirus Pulmonary Syndrome—United States: Updated Recommendations for Risk Reduction." *MMWR. Recommendations Report* 51 (2002) (RR-9).

———. *Malaria Parasites*. Atlanta, GA: Author, November 9, 2012. Accessed December 16, 2013. http://www.cdc.gov/ malaria/about/biology/parasites.html.

———. "Methicillin-resistant *Staphylococcus aureus* Infections among Competitive Sports Participants—Colorado, Indiana, Pennsylvania, and Los Angeles County, 2000–2003." *MMWR* 52 (2003): 793–95.

———. "Questions and Answers about Anthrax." Atlanta, GA: Author, 2008. Accessed June 2, 2011. http://emergency. cdc.gov/agent/anthrax/faq.

———. "Vaccinia (Smallpox) Vaccine: Recommendations of the Immunization Practices Advisory Committee (ACIP)." *MMWR* 40 (1991): 1–40.

Chad, S. *Briefing Paper. Silent Killer, Economic Opportunity: Re-thinking Non-communicable Disease*. London, England: Centre on Global Health Security, 2012.

Chaput, J. P., and A. M. Sharma. "Is Physical Activity in Weight Management More about 'Calories in' than 'Calories out'?" *British Journal of Nutrition* 106, no. 1 (December 2011): 1768–69.

Chin, J. E. *Control of Communicable Diseases Manual*. 17th ed. Washington, DC: American Public Health Association, 2000.

Coalition for DSM-5 Reform. *Coalition for DSM-5 Open Letter*. Accessed December 9, 2013. http://dsm5-reform.com/.

Coleman, P. G., E. M. Fevre, and S. Cleaveland. "Estimating the Public Health Impact of Rabies." *Emerging Infectious Diseases* 10 (2004): 140–42.

Collinge, J., J. Whitfied, E. McKintosh, J. Beck, S. Mead, D. J. Thomas, and M. P. Alpers. "Kuru in the 21st Century—An Acquired Human Prion Disease with Very Long Incubation Periods." *Lancet* 367 (2006): 2068–74.

Commission on the Social Determinants of Health. *Closing the Gap in a Generation. Health Equity through Action on the Social Determinants of Health*. Geneva, Switzerland: World Health Organization, 2008. ISBN 978-92-4-156370-3.

Cowell, A., and W. Neuman. "*E. coli* 'Disaster' Rocks Germany." *The Toronto Star*, June 2, 2011. Toronto, ON. A 25.

Cosgrove, L., and L. Drimsky. "A Comparison of DSM-IV and DSM-5 Panel Members' Financial Association with Industry: A Pernicious Problem Persists." *PLoSMedicine* 9, no. 3 (March 2012): 1–5.

Cosgrove, L., S. Krimsky, M. Vijayaraghavan, and L. Schneider. "Financial Ties between DSM-IV Panel Members and the Pharmaceutical Industry." *Psychotherapy and Psychosomatics* 75, no. 3 (April 2006): 154–60.

Crockett, M., L. Ford-Jones, C. Hui, J. Keystone, and S. Kuhn, S. "Travel-related Illnesses in Paediatric Travelers Who Visit Friends and Relatives Globally." *Canadian Paediatric Surveillance Program: Protocols*, March, 2009 and February, 2011. Accessed May 28, 2011. http://www.cps.ca/English/surveillance/cpsp/studies/TRIP.pdf.

Espinal, M. A., A. Laszlo, L. Simonsen, F. Boulahbal, S. J. Kim, A. Reniero, S. Hoffner, H. L. Rieder, N. Binkin, C. Dye, R. Williams, M. C. Raviglione. "Global Trends in Resistance to Antituberculosis Drugs. World Health Organization—International Union against Tuberculosis and Lung Disease Working Group on Anti-Tuberculosis Drug Resistance Surveillance." *New England Journal of Medicine* 344, no. 17 (2001): 1294–1303.

Davitz, L. L., and J. R. Davitz. "Cross-cultural Inferences of Physical Pain and Psychological Distress." *Nursing Times* 73 (1977): 521–23 and 556–58.

Deer, B. *Interview: Dr. Andrew Wakefield, Research Team Leader, Royal Free Hospital School of Medicine.* 1998. Accessed May 26, 2011. http://www.briandeer.com/wakefield/royal-video.htm.

de Leon, J. "Is Psychiatry Scientific? A Letter to a 21st Century Psychiatry Resident." *Psychiatry Investigations* 10, no. 3 (September 10, 2013): 205–17.

Demicheli, V., T. Jefferson, A. Rivetti, and D. Price. "Vaccines for Measles, Mumps and Rubella in Children." *Cochrane Database of Systematic Reviews* 19, no. 4 (2005). doi:10.1002/14651858.CD004407.pub.2.

de Silva, N. R., S. Brooker, P. J. Hotez, A. Montresor, D. Engels, and L. Savioli. "Soil-transmitted Helminth Infections: Updating the Global Picture." *Trends in Parasitology* 19, no. 12 (2003): 547–51.

Donatelle, R. J. *Access to Health.* Green Ed. Toronto, ON: Benjamin Cummings, 2010.

Donnelly, C. A. "Bovine Spongiform Encephalopathy in the United States: An Epidemiologist's View." *New England Journal of Medicine* 350, no. 6 (2004): 539–42.

Dubos, R., and J. Dubos. *The White Plague: Tuberculosis, Man, and Society.* Boston, MA: Little, Brown, and Company, 1952.

Durando, J. "Paris Terror Attack: What We Know." *USA Today Network*, January 9, 2015. Accessed January 6, 2016. http://www.usatoday.com/story/news/nation-now/2015/01/09/paris-terror-attack-charlie-hebdo/21490645/.

Dye, C., and N. Gay. "Modelling the SARS Epidemia." *Science* 300 (2003): 1884–85.

Ena, J. "Infections Spread by Close Personal Contact." In *Public Health and Preventive Medicine.* 5th ed., edited by R. B. Wallace, N. Kohatsu, and J. M. Last, 201–11. Toronto, ON: McGraw Hill Medical, 2008.

Fantz, A., and C. E. Schoichet. "'Terrorists murdered soldier in cold blood,' Canada's Prime Minister says." CNN, October 31, 2014. Accessed January 4, 2016. http://www.cnn.com/2014/10/22/world/americas/canada-ottawa-shooting/index.html.

Findlay, D. "The Body Perfect: Appearance Norms, Medical Control, and Women." In *Social Control in Canada: Issues in the Social Construction of Deviance*, edited by B. Schissel and L. Mahood, 174–200. Don Mills, ON: Oxford University Press, 1996.

Feikin, D. R., D. C. Lezotte, R. F. Hamman, D. A. Salmon, R. T. Chen, and R. E. Hoffman. "Individual and Community Risks of Measles and Pertussis Associated with Personal Exemptions to Immunization." *Journal of the American Medical Association* 284, no. 3 (2000): 145–50.

FitzGerald, J., L. Wang, and R. Elwood. "Tuberculosis 13: Control of Disease among Aboriginal People in Canada." *Canadian Medical Association Journal* 162, no. 3 (2000): 351–55.

Forge, F., and J-D. Frechette. *Mad Cow Disease and Canada's Cattle Industry.* Ottawa, ON: Parliamentary Information and Research Service, July 2005.

Friedman, M. J., P. A. Resick, R. A. Bryant, J. Strain, M. Horowitz, and D. Spiegel. "Classification of Trauma and Stressor-related Disorders in DSM-5." *Depression and Anxiety* 28, no. 9 (2011a): 737–49.

Friedman, M. J., P. A. Resick, R. A. Bryant, and C. R. Brewin. "Considering PTSD for DSM-5." *Depression and Anxiety* 28, no. 9 (2011b): 750–69.

Friis, R. H., and T. A. Sellers. *Epidemiology for Public Health Practice.* Toronto, ON: Jones and Bartlett Publishers, 2009.

Garner, J. S. "Guidelines for Isolation Precautions. Hospital Infections Control Practices Advisory Committee." *Infection Control and Hospital Epidemiology* 17 (1996): 53–60.

Goodwin Veenema, T. *Disaster Nursing and Emergency Preparedness for Chemical, Biological, and Radiological Terrorism and Other Hazards.* 2nd ed. New York: Springer Publishing, 2007.

Gordis, L. *Epidemiology.* Philadelphia, PA: W. B. Sauders, 1996.

Government of Canada. *Justice Laws Website*. Ottawa, ON: Author, 2013. Accessed December 13, 2013. http://laws-lois. justice.gc.ca/eng/acts/P-9.01/.

Groesz, L. M., M. P. Levine, and S. K. Murnen. "The Effect of Experimental Presentation of Thin Media Images on Body Satisfaction: Meta-analytic Review." *International Journal of Eating Disorders* 31, no. 1 (2002): 1–16.

Guris, D., M. Marin, and J. F. Seward. "Varicella and Herpes Zoster." In *Public Health and Preventive Medicine*. 5th ed., edited by R. B. Wallace, N. Kohatsu, and J. M. Last, 127–33. Toronto, ON: McGraw Hill Medical, 2008.

Haddow, G. D., J. A. Bullock, and D. Coppola. *Introduction to Emergency Management*. 4th ed. Burlington, MA: Elservier, Inc., 2011.

Hahn, D. B., W. A. Payne, M. Gallant, and P. C. Fletcher. *Focus on Health*. 2nd Canadian ed. Toronto, ON: McGraw-Hill Ryerson, 2006.

Hales, D., and L. Lauzon. *An Invitation to Health*. 1st Canadian ed. Toronto, ON: Thomson Nelson, 2007.

Hall, J. "New Superbug Threatens Ontario." *The Toronto Star*, May 31, 2011. Toronto, ON.

Harlem Brundtland, G. "The Future of the World's Health." In *Critical Issues in Global Health*, edited by C. E. Koop, C. E. Pearson, and M. R. Schwarz, 3–11. San Francesco, CA: Jossey-Bass, 2002.

Hartog, J., and E. A. Hartog. "Cultural Aspects of Health and Illness Behavior in Hospitals." *Western Journal of Medicine* 139 (1983): 911–16.

Health Canada. *Canada's Food and Drugs Act and Regulations*. Ottawa, ON: Author, 2007. Accessed December 12, 2013. http://www.hc-sc.gc.ca/fn-an/legislation/acts-lois/act-loi_reg-eng.php.

———. *First Nations and Inuit health: Summary of Epidemiology of Tuberculosis in First Nation's Living on-reserves in Canada, 2000–2008*. Ottawa, ON: Author, May 15, 2012a. Accessed December 17, 2013. http://www.hc-sc.gc.ca/ fniah-spnia/pubs/diseases-maladies/_tuberculos/tuberculos-epidemio/index-eng.php.

———. *First Nations and Inuit health: Tuberculosis (TB)*. Ottawa, ON: Author, December 7, 2012b. Accessed December 17, 2013. http://www.hc-sc.gc.ca/fniah-spnia/diseases-maladies/tuberculos/index-eng.php.

———. *Food Safety*. Ottawa, ON: Author, November, 2011. Accessed December 12, 2013. http://www.hc-sc.gc.ca/fn-an/ securit/index-eng.php.

———. *Notifiable Diseases Online: Glossary*. Ottawa, ON: Author, 2003. Accessed April 15, 2011. http://dsol-smed .phac-aspc.gc.ca/dsol-smed/ndis/gloss_e.html.

———. *Search A-Z index: Influenza; SARS*. Ottawa, ON: Author, n.d. Accessed April 17, 2011. http://www.hc-sc.gc.ca/ index_e.html.

Health Council of Canada. "A Citizen's Guide to Health Indicators. A reference Guide for Canadians." Ottawa, ON: Health Council of Canada, January, 2011. Accessed January 2, 2013. http://www.healthcouncilcanada.ca/rpt_det_gen. php?id=130.

Heymann, D. L. *Control of Communicable Diseases Manual: An Official Report of the American Public Health Association*. 19th ed. Washington, DC: American Public Health Association, 2008.

Hiramatsu, K., L. Cui, M. Kuroda, and T. Ito. "The Emergence and Evolution of Methicillin-resistant *Staphylococcus aureus*." *Trends in Microbiology* 9, no. 10 (2001): 486–93.

Honda, H., Y. Schimizu, and M. Rutter. "No Effect of MMR Withdrawal on the Incidence of Autism: A Total Population Study." *The Journal of Child Psychology and Psychiatry* 46, no. 6 (2005): 572–79.

Hornick, D. B. "Tuberculosis." In *Public Health and Preventive Medicine*. 5th ed., edited by R. B. Wallace, N. Kohatsu, and J. M. Last, 248–74. Toronto, ON: McGraw Hill Medical, 2008.

Hopkins, D. R. "Dracunculiasis." In *Public Health and Preventative Medicine*. 15th ed., edited by R. B. Wallace, 320–22. Toronto, ON: McGraw Medical, 2008.

Hotez, P. J., S. Brooker, J. M. Bethony, M. E. Bottazzi, A. Loukas, and S. Xiao. "Hookworm Infections." *New England Journal of Medicine* 351 (2004): 799–807.

Human Resources and Skills Development Canada. "Federal Disability Report. Ottawa, ON: Author, 2010. Accessed December 14, 2013. http://www.hrsdc.gc.ca/eng/disability_issues/reports/fdr_2010.pdf.

———. *Indicators of Well-being in Canada. Canadians in Context—People with Disabilities*. Ottawa, ON: Author, 2007. Accessed December 12, 2013. http://www4.hrsdc.gc.ca/.3ndic.1t4r@-eng.jsp?iid=40.

———. *Indicators of Well-being. Work. Work-related Injuries*. Ottawa, ON: Author, 2013. Accessed December 14, 2013. http://www4.hrsdc.gc.ca/.3ndic.1t.4r"-eng.jsp?iid=20.

Hyman, I., and G. Dussault. "Negative Consequences of Acculturation: Low-birth-weight in a Population of Pregnant Immigrant Women." *Canadian Journal of Public Health* 91, no. 5 (2000): 357–61.

International Obesity Task Force. *Overweight and Obesity.* Atlanta, GA: Center for Disease Control, 2006. Accessed May 5, 2011. http://www.iotf.org/popout.asp?linkto+httP;//www.cdc.gov/nccdphp/dnpa/obesity/.

Jackson, A. C. "Rabies Pathogenesis." *Journal of Neurovirology* 8 (2002): 267–69.

Jackson, R. *Statement of Richard Jackson, Director, National Center for Environmental Health Centers for Disease Control and Prevention, Department of Health and Human Services before the Subcommittee on Labor, Health and Human Services, and Education Committee on Appropriations, US. Senate on June 1, 1998.* Washington, DC: CDC, 1998. Accessed May 30, 2011. http://www.cdc.gov/ncidod/diseases/jackson/htm.

Jacobsen, K. H. *Introduction to Global Health.* Toronto, ON: Jones and Bartlett Publishers, 2008.

Jerschow, E., A. P. McGinn, G. de Vos, N. Vernon, S. Jariwala, G. Hudes, and D. Rosenstreich. "Dichlorophenol-containing Pesticides and Allergies: Results from the US National Health and Nutrition Examination Survey 2005–2006." *Annuals of Allergy, Asthma, and Immunology* 109, no. 6 (December, 2012): 420–25. doi:10.1016/j.anai.2012.09.005.

Jamoulle, M., and M. Roland. *Quaternary Prevention. Wonca Classification Committee, Hong Kong.* Bruxelles, Belgium: Research group Fédération des Maisons Médicales, June 6–9, 1995. Ch. De Waterloo 255/12 B-1060. Accessed December 17, 2013. http://www.ph3c.orgPH3C/docs/27/000103/0000261.pdf.

Jo Damazo, and W. J. Bartfay. "Communicable Diseases: Current Perspectives and Challenges." In *Community Health Nursing: Caring in Action.* 1st Canadian ed., edited by J. E. Hitchcock, P. E. Schubert, S. A. Thomas, and W. J. Bartfay, 191–215. Toronto, ON: Nelson Education, 2010.

Joint Task Group on Public Health Human Resources. *The Federal/Provincial/Territorial Joint Task Group on Public Health Human Resources: Building the Public Health Workforce for the 21st Century.* Ottawa, ON: Author, 2006.

Kachur, S. P., A. M. de Oliveria, and P. B. Bloland. In *Public Health and Preventive Medicine.* 5th ed., edited by R. B. Wallace, N. Kohatsu, and J. M. Last, 373–86. Toronto, ON: McGraw Hill Medical, 2008.

Kain, K. C., D. W. MacPherson, T. Kelton, J. S. Keystone, J. Mendelson, and J. MacLean. "Malaria Deaths in Visitors to Canada and in Canadian Travelers: A Case Series. *Canadian Medical Association Journal* 164 (2001): 654–59.

Kazakova, S. V., J. C. Hageman, M. Matava, A. Srinivasan, L. Phelan, B. Garfinkel, T. Boo, S. McAllister, J. Anderson, B. Jensen B, D. Dodson, D. Lonsway, L. K. McDougal, M. Arduino, V. J. Fraser, G. Killgore, F. C. Tenover, S. Cody, D. B. Jernigan. "A Clone of Methicillin-resistant *Staphylococcus aureus* among Professional Football Players." *New England Journal of Medicine* 352, no. 5 (2005): 468–75.

Kemp, M., and B. Hart. "Critically Appraised Topic: MMR Vaccine and Autism: Is There a Link?" *Journal of the American Academy of Physicians* 23, no. 6 (2010): 48–50.

Kindig, D. *Have You Heard of "Primordial Prevention"?* Blog in Population Health Basics, 2011. Accessed December 17, 2013. http://www.improvingpopulationhealth.org.blog/2011/05/primordial_prevention.html.

Kirby, M. *Reforming Health Protection and Promotion in Canada: Time to Act. 14th Report on the Standing Senate Committee on Social Affairs, Science and Technology.* Ottawa, ON: Government of Canada, 2003.

Klaas, D., and W. J. Bartfay. "Care of Young, Middle, and Older Adults." In *Community Health Nursing: Caring in Action.* 1st Canadian ed., edited by J. E. Hitchcock, P. E. Schubert, S. A. Thomas, and W. J. Bartfay, 374–416. Toronto, ON: Nelson Education, 2010.

Kleinman, A. *The Illness Narratives: Suffering, Healing, and the Human Condition.* New York: Basic Books, 1988.

Kleinman, A., L. Eisenberg, and B. Good. "Culture, Illness and Care. Clinical Lessons from Anthropologic and Cross-cultural Research." *Annuals of Internal Medicine* 88 (1978): 251–58.

Kobayashi, K. M. "Immigration, Ethnicity, Aging and Health." In *Health, Illness, and Health Care in Canada.* 4th ed. 205–19. Toronto, ON: Nelson, 2009.

Konner, M. "Epidemic of Panic." *Nature* 469, no. 7331 (2011). Accessed May 26, 2011. http://www.nature.com.uproxy.library.dc-uoit.ca/nature/journal/v469/n7331/full/469468a.html.

Kowa, S., and J. Giordano. "A Brief Historicity of the Diagnostic and Statistical Manual of Mental Disorders: Issues and Implications for the Future of Psychiatric Canon and Practice." *Philosophy, Ethics, Humanities and Medicine* 13 no. 72 (January 2012). doi:10.1186/1747-5341-7-2.

Kuehlein, T., D. Sghedoni, G. Visentin, J. Gérvas, and M. Jamoule. "Quaternary Prevention: A Task of the General Practitioner." *Primary Care* 10, no. 18 (2010): 350–54.

LaMar, J. E., R. B. Carr, C. Zinderman, and K. McDonald. "Sentinel Cases of Community-acquired Methicillin-resistant *Staphylococcus aureus* Onboard a Naval Ship." *Military Medicine* 168, no. 2 (2003): 135–38.

Landesman, L. Y. *Public Health Management of Disasters: The Practice Guide.* 3rd ed. Washington, DC: American Public Health Association, 2012.

Larson, E. "Community Factors in the Development of Antibiotic Resistance." *Annual Review of Public Health* 28 (2007): 435–37.

LeDuc, J. W. "Epidemiology of Viral Hemorrhagic Fevers." In *Public Health and Preventive Medicine.* 5th ed., edited by R. B. Wallace, N. Kohatsu, and J. M. Last, 352–62. Toronto, ON: McGraw Hill Medical, 2008.

Leitch, K. K. *Reaching for the Top: A Report by the Advisor on Healthy Children and Youth.* Ottawa, ON: Health Canada, 2007.

Levy, S. B., and B. Marshall. "Antibacterial Resistance Worldwide: Causes, Challenges and Responses." *Nature and Medicine* 10 (2004): S122–S129.

Loriggio, P. "Ringleader of 'Toronto 18' Terror Plot Denied Parole." *The Canadian Press.* 2014 Accessed January 4, 2016. http://www.ctvnews.ca/canada/ringleader-of-toronto-18-terror-plot-denied-parole-1.2021698.

MacLean, J. D., A. M. Demers, M. Ndao, E. Kokskin, B. J. Ward, and T. W. Gyorkos. "Malaria Epidemics and Surveillance Systems in Canada." *Emerging Infectious Diseases* 7, no. 10 (2004). http://www.cdc.gov/ncidod?EID/vol10no7/03-0826.htm.

MacMahon, B., and T. F. Pugh. *Epidemiology: Principles and Methods.* Boston, MA: Little Brown, 1970.

Madsen, K., A. Hivid, D. Vestergaard Schendel, J. Wohfart, P. Thorsen, J. Olsen, and M. Melbye. "A Population-based Study of Measles, Mumps, and Rubella, Vaccination and Autism." *The New England Journal of Medicine* 347, no. 19 (2002): 1477–82.

Mandleco, B., and W. J. Bartfay. "Care of Infants, Children, and Adolescents." In *Community Health Nursing: Caring in Action,* 1st Canadian ed., edited by J. E. Hitchcock, P. E. Schubert, S. A. Thomas, and W. J. Bartfay, 325–73. Toronto, ON: Nelson Education, 2010.

Marchant-Short, S., and L. L. Whitney. "Communicable Diseases." In *Community Health Nursing: A Canadian Perspective,* 3rd ed., edited by L. Leeseberg Stamler and L. Yiu, 189–212. Toronto, ON: Pearson Canada, 2012.

Marks, J. S., and D. V. McQueen. "Chronic Disease." In *Critical Issues in Global Health,* edited by C. E. Koop, C. E. Pearson, and M. R. Schwarz, 117–26. San Francisco, CA: Jossey-Bass, 2002.

McDade, J., and D. Franz. "Bioterrorism As a Public Health Threat." *Emerging Infectious Diseases* 4, no. 3 (1998). Accessed May 30, 2011. http://www.cdc.gove/ncidod/eid/vol4no3/mcdade.htm.

McDiarmid, J. "Firms Scramble to Deal with Flu." Toronto, ON: *The Star.com,* January 18, 2013. Accessed January 19, 2013. http://www.thestar.com/business/article/1317129--business-scrambles-to-deal-with-flu-outbreak.

McKeown, T. "Determinants of Health." In *The Nation's Health.* 4th ed., edited by P. R. Lee and C. L. Estes, 6–13. Boston, MA: Jones and Bartlett, 1994.

McManus, P. "Malaria in Canada? Mysteries of Canada." ZIZCAN Systems Corporation, 2011. Accessed June 3, 2011. http://www.mysteriesofcanada.com/Canada/malaria_in_canada.htm.

Meslin, F. X. "The Challenge to Provide Affordable Rabies Post-exposure Treatment." *Vaccine* 21 (2003): 4122–23.

Mikkonen, J., and D. Raphael. *Social Determinants of Health: The Canadian Facts.* Toronto, ON: York University School of Health Policy and Management, 2010. Accessed December 14, 2013. http://www.thecanadianfacts.org/The_Canadian_Facts.pdf.

Ministry of Agriculture, Food and Rural Affairs. "Ontario Weeds: Common Ragweed. Ottawa, ON: Government of Ontario, 2015. Accessed October 16, 2015. http://www.omafra.gov.on.ca/english/crops/facts/ontweeds/common_ragweed.htm.

Mitty, E. "Iatrogenesis, Frailty, and Geriatric Syndromes." *Geriatric Nursing* 31, no. 5 (2010): 368–74. doi:10.1016/j.gerinurse.2010.08.004.

Mosley, B. "Striking the Balance." *Women's Sport and Fitness* 19 (1997); 29.

Muntaner, C., E. Ng., and H. Chung. *Better Health: An Analysis of Public Policy and Programming Focusing on the Determinants of Health and Health Outcomes that are Effective in Achieving the Healthiest Populations.* Ottawa, ON: Canadian Health Services Research Foundation and Canadian Nurses Association, 2012.

Murray, C. J. L., and A. D. Lopez. *The Global Burden of Disease: A Comprehensive Assessment of Mortality and Disability from Diseases, Injuries and Risk Factors in 1990 and Projected to 2020.* Vol. 1. Geneva, Switzerland: WHO, 1996.

National Aboriginal Health Organization (NAHO) First Nations Centre. *First Nations Regional Longitudinal Health Survey 2002/2003: Report on Selected Indicators by Gender*. Ottawa, ON: Author, 2006. Accessed May 21, 2011. http://rhs-ers.ca/English/pdf/rhs2002-03reports/rhs-report_on-selected_indicators_by_gender.pdf.

National Expert Commission Canadian Nurses Association. *The Health of Our Nation, the Future of Our Health System. A Nursing Call to Action*. Ottawa, ON: Canadian Nurses Association, 2012. ISBN 978-1-55119-387-8.

National Center for Infectious Diseases. *vCJD (Variant Creutzfeldt-Jakob Disease)*. Washington, DC: Author, 2007. Accessed May 20, 2011. http://www.cdc.gov/ncidod/dvrd/vcjd/index.htm.

Naylor, D. *Learning from SARS: Renewal of Public Health in Canada: A Report to the National Advisory Committee on SARS and Public Health*. Ottawa, ON: Health Canada, 2003.

Nemeroff, C. B., D. Weinberger, M. Rutter, H. L. Macmillan, R. A. Bryant, S. Wessely, D. J. Stein, C. M. Pariantc, F. Seemuller, M. Berk, G. S. Malhi, M. Preisig, M. Brunc, and P. Lysaker. "DSM-5: A Collection of Psychiatrist Views on the Changes, Controversies, and Future Directions." *BMC Medicine* 12, no. 11 (September 12, 2013): 202. doi:10.1186/1741-7015-11-202.

Nicasio, A. M., J. L. Kuti, and D. P. Nicolau. "The Current State of Multidrug-resistant Gram-negative Bacilli in North America." *Pharmacotherapy* 28 (2008): 235–49.

Norrby, S. R., C. E. Nord, and R. Finch. "Lack of Development of New Antimicrobial Drugs: A Potential Threat to Public Health." *Lancet Infectious Diseases* 5 (2005): 115–19.

North Bay Parry Sound District Health Unit. "Investigative Summary of the *Escherichia coli* Outbreak Associated with a Restaurant in North Bay, Ontario: October to November 2008. (North Bay: NBPSDHU, June 2009)." North Bay, ON: Author, June, 2009. Accessed May 19, 2011. http://www.healthunit.biz/docs/Ecoli%20Outbreak/2008%20NBPSDHU%20Ecoli%20Report_June%202009_Formatted.pdf.

Obesity HQ. *Overweight and Obesity in South America*, 2012–2013. Accessed December 17, 2013. http://www.obesityhq.com/global-obesity/south-america/.

O'Conner, D. B. *Part One: A Summary of the Walkerton Inquiry: The Events of May 2000 and Related Issues*. Ontario Ministry of the Attorney General. Toronto, ON: Publications Ontario, 2002.

Ontario Association of Community Care Access Centres, Ontario Federation of Community Mental Health and Addiction Programs and Ontario Hospital Association. *Ideas and Opportunities for Bending the Health Care Cost Curve*. Toronto, ON: Author, 2010.

Ontario Association of Food Banks. *The Cost of Poverty. An Analysis of the Economic Costs*, 2008. Toronto, ON: Author, 2008.

Ontario Ministry of Health and Long-Term Care. (MOHLTC). *Screening Tool for Influenza-like Illness in Health Care Settings*. Toronto, ON: MOHLTC, 2009. Accessed April 15, 2011. http://www.health.gov.on.ca/english/providers/progra/emu/health_notices/screening_tool_20090519.pdf.

Ontario Ministry of Labour. *Profile of Ontario's Mining Sector*. Ottawa, ON: Author, September 10, 2014. Accessed October 15, 2015. http://www.labour.gov.on.ca/english/hs/pubs/miningprogress/profile.php.

Ontario Ministry of Natural Resources. *State of Resources Report: Rabies*. Ottawa, ON: Queen's Printer for Ontario, 2013. Accessed January 3, 2013. http://www.mnr.gov.on.ca/en/Business/SORR/2ColumnSubPage/STEL02_165925.html.

Ontario Poison Centre. *Statistics: 2005 Annual Report*. The Hospital for Sick Children, Toronto, ON: Author, march, 2007. Accessed December 13, 2013. http://www.ontariopoisoncentre.com/ontariopoisoncentre/section.asp?s=StatisticsandsID=7936.

Overbye, K. M., and J. E. Barrett. "Antibiotics: Where Did We Go Wrong?" *Drug Discovery Today* 1 (2005): 45–52.

Pan, E. S., B. A. Diep, H. A. Carleton, E. D. Charlebois, G. F. Sensabaugh, B. L. Haller, and F. P. Remington. "Increasing Prevalence of Methicillin-resistant *Staphylococcus aureus* Infections in California Jails." *Clinical and Infectious Diseases* 37, no. 10 (2003): 1384–88.

Parliament of Canada. *Healthy Weights for Healthy Kids: Report on the Standing Committee on Health*. Ottawa, ON: Government of Canada, 2007. Accessed May 6, 2011. http://www.ccfn.ca/pdfs/healthyweightsforhealthykids.pdf.

Piemann, C., and D. Cliver. *Foodborne Infections and Intoxications*. 3rd ed. New York: Academic Press, 2006.

Pereira, J. A., S. Quach, J. S. Hamid, S. D. Quan, A. J. Diniz, R. Van Exan, J. Malawski, M. Finkelstein, S. Samanani, and J. C. Kwong, for the Public Health Agency of Canada and Canadian Institutes of Health Research Influenza Research Network (PCIRN) Program Delivery and Evaluation Group. "The Integration of Barcode Scanning Technology into Canadian Public Health Immunization Settings." *Vaccine.* pii: S0264-410X(13)01532-6 (November 17, 2013). doi:10.1016/j.vaccine.2013.11.015.

Piesman, J., and L. Gern. "Lyme Borreliosis in Europe and North America." *Parasitology* 129 (2004): S191–S220.

Plotkin, S. A. "Vaccines: Past, Present and Future." *Nature and Medicine* 11 (2005): S5–S11.

Plotkin, S. A., and W. A. Orenstein. *Vaccines.* 5th ed. Philadelphia, PA: W. B. Saunders, 2008.

Porter, M., ed. *A Dictionary of Epidemiology.* 5th ed. (Edited for the International Epidemiological Association). Toronto, ON: Oxford University Press, 2008.

Preston, S. H. "Human Mortality through History and Prehistory." In *The State of Humanity,* edited by J. Simon. London, England: Blackwell, 1995.

Preston, S. H. "Mortality Trends." *Annual Review of Sociology* 3 (1977): 163–78.

Price, C., W. W. Thompson, B. Goodson, E. S. Wentraub, L. A. Croen, V. L. Hinrichsen, M. Marcy, et al. "Prenatal and Infant Exposure to Thimerosal from Vaccines and Immunoglobins and Risk of Autism." *Pediatrics.* September 13, 2010. doi:10.1542/peds.2010-0309.

Projan, S. J., and D. M. Shales. "Antibacterial Drug Discovery: Is it All Downhill from Here?" *Clinical and Microbiology Infections* 10 (2004). 18–22.

Public Health Agency of Canada (PHAC). *Act to Establish Public Health Agency Outcomes into Force.* Ottawa, ON: Author, 2006a. Accessed April 19, 2008. http://www.phac-aspc.gc.ca/media/nr-rp?2006/2006_11_e.html.

———. *Archieved-national Notifiable Diseases.* Ottawa, ON: Author, March, 2010a. Accessed December 10, 2013. http://www.phac-aspc.gc.ca/bid-bmi/dsd-dsm/duns-eng.php.

———. *Backgrounder: United Nations NCD Summit—Chronic Diseases. Most Significant Cause of Death Globally.* Ottawa, ON: Author, 2011a. Accessed December 17, 2013. http://www.phac-aspc.gc.ca/media/nr-rp/2011/2011_0919-bg-di-eng.php.

———. *Bioterrorism and Emergency Preparedness.* Ottawa, ON: Author, 2005. Accessed June 3, 2011. http://www.phac-aspc.gc.ca/ep-mu/bioem-eng.php.

———. "Bioterrorism and Public Health." *Canada Communicable Disease Report* 27, no. 4 (2001a).

———. *Canada's Aging Population. Division of Aging Seniors,* Ottawa, ON: PHAC, 2008. Accessed April 2, 2011. http://www.phac-aspc.gc.ca/seniors-aines/publications/public/various-varies/papier-fed-paper/index-eng.php.

———. *Canadian Immunization Guide.* Ottawa, ON: Author, 2013a. Accessed December 10, 2013. http://www.phac-aspc.gc.ca/publicat/cig-gci/p01-eng.php.

———. *Canadian Immunization Guide.* 7th ed. Ottawa, ON: Government Services Canada, 2006b.

———. *Canadian Integrated Public Health Surveillance (CIPHS).* Ottawa, ON: Author, 2007a. Accessed April 16, 2011. http://www.phac-aspc-gc.ca/php-psp/ciphs-eng.php#wiphis.

———. *Canadian Network for Public Health Intelligence. Fostering Collaboration and Consultation through Innovation in Disease Surveillance, Intelligence Exchange, Research, and Response to Protect, Promote and Support Public Health.* Ottawa, ON: PHAC, February, 2013b. Accessed December 17, 2013. http://www.ncceh.ca/sites/default/files/Surveillance_Workshop_Feb_2013-Beattie.pdf.

———. *Core Competencies for Public Health in Canada: Release 1.1.* Ottawa, ON: Author, 2007a.

———. *Creutzfeldt-Jakob Disease (CJD).* Ottawa, ON: Author, 2009a. Accessed May 21, 2011. http://www.phac-aspc.gc.ca/hcai-iamss/cjd-mcj-cjdss-ssmcj/stats_e.html#canada.

———. *Diseases Under National Surveillance (as of January, 2009).* Ottawa, ON: PHAC, 2010b. Accessed April 23, 2011. http://www.phac-aspc.gc.ca/bid-bmi/dsd-dsm/duns.eng.php.

———. *Frequently Asked Questions: Malaria.* Ottawa, ON: Author, 2004. Accessed June 3, 2011. http://www.phac-aspc.gc.ca/media/advisories_avis/mal_faq-eng.php.

———. *General Information.* Ottawa, ON: Author, 2012. Accessed September 12, 2012. http://www.phac-aspc.gc.ca/wn-no/gen-eng.php.

———. *Hantaviruses.* Ottawa, ON: Author, 2009b. Accessed June 6, 2011. http://www.hc-sc.gc.ca/hl-vs/iyh-vsv/diseases-maladies/hantavirus-eng.php.

———. *Injury Prevention Funding to Promote Active and Safe Play.* Ottawa, ON: Author, 2013c. Accessed December 14, 2013. http://www.phac-aspc.gc.ca/inj-bles/fs-fr/2013_0121-eng.php.

———. *Lyme Disease*. Ottawa, ON: Author, 2011b. Accessed June 2, 2011. http://www.phac-aspc.gc.ca/id-mi/lyme-eng.php.

———. *Lyme Disease Fact Sheet*. Ottawa, ON: Author, 2010c. Accessed June 2, 2011. http://www.phac-aspc.gc.ca/id-mi-lyme-fs-eng.php.

———. *Mental Illness*. Ottawa, ON: Author, 2013d. Accessed December 14, 2013. http://www.phac-aspc.gc.ca/cd-mc/mi-mm/.

———. *National Notifiable Diseases*. Ottawa, ON: PHAC, 2009c. Accessed April 18, 2011. http://dsol-smed.phac.aspc.gc.ca/dsol.smed.ndis/list_e.html.

———. *Number of Cases of Lyme Disease*. Ottawa, ON: Author, 2009d. Accessed June 2, 2011. http://www.phac-aspc.gc.ca/id-mi/lyme-eng.php.

———. *Obesity in Canada—Snapshot*. Ottawa, ON: Author, 2009e. Accessed May 26, 2011. http://www.phac-aspc.gc.ca/publicat/2009/oc/index-eng.php.

———. *Surveillance*. Ottawa,ON: Author, November 14, 2013e. Accessed December 16, 2013. http://www.phac-aspc.gc.ca/surveillance-eng.php.

———. *The Canadian Nosocomial Infection Surveillance Program*. Ottawa, ON: Author, 2007b. Accessed May 21, 2011. http://www.phac-aspc.gc.ca/nois-sinp/survprog-eng.php.

———. *The Chief Public Health Officer's Report on the State of Public Health in Canada, 2013. Infectious Diseases. The Never-ending Treat*. Ottawa, ON: Author, 2013f. Accessed October 21, 2015. http://www.phac-aspc.gc.ca/cphor-sphc-respcacsp/2013/infections-eng.php.

———. *Waterborne Cryptosporidiosis Outbreak, North Battleford, Saskatchewan. Canada Communicable Disease Report (CCDR)*. Ottawa, ON: Author, 2001a. Accessed May 19, 2011. http://www.phac.aspc.gc.ca/publicat/ccdr-rmtc/01vol27?dr2722ea.html.

———. *Waterborne Outbreak of Gastroenteritis Associated with Municipal Water Supply*. Walkerton, Ontario. Communicable Disease Report (CCDR). Ottawa, ON: Author, 2000. Accessed May 19, 2011. http://www.phac-aspc.gc.ca/publicat/ccdr-rmtc/00vol26/dr2620eb.html.

———. *West Nile Virus MONITOR: Human Surveillance (2002–2008)*. Ottawa, ON: PHAC, 2009f. Accessed April 18, 2011. http://www.phac-aspc.gc.ca/wnv.vwm/index-eng.php.

———. *West Nile virus MONITOR: Human Surveillance (2003–2005)*. Ottawa, ON: Author, 2006c. Accessed May 2010. http://www.phac-aspc.gc.ca/wnv-vwn.monhumunsurv-archieve_e.html.

Public Safety Canada. *Impact of West Nile Virus on Canada's health Infrastructure*. Ottawa, ON: Author, September 17, 2003. Accessed April 17, 2011. http://www.publicsafety.gc.ca/prg/em/ccirc/2003/in03-002-eng.aspx.

Quinlan, E., and H. D. Dickinson. "The Emerging Public Health System in Canada." In *Health, Illness, and Health Care in Canada*, 4th ed., edited by B. Singh Bolaria, and H. D. Dickinson, 42–55). Toronto, ON: Nelson Education, 2009.

Ragucci, A. T. "Italian Americans." In *Ethnicity and Medical Care*, edited by A. Harwood, 56–84. Cambridge, Massachusetts: Harvard University Press, 1981.

Ramaswamy, V., and V. M. Cresence. "*Listeria*: Review of Epidemiology and Pathogenesis." *Journal of Microbiology, Immunology and Infections* 40 (2007): 4–13.

Raphael, D. *Social Determinants of Health*. 2nd ed. Toronto, ON: Canadian Scholars' Press Inc., 2009.

Reed, K. D. "Laboratory Testing for Lyme Disease: Possibilities and Practicalities." *Journal of Clinical Microbiology* 40, no. 2 (2002): 319–24.

Regional Infection Control Networks (RICN). *Giving a Helping Hand. Annual Report 2009–2010*. RICN: Charterhouse Printing Services, 2010. Accessed May 16, 2011. http://www.ricn.on.ca.

———. *Mantoux Tuberculin Skin Test: An Independent Learning Module on Administration, Reading and Interpretation* (CD). RICN, 2009. Accessed May 17, 2011. http://www.ricn.on.ca.

Ritterman, J. "Preventing Microbial Resistance: The Next Step." *Permanent Journal* 10, no. 3 (2006): 22–24.

Rodnick, J. E., and J. Gude. "Pulmonary Infections." In *Family Medicine: Principles and practice*, 5th ed., edited by R. B. Taylor, 734–60. New York: Springer Publishing, 1998.

Rodriguez, D., and C. O. Long. "Emergency Preparedness for the Home Healthcare Nurse." *Home Healthcare Nurse* 24, no. 1 (2006): 21–27.

Romanow, R. J. *Building on Values: The Future of Health Care in Canada—Final Report. Commission on the Future of Health Care in Canada*. Ottawa, ON: Government of Canada, 2002. (Cat. No. CP32-85/2002E-IN).

Ross, O. "Andrew Wakefield's Fraudulent Vaccine Research." *The Star*, 2011 Accessed May 26, 2011. http://www.thestar.com/news/insight/article/918362--andrew-wakefield-s-fraudulent-research.

Rupprecht, C. E., C. A. Hanlon, and D. Slate. "Oral Vaccination of Wildlife against Rabies: Opportunities and Challenges in Prevention and Control." *Developmental Biology* (Basel) 119 (2004): 173–84.

Rybak, M. J., and K. L. LaPlante. "Community Associated Methicillin-resistant *Staphylococcus aureus*: A Review." *Pharmacotherapy* 25, no. 1 (2005): 74–85.

Safe Kids Canada and Alberta Centre for Injury Control and Research. *White Paper on the Prevention of Poisoning of Children in Canada*. Calgary, AL: Authors, October, 2011. Accessed December 12, 2013. http://www.parachutecanada.org/downloads/policy/WhitePaper_Poisoning.pdf.

Salvation Army. *Canada Speaks: Exposing Myths about the 150,000 Canadians Living on the Street*. Toronto, ON. Author, May, 2011. Accessed December, 17, 2013. http://vcu.visioncritical.com/wp-content/uploads/2012/09/REP_TheDignityProject_CanadaSpeaks_01.05.12.pdf.

Scheider, D., and P. Pautler. "Field Trip: Poisonous Plants. *Nature Magazine*, November 29, 2010. Accessed October 12, 2015. http://onnaturemagazine.com/field-trip-poisonous-plants.html.

Schissel, B. "The Pathology of Powerlessness: Adolescent Health in Canada." In *Health, Illness, and Health Care in Canada*. 4th ed., edited by B. S. Bolaria, and H. D. Dickinson, 300–30. Toronto, ON: Nelson, 2009.

Sharma, A. M., and D. C. Lau. "Obesity and Type 2 Diabetes." *Canadian Journal of Diabetes* 37, no. 2 (April, 2013): 63–64. doi:10.1016/j.cjd.2013.03.360.

Shaw Media. "Canadian Mine Safety in the Global Context." Regina, AB: *Global Regional News*, June 9, 2011. Accessed December 17, 2013. http://www.republicofmining.com/2011/06/10/canadian-mine-safety-in-a-global-context-global-regina-news-june-9-2011/.

Sheldon, A. "Antibiotic Resistance: A Survival Strategy." *Clinical Laboratory Science* 18 (2005): 170–81.

Shields, M. "Overweight and Obesity among Children and Youth." *Health Reports*. Ottawa, ON: Statistics Canada (Catalogue No. 82-003-XIE). 17, no. 3 (2006): 27–42.

Shine, K. I. "Reinventing Medicine and Public Health." In *Critical Issues in Global Health*, edited by C. E. Koop, C. E. Pearson, and M. R. Schwarz, 305–13. San Francisco, CA: Jossey-Bass, 2002.

Slinger, R., A. Giulivi, M. Bodie-Collins, F. Hindieh, R. S. John, G. Sher, M. Goldman, M. Ricketts, and K. C. Kain. "Transfusion-transmitted Malaria in Canada." *Canadian Medical Association Journal* 164 (2001): 377–79.

Smartrisk. *The Economic Burden of Injury in Canada*. Toronto, ON: SMARTRISK, 2009. Accessed December 12, 2013. http://www.phac-aspc.gc.ca/injury-bles/ebuic-febnc/.

Smeeth, L., C. Cook, E. Fambone, L. Heavey, L. Rodriguez, P. Smith, and A. Hall. "MMR Vaccination and Pervasive Developmental Disorders: A Case Control Study." *The Lancet* 64 (2004): 963–69.

Snow, R. W., E. L. Korenromp, and E. Gouws. "Pediatric Mortality in Africa: *Plasmodium falciparum* Malaria as a Cause or Risk?" *American Journal of Tropical Medicine and Hygiene* 71, Suppl. 2 (2004): 16–24.

Statistics Canada. *Canada's Population Estimates; Age and Sex 2014*. Ottawa, ON: Author, 2014. Accessed November 10, 2015. http://www.statcan.gc.ca/daily-quotidien/140926/dq140926b-eng.htm.

———. *Canadian Community Health Survey, 2009–2010*. Ottawa, ON: Author, 2010a.Accessed September 12, 2012. http://www.statcan/gc.ca/search-recherche/bb/info/obesity-obesite-eng.htm.

———. *Canadian Community Health Survey, 2011–2012*. Ottawa, ON: Author, 2013. Accessed December 14, 2013. http://www.statcan.gc.ca/health-sante/index-eng.htm.

———. *Causes of Death*. Ottawa, ON: Author, 2000. Catalogue #'s 84-208-XPB; 84F0208; 84F0208XPB and 84-208-XIE.

———. *Dynamics of Immigrant's Health in Canada. Evidence from the National Population Health Survey. The Daily*. Ottawa, ON: Author, 2005a. Accessed May 4, 2011. http://www.statcan.ca/Daily/English/050233/d/5050223c.htm.

———. *Health Indicators (1)*. Ottawa, ON: Author, 2003 (Catalogue No. 82221XIE).

———. *Nutrition: Findings from the Canadian Community Health Survey. Measured Obesity. Adult Obesity in Canada: Measured Height and Weight*. Ottawa, ON: Author, 2005b. Accessed May 6, 2011. http://www.statcan.ca/english/research/82-620-MIE/2005001/articles/adults/aobesity.htm.

———. *Participation and Activity Limitation Survey 2006: Tables*. Ottawa, ON: Author, December, 2007. Catalogue number 89-628-XIE-No. 003.

———. "Population Projections: Canada, the Provinces and Territories." *The Daily,* Ottawa, ON: Author, 2010b. Accessed December 17, 2013. http://www.statcan.gc.ca/daily-quoitidien/100526/dq100526b-eng.htm.

———. *Population Projections of Visible Minority Groups, Canada, Provinces and Regions, 2001–2007*. Ottawa, ON: Author (Demography Division), 2005c. Accessed May 4, 2011. http://www12.statcan.ca/english/census01/Products/Analytic/companion/etoimm.provs.cfm.

———. *2006 Census*. Ottawa, ON: Government of Canada, 2006. Accessed May 5, 2011. http://www.12statcan.ca/english/Census/Index.cfn.

Steafel, E. "Paris Terror Attack: Everything We Know on Saturday Afternoon." *The Telegraph*, November 21, 2015. Accessed January 6, 2015. http://www.telegraph.co.uk/news/worldnews/europe/france/11995246/Paris-shooting-What-we-know-so-far.html.

Strausbaugh, L. J. "Emerging Infectious Diseases: A Challenge to All." *American Family Physician* 55, no. 1 (January, 1997): 111–18.

Sullivan, P. "Safety of Drinking Water Remains a Crucial Health Issue: CMA President Says." *Canadian Medical Association*, 2004. Accessed March 2, 2011. http://www.cma.ca/index.cfm/ci_id/10013192/la_id/1.html.

Swanson, J. M., and M. Albrecht. *Community Health Nursing: Promoting the Health of Aggregates*. Toronto, ON: WB Sunders Company, 1993.

Talbot, G. H., J. Bradley, J. E. Edwards Jr., D. Gilbert, M. Scheld, and J. G. Bartlett. "Bad Bugs Need Drugs: An Update on the Development Pipeline from the Antimicrobial Availability Task Force of the Infectious Diseases Society of America." *Clinical Infectious Diseases* 42 (2006): 657–68.

Teutsch, S., R. Churchill, and R. Elliot. *Principles and Practice of Public Health Surveillance*. New York: Oxford University Press, 1994.

The Lung Association. *Tuberculosis: Information for Health Care Providers*. 4th ed. Toronto, ON: Author, 2009.

Thomas, S. A., and W. J. Bartfay. "Global Health Perspectives for Community Health Nurses." In *Community Health Nursing: Caring in Action*, 1st Canadian ed., edited by J. E. Hitchcock, P. E. Schubert, S. A. Thomas, and W. J. Bartfay, 143–72. Toronto, ON: Nelson Education, 2010.

Thompson, N. "'Toronto 18' Convicted Granted a Day Parole." *The Globe and Mail*, January 2, 2016. Accessed January 4, 2016. http://www.theglobeandmail.com/news/national/toronto-18-convict-granted-day-parole/article27987280/.

Thompson, V. D. *Health and Health Care Delivery in Canada*. Toronto, ON: Mosby Elsevier, 2010.

Twaddle, A. C. "Sickness and Sickness Career: Some Implications." In *The Relevance of Social Science for Medicine*, edited by Eisenberg, and A. Kleinman, 111–33. Dordrecht: Reidel, 1981.

Tripp-Reimer, T., and L. A. Afifi. "Reconceptualizing the Construct of Health: Integrating Emic and Etic Perspectives." *Research in Nursing and Health* 7 (1984): 101–109.

Tucker, E. "Soldier Killed in What Harper Calls 'Terrorists' Attack in Ottawa." *Global News*, October 22, 2014. Accessed January 4, 2016. http://globalnews.ca/news/1628313/shots-fired-at-war-memorial-in-ottawa-says-witness/.

UNICEF. *Innocenti Report Card 10: Measuring Child Poverty. New League Tables on Child Poverty in the Worlds Rich Countries*. Florence, Italy: Innocenti Research Centre, 2012. ISBN 978-88-8912-965-4.

Vergidis, P. I., and M. E. Falagas. "Multidrug-resistant Gram-negative Bacterial Infections: The Emerging Threat and Potential Novel Treatment Options." *Current Opinions in Investigative Drugs* 9 (2008): 176–83.

Wakefield, A., S. Murch, A. Anthony, J. Linnell, D. M. Casson, M. Malik, M. Berelowitz, A. P. Dhillon, M. A. Thompson, P. Harvey, A. Valentine, S. E. Davies, and J. A. Walker-Smith. "Illeal-lymphoid-nodular Hyperplasia, Non-specific Colitis, and Pervasive Development Disorder in Children. *Lancet* 351, no. 9103 (1998): 637–41.

Wallace, R. B. "Epidemiology and Public Health." In *Public Health and Preventive Medicine*. 5th ed., edited by R. B. Wallace, N. Kohatsu, and J. M. Last, 5–26. Toronto, ON: McGraw Hill Medical, 2010.

Walker, D. *For the Public's Health: A Plan for Action. Final Report of the Ontario Expert Panel on SARS and Infectious Disease Control*. Toronto, ON: Ministry of Health and Long-Term Care, 2004. Accessed April 11, 2011. http://www.health.gov.on.ca/english/public/pub/ministry_reports/walker04/walker04_mn.html.

Waller, G. "Perceived Control in Eating Disorders: Relationship with Reported Sexual Abuse." *International Journal of Eating Disorders* 23, no. 2 (1998): 213–16.

Warrell, M. J., and D. A. Warrell. "Rabies and Other Lyssavirus diseases." *Lancet* 363 (2004): 959–69.

Waxler-Morrison, N., J. M. Anderson, E. Richardson, and N. A. Chambers. *Cross-cultural Caring: A Handbook for Health Professionals.* 2nd ed. Vancouver, BC: University of British Columbia Press, 2005.

Weber, C. "Update on Antimicrobial Resistance." *Dermatology Nursing* 18 (2006): 15–19.

Weigel, L. M., D. B. Clewell, S. R. Gill, N. C. Clark, L. K. McDougal, S. E. Flannagan, J. F. Kolonay, J. Shetty, G. E. Killgore, and F. C. Tenover. "Genetic Analysis of a High-level Vancomycin-resistant Isolate of *Staphylococcus aureus*". *Science* 302, no. 5650 (2003): 1569–71.

Weinstein, R. A. "Controlling Antimicrobial Resistance in Hospitals: Infection Control and Use of Antibiotics." *Emerging Infectious Diseases* 7, no. 2 (2001): 188–92.

Wenzel, R. "The Antibiotic Pipeline—Challenges, Costs and Values." *New England Journal of Medicine* 351 (2004): 523–26.

Wilkins, K., and S. G. Mackenzie. *Work Injuries.* Ottawa, ON: Statistics, November, 2008.

Canada. Retrieved December 14, 2013. http://www.statcan.gc.ca/pub/82-003-x/2006007/article/10191-eng.htm.

White, J. "The Prevention of Eating Disorders: A Review of the Research on Risk Factors with Implications for Practice." *Journal of Child and Adolescent Psychiatric Nursing* 13, no. 2 (April 2000): 28–35.

Wolf, N. *The Beauty Myth.* Toronto, ON: Vintage Books.op, 1990.

Wopfner, N., G. Gadermaier, M. Egger, R. Asero, C. Ebner, B. Jahn-Schmid, and F. Ferreira. "The Spectrum of Allergens in Ragweed and Mugwort Pollen." *International Archives of Allergy and Immunology* 138, no. 4 (2005): 337–46. doi:10.1159/000089188.

World Health Organization (WHO). *Anti-tuberculosis Drug Resistance in the World. Report 3 of the WHO/IUATLD Global Project on Anti-Tuberculosis Drug Resistance Surveillance.* Geneva, Switzerland: Author, 2003.

———. "Communicable Diseases 2000: Highlights of Activities in 1999 and Major Challenges for the Future." 2000a. Accessed April 16, 2011. http://www.who.int/infectious-disease-news/CDS2000/PDF/cd2000.pdf.

———. *Communicable Diseases: Highlights of Communicable Disease Activities, Major Recent Achievements.* Switzerland, Geneva: Author, 2009a. Accessed May 18, 2011. http://www.searo.who.int/EN/Section10.htm.

———. *Confirmed Human Cases of Avian Influenza A (H5N1).* Geneva, Switzerland: Author, 2008. Accessed May 20, 2011. http://www.int/scr/disease/avian_influenza/country/en.

———. *Fact Sheet. HIV, TB, and Malaria: Three Major Infectious Disease Threats. Back 001.* Geneva, Switzerland: Author, 2000b. Accessed May 18, 2011. http://www.who.int/inf-fs/en/back001.

———. *Fact Sheet. Tuberculosis F-S 104.* Geneva, Switzerland: Author, 2000c. Accessed May 18, 2011. http://www.who.int/inf-fsfact104.

———. *Five Keys to Safer Food.* Geneva, Switzerland: Author, 2009b. Accessed May 19, 2011. http://www.int/foodsafety/consumer/5keys/en/.

———. "International Health Regulations, 2010a. Geneva, Switzerland: Author, 2010b. Accessed April 16, 2011. http://www.who.int.csr.ish/en.

———. *International Statistical Classification of Disease and Related Health Problems.* 2nd ed., 10th revision. Geneva, Switzerland: WHO, 2004a.

———. *Multidrug Resistant—Tuberculosis (MDR-TB). October 2013 Update (GTB No. 17).* Geneva, Switzerland: Author, October, 2013a. Accessed December 17, 2013. http://www.who.int/tb/challenges/mdr/mdr_tb_factsheet.pdf.

———. *NCD Country Profiles, 2011. Canada.* Geneva, Switzerland: Author, 2011a. Accessed December 17, 2013. http://www.who.int/nmh/countries/can_en.pdf.

———. *Neurological Disorders: Public Health Challenges.* Geneva, Switzerland: WHO, 2006. Accessed December 13, 2013. http://www.who.int/mental_health/neurology/neurodiso/en/.

———. *Obesity and Overweight.* Geneva, Switzerland: Author, 2013b. Accessed December 19, 2013. http://www.who.int/mediacentre/factsheets/fs311/en/.

———. *Report of a Technical Consultancy to Review the Role of Parasitologic Diagnosis to Support Malaria Disease Management: Focus on Use of RDT in Areas of High Transmission Deploying ACT.* Geneva, Switzerland: Author, 2004b.

———. *Report of the Director General. 1998 World Health Report: Health in the 21st Century. A Vision for All.* Geneva, Switzerland: Author, 1998.

————. *Schistosomiasis.* Geneva, Switzerland: Author, 2014. Accessed October 21, 2015. http://www.who.int/schistosomiasis/en/.

————. "WHO Mortality Data." Geneva, Switzerland: Author, 2010b. Accessed April 16, 2011. http://www.who.int.who.sis.mort.en.

————. *World Health Organization, World Health Report 2001: Mental Health: New Understanding, New Hope.* Geneva, Switzerland: WHO, 2004c.

————. *World Health Statistics 2011.* Geneva, Switzerland: Author. June, 2011b. ISBN 978-92-4-156419 9.

World Health Organization and UNICEF. *World Malaria Report, 2005.* Geneva, Switzerland: Author, 2005.

World Health Organization (WHO) World Mental Health Survey Consortium. "Prevalence, Severity, and Unmet Need for Treatment of Mental Disorders in the World Health Organization World Mental Health Survey." *JAMA* 291 (2004) 2581–90.

Worldwatch Institutes. *Obesity Epidemic Threatens Health in Exercise Deprived Societies.* Worldwatch Issue Alert. Washington, DC: Author, 2000. Accessed May 6, 2011. http://www.worldwatch.org/charimain/issue.

Young, T. "Review of Research on Aboriginal Populations in Canada: Relevance to Their Health Needs." *British Medical Journal* 327 (2003): 419–22.

Young, T., J. Reading, B. Elias, and J. D. O'Neil. "Type 2 Diabetes Mellitus in Canada's First Nations: Status of an Epidemic in Progress." *Canadian Medical Association Journal* 163, no. 5 (2000): 127–29.

Zinderman, C. E., B. Conner, M. A. Malakooti, J. E. LaMar, A. Armstrong, and B. K. Bohnker. "Community Acquired Methicillin-resistant *Staphylococcus aureus* among Military Recruits." *Emerging Infectious Diseases* 10, no. 5 (2004): 941–49.

Zinner, S. H. "The Search for New Antimicrobials: Why We Need New Options." *Expert Review of Antimicrobial and Infectious Therapies* 3 (2005): 907–13.

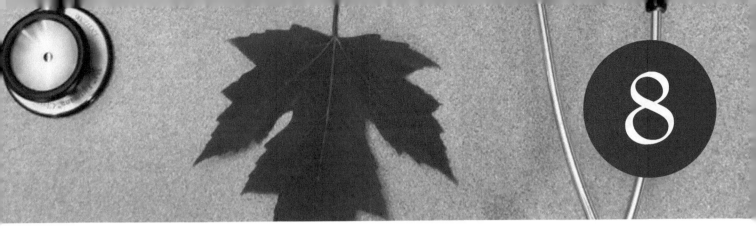

Environmental and Occupation Health and Safety

Health is not a single lineal destination. It is a dynamic and complex interactive journey through one's physical, biochemical, social-political, cultural and spiritual environments.

—Wally J. Bartfay (2011)

Learning Objectives

After completion of this chapter, the student will be able to:

- Define the terms environmental health, occupational health, and toxicology,
- Describe the scope of environmental and occupational health and safety as a key determinant of public health practice and research in Canada and abroad,
- Explain the interdependence between human health and the health of global ecosystems,
- List and describe potential social, cultural, and political determinants affecting one's living and work environments and their impact on health,
- Explain the current and predicted outcomes of global warming and climate change on the environment and threats to the health and safety of individuals, families, communities, and entire nations,
- List and describe actual or potential environmental and occupational health hazards,
- Describe the importance of maintaining a safe and healthy work environment for the preservation and promotion of the health of workers in Canada,
- Describe the role of public health professionals and workers for planning and implementation strategies which seek to promote and/or preserve health via environmental/occupational influences, and
- Identify and describe current barriers and challenges for preserving and maintaining healthy environments in Canada and abroad.

Core Competencies addressed in Chapter 8

Core Competencies	Competency Statements
1.0 Public Health Sciences	1.1, 1.2, 1.4
2.0 Assessment and Analysis	2.1, 2.2, 2.3, 2.4, 2.5, 2.6
3.0 Policy and Program Planning, Implementation, and Evaluation	3.1, 3.6, 3.7, 3.8
4.0 Partnerships, Collaboration, and Advocacy	4.1, 4.2, 4.3, 4.4
5.0 Diversity and Inclusiveness	5.1, 5.2
6.0 Communication	6.2, 6.3
7.0 Leadership	7.1, 7.2, 7.3, 7.5, 7.6

Note: Please see the following document or web-based link for a detailed description of these specific competencies. Public Health Agency of Canada (2007).

Introduction

The environment is a complex and dynamic system of living organisms and natural processes, and within which the human species is just one of many living organisms in the web of life and nature. Although, we are a species that have a disproportionate magnitude of negative ripple effects on the environment and on our health and well-being globally. Our *environment* is more than one's physical or geographical location, but is currently regarded as a critical social determinant of health that consists of interdependent and interconnected components of one's physical, biochemical, social-political, cultural, and spiritual milieus and situations (Bartfay and Bartfay 2015). If we support the view that the environment is a critical social determinant of health (Commission on the Social Determinants of Health, World Health Organization 2008; Raphael 2009), then one's work or living environments are mutually interdependent and inseparable and cannot be divided or examined by artificial boundaries.

Environmental health is defined as a branch of public health which examines both positive and negative factors and influences on the environment and ecosystems on human health (Bartfay and Bartfay 2015). Environmental health is also the study of the ecosystems in which we live in and the impact of science and technology to use energy sources (e.g., fossil and nuclear) to transform raw materials into commercial goods and their by-products. A growing body of research in recent years had greatly added to our understanding of how the environment can protect and sustain life or contribute to disability, suffering, and/or premature death.

For example, on October 4, 2010, a toxic sludge dam burst from the Ajkai Timfodgyar

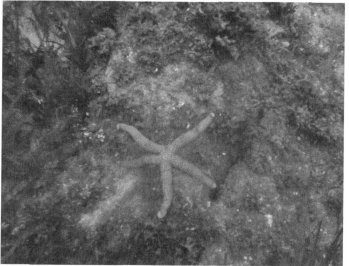

Source: Photo by Wally J. Bartfay

Photo 8.1 The environment is now recognized as a critical social determinant of health in Canada and globally. The Great Barrier Reef in Australia is approximately 2300 kilometres in length and supports over 1500 species of fish, 400 species of coral and 4000 species of molluscs just to name a few. Due to climate change and global warming, coral in the reef is slowing dying.

aluminum plant reservoir in the Veszprém County located in western Hungary, and released approximately 35.3 million cubic feet of toxic red sludge (Enserink 2010; Gura 2010; Murphy 2010; The Sofia Echo Staff 2010). The toxic sludge was released as a 1–2 m wave which was powerful enough to move cars in its path, flooding several nearby localities, and at least 9 people were killed and 122 were injured as a consequence of this *regionalized environmental disaster*. Analysis of the toxic red sludge showed that it contained levels of chromium at 660 mg/kg, arsenic at 110 mg/kg, and mercury at 1.2 mg/kg (The Independent 2010). The characteristic red colour of the mud originated from hydrated iron (III) oxide (ferrihydrite), which was a main component of the sludge.

According to Murphy (2010), more than 120 individuals were injured as a result of this ecological disaster in Hungary, and it also affected the surrounding countries because the toxic sludge leaked into the Danube River and other critical water supplies. Several surrounding towns were engulfed in 35.3 million cubic feet of red toxic sludge when the reservoir burst and several victims had chemical burns when they came into contact with this toxic spill. Although several hundred tonnes of plaster were poured into the Marcal River in an attempt to stop the flow of the red toxic sludge, it eventually entered the Danube River and other water supplies in surrounding districts and countries (Murphy 2010). In fact, the chemicals present in the toxic spill extinguished all life (e.g., fish, water birds, frogs) in the Marcal River and the toxic sludge reached the Danube River on October 7, 2010, despite efforts by local authorities to contain the spill. This prompted countries such as Slovakia, Croatia and Serbia, Romania, Bulgaria and the Ukraine to develop public emergency plans in response to this environmental disaster in Hungary. Hence, a single chemical spill can have wide-spread negative environmental ripple effects and pose a potential health risk for all exposed individuals well beyond the area where the environmental disaster transcribed.

If we accept the notion that humans are living beings who subsist, live, and work in a variety of interconnected and interdependent environments; then we must also examine the impact of the environment as a critical social determinant of health from the holistic care perspective (Bartfay and Bartfay 2015). This is also critical in terms of evidence-informed public health (EIPH) practice in a variety of environmental contexts and/or occupational health settings. The reader is referred to Chapter 1 for detailed discussions on EIPH; the social determinants of health, and the holistic care paradigm.

In this chapter, we shall explore the impact of various environmental factors and influences on the health of individuals in Canada and globally. We shall also examine the importance of occupational work environments in terms of preserving and promoting the health and safety of workers. Selected historical and recent examples are utilized to reinforce salient environmentally and occupationally linked concepts and themes of relevance to public health in this chapter.

As a branch or component of public health, the fields of environmental and occupation health are not only concerned with the health and well-being of individuals, but also the health of families, groups, communities, and/or entire populations. This perspective encompasses a broad range of potential environmental/occupational hazards including chemical and physical toxicants, to biological agents of infectious disease, and interactions with genetic and social factors (Bartfay and Bartfay 2015). Environmental and occupational risk assessments are critical for preserving the health and well-being of residents in Canada and those abroad. Indeed, the negative ripple effects of a so-called "regionalized environmental disaster" can quickly spread and affect adjacent communities or even nations.

A growing body of research in recent decades has greatly added to our understanding of how the environment can either sustain and protect human life and health; or contribute to disability, morbidity, or premature death and decreased quality of life (Bartfay and Bartfay 2015; Schubert and Bartfay 2010). Griffiths and Stewart (2009) argue that climate change is the most important public health challenge of the twenty-first century because it threatens the basic elements of our existence. These elements include the availability and quality of our food supplies, the air we breathe, and quality of our water supplies. In addition, climate changes during the past decades have resulted in increased temperature associated morbidity and mortalities globally; increased the magnitude and frequency of severe weather-related natural events (e.g., severe floods, hurricanes, droughts), and have changed the distribution and patterns of various diseases transmitted by mosquitoes, ticks, rodents, and various animals (CDC 2015). It is a public health priority to develop and implement effective strategies to minimize the damage already done, not only for our own health but that of future generations; especially given that the global population is predicted to rise to over 9 billion in 2050 (CDC 2015; Griffiths and Stewart 2009).

The relationship between the environment and human health has been known for centuries. For example, the Greek physician Hippocrates (460–377 BC) detailed his observations between various diseases and environmental conditions (e.g., water sources, swamps, air quality, and seasons) in his books *Epidemic I*, *Epidemic III*, and *On Airs, Waters and Places* (Aschengrau and Seage III 2003; Franco and Williams 2000; Gallin and Ognibene 2007; Jones 1923).

> Whoever wishes to investigate medicine properly should proceed thus; in the first place consider the season of the year, and what effects each of them produces…One should consider most attentively the waters which inhabitants use, whether they be marshy and soft, or hard and running… and the mode in which the inhabitants live, and what are their pursuits, whether they are fond of drinking and eating to excess, and given to indolence, or are fond of exercise and labor.
>
> (Hippocrates 1938, 19)

Also consistent with Hippocrates' belief that air is a critical factor in diseases is seen in the origin of the term "malaria" or bad air, a disease which we currently know is transmitted by certain female mosquitoes that breed in standing pools of water.

According to Naidoo and Wills (2000), the impact of modern medicine in reducing global mortality and morbidity has been minor in comparison to the major impact of improved environmental conditions, such as clean and safe water supplies and improvements in sanitation. It is estimated that approximately 75% of "good health" is the result of factors that are beyond direct episodic health care services received in acute care facilities (National Expert Commission Canadian Nurses Association 2012; Standing Senate Committee on Social Affairs, Science and Technology, Subcommittee on Population Health 2009). For example, it has been estimated that only 5 of 30 years in life expectancy increases during the past century can been directly attributed to curing agents such as antibiotics (Bunker, Frazier, and Mosteller 1994); whereas the vast majority are due to the improvements in living conditions, improved nutrition, water quality, and sanitation (Bartfay and Bartfay 2015; Schubert and Bartfay 2010).

There is a growing body of research that indicates that environmental changes triggered by human activities and technology (e.g., use of fossil fuels, chemical by-products, nuclear waste) during the past few decades have profoundly changed our planet and are threatening the health and very existence of all living organisms worldwide (Maxwell 2009; Merrill 2008; Schubert and Bartfay 2010). A growing awareness of the importance for protecting our environment by both children and adults and the negative effects of climate change has increased via popular culture, the mass media (e.g., news broadcasts, television, radio, newspapers), and social medias (e.g., Twitter, Facebook, YouTube) during the past few decades.

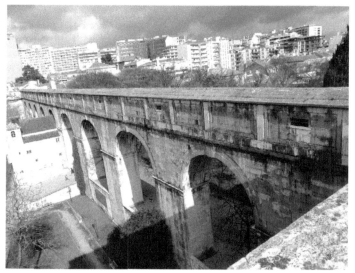

Source: Wally J. Bartfay

Photo 8.2 The Mãe d'Áqya das Amoreiras covered aqueduct was built during the eighteenth century, and continues to bring critical fresh drinking water to a large portion of the City of Lisbon, Portugal. Currently, it is widely known that polluted water supplies are associated with several types of waterborne infections including cholera, campylobacteriosis, typhoid fever, and cryptosporidiosis.

Group Activity-Based Learning Box 8.1

Environmental Factors or Issues in Your Community

It is designed to stimulate classroom discussion and debates related to current environmental factors or issues in your community, and the role of public health. Working in small groups of three to five students, discuss and answer the following questions:

1. What are some of the current environmental factors or issues affecting your community or region?

2. How may these environmental factors or issues affect the health and well-being of residents of your community?

3. What public health efforts are currently in place to help individuals, families, or groups manage these environmental factors or issues?

4. How can published environmental research be better utilized to promote the health and well-being of residents in your community or region?

For example, the publication of the children's classic *The Lorax* by Dr. Seuss (1971) was instrumental in bringing environmental awareness to the negative ripple effects associated with clear cutting forests and industrial pollution to children and adults alike. The book's significance and warnings related to the perils of unsustainable development and its negative effects on human health and ecosystems remain relevant to this very day (Marris 2011; Morgan and Morgan 1985). This children's environmental book continues to generate wide discussions and debate related to industrialization, clear cutting forestry practices and their impact on ecosystems globally (Time 1989). For example, the line in *The Lorax*, "*I hear things are just as bad up in Lake Erie*" was subsequently removed more than 14 years after the story was first published after research associates from the Ohio Sea Grant Program wrote to Dr. Seuss about their environmental clean-up efforts undertaken for Lake Erie (Morgan and Morgan 1995). On April 7, 2010, Amnesty International USA noted in their blog that the story of *The Lorax* by Dr. Seuss (1971) "amazing*ly parallels that of the Dongria Kondh peoples of Orissa*" *in present day India* "*where Vedanta Corporation is wrecking the environment of the Dongria Kondh people*" (Acharya 2011).

What Is Global Warming and Climate Change?

Global warming is defined as the increase in the earth's overall temperature as a result of both human and natural causes including greenhouse gas emissions through carbon-based fuel combustion, industrial pollution, depletion of the protective ozone layer, deforestations, and volcanic emissions into the atmosphere (Bartfay and Bartfay 2015). *Climate change* is defined as significant and dramatic changes in the frequency, intensity, spatial extent, duration, timing of extreme weather (e.g., hurricanes, tornadoes), and climate-associated events (e.g., draught, ice storms, flooding), which can result in unprecedented extreme weather and climatic events that threaten human societies, infrastructures, health, and human survival (Bartfay and Bartfay 2015).

For example, hurricane Sandy in 2012 was described as a "superstorm" which had furious winds of over 100 km/h and was over 1,600 km in diameter, which is larger than the province of Ontario in width (Freeman 2012). As of November 1, 2012 the death toll associated with hurricane Sandy was 74 in the United States, and 2 deaths in Ontario including a woman who was hit by a Staples commercial outlet sign and a hydroelectric worker in Sarnia (Cortez 2012; The Associated Press 2012). The economic costs associated with hurricane Sandy includes the loss of property and damage to infrastructures (e.g., bridges, roads, sewers, gas lines) and lost wages combined was estimated to be between \$50 and \$60 billion (US) (Rugaber and Crustsinger 2012). Approximately 6.5 million residents in the United States were without power including 4 million in the states of New York and Jersey. At the height of the storm in Ontario, nearly 150,000 customers were without power (Cortez 2012; Freeman 2012). Hurricane Sandy also resulted in massive flooding in several coastal regions in the United States. Massive flooding also struck the country of Haiti and health officials were worried about a possible cholera outbreak in early November, 2012 resulting from this single extreme weather event. Hence, a single climatic event such as hurricane Sandy can have significant negative ripple effects over large geographical areas, which includes the loss or damage to property and infrastructure (e.g., homes, businesses, bridges, sea walls),

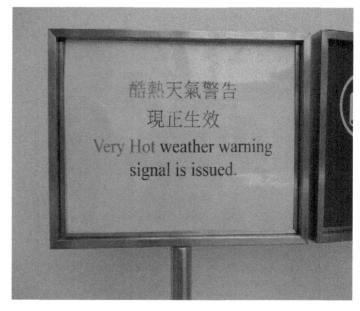

Source: Wally J. Bartfay

Photo 8.3 An extreme weather warning sign posted by public health officials in Hong Kong.

lost wages, mental distress and anxiety, health and safety issues (e.g., broken gas lines, contaminated water supplies), and mortality.

Shepherd Marshall and Knox (2012) note that the *United Nations Intergovernmental Panel on Climate Change* and other scientific reports suggest that the intensity of hurricanes (aka tropical cyclones) will increase over the next few decades due to the warming of sea waters linked to global warming. In fact, the surface temperature along the east cost of the United States is approximately 2.8°C above average, which helped to intensify hurricane Sandy. Moreover, the sea levels along these cost lines are rising up to four times faster than the global average, making this region of the world more vulnerable to severe storms and associated flooding (Reguly 2015; Shepherd Marshall and Knox 2012). For example, the Maldives are composed of approximated 1,200 islands located off the south-west coast of India. The Maldives realized that something was terribly wrong as far back in 1987 when tidal waves inundated their capital city of Malé (Ruguly 2015). Islanders fear that the atoll may slip beneath the waves due to rising sea levels linked to global warming and climate change. Indeed, more than 80% of the total land area for the islands of the Maldives lie less than 1 m above sea level (Ruguly 2015).

Canada alone produces approximately 700 megatonnes of greenhouse gases per year, and the average Canadian produces approximately four times the global average level of emissions or 23.6 tonnes per person per year (David Suzuki Foundation, n.d.). Merrill (2008) reports that measures of carbon dioxide (CO_2) begun in the year 1957 and since that time 7.1 gigatonnes of CO_2 are released into the atmosphere each year by human activities, and 3.2 gigatonnes remain in the atmosphere.

Greenhouse Effect

The *greenhouse effect* is defined as the trapping of infrared radiation from the earth by greenhouse gases in the earth's atmosphere, which results in the warming of the surface temperature of the earth (Bartfay and Bartfay 2015). The collective effects of these natural and human causes have resulted in a 0.6°C–0.8°C increase in the earth's temperature over the past century, with approximately half of this noted increase occurring during the past 25–30 years (Brohan et al. 2006; Dai 2006; Haines, McMichael, and Epstein 2006; International Panel on Climate Change 2005). Based on numerous computer-based climate models, it is predicted that the average temperature of the earth could rise an additional 1.5°C–5.8°C (International Panel on Climate Change 2005; Merrill 2008). Borenstein (2011a) reports that massive amounts of greenhouse gases trapped below the thawing permafrost in the Arctic will likely seep into the air over the next three decades, accelerating and amplifying global warming.

Computer models predict that these heat-trapped gases under the Arctic may, in fact, be a bigger contributor to global warming than the cutting down of forests. It is predicted that over the next 30 years, approximately 45 billion metric tonnes of carbon from the gases methane and CO_2 will be swept into the atmosphere during summer thaws. Comparatively, this is equivalent to the amount of heat-trapping gases spewed by burning fossil fuels such as coal and gas during a 5-year period combined. If we take this Arctic thawing effect into consideration, it is predicted that global warm-

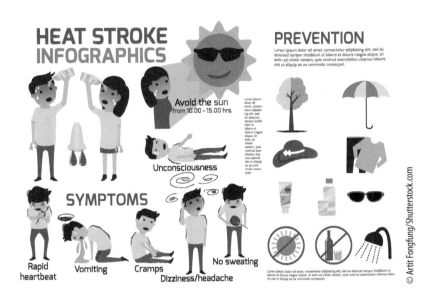

Photo 8.4 Common signs and symptoms of heat stroke. Climate change and global warming are increasingly being associated with negative health consequences and outcomes.

ing will be accelerated by 20%–30%, in comparison to fossil fuel emissions alone. When the panel of climate scientists issued their last comprehensive report on global warming in 2007, they did not factor in trapped methane and CO_2 from beneath the permafrost (Borenstein 2011a).

According to a recent report released by the United Nations and the World Meteorological Organization, which is based on an international panel of climate experts who met in November 2011; extreme weather is predicted to overwhelm many countries of the world including developed northern regions such as Canada and make certain regions unlivable (Borenstein 2011a). It is notable that more than 95% of fatalities associated with global warming and climate changes since the 1970s have been in the developing regions of the world, and the economic losses are predicted at over $200 billion a year. The report predicts that heat waves, for example, used to occur approximately every 20 years during the past mid-century will occur every 5 years by the end of the current century.

For example, in January, 2013 a heat wave hit the continent of Australia and record breaking temperatures that reached 52°C and more were recorded. Extreme temperatures such as these threaten the health and safety of all individuals especially those with heart or respiratory conditions, young infants and children, and the elderly. Moreover, there is at least a two-in-three chance that heavy downpours will increase, both in the tropics and northern regions, and from tropical cyclones. In some developed northern regions of the world, such as Canada, Russia, and Greenland, coastal cities will be increasingly vulnerable because of weather extremes and rises in the sea level attributed to human activities (Borenstein 2011b).

International Frameworks and Protocols for Climate Change

The ozone layer can be damaged when synthetic chemicals such as halons and chlorofluorocarbons (CFCs) are released into the atmosphere and react with the ozone in the presence of sunlight (Schubert and Bartfay 2010; World Meteorological Organization 2006). In 1987, an international treaty known as the *Montréal Protocol on Substances That Deplete the Ozone Layer* was signed by delegates at a conference in Montréal, Québec to protect the ozone layer by stopping the emission of halocarbon gases and other harmful substances. It has been estimated that without the Montréal protocol in place, ozone depletion associated with CFCs alone would be approximately tenfold greater by 2050, in comparison to 1987 levels (Gindi 1992; United Nations Environmental Programme 2002; World Meteorological Organization 2006). In 1998, Canada also established the *Ozone-Depleting Substances Regulations*, which regulate the manufacturing, transport, import, and export of known ozone-depleting substances (Bartfay and Bartfay 2015; Schubert and Bartfay 2010). Other Canadian initiatives include the conservation, recovery, and recycling of ozone-depleting chemicals (Environment Canada 1996, 2000; Shah 2003).

In 1992, delegates from 154 nations met in Rio de Janeiro, Brazil at the United Nations Conference on Environment and Development to discuss growing international concerns related to global warming and climate change (Merrill 2008; United Nations Framework Convention on Climate Change 2006a, 2006b). Delegates at the conference acknowledged that climate change was affected by human activities globally and influenced by each country collectively, as detailed in the treaty known as the *United Nations Framework Convention on Climate Change*.

On December 11, 1997, delegates from the United Nations met once again to discuss global warming and climate change in Kyoto, Japan. During this international conference, the *Kyoto Protocol* was formulated, which sets standards and targets for decreasing greenhouse emissions among the countries that ratified the protocol. The Kyoto Protocol (1997) is

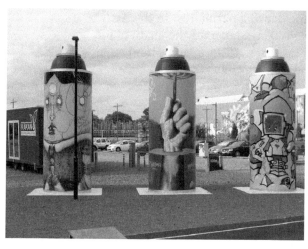

Source: Photo by Wally J. Bartfay

Photo 8.5 Aerosol cans, refrigerators, and air-conditioning units containing CFC's have now been banned. Chlorofluorocarbons (CFCs) are fully halogenated paraffin hydrocarbons that contain only carbon, chlorine, and fluorine, produced as volatile derivative of methane, ethane, and propane. Because CFCs contribute to ozone depletion in the upper atmosphere, the manufacture of such compounds has been phased out under the Montreal Protocol.

an example of a multilateral agreement that set forth international policies to help limit and reduce greenhouse gas emissions by several developed and industrialized nations (Friis 2012; United Nations Framework Convention on Climate Change 2006a, 2006b). By February 2005, 141 nations had ratified the Kyoto Protocol (The Woods Hole Research Center, n.d.). Currently, 165 nations have ratified the Kyoto Protocol (United Nations Framework Convention on Climate Change 2006b).

It is noteworthy that the United States, the world's current leading producer of CO_2, withdrew its support in 2001 under George W. Bush's administration. Bush's rationale for withdrawing his country's support for the Kyoto Protocol was that it was too costly from an economic perspective and that the science behind global warming was questionable and flawed in nature (Merril 2008). In addition to the United States, Australia has also declined to support the tenets of the Kyoto Protocol. Unfortunately, in December 2011, Canada announced that it would not resign the Kyoto accord under the Harper government due to concerns about the stability and recovery of the economy following the 2008–2009 global economic recession.

In 2009, delegates from 192 countries assembled in Copenhagen, Denmark with the goal of reaching a new international agreement to deal with global warming (The Guardian 2010; World Business Council for Sustainable Development 2010). Delegates at this international meeting proposed in an agreement known as the *Copenhagen Accord* that any increase in global temperatures between the years 2010 and 2050 should be kept to less than 2°C. It is not surprising that this agreement was not opposed by many countries, including developing nations, because it was not deemed legally binding in nature. Nonetheless, this international conference has resulted in positive ripple effects in terms of increasing the awareness of the general public globally related to the need to manage and control greenhouse gases and associated predicted negative environmental, economic, political, and health consequences.

During the December, 2012 emission talks in Doha, Qatar, it was reported that 38.2 billion tonnes of CO_2 (or approximately 1.1 million kilograms released every second) were being released into the atmosphere by all the world's nations combined annually from the burning of fossil fuels such as coal and oil (Ritter 2012). According to the reports by the Global Carbon Project, worldwide CO_2 levels are 54% higher currently, in comparison to 1990 baseline values. Of the planets top polluters, Germany and the United States were the only countries that reduced their emissions in 2011; whereas Canada increased emissions by 2%. Developing nations such as China argue that they must be allowed to increase its emissions as their economy expands, lifting millions of individuals out of poverty (Ritter 2012).

On December 12, 2015, the United Nations (2015) announced that 195 countries have agreed to adopt the 31 page *Paris Agreement* on climate change. The Paris Agreement consists of five key points which requires countries to fulfil their national carbon-reduction plans they submitted prior to the commence of the conference, and calls for 5 year reviews of the plants to keep countries obligated and on track (Reguly 2015; United Nations 2015; Walters 2015). The first point is to limit global temperature increases to "well below" 2°C, while pursing efforts to limit temperature increases to preindustrial levels of 1.5°C. Second, the Paris Agreement is

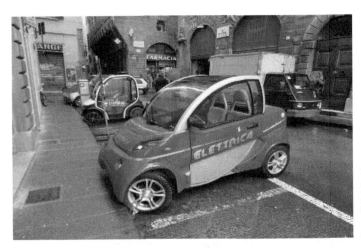

Source: Wally J. Bartfay

Photo 8.6 Electric cars lined-up at a charging station in Florence, Italy. In an attempt to help decrease greenhouse emissions, several automobile manufacturers have already developed more efficient and environmentally friendly electric and hybrid (gas and electric) cars.

considered the world's first universal climate agreement, which includes both developed and developing nations. Previous emission treaties, such as the 1997 Kyoto Protocol, only included wealthy developed nations. The third point involves helping the poorer developing nations. Specifically, developed nations will provide $100 billion (US) annually to developing nations by 2020 to help combat climate change and foster the development of greener economies. The fourth point involves publishing individual greenhouse gas reduction targets for each committed country. Countries will be tasked with preparing, maintaining, and publishing their own greenhouse gas reduction targets, which shall be reviewed and revised every 5 years. This is perhaps the most controversial point because there are no quality assurance checks and balances to ensure that countries such as China and India, are in fact, reporting accurate figures. The fifth point seeks to obtain a carbon neutral world by 2050. Specifically, the accord sets the goals of a carbon neutral planet sometime after the year 2050, but before 2100. This means a commitment to limiting the amount of greenhouse gases emitted by human activities globally to levels that can be absorbed naturally by trees, vegetation, soils, and the oceans.

In an attempt to help decrease greenhouse emissions, several major automobile manufacturer's in developed nations such as Canada, the United States, Japan, and Germany have already developed more efficient electric and hybrid (gas and electric) cars. In addition, provincial governments such as those in the province of Ontario are requiring that all cars and light trucks meet current provincial emission standards in order to be licensed for operation (Bartfay and Bartfay 2015). Municipalities in Canada are encouraging individuals to recycle and plant more trees, and researchers are developing new technologies to capture CO_2 for further use or sequestration. Additional innovations include polymer-metallic membranes used to separate out and capture CO_2 from industrial gas by-products; liquid absorbents or solid sorbents that trap CO_2 from mixed-gas streams and then release CO_2 into a separate gas stream; and refrigeration or liquefying separations that require cooling of gases to liquid followed by distillation (Merrill 2008).

How Does Global Warming and Climate Change Affect Human Health?

The World Health Organization reports that there are over 150,000 deaths annually associated with global climate change, and this number is expected to double by the year 2030 (Wilson 2007). A growing number of studies have linked global warming and climate change with adverse health effects including disruptions in food production and availability, illness, morbidity, and increased mortality associated with more extreme temperatures, flooding, severe storms, droughts, emergence and resurgence of a number of diseases, increases in the number and distribution of waterborne, foodborne, vector-borne, and rodent-borne diseases (Frumkin 2008; Maxwell 2009; Merrill 2008; Pascual et al. 2006; Schubert and Bartfay 2010; World Health Organization 2006).

For example, on August 25, 2005, hurricane Katrina hit the shores of the southern Louisiana coast and submerged parts of New Orleans under water. Hurricane Katrina was responsible for 1,836 deaths and an estimated $108 billion (2005, US) in damage to homes, property, and infrastructure (Freeman 2012; Merrill 2008). Public Safety and Emergency Preparedness Canada (2005) reports that the 2005 flood in Alberta attributed to global climate change, affected more than 14 communities; resulted in the need to evacuate more than 7,000 residents; severely damaged more than 4,000 homes, and resulted in the death of 2 victims of the flood.

Over the past decade, over 2.6 billion individuals in more than 45 countries worldwide have experienced negative health effects resulting from natural disasters and/or economic crisis (World Health Organization 2007a, 2014). Disasters are typically acute in nature, they occur suddenly and unexpectedly, and can be caused by human error, earthquakes, floods, fires, hurricanes, cyclones, volcanic eruptions, air crashes, biological hazards, food shortages, droughts, infectious diseases, and extreme weather conditions (Haddow, Bullock, and Coppola 2011; Landesman 2005, 2012). For example, the environmental conditions following natural disasters increase the risk for infectious diseases due to a lack of proper sanitation, an increase in exposure to waterborne agents and vectors like mosquitoes, infections resulting from wounds and injuries, and crowding due to a lack of proper housing or shelters (e.g., evacuation camps or shelters) (Centers for Disease Control and Prevention 2002, 2005; Guha-Sapir, Hargitt, and Hoyais 2004). According to Merrill (2008), in the year 2005 alone there were 156 episodes of extreme flooding globally that resulted in 8,000 deaths; approximately 18 million people were displaced from their homes, and almost $82 billion (US) in damage or loss of property. According to the Canadian Disaster Database, chemical and fuel spills, floods, snowstorms, and forest fires were the most common disasters reported in Canada over the past decade (Public Safety Canada 2013).

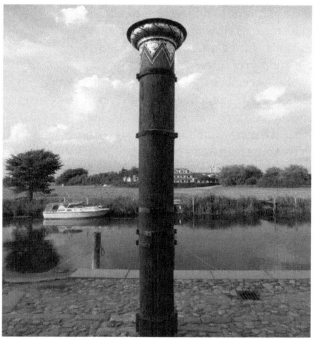

Source: Wally J. Bartfay

Photo 8.7 A flood pole in Ribe, Denmark marking major floods since 1672 (ring at the top of pole), which devastated homes, businesses and resulted in injuries, disabilities, and the loss of life in this low-lying European country. Denmark has subsequently built various flood levies and dikes which extend to neighbouring Netherlands.

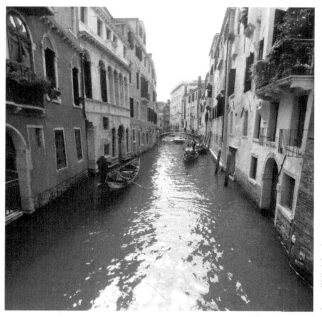

Source: Wally J. Bartfay

Photo 8.8 Flooding has been linked to global climate changes and the melting of polar ice caps and is a growing public health concern globally. The "acqua alta" flooding in Venice, Italy occurs annually and is associated with high water levels and tides in the northern Adriatic Sea. On February 12, 2013, flood water levels reached 143 cm in Venice.

Based on a recent report by the National Roundtable on the Environment and the Economy released in September, 2011, climate change will cost an estimated $5 billion a year by 2020 and will continue to climb steeply to between $21 billion and $43 billion per year to 2050 (Scoffield 2011a, 2011b). This report is the first attempt to put a price tag on the impact of climate change in Canada, and is based on the assumption that our planet will be able to contain global warming to about 2°C until 2050.

By 2050, the effects of global climate change will result in warmer weather impacting our forests, increased forest fire risks and pests especially in the western provinces, and will cost the lumber industry between $2 billion and $17 billion a year in lost revenues. According to Scoffield (2011a, 2011b), flooding along the coasts in Canada and rising sea levels will cost us between $1 billion and $8 billion annually within the next four decades. The coasts of Prince Edward Island, Nunavut, and British Columbia are most vulnerable. Global warming will also have negative ripple effects in terms of health care costs. For example, the City of Toronto alone will see an increase in associated health care costs of between $3 million to $8 million by 2050. This report also predicts that global warming will lead to between 5 and 10 additional deaths per 100,000 residents in Canada per year by 2050 (Scoffield 2011a, 2011b).

Public Safety and Emergency Preparedness Legislation in Canada

Disasters, be they natural (e.g., flooding, forest fires, earthquakes, hurricanes, pandemics) or man-made (e.g., chemical spills, bombings, train derailments, bioterrorism), typically occur suddenly and with little or no warning. These events can often result in injury, disability, and/or mortality and can also leave communities or entire regions with long-term negative ripple effects including adverse environmental, socioeconomic, environmental, and/or health outcomes (Beach 2010; Haddow, Bullock, and Coppola 2011; Landesman 2005, 2012; Public Safety Canada 2013a; Rebmann, Carrico, and English 2008). An example of a natural disaster is the 2011 tornado that tore across the Huron country in Ontario. This tornado was rated a F3 tornado on the Fujita scale that was caused by a single supercell that killed 1 man in Goderich, Ontario, 37 were injured, 1,000 trees were destroyed, and an estimated $100 millions of damage were done to homes and businesses (McCabe 2011; Robins 2011). An example of a man-made disaster is the 2013 Lac-Mégantic train derailment that resulted in 6 million litres of volatile crude oil spilling-out into the environment that subsequently resulted in a massive explosion and fire in Québec. This single preventable man-made disaster resulted in the death of 42 residents, 5 missing individuals still, contamination of the surrounding environment with crude oil, and millions of dollars damage to homes and businesses (Chiasson 2015; Mackrael 2014).

Disaster preparedness at the local, provincial and territorial, and national levels helps to ensure support for public health authorities and organizations during and after the occurrence of a natural or man-made disaster. Emergency preparedness responses in Canada typically occur at the local or community level where municipalities have the first responsibility in managing the disaster. If their local expertise and resources are exceeded beyond their means or needs, then provincial/territorial and/or federal assistance are typically sought to deal with the specific disaster and its aftermath. Hence, emergency management preparedness plans are critical to successfully manage public health emergencies and disasters to engage and guide coordinated and comprehensive efforts by various levels of governments, nongovernmental and voluntary organizations (e.g., Red Cross), public health officials, and private agencies (Beach 2010; Haddow, Bullock, and Coppola 2011; Landesman 2005, 2012; Public Safety Canada 2013a; Rebmann, Carrico, and English 2008).

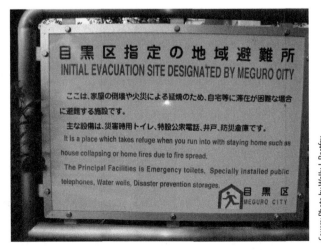

Source: Photo by Wally J. Bartfay

Photo 8.9 A civilian disaster evacuation sign in Meguro City, Japan. Emergency preparedness and disaster management are critical components of public health following disasters such as chemical spills, bioterrorism, earthquakes, tornadoes, floods, and tsunamis to name but a few.

There are three complementary federal legislations that deal with emergencies and emergency preparedness. The first is the *Emergencies Act,* which replaced the War Measures Act as the source of the federal government's authority to act during a national crisis or emergency to ensure the safety and security of all Canadians. This Emergencies Act defines a *national emergency* as

> an urgent and critical situation of a temporary nature that seriously endangers the lives, health or safety of Canadians and is of such proprotions or nature as to exceed the capacity of a province to deal with it, or seriously threatens the sovereignty, security and territorial integrity of Canada, and cannot be effectively dealt with under any other law of Canada. (Ministry of Justice 2014a, 8)

There are four categories of so-called "national emergencies": (a) public welfare emergencies (e.g., major natural disasters), (b) public order emergencies (e.g., serious national security treat), (c) international emergencies (e.g., acts of force or violence), and (d) a state of war (i.e., either active or imminent involving Canada and/or its allies).

The second legislation is the *Emergency Preparedness Act* which provides a basis for the planning and programming to deal with disasters, and addresses the need for cooperation between the provinces and territories and the federal government. This Act also addresses the need for public awareness, and provides a structure or legislative framework for the necessary training and education of public health professionals and workers and first responders to disasters and emergencies (Ministry of Justice 2014b).

The third federal legislation is the *Emergency Management Act* which defines the specific roles and responsibilities for all federal ministers, and provides direction for critical infrastructure protection which is a major challenge during a major disaster or national emergency (Ministry of Justice 2014c). This Act also replaces specific sections of the Emergency Preparedness Act and enhances and promotes communication and information exchange between various levels of government. Public Safety Canada (2013b) defines *critical infrastructures* as physical or information technology facilities, networks, services, and/or assets that are deemed vital and essential for the health, safety, or economic well-being of Canadians across the life span, and for the effective functioning of governments.

Emergency Management and Incident Management Systems

Emergency management is defined as a critical component of all public health systems in Canada and abroad which involves a diverse group of highly skilled professionals and government officials to protect the health and safety of the public at large during a crisis or emergency that requires immediate and coordinated action. Emergency management involves plans, institutional arrangements, and legislations (see the Emergency Management Acts above) to engage and guide governmental agencies, nongovernmental agencies (e.g., Red Cross), volunteers, and other agencies to deal with crisis and emergencies in an effort to attempt to avoid a massive disaster or catastrophe (Haddow, Bullock, and Coppola 2011; Landesman 2012). Emergency management consists of a process or life cycle of four main events (Beach 2010; Hogan 2007; Veenema 2013):

  i. Preventing or mitigating the effects of a crisis or emergency
  ii. Preparing for the event of an emergency, crisis or disaster
  iii. Responding to an emergency, crisis, or disaster to reduce its impact on the public at large
  iv. Recovering from an emergency, crisis, or disaster by assisting communities to return to normal

We argue that public health systems need to be properly funded and should have the needed highly skilled and trained health care professionals and workers to plan and deliver public health programs and emergency health care services during such events. In certain provinces in Canada, such as Ontario, emergency management programming is organized into the following five stages (Ontario Ministry of Health and Long-Term Care 2015):

i. *Prevention stage*: Involves activities undertaken to prevent or avoid a public health emergency or disaster (e.g., eradication of smallpox, treating, and monitoring community drinking water supplies).

ii. *Mitigation stage*: Involves actions undertaken to decrease or reduce the impact of an emergency, crisis, or disaster (e.g., infection control and prevention measures).

iii. *Preparedness*: Involves developing action plans and protocols to deal with various public emergencies, crisis, or disasters to enhance the effectiveness of responses and recovery activities (e.g., conducting training and mock disaster management drills).

iv. *Response*: Involves the actual undertaking of the planned and coordinated actions necessary to deal with the emergency, crisis, or disaster (e.g., acquisition and mobilization of health care professionals and equipment to the site).

v. *Recovery*: Involves activities that assist communities and individuals to recover from an emergency, crisis, or disaster and return to a state of normalcy (e.g., rebuilding critical infrastructures such as bridges and roads, administering ongoing treatments and care to the sick and injured).

The goal of all public health emergency preparedness programs is to enable and ensure a consistent, coordinated, and effective response to a public health emergency, crisis or disaster. Figure 8.1 shows the Public Health Preparedness and Response Competency Map developed by the Association of Schools and Programs of Public Health (2010).

The *Incident Management System (IMS)* is a standardized function-driven model employed throughout North America to manage and response to emergencies, crisis, and disasters, and provides the framework for all levels of government in Canada to develop emergency response plans regardless of the nature of the incident or its level of complexity. The basis IMS structure consists of five components: (a) command, (b) operations, (c) planning, (d) logistics, and (e) finance and administration. This structure and framework allows personnel to communicate directly

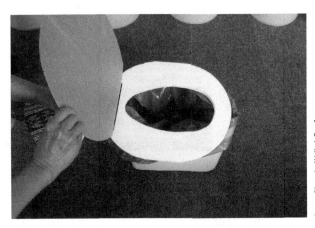

Source: Photo by Wally J. Bartfay

Photo 8.10 A disposable and portable toilet kit. Access to quick sanitation and disposal of waste products is critical following a disaster where water and santitation facilities may be damaged or compromised.

with other health care jurisdictions and other emergency response organizations in a coordinated manner to distribute medical and other supplies from federal and provincial stock piles to frontline health care professionals and workers (e.g., preparing for Pandemic Influenza in Manitoba plan, see http://www.gov.mb.ca/health/publichealth/pandemic.html). Similarly, the *Incident Command System (ICS)* is a management system that is employed by first responders for on-site emergencies and consists of a formalized command structure with specific areas of responsibility assigned to individuals as needed. The ICS typically consists of one incident commander (IC), who has centralized authority and decision making on-site, although there may be additional command staff as warranted by the specific emergency or crisis (e.g., media relations officer, safety officer) (Beach 2010; Hogan 2007). The IC overseas operations, planning, and logistics needed to meet the on-site needs.

Infectious Diseases

There is a growing body of evidence linking global warming and climate change to increased numbers of infectious diseases (Haines, McMichael, and Epstein 2006; Kovats et al. 2003; Merrill 2008). In 1998, which was one of the hottest years recorded in the past century on our planet, storms associated with El Niño (warming of the surface of the ocean off the western coast of South America) and hurricanes were abnormally frequent and intense, and which caused massive flooding, forest fires, and deforestation in affected regions. As

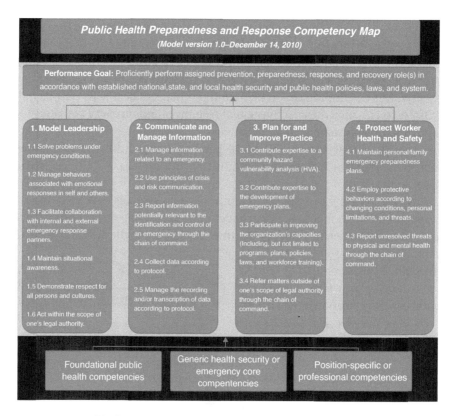

Figure 8.1 Public health preparedness and response competency map.

Source: Association of Schools and Programs of Public Health (2016).

a consequence of these intense storms, Indonesia and Brazil reported an epidemic of respiratory illnesses and Central America experienced a dramatic increase in the number of water and insert-borne diseases including malaria and cholera (Haines, McMichael, and Epstein 2006; Kovats et al. 2003; Merrill 2008).

Over the past two decades, deforestation rates have been estimated to range between 12 and to 16- million hectares per year, and forests have virtually disappeared in 25 countries (Frumkin 2005; Millennium Ecosystem Assessment 2005; Vajpeyi 2001). The ecosystems of forests are critical for managing the availability and spread of pathogens that can affect human health and well-being. For example, during 1997–1998 when Indonesia deforested 10 million hectares via burning, it directly affected 20 million residents and cost $9.3 billion in increased health care costs for residents of this nation and lost economic productivity (Merrill 2008). Indeed, deforestation can result in the decreased availability of medicinal plant sources and entire plant and animal species, which can result in ecological imbalances and the subsequent spread of infectious diseases such as Chagas disease, cholera, Lyme disease, malaria, meningitis, encephalitis, dengue fever, lymphatic filariasis, Schistosomiasis, and West Nile virus to name but a few (Frumkin 2005; Millennium Ecosystem Assessment 2005).

Deforestation also results in a loss of habit for certain species and predators, which causes a disruption in the food chain and increases the potential for the amount of disease-carrying prey. Small animals, for example, can carry a variety of diseases such as HIV-1, Junin virus, Marburg virus, and Lyme disease (Merrill 2008; Vajpeyi 2001). The negative ripple effects of deforestation on human health also have to be considered when considering all-inclusive holistic definitions of health and well-being (e.g., spiritual, emotional, physical, social, environmental). Hence, deforestation can negatively affect individuals, families, groups, or entire communities in Canada and abroad (Bartfay and Bartfay 2015).

As the surface temperature of our planet slowly continues to increase, infectious diseases transmitted by mosquitoes (e.g., dengue fever, encephalitis, yellow fever, malaria) are likely to migrate to more northern regions that were previously considered too cold for these insects to survive (Hodge, Anthony, and Longo 2002; Watson 2007). In fact, the West Nile virus was previously only found in warm temperate regions of the world (i.e., Northern Africa) and transmitted by infected female mosquitoes to birds and humans. The first case of West Nile virus was isolated in a woman living in the West Nile region of Uganda in 1937 (World Health Organization 2011). As a result of global warming and climate change, mosquitoes responsible for the transmission of the West Nile virus have migrated out of Africa into Europe, the United States, Canada, and other parts of the world.

The West Nile virus first appeared in Canada in 2001, and public health officials responded by including the surveillance of dead birds (e.g., crows, blue jays), mosquitoes, and affected humans (Quinlan and Dickinson 2009; Schubert and Bartfay 2010). One year later, Canadian public health officials documented the West Nile virus in Saskatchewan, Manitoba, Ontario, Québec, and Nova Scotia. In Canada, there are 74 known species of mosquitoes and the West Nile virus has been found to be present in 10 of these species (Ontario Ministry of Health and Long-Term Care 2012). The Public Health Agency of Canada (2006, 2012) reports that 1,300 human confirmed cases of West Nile virus were identified in 2003; 29 in 2004; 224 in 2005, and 421 cases and asymptomatic infections as of October, 2012.

Ozone Depletion and UV Radiation

Depletion of the protective stratospheric ozone layer results in higher levels of ultraviolet-B (UVB with wavelength of 290–320 nm) radiation reaching the earth's surface, which is associated with an increased risk for developing skin damage (e.g., actinic keratosis) and cancer, cataracts, and suppression of the body's immune system (Armstrong and Kricker 2001; McCarty 2002; Sleijiffers, Garssen and Van Loveren 2002; World Health Organization 2007b). The World Health Association (2007b) estimates that up to 20% of cataracts worldwide are attributable to exposure to UV radiation, and this number is likely to increase as a result of the depletion of the ozone layers. Moreover, increased exposure to UV radiation can suppress the functioning of the immune system in humans, making individuals more susceptible to infectious diseases (Maxwell 2009; Sleijffers, Garssen, and Van Loveren 2002).

The Environmental Protection Agency (EPA) (2006) reports that increases in UV radiation also adversely affect terrestrial and aquatic ecosystems (e.g., damage to plankton, fish, shrimp, crab, amphibians and other species) and biogeochemical cycles, which result in altering sources and sinks of greenhouse gases; and thus, negatively results in increases in atmospheric levels of greenhouse gases. In 1992, scientists from Environment Canada were the first to develop a method to predict the strength of the sun's UV rays based on day-to-day changes in the ozone layer. Canada became the first country to issue nationwide daily predictions of UV radiation levels, which first began in 1992. The UV index rating is now a common feature of daily weather forecasts in many developed nations around the world (Robinson Vollman, Anderson, and McFarlane 2004). Table 8.1 provides the reader with a description of the UV index rating, and recommended sun protection actions associated with each categorical ranking by public health professionals.

Air Quality and Pollution

Air is a mixture of a variety of gases that surrounds our planet and makes up our atmosphere, and comprises approximately 78% nitrogen and 21% oxygen by volume and a variety of other gases (e.g., CO_2, carbon monoxide, helium, argon) and water vapor

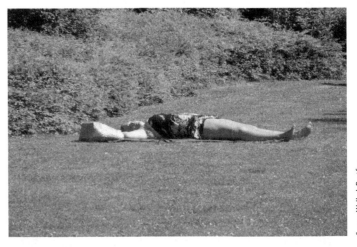

Source: Wally J. Bartfay

Photo 8.11 Despite public health campaigns warning against the hazards of excessive exposure to UV light sources from the sun and tanning salons, there remains a popular myth in Canada and internationally that a "glowing tan is healthy."

Table 8.1 UV Index Rating and Recommended Sun Protection Actions by Public Health Professionals

UV Index Category	Description of Risk Rating	Sun Protection Actions
0–2	Low	–Wear sunglasses and rimed hat on clear bright days –Use sunscreen (SPF 14+ with UVA and UVB sun protection) and cover-up if outdoors for more than 1 h
3–5	Moderate	–All actions for low risk apply here –Use sunscreen and cover-up if outdoors for more than 30 min –Try to stay in shaded areas near midday
6–7	High	–This UV rating may damage the skin and cause sunburn –All actions for moderate risk apply here –Limit direct exposure to the sun between 11 a.m. and 4 p.m.
8–10	Very high	–Extreme precautions should be taken with this UV rating as unprotected skin can quickly burn and be damaged –All actions for high risk apply here
11+	Extreme	–Unprotected skin may burn and become damaged in minutes –All actions for very high risk apply here –Avoid the outdoors unless absolutely necessary to be outside, especially between the hours of 11 a.m. and 4 p.m. and/or seek shaded areas whenever possible

(Bartfay and Bartfay 2015). The five most prominent or common pollutants in the air are carbon monoxide, sulphur oxides, nitrogen oxides, suspended particles, and hydrocarbons (Beckmann Murray et al. 2006; Maxwell 2009; Merrill 2008).

For example, Edwards (2001) notes that approximately two-thirds of Canadians surveyed report that air pollution has made their personal health worse, and approximately half have expressed concern about the air quality in their community. Similarly, researchers in Windsor, Ontario employed a time-stratified case-crossover design study to assess the relationship between ambient air pollution levels (i.e., increased levels of sulphur dioxide, nitrogen dioxide, and carbon monoxide) and visits to emergency departments by children aged 2–14 years of age (Lavigne, Villeneuve, and Cakmak 2012). Windsor is a city known for poor air quality. The researchers concluded that ambient air pollution significantly increased the risk of visits to emergency departments for treatment of asthma in children.

The Honourable Rona Ambrose, Canada's federal Minister for the Environment, stated that there were 53 smog advisory days in Ontario, 24 in Québec, and 3 in the Atlantic provinces during the summer of 2005 alone (Minister of Public Works and Government

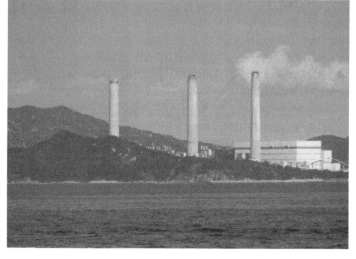

Source: Wally J. Bartfay

Photo 8.12 The effects of air pollution due to the burning of fossil fuels such as coal and its link to global warming, and the associated negative ripple effects on human health, are a growing public health concern in Canada and internationally.

Services Canada 2007). Moreover, there were 10 smog advisor issues in Québec and 5 in Ontario during the winter of 2005. According to Minister Ambrose, the direct and indirect costs associated with air pollution in the province of Ontario alone in 2005 were estimated to be $374 million due to lost productivity and work time; $507 million in pain and suffering, and a whopping $6.7 billion in social welfare costs associated with premature mortality (Minister of Public Works and Government Services Canada 2007).

Outdoor air contaminants include a variety of particles and fumes from industry, smoke from forest fires, dust from volcanoes, fungi, spores, and bacteria that may become airborne. Due to increased public awareness of these hazards, industry has begun to respond to these concerns (Bartfay and Bartfay 2015). For example, the oil and gas industry in Western Canada has taken measures to decrease and control emissions due to sour gas well flaring over the past two decades, which involves the burning of small amounts of natural gas that is found in the oil pumped from gas wells (Petroleum Communication Foundation 2000ab).

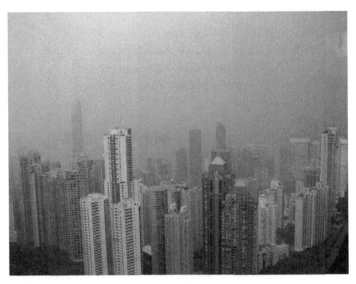

Source: Wally J. Bartfay

Photo 8.13 Heavy smog as seen from Victoria Peak in Hong Kong derived from mainland China. Smog is a mixture of air pollutants, nitrogen oxides, and various volatile organic compounds and sunlight that occurs with high temperatures and calm winds. In urban settings, at least 50% of precursors for smog are derived from cars, buses, trains, boats, and aircraft that use fossil fuels (e.g., gasoline, diesel), and the remaining 50% is often from industrial sources or natural sources (e.g., forest fires). Smog is a major public health concern that can result in respiratory distress, breathing difficulties, burning eyes, and a variety of respiratory diseases.

The potential adverse effects of air pollution on human health (e.g., lung disease, certain cancers) and on the environment (e.g., acid rain and global warming) are numerous. According to one report, the estimated number of cases of mortality directly associated with air pollution globally ranges from 200,000 to 570,000 per year (World Resources Institute 2010). Mann et al. (2002) reported that individuals with ischemic heart disease combined with arrhythmias or congestive heart failure had increased sensitivity to pollutants emitted from motor vehicles. Similarly, a group of Swedish researchers reported that vehicle exhaust emissions, especially NO_2, are associated with an increased risk of developing lung cancer (Nyberg et al. 2000).

Henderson et al. (1975) utilized census tracts in Los Angeles, California to examine the effects of air pollutants on lung cancer rates for these residents. The researchers aggregated the census tracts into 14 study areas that represented homogeneous air pollution profiles in the region. The study found a significant correlation between the geographical distribution of lung cancer cases and the general location of emission sources for noted hydrocarbons into the atmosphere. Similarly, Pope and associates (2002) utilized a prospective study to examine air pollution levels and mortality on approximately 500,000 adults who resided in metropolitan areas in the United States. The researchers found that exposure to fine particulate matter in the air over extended periods of time was a significant risk factor for both lung cancer and cardiopulmonary mortality.

Manfreda et al. (2001) investigated the variability of asthma-related manifestations and medication use in Vancouver, Winnipeg, Hamilton, Montréal, Halifax, and Prince Edward Island. The results of this pan-Canadian study showed that air quality was directly associated with the incidence of reported asthma and associated medication use in adults aged 20–40 years.

Canada's *National Ambient Air Quality Objectives* are dynamic national goals for improving outdoor air quality and reducing air pollution (Health Canada 1999; Schubert and Bartfay 2010). Accordingly, air quality is monitored by both federal and provincial/territorial governments in Canada. The *Air Quality Index*, which is also commonly referred to as the *Index of the Quality of Air,* has been developed to help inform the general public, public health care professionals and workers, and researchers of the prevailing air quality in their communities (Health Canada 1998). It is important to note that these aforementioned indexes do not measure the air quality per se, but only evaluate the presence or levels of certain airborne pollutants present (e.g., ozone, smog) (Bartfay and Bartfay 2015; Schubert and Bartfay 2010; Health Canada 1998, 1999).

Indoor contaminants (e.g., tobacco, molds and bacteria, cleaning products) can also pose health risk to Canadians either through their direct inhalation or indirectly through their effects on the environment. Young children, the elderly, and individuals with respiratory diseases (e.g., asthma, chronic obstructive pulmonary disease) are more susceptive to the negative effects of air pollution and/or smog in their environments (Bartfay and Bartfay 2015).

For example, passive smoking or exposure to second-hand smoke (e.g., in homes, taverns, restaurants or other public places) is a major indoor environmental pollutant that has been linked to negative health effects including lung cancer in adults and asthma among children (Perez 2004; Shields 2007). Statistics Canada (2011d) reports that the proportion of nonsmokers aged 12 and older who were regularly exposed to second-hand

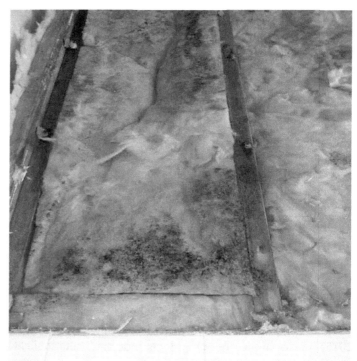

Source: Wally J. Bartfay

Photo 8.14 Black mold (aka *Stachybotrys*) in a home may be potentially toxic to humans via the production of mycotoxins, which may damage internal organs, result in respiratory problems, skin inflammations, nauseas, fatigue, and the suppression of the immune system.

smoke in home environments has steadily declined due to public awareness and public health promotion campaigns related to the negative health effects since 2003, and reached 5.9% in the year 2010. Young Canadians aged 12–19 made-up one-third of the 1.3 million nonsmokers who were regularly exposed to second-hand smoke at home. In 2010, 14.9% of young Canadians aged 12–19 were exposed to second smoke at home falling from 23.4% in 2003 to 15.5% (Statistics Canada 2011d).

There are a variety of air fresheners on the market in Canada and abroad which range from aerosol sprays, electronically programmable metered mist dispensers, and/or solid blocks from which potentially toxic chemicals may volatilized into the air of a home. Some air fresheners contain trace amounts of formaldehyde which can trigger asthmatic attacks and this chemical is also a known carcinogen to humans (e.g., nasopharyngeal cancer) (U.S. Environmental Protection Agency 2007a, 2007b; Arts, Rennen and De Heer 2006; Pinkerton, Hein, and Stayner 2004; Hester et al. 2003; International Agency for Research on Cancer, n.d.). Paradicholorobenzene is also found in some air fresheners and is a respiratory irritant that can also trigger an asthma attack (U.S. Agency for Toxic Substances and Disease Registry 2005). Moreover, paradicholorobenzene is a key ingredient present in moth balls along with naphthalene, which can damage red blood cells in vitro. Solid air fresheners are also a public health concern because they can be potentially fatal if eaten by a small child or family pet (Maxwell 2009; U.S. Environmental Protection Agency 2007a, 2007b).

Sick-Building Syndrome

Sick-building syndrome (SBS) was first recognized as a clinical condition in 1982 and has been a growing public health concern over the past few decades. In 1984, a report commissioned by the World Health Organization suggested that up to 30% of new and remodelled buildings worldwide may be linked to symptoms associated with SBS by workers and/or inhabitants (Burge 2004; Godish 2001; Martin-Gil et al. 1997; Murphy 2006; US Environmental Protection Agency 2010). These buildings affected may include places of business or work, schools, colleges and universities, libraries, community centres, private homes, apartments, hospitals, and long-term care facilities. The signs and symptoms associated with SBS may be localized to specific rooms or zones in a building, or may be widespread throughout the building. Affected occupants of these buildings may complain of a variety of signs and symptoms including irritation of the eyes, nose or throat; dry cough; dizziness and nausea; difficulty concentrating and generalized fatigue; neurotoxic or general health problems; skin irritations and rashes; nonspecific hypersensitivity reactions, headaches; odour; and altered taste sensations. These signs and symptoms typically fade or disappear once the individual leaves the particular room, zone, or building affecting them. For example, an individual may suffer with these symptoms at work, but often fade overtime when they

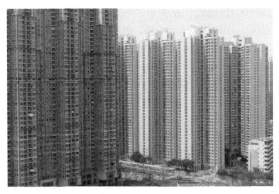

Photo 8.15 A densely populated high rise complex in New Territories, Hong Kong. A 1984 World Health Organization report suggested that up to 30% of new and remodeled apartment and office buildings worldwide may be subject to complaints of Sick-building syndrome, which is often associated with poor indoor air quality and circulation.

return home. Hence, this example illustrates the importance of examining both living and work environments collectively and their negative and positive impacts as the individual moves from one environment to another.

The United States EPA reports that during the early and mid-1900s, building ventilation standards were approximately 15 cubic feet per minute (cfm) of outside air for each building occupant, primarily to dilute and/or remove body odours. As a result of the 1973 oil embargo in the United States, national energy conservation measures called for a reduction in the amount of outdoor air ventilation to 5 cfm per occupant. Research has shown that this reduced standard is inadequate and has been linked to an increased incidence of SBS. Consequently, outdoor air ventilation standards have been revised to a minimum of 15 cfm of outdoor air per person in private dwellings and 20 cfm per person in office spaces (US EPA 2010). Other sources linked to SBS include indoor air pollutants such as tobacco smoke, mold and mildew, bacteria and viruses, adhesives, carpets, upholstery, manufactured wood products, copy machines, pesticides, cleaning agents, and other volatile organic compounds (VOCs), including formaldehyde (Burge 2004; Godish 2001; Martin-Gil et al. 1997; Murphy 2006; US EPA 2010).

A closely associated term to SBS is "building-related illness" (BRI). *BRI* is employed when signs and symptoms are present for a specific clinically diagnosable illness which can be directly attributed to airborne building contaminates. Individuals with BRI often present with clinical signs and symptoms including cough, chest tightness, fever, chills and muscle aches, mucus membrane irritation, and upper respiratory congestion which can be clinically defined and have a clearly identifiable cause. Moreover, unlike victims affected with SBS, the signs and symptoms for individuals with BRI are often prolonged in nature and do not subside or fade after leaving the building (Burge 2004; Godish 2001; US EPA 2010). For example, one indoor bacterium, *Legionella*, has caused both Legionnaire's Disease and Pontiac Fever.

Water Quality and Pollution

Improving access to clean and safe drinking water supplies could increase life expectancy in developing countries by more than 15 years (Schubert and Bartfay 2010). Domestically, the quality of our drinking water has been shown to profoundly affect the health of our residents. For example, during the summer of 2000, the water supply in Walkerton, Ontario became contaminated with *Escherichia coli 0157:57* (Ali 2004; O'Connor 2002). As a consequence, 2,300 residents of Walkerton became severely ill, 7 died, and the economic impact was estimated to be in excess of $64.5 million (Sullivan 2004). Hence, a safe source of drinking water and efficient sewage treatment infrastructures are vital to the health and safety of all residents of Canada and internationally, and are vital components of all public health systems globally (Quinlan and Dickinson 2009; Schubert and Bartfay 2010).

Health Canada (2004) has developed specific guidelines for all public and privately owned drinking water supplies. Indeed, approximately 25% of individuals in Canada rely on private wells, cisterns, or other sources of drinking water, and assume responsibility for their overall purity and quality (Canadian Water and Wastewater Association, n.d.). Bacteriological testing of public and private water supplies is typically done by designated provincial health laboratories and/or privately contracted laboratories (Health Canada 2008). Drinking water supplies should not contain more than 10 total coliform bacteria per 100 mL of water (Health Canada 2008). This often results from surface water infiltration or seepage from a nearby septic system into a well. The presence of *E. coli* suggests that it has been contaminated with faecal matter and should not be consumed. The maximum acceptable concentration of *E. coli* is 0 per 100 mL of water (Health Canada 2008).

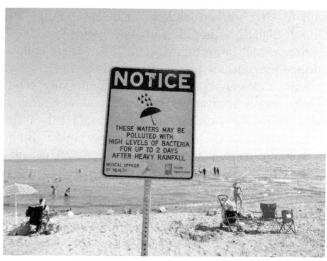

Source: Wally J. Bartfay

Photo 8.16 A public health warning sign by the Medical Officer of Health for the Durham Region of Ontario notifying beach goers and swimmers that the water in Lake Ontario may be contaminated with potentially harmful bacteria after heavy rainfalls.

Canada contains approximately 15% of the global fresh water supply; however, 60% of our water sources exist far away from urban and populated areas (Robinson Vollman, Anderson, and McFarlane 2004). The estimated health care costs associated with water pollution in Canada are $300 million per year. Recent outbreaks of waterborne diseases such as *E. coli* and *cryptosporidium* in Kitchener-Waterloo, Collingwood, and Walkerton, Ontario; Kelowna, British Columbia, and North Battleford, Saskatchewan over the past decade have affected thousands of residents and have also resulted in mortality. Approximately 87% of Canadians (mostly urban) receive treated (e.g., chlorinated) municipal tap water and the remaining 13% rely on private cisterns or wells (Robinson Vollman, Anderson, and McFarlane 2004). Diarrhea due to infectious (waterborne) microbes is responsible for over 34,000 deaths each year, which is more than those attributed to HIV/AIDS and cancer combined. To put this into another perspective, this number is equivalent to 100 jumbo jets crashing daily.

The federal government passed the *Canada Water Act* in 1970, and created the Department of the Environment in 1971 (Schubert and Bartfay 2010). The federal government maintains responsibility for such things as navigation on our oceans and waterways and for fisheries. According to the British North American Act of 1867, the provinces are the *owners* of the water resources and assume responsibility for their day-to-day management.

The Great Lakes provides drinking water, recreation, and industry to more than 40 million individuals in eight states and two Canadian provinces (Alliance for the Great Lakes 2010). In 1985, the *Great Lakes Water Quality Board* identified 11 pollutants resulting from industrial production in the area that have the potential to result in negative health effects on humans and other species (Shah 2003). These pollutants include polychlorinated bisphenols (PCBs); Dichlorodiphenyltrichloroethane (DDT) and its breakdown products aldrin and dieldrin; toxaphene; dioxins (2.3.7.8-TCDD), furans (2.3.7.8-TCDF); mirex, mercury; alkylated lead, benzopyrene, and hexachlorobenze. All of these chemicals have been shown to be present in the ecosystem of the Great Lakes. For example, chemicals such as mercury or PCB can accumulate in herring gull eggs and fish that are consumed by other animal species or humans.

According to a study by the Center for Public Integrity in Washington, DC, at least 9 million Americans living near the Great Lakes basin may be in danger from high levels of chemical pollution; and there are numerous so-called "areas of concern" (AOC) where chemical contamination of sediments from the lakes has seriously endangered the quality of life for people and their health, and threatens the survival of various wildlife (Environment Canada 2011; Ottawa Citizen 2008). This study found elevated infant mortality rates in 26 areas; premature births in 4 of the areas, and identified 108 hazardous waste sites; of which 71 pose a potential health hazard to public health and safety. This study echoes a series of reports done by Health Canada in the 1990s that revealed 17 Canadian AOC where there were elevated levels of illnesses that have been linked to pollution in the Great Lakes basin (The Ottawa Citizen 2008). In Lake Superior, the levels of polybrominated diphenyl ethers, a persistent, bioaccumulative, and toxic chemical, doubled every 3–4 years between 1980 and 2000 (Zhu and Hites 2004).

All of the Great Lakes and their connecting channels are currently under fish consumption advisories for one or more toxic chemicals; which include mercury,

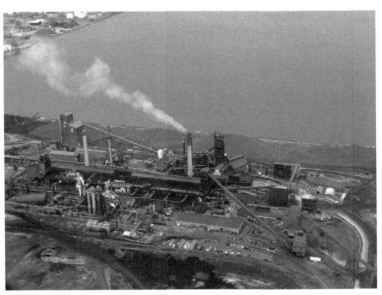

Source: SF photo/Shutterstock.com

Figure 8.2 Aerial view of a steel mill located along the shores of Lake Ontario in Hamilton. Studies of the Great Lake Basin reveal that there are several polluted areas of concern that have been lined to increased illness, premature deaths, and increased infant mortality.

PCBs, dioxins, and chlordane, and there have been over 1,500 advisories of such to date. Mackenzie, Lockridge, and Keith (2005) reports that the sex ratio of males to females in a First Nation community near Sarnia, Ontario has dropped to fewer than 35% boys. The First Nation's community is located in close proximity to large petrochemical companies that have released toxic chemicals (e.g., endocrine disruptors, mercury) into the water supplies over the years. Researchers hypothesize that chemical exposure may be contributing to the decline in males in this First Nation community (See Group Review Exercise entitled "The disappearing male").

Following amendments to the 1987 *Great Lakes Water Quality Agreement*, the *Canadian-Ontario Agreement Respecting Great Lakes Water Quality* was revised to provide more specific directives and frameworks for restoring these noted AOC. These agreements help provide guidelines for controlling pollution in the Great Lakes, conserving fragile ecosystems, and to help preserve and protect human health (Environment Canada 2011). Of the 43 original AOC in Canada and the United States, 4 have currently been delisted: Collingwood Harbour, Severn Sound and Wheatley Harbour in Canada, and the Oswego River in the United States (Environment Canada 2011).

CanWest MediaWorks Publications Incorporated (2008) reports that three Vancouver sewage treatment plants have been failing federal environmental tests for several years, while dumping billions of liters of partly treated waste waters into the Fraser River, Burrard Inlet, and Strait of Georgia in British Columbia. The three treatment plants are the Iona Island plant in Richmond, Lions Gate plant in West Vancouver, and the Annalis Island plant in Delta. The standard toxicity test was originally developed by Environment Canada (1990), as is performed by contracted outsourced laboratories at arm's length. A sample is taken from a treated waste water plant before it is discharged into the environment. Rainbow trout are employed for this test and placed in the water sample collected for a total of 96 h. If half (50%) of the test sample perishes, the test is considered a failure (Environment Canada 1990). In the metro Vancouver area, 21 documented test failures occurred in 2006; 18 in 2005 and 13 in 2004, although no penalties were issued by Environment Canada (CanWest MediaWorks Publications Inc. 2008).

Table 8.2 shows a breakdown of the total number of major reported spills (>100 tonnes) of sewage and effluent by environmental regions in Canada. Environment Canada's five environmental regions are: (a) Pacific and Yukon—which includes British Columbia and the Yukon Territory; (b) Prairie and Northern regions—which includes Alberta, Saskatchewan, Manitoba, and the Northwest Territories; (c) Ontario;

Table 8.2 Reported Major Spills (>100 tonnes) of Sewage and Effluent in Canada by Environmental Regions (1984–1995)

Environmental Regions	Quantity per Reported Spill (Tonnes)	Sector or Industry	Comments Related to Causes	Totals per Region
1. Pacific and Yukon	–100,000 –27,000 –21,300 –13,500 –11,000 –4,800 –4,500	–Municipal government –Pulp and paper –Municipal government –Municipal government –Municipal government –Pulp and paper –Municipal government	–Pipeline leak, discharged into a river –Discharge from pulp and paper mill into a lake due to equipment failure –Spill to a river due to equipment failure –Overflow discharged into a river –Discharge into marine environment due to equipment failure –Discharge from pulp and paper mill on land due to equipment failure –Discharge into a river due to equipment failure	182,100
2. Prairie and Northern	–84,000	–Municipal government	–Spill from municipal sewage treatment plant	84,000
3. Ontario	–980,000 –875,000 –300,000 –250,000 –160,000 –145,000 –100,000 –80,000 –72,000 –65,000	–Metallurgy –Provincial government –Municipal government –Municipal government –Municipal government –Metallurgy –Municipal government –Municipal government –Municipal government –Municipal government	–Dirty water discharge from a steel mill to harbour via storm sewer –By-pass of chlorinated sewage due to storm –Sewage by-pass due to rain –Sewage by-pass due to rain –Sewage by-pass due to rain –Discharge of dirty water from steel mill filtration plant into a lake –Sewage by-pass due to rain –Sewage by-pass due to rain –Sewage by-pass due to rain –Sewage by-pass due to melting snow	3,027,000

(Continued)

Table 8.2 Reported Major Spills (>100 tonnes) of Sewage and Effluent in Canada by Environmental Regions (1984–1995) (*Continued*)

Environmental Regions	Quantity per Reported Spill (Tonnes)	Sector or Industry	Comments Related to Causes	Totals per Region
4. Québec	–None reported			0
5. Atlantic	–132,000 –4,550 –3,200 –2,300	–Municipal government –Construction –Municipal government –Federal government	–Discharge into harbour from sewage treatment plant –Intentional dumping of sewage into a river from a construction site –Discharge into a river from a sewage treatment plant –Sewage escaped to a National Park from hole in lagoon	142,050
			National total	**3,435,150 tonnes**

Source: Adapted from Environment Canada (2006).

(d) Québec, and (e) the Atlantic region—which includes New Brunswick, Nova Scotia, Prince Edward Island, and Newfoundland. Alarmingly, a total of 3,435,150 tonnes of sewage and effluent were spilled into our environment in Canada between the years 1984 and 1995 alone (Environment Canada 2006).

Sewage and effluents are spilled in high quantities nationwide due to a variety of reasons including human error, aging sewage infrastructures, and excessive downpours of rain. For example, Puddicombe (2009) reported that 8.7 million liters of raw sewage was released into the Ottawa River on April 25, 2009 due to a heavy rainfall, which brought the total amount of raw sewage released since February of that year to approximately 125 million liters. The City of Ottawa was fined $500,000 after approximately 1 billion liters of raw sewage flowed into the Ottawa River for a period of over 2 weeks in August, 2006 (Puddicombe 2009). There are a large number

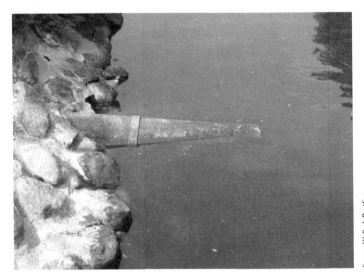

Photo 8.17 Sewage and effluents are spilled in high quantities into our water sources nationwide due to a variety of factors including human error, aging sewage infrastructures and excessive downpours of rain water associated with extreme weather conditions and climate change.

of spills at the municipal level and one may predict that the frequency and quantity of spills will increase in the next decade due to the aging municipal water and sewage infrastructures and treatment facilities (Bartfay and Bartfay 2015).

Health Canada (2002, 2004) reports that approximately 40% of individuals drink fluoridated water, and they have also set standards for labelling requirements for this chemical in household products such as toothpaste.

The recommended level of fluoride in drinking water is 0.8–1.0 mg/L (Federal-Provincial Subcommittee on Drinking Water of the Federal-Provincial Committee on Environment and Occupational Health 2002). Although the associated risk of using fluoride to threat municipal drinking water supplies is minimal, public health care professionals should be aware that young children under the age of 6 years who ingest fluoride are at increased risk of developing dental fluorosis (Shah 2003). Although dental fluorosis does not damage the teeth per se, it does result in a brownish discolouration (Schubert and Bartfay 2010). In addition, excess consumption of fluoride may result in an increased risk of bone loss and fractures in peri and postmenopausal women (Hales 2009; Hales and Lauzon 2007).

The City of Toronto Department of Public Health (1990) conducted a study to assess the quality of drinking water from municipal tap sources versus bottled water. Interestingly, findings from this study revealed no bacterial contamination from its municipal water sources taken from household taps, but bacteria was present in both device-treated and commercially sold bottled water. Weldon (1999) notes that expiration dates are not required on bottle water in Canada and may consequently harbour the growth of bacteria overtime. In addition, traces of bisphenol A (BPA), a known endocrine disrupter, has been reported after 39 weeks in large polycarbonate containers that are typically found in homes or offices at room temperature (Weldon 1999). Add to your knowledge of water quality guidelines and treatments by accessing the following websites and resources.

Web-Based Resource Box 8.1 Water Quality Guidelines and Treatments

Learning Resource	Website
Health Canada: What's in your well? A guide to well water treatment and maintenance (2008) This user-friendly guide provides an overview of basic well water treatments if contamination occurs and how to safely monitor private water supplies	http://www.hc-sc.gc-ewh-semt/pubs/water-eau/well-puits_e.html
Health Canada: Guidelines for Canadian drinking water quality: Supporting documents (March 1, 2004) This resource describes water quality standards for drinking water in Canada and how to manage various drinking water supplies	http://www.hc-sc.gc.ca/ewh-semt/water-eau/drink-potab/guide/index-eng.php
Health Canada: Drinking water chlorination (May 22, 2003) This resource describes the public health benefits and rational for treating water supplies with chlorine	http://www.hc-sc.gc.ca/english/iyh/environment/chlorine.html
Health Canada: Fluorides and human health (October, 3, 2002a) This resource describes the public health benefits and rational for treating water supplies with fluorides	http://www.hc-sc.gc.ca/english/iyh/environment/fluorides.html
Health Canada: Questions and answers on bottled water (November 23, 2000) This resource describes possible contaminates associated with bottled water sources sold and distributed in Canada	http://www.hc-sc.gc.ca/fn-an/securit/facts-faits/faqs_bottle_water-eau_embouteille-eng.php

Chlorine remains the most widely utilized additive to drinking water supplies in Canada, which is used to reduce or eliminate a variety of microorganisms such as bacteria and viruses (Health Canada 2003, 2008). Although the associated health risks are minimal, the addition of chlorine to drinking water may cause it to react with organic matter present in water supplies and produce trihalomethanes, which are potential carcinogenic and mutagenic compounds (Hales and Lauzon 2007; Shah 2003). Currently, a growing number of communities across Canada are using ozone to disinfect their municipal water supplies due to growing public health concerns related to chlorine (Bartfay and Bartfay 2015; Schubert and Bartfay 2010).

What Is Toxicology?

Toxicology is defined as the study of the adverse effects of synthetic chemical substances, products and natural toxins, which includes their cellular, biochemical, and molecular mechanisms of action, and the actual or potential ability of these chemicals to cause harm, ill effects, disease, and/or mortality in living organisms including humans (Bartfay and Bartfay 2015). Various subspecialty areas have emerged in the discipline including ecoenvironmental, regulatory, forensic, clinical, reproductive, and developmental toxicology.

Each and every day, we are exposed to a multitude of natural and man-made (synthetic) chemicals in the air we breathe, the food and beverages we consume, and the various consumer products we use including cell phones, computer terminals, chairs we sit on and hair combs to name but a few. These chemicals can enter the body through ingestion, inhalation, or through contact with our skin or mucous membranes. Some may be essential nutrients (e.g., vitamins), while others may be potentially toxic compounds (e.g., BPA in the lining of aluminum cans).

The field of toxicology has been in existence for centuries and its historical origins can be traced back to the study of poisons (Gochfeld 2008; Maxwell 2009; Merrill 2008). In ancient Greece and Rome, poisons were employed for political aims and ambitions and also to accomplish personal suicide. Indeed, it is widely reported that Socrates (470–399 BC) and Theophrastus (370–286 BC) were both executed via poison. Friis (2012) notes that around the fourth century BC, poisoning by use of arsenic and other means grew more frequent during the Roman Empire. Nero, for example, is believed to have used arsenic to poison Claudius to serve his political aspirations. Poisonings were also employed frequently during the middle ages to do away with rivals including politicians, wealthy patrons, nobility, and spouses (Friis 2012).

One of the founders of the science of toxicology was Paracelsus (1493–1541), who was born Phillippus Tehophrastus Aureolus Bombastus von Hohemheim (Borzelleca 2000). Paracelsus made several contributions to the science of toxicology including the importance of establishing a dose–response relationship and the notion of target organ specificity for chemicals. In 1813, Mathieu Orfila authored a book entitled *Trait des poisons* in which he detailed various types of poisons and their effects on the body, and also made a significant contribution to the field of forensic toxicology (Friis 2012).

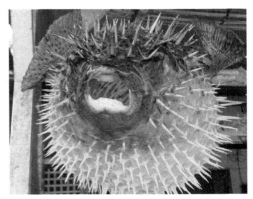

Source: Wally J. Bartfay

Photo 8.18 The blowfish, a type of puffer fish is considered a delicacy in Japan (i.e., Fugu), but may be deadly dangerous if not prepared by qualified and experienced sushi chefs. The tissues of the fish, which could include the reproductive organs, liver, intestines and skin contain the poison tetrodotoxin. In fact, Fugu poison is 1200 times stronger than cyanide.

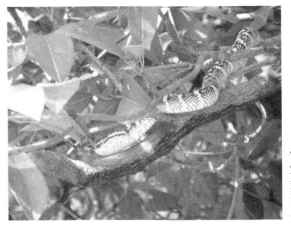

Source: Wally J. Bartfay

Photo 8.19 *Trimeresurus* is a genus of venomous green tree pit vipers found in Asia and the Indian Subcontinent that produces a haemotoxin that destroys red blood cells via rapid hemolysis, disrupts blood clotting, and causes tissue and/or organ degeneration and damage. Injury from a hemotoxic agent is often very painful and can cause permanent damage and mortality. Loss of an affected limb is possible even with prompt treatment with anti-venom.

Chemical toxicity occurs when a chemical agent or substance produces detrimental effects on living organisms in the environment, including humans (Bartfay and Bartfay 2015). There are approximately 60,000 different chemical substances that are employed for commercial and industrial activities in Canada and the United States (Robinson Vollman, Anderson, and McFarlane 2004). In 1988, the first year that the *EPA Toxic*

Release Inventory was released, 20,458 manufacturing facilities in the United States alone released 2.18 billion pounds of toxic waste substances directly into the atmosphere and 164 million pounds were directly discharged to surface water sources.

Industrial cities such as Sarnia, Ontario, which produces approximately 40% of all chemicals in Canada, must effectively plan for potential spills of toxic chemicals into the environment (see the Group Review Exercise entitled "The Disappearing Male"). It is estimated that over 150 million kilograms of toxic chemicals are released by manufacturing facilities into Canada's environment each year, which includes 7 million kilograms of chemicals that are known carcinogens (Pearson Education 2011). Furthermore, the *International Agency for Research on Cancer* lists approximately 60 workplace chemicals as known or probable carcinogens (Canadian Breast Cancer Foundation 2011). The Research Focus Box 8.1describes a study which examined exposure to various chemicals in Canadian work environments and their association with the development of bladder cancers.

Human bio-monitoring is an effective way to provide baseline information about levels of exposure to environmental chemicals, and can help determine usual exposure and changes over time (Bushnik et al. 2010). Chemicals are typically classified based on their mechanism of action; target organ, structure, source, use or economic role (Gochfeld 2008; Maxwell 2009; Merrill 2008). Table 8.3 provides the reader with common classifications or taxonomies employed by toxicologist and examples of each, but the list is not intended to be exhaustive in nature. A basic understanding of these classifications is critical for all public health care professionals and workers dealing with environmental and occupational chemicals and agents.

Research Focus Box 8.1

A Case-Control Study of Occupational Risk Factors for Bladder Cancer in Canada

Study Aim/Rationale
Exposure to certain chemicals and substances in work environments may be associated with an increased risk for the development of bladder cancer for certain occupations. This case-control study sought to determine the occupational risk factors associated with the development of bladder cancer in seven Canadian provinces.

Methodology/Design
This was a population-based case-control study that employed a dataset of 887 workers with the incidence of histologically confirmed bladder cancer between the years 1994 and 1997. These workers were matched by age and sex for 2,847 controls surveyed in 1996. Questionnaires were distributed and completed by approximately 60% of the respondents. The odds ratios (ORs) for the various occupations and self-reported exposures in their work environments were adjusted for age, race, smoking, province, and several dietary factors via unconditional logistic regression analysis.

Major findings
The investigators reported a statistically significant increased risk among males who were hairdressers (OR = 3.42, 1.09–10.8), primary metal workers (OR = 2.40, 1.29–4.50), miners (OR = 1.94, 1.18–3.17), and those who were automechanics (OR = 1.69, 1.02–2.82). A duration-respond trend was noted in both primary metal workers and automechanics. For female workers, significant increased risks were observed among lumber processors (OR = 8.78, 1.28–60.1), general labourers (OR = 2.18, 1.05–4.52), nurses (OR = 1.54, 1.03–2.31), and general office clerks (OR = 1.48, 1.01–2.17).

Implications for Public Health
Results from this preliminary study suggest that certain occupations in Canada pose an increased health risk associated with the development of bladder cancer through environmental exposure in their workplaces. Further investigations are warranted to ascertain the suspected causative factors in the work environment (e.g., chemotherapeutic agents for nurses, petroleum products for automechanics, fumes for metal workers) and their association with the development of bladder cancer.

Source: Gaertner, Trpeski, and Johnson (2004).

Table 8.3 Common Classification or Taxonomies of Toxic Agents

Classification or Taxonomy of Toxic Agents	Common Examples
1. By use	Solvents, pharmaceutical agents, acid, bases, pesticides, detergents and cleansers, paints and dyes
2. By target organ	Carcinogen (initiators and promoters), immunotoxin, cardiotoxin, endocrine toxin, dermatotoxin, genotoxin (mutagens), hematoxin, hepatotoxin, neurotoxin, pulmonary toxin
3. By mechanism of action	Cell membrane disruption (e.g., lipid peroxidation), competitive binding of active sites or receptors, enzyme induction or inhibition, formation of oxygen-free radicals, redox reactions (e.g., antioxidants), metabolic poisons, macromolecular binding, hormone activity (e.g., synthesis or receptor regulation), immune effects, irritants
4. By source	(a) *Natural or biological toxins*: Plant, bacterial, invertebrate and vertebrate (b) *Synthetic (man-made) chemicals*: Pharmaceutical agents, industrial raw materials, by-products and wastes
5. By structure	(a) *Organic chemicals*: Aliphatics (e.g., ethanes, ethenes), aromatics (e.g., phenols, benzene), chlorinated hydrocarbons (e.g., chlorinated alkanes and alkenes), chlorinated polyaromatics (e.g., gioxins, furnas, PCBs), ethers, ketones, aldehydes, alcohols, organic acids, amines and nitriles (b) *Inorganic chemicals*: Acids and bases, anions and cations, heavy metals, metalloids (e.g., arsenic, selenium) and salts

Acute toxicity studies employing various animal models are undertaken to assess for any adverse effects observed within a 24-h period following a single dose (exposure) to a specific chemical (Bartfay and Bartfay 2015). By contrast, chronic toxicity animal studies occur after repeated dosing (exposure) of the animals for more than 10% of their typical life span (Chan, O'Hara, and Hayes 1982; Gochfeld 2008; Stevens and Gallo 1982). Figure 8.3 shows the dose–response curve estimates for a suspected chemical and the observed toxic effect. The TD 50 represents the toxic dose in 50% of the test animals and the ED describes the specific dose of a chemical that produces a specific observed effect in 50% of the cases.

The *dose–response* is defined as a quantitative estimate between the relationship between a suspected chemical and the observed toxic effect (e.g., cancer slope factor or weight-of-the-evidence classification for carcinogenicity) (Bartfay and Bartfay 2015). The dose–response is typically summarized in the form a graph which plots dose on the *x* axis against the response on the *y* axis (see Figure 8.3). The *threshold dose* is defined as the highest dose at which no toxic effects are observed (Bartfay and Bartfay 2015). For example, if the threshold dose is zero, then from a practical standpoint there is no safe dose for that specific chemical (Maxwell 2009).

A researcher may also be interested in determining the lethal acute oral dose of a chemical in an experimental rodent model. The researcher will typically administer several dosage levels of the chemical orally, including some which are believed to be lethal. Data from this investigation are then employed to calculate the acute oral dose that is lethal in 50% of the test rodents, and this is typically reported as the LD_{50} for that

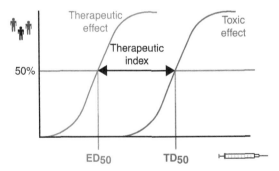

Figure 8.3 Graph depicting the dose–response curves for a suspected chemical.

Source: PharmacologyCorner.com retrieved December 15, 2015 from http://pharmacologycorner.com/wp-content/uploads/2011/01/therapeutic-index1.gif

chemical expressed in units of milligrams of chemical per kilogram of body weight (Friis 2012; Gochfeld 2008). Similarly, when a researcher seeks to determine the lethal dose for 50% of exposed rodents to a chemical inhaled, this would be expressed as the LC_{50}. The LC_{50} is the regarded as the concentration of chemical in the air that is acutely lethal in this experimental rodent mode. The ED_{50} may also be reported and is regarded as a general concept which describes the specific dose of a chemical that produces a specific observed effect in 50% of the test animals (e.g., development of a cancerous tumour) (Bartfay and Bartfay 2015).

It is important to note that these measures of lethality may not describe a chemical's full spectrum of toxicity in living organisms and/or ecosystems per se (Gochfeld 2008; Scientific Group on Methodologies for the Safety Evaluation of Chemicals 1998; Snodin 2002). For example, chemicals that have low acute toxicity may have other effects such as carcinogenicity or teratogenicity due to long-term exposure. Toxicologists, therefore, often take into consideration the total dose of exposure, how often each specific dose occurs, and the time period during which the exposure took place in order to develop a better understanding of the effects of the chemical under investigation. Infants and young children who have smaller body sizes and weight and who are developing are typically more susceptible to chemicals, in comparison to adults who may be given the same dose of a chemical (Bartfay and Bartfay 2015). In addition, the elderly who often have decreased liver and renal function essential for the metabolism and excretion of substances from the body may be more susceptible to chemical exposure (Amendola and Wilkinson 2000; Landrigan and Carlson 1987; Russell and Gruber 1987).

The toxicity of many ingredients has not been well characterized or empirically evaluated for their potential impact on human health and well-being. Phthalates, for example, have been used as plasticizers by the cosmetic industry for many decades in nail polish, hair spray products, and fragrances, but have only been investigated as possible endocrine disruptors (LoSasso, Rapport, and Axelrod 2001; Maxwell 2009; U.S. Food and Drug Administration 2006). During the 1950s and 1960s, hexachlorophene was aggressively marketed to African-American and Canadian women in magazines as a bleaching cream. Specifically, this ingredient was utilized in underarm deodorant products as ammoniated mercury, which is a known neurotoxic substance.

During May 2011, Environmental Defense Canada (EDC) urged Health Canada to improve its current cosmetic regulation guidelines by making companies list all metals on their product labels (EDC 2011; Mehta 2011). Currently, the guidelines for metals in cosmetics employ the same standards that are applied for ingestible pharmaceuticals in Canada. This report asked women of various ages across Canada to identify five common pieces of face makeup they applied on a regularly basis. These findings were disputed by the *Canadian Cosmetics, Toiletries and Fragrances Association*, which argues that the report "lacks context" since the metals are not necessary ingredients, but impurities and/or unintentional contaminants that result from the manufacturing process.

Group Activity-Based Learning Box 8.2

How Are Toxic Substances Managed in Your Community?
It seeks to explore major toxicological issues or concerns and how they are currently being managed to preserve and maintain the health of residents in your community or region. Working in small groups of three to five students, discuss and answer the following questions:

1. What are some of the major toxicological issues or concerns in your community or region?

2. How are toxic substances and materials stored and/or disposed of in your community or region?

3. What are the actual or potential public health issues related to the storage and/or disposal of these toxic substances and materials?

4. How can published research in the fields of toxicology be employed by public health care professionals and workers to preserve and promote the health and well-being of residents in your community or region?

EDC (2011) subsequently chose 5 additional products and 49 different items to test for trace amounts of nickel, lead, and beryllium. The items tested included a variety of powders, foundations, concealers, blushes, mascaras, eyeliners, and lip glosses. The findings revealed that these test samples on average contained four out of eight metals of concerns and all but one of the products contained metals within the draft guidelines recommended by Health Canada. There is certainly no safe level of lead, for example. Nonetheless, the cosmetic industry argues that mandatory labelling of these metal impurities for their products would create unnecessary concern among consumers with a lack of context, and would eventually lead to a desensitizing by consumers toward real health hazards (EDC 2011; Mehta 2011).

Examples of Commonly Known Toxic Heavy Metals and Chemicals

Mercury

In the classic children's book, *Alice in Wonderland* written in 1865, Lewis Carroll portrays the "Mad Hatter" as a zany character, which had grounding in reality. In fact, mercury-containing compounds were often applied during the process of converting furs, such as beaver pelts from Canada, into a stiff felt product used to manufacture hats for men during the eighteenth and nineteenth centuries (Friis 2012). Millinery workers who were chronically exposed to mercury fumes in poorly ventilated factories were more prone to develop the neuropsychiatric syndrome known as mercurial erethism or *mad hatter's disease*, in comparison to other workers not exposed to mercury fumes. This clinical condition is characterized by personality changes, irritability, memory loss, decreased ability to concentrate and perform simply tasks, loss of self-confidence, and depression.

Mercury is a naturally occurring heavy metal that can exist in three forms: (a) elemental; (b) inorganic, and (c) organic (Statistics Canada 2011a). The most common form of mercury exposure is in the form of methylmercury through the consumption of fish and seafood, and through a lesser extent inorganic mercury through dental fillings. Statistic Canada (2011a) reports that chronic exposure to high levels of methylmercury may cause numbness and tingling in the extremities, blurred vision, deafness, lack of muscle coordination, and intellectual impairment, as well as adverse effects on the cardiovascular, gastrointestinal, and reproductive systems. In addition, prenatal exposure to mercury may interfere with the normal development of the central nervous system and may result in neurological and developmental delays in children.

Mercury and other heavy metal contaminants and pharmaceuticals disposed of in the Great Lakes Basin and other Canadian water sources are a growing concern, and some of these substances have been linked to alternations to human health (Alliance for the Great Lakes 2010; Koch 2011). One Canadian study, for example, found a series of outbreaks of Minamata disease in Thunder Bay, Collingwood, Sarnia, and Cornwall. Minamata disease, which includes cerebral palsy as one of its associated clinical symptoms, is caused by mercury poisoning. Each of the noted affected areas had large chlor-alkali plants that use mercury for making chlorine. Between 1948 and 1995, it is estimated that these plants released 742 tonnes of mercury into the Great Lakes. Similarly, mercury dumped in Sarnia, Ontario eventually ended up in the St. Claire River; which then flowed into Lake St. Claire, and then flowed down the Detroit River to Lake Erie (The Ottawa Citizen 2008).

Although the use of mercury has been gradually phased out in consumer products such as thermometers and gauges, it is still employed in some medical devices and dental fillings in certain developing countries, button-cell batteries for small electronic appliances (e.g., hearing aids) and compact fluorescent bulbs (Bartfay and Bartfay 2015). Mercury is present throughout all regions of Canada, especially in the remote Arctic regions due to its persistence, mobility, and tendency to accumulate in colder climates. Health Canada recommends a clinical blood guidance value for total mercury (i.e., all forms) of 20 µg/L for adults; and a revised value of 8 µg/L for children, pregnant women, and women of childbearing age (Statistics Canada 2011a).

Mercury contamination in Canada was first reported during the 1970s (Robinson Vollman, Anderson, and McFarlane 2004), and the level of mercury in the blood and hair of First Nations and Inuit peoples have dropped significantly over the past four decades. Nonetheless, despite this noted drop, the threat of mercury in the environment has severely altered or disrupted traditional, social, and cultural practices in these Indigenous communities. For examples, traditional fishing, hunting, and trapping practices and enterprises, and the gathering of food from land and water sources have been restricted as a result of environmental contaminants (e.g., mercury, PCB, dioxins). This has often forced Indigenous communities to import foods at increased costs; impose new western-style diets on residents that have contributed to obesity and the growing rates of type-2 diabetes, and find new ways to support themselves through new economic means (Robinson Vollman, Anderson, and McFarlane 2004). The reader is referred to Chapter 4 for a detailed discussion on Indigenous definitions of health and well-being and their critical link to the environment.

The *Canadian Health Measures Survey* (CHMS) is the most comprehensive direct health measures survey ever undertaken on a national scale in Canada, and includes blood levels of various toxic heavy metals including mercury, cadmium, and lead for the years 2007–2009 (Wong and Lye 2009; Statistics Canada 2011a, 2011b). The CHMS consisted of an in-home interview which collected demographic and socioeconomic data, information about their medical history, current health status and lifestyle, environment, and housing characteristics. In addition, various physical measurements (e.g., blood pressure, weight, height and physical fitness) and blood and urine samples were also obtained from participants at a mobile clinic.

The findings revealed that 88% of Canadians aged 6–79 (geometric mean = 0.69 µg/L) had detectable mercury in their blood samples, and fewer than 1% of Canadian adults have total blood concentrations of mercury above the Health Canada guidance value of 20 µg/L (Wong and Lye 2008). The *geometric mean* is a type of average that is less influenced by extreme values, in comparison to the traditional arithmetic mean and provides a better estimate of central tendency for highly skewed data, and is a common measure employed in the measurement of environmental chemicals found in human blood or urine (Statistics Canada 2011c). Children aged 6–11 years had a geometric mean concentration of 0.27 µg/L, similar to that of teens aged 12–19 (0.31 µg/L); and these concentrations increased with age reaching 1.02 µg/L for those aged 40–59, before decreasing to 0.87 µg/L in the 60–79 age group. These concentrations were similar for males and females across all groups, with no noted significant differences between the two sexes (Statistics Canada 2011a).

Lead

Lead occurs naturally in the environment and individuals can be exposed to this toxic heavy metal from contaminated water supplies, food, dust, air, consumer products (e.g., children toys, jewellery, mini-blinds, crystal alcohol decanters containing lead) and certain occupations (e.g., plumbers, mechanics), and hobbyist (e.g., stain-glass making) (Statistics Canada 2011b). In Canada, the current blood clinical intervention level is 10 µg/dL; however, some studies have shown that young children may experience adverse health effects with blood levels below this current national standard (e.g., neurological damage) (Statistics Canada 2011b).

Since the 1970s, lead concentrations in our environment and in humans have been declining significantly, including its use as a solder in food cans and for plumbing fixtures. In 1922, a General Motors chemist found that the addition of tetraethyl lead to gas could decrease the knocking noises in the engine and make for a smoother ride. Health Canada (2007) reports that leaded gasoline was officially banned in 1990. Given that this heavy metal does not break down over time, lead from previous sources (e.g., lead-acid car batteries in land-fills, solder used in food cans, plumbing or electronics, lead used in older paint products) can continue to be a source of exposure.

The CHMS measured blood lead concentrations in the Canadian population from 2007 to 2009, and found this heavy metal in 100% of the population aged 6–79 years, but less than 1% had blood concentration levels (geometric mean = 1.34 µg/dL) at or above the clinical intervention level of 10 µg/dL (Statistics Canada 2011a, 2011b). By comparison, the clinical intervention level was 27% three decades ago. In general, males had higher blood concentrations than females, and individuals with the lowest household incomes had higher blood lead concentrations than those with highest household incomes. This finding highlights the importance of employment and income as important social determinants of health in Canada. In addition, individuals who were born outside of Canada had higher blood lead concentrations than those born in Canada. People who lived in homes built more than 50 years ago had higher blood lead concentrations than those who lived in homes less than 20 years old. It is also interesting to note that blood lead concentrations were higher in individuals who were current or former smokers, and in people who drank alcohol once or more per week (Statistics Canada 2011b).

Dichlorodiphenyltrichloroethane

It may be argued that the current environmental health movement began when Rachel Carson (1962), a marine biologists, published her influential book entitled *Silent Spring*, in which she detailed the devastating environmental and health impacts of the pesticide DDT (Schubert and Bartfay 2010). This synthetic pesticide was widely employed globally after the Second World War for the control of a wide range of insects, especially mosquitoes that were responsible for the transmission of malaria (Harris Ali 2009).

For example, it has been estimated that over 80 million pounds of DDT were applied in the United States in 1959 alone (Hales and Lauzon 2007). Carson (1962) carefully detailed how DDT was widespread in the

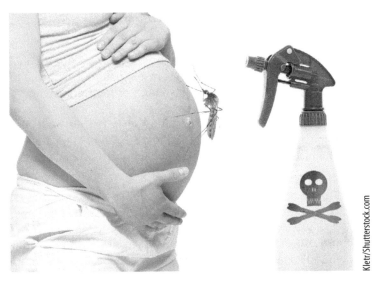

Photo 8.20 DDT is a banned chemical in Canada previously used for insect control which has been linked to a variety of birth defects, reproductive dysfunctions and certain types of cancer.

environment and food chain, and that it remained there for up to 15 years before being degraded. The work of Carson and other scientists eventually leads to the restricted use of DDT in 1969, and its eventual ban in 1972 in the United States (Hales and Lauzon 2007; Jaga and Dharmani 2003). Exposure to DDT has been associated with an increased risk of birth defects, still births and spontaneous abortions, and reproductive dysfunctions in men, and cancer (Ayotte et al. 2001; Beard 2006; Korrick et al. 2001; Longnecker et al. 2002; Salazar-Garcia et al. 2004).

Although DDT was never manufactured in Canada, it was first registered as a pesticide in 1946 and widely employed in pest control products in Canada until the 1960s (Commission for Environmental Cooperation [CEC] 1997; Government of Canada 2005). Provincial legislation in Canada provides additional regulatory powers to control the transportation, storage, disposal, and use of pest control products. For example, during the period of 1991–1992, the Ontario Ministry of Agriculture and Food and Rural Affairs conducted a waste agricultural pesticide collection program that collected approximately 1,180 kg of DDT (CEC 1997).

The Government of Canada (2005) reports that in response to increasing environmental and safety concerns, most uses of DDT in Canada were phased out by the mid-1970s. The registration of all uses of DDT was discontinued in 1985, with the understanding that existing stocks would be sold, used, or disposed of by December 31, 1990. Currently, the purchase, sale, or use of DDT in Canada constitutes a violation of the *Pest Control Products Act* (Government of Canada 2005). The Research Focus Box 8.2 provides the reader

---

Research Focus Box 8.2

Reproductive Effects of Occupational DDT Exposure Among Male Malaria Control Workers

Study Aim/Rationale
The aim of this investigation was to assess the potential occupational health effects of exposure to DDT on the reproductive health of antimalaria campaign workers in Mexico.

Methodology/Design
The researchers employed a population-based study to examine the association between occupational exposures to the pesticide DDT on the reproductive history of 2,033 workers. Data on occupational exposure levels

(Continued)

Research Focus Box 8.2 (*Continued*)

and reproductive outcomes were assessed via a questionnaire and subjects provided information on 9,187 pregnancies. The researchers estimated paternal exposure to DDT levels before each pregnancy using three approaches: (a) a dichotomous indicator for pregnancies before and post exposure, (b) a qualitative index comprised four exposure categories, and (c) an estimation of the DDT metabolite DDE [1-1-dichloro-2, 2-bis (p-chlorophenyl) ethylene] accumulated in fat. The researchers employed logistic regression analysis to determine associations and adjusted for the parents' age at each child's birth, exposure to other pesticides and chemical substances at work, smoking, and alcohol consumption.

Major Findings
The reported OR for birth defects comparing pregnancies after and before the first exposure was 3.77 [95% confidence interval (CI), 1.19–9.52]. In comparison to the lowest quartile of estimated DDE in fat, the ORs were 2.48 (95% CI, 0.75–8.11); 4.15 (95% CI, 1.38–12.46), and 3.76 (95% CI, 1.23–11.44) for quartiles 2 (equal to 50 μ/g DDE in fat), 3 (equal to 82 μ/g DDE in fat), and 4 (equal to 298 μ/g DDE in fat), respectively. The researchers found an increased risk of birth defects associated with high occupational exposures to DDT in the group of Mexican subjects.

Implications for Public Health
These findings provide evidence that occupational exposure to DDT in Mexican antimalaria workers is associated with an increased risk of birth defects. Although the use of the pesticide DDT has been shown to be effective for controlling mosquitoe populations in Mexico associated with the transmission of malaria, parental occupational or environmental exposure to this pesticide possess negative health effects for the foetus in utero including associated birth defects.

Source: Salazar-Garcia, et al. (2004).

with a study that examined the negative health effects associated with occupational DDT exposure among male malaria control workers in Mexico. Although the DDT has been shown to be effective for the control of various mosquitoes known to transmit malaria and other diseases, exposure to this pesticide has been linked to various negative health outcomes including birth defects in utero.

Bisphenol A

BPA is an industrial chemical used primarily in the manufacturing of polycarbonate plastic (e.g., food containers and water bottles) and epoxy resins, which are employed as protective linings for canned foods and beverages, the metal lids for glass jars and bottles, and dental sealants (Statistics Canada 2011c). Individuals are primarily exposed to BPA through dietary means, although some consumer products may be sources of BPA (e.g., plastic containers, aluminum cans). This chemical can migrate from food

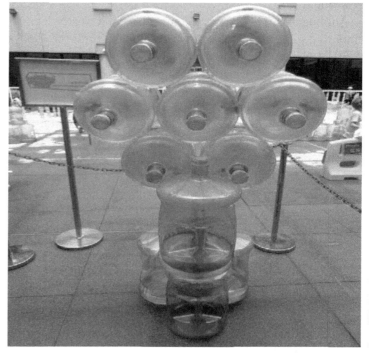

Source: Wally J. Bartfay

Photo 8.21 Traces of BPA, a known endocrine disrupter, have been reported after several weeks for certain water sources stored in large polycarbonate containers that are typically found in homes and offices worldwide. Canada was the first country to declare BPA a toxic substance used to harden plastic products in September, 2010.

packaging, particularly when heated (e.g., TV dinners), as well as from repeat-use plastic containers placed into microwave ovens. Certain animal-based studies suggest that low levels of exposure to BPA early in the life cycle can negatively affect neural development and behaviour. The *National Health and Nutrition Examination Survey* in the United States detected BPA in 93% of the American population aged 6 and older. Similarly, the *German Environmental Survey* detected BPA in 99% of 3–14 year olds. Taken together, these data suggest continual and widespread exposure to BPA (Statistics Canada 2011c).

Based on data from the 2007 to 2009 CHMS, BPA was detected in 91% of the urine samples with a geometric mean concentration of 1.16 μg/L (or 1.40 μg/g creatinine), and children had significantly higher concentrations (Bushnik et al. 2010; Statistics Canada 2011c). Children aged 12–19 years old were found to have a geometric mean concentration of 1.50 μg/L, compared to 1.30 μg/L for those aged 6–11 years (Statistics Canada 2011c). These Canadian findings are consistent with results for international studies reporting mean or median urine concentrations of 1–3 μg/L (Statistics Canada 2011c). Given the short half-life of orally ingested BPA and high frequency of detection, data from the CHMS suggest continual widespread exposure to this chemical by Canadian residents (Bushnik et al. 2010).

BPA has been known to be estrogenic since the mid-1930s, but concerns of the use of BPA in consumer products began to surface in 2008 after the release of several scientific reports that questioned its safety. Tests on rodents indicate that BPA mimics estrogen and may result in abnormalities in their chromosomes. The United States Food and Drug Administration (2010) raised further concerns regarding exposure of fetuses, infants, and young children to BPA. It has also been linked to an increased risk of developing breast cancer in women; prostate cancer and decreased testosterone levels in men, and birth abnormalities and developmental problems in children (Andrews 2008). In April 2008, the federal Minister of Health Tony Clement, declared that his government intended to ban baby bottles containing BPA. During a national press conference, Minister Clement stated:

We have concluded the early [childhood] development is sensitive to the effects of bisphenol A… Although our science tells us that exposure levels to newborns and infants are below the levels that cause effects, we believe that the current safety margin needs to be higher. We have concluded that it is better to be safe than sorry.

(Andrews 2008, 1)

In September 2010, Canada became the first country to declare BPA as a toxic substance. Subsequently, the European Union has also banned BPA in plastic baby bottles (Mittelstaedt 2010). In spite of this prudent public health ban, BPA is still permitted to be utilized in the lying of metal cans in Canada and certain plastic food containers.

Canadian Legislation to Preserve and Protect the Environment

The *Canadian Environmental Protection Act* (CEPA or Bill C-32) was enacted by Parliament in 1988 to provide legislative standards for assessing, identifying, evaluating, and managing various toxic chemicals and substances in Canada (Government of Canada 1999). The primary aim of the Act was to preserve and protect human health and well-being and our environments through the reduction and elimination of known toxic chemicals and substances. Moreover, the Act sought to regulate and control the entry of new substances into Canada that could pose a risk to human health. In 1992, the *National Pollutant Release Inventory* (NPRI) was established and is mandated under CEPA (Bill C-32) (Environment Canada 1992, 2000). The NPRI serves as a national database for information related to a variety of chemicals and substances that are annually released into water sources, on land or into the atmosphere. The NPRI database maintains records of off-site transfers for disposal or recycling purposes, and requires manufacturers and companies to report detailed information about the release and/or transfer of toxic pollutants to the federal government on a yearly basis.

In 1994, the *House of Commons Standing Committee on the Environment and Sustainable Development* was given the task of reviewing the CEPA. The committee recommended that the primary focus of the CEPA be redirected from the management of toxic chemicals and substances to the prevention of environmental pollution. The CEPA also provides the federal government with the legal authority to confront environmental polluters on water, land, or through the various layers of the atmosphere.

In 1999, the *New Substance Notification Regulations* was enacted and requires that all relevant information regarding new substances be disclosed and provided if they are intended to be manufactured or imported into Canada (Schubert and Bartfay 2010). A variety of federal legislations have also been introduced to protect our environment and the health and well-being of residents of Canada. For example, the *Motor Vehicle Safety Act* provides legislation and national

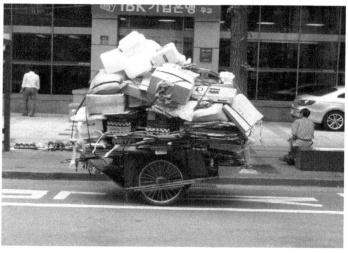

Source: Wally J. Bartfay

Photo 8.22 A cart stacked with cardboard and plastic products to be sold as recyclable materials in Seoul, Korea. The "4 Rs" of waste reduction consists of "reducing, reusing, recycling, and rethinking" how we use various materials and products and dispose of our trash in landfills. Canadians produce more garbage (777 kg per person per year) than any other industrialized nation in the world, and waste twice as much fresh drinking quality water (Cassese 2013).

standards on emissions permitted by gasoline and diesel-powered motor vehicles in Canada (Dickinson et al. 1996). In addition, the *Fishers Act, Canadian Shipping Act*, and the *Arctic Waters Pollution Prevention Act* prohibit the dumping or deposition of harmful substances such as oil and other petroleum products and garbage into our waterways and supplies (Beckman Murray et al. 2006; Dickinson et al. 1996).

In sheer numbers, as well as their potential to cause harm to humans and other species, old or inadequate waste disposal sites in Canada and abroad are among the principle sources of soil and groundwater contamination. In Canada alone, and if we exclude privately owned landfills, there are over 10,000 active, closed, or abandoned waste disposal sites and approximately 10% of these are believed to pose a potential risk to human health (Robinson Vollman, Anderson, and McFarlane 2004). In addition, the number of large spills exceeding 100 tonnes in Canada increased for the years 1984–1992 and the sectors reporting large spills include chemical, government, metallurgy, mining, petroleum, pulp and paper, and service industry (Environment Canada 2006).

For example, Table 8.4 shows the number of major reported spills for each of Environment Canada's five regions for petroleum, oil, or gasoline. It is worthy to note the alarming number of major spills, defined as those over a 100 tonnes, attributed to human error or oversight. Between the years 1984 and 1995 alone, 61,380 reported tonnes of oil, petroleum, or gasoline were spilled into the environment in Canada (Environment Canada 2006). These petroleum-based products may be potentially carcinogenic in nature, and exposure has also been linked to a variety of birth defects and respiratory diseases such as asthma (e.g., Eisen et al. 2001; Jarvholm et al. 1982; Lillienberg et al. 2010; Robertson, Weir, and Sherwood Burge 1988).

Major oil spills such as the March 24, 1989 Exxon Vladez shipping spill in Alaska and the British Petroleum (BP) Deepwater Horizon oil rig spill from April 20 to July 15, 2010 in the Gulf of Mexico are recent examples of how crude oil and other petroleum products can have both acute and chronic negative ripple effects on entire ecosystems, a variety of wildlife species and human health (Friis 2012; Institute of Medicine 2010; Lyons et al. 1999; Morita et al. 1999; San Sebastian, Armstrong, and Stephens 2002). On November 15, 2012, after a lengthy 2.5-year court battle, BP agreed to pay a record $4.5 billion (US) settlement with the United States Government and includes $2.4 billion to the National Fish and Wildlife Foundation, $350 million to the National Academy of Sciences, and approximately $500 million to the Securities Exchange Commission (Kunzelman 2012).

Table 8.4 Reported Major Spills (>100 tonnes) of Petroleum, Oil, or Gasoline in Canada by Environmental Regions (1984–1995)

Environmental Regions	Quantity per Reported Spill (Tonnes)	Sector or Industry	Comments Related to Causes	Totals per Region
1. Pacific and Yukon	– 750 – 190	– Petroleum – Petroleum	– Pipeline spill on land – Pipeline failure, spilled on land	940
2. Prairie and Northern	– 13,075 – 6,200 – 2,150 – 1,045	– Mining – Petroleum – Petroleum – Petroleum	– Spill in production field, overflow due to human error – Pipeline spill due to equipment failure – Pipeline lead due to material failure – Pipeline spill due to corrosion	22,470
3. Ontario	– 4,050 – 3,475 – 3,060	– Petroleum – Metallurgy – Metallurgy	– Dyke failure – Discharge of oil and water mixture from steel mill into a lake – Discharge of oil and water mixture from steel mill into a lake	10,585
4. Québec	– 5,580 – 715 – 400 – 395 – 295 – 250 – 235 – 155	– Petroleum – Petroleum – Petroleum – Mining – Petroleum – Petroleum – Petroleum – Transportation	– Above-ground tank failure in a refinery due to overstressed material – Ship collision – Ship collision due to human error – Failed valve fitting due to vandalism – Above-ground tank spill due to human error – Pipeline spill due to human error – Ship grounding due to storm floods – Valve failure due to human error in rail transport	8,025
5. Atlantic	–17,200 –910 –440 –410 –400	–Petroleum –Petroleum –Petroleum –Petroleum –Federal government	–Shipping accident due to severe storm –Ship collision –Ship grounding –Ship grounding –Pipeline leak to a lagoon	19,360
			National total	**61,380 tonnes**

Source: Adapted from Environment Canada (2006).

A more recent example in Canada involves the James Cree Nation community of approximately 1,600 people in Saskatchewan, which felt abandoned with poisoned waters in the wake of a major crude oil pipeline spill (McSheffrey 2016). Husky Energy has been under fire since one of its pipelines failed early on July 21, 2016 releasing up to 1,570 barrels or approximately 250,000 litres of crude oil and other toxins into the North Saskatchewan River, a drinking water source for thousands of Canadians. The disaster prompted emergency water restrictions in several municipalities, killed more than 140 animals, and is the subject of an ongoing federal and provincial investigation by authorities (McSheffrey 2016).

In March 2000, Joe Jordan introduced his private members Bill C-268, the *Canada Well-being Measurement Act* to the House of Commons in Ottawa (Schubert and Bartfay 2010). This bill proposed replacing the gross domestic product (GDP) indicator with the genuine progress indicator (GPI). In brief, the GPI seeks to encourage the development of a national set of standards for the economic, social, and environmental well-being of residents of Canada. During his address to the House of Commons, he stated:

> When pollution makes people sick, the cost of their medical care is added to the GDP. When the insurance industry has to repair or replace billions of dollars' worth of property because of increasingly violent weather events, the GDP goes up. These things are added into the GDP where they are mistaken for progress. In each case, the expenses are incurred because we have failed to prevent problems. These expenses are a sign of distress, not increased well-being. (Jordan 2000)

It is notable that although Bill C-268 was subsequently passed by Parliament by a vote of 185 to 46, there has been little movement by federal governments during the past decade to generate annual GPI measures for Canada. The reader is referred to the Web-Based Resource Box 82 for additional resources related to the environmental and its association with health.

Web-Based Resource Box 8.2 Environmental Health

Learning Resources	Website
Environment Canada: Clean air online This resource provides information related to air pollution standards and associated health risks	http://www.ec.gc.ca/air/acid-rain_e.html
Environment Canada: Ecosystem information This resource provides an overview of what an ecosystem is and why it is important to both humans and animals	http://www.ecoinfo.org
First Nations Environmental Network This website highlights various environmental issues and concerns by Indigenous peoples in Canada and discusses the importance of the environment for their heritage, lifestyle, and health	http://www.fnen.org
National Institute of Environmental Health Sciences This resource highlights scientific investigations related to the environment and ecosystems and their impact on humans and other life forms	http://www.niehs.nih.gov

Work Environments and Occupational Health and Safety

In order to view health from a holistic perspective, we have to examine both the living and work environments of humans collectively as a critical determinant of health (Bartfay and Bartfay 2015). Indeed, workers must shuttle to and from their living and work environments. For example, both the ancient Greeks and Romans recognized that certain mercury-based chemicals used in the production of metals could be poisonous to workers and its negative effects remained even after leaving the work environment (Lippman, Cohen, and Schlesinger 2003; US Department of Labour, Occupational Safety and Health Administration 2010).

Hippocrates (460–370 BC) described the toxic properties of the heavy metal lead on human health. Similarly, the toxic properties of zinc and sulphur were detailed by the Roman scholar Phiny the Elder (29–79 AD) during the first century AD (Friis 2012; Gochfield 2005). Phiny also invented one of the earliest workplace safety equipment, which consisted of a simple mask constructed from the bladder of sheep and/or other animals to help protect workers from inhaling toxic dust particles and metal fumes. Protective devices, such as masks, remain as critical implements to help defend workers against various hazards when they move between their living and work environments.

Occupational health and safety (OHS) is a branch or subspecialty of public health which examines both positive and negative health outcomes that are influenced or associated with exposure to general work conditions and/or specific known hazards that are encountered in work environments, and which seeks to preserve, promote, and/or restore the health and safety of workers (Bartfay and Bartfay 2015). There are over 2.8 million work-related occupational injuries and illnesses each year globally, of which 350,000 deaths are due to fatal work-related injuries (International Labour Organization 2005; Pruss-Ustun, Rapiti, and Hutin 2005).

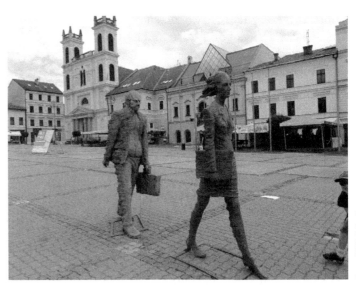

Source: Wally J. Bartfay

Photo 8.23 Growing fears of job insecurity, lay-offs, and global economic downfalls are contributing to increased hours spent at work by Canadians. In 1986, 23% of Canadian workers spent 6 or more hours per day doing leisure activities with their spouse or family, while only 14% reported the same in 2005 (Turcotte 2014).

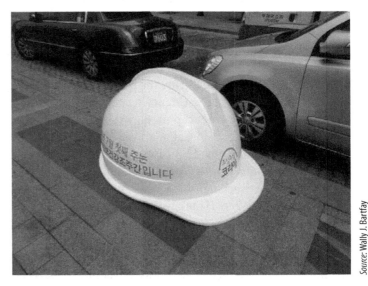

Source: Wally J. Bartfay

Photo 8.24 Safety equipment such as hard hats, breathing masks, and safety glasses and goggles are critical for the prevention of work-related injuries and disabilities in Canada and abroad.

Nelson et al. (2005) estimate that approximately 270 million workers suffered from nonfatal injuries and 160 work-related diseases annually. Moreover, only 10%–15% of workers globally have access to basic OHS services (e.g., safety officers, occupational nurse, and mandatory safety training workshops for new employees).

Since 1941, the International Labour Organization (ILO) has been collecting statistics on occupational injuries for publication in the *Yearbook of Labour Statistics*. Data provided by sex and by economic activity are available for only approximately 40% of the countries with data on occupational injuries based on the most recent version of the International Standard Industrial Classification of All Economic Activities (ILO 2013a). The ILO reports that every 15 sec, a workers dies from a work-related accident or disease; and every 15 sec, 160 workers have a work-related accident somewhere in the world (ILO 2013b).

According to *Canadian Community Health Survey* (CCHS), an estimated 630,000 Canadian workers experienced at least one activity-limiting occupational injury based on cross-sectional estimates of the proportion of workers injured on the job by occupational category, and selected work-related and sociodemographic characteristics (Wilkins and Mackenzie 2008). Of people in the trades (e.g., plumber, carpenter, electrician, welder, automechanic), transport (e.g., trucking, railway), and equipment operators (e.g., bulldozer operators, heavy diggers, forklifts), 9% of workers sustained an on-the-job injury, compared with only 2% of workers in the white-collar sector (e.g., office workers, bankers, accountants, teachers, architects).

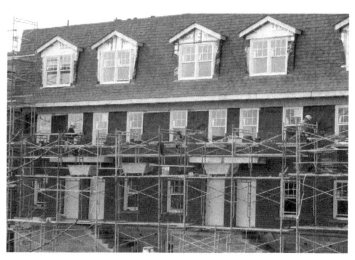

Source: Wally J. Bartfay

Photo 8.25 Individuals working in the construction industry in Canada continue to have the highest rates of injuries at 24.5 cases per 1,000 workers (Human Resources and Skills Development Canada 2013).

In the years 2002–2004, acute injuries occurring on the job resulted in an average of 465 deaths annually, and close to 300,000 compensated time-loss claims. The consequences of occupational injuries can be appreciable. These include lost incomes, time away from work or training, health care expenses, compensation costs, possible long-term health problems or disability, and a burden on the family of the injured worker (Wilkins and Mackenzie 2008). It is notable that the CCHS only asked respondents about how many activity-limiting injuries they had sustained during the past year, and were not asked to provide details regarding the *most serious* injuries per se. Hence, estimates related to so-called minor or less severe injuries (e.g., minor laceration requiring stitches) were not captured by this cross-sectional national survey. Figure 8.4 shows the number of work-related injury cases in Canada from 1982 to 2010. We observe that the number of work-related injuries in Canada increased from 43.8 cases per 1,000 employed in 1982 to 48.9 in 1987. Following 1987, the rate declined continuously to 14.7 per 1,000 employed in 2010.

In 2008, those working in the construction industry in Canada had the highest rates of injuries at 24.5 cases per 1,000 workers (Human Resources and Skills Development Canada, (2013). Human Resources and Skills Development Canada (2013) reports that in 2010, one out of every 68 employed workers was injured or harmed on the job and received workers compensation as a result. Moreover, men experienced a higher rate of injury (18.8 cases per 1,000), in comparison to their female counterparts (11.2 cases per 1,000 workers). The highest rate of injury in 2010 was in Manitoba (24.4 cases per 1,000 workers), and the lowest rate was in Ontario (9.1 cases per 1,000 workers). Workers in construction (24.5 cases per 1,000 workers) and in manufacturing (24.0 cases per 1,000 workers) had the highest rates. By contrast, the rate in the financial sector was a little less than one (0.6 case) per 1,000 employees (Human Resources and Skills Development Canada 2013).

According to Human Resources and Skills Development Canada (2013), one in every 68 employed workers in 2010 was injured or harmed on the job and received workers compensation as a result. The highest rate of injury occurred in the province of Manitoba with 24.4 cases per 1,000 employed workers; the lowest rate occurred in Ontario with 9.1 cases per 1,000 employed workers, and the national average was reported to be 14.7 cases per 1,000 employed workers (Association of Workers' Compensation Boards of Canada and Statistics Canada 2012).

Occupational exposure to various chemicals (e.g., pesticides, solvents) and radiation have been shown to pose serious health risks for women in Canada and abroad, including an increased risk of developing breast

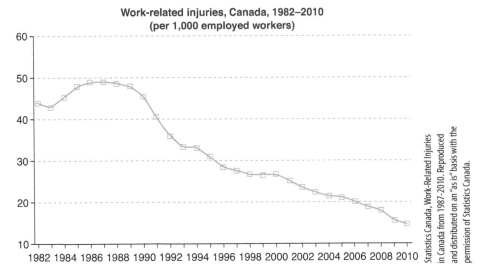

Work-related injuries, Canada, 1982–2010
(per 1,000 employed workers)

Statistics Canada, Work-Related Injuries in Canada from 1987-2010. Reproduced and distributed on an "as is" basis with the permission of Statistics Canada.

Figure 8.4 Work-related injuries in Canada from 1987 to 2010.

Source: HRSDC calculations based on data from Association of Workers' Compensation Boards of Canada. Available from: Association of Workers' Compensation Boards of Canada and Statistics Canada (July 2012).

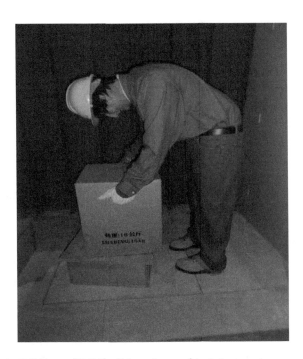
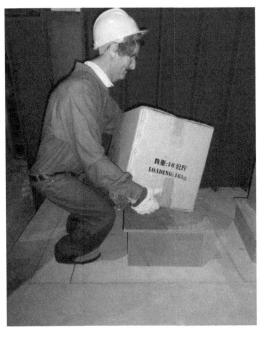

Source: Wally J. Bartfay

Photo 8.26a and 8.26b Education and training sessions, such as how to safely and properly lift heavy objects, are keys to the prevention of work-related injuries and disabilities. The worker on the left (Photo 18a) is not using a proper technique for lifting and is at increased risk for injury or strain of the back. Conversely, the worker on the right (Photo 18b) is using proper lifting technique and is less prone to back injury or strain.

cancer. The Canadian Breast Cancer Foundation (2011) reports an almost tripling of the breast cancer risk among women with an occupational history of farming because they were more likely to be exposed to pesticides–chemicals, many of which are now known carcinogens. In addition, women who went from farming environments to the auto industry to work had an even greater risk for developing breast cancer. The relative risk doubled for workers in solvent-using industries, those in metal production, and for those involved in the fabrication of furniture, chemicals, printing materials, textile, and clothing. Health care professionals and workers including female nurses and dental hygienists who are routinely exposed to radiation or those who perform X-rays also had an increased risk (Canadian Breast Cancer Foundation 2011).

Bernardino Ramazzini (1633–1714)

Bernardino Ramazzini (1633–1714) is credited as writing the first book on occupational health and industrial hygiene in 1700 entitled *De morbis articicum diatribe* (or *The Diseases of Workers*) and is regarded as the father of occupational medicine (Franco 1999; Friis 2012; Gochfield 2005). Ramazzini identified and detailed several negative health outcomes associated with environmental contaminates that a variety of workers were exposed to including chemicals, dust, metals, and abrasive agents (Garrison 1926; Rosen 1958).

His descriptions covered a large variety of occupations from miners, to fabric workers, to workers who cleaned privies. He is also regarded as a pioneer in the field of ergonomics and he described various hazards associated with different postures assumed by a variety of workers. He described the occupational health hazards of workers exposed to lead and lead poisoning from the glaze used by potters and the dangers of mercury exposure in the work environments of mirror-makers and goldsmiths. He reported that individuals in these reported occupations seldom reached old age, and if they did their health was often severely compromised. For example, many workers had palsy of the neck and hands, loss of teeth, vertigo, asthma, and other respiratory ailments and paralysis.

Percival Pott (1714–1788)

Sir Percival Pott was an eighteenth century surgeon in London, England who made a significant contribution to our understanding of the impact of work environments on the health of workers (Doll 1975; Merrill 2008; Pott 1775). In a short chapter in his 725 pages book (Pott 1775) entitled *A Short Treatise of the Chimney Sweeper's Cancer*, he was the first to describe chimney soot as the first known environmental carcinogen and as an occupational hazard for chimney sweeps. Pott (1775) described the plight of chimney sweeps, who were often young boys, during the eighteenth century in England as follows in his book:

> The fate of these people seems singularly hard; in their early infancy, they are most frequently treated with great brutality, and almost starved with cold and hunger; they are thrust up narrow, and sometimes hot chimnies, where they are bruised, burned, and almost suffocated; and when they get to puberty, become perculiary [sic] liable to a noisome, painful and fatal disease…Other people have cancers of the same part; and so have others besides lead-workers, the Poictou colic, and the consequent paralysis; but it is nevertheless a disease to which they are particularly liable; and so are chimney sweepers to the cancer of the scrotum and testicles. The disease, in these people…seems to derive its origins from a lodgment of soot in the rugae of the scrotum.
>
> (Pott 1775, 521–2)

Pott's detailed observations are often regarded as the foundation on which carcinogenic chemical by-products may be identified and on which the knowledge of cancer prevention has been built (Friis 2012; Merrill 2008). Following his scientific conclusions related to the observed association between the development of scrotal cancer and the occupational hazards of being exposure to soot by chimney sweeps, Pott (1775) established one of the earliest occupational hygiene control measures. Namely, that chimney sweeps bathe at least once per week.

Pott's observation linking occupational exposure to soot and smoke and their association with prostate cancer remains relevant today. Indeed, there is a growing body of scientific literature that has linked occupational exposure to soot, ash, chemicals, and smoke in firefighters with an increased risk of developing various cancers including cancers of the prostate, bladder, testicles, colon, kidneys, breast, brain, leukaemia and non-Hodgkin's lymphoma, and increased risk of mortality (e.g., Ahn, Jeong and Kim 2012; Austin, Dussault and Ecobichon 2001; Gaertner et al. 2004; Youakim 2006; Zeig-Owens et al. 2011). In 2002, Manitoba became the first Canadian province to recognize cancer as an occupational health risk associated with firefighting (Kusch 2010). Firefighters in British Columbia, Alberta, Saskatchewan, Manitoba, Ontario, and Nova Scotia now have presumptive legislation, which now places the onus on workers' compensation boards (WCB) to bring forward proof to establish why a disabled firefighter should not be eligible for compensation, rather than placing the burden of proof on the sick firefighter (Constant 2008).

For example, in 2008, the provincial government of British Columbia moved forward with the *Firefighters Occupational Disease Regulation* under the *Worker's Compensation Act* (Constant 2008). This legislation states that a worker with at least 20 years of employment as a firefighter who is disabled on or after May 27, 2008 from testicular or lung cancer will now be covered. These additions follow seven primary site cancers already listed as of April 11, 2005: Leukaemia (covered after 5 years of employment), non-Hodgkin's lymphoma (20 years), bladder cancer (15 years), brain cancer (10 years), colorectal cancer (20 years), kidney cancer (20 years), and ureter cancer (15 years).

Kusch (2010) reports that there are more than 200 carcinogens that have been linked to the development of breast cancer that are present at fires in Canada, making it one of the most susceptible cancers for female firefighters. Female firefighters have three to five times the risk of being diagnosed with breast cancer, in comparison to those in other occupations. In Manitoba, 43 of the 950 active firefighters are women. In 2010, Jennifer Howard, the Minister responsible for the Workers Compensation Board in Manitoba introduced Bill 6. This legislation adds breast cancer and three other cancers (multiple myeloma, primary site prostate, and skin cancer) to 10 other illnesses already covered for firefighters by workers compensation in the province of Manitoba (Kusch 2010). Similarly, in May 4, 2011 the province of Alberta added four additional cancers (prostate, breast, skin, and multiple myeloma) to their presumptive coverage by workers compensation boards, bringing the total to 14 now covered (Wells 2011). The Research Focus Box 8.3 provides an example of a study which examined the negative health effects associated with exposure to dust, ash, soot, and other materials by first responders following the 9/11 attacks by terrorists on New York City in 2001.

Research Focus Box 8.3

Early Assessment of Cancer Outcomes in New York City Firefighters After 9/11 Attacks: An Observational Cohort Study

Study Aim/Rationale

The attacks on the World Trade Center (WTC) in New York City on September 11, 2001 resulted in the exposure of first responders, including firefighters, to dust, fumes, ash, soot, and a variety of suspected carcinogens. This aim of this observational study was to determine the incidence of cancer among firefighters who responded to the WTC disaster 7 years after the disaster.

Methods

An observational cohort study was employed to assess 9,853 males who were employed as firefighters on January 1, 1996. On and after 9/11, person-time for 8,927 firefighters were classified as WTC-exposed, and all person-time non-WTC after 9/11 for 926 firefighters were classified as non-WTC exposed for comparison purposes. Cancer cases were confirmed by matches from state tumour registries or through appropriate clinical documentation. Incidence rates for WTC-exposed and non-WTC exposed were adjusted for age, race, ethnic origin, secular trends with the United States National Cancer Institute Surveillance Epidemiology and End Results reference population.

Major Findings

The standardized incidence ratios (SIRs) for the incidence of cancer among WTC-exposed firefighters was 1.10 (95% CI 0.98–1.25) compared with an SIR for the WTC for the nonexposed firefighters was 1.19 (95% CI

(Continued)

Research Focus Box 8.3 (*Continued*)

0.96–1.47) corrected for possible surveillance bias and 1.32 (1.07–1.62) without correction for surveillance bias. Secondary analyses of the data produced similar findings.

Implications for Public Health
These findings suggest that firefighters who were in the WTC-exposed cohort had a modest increased risk for the development of cancer, and were not limited to specific organ types due to the limited exposure follow-up time for this study. As with any observational study, we cannot rule out the possibility that the effects observed in the exposed cohort might be due to unidentified confounders. These preliminary results also suggest that firefighters who attended the 9/11 disaster in New York City may be at increased risk for developing cancer over time. Additional studies are warranted to examine the effects of time on the development of specific cancer types in this exposed cohort.

Source: Zeig-Owens et al. (2011).

Alice Hamilton (1869–1970)

Dr. Alice Hamilton's description of *phossy jaw* or phosphorus necrosis of the jaw, is a painful and disfiguring condition that occurred among the workers who manufactured matches during the late 1900s, and was linked to exposure to white or yellow phosphorus paste (Friis 2012; Gochfeld 2005; Hamilton 1943). Many of the workers during this time period were young children who worked in vapour-filled and poorly ventilated factories. The condition developed over years of exposure that resulted in various clinical manifestations including debilitation, neurological disturbances, and hemorrhages of the lung. Phosphorous dust inhaled or injected by match workers is able to penetrate into a defective tooth and travel down into the roots to the jawbone, which subsequently kills the tissue cells and makes the victim prone to infections and abscesses. The jaw swells and causes severe and intense pain for the victim and penetrates into the area of the orbit of the eye, often resulting in loss of an eye. Hamilton, who crusaded against industrial hazards encountered by match workers, wrote the following description of this condition:

> In severe cases one lower jawbone may have to be removed, or an upper jawbone – perhaps both. There are cases on record of men and women who had to live all the rest of their days on liquid food. The scars and contractures left after recovery were terribly disfiguring, and led some women to commit suicide. Here was an industrial disease which could be clearly demonstrated to the most skeptical. Miss Adams told me that when she was in London in the 1880's, she went to a mass meeting of protest against phossy jaw and on the platform were a number of pitiful cases, showing their scars and deformities. (Hamilton 1943, 4)

Occupational Health and Safety in Canada

According to Storey (2009), workers' compensation payments made by compensation boards in Canada for various direct costs associated with occupational injuries are in excess of $4.7 billion annually. When indirect costs are included, WCB payments cost the Canadian economy in excess of $9.3 billion annually. In Canada, each province and territory has legislated standards for health and safety in the workplace. For example, employers in the province of Alberta must comply with their OHS code, which came into effect on April 30, 2004 (Alberta Government 2004).

Health Canada (2004) notes that research on the Canadian workforce consistently indicates that health care professionals and workers such as nurses, have a greater risk of workplace injuries and more mental health issues in comparison to all other occupational groups. Moreover, health care professionals, especially nursing personnel, have considerably more sick time than those employed in other occupations. Although the labour force increased by 18.5% in Canada between the years 1996 and 2002; the average number of injuries per year for health care workers increased by 7.8% (Health Canada 2004).

For example, in the province of Ontario, 58% of all stress-related claims were directly related to violence, with a steady increase in post-traumatic stress between the years 1996 and 2002. The prevalence of musculoskeletal symptoms in nursing personnel was 60%–72% for upper-body and lower-body symptoms, respectively. Psychological distress is common in health care professionals and workers as a result of patient violence, aggression, high workloads, mandatory shift-work, and other factors. Infectious diseases are also a growing concern, as highlighted by the emergence of Severe Acute Respiratory Syndrome in 2003 in Canada and blood and body fluid exposure, which carries the risk of HIV/AIDS and hepatitis transmission (Health Canada 2004).

Several Canadian organizations, which include the *Canadian Centre for Occupational Health and Safety* (CCOHS); the WCB) and the *Workplace Hazardous Materials Information System* (WHMIS) strive to preserve the health, safety, and well-being of all workers in Canada (Thompson 2010). In Canada, OHS is divided among 14 jurisdictions which comprised 10 provincial; 3 territorial and 1 federal. The federal government deals with labour affairs for certain sections of their workforce including employees of the federal government (e.g., public sector workers) or federal corporations, and also has jurisdictions over workers in occupations that cross provincial or territorial lines (e.g., communication, transportation industry). In addition, each province and territory in Canada has its own OHS agency, which enacts and enforces its own work-related legislations (see Table 8.5).

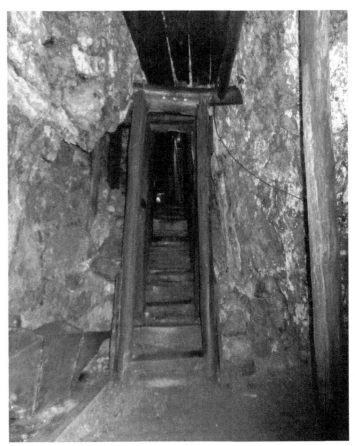

Source: Wally J. Bartfay

Photo 8.27 Over 380,000 individuals in Canada work in the mining and mineral processing industries, which contributed $54 billion toward our GDP in 2013 alone (The Mining Association of Canada 2014). Mining remains one of the most dangerous occupations in Canada and abroad. For example, the Springhill Mining Disasters in Nova Scotia collectively killed over 138 men and boys working in the coal mines over a span of 65 years. The Westray Mine disaster of 1992 in Nova Scotia killed 26 miners due to an underground methane explosion.

These provincial and territorial OHS legislations seek to preserve and ensure a safe working environment for all individuals; support the rights of workers through legislation; set guidelines; provide a mechanism for enforcement, and outline the rights of employees, which include the: (a) right to be aware of potential safety and health hazards in their workplaces, (b) right of employees to partake in activities (e.g., serve on health and safety committees, training sessions) aimed at preventing occupational accidents or diseases, and (c) the right of employees to refuse to engage in dangerous work or activities without the fear of losing their job.

Various occupational-related diseases can result from exposure to various chemicals, products or materials that are unique to workplace settings and tend not to be present in concentrated forms in daily life (e.g., asbestos, benzene, ionizing radiation). For example, between the years 1988 and 2012, WorkSafeBC (2013) reported 86 deaths due to occupational disease and 63 fatalities due to on-site injuries.

For example, a worker in the automanufacturing industry exposed to paint fumes may currently refuse to work if their employers do not provide them with proper safety masks and ventilation to protect them against potentially harmful fumes. A report by the Canadian Breast Cancer Foundation (2011) describes the story of

Table 8.5 Provincial and Territorial Health and Safety Legislations in Canada

Province or Territory	Legislation
Newfoundland and Labrador	Occupational Health and Safety Act and WHMIS
Prince Edward Island	Occupational Health and Safety Act and WHMIS
Nova Scotia	Occupational Health and Safety Act and WHMIS
New Brunswick	Occupational Health and Safety Act and WHMIS
Québec	Act Representing Occupational Health and Safety and WHMIS
Ontario	Occupational Health and Safety Act and WHMIS
Manitoba	Workplace Safety and Human Act and WHMIS
Saskatchewan	Occupational Health and Safety Act and Occupational Health and Safety Regulations, Part XXII
Alberta	Occupational Health and Safety Code, Part 29 and WHMIS—Sections 395–414
British Columbia	Worker's Compensation Act and Occupational Health and Safety Regulation, Part 5
Yukon	Occupational Health and Safety Act and WHMIS
Northwest Territories	Safety Act and WHMIS
Nunavut	Safety Act and WHMIS

Note: WHMIS, Workplace Hazardous Materials Information System regulations.

Source: Adapted from Canadian Centre for Occupational Health and Safety (2005), http://www.ccohs.ca/.

Ms. Sandy Knight aged 52, who spent 20 years working in the auto industry in Windsor, Ontario. She started work at the age of 19 where she was required to paint, and assemble auto parts. She notes that paint fumes and smoke from cooling plastic parts were often present on the factory floor where dashboards, taillights, and other car parts were made. Ms. Knight and her co-workers did not wear protective masks because they were not mandatory at the time. Protective masks in this auto plant only became mandatory 10 years after she started to work as a spray painter, and her job ended in 1998 when the plant closed. Two years later she was diagnosed with breast cancer and believes it is attributed to her work environment. She maintains that many women are still not wearing masks and still dealing with poor or inadequate ventilation in workplace settings and that during economic downturns, individuals are often more reluctant to speak up for better working conditions (Canadian Breast Cancer Foundation 2011).

Prior to March 1996, Statistic Canada managed the *National Work Injuries Statistics Program* (NWISIP), and collected data from all the provincial and territorial workers' compensation boards (Canadian Centre for Occupational Health and Safety 2011). After March 1996, the *Association of Workers' Compensation Boards of Canada* (AWCBC) assumed responsibility of the NWISIP. WCBs and commissions across Canada collect data related to accepted time-loss injuries and fatality reports that are published under the NWISP according to the following eight main categories (Canadian Centre for Occupational Health and Safety 2011, 1):

1. Nature of the injury (specific type of injury or disease)
2. Part of the human body affected by the specific injury or disease

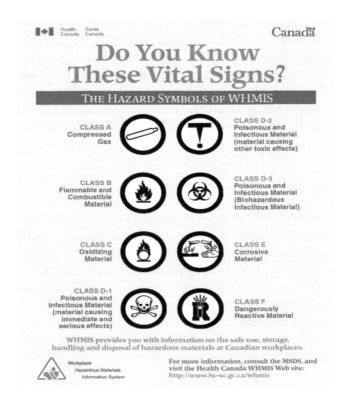

Figure 8.5 The primary aim of the Workplace Hazardous Materials System (WHMIS) is to decrease the number of work-related injuries, illness, disabilities, and death through comprehensive workplace communication and education regarding various hazardous materials and products. *Source*: Health Canada, Ottawa, Ontario. http://img.docstoccdn.com/thumb/orig/55040754.png or http://alsehha.gov.sa/dpcc/en/topics.asp?tid=3 or http://alsehha.gov.sa/dpcc/images/wp_hazard.gif.

3. Source or immediate cause of the injury
4. Type of event or accident that resulted in the injury (e.g., fall, operating a machine)
5. The specific type of industry (e.g., mining, health care services, manufacturing) that the worker was employed at during the time of injury
6. Specific occupation of the injured or ill worker
7. Province or territory in which the injury, disease, or fatality occurred
8. Age and sex of the worker

The CCOHS oversees WHMIS, which became law through complementary federal, provincial, and territorial legislation in Canada in October, 1988, and operates as a separate division within Health Canada (Thompson 2010). The CCOHS was first established in 1978 and is governed by a council of representatives from three key stakeholders: (a) government (federal, provincial/territorial), (b) employers, and (c) workers (Shah 2003; Stafanson and Bartfay 2010).

The WHMIS is a comprehensive federally legislated system to ensure the safe use and handling of hazardous materials and substances in Canadian workplaces (Bartfay and Bartfay 2015; Shah 2003; Stafanson and Bartfay 2010).

The national standards for WHMIS were established based on the federal *Hazardous Products Act* and the *Controlled Products Regulations*, and applies to all Canadian workplaces (e.g., industrial, health care settings) in which hazardous materials (e.g., radioactive products, chemotherapeutic agents, combustible agents, infectious materials, medical waste products) are present. This includes the notification of workers regarding the nature of the specific hazard(s) that they may encounter in their workplace; the appropriate labelling of these hazardous materials, and a material safety sheet which details the nature, properties, toxicities, and associated first aid treatments. The Web-Based Resource Box 8.3 provides the reader with additional resources related to OHS in Canada.

Work-Related Stress

Stress is a normal part of everyday life, which can have negative or positive effects on individuals depending on the nature of the stressor; its magnitude or degree; whether it is acute or chronic in nature, and the coping skills and resources available to effectively manage or deal with the stressor. *Stress* is defined as any physical, social, political, economic, or cultural force which creates an imbalance and which can have either a negative or positive influence on an individual or group (Bartfay and Bartfay 2015). Certain levels of stress related to one's family, occupation, and life in general in expected and normal (Health Canada 2000; Statistics Canada 2010). Indeed, stress is often what provides us with the motivation and energy to meet our daily challenges at home and in the workplace. However, if stress levels are not properly managed, they can lead to the development of a variety of mental and physical conditions and diseases including anxiety, insomnia, depression, and cardiovascular disease. When stress turns into feelings of unwanted pressure, anxiety, frustration, or dissatisfaction, stress can manifest itself as a negative ripple effect in both the home and work environments (Bartfay and Bartfay 2015).

Table 8.6 lists potential stressors with examples of each that can contribute to increased levels of workplace stress and alterations to health overtime (e.g., Canadian Centre for Occupational Health and Safety 2012; Karasek 1979; Shields 2002, 2004; Statistics Canada 2010, 2012; Wilkins 2007; Williams 2003).

Statistics Canada (2010) notes that in the year 2008, 21.2% of males (or 2.8 million individuals) and 23.4% of females (or 3.2 million individuals) aged 15 years and older reported that most days were *quite a bit* or *extremely stressful*. Moreover, males and females aged 35–54 and males aged 25–34 were most likely to report

Web-Based Resource Box 8.3 Occupational Health and Safety

Learning Resources	Website
Association of Workers' Compensation Boards of Canada (AWCBC) This board provides details related towork-related legislations in Canada and provides statistics related to workplace injuries and the number of individuals receiving workers compensation by sex and occupation in Canada	http://www.awcbc.org/en/index/asp
Board of Canadian Registered Safety Professionals This website describes the activitiesand mandates of workplace safety officers	http://www.bcrsp.ca
Canadian Centre for Occupational Health and Safety This resource highlights the Centre's aims and mandates related to the promotion of safe and healthy workplaces in Canada	http://www.ccohs.ca
Canadian Occupational Health Nurses Association This voluntary association for nurses promotes the practice of occupational nursing in a variety of work settings in Canada	http://www.cohna-aciist.ca

Table 8.6 Potential Stressors That can Contribute to Increased Levels of Workplace Stress and Alterations to Health

Potential Stressors	Examples
Work/family imbalance	Children (e.g., hockey practice, swimming classes)
	Aging parents (e.g., need to drive to primary health care provider appointments, house, or yardwork)
	Caregiver burden (e.g. looking after an ill spouse, child, or parent)
	Lack of personal time to exercise
	Lack of time to prepare healthy family meals and reliance on high caloric, fat, and salty drive-thru meals
	Lack of time to sleep or insomnia
Technology/mobile electronic and digital devices	E-mails, Internet access at home 24/7
	Nomophobia or the fear of not being permanently "wired" and available to all including work colleagues and supervisors (e.g., even on weekends, holidays, etc.)
	Commuting times with cars, buses, subways, etc. and delays (e.g., traffic jams)
	Expectation to keep up to date with new software and hardware products on own without in-service training opportunities
Lack of job security	Economic downturns
	Fear of outsourcing
	Contract work with no benefits
	Fear of lay-off during economic downturns
	Lack of seniority in organization
Nature of work and job dissatisfaction	Shift-work (e.g., health care professionals, factory workers, police officers)
	Fear of infectious diseases by health care professionals/lab personnel
	High levels of noise, heat, poor air quality, etc.
	Risk of personnel injury (e.g., construction workers, miners)
	Sedentary nature of office work
	Lack of intellectual challenge
	Monotonous work (e.g., assembly-line work, cashier)
	Being over qualified for current job (e.g., PhD prepared engineer working in a call centre or as an office clerk)
	Lack of career development opportunities (e.g., in-service training, certifications)
	Expectation to train new recruits or junior personnel without extra time allotted or recognition for your efforts
Financial stressors	Mortgages and loans
	Repair to home or car
	Cost of prescription medications
	Household debt (e.g., maxed-out credit cards)
	Daycare costs for children
	Costs to provide care to aging parents (e.g., nursing, personal care assistants)

(Continued)

Table 8.6 Potential Stressors That can Contribute to Increased Levels of Workplace Stress and Alterations to Health (*Continued*)

Potential Stressors	Examples
Low job control/input	Limited opportunities for career advancements Little or no nonmonetary recognition/feedback from supervisors or peers Lack of opportunities to be creative or engage in self-directed work Over qualified/educated for current job Being bullied by managers or co-workers
High job demands	Being over-promoted and ill-qualified for current position (e.g., lack of education or training) Heavy workloads Long working hours with few breaks Expectation to work overtime and on weekends/holidays to meet required deadlines (no down time) Conflicting priorities
Office politics/hostile work environment	Favouritism by manager or supervisors Lack of available time to socialize outside of office hours with so-called "movers-and-shakers" at work Having to split credit for group work completed mostly by one or more individuals Being harassed by supervisor or co-worker Lack of organizational systems/mechanisms to deal with concerns of workers Autocratic management styles Nonparticipation in decision-making processes Lack of perceived fairness (e.g., who gets what and when such as preferred holiday times)

high levels of daily stress. Females aged 15–24 and 35–44 were more likely to report that most of their days were *extremely stressful*, and these age groups correspond to the time when most individuals have to manage multiple roles and responsibilities associated with families and careers. Health care expenditures are approximately 50% greater for workers who report high degrees of stress in their life, and stress-related absences cost employers in excess of $3.5 billion annually (Duxbury and Higgins 2001; Williams 2003).

If we exclude women who were on maternity leave or holidays, 7.0% of full-time employees (defined as worked 30+ hours/week) were absent from work for all or part of the week for personal reasons in 2001 (Statistics Canada 2012). By 2011, this figure had risen to 8.1% (*N* = 913,000). Extrapolated over the entire work year, work time lost for personal reasons increased from 8.5 days per worker in 2001, to 9.3 days in 2011 (Statistics Canada 2012). Experiencing stress for long or chronic periods of time, although they may be perceived as mild or at lower degree or level, will also activate the *fight or flight* response in individuals. This can result in increased blood pressure and heart rates, increased cholesterol and fatty acids in the blood, faster blood clotting times, increased production of stomach and digestive enzymes and acids, decreased protein synthesis, anxiety, nervousness, difficulty in concentrating, mood swings, and insomnia to name but a few (Health Canada 2000; Statistics Canada 2012; Wilkins 2007; Williams 2003).

Since the causes of workplace-related stress can vary from individual to individual, so do the strategies to prevent, manage, and/or reduce the identified stressor(s) (Bartfay and Bartfay 2015). For example, if the workplace is too noisy, control measures such as physical barriers (e.g., sound-dampening doors, earplugs) should be implemented where ever possible. If the worker is experiencing pain and discomfort associated with repetitive types of jobs (e.g., assembly-line work, cashier), mandatory breaks could be implemented

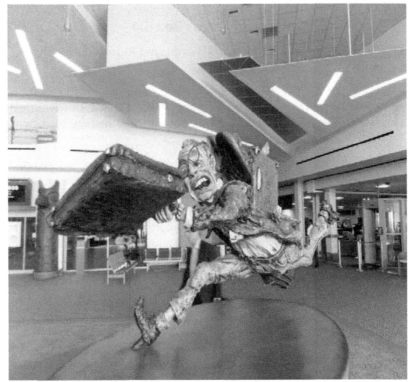

Source: Wally J. Bartfay

Photo 8.28 Work-related stress is a growing occupational health concern in Canada and globally. Statistics Canada reports that more than 1 in 4 adult workers (27% or 3.7 million workers) described their lives as highly stressful, and mental health issues alone are estimated to cost employers in excess of $20 billion annually and account for 3-out-of-4 short-term work-related disability claims (Crompton 2014). Health care expenditures in Canada are approximately 50% greater for workers who report high degrees of stress in their lives and stress-related absences cost employers in excess of $3.5 billion annually.

along with ergometric redesigns of the workstations. Workplace health and safety programs that target the source(s) of the stress or stressors in the workplace should be implicated by health care professionals (e.g., occupational health nurse). Managers and supervisors should keep job demands reasonable by providing realistic deadlines, hours of work, and feedback regarding performance expectations and outcomes achieved. Stress management training and confidential counselling services should be made available to all workers to help address the root causes of the stress and coping skills, as well as issues surrounding bullying and/or harassment in the workplace (Canadian Centre for Occupational Health and Safety 2012; Health Canada 2000; Shields 2004; Williams 2003).

In addition to the above, being unemployed is regarded as one of the greatest single stressors that an individual or family can face (Bartfay, Bartfay, and Wu 2013; Bezrucka 2009; Stuckler et al. 2011). For example, Strully (2009) reported that losing one's job was associated with a 54% chance of reporting fair or poor health and, for an individual with no pre-existing health conditions, the chances of reporting a new state of ill health increased by 83%. Struckler et al. (2011) examined the negative health effects associated with the recent global recession in 2008–2009 and government expenditures for 26 countries in the European Union (EU). The investigators found that every 1% increase in unemployment was associated with a 0.79% increase in the rates of suicide and homicide in the EU. The Research Focus Box 8.4 highlights a Canadian study which examined the impact of this global economic recession on the health of unemployed blue-collar autoworkers in the province of Ontario. All participants reported high levels of stress, anxiety, and depression. In addition, approximately 30% of unemployed workers reported that they suffered from alterations to sexual function, intimacy, and insomnia due to high levels of emotional stress.

Research Focus Box 8.4

Impact of the Global Economic Crisis on the Health of Unemployed Autoworkers

Study Aim/Rationale

To determine the impact of the 2008–2009 global economic recession on the health of unemployed blue-collar workers in the automotive manufacturing sector in Ontario, Canada. This investigation also sought to examine the lived experiences of unemployed blue-collar workers and their current health service needs.

Methodology/Design

A phenomenological investigation was undertaken between September and November, 2009. A total of 22 male and 12 females were recruited for this investigation, which employed purposive sampling techniques. Participants were asked to complete a quantitative demographic and financial questionnaire related to their sex, age, highest level of formal education completed, monthly household income, number of dependents, number of years employed in the automotive sector, and the number of months laid off at the time of the interview. The qualitative component of the study consisted of semistructured interviews conducted in focus group sessions that lasted from 2 to 2.5 hours in duration. The narrative responses were recorded and transcribed verbatim, categorized, and thematically analyzed. Quality assurance checks for data completeness and accuracy were performed on 40% of the raw data transcribed.

Major Findings

Reported monthly household income while employed ranged from $2,450 to $8,000 with a mean of $4,026.9 (±1550.8). Monthly household income while unemployed decreased significantly (mean = $1,596.6 ± $1,550.8, $p = 0.001$), in comparison to monthly employed incomes. The total number of years employed ranged from 2 to 31.7 with a mean of 15 ± 8. The total number of months laid off during the data collection period ranged from 1 to 39 with a mean of 13.9 ± 10.1. High levels of stress, anxiety, and depression were reported in all participants (100%). Approximately three-quarters of respondents reported that they suffered from chronic neck, knee, shoulder, or back pain attributed to the repetitive nature of assembly-line work. 61.8% of respondents also reported that since being laid off they had ceased going to dentists, physiotherapists, massage therapists, acupuncturists, and chiropractors to help manage their work-related pain and discomfort because their work-related benefits were cut-off. 32.4% of respondents indicated that filling prescription medications were a financial challenge, and 21.9% had to make alternative housing arrangements (e.g., move in with relatives, live in their car) due to their inability to meet rent or mortgage obligations. Lastly, 29.4% of respondents identified that they suffered from alterations to sexual function, intimacy, and problems sleeping due to high levels of emotional stress.

Implications for Public Health

These findings suggest that unemployed blue-collar autoworkers in Ontario and their families experience various negative health effects due primarily to financial constraints and the termination of employee-based health benefits (e.g., drug and dental plans). These findings also indicate that unemployed workers are reluctant to access private or public health services due to financial constraints (e.g., inability to pay for prescription medications). The authors argue that to obtain a better understanding of how major economic recessions and associated unemployment affects the health of various workers and regional populations requires an examination of the social determinants of health, including how communities share various resources among their members.

Source: Bartfay, Bartfay, and Wu (2013).

Environmental and Occupational Risk Assessments for Public Health

An *environmental and occupational risk assessment* is defined as a formalized process for characterizing and estimating the impact or magnitude of harm to human health and/or damage to natural or artificial ecosystems resulting from exposure to one or more hazardous chemicals or substances on a specific target population or community, and are intended to provide objective information to help establish or inform public health policy and planning decisions (Bartfay and Bartfay 2015). Risk assessments are now commonly done for a variety of purposes including the impacts of construction for a new dam or bridge, finance and investments, medical errors, and more recently to determine the threat of a biological, chemical or radioactive act of terrorism on public health and well-being (e.g., Apostolakis and Lemon 2005; Elad 2005; Gochfeld and Burger 2008; Lin, Tokai, and Nakanishi 2005; Meinhardt 2005; Tanaka 2003). Risk assessments take into account a variety of human values related to health and well-being, safety, environmental and ecological concerns, and fiscal concerns as well.

Governments in Canada and internationally as well as the general public have been increasingly aware of the importance of conducting nonbiased risk assessments to protect and preserve their own health and values as well as ecosystems and the environment (e.g., safe drinking water, clean air, unpolluted waters for fishers, erosion control, recreational pursuits, sediment quality standards, preservation of wildlife and at risk species). However, protecting human health does not necessarily protect the environment or ecosystems and their component communities and living organisms from harm (Gochfeld and Burger 2008). Indeed, humans may be more or less susceptible to certain chemicals introduced into the environment than experimental or wild animals. Furthermore, the potential identified risks and benefits may not be uniform in nature. For example, there is an extensive literature which details the benefits for adults eating a diet rich in fish which is high in protein and rich in beneficial omega-3 fatty acids (PUFAs). Nonetheless, certain types of fish (e.g., tuna, sword fish) are also high in mercury (MeHg, a neurotoxin), and pregnant women are advised to limit their consumption (Burger et al. 2005; Friis 2012; Gochfeld and Burger 2005; Mahaffey 2005; Merrill 2008).

There are several approaches for applying environmental risk assessments in making policy decisions in the context of public health, well-being, and safety (e.g., Gochfeld and Burger 2008; Lin Tokai, and Nakanishi 2005; Meinhardt 2005; Tanaka 2003). For example, one can employ mathematical models to estimate the risk associated with various chemical hazards stored on site by a factory located near a community, starting with a list of chemicals stored that pose the greatest health hazards. One may also compare and contrast the risk and

benefits from two or more alternative proposals. For example, the decision to ban or not ban a particular chemical (e.g., pesticide or herbicide) in a community, and then choose the proposal with the lowest risk to public health, safety, or well-being.

Figure 8.6 shows a framework which depicts some of the critical steps for conducting a risk assessment for public health in terms of its predicted impact on a defined target population or community (Bartfay and Bartfay 2015). The first step is to clearly define the problem or aim of the proposal and the specific environmental/occupational context, which may be biological, chemical, or radioactive in nature. It is critical to clearly define the known

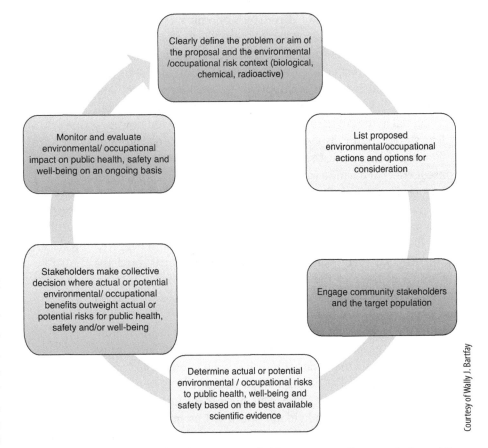

Figure 8.6 Environmental and occupational risk assessment framework for public health.

Courtesy of Wally J. Bartfay

hazard(s) and establish the specific endpoints or health outcomes (e.g., lung cancer, birth defects, increased mortality) that will be employed in the environmental/occupational risk assessment.

In regards to cancer, for example, it has become common to state that an exposure to an environmental hazard is *acceptable* if it does not cause an increase in the overall lifetime death rate of cancer greater than one-in-one-million (or 10^{-6} elevated risk) exposed individuals (Gochfeld and Burger 2008). By comparison, regulations regarding occupational or natural hazards exposure for radon are on the order of 10^{-4} for radon; a 1 in 10 lifetime risk of developing lung cancer for chromate workers, and a 30% lifetime risk of developing lung cancer by asbestos miners and workers (Brenner and Sachs 2006; Hazelton et al. 2006; Joshi and Gupta 2004; Park et al. 2004; Selikoff and Seidman 1991; U.S. Centers for Disease Control and Prevention 2002). Hence, we need to recognize that various numerical risks that have been previously utilized by industry, governments, or health agencies are arbitrary and theoretical in nature, as opposed to practical in reference to acceptable nonoccupational-related exposures.

There is a tendency to treat mortality, which appears at the end of the spectrum of possible outcomes, as the gold standard currently in Canada and globally (Bartfay and Bartfay 2015). Nonetheless, we should also consider other possible negative health ripple effects and outcomes along this risk assessment spectrum (e.g., physical and social disabilities, stress and anxiety, health related quality of life, caregiver burden, etc.) associated with exposure to the identified environmental/occupational hazard(s). If we accept the notion that health is a holistic entity and resource, then we argue that it is also imperative to utilize a holistic approach to make informed decisions. However, the process for determining a so-called "acceptable environmental health risk" by all identified stakeholders is often a social–political decision in Canada, as opposed to a purely scientific one per se (Bartfay and Bartfay 2015). Unfortunately, in both developed and developing nations around the world this is often driven by economic interests (Everett Kopp, Pearson, and Schwarz 2002; Merson, Black, and Mills 2012).

Second, it is critical to list all of the proposed environmental/occupational actions and options for examination and consideration. During this step, it is important to consider the type and quantity of the known hazard, projected exposure levels, its mobility potential in the environment (e.g., soil, air, water), and how they will be stored and/or disposed of in the surrounding environment.

For example, we must consider both the acute- and long-term consequences of having a waste disposal and storage site for nuclear wastes near a community. In fact, it may take up to 300,000 years for spent radioactivity fuel rods to become comparable to levels of the natural occurring uranium ore when they were first mined (Maxell 2009; Ryskamp 2003). In March 2011, a tsunami triggered by the Tokoku earthquake near Fukushima Japan triggered the meltdown of three of the Fukushima Daiichi nuclear plant's six reactors. Over 300,000 people living in the area had to be evacuated and large amounts of radioactive ground water continues to leak into the ocean affecting aquatic species and wildlife in the region. In addition, nuclear power plants, once decommissioned, must also be treated as a major environmental radioactive waste hazard that may pose potential negative ripple health effects in a region for thousands of years to come. This nuclear explosion in Japan left 15,883 dead, 9,500 individuals still listed as missing, 26,992 injured, and 185,000 people displaced from their homes and communities that may last 30 or more years (CNN 2013). According to Maxwell (2009), this long time frame amplifies the technical challenges of finding a suitable location where the repository will not

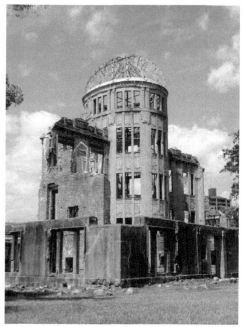

Source: Photo by Wally J. Bartfay

Photo 8.29 The A-bomb Dome Building located in Peace Park, Hiroshima, Japan. During the final stage of World War II, the United States detonated two nuclear weapons over the Japanese cities of Hiroshima and Nagasaki on August 6 and 9, 1945, respectively. The two bombings killed at least 129,000 people and several individuals later died from radiation poisoning and various cancers, and children of survivers have high rates of genetic diseases and mutations.

be compromised due to erosion, hydrologic changes or even earthquakes, and tsunamis. Hence, communicating the actual known or potential hazards to people in the distant future is a major public health challenge.

Third, it is critical to engage all stakeholders involved including the target population and/or community or region that will be ultimately affected. As highlighted in the chapter entitled *Introduction to Public Health*, there are critical values and principles for delivering public health in Canada which include social justice, sustainable development, recognition of the importance of both individuals and the community as a whole, self-determination, empowerment, and community participation (Public Health Agency of Canada, [PHAC] 2007). Hence, the primary aim of public health during this process is to empower all stakeholders and communities to make informed decisions and partake in interventions which seek to preserve, promote, and/or restore their health (PHAC 2007). The responsibility for the promotion and preservation of health is multisectorial and shared among all citizens and residents, community members, health care professionals and workers, health service institutions and organizations, industry, and all levels of government in Canada.

Fourth, it is critical to determine actual and/or potential environmental/occupational risks and benefits to public health, safety, and well-being across the life span based on the best available evidence. EIPH "is the process of distilling and disseminating the best available evidence from research, practice, and experience and using the evidence to inform and improve public health policy and practice"(National Collaborating Centres for Public Health 2011, 1). Establishing what the best available evidence is requires judgment on its suitability and quality, formal debate, and consensus that it should be utilized by all stakeholders concerned. This involves both qualitative and quantitative estimates of the impact of the identified environmental hazard(s) on individuals across the life span. In addition, it is critical to consider the potential effects of natural disasters (e.g., flooding, earthquakes, tsunamis, forest fires), bioterrorist threats, and human error. The reader is referred to Chapter 1 entitled for a detailed discussion of what evidence is, how it should be gathered, evaluated, and employed the context of public health. The reader is referred to Chapter 7 for additional discussions and information related to bioterrorism.

For example, on April 26, 1986, a large explosion and fire occurred at the Chernobyl nuclear plant located in the Ukraine due to human error (Friis 2012; Maxwell 2009). In fact, a series of human errors resulted in a power surge in the core at the time when the emergency cooling system for the core had been turned off as part of the test. The design of the Soviet built reactor at Chernobyl differed from that of Canadian reactors including the lack of a containment building and the use of graphite to absorb neutrons in the core. Consequently, the nuclear fuel rods melted, ruptured, and exploded releasing large quantities of radioactive steam high into the atmosphere. Radioactive materials, including iodine and cesium, were deposited over wide parts of Europe including Russia, Austria, Germany, Switzerland, and northern Italy. Some of the noted acute negative ripple effects of this nuclear disaster attributed to human error included the release of half the reactor's caesium 137 and iodine 131 into the atmosphere. This nuclear meltdown attributed to human error resulted in the deaths of 31 individuals, 209 suffered from acute radiation poisoning, and approximately 185,000 individuals in the surrounding region received radiation doses that were four times the internationally accepted limit (Carlisle 1996). Some of the

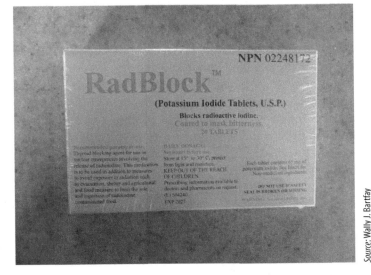

Source: Wally J. Bartfay

Photo 8.30 Potassium iodine tablets, a thyroid blocking agent, for use during nuclear emergencies involving the release of radioiodine into the atmosphere, and distributed by Durham Public Health to residents who reside near a nuclear power generating plant in the region.

more chronic or long-term negative health ripple effects following this nuclear accident were only detected 4–5 years after the nuclear accident occurred.

For example, in the Gomel region of Belarus, which is located north of the Chernobyl reactor, a shape increase in the number of thyroid cancer cases in children was noted from 1% to 2% per year during the time period of 1986–1989; to 38 in 1991 (Kazakov, Demidchik, and Astakhova 1992). Subsequent studies have also demonstrated increases in the number of thyroid cancer cases in three countries affected by the radioactive fallout (Belarus, Ukraine, and western parts of Russia) (Cardis et al. 2006; Dolk and Lechat 1993; Friis 2012; Reiners 2009). The number of cases had totalled over 5,000 by 2010, with an estimated 15,000 more cases to surface during the next 50 years among exposed children in the region (Dolk and Lechat 1993; Reiners 2009). Hence, research provides the essential knowledge base that enables health care professionals and workers and community stakeholders with the necessary information to make evidence-informed decisions (Bartfay 2010a; Friis 2012; Gochfeld and Burger 2008).

Fifth, all identified stakeholders should make a collective and democratic decision where actual or potential environmental/occupational benefits out-weigh all identified risks to public health, safety, or well-being. This may include a formal vote on the proposal and the official recording of the outcomes.

Lastly, it is critical to monitor and evaluate the environmental/occupational impact on public health, safety, and well-being on an ongoing or prospective basis. This should include the tracking of exposed individuals and workers for any early detectable adverse health effects, and compare them with similar individuals and workers (i.e., controls) who are not exposed. A variety of assessments (e.g., physical exams, blood tests, questionnaires and surveys) and research approaches can be utilized for this purpose.

Future Directions and Challenges

Although Canada is often viewed as a leader in environmental sustainability and as a strong advocate for global sustainable development, there remains a number of challenges associated with preserving and protecting our environment and the health of our residents and workers (Schubert and Bartfay 2010). For example, Rona Ambrose, the federal minister of the environment, reported that since our ratification of the Kyoto Protocol (1997), Canada ranks 29th overall out of 30 countries in regard to both water consumption use and environmental indicators; 27th in reference to sulphur oxide pollution, and 26th for both species at risk and greenhouse gas emissions (Minister of Public Works and Government Services Canada 2007).

There is a growing need for public health care professionals and workers to become cognizant of current and emerging environmental conditions that may threaten the health and well-being of citizens and residents across the life span in Canada and globally. Health Canada (1998), for example, has prepared a comprehensive handbook for public health care professionals entitled *Environment and Health: A Handbook for Health Professionals* which is an excellent resource guide. In addition, professional schools (e.g., medicine, nursing) in Canada need to teach future generations of public health care professions the intricate links between human health and disease and associated environmental determinants.

Health Canada (1997) reports that one of the greatest challenges we face as a nation is to ensure that the long-term health of our residents encompasses the notion of a sustainable environment in the new millennium. This will include the need to embrace the concept of sustainable development and includes the integration of economic, social, and environmental goals and their potential impact on health. Sustainable development also reflects an inherent understanding that development is essential to meet the growing demands of our society and to improve our quality of life. Nonetheless, it must be based on the efficient and environmentally responsible use of all society's scarce resources (i.e., natural, human, and economic) (Health Canada 1997).

Although the scope of actual and potential hazards encountered in work environments is enormous, there is currently a dearth of empirical research to examine both the acute- and long-term effects of exposure to these hazards by workers. Furthermore, little comparative research exists to assess the impact of these environmental hazards on the health and well-being of workers across different occupations with similar exposure risks. A classic statement made over four decades ago by Wallick (1972) remains valid today in terms of the lack of scientific progress made in reference to environmental hazards encountered by workers in the various occupations in Canada and abroad. Indeed, few studies have been conducted to measure the full impact and dimensions of occupational illness, occupational pollution, and exposures to various agents in the work environment and their impact on human health. For example, although we can estimate the rate of specific kinds of cancer for different occupations, there are only a few epidemiological studies which have examined the negative health effects of specific chemicals, noise pollution, stress, and other variables on groups of workers due to both acute and chronic exposure (Bartfay and Bartfay 2015).

Lastly, we must acknowledge the fact that Western-style development patterns are not sustainable on the global environmental scale for our planet. Indeed, the global average ecological footprint was 54.1 acres per capita in 2001, which has already exceeded the global carrying capacity of 38.8 acres per capita (Venetoulis and Talberth 2006). In other words, the global impact was already 39% greater than the capacity of our planet to sustain human populations. This is also reflected in other statistics such as the inability of countries to grow enough food to sustain their own populations. For example, it is estimated that more than 8 million people have died as a consequence of hunger in sub-Saharan Africa and South Asia alone (United Nations Secretariat 2004). We shall examine global health in greater detail in Chapter 9. In light of these environmental and ecological realities, our planet faces a difficult challenge in devising a global future that is both sustainable and more equitable than the present, without comprising our health and well-being. Indeed, the health of all citizens of this planet depends on continued stability and functioning of the Earth's environment and its atmosphere that supports life for its entire species, including humans. The reader is referred to Chapter 9 for a detailed discussion on how various environmental and other social determinants of health are affecting the health of various populations around the world.

Group Review Exercise Box 8.1 "The Disappearing Male"

Overview of This Investigative Documentary
This Canadian Broadcasting Corporation television (CBC-TV) investigative documentary examines the link between toxic chemicals known as "endocrine disruptors" or "hormone mimicking chemicals" present in our ecosystem and environment and their association to negative health outcomes and the male reproductive system in particular. These hormone mimicking chemicals are present in a variety of products including sunglasses, carpets, cosmetics and certain plastic bottles and containers, shampoo, and meat and dairy products routinely consumed by humans. This documentary argues that the continued presence of these toxic chemicals threatens the very survival of the human species because of their negative effects on the male reproductive system. In the past decade, there has been a dramatic increase in the incidence of young males suffering from genital deformities, decreased sperm counts and abnormalities, and testicular cancer. Moreover, we also observe that males are at greater risk of suffering from ADHD, autism, Tourette's syndrome, cerebral palsy, and dyslexia.

Instructions
This assignment may be done alone, in pairs or in groups of up to 5 people (note: if you are doing this assignment in pairs or groups, please only submit one hard or electronic copy to your instructor). The assignment should be type-written and between 4 and 6 pages maximum in length (double-spaced please). View the documentary entitled "The disappearing male" which aired on CBC-TV investigative program "DocZone". See link: http://www.cbc.ca/documentaries/doczone/2008/disappearingmale/ Or http://www.cbc.ca/documentaries/doczone/2008/disappearingmale/endocrine.html or http://www.cbc.ca/player/Shows/Shows/Doc+Zone/2008-09/ID/1233750780/.

(Continued)

Group Review Exercise Box 8.1 (*Continued*)

View this documentary and take detailed notes during the presentation:

   i. Provide a brief overview of the salient environmental links between endocrine disruptors and human health highlighted in this documentary.

   ii. What are some of the environmental determinants of health addressed in this investigative documentary?

   iii. Briefly discuss how these hormone mimicking environmental chemicals are threatening the survival of the species, and why males appear to be especially at risk.

   iv. Briefly discuss how these chemicals released into the environment are impacting communities including Indigenous populations who reside in the so-called "chemical valley" region near Sarnia, Ontario.

   v. What are some of the current and future implications and challenges for public health in Canada addressed in this documentary?

Summary

- The environment is more than one's physical or geographical location, but is currently regarded as a critical social determinant of health that consists of interdependent and interconnected components of one's physical, biochemical, social–political, cultural and spiritual milieus, and situations.
- One's work and living environments are mutually interdependent and inseparable and therefore should be examined collectively in the context of a critical social determinant of health.
- Environmental health is defined as a branch of public health which examines both positive and negative factors and influences on the environment and ecosystems on human health.
- There is a growing body of evidence to indicate that environmental changes including human activities and technologies are threatening ecosystems and the existence of living organisms.
- An ecosystem is defined as a local or regional community or area of living organisms which include humans, plants and microorganisms, and the physical settings in which they occupy and live their lives within.
- Global warming is an increase in the earth's overall temperature as a result of both human (e.g., industrial pollution, fossil-based fuels) and natural cases (e.g., volcanoes).
- The greenhouse effect was defined as the trapping of infrared radiation from the earth by greenhouse gases in the earth's atmosphere, which results in the warming of the surface temperature of the earth.
- Toxicology is the study of the adverse effects of synthetic chemical substances and products and natural toxins, which includes their cellular, biochemical, and molecular mechanisms of action, and the actual or potential ability of these chemicals to cause harm, ill effects, disease, and/or mortality in living organisms including humans.
- CEPA (Bill C-32) was enacted by Parliament in 1988 to provide legislative standards for assessing, identifying, evaluating, and managing various toxic chemicals and substances in order to preserve and protect human health.
- In 1992, the NPRI was established and serves as a national database for information related to a variety of chemicals and substances that are annually released into water sources, on land, or into the atmosphere in Canada.
- Occupational health and safety is a branch or subspecialty of public health which examines both positive and negative health outcomes that are influenced or associated with exposure to general

work conditions and/or specific known hazards that are encountered in work environments, and which seeks to preserve, promote, and/or restore the health and safety of workers.

- Stress is defined as any physical, social, political, economic, or cultural force which creates an imbalance and which can have either a negative or positive influence on an individual or group.
- Since the causes of workplace-related stress can vary from individual to individual, strategies to prevent, manage, and/or reduce the identified stressor(s) will also vary according to the identified need or situation.

Critical Thinking Questions

1. Identify a major industry in your community or surrounding region and identify a potential occupational risk and a potential environmental hazards associated with this industry. Describe at least one public health intervention that may reduce or eliminate these noted occupational risks and environmental hazards.
2. Identify regional, provincial/territorial, and/or national policies and legislations associated with occupational and/or environmental health which have a positive influence of individuals in your community.
3. Describe social determinants of health in your community which directly influence occupational and/or environmental health.
4. Propose ways of incorporating environmental and occupational health principles into public health practice, education, and policy.

References

Acharya, G. "They Are the Lorax, They Speak for the Trees." *Amnesty International USA*, July 4, 2010. Retrieved November 26, 2011. http://blog.amnestyusa.org/business/they-are-the-lorax-they-speak-for-the-trees/.

Ahn, Y. S., K. S. Jeong, and K. S. Kim. "Cancer Morbidity of Professional Emergency Responders in Korea." *American Journal of Industrial Medicine* 55, no. 9 (September 2012): 768–78.

Alberta Government. *Human Resources and Employment: Workplace Health and Safety.* Edmonton, AL: Author, April 30, 2004. Retrieved November 1, 2011. http://investincanada.ic.ca.

Ali, S. H. (2004). "A Socio-Ecological Autopsy for the *E. coli* 0157:H7 Outbreak in Walkerton, Ontario, Canada." *Social Science and Medicine* 58 (2004): 2601–12.

Alliance for the Great Lakes. *Protecting the Great Lakes From Pharmaceutical Pollution.* Chicago, IL: Author, 2010. Retrieved November 8, 2011. http://www.greatlakes.org.

Amendola, A., and D. R. Wilkinson. "Risk Assessment and Environmental Policy Making." *Journal of Hazardous Materials* 78 (2000): ix–xiv.

Andrews, M. "Baby Bottles Containing BPA to be Banned in Canada." Vancouver, BC: *The Vancouver Sun*, April 19, 2008. Retrieved November 1, 2011. http://www.canada.com/vancouversun/news/business/story.html?id=b6f39f37-6194-4aa5.

Apostolakis, G. E., and D. M. Lemon. "A Screening Methodology for the Identification and Ranking of Infrastructure Vulnerabilities Due to Terrorism." *Risk Analysis* 25 (2005): 361–76.

Armstrong, B. K., and A. Kricker. "The Epidemiology of UV Induced Skin Cancer." *Journal of Photochemicals and Photobiology* B(63) (2001): 8–18.

Arts, J., M. Rennen, and C. De Heer. "Inhaled Formaldehyde: Evaluation of Sensory Irritation in Relation to Carcinogenicity." *Regulatory Toxicology and Pharmacology* 44, no. 2 (2006): 144–60.

Aschengrau, A., and G. R. Seage III. *Essentials of Epidemiology in Public Health.* Toronto, ON: Jones and Bartlett Publishers, 2003.

Association of Schools and Programs of Public Health. *Public Health Preparedness and Response Core Competency Model*, 2. December 17, 2010, Accessed January 6, 2016. http://tools.niehs.nih.gov/wetp/1/12TrainersExchange/3_Handouts_Developing_and_Implementing_Preparedness.pdf.

Association of Workers' Compensation Boards of Canada and Statistics Canada. *Labour Force Survey Estimates (LFS), by Sex and Detailed Age Group, Annual (CANSIM Table 282-0002)*. Ottawa, ON: Statistics Canada, 2012.

Austin, C. C., G. Dussault, and D. J. Ecobichon. "Municipal Firefighter Exposure Groups, Time Spent at Fires and Use of Self-Contained-Breathing-Apparatus." *American Journal of Industrial Medicine* 40, no. 6 (December 2001): 683–92.

Ayotte, P., S. Giroux, E. Dewailly, A. M. Hernandez, P. Farias, R. Danis, and C. Villanueva Díaz. "DDT Spraying for Malaria Control and Reproductive Function in Mexican Men." *Epidemiology* 12, no. 3 (May 12, 2001): 366–7.

Bartfay, W. J. "Environmental Perspectives on Health." In *Community Health Nursing: Caring in Action*, 116–42, Edited by J. E. Hitchcock, P. E. Schubert, S. A. Thomas, and W. J. Bartfay. Toronto, ON: Nelson Education, 2010a.

———. "Global Health Perspectives for Community Health Nurses." In *Community Health Nursing: Caring in Action* 143–72, edited by J. E. Hitchcock, P. E. Schubert, S. A. Thomas, and W. J. Bartfay. Toronto, ON: Nelson Education, 2010b.

Bartfay, W. J., and E. Bartfay. *Public Health in Canada*. Boston, MA: Pearson Learning Solutions, 2015. (ISBN:13:978-1-323-01471-4).

Bartfay, W. J., E. Bartfay, and T. Wu. "Impact of the Global Economic Crisis on the Health of Unemployed Autoworkers." *Canadian Journal of Nursing Research* 45, no. 10 (September 2013): 66–79.

Beach, M. *Disaster Preparedness and Management*. Philadelphia, PA: F. A. Davis Company, 2010.

Beard, J. "DDT and Human Health." *Science and Total Environment* 355, no. 1–3 (February 15, 2006): 78–89.

Beckmann Murray, R., J. Proctor Zentner, V. Pangman, and C. Pangman. *Health Promotion Strategies Through the Lifespan*. Canadian ed. Toronto, ON: Pearson Prentice Hall, 2006.

Bezrucka, S. "The Effect of the Economic Recession on Population Health." *Canadian Medical Association Journal* 181, no. 5 (2009): 499–510.

Borenstein, S. "Thawing Permafrost Could Worsen Global Warming. *Toronto Star*. Toronto, ON. A33, December 1, 2011a.

———. "Why World's Weather Will Be Going to Extremes." *Toronto Star* A24, November 19, 2011b. Toronto, ON.

Borzelleca, J. F. "Profiles in Toxicology. Paracelsus: Herald of Modern Toxicology." *Toxicological Science* 53 (2000): 2–4.

Brenner, D. J., and R. K. Sachs. "Estimating Radiation-Induced Cancer Risk at Very Low Doses: Rationale for Using a Linear No-Threshold Approach." *Radiation and Environmental Biophysics* 44, no. 4 (2006): 253–56.

Brohan, P., J. J. Kennedy, I. Harris, S. B. Tett, and P. D. Jones. "Uncertainty Estimates in Regional and Global Observed Temperature Changes: A New Dataset From 1850." *Journal of Geophysical Research* 111 (2006): D12106.

Bunker, J. P., H. S. Frazier, and F. Mosteller. "Improving Health: Measuring Effects of Medicare Care." *Millbank Quarterly* 72 (1994): 225–58.

Burge, P. S. "Sick Building Syndrome." *Occupational and Environmental Medicine* 34 (February 2004): 185–91.

Burger, J., A. H. Stern, and M. Gochfeld. "Mercury in Commercial Fish: Optimizing Individual Choices to Reduce Risks." *Environmental Health Perspectives* 113 (2005): 266–71.

Bushnik, T., D. Haines, P. Levallois, J. Levesque, J. Van Oostdam, and C. Viau. *Lead and Bisphenol A Concentrations in the Canadian Population*. Ottawa, ON: Statistics Canada, 2010. Retrieved October 16, 2011. http://www.statcan.gc.ca/pub/82-003-x/2010003/article/11324-eng.htm.

Canada Press. *Sandy Claims Second Canadian Victim After Ontario Hydro Workers Dies Repairing Damage*. Toronto, ON: Author, October 31, 2012. Retrieved November 2, 2012. http://news.nationalpost.com/2012/10/13/sandy-claims-second-canadian-victim-after-ontario.

Canadian Breast Cancer Foundation (CBCF). *Cleaning the Air*. Toronto, ON: The Toronto Star, November 19, 2011.

Canadian Centre for Occupational Health and Safety. *Work Injury Statistics*. Ottawa, ON: Author, 2011. Retrieved November 4, 2011. http://www.ccohs.ca/oshanswers/information/injury_statistics.html.

———. *Workplace Stress-General*. Ottawa, ON: Author, 2012. Retrieved January 27, 2013. http:www.ccohs.ca/oshanswers/psycholsocial/stress.html.

CanWest MediaWorks Publications Inc. "Metro Sewage Plants Failing Federal Tests. Three Metro Vancouver Sewage Treatment Plants Have Been Failing Federal Environmental Tests at least Seven Years while Dumping Billions of Litres of Partly Treated Waste into the Fraser River, Burrard Inlet and the Strait of Georgia without Penalty." May 3, 2008. http://www.canada.com/vancouversun/news/story.html?id=d8b754dd-caee-4139-ba74-8d1b62148650.

Cardis, E., D. Krewski, M. Boniol, V. Drozdovitch, S. C. Darby, E. S. Gilbert, S. Akiba, J. Benichou, J. Ferlay, S. Gandini, C. Hill, G. Howe, A. Kesminiene, M. Moser, M. Sanchez, H. Storm, L. Voisin, and P. Boyle. "Estimates of the Cancer Burden in Europe from Radioactive Fallout from Chernobyl Accident." *International Journal of Cancer* 119 (2006): 1224–35.

Carlisle, D. (1996). "Bitter Rain." *Nursing Times* 92, no. 16 (1996): 16–17.

Carson, R. *Silent Spring*. Boston, MA: Houghton Mifflin, 1962.

Cassese, M. "Canadians Produce More Garbage than Anyone Else. Conference Board Calls Canada an 'Environmental Laggard.'" *CBC News and Reuters*, January 17, 2013. Toronto, ON. Retrieved January 6, 2016. http://www.cbc.ca/news/business/canadians-produce-more-garbage-than-anyone-else-1.1394020.

Centers for Disease Control and Prevention (CDC). *Climate Effects on Health*. Atlanta, GA: CDC, 2015. Retrieved January 7, 2016. http://www.cec.gov/climateandhealth/effects.

———. "Infectious Disease and Dermatologic Conditions in Evacuees and Rescue Workers after Hurricane Katrina—Multiple States, August–September, 2005." *MMWR* 54 (2005): 1–4.

———. "Tropical Storm Allison Rapid Needs Assessment—Houston, Texas, June 2001." *MMWR* 51 (2002): 365–68.

Chan, P. K., G. P. O'Hara, and A. W. Hayes. "Principles and Methods for Acute and Subacute Toxicity." In *Principles and Methods of Toxicology*, 1–51, edited by A. W. Hayes. New York: Raven Press, 1982.

Chiasson, P. "Lac-Mégantic Somber Record Anniversary of Rail Disaster." *The Canadian Press*, July 6, 2015. Retrieved December 29, 2015. http://www.thestar.com/news/canada/2015/07/06/lac-megantic-marks-somber-second-anniversary.html.

City of Toronto Department of Public Health. *The Quality of Drinking Water in Toronto: A Review of Tap Water, Bottled Water and Water Treated by a Point-of-Use Device*. Toronto, ON: City of Toronto, 1990.

Commission for Environmental Cooperation (CEC). *North American Regional Action Plan on DDT, North American Working Group for the Sound Management of Chemicals Task Force on DDT and Chlordane*. Montréal, QC, 1997.

Commission on the Social Determinants of Health, World Health Organization. *Closing the Gap in a Generation. Health Equity Through Action on the Social Determinants of Health*. Geneva, Switzerland: World Health Organization, 2008. ISBN:978924156370-3.

Constant, J. "Additional Firefighter Cancers Now Covered." *Canada's Occupational Health and Safety Magazine*, September 1, 2008. Retrieved November 2, 2012. http://www.ohscanada.com/news/additional-firefighter-cancer-now-covered/10000228793/.

Cortez, J. *East Coasts Faces Daunting Rebuild*, A25. Toronto, ON: Toronto Star, November 1, 2012.

CNN. *2011 Japan Earthquake-Tsunami Fast Facts*. September 20, 2013. Retrieved December 15, 2015. http://www.cnn.com/2013/07/17/world/asia/japan-earthquake—tsunami-fast-facts/index.html.

Crompton, S. (2014). "What's Stressing the Stressed? Main Sources of Stress Among Workers." *Statistics Canada*. Ottawa, ON. Retrieved January 7, 2016. http://www.statcan.gc.ca/pub/11-008-x/2011002/article/11562-eng.htm.

Dai, A. "Recent Climatology, Variability and Trends in Global Surface Humidity." *Journal of Climate* 19 (2006): 3589–606.

Davis, H. W., K. Teschke, S. M. Kennedy, M. R. Hodgson, C. Hertzman, and P. A. Demers. "Occupational Exposure to Noise and Mortality From Acute Myocardial Infarction. *Epidemiology* 16, no. 1 (2005): 25–32.

Dickinson, G., M. Liepner, S. Talos, and D. Buckingham. *Understanding the Law*. 2nd ed. Toronto, ON: McGraw-Hill Ryerson Ltd, 1996.

Dolk, H., and M. F. Lechat. "Health Surveillance in Europe: Lessons From EUROCAT and Chernobyl." *International Journal of Epidemiology* 22 (1993): 363–8.

Doll, R. "Pott and the Path to Prevention." *Archieves Geschwulstforsch* 45 (1975): 521–31.

Duxbury, L., and C. Higgins. *Work-Life Balance in the New Millennium: Where Are We? Where Do We Need to Go?* Canadian Policy Research Networks (CPRN). Discussion paper No. W/12. Ottawa, ON: Author, 2001.

Edwards, P. "Climate Change: Air Pollution and Your Health." *Canadian Journal of Public Health* 92, no. 3 (2001): 108–12.

Eisen, E. A., T. J. Smith, D. Kriebel, S. Woskie, D. J. Myers, S. M. Kennedy, S. Shalat, and R. R. Monson. "Respiratory Health of Automobile Workers and Exposure to Metal-Working Fluid Aerosols: Lung Spirometry." *American Journal of Industrial Medicine* 39 (2001): 443–53.

Elad, D. (2005). "Risk Assessment of Malicious Biocontamination of Food." *Journal of Food Protection* 68 (2005): 1302–05.

Environment Canada. "Biological Test Method. Acute Lethality Test Using Rainbow Trout." *Government of Canada Publication*. Environment Canada and Environment Technology Centre, Ottawa, ON, July, 1990 (Cat. No. ISBN 0-662-18074-7). Retrieved December 14, 2015. http://publications.gc.ca/site/eng/453449/publication.html.

———. *National Pollutant Release Inventory (NPRI)*. Ottawa, ON: Author, 1992. Retrieved November 1, 2011. http://www.ec.gc.ca/pdb/npri/npri_home_e.cfm.

———. *Canada's Ozone Layer Protection Program: A Summary*. Ottawa, ON: Author, 1996.

Environment Canada. *Great Lakes Areas of Concern*. Ottawa, ON: Author, 2011. Retrieved January 25, 2013. http://www.ec.gc.ca/raps.pas/.

———. *Informing Canadians on Pollution 2002. Highlights of the 2000 National Pollutant Release Inventory (NPRI)*. Ottawa, ON: Author, 2000.

———. *National Spill Statistics and Trends*. Ottawa, ON: Author, 2006. Retrieved November 30, 2011. http://www.ec.gc.ca/ee-ue/default.asp?lang=enandn=1C33E5B4.

Environmental Defense Canada. "Heavy Metal Hazard: The Health Risks of Hidden Heavy Metals in Face Makeup." Toronto, ON: Author, May 2011. Retrieved January 28, 2013. http://environmentaldefence.ca/reports/heavy-metal-hazard-health-risks-hidden-heavy-metals-in-face-makeup.

Everett Koop, C., C. E. Pearson, and M. R. Schwarz. *Global Issues in Global Health*. San Francisco, CA: Jossey-Bass, 2002.

Federal-Provincial Subcommittee on Drinking Water of the Federal-Provincial Committee on Environmental and Occupational Health. *Guidelines for Canadian Drinking Water Quality*. 6th ed. Ottawa, ON: Health Canada, 2002. Retrieved November 8, 2011. http://www.hc-sc.gc.ca/ehp/ehd/catalogue/bch_pubs/dwgsup_doc/dwsgsup_doc.htm.

Franco, D. A., and C. E. Williams. "'Airs, Waters, Places' and Other Hippocratic Writings: Inferences for Control of Foodborne and Waterborne Diseases." *Journal of Environmental Health* 62, no. 10 (2000): 9–14.

Franco, G. "Ramazzini and Worker's Health." *Lancet* 354 (1999): 858–61.

Freeman, S. *Hurricane Sandy: Canadian Insurers Could Take Financial Hit*. Montréal, QC: The Montréal Gazette, 2012. Retrieved November 2, 2012. http://www.montrealgazette.com/business/Hurrican+Sandy+Canadian+reinsurers+could+take+hit//

Friis, R. H. *Essential of Environmental Health*. 2nd ed. Toronto, ON: Jones and Bartlett Learning, 2012.

Frumkin, H. *Environmental Health: From Global to Local*. San Francisco, CA: John Wiley and Sons, Inc., 2005.

Gaertner, R. R., L. Trpeski, K. C. Johnson, and Canadian Cancer Registries Epidemiology Research Group. *Cancer Causes and Control* 15, no. 10 (December, 2004): 1007–9.

Gallin, J. I., and F. P. Ognibene. *Principles and Practice of Clinical Research*. 2nd ed. Burlington, MA: Academic Press/Elsevier, 2007.

Garrison, F. H. *History of Medicine*. Philadelphia, PA: Saunders, 1926.

Gindi, M. "Ultraviolet Radiation: A Public Health Perspective." *Public Health and Epidemiology Reports Ontario* 3, no. 9 (1992): 136–40.

Gochfeld, M. "Chronologic History of Occupational Medicine." *Journal of Occupational and Environmental Medicine* 47 (2005): 96–114.

———. "Principles of Toxicology." In *Public Health and Preventive Medicine*. 15th ed., edited by R. B. Wallace and N. Kohatsu, 505–23. Toronto, ON: McGraw Hill Medical, 2008.

Gochfeld, M., and J. Burger. "Environmental and Ecological Risk Assessment." In *Public Health and Preventive Medicine*. 15th ed., edited by R. B. Wallace and N. Kohatsu, 545–62. Toronto, ON: McGraw Hill Medical, 2008.

———. "Good Fish/Bad Fish: A Composite Benefit-Risk by Dose Curve." *Neurotoxicology* 26, no. 4 (2005): 511–20.

Godish, T. *Indoor Environmental Quality*. New York: CRC Press, 2001. ISBN:1566704022.

Government of Canada. *Bill C-32: The Canadian Environmental Protection Act, 1999*. Ottawa, ON: Author, 1999. Retrieved November 1, 2011. http://www.ec.gc.ca/CEPARegistry/the_act.

———. *Order Adding a Toxic Substance to Schedule 1 to the Canadian Environmental Protection Act, 1999*. Ottawa, ON: Author, February 15, 2005. Retrieved November 1, 2011. http://www.gazette.gc.ca/archieves/p2/2005/2005-03-09/html/sor-dors40-eng.html.

Griffiths, J., L. Stewart. *Sustaining a Healthy Future. Taking Action on Climate Change (Special Focus on the NHS)*. London, UK: The UK Faculty of Public Health, 2009. ISBN:1-900273-36-5.

Guha-Sapir, D., D. Hargitt, and P. Hoyois. *Thirty Years of Natural Disasters 1974–2003: The Numbers.* Centre for Research on the Epidemiology of Disasters and Universitaries De Louvain: UCL Presses, 2004. Retrieved November 2, 2011. http://www.emdat.net/documents/Publication/publication_2004_emdat.pdf.

Gura, D. "Toxic Red Sludge Spill From Hungarian Aluminum Plant 'An Ecological Disaster.'" *NPR,* October 5, 2010. Retrieved November 20, 2011. http://www.npr.org/blogs/thetwo-way/2010/10/05/130351938/red-sludge-from-hungarian-aluminum-plant-spill-an-ecological-disaster.

Haddow, G. D., J. A. Bullock, and D. Coppola. *Introduction to Emergency Management.* 4th ed. Burlington, MA: Elservier, Inc., 2011.

Haines, A., A. McMichael, and P. Epstein. (2006). "Environment and Health: Global Climate Change and Health." *Journal of the Canadian Medical Association* 163 (2006): 729–34.

Hamilton, A. *Exploring the Dangerous Trades: The Autobiography of Alice Hamilton.* Boston, MA: Little, Brown and Company, 1943.

Hales, D. *An Invitation to Health.* 2009–2010 ed. Belmont, CA: Wadsworth Cengage Learning, 2009.

Hales, D., and L. Lauzon. *An Invitation to Health.* 1st Canadian ed. Toronto, ON: Thomson/Nelson, 2007.

Harris Ali, S. "Environmental Health and Society." In *Health, Illness and Health Care in Canada.* 4th ed. edited by B. Singh Bolaria and H. D. Dickinson, 370–87. Toronto, ON: Nelson Education, 2009.

Hazelton, W. D., S. H. Moolgavkar, S. B. Curtis, J. M. Zielinski, J. P. Ashmore, and D. Krewski. "Biologically Based Analysis of Lung Cancer Incidence in a Large Canadian Occupational Cohort With Low-Dose Ionizing Radiation Exposure, and Comparison With Japanese Atomic Bomb Survivors." *Journal of Toxicology and Environmental Health Analysis* 69, no. 11 (2006): 1013–38.

Health Canada. *Health and Environment—Partners for Life.* Ottawa, ON: Public Works and Government Services Canada, 1997 (Cat. No. H49-112/1007E, ISBN 00662-26149-6).

———. *Health Environment: The Health and Environmental Handbook for Health Professionals.* Ottawa, ON: Minister of Public Works and Government Services, Canada, 1998.

———. *National Ambient Air Quality Objectives for Ground-Level Ozone. Part I: A Report by the Federal-Provincial Working Group on Air Quality Objectives and Guidelines.* Ottawa, ON: Author, 1999.

———. *Best Advice on Stress Risk Management in the Workplace (Parts 1 and 2).* Ottawa, ON: Author, 2000 (Catalog No. H39-546/2000E, ISBN 0-662-29236-7).

———. *Fluorides and Human Health.* Ottawa, ON: Author, 2002. Retrieved November 8, 2011. http://www.hc-sc.gc.ca/english/iyh/environment/fluorides.html.

———. *Drinking Water Chlorination.* Ottawa, ON: Author, 2003. Retrieved November 8, 2011. http://www.hcsc.gc.ca/english/iyh/environment/chlorine.html.

———. *Lead and Health.* Ottawa, ON: Author, 2007. ISBN:978-0-662-44815-0. (Catalog No. H128-1/07-496-4E).

———. *What's in Your Well? A Guide to Well Water Treatment and Maintenance.* Ottawa, ON: Author, 2008. Retrieved November 8, 2011. http://www.hc-sc.gc.ca/ewh-semt/pubs/water-eau/wellpuits_e.html.

———. *Guidelines for Canadian Drinking Water Quality. Supporting Documents.* Ottawa, ON: Author, 2004a. Retrieved November 8, 2011. http://www.hc.sc.gc.ca/ewh-sempt/pubs/water-eau/doc_sup-appui/index_e.html.

———. "Trends in Workplace Injuries, Illnesses, and Policies in Healthcare Across Canada." Ottawa, ON: Author, 2004b. Retrieved November 4, 2011. http://www.hc-`sc.gc.ca/hcs-sss/pubs/nurs0infirm/2004-hwi-ipsmt/index-eng.php.

Henderson, B. E., R. J. Gordon, H. Menck, J. Soohoo, S. P. Martin, and M. C. Pike. "Lung Cancer and Air Pollution in South-Central Los Angeles Country." *American Journal of Epidemiology* 101 (1975): 477–88.

Hester, S. D., G. B. Benavides, L. Yoon, K. T. Morgan, F. Zou, W. Barry, and D. C. Wolf. "Formaldehyde-Induced Gene Expression in F344 Rat Nasal Respiratory Epithelium." *Toxicology* 187, no. 1 (2003): 13–14.

Hippocrates. "On Airs, Waters, and Places." *Medical Classics* 3 (1938). 19–42.

Hodge, R., R. Anthony, and J. M. J. Longo. "International Monitoring for Environmental Health Surveillance." *Canadian Journal of Public Health* 93, no. 1 (2002): S16–23.

Hogan, D. M. *Disaster Medicine.* 3rd ed. Philadelphia, PA: Lippincott, 2007.

Human Resources and Skills Development Canada. *Indicators of Well-Being. Work. Work-Related Injuries.* Ottawa, ON: Author, 2013. Retrieved January 30, 2013. http://www4.hrsdc.gc.ca/.3ndic.1t.4r@-eng.jsp?iid=20.

Institute of Medicine. *Assessing the Effects of the Gulf of Mexico Oil Spill on Human Health*. Washington, DC: The National Academies Press, 2010.

International Agency for Research on Cancer. *Agents reviewed by the IARC Monographs*. n.d. Retrieved October 14, 2011. http://monographs.iarc.fr/ENG/Classification/Listagentsalphorder.pdf.

International Labour Organization. *Decent Work-Safe Work. Introductory Report to the XVIIth World Congress on Safety and Health at Work*. ILO. 2005. http://www.ilo.org/safework/lang-en/index.htm.

———. "Safety and Health Statistics." Geneva, Switzerland: ILO, 2013a. Retrieved November 12, 2013. http://www.//ilo.org/global/statistics-and-databases/statistics-overview-and-topics/ssafety-a.

———. "Safety and Health at Work." Geneva, Switzerland: ILO, 2013b. Retrieved November 12, 2013. http://www/ilo.org/global/topics/safety-and-health-at-work/lang—en/index.htm.

International Panel on Climate Change. "Carbon Dioxide Capture and Storage," 2005. Retrieved November 2, 2011. http://arch.rivm.nl/env/int/ipcc/pages_media/SRCC-final/SRCC_TechnicalSummary.pdf.

Jaga, K., and C. Dharmani. "Global Surveillance of DDT and DDE Levels in Human Tissues." *International Journal of Occupational Medicine and Environmental Health* 19, no. 1 (2003): 83.

Jarvholm, B., B. Blake, B. Lavenius, G. Thiringer, and R. Vokmann. "Respiratory Symptoms and Lung Function in Oil Mist-Exposed Workers." *Journal of Occupational Medicine* 24 (1982): 473–79.

Jones, W. H. S. *Hippocrates* (translation). Vol. I, 71–137. London, UK: William Heinemann, 1923.

Jordan, J. The Canada Well-being Measurement Act. Presentation to the House of Commons. Ottawa, ON, March 27, 2000. Retrieved November 2, 2011. http://www.cyberus.ca/choose.sustain/7GI/Joe-intro.shtml.

Joshi, T. K., and R. K. Gupta, (2004). "Asbestos in Developing Countries: Magnitude of Risk and Its Practical Implications." *International Journal of Occupational Medicine and Environmental Health* 17, no. 1 (2004): 179–85.

Karasek, R. (1979). "Job Demands, Job Decisions Latitude and Mental Strain: Implications for Job Redesign." *Administrative Science Quarterly* 24 (1979): 285–306.

Kazakov, V. S., E. P. Demidchik, and L. N. Astakhova. "Thyroid Cancer After Chernobyl." [Letter]. *Nature* 359 (1992): 21.

Koch, W. "Study: Great Lakes' Mercury Pollution Poses Health Risks." *USA Today*, October 12, 2011. Retrieved November 8, 2011. http://content.usatoday.com/communities/greenhouse/post/2011/10/greak-lakes-mercury-poses-health-risks.

Korrick, S. A., C. Chen, A. I. Damokosh, J. Ni, X. Liu, S. I. Cho, L. Altshul, L. Ryan, and X. Xu. "Association of DDT with Spontaneous Abortion: A Case-Control Study." *Annuals of Epidemiology* 11, no. 7 (October 2011): 491–6.

Kovats, R., M. Bouma, S. Hajat, E. Worrall, and A. Haines. "El Niño and Health." *Lancet* 362 (2003): 1481–89.

Kunzelman, M. BP to pay $4.5 B for spill. Toronto, ON: *The Toronto Star*, A3, November 16, 2012.

Kusch, L. *More Protection for Firefighters: Bill 6 Adds Cancers to Occupational Illness List*. Winnipeg, Canada: Winnipeg Free Press, August 8, 2010. Retrieved November 2, 2012. http://www.winnipegfreepress.com/local/more-protection-for-firefighters-111511564.html.

Landesman, I. Y. *Public Health Management of Disasters: The Practice Guide*. 2nd ed. Washington, DC: American Public Health Association, 2005.

———. *Public Health Management of Disasters: The Practice Guide*. 3rd ed. Washington, DC: American Public Health Association, 2012.

Landrigan, P. J., and J. E. Carlson. "Environmental Policy and Children's Health." *The Future of Children* 5, no. 2 (1995): 34–52.

Lavigne, E., P. Villeneuve, and S. Cakmak. (2012). "Air Pollution and Emergency Department Visits for Asthma in Windsor, Canada." *Canadian Journal of Public Health* 103, no. 1 (2012): 4–8.

Lillienberg, L., E. M. Andersson, B. Jarvholm, and K. Toren. "Respiratory Symptoms and Exposure-Response Relations in Workers Exposed to Metalworking Fluid Aerosols." *Annuals of Occupational Hygiene* 54, no. 4 (2010): 403–11.

Lin, B. L., A. Tokai, and J. Nakanishi. "Approaches for Establishing Predicted-No-Effect Concentrations for Population-Level Ecological Risk Assessment in the Context of Chemical Substances Management." *Environmental Science and Technology* 39 (2005): 4833–40.

Lippman, M., B. S. Cohen, and R. B. Schlesinger. *Environmental Health Science: Recognition, Evaluation, and Control of Chemical and Physical Health Hazards*. New York: Oxford University Press, 2003.

Longnecker, M. P., M. A. Kiebanoff, J. W. Brock, H. Zhou, K. A. Gray, L. L. Needham, and A. J. Wilcox. "Maternal Serum Level of 1,1-dichloro-2,2-bis(p-chlorophenyl) Ethylene and Risk of Cryptorchidism, Hypospadias, and Polythelia Among Male Offspring." *American Journal of Epidemiology* 155, no. 4 (February 2002): 313–22.

LoSasso, G. L., L. J. Rapport, and B. N. Axelrod. "Neuropsychological Symptoms Associated with Low-Level Exposure and (Meth)acrylates Among Nail Technicians." *Neuropsychiatry Neuropsychology and Behavioral Neurology* 14, no. 3 (2001): 183–89.

Lyons, R. A., J. M. Temple, D. Evans, D. L. Fone, and S. R. Palmer. "Acute Health Effects of the Sea Empress Oil Spill." *Journal of Epidemiology and Community Health* 53 (1999): 306–10.

Mackenzie, C. A., A. Lockridge, and M. Keith. "Declining Sex Ratio in a First Nation Community." *Environmental Health Perspectives* 113 (2005): 1295–98.

Mackrael, K. (August 19, 2014). "Lac-Mégantic Derailment: Anatomy of a Disaster." *The Globe and Mail.* Retrieved December 29, 2015. http://www.theglobeandmail.com/news/national/lac-megantic-derailment-anatomy-of-a-disaster/article20129764/.

Mahaffey, K. R. "Mercury Exposure: Medical and Public Health Issues." *Trans-American Clinical Climatological Association* 116 (2005): 127–53; Discussion 153–54.

Manfreda, J., M. R. Becklake, M. R. Sears, M. Chan-Yeung, H. Dimich-Ward, H. C. Siersted, P. Ernst, L. Sweet, L. Van Til, D. M. Bowie, N. R. Anthonisen, and R. B. Tate. "Prevalence of Asthma Symptoms Among Adult Aged 20–40 Years in Canada." *Canadian Medical Association Journal* 164, no. 7 (2001): 995–1001.

Mann, J. K., I. B. Tager, F. Lurmann, M. Segal, C. P. Quesenberry, Jr., M. M. Lugg, J. Shan, and S. K. Van Den Eeden. "Air Pollution and Hospital Admissions for Ischemic Heart Disease in Persons With Congestive Heart Failure or Arrhythmia." *Environmental Health Perspectives* 110 (2002): 1247–52.

Marris, E. "In Retrospect: The Lorax." *Nature* 476 (2011): 148–49.

Martin-Gil, J., M. C. Yanguas, J. F. San Jose, F. Rey-Martinez, and F. J. Martin-Gil. "Outcomes of Research into a Sick Hospital." *Hospital Management International*, 80–2. New York: Sterling Publications Limited, 1997.

Maxwell, N. I. "Social Differences in Women's Use of Personal Care Products: A Study of Magazine Advertisements, 1950-1994." *Silent Spring Institute*, 2000. Retrieved October 12, 2011. http://library.silentspring.org/publications/pdfs/magazinestudy.pdf.

———. *Understanding Environmental Health: How We Live in the World.* Toronto, ON: Jones and Bartlett Publishers, 2009.

McCabe, L. J. "Goderich Tornado August 21, 2011." *Disaster Planning and Rebuild.* City of Goderich, ON, August 2011. Retrieved December 29, 2015. http://www.goderich.ca/en/Heritage/resources/Larry-Goderich_Tornado-Spring_2013.pdf.

McCarty, C. A. "A Review of the Epidemiologic Evidence Linking Ultraviolet Radiation and Cataracts." *Develops in Ophthalmology* 35 (2002): 21–31.

McSheffrey, E (August 24, 2016). *First Nations with Poisoned Waters Feels Abandoned After Husky Oil Spill. National Observer.* Retrieved April 15, 2017, http://www.nationalobserver.com/2016/08/24/news/first-nation-poisoned-waters-feels-abandoned-after-husky-oil-spill.

Mehta, D. "Regulate Metals in CDN Cosmetics: Report." *The Canadian Press*, May 15, 2011. Retrieved May 15, 2011. http://news.ca.msn.com/health/regulate-metals-in-cdn-cosmeticsreport.

Meinhardt, P. L. "Water and Bioterrorism: Preparing for the Potential Threat to U.S. Water Supplies and Public Health." *Annual Review of Public Health* 26 (2005): 213–17.

Merrill, R. M. *Environmental Epidemiology: Principles and Methods.* Toronto, ON: Jones and Bartlett Publishers, 2008.

Merson, M. H., R. E. Black, and A. J. Mills. *Global Health: Diseases, Programs, Systems Policies.* 3rd ed. Toronto, ON: Jones and Bartlett Publishing, 2012.

Millennium Ecosystem Assessment. *Ecosystems and Human Well-Being: A Framework for Assessment.* Washington, DC: Island Press, 2005.

Ministry of Justice. *Emergency Preparedness Act R.S.C. 1985, C.6 (4th Suppl.).* Ottawa, ON: Author, 2014a. Retrieved December 29, 2015. http://laws.justice.gc.ca/eng/acts/E-4.6/20021231/P1TT3xt3.html.

———. *Emergency Preparedness Act, Repealed, 2007, c15, s13.* Ottawa, ON: Author, 2014b. Retrieved December 29, 2015. http://laws.justice.gc.ca/PDF/E-4.5.pdf.

————. *Emergency Preparedness Act. S.C. 2007, C.15.* Ottawa, ON: Author, 2014c. Retrieved December 29, 2015. http://laws-loins.justice.gc.ca/PDF/E-4.5.pdf.

Minister of Public Works and Government Services Canada. "A Breath of Fresh Air: Made in Canada Solutions to Meet Canada's Environmental Challenge. Speaking Notes for an Address by the Honourable Rona Ambrose, Minister of the Environment of Canada." Vancouver, BC (March 31, 2006), 2007. Retrieved November 7, 2011. http://www.ec.gc.ca/minister/speeches/2006;060331_s_e.htm.

Mittelstaedt, M. "Canada the First to Declare Bisphenol a Toxic." *The Globe and Mail.* Toronto, ON, October 13, 2010. Retrieved November 1, 2011. http://www.theglobeandmail.com/news/national/candaa-first-to-declare-bisphenol-a-toxic/article1755272.

Morgan, J., and N. Morgan. *Dr. Seuss and Mr. Geisel: A Biography.* New York: Random House, 1995. ISBN:978-0679416869.

Morita, A., Y. Kusaka, Y. Deguchi, A. Moriuchi, Y. Nakanaga, M. Iki, S. Miyazaki, and K. Kawahara. "Acute Health Problems Among the People Engaged in the Cleanup of the Nakhodka Oil Spill." *Environmental Research* 81 (1999): 185–94.

Murphy, M. *Sick Building Syndrome and the Problem of Uncertainty: Environmental Politics, Technoscience, and Women Workers.* Duke University Press, 2006. ISBN:978-0-8223-3671-6.

Murphy, V. "Hungarian Chemical Spill is Eco Disaster. *The Mirror,* UK, 2010. Retrieved November 20, 2011. http://www.mirror.co.uk.news/top-stories/2010/10/06/.

Naidoo, J., and J. Wills. *Health Promotion: Foundations for Practice.* 2nd ed. Toronto, ON: Bailliere Tindall/Elsevier Limited, 2000.

National Collaborating Centres for Public Health (NCCCPH). "What Is Evidence-Informed Public Health? Fact Sheet." November 2011. Retrieved November 13, 2013. http://www.nccmt.ca/eiph/.

National Expert Commission Canadian Nurses Association. *A Nursing Call to Action. The Health of Our Nation, the Future of Our Health System.* Ottawa, ON: Canadian Nurses Association, 2012. ISBN:978-1-55119-387-8.

Nelson D, M. Concha-Barrientos, T. Driscoll, K. Steenland, M. Fingerhut, L. Punnett, A. Pruss-Ustun, J. Leigh, and C. Corvelan. "The Global Burden of Selected Occupational Diseases and Injury Risks: Methodology and Summary." *American Journal of Industrial Medicine* 48, no. 6 (2005): 400–18.

Nyberg, F., P. Gustavsson, L. Jarup, T. Bellander, N. Berglind, R. Jakobsson, and G. Pershagen. "Urban Air Pollution and Lung Cancer in Stockholm." *Epidemiology* 11 (2000): 487–95.

O'Connor, D. R. *Walkerton Commission of Inquiry Reports: A Strategy for Safe Drinking Water.* Toronto, ON: Ontario Minister of the Attorney General, 2002. ISBN:0-7794-2621-5. http://health.gov.on.ca/en/pro/programs/publichealth/oph_standards/ophsprotocols.aspx.

Ontario Ministry of Health and Long-Term Care. *West Nile Virus.* Toronto, ON: Author, 2012. Retrieved October 24, 2012. http://health.gov.on.ca/en/public/programs/publichealth/wnv/default.aspx/wnv_mn.html.

————. *Ontario Public Health Standards.* Toronto, ON: Author, 2015. Retrieved January 6, 2016.

Park, R. M., J. F. Bena, L. T. Stayner, R. J. Smith, H. J. Gibb, and P.S. J. Lees. "Hexavalent Chromium and Lung Cancer in the Chromate Industry: A Quantitative Risk Assessment." *Risk Analysis* 24 (2004): 1099–108.

Pascual, M., J. A. Ahumada, L. F. Chaves, X. Rodo, and M. Bouma. "Malaria Resurgence in the East African Highlands: Temperature Trends Revisited." *Proceedings of the National Academy of Science USA* 103 (2006): 5829–34.

Pearson Education. *Toxic Chemical Spills.* Toronto, ON: Author, 2011. Retrieved November 23, 2011. http://www.pearsoned.ca/school/science11/chemistry11/matter_and_bonding/toxic_chemical.

Perez, C. E. "Second-Hand Smoke Exposure: Who's at Risk?" *Health Reports* 16, no. 1 (2004): 9–17.

Petroleum Communication Foundation. *Flaring: Questions and Answers.* Calgary, Alberta: Author, 2000a.

————. *Sour Gas: Questions and Answers.* Calgary, Alberta: Author, 2000b.

Pinkerton, L. E., M. J. Hein, and L. T. Stayner. "Mortality Among a Cohort of Garmet Workers Exposed to Formaldehyde: An Update." *Environmental Medicine* 61, no. 3 (2004): 193–200.

Pope, C. A., III, R. T. Burnett, M. J. Thun, E. E. Calle, D. Krewski, K. Ito, and G. D. Thurston. "Lung Cancer, Cardiopulmonary Mortality, and Long-Term Exposure to Fine Particulate Air Pollution." *JAMA* 287 (2002): 1132–41.

Pott, P. *Chirurgical Observations Related to the Cataract, the Polypus of the Nose, the Cancer of the Scrotum, the Different Kinds of Ruptures, and the Mortification of the Toes and Feet. Volume 3—A Short Treatise of the Chimney Sweeper's Cancer,* edited by L. Hawes, W., Clark, R., and Collins. London, UK, 1775.

Pruss-Ustun, A., E. Rapiti, and Y. Hutin. "Estimation of the Global Burden of Disease Attributable to Contaminated Sharps Injuries Among Health-Care Workers." *American Journal of Industrial Medicine* 48, no. 6 (2005): 482–49.

Public Health Agency of Canada. *Core Competencies for Public Health in Canada: Release 1.1.* Ottawa, ON: Author, September 2007.

———. "*West Nile Virus MONITOR: Human Surveillance (2003–2005)*," 2006. Retrieved November 2, 2011. http://www.phac-aspc.gc.ca/wnv-vwn.mon-humunsurv-archive_e.html.

———. *General Information.* Ottawa, ON: Author, 2012. Retrieved October 24, 2012. http://www.phac-aspc.gc.ca/wn-no/gen-eng.php.

Public Safety Canada. *Canadian Disaster Database.* Ottawa, ON: Government of Canada, 2013a. Retrieved December 15, 2015. http://www.publicsafety.gc.ca/cnt/rsrcs/cndn-dsstr-dtbs/index-eng.aspx.

———. *Emergency Management.* Ottawa, ON: Author, 2013b. Retrieved December 29, 2015. http://www.publicsafety.gc.ca/cnt/mrgnc-mngmnt/index-eng.aspx or http://publications.gc.ca/site/archivee-archived.html?url=http://publications.gc.ca/collections/collection_2013/sp-ps/PS1-7-2013-eng.pdf.

Public Safety and Emergency Preparedness Canada. *Canadian Disaster Database.* Ottawa, ON: Author, 2005. Retrieved November 7, 2011. http://www.psepc-sppcc.gc.ca/res/em/cdd/search-en.asp.

Puddicombe, D. "Rain Delivers Another Sewage Spill." *Ottawa Sun,* April 27, 2009. Ottawa, ON.

Quinlan, E., and H. D. Dickinson. "The Emerging Public Health System in Canada." In *Health, Illness, and Health Care in Canada.* 4th ed., edited by B. Singh Bolaria and H. D. Dickinson, 42–55. Toronto, ON: Nelson Education, 2009.

Raphael, D. *Social Determinants of Health,* 2nd ed. Toronto, ON: Canadian Scholars' Press Inc., 2009.

Rebmann, T., R. Carrico, and J. F. English. "Lessons Public Health Professionals Learned From Past Disasters." *Public Health Nursing* 25, no. 4 (2008): 344–52.

Reguly, E. "Paris Climate Talks. Small Island States Make Waves at Paris Conference." *The Globe and Mail.* Toronto, ON, December 13, 2015. Retrieved December 14, 2015. http://www.theglobeandmail.com/news/world/small-island-states-make-waves-at-paris-climate-conference/article27742043/.

Reiners, C. "Radioactivity and Thyroid Cancer." *Hormones* 8, no. 3 (2009): 185–91.

Ritter, K. *New Zealand Calls Kyoto Pact 'Outdated,'* A18. Toronto, ON: Toronto Star, December 3, 2012.

Robertson, A. S., D. C. Weir, and P. Sherwood Burge. "Occupational Asthma Due to Oil Mists." *Thorax* 43 (1988): 200–05.

Robins, G. "Powerful Tornado Kills Man in Goderich, Ontario." *The Canadian Press,* 2011. Retrieved December 29, 2015. http://www.cbc.ca/news/canada/toronto/powerful-tornado-kills-man-in-goderich-ontario-1.979470.

Robinson Vollman, A., E. T. Anderson, and J. McFarlane. *Canadian Community as Partner: Theory and Practice in Nursing.* New York: Lippincott William and Wilkins, 2004.

Rosen, G. *A History of Public Health.* New York: MD Publications, 1958.

Rugaber, C. S., and M. Crutsinger. *Hurricane Sandy Estimated to Cost $60 Billion.* New York: Associated Press-Business Time, 2012. Retrieved November 2, 2012. http://business.time.com/2012/10/13/hurrican-sandyu-estimated-to-cost-60-billion/.

Russell, M., and M. Gruber. "Risk Assessment in Environmental Policy Making." *Science* 236 (1987): 286–90.

Salazar-Garcia, F., E. Gallardo-Diaz, P. Ceron-Mireles, D. Loomis, and V. H. Borja-Aburto.(April 1,). "Reproductive Effects of Occupational DDT Exposure Among Male Malaria Control Workers." *Environmental Health Perspectives* 112, no. 5 (2004): 542–47.

San Sebastian, M., B. Armstrong, and C. Stephens. "Outcomes of Pregnancy Among Women Living in the Proximity of Oil Fields in the Amazon Basin of Ecuador." *International Journal of Environmental Health* 8 (2002): 312–19.

Schubert, P. E., and W. J. Bartfay. "Environmental Perspectives on Health." In *Community Health Nursing: Caring in Action,* 1st Canadian ed., edited by J. E. Hitchcock, P.E. Schubert, S.A. Thomas, and W. J. Bartfay, 117–42. Toronto, ON: Nelson Education, 2010.

Scientific Group on Methodologies for the Safety Evaluation of Chemicals. "Alternative Testing Methodologies (SGOMSEC 13-IPCS 29)." *Environmental Health Perspectives* 106, no. 2 (1998): 405–12.

Scoffield, H. *Climate Change Costly for Canada: Research.* Toronto, ON: The Canadian Press, 2011a. Retrieved September 29, 2011. http://news.ca.msn.com/health/climate-change-costly-for-canada-research-158.

———. Price of Climate Change Climbs. *Toronto Star,* A4, September 30, 2011b.

Selikoff, I. J., and H. Seidman. "Asbestos-Associated Deaths Among Insulation Workers in the United States and Canada, 1967–1987." *Annuals of the New York Academy of Science* 643 (1991): 1–14.

Shah, C. P. *Public Health and Preventative Medicine in Canada*. 5th ed. Toronto, ON: Elsevier Canada, 2003.

Shepherd Marshall, J., and J. Knox. "Hurricane Sandy and Climate Change." Toronto, ON: The Star, 2012. Retrieved November 2, 2012. http://www.thestar.com/opinion/editoiralopinion/article/1280681–hurricane-sandy-and-climate-change.

Shields, M. "Shift Work and Health." *Health Reports* 13, no. 4 (2002): 11–33. Ottawa, ON: Statistics Canada (Catalogue No. 82-003).

———. "Smoking-Prevalence, Bans and Exposure to Second-Hand Smoke." *Health Reports* 18, no. 3 (2007): 67–85.

———. "Stress, Health and the Benefit of Social Support." *Health Reports* 15, no. 1 (2004): 9–38. Ottawa, ON: Statistics Canada (Catalogue No. 82-003).

Sleijffers, A., J. Garssen, and H. Van Loveren. "Ultraviolet Radiation, Resistance to Infectious Diseases, and Vaccination Responses." *Methods* 28 (2002): 111–21.

Snodin, D. J. "An EU Perspective on the Use of In Vitro Methods in Regulatory Pharmaceutical Toxicology." *Toxicology Letters*, 127 (2002): 161–68.

Stafanson, D., and W. J. Bartfay. "Varied Roles and Practice Specialties in Community Health Nursing." In *Community Health Nursing: Caring in Action*. 1st Canadian ed., edited by J. E. Hitchcock, P.E. Schubert, S.A. Thomas, and W. J. Bartfay, 59–97. Toronto, ON: Nelson Education, 2010.

Standing Senate Committee on Social Affairs, Science and Technology, Subcommittee on Population Health. *A Healthy, Productive Canada: A Determinant of Health Approach*. Ottawa, ON: Author, 2009. Retrieved November 3, 2013. http://www.parl.gc.ca/Content/SEN/Committee/402/popu/rep/rephealth1jun09-e.pdf.

Statistics Canada. *Mercury Concentrations in the Canadian Population, 2007 to 2009*. Ottawa, ON: Author, 2011a. Retrieved October 16, 2011. http://www.statcan-gc.ca/pub/82-625-x/2010002/article/11329-eng.htm.

———. *Lead Concentrations in the Canadian Population, 2007–2009*. Ottawa, ON: Author, 2011b. Retrieved October 16, 2011. http://www.statcan.gc.ca/pub/82-625-x/2010002/article/11328-eng.htm.

———. *Bisphenol A Concentrations in the Canadian Population, 2007 to 2009*. Ottawa, ON: Author, 2011c. Retrieved October 16, 2011. http://www.statcan.gc.ca/pub/82-625-X/2010002/article/11327-eng.htm.

———. *Exposure to Second-Hand Smoke at Home, 2010*. Ottawa, ON: Author, 2011d. Retrieved November 8, 2011. http://ww.statcan.gc.ca/pub/82-626-x/2011001/article/11460-eng.htm.

———. *Work Absences in 2011*. Ottawa, ON: Author, 2012. Retrieved January 27, 2013. http://www.statcan.gc.ca/pub/75-001-x/2012002002/article/11650-eng.htm.

———. *Perceived Life Stress*. Ottawa, ON: Author, 2010. Retrieved January 27, 2013. http://www.statcan.gc.ca/pub/82-229-x/2009001/status/pls-eng.htm.

Stevens, K.P., and M. A. Gallo. "Practical Considerations in the Conduct of Chronic Toxicity Studies." In *Principles and Methods of Toxicology*, edited by A. W. Hayes, 53–77. New York: Raven Press, 1982.

Storey, R. "Don't Work Too Hard: Health and Safety Workers' Compensation in Canada." In *Health, Illness and Health Care in Canada*, 4th ed., edited by B. Singh Bolaria and H. D. Dickinson, 388–411. Toronto, ON: Nelson Education, 2009.

Strully, K. W. "Joss Loss and Health in the US Labor Market." *Demography* 46 (2009): 221–26.

Stuckler, D., S. Basu, M. Suhreke, A. Coutts, and M. McKee. "Effects of the 2008 Recession on Health: A First Look at European Data." *Lancet* 378, no. 9786 (2011): 124–25.

Seuss, Dr. *The Lorax*. New York: Random House, 1971. ISBN:978-0-375-86136-9.

Sullivan, P. "Safety of Drinking Water Remains a Crucial Health Issue, CMA President Says." *Canadian Medical Association*, 2004. Retrieved November 8, 2011. http://www.cma.ca/index.cfm/ci_id/10013192/la_id/1.html.

Tanaka, Y. "Ecological Risk Assessment of Pollutant Chemicals: Extinction Risk Based on Population-Level Effects." *Chemosphere* 53 (2003): 421–25.

The Associated Press. "Hurricane Sandy Death Tolls Reaches 74 in U.S." *New York Daily News*, November 1, 2012. Retrieved November 2, 2012. http://www.nydailynews.com/new-york/hurrican-sandy-death-toll-reaches-74-article-1.1.

The Guardian. "Climate Change Talks Yield Small Chance of Global Treaty." *The Guardian* April 11, 2010. Retrieved November 1, 2011. http://www.guardian.co.uk/environment/2010/apr/11/climate-change-talks-deal-treaty.

The Independent. "Danube 'Neutralizing Toxic Sludge.'" *The Independent, UK,* 2010. Retrieved November 20, 2011. http://www.independent.co.uk.news/world/europe/danube-neutralizing-toxic-sludge-2101531.html.

The Mining Association of Canada. *Mining Facts.* Ottawa, ON: Author, 2014. Retrieved January 7, 2016. http://mining.ca/resources/mining-facts.

The Ottawa Citizen. "Great Lakes Basin Chemical Pollution Threatens Millions." Ottawa, ON, 2008. Retrieved November 8, 2011. http://www.canada/com/ottawacitizen/news/story/html?id=9a3b7363-1935-4046-817d-f86.

The Sofia Echo Staff. "Fears of Regional Contamination After Chemical Spill in Hungary." *The Sofia Echo Staff,* 2010. Retrieved November 20, 2011 from http://www.sofiaecho.com/2010/10/05/971794_fears-of-regional-contamination-after-chemical-spill-in-Hungary.

The Woods Hole Research Center. (n.d.). *The Kyoto Protocol,* n.d. Retrieved November 1, 2011. http://www.shrc.org/resources/online_publications/warming_earth/hyoto.htm.

Thompson, V. D. *Health and Health Care Delivery in Canada.* Toronto, ON: Mosby/Elsevier, 2010.

Time. "California: Chopping Down Dr. Seuss." *Time,* October 2, 1989. Retrieved November 28, 2011. http://www.time.com/time/magazine/article/0,9171,958654,00.html?iid=chix-sphere.

Turcotte, M. *Time Spent with Family During a Typical Workday, 1986 to 2005.* Ottawa, ON: Statistics Canada, 2014. Retrieved January 7, 2016. http://www.statcan.gc.ca/pub/11-008-x/2006007/9574-eng.htm.

U.S. Agency for Toxic Substances and Disease Registry. (2005). *ToxFAQs: Naphthalene.*

U.S. Centers for Disease Control and Prevention. *Work-Related Lung Disease Surveillance Report 2002.* Washington, DC: Author, 2002. Retrieved September 22, 2011. http://www.cdc.gov/niosh/docs/2003-111/2003-111.html.

U.S. Department of Labour, Occupational Safety and Health Administration. *Industrial Hygiene.* Washington, DC: Author, 2010. Retrieved September 11, 2011. http:///actrav.itcilo.org/actrav-english/telearn/osh/hazard/hyg.htm.

U.S. Environmental Protection Agency. *An Introduction to Indoor Air Quality: Formaldehyde,* 2007a. Retrieved October 14, 2011. http://www.epa.gov/iag/formalde.html.

———. *Learn About Chemicals Around Your House: Air Fresheners.* 2007b. Retrieved October 14, 2011. http://www.epa.gov/kidshometour/products/airf.htm.

———. *Indoor Air Facts No. 4 (Revised): Sick Building Syndrome.* Washington, DC: Author, 2010. Retrieved November 4, 2011. http;//epa.gov/iaq/pubs/sbs.html.

U.S. Food and Drug Administration. "Ingredients Prohibited and Restricted by FDA Regulations, 2006." 2006. Retrieved October 14, 2011. http://www.cfsan.fda.gov/-dms/cos-210.html.

United Nations. "Adoption of the Paris Agreement. Framework Convention on Climate Change." *Conference of the Parties, Twenty-First Reunion,* Paris, 30 November to 11 December 2014. Paris, France, 2015. Retrieved December 14, 2015. http://unfccc.int/resource/docs/2015/cop21/eng/l09.pdf.

United Nations Environment Programme. *Scientific Assessment of Ozone Depletion: Executive Summary,* 2002. Retrieved November 2, 2011. http://ozone.unep.org/pdfs/Scientific_assess_depletion/05-Executivesummary.pdf.

United Nations Framework Convention on Climate Change. *Kyoto Protocol,* 2006a. Retrieved November 2, 2011. http://unfccc.int/Kyoto_protocol/background/items3145.php.

———. *The United Nations Framework Convention on Climate Change: Essential Background,* 2006b. Retrieved November 2, 2011. http://unfccc.int/essential_background/convention/items/2627.php.

United Nations Secretariat. *Bulletin on the Eradication of Poverty,* 2004. Retrieved November 8, 2011. http://www.un.org.esa/socdev/poverty/documents/boep_10_2003_EN.pdf.

Vajpeyi, D. K. *Deforestation, Environment, and Sustainable Development: Comparative Analysis.* Westport, CT: Greenwood Publishing Group, 2001.

Veenema, T. G. *Disaster Nursing and Emergency Preparedness for Chemical, Biological, and Radiological Terrorism and Other Hazards.* 3rd ed. New York: Springer, 2013.

Venetoulis, J., and J. Talberth. *Ecological Footprint of Nations: 2005 Update: Redefining Progress,* 2006. Retrieved November 7, 2011. http://www.rporgress.org/publications2006/Footprint%2-of%20Nations%202005.pdf.

Wallick, F. *The American Worker: An Endangered Species*. New York: Ballantine Books, 1972.

Walters, H. "5 Key Points in Paris Agreement on Climate Change." *CBC News*, December 12, 2015, Toronto, ON. Retrieved December 14, 2015. http://www.cbc.ca/news/world/paris-agreement-key-climate-points-1.3362500.

Watson, R. "Climate Change Is Likely to Affect the Health of Millions, Report Warms." *British Medical Journal* 334, no. 7597 (April 14, 2007): 768.

———. *Introduction to Atmospheric Chemistry*. Toronto, ON: York University, 1999. Retrieved November 1, 2011. http://cac.yorku.ca.

Wells, J. *Firefighters Get Increased Cancer Coverage*. Calgary, Alberta: Calgary Sun, 2011. Retrieved November 2, 2012. http://www.calgarysun.com/2011/05/04firefighters-get-increased-cancer-coverage.

Wilkins, K. "Work Stress Among Health Care Providers." *Health Reports*. Ottawa, ON: Statistics Canada 18, no. 4 (2007): 33–36. (Catalogue No. 82-2003).

Wilkins, K., and S. G. Mackenzie,. *Work Injuries*. Ottawa, ON: Statistics Canada, 2008. Retrieved October 16, 2011. http://www.statcan.gc.ca/pub/82-003-x/2006007/article/10191-eng.htm.

Williams, C. "Sources of Workplace Stress." *Perspectives on Labour and Income* 4, no. 6 (June 2003): 1–11 (Online edition).

Wilson, J. "Facing an Uncertain Climate." *Annuals of Internal Medicine* 146, no. 2 (January 2007): 153–56.

Wong, S. L., and E. J. D. Lye. *Lead, Mercury and Cadmium Levels in Canadians*. Ottawa, ON: Statistics Canada, 2008. Retrieved October 16, 2011. http://www.statcan.gc.ca/pub/82-003-x/2008004/article/6500106-eng.htm.

WorkSafeBC. *Occupational Disease Data by Type of Disease and Five-Year Period: 1988–2012*. British Columbia, Canada, 2013. Retrieved January 8, 2016. http://www.worksafebc.com/publications/reports/statistics_reports/occupational_disease/1988-2012/assets/Table1.pdf.

World Business Council for Sustainable Development. (2010). "Climate: Is the Copenhagen Accord Already Dead?" Retrieved November 1, 2011. http://www.wbcsd.org/plugins/DocSearch/details.asp?type=DocDetandObjectID=MzcOnzE.

World Health Organization. *Using Climate to Predict Infectious Disease Epidemics*. Geneva, Switzerland: Author, 2006. Retrieved November 2, 2011. http:///www.who.int/globalchange/publications/infectdiseases.pdf.

———. *Health Effects of UV Radiation*. Geneva, Switzerland: Author, 2007a. Retrieved November 2, 2011. http://www.who.int/uv/health/en/.

———. *Working for Health: An Introduction to the World Health Organization*. Geneva, Switzerland: Author, 2007b. Retrieved December 15, 2015. http://www.who.int/about/borchure_en.pdf?ua=1.

———. *Good Practice in Occupational Health Services: A Contribution to Workplace Health*. Geneva, Switzerland: Author, 2008. Retrieved November 2, 2011. http://www.euro.who.int/document/e77650.pdf.

———. *West Nile Virus*. Geneva, Switzerland: Author, 2011. Retrieved October 24, 2012. http://www.who.int/mediacentre/factsheet/fs354/en/index.html.

———. *Emergency and Essential Surgical Care*. Geneva, Switzerland: Author, 2014. Retrieved December 15, 2015. http://www.who.int/surgery/en.

World Meteorological Organization. *Scientific Assessment of Ozone Depletion: 2006*, 2006. Retrieved November 2, 2011. http://www.esrl.noaa.gov/csd/assessments/2006/executivesummary.html.

World Resources Institute. "Urban Air: Health Effects of Particulates, Sulfur Dioxide, and Ozone," 2010. Retrieved November 7, 2011. http://health.allrefer.com/health/hemoglobin-derivates-info.html.

Youakim, S. "Risk of Cancer Among Firefighters: A Quantitative Review of Selected Malignancies." *Archives of Environmental and Occupational Health* 61, no. 5 (2006): 223–31.

Zeig-Owens R., M. P. Webber, C. B. Hall, T. Schwartz, N. Jaber, J. Weakley, T. E. Rohan, H. W. Cohen, O. Derman, T. K. Aldrich, K. Kelly, and D. J. Prezant. "Early Assessment of Cancer Outcomes in New York City Firefighters After 9/11 Attacks: An Observational Cohort Study." *Lancet* 3, no. 378(9794) (2011): 898–905.

Zhu, L. Y., and R. A. Hites. "Temporal Trends and Spatial Distributions of Brominated Flame Retardants in Archived Fishes From the Great Lakes." *Environmental Science and Technology* 38, no. 10 (2004): 2779–84.

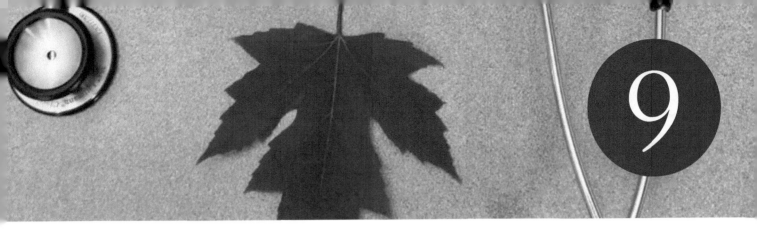

Global Health: A Primer

A single chopstick is weak and can be easily broken. However, when you bundle a handful of chopsticks together, they are strong and unbreakable.

—Old Chinese proverb

Learning Objectives

After completion of this chapter, the student will be able to:
- Define the terms global health and globalization,
- Describe the scope and significance of examining health and well-being from a global perspective,
- List and describe the United Nations 15 Millennium Development Goals (MDGs) and the 17 Sustainable Development Goals (SDGs),
- List and describe various population-based measures of health burden and how they are utilized to examine the impact and effectiveness of public health initiatives,
- Recognize and describe potential social, cultural, economic, and political factors affecting global health outcomes in terms of leading causes of mortality and morbidity in developed and developing countries and/or regions of the world,
- List and describe two neglected tropical diseases (NTDs) and the current challenges facing their surveillance and management from the regional and global perspectives,
- Explain the current and predicted outcomes of population growth from a national and global perspective, and
- Describe the role of public health professionals and workers for planning and implementing strategies which seek to promote and/or preserve the health of all citizens of our planet.

Core Competencies addressed in Chapter 9

Core Competencies	Competency Statements
1.0 Public Health Sciences	1.1, 1.2, 1.4, 1.5
2.0 Assessment and Analysis	2.1, 2.4, 2.5
3.0 Policy and Program Planning, Implementation, and Evaluation	3.1, 3.2, 3.6
4.0 Partnerships, Collaboration, and Advocacy	4.3, 4.4
5.0 Diversity and Inclusiveness	5.1, 5.2, 5.3
6.0 Communication	6.2, 6.3
7.0 Leadership	7.2, 7.3

Note: Please see the following document or web-based link for a detailed description of these specific competencies. Public Health Agency of Canada (2007).

Introduction

The term "global health" is an evolving one which embraces a wide range of health-promoting and health-preserving activities and challenges that span international borders and boundaries (Bartfay and Bartfay 2015; Thomas and Bartfay 2011). The *Ottawa Charter* was the first global acknowledgement to declare that caring for one's self and others is conducive to health and the well-being of our citizens, and it identified the importance of caring, holism, and the environment as essential concepts for health promotion (World Health Organization [WHO] 1986, 2014d). The *Bangkok Charter of Health Promotion* has explicated the link among health, society, and globalization, and the need for action to improve the health of all citizens based on these interrelationships (WHO 2005a). The Bangkok Charter argued that health promotion must become an integral component of both domestic and foreign policy and international relations (WHO 2005a).

Global health is defined as an area of research and practice that seeks to improve the health via the social determinants of health (SDH) by promoting social justice and equity, human rights, and sustainable development both on the national and on the international scale and by fostering and promoting the availability and access to healthcare professionals, healthcare financing, and delivery of primary healthcare services to all citizens of this planet (Bartfay and Bartfay 2015). In other words, global health can be utilized as a framework or vehicle to achieve *health for all* citizens of this planet, and it transcends national borders or individual national concerns per se (Messias 2001; Seear 2007; WHO 1978, 2005a, 2009). For example, the cholera epidemic that took an estimated 20,000 lives in Egypt during the years 1947 and 1948 served as the impetus for various countries to offer their assistance with this epidemic.

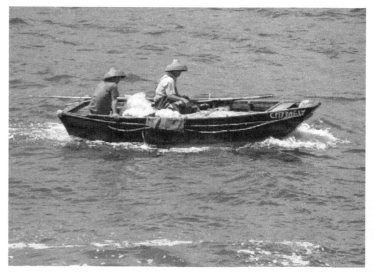

Photo 9.1 Fisher persons in Hong Kong harbour. Having a stable and reliable source of income is critical to obtain other necessities associated with health including proper shelter and housing, food sources and supplies, access to certain healthcare services, medications and recreational activities and pursuits.

Source: Wally J. Bartfay

Important international health agencies include the Canadian International Development Agency (CIDA), Canadian Council for International Co-operation (CCIC), WHO, Pan American Health Organization (PAHO), United Nations Children's Emergency Fund (UNICEF), World Food Programme (WFP), and the World Bank that places a priority on achieving equity in health for all citizens of our planet, reducing disparities and protecting against global threats that disregard national borders.

The recent outbreak of Ebola virus in West Africa in 2014 and beyond its borders (e.g., the United States, the United Kingdom) highlights the critical need to examine health from a global context and perspective (WHO 2014b, 2016a). The most severely affected countries included Guinea, Sierra Leone, and Liberia that have relatively weak public health systems, few healthcare personnel and healthcare infrastructures to deal with the epidemic. On August 8, 2014, the WHO Director General declared this Ebola outbreak a public health emergency of international concern (WHO 2014a). Ebola entered the United States in October 2014, via Mr Thomas Eric Duncan, a victim who was infected with Ebola while visiting West Africa. Duncan was treated at the Texas Health Presbyterian Hospital, but later died due to complications. Two nurses who cared for Mr Duncan, Amber Joy Vinson, and Nina Pharm also tested positive for the Ebola virus and were placed under strict isolation (Poladian 2014).

Ebola virus disease (EVD), which is also called *ebola hemorrhagic fever* is a disease which affects humans and other primates, and is caused by the Ebola virus. EVD was first identified in 1976 in Nzara, South Sudan, and in Yambuku, the Democratic Republic of Congo (formally Zaire), and received its name based on the Ebola River were victims were first identified (WHO 2014a). Five species of Ebola have been identified to date: (a) Zaire, (b) Bundibugyo, (c) Sudan, (d) Reston, and (e) Taï Forest. The exposed victim typically begins to experience signs and symptoms between two and three weeks after coming into direct contact with the virus (e.g., a dead relative, patient with EVD). EVD is not transmitted via an air-borne mechanism, but requires direct contact with an infected victim showing signs or symptoms or a deceased individual. Signs and symptoms of EVD include high fever, sore throat, skin rash, muscle aches and pain, headaches, nausea and vomiting, diarrhea, decreased liver and kidney function, and bleeding (e.g., eyes, nose, mouth). Death is usually attributed to low blood pressure and severe loss of body fluids or blood. There is no specific cure for EVD, but rest and oral and intravenous hydration appears to improve survival outcomes. On October 20, 2014, Nigeria and Senegal were declared Ebola-free by the WHO (Lunn 2014). There are currently no licensed Ebola vaccines available at publication of this textbook. Nonetheless, two potential candidates, including one Canadian vaccine developed in Winnipeg, Manitoba, are undergoing human clinical trials in Africa. From 1976 to January 17, 2016, there have been 28,638 cases of EVB, and 11,316 death worldwide (WHO 2016a).

Web-Based Resource Box 9.1 Canadian and International Organizations and Agencies for Promoting and Preserving Global Health

Learning resource	Website
Canadian Council for International Cooperation (CCIC) This council is a collation of various Canadian voluntary sector organizations.	http://www.ccic.ca
Canadian International Development Agency (CIDA) The mandate of this federal agency includes managing Canada's support and resources effectively and accountably to achieve meaningful, sustainable results, and engaging in policy development in Canada and internationally.	http://www.acdi-cida.gc.ca
Canadian Society for International Health (CSIH) Is a national non-governmental organization that works domestically and internationally to reduce global health inequities and strengthen health systems.	http://www.csih.org/en/index.asp

(Continued)

Web-Based Resource Box 9.1 Canadian and International Organizations and Agencies for Promoting and Preserving Global Health (*Continued*)

Learning resource	Website
Global Health Council (GHC) Is a member network dedicated to saving lives and improving the health of the 2 billion people living on less than $2 (U.S.) per day.	http://globalhealth.org
Pan American Health Organization (PAHO) This non-profit organization provides technical co-operation and mobilizes partnerships to improve health and quality of life in the countries of the Americas.	http://www.new.paho.org

Developing an understanding and need to examine health and public primary healthcare challenges from an international perspective is critical for all public healthcare professionals and workers in Canada and abroad. Indeed, the emergence of severe acute respiratory syndrome (SARS), West Nile virus, H1N1, Ebola, and the Zika virus are recent examples of how quickly diseases can spread and the global challenges faced by public healthcare professionals and officials in terms of their surveillance, tracking, and management (Campbell 2006; Quinlan and Dickinson 2009). This chapter provides the reader with an overview of global health and selects current and emerging international public healthcare issues.

Group Activity-Based Learning Box 9.1

Thinking About Health From a Global Context

This Group Activity-Based Learning Box 9.1 provides the student with an opportunity to begin to think about health from an international or global health context. Select a country or region of the world outside of North America that is of interest to your group. Working in small groups of three to five students, discuss and answer the following questions:

1. What resources would you employ to find out about current health challenges in your selected country or region?

2. How is public health being administered to those in need and what are the noted barriers and facilitators?

3. Which international health organizations are currently involved in assisting with healthcare delivery or services in your chosen country or region?

4. What questions would you need to ask to evaluate the impact of primary healthcare and/or health promotion initiatives in your chosen country or region?

5. How can published research be better utilized to promote the health and well-being of individuals, families, groups, or entire populations in your chosen country or region?

Global warming and its associated environmental affects (e.g., drowning due to flooding, mud slides, extreme heat, drought) is predicted to cause between 150,000 and 300,000 deaths annually and 5 million illnesses, and these numbers are expected to double by the year 2030 (CDC 2015; Vidal 2009; Wilson 2007; West 2015). Flooding as a result of coastal storm surges will affect the lives of up to 200 million people globally by 2080.

Moreover, natural disasters, such as an earthquake and associated tsunamis can affect large regions, result in damage to infrastructures (e.g., buildings, supply roads, bridges, electrical power grids), injury or death, and strain and/or overwhelm already heavily burdened public healthcare systems.

For example, the December 26, 2004, tsunamis that hit the coasts of India, Thailand, Malaysia, Indonesia, Somalia, Kenya, Maldives, Bangladesh, Burma, Mauritius, and Tanzania resulted in over $10 billion in damage to infrastructures (e.g., power lines, bridges, roads, sewers), additional strain on already heavily burdened public health systems even with disaster emergency relief from other regions of the world, loss of property, at least 230,000 fatalities, 500,000 injuries, and it is estimated that 5 million people lost their homes or access to food and clean water supplies (Landsman 2005; Paris et al. 2007). The reader is

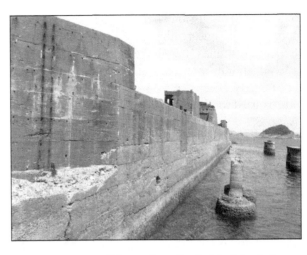

Photo 9.2 Seawall located on Battleship Island, Japan. Seawalls are critical in earthquake prone regions of the world like Japan, where tsunamasis can be triggered and devastate entire communities.

referred to the chapter entitled *Environmental and Occupational Health and Safety* for a detailed discussion related to global warming and climate change and their impact on health and disease.

The United Nations avowed that by the year 2000, health would be a possibility for all citizens of our planet (WHO 1978, 2014b). This *Health for All* objective requires that access to and the availability of essential healthcare resources be made available to all those in need, despite their social standing or financial resources. Although this noble objective is still let to be realized, it did set in motion the need to address health equity policies and healthcare planning and delivery from a global needs perspective. Ruckert and Labonté (2014) report that health equity during economic downturns is primarily impacted through austerity budgets and associated program cutbacks in areas crucial to addressing the inequitable distribution of SDH, which includes social assistance to those in need, adequate housing, education, and the qualitative transformation of labour markets and employment. The concept of global health is one that is constantly evolving with a growing recognition that international social, cultural, political, economic, and environmental issues directly affect health outcomes and how primary healthcare services are provided and delivered around the world. Health is not a tradable commodity, but is a matter of basic human rights and a public sector duty (Commission on the Social Determinants of Health 2008). For example, Bill and Melinda Gates (2006) have highlighted the importance of examining health issues from a global perspective, for improving the quality of life of individuals and the productivity of nations, and as a cornerstone of humanity.

> We believe health is the cornerstone of human development. When health takes hold, life improves by all measures. Conversely, poor health aggravates poverty, poverty deepens disease, and nations trapped in this spiral will not escape without the world's help. In Africa, the cost of malaria in terms of treatment and lost productivity is estimated to be $12 billion a year. The continent's gross domestic product could be $100 billion higher today if malaria had been eliminated in the 1960s. And if HIV infection rates continue at their present levels, the world will likely see 45 million new infections by 2010 and lose nearly 70 million people by 2020. That's 70 million of the most productive members of society—health workers, educators, and parents. (Gates and Gates 2006).

What Are the Millennium Development Goals?

The United Nations had developed goals for the new millennium (United Nations 2008, 2013; United Nations Development Program [UNDP] 2009) that sought to address a variety of global SDH and well-being such as poverty, education, clean water, gender equality, and maternal and child health. The reader is referred to Chapter 1 for a detailed discussion on the 15 SDH. For example, UNICEF (2012) reported that child poverty was a growing global health concern that also affected developed nations of the world including Iceland (4.7%), Germany (8.51%), Australia (10.9%), the United Kingdom (12.1%), Spain (17.1%), the United States (23.1%), and Canada (13.3%), and the international average is 11%. Similarly, the Ontario Association of food Banks (2008) reported that poverty affected over 3 million Canadians, including 600,000 children per year. In 2012, 882,188 individuals used food banks in Canada which represented a 30.6% increase in comparison to March 2008 figures ($N = 675,735$), and 38.4% of users were children (Food Banks Canada 2012). The Salvation Army (2011) reported that at any given time in Canada, over 150,000 individuals were homeless and living on the street.

UNICEF Canada (2013) measured child well-being in 29 of the world's richest countries, including Canada. Canada ranked in a middle position (17 out of 29 nations) overall; 15 out of 19 in terms of maternal well-being, 14 out of 29 for education, 16 out of 29 for behaviours and risks, 11 out of 29 for housing and environment, and an alarming 27 out of 29 for health and safety. Based on 2013 data from 29 countries with similar health-care accounting systems in the *Organization for Economic Co-operation and Development*, per capita spending (U.S. dollars) on health care remained highest in the United States ($9086, 17.1% of GDP) followed by France ($4361, 11.6% GDP), Germany ($4920, 11.2% of GDP), Denmark ($4847, 11.1% of GDP), Canada ($4569, 10.7 GDP), Australia ($4115, 9.4% of GDP), Japan ($3713, 10.2% of GDP), Finland ($3645, 9.1% of GDP), and the United Kingdom ($3364, 8.8% of GDP) (Canadian Institute for Health Information [CIHI] 2015).

In September 2000, 189 heads of state adopted the United Nations Millennium Declaration and endorsed this global framework for developing and fostering partnerships to work collectively to reduce poverty and hunger, tackle ill-health, gender inequality, lack of education, lack of access to clean water supplies, and environmental degradation (WHO 2012). This declaration consisted of eight major priority MDGs, and a number of indicators to monitor progress with a targeted year of 2015 for completion and evaluation (see Figure 9.1). The MDGs were a profound statement of the concerted will of the global community to act decisively and reflected an international consensus on the need for global actors to

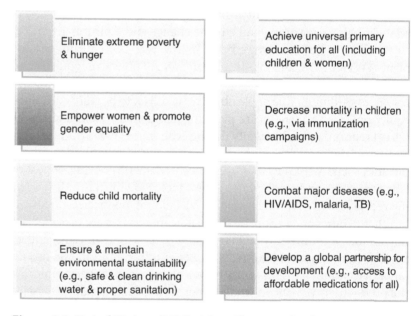

Figure 9.1 United Nations (2008) eight millennium development goals.

Source: Adapted from United Nations (2008).

work together for coherent social and economic development based on the SDH (Commission on the Social Determinants of Health 2008). By adopting SDH as targets for collaborative action, relevant stakeholders and multilateral agencies and organizations had a mechanism to work towards common thematic goals (e.g., early child development, gender equity, employment and working conditions, healthcare systems) and how to evaluate progress made.

James Wolfensohn (2002), the former World Bank President, estimated that it would take an additional $40–$60 billion a year to fulfil all of the eight proposed MDGs. UNICEF estimated that it would cost approximately $63 billion and $29 billion to achieve the water and sanitation targets over a period of 10 years (2005–2015), respectively (Lenton et al. 2005). The WHO (2006c) estimated that it would cost approximately $56 billion over 10 years to implement the *Global Plan to Stop TB*. However, it would only costs an estimated $150 million to develop one new anti-malarial drug (Medicines for Malaria Venture 2007). None of these noted additional

Table 9.1 Average Annual Rate of Decline (%) in Mortality in Children Under the Age of 5 Years, 1990–1999 and 2000–2009 by WHO Regions of the World.

WHO Region	1990–1999	2000–2009
(i) African region	1.0	2.5
(ii) Region of the Americas	4.2	4.3
(iii) South-East Asia region	2.7	4.0
(iv) European region	3.7	5.6
(v) Eastern Mediterranean region	1.8	2.1
(vi) Western Pacific region	2.4	5.4
Global	**1.3**	**2.7**

Source: Adapted from the World Health Organization (2011), 13.

estimated costs are beyond our grasps. Indeed, for comparison purposes, the U.S. Bureau of the Census (2006) estimated that $20 billion dollars' worth of candies and chocolate and over $40 billion worth of soft drinks (pop) was produced in the United States in 2005 alone.

In January 2012, the WHO (2012b) reported on the progress made to date in reference to the MDGs first outlined in September 2000. Table 9.1 shows the average percentage annual rate of decline for mortality for children under the age of 5 years by WHO regions of the world. In sum, annual global deaths of children under the age of 5 years fell to 8.1 million in 2009, compared to 12.4 million in 1990. The deaths of nearly 3 million children can be attributed to diarrhea and pneumonia annually and it is estimated that 40% of children die in the first month of life (WHO 2011, 2012b). Hence, improving the care received by newborns globally requires greater efforts. The estimated percentage of underweight children under the age of 5 years dropped from approximately 25% in 1990 to 16% in 2010. Nonetheless, a staggering 104 million children are still undernourished.

The WHO (2012b) reported that the number of women dying as a consequence of giving birth and/or complications experienced during pregnancy has decreased by 34% from 546,000 in 1990, compared to 358,000 in 2008. Although the progress is notable, the annual death rate of decline is 2.3% less than half of the 5.5% needed to achieve the desired target. It is notable that almost all of the maternal deaths reported (99%) in 2008 occurred in developing nations (WHO 2012b). Moreover, approximately half of all pregnant women made the WHO-recommended minimum of four antenatal visits during the period of 2000–2010. It is notable that fewer than half of all births in WHO regions of Africa and South-East Asia occurred with skilled assistance from a health-care worker or professional (e.g., formally trained

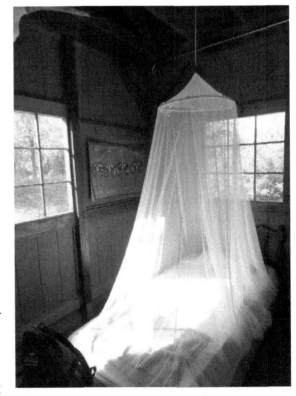

Source: Wally J. Bartfay

Photo 9.3 Photo of an insecticide-treated mosquitoe net, which costs approximately $10.00 (Canadian), has been shown to be a cost-effective means to help limit the spread of malaria in high-risk regions of the world.

midwife, physician, registered nurse). Contraceptive use has been increasing globally by 0.2% per year since the year 2000, and between 2000 and 2008 there were 48 births per 1,000 adolescent girls aged 15–19 years of age (WHO 2012b).

The number of HIV infections has declined by 17% globally from 2001 and 2009 (WHO 2012b). In 2009, 2.6 million individuals contracted a HIV infection and there were 1.8 million HIV/AIDS-related deaths globally. Tuberculosis (TB) mortality among HIV-negative individuals has dropped from approximately 30 deaths per 100,000 in 1990 to 20 deaths per 100,000 in 2009. It is notable that HIV-associated TB and multidrug-resistant TB are typically more clinically challenging to diagnosis and treat successfully.

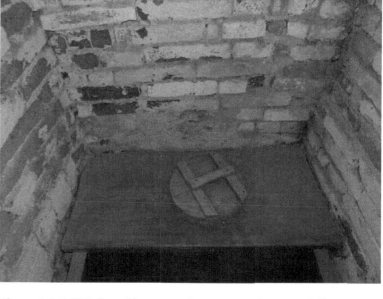

Source: Wally J. Bartfay

Photo 9.4 WHO (2012b) reports that in 2008 alone, 2.6 billion people had no access to a hygienic toilet or latrine and 1.1 billion individuals were defecating in the open.

The WHO (2012b) reported that 42 countries were on course to meet the MDG target for reducing malaria. In the year 2009 alone, an estimated 225 million cases of malaria resulted in 781,000 deaths globally, and most of these occurred in children under the age of 5 years. Although the supply of insecticide-treated mosquitoe nets employed increased, the demand unfortunately for these protective mosquitoe nets was outweighed by the available supply in most jurisdictions. Similarly, although access to anti-malarial medicines (especially artemisinin-based combination drugs) has increased, there availability was inadequate in all countries surveyed in 2007 and 2008.

The percentage of individuals with access to a safe public drinking water supply increased from 77% to 87%, which was sufficient to meet the MDG target set (WHO 2011, 2012b). Nonetheless, significant gaps still exist between urban and rural areas in many countries. The slowest improvement has been in the WHO African Region, where the percentage of the population using toilets or latrines increased from 30% in 1990 to 34% in 2008. The lack of proper sanitation and toilets significantly increases the risk for infections such as schistosomiasis, trachoma, viral hepatitis, and cholera.

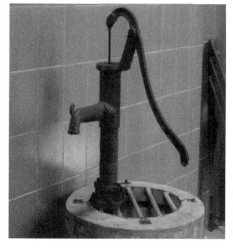

Source: Wally J. Bartfay

Photo 9.5 Approximately 1.1 billion individuals around the world currently do not have access to a safe and clean water supply. Although Canada contains approximately 15% of the world fresh water supply, approximately 60% of our water sources exist far away from populated or urban centres with designated infra-structures for delivering fresh water supplies to homes, businesses and industry.

What Are the Sustainable Development Goals?

During the 2010 MDG Summit, an outcomes document requested that the Secretary General of the United Nations begin to make plans beyond the 2015 deadline (United Nations Secretary General 2010). This stimulated further discussions at the 2012 Rio+20 Conference on Sustainable Development to begin designing a new global plan and framework. Stakeholders included not only internal member states, but broad participation from external stakeholders including non-governmental organizations (NGOs), private sector members, businesses, academics, and scientists. Their goal was to stimulate governments, UN agencies, and the public to find practical and realistic solutions surrounding the global issue of sustainable development based on the following three dimensions: (a) environment; (b) social, and (c) economic. The following 12 thematic areas or priority areas were identified (United Nations Sustainable Development Network 2013; UNDP 2015):

1. Macroeconomics, population dynamics, and planetary boundaries,
2. Reducing poverty and building peace in fragile regions of the world,
3. Addressing challenges of social inclusion (e.g., gender inequalities and human rights),
4. Early childhood development, education, and transition to the work world,
5. Health for all,
6. Promoting development and use of low-carbon energy sources and sustainable industries,
7. Sustainable agricultural practices and food systems,
8. Preserving forests, oceans, biodiversity, and ecosystem services,
9. Sustainable cities including the concepts of inclusiveness, resiliency, and connectiveness,
10. Good governance of extractive and land resources,
11. Global governance and norms for sustainable development, and
12. Redefining the role of business for sustainable development.

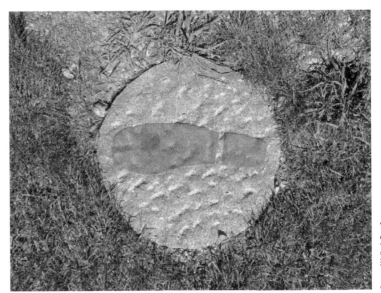

Source: Wally J. Bartfay

Photo 9.6 According to a World Wildlife Foundation report, if the entire planet lived liked Canadians do, it would take 3.5 Earth's to support the demand. Canada and the United States are among the top 10 countries in the world with the largest "ecological footprints" per capital (CBC News 2012).

Subsequently 17 SDGs were formulated from these 12 aforementioned thematic areas and are listed in the following (United Nations 2014; UNDP 2015):

- Goal 1: End poverty in all forms everywhere.
- Goal 2: End hunger, achieve food security and improved nutrition, and promote sustainable agriculture.
- Goal 3: Ensure healthy lives and promote well-being for all across the lifespan.
- Goal 4: Ensure inclusive and equitable quality education and promote lifelong learning opportunities for all.
- Goal 5: Achieve gender equality and empower women and girls.
- Goal 6: Ensure availability and sustainable management of water and sanitation for all.
- Goal 7: Ensure access to affordable, reliable, sustainable, and modern energy for all.
- Goal 8: Promote sustained, inclusive, and sustainable economic growth; full and productive employment; and decent work for all.
- Goal 9: Build resilient infrastructure, promote inclusive and sustainable industrialization, and foster innovation.
- Goal 10: Reduce inequality within and among countries.

- Goal 11: Make cities and human settlements inclusive, safe, resilient, and sustainable.
- Goal 12: Ensure sustainable consumption and production patterns.
- Goal 13: Take urgent action to combat climate change and its impacts.
- Goal 14: Conserve and sustainable use of oceans, seas, and marine resources for sustainable development.
- Goal 15: Protect, restore, and promote sustainable use of terrestrial ecosystems; sustainably manage forests; and halt and reverse land degradation, and halt biodiversity loss.
- Goal 16: Promote peaceful and inclusive societies for sustainable development; provide access to justice for all; and build effective, accountable, and inclusive institutions at all levels.
- Goal 17: Promote the means of implementation and revitalize the global partnership for sustainable development.

What Is Globalization?

Globalization is defined as a fundamental and relatively accelerated change to human societies and social–cultural–political and geographical environments around our world due to a variety of processes by which individuals, groups, and entire nations or regions are becoming increasingly more connected and interdependent via commerce and trade, information technology, knowledge and communication exchanges, migration and cultural diffusion, and healthcare issues (Bartfay and Bartfay 2015). Globalization presents public healthcare professionals and workers with the challenge and ethical responsibility of being competent healthcare providers for a "global village of citizens." Providing primary healthcare services in an increasingly dynamic, fluid, and diverse global society requires public healthcare professionals and workers to address complex and diverse healthcare challenges across the lifespan. Globalizing has a direct effect on the broad SDH such as the availability of housing, clean water supplies and sanitation, employment, education and access to healthcare facilities and professionals, and the availability of safe food supplies (Lee, Yach, and Kamradt-Scott 2012; Seear 2007; Taylor 2009; Woodward et al. 2001).

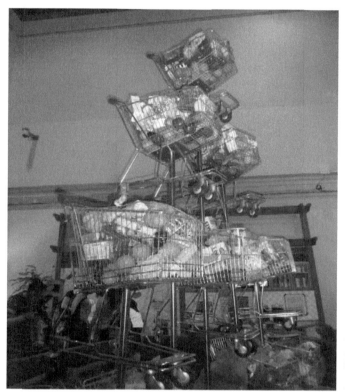

Source: Wally J. Bartfay

Photo 9.7 Access to safe and affordable food supplies is a basic social determinant of health. It is estimated that 51% or $27 billion of food purchased by Canadians is wasted and throw out into the trash every year (McGuinn 2012; Neibergall 2012). This is especially alarming given that an estimated 1.02 billion people are malnourished globally.

The United Nations Food and Agricultural Organization (2011) estimates that approximately one-third of all food produced is wasted or lost, which accounts for approximately 1.3 billion tons of food wasted per year.

For example, in July 2008, China was struck with a tainted baby infant milk formula scandal (Ramzy and Yang 2008). This scandal resulted in the death of six children due to kidney failure, an estimated 54,000 infants had to be hospitalized, and more than 300,000 became seriously ill (Branigan 2008; Scott 2008; Zhu 2009). This national scandal is known as the "big-headed babies" scandal in China because malnourished infants developed swollen heads, touched-off domestic demands for greater scrutiny of Chinese food products and exports internationally. According to Chinese authorities, infant milk powder produced by the Chinese Shijiazhuang-based dairy giant Sanlu Group was contaminated with melamine. Melamine a chemical employed in the plastics manufacturing sector to manufacture melamine–formaldehyde resin, a type of plastic known for its flame-retardant properties and is commonly employed in the manufacturing of dry erase boards and kitchen countertops. Melamine is rich in nitrogen and has been apparently added to a variety of food products in China to increase their protein content, including a widely publicized case in 2007 which resulted in the poisoning of thousands of dogs and cats in the United States (Ramzy and Yang 2008). Melamine adulteration of food supplies and products may result in renal failure and/or urinary problems in both humans and animals when it reacts with cyanuric acid inside the body.

A number of criminal prosecutions occurred, including the execution of two men (Geng Jinping and Zhang Yujun) by the authority of the Chinese Supreme People's Court for their roles in the tainted milk scandal, another given a suspended death penalty, three others receiving sentences of life imprisonment, two receiving 15-year jail terms, and seven local government officials as well as the Director of Administration of Quality Supervision, Inspection, and Quarantine being fired or forced to resign (Zhu 2009). This issue has raised international concerns about food safety and political corruption in China, and has damaged the reputation of China's food exports with at least 11 countries banning all imports of dairy products from China (Chen 2008; Wong 2008).

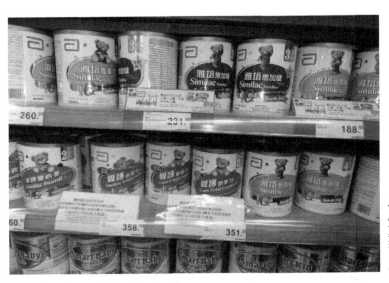

Photo 9.8 Hong Kong has placed caps on the amount of baby formula that can be exported to mainland China due to fears by mainland residents flocking to Hong Kong to buy "safe" baby formula for their infants.

In recent years, under globalization, market integration has increased. This is manifested in new production arrangements, including significant changes in labour, employment, and working conditions, expanding areas of international and global economic agreements, and accelerating commercialization of goods and services—some of them undoubtedly beneficial for health, some of them disastrous.

—(Commission on the Social Determinants of Health 2008, 14).

These interdependent trends and processes are resulting in far-reaching ripple effects both within and between countries and entire regions on this planet. Although globalization has resulted in positive ripple effects in terms of trade and commerce and communication of scientific findings; for example, it has also resulted in negative ripple effects in terms of the spread of communicable diseases (e.g., HIV/AIDS, SARS, H1N1), increased poverty and malnutrition, and a decrease in housing and living conditions for many individuals in both developed and developing nations (Skolnik 2008; Walraven 2010).

The WHO Commission on the Social Determinants of Health (2008) views certain goods and services as basic human rights and societal needs including access to clean and safe water supplies and access to healthcare services, regardless of the ability of individuals to pay for these. In such instances, it is the public sector rather than the marketplace that should determine and underwrite adequate supply and access by all individuals with respect to health. It should also be the public sectors responsibility to ensure decent and safe working conditions (e.g., legislative labour standards) and to monitor and/or control the circulation of health damaging commodities (e.g., tobacco products, alcohol). Moreover, global governance

Research Focus Box 9.1

Age-Specific and Sex-Specific Mortality in 187 Countries, 1970–2010: A Systematic Analysis for the Global Burden of Disease Study 2010.

Study Aim/Rationale

The aim of the study was to estimate global life tables and annual death rates for 187 countries for the years 1970–2010 inclusive. The researchers estimated mortality trends in children under the age of 5 years and the probability of mortality in adults aged 15–59 years for each country based on the available data.

Methodology/Design

Death registration data were available for more than 100 countries and the researchers corrected for under-count with improved death distribution methods. The investigators applied refined methods to survey data on sibling survival that corrected for survivor, zero-sibling, and recall bias, and separated estimated mortality from natural disasters (e.g., hurricanes, flooding, earthquakes) and wars. Final estimates of mortality for children under 5 years of age and for adults (15–59 years) were generated via Gaussian regression analysis. The researchers used these results as input parameters in a relational model life table system, and all mortality rates and numbers were estimated with 95% uncertainty intervals.

Major Findings

From 1970 to 2010, the global life expectancy for males at birth increased from 56.4 years to 67.5 years. Similarly, the global female life expectancy at birth increased from 61.2 to 73.3 years. Life expectancy rose approximately 3–4 years every decade from 1970 onwards, with except for the 1990s. Substantial reductions in mortality occurred in eastern and southern sub-Saharan Africa since 2004, which is attributed to increased coverage of antiretroviral therapy and preventative measures against malaria. Globally, 52.8 million deaths occurred in 2010, which is approximately 13.5% more in comparison to 1990 figures (46.5 million), and 21.9% more than death rates in 1970 (43.3 million). Proportionally more deaths occurred at age 70 or older, in comparison to 1990 figures (42.8% versus 33.1%). Deaths in children under the age of 5 years declined by approximately 60% since 1970 figures (6.71 million versus 16.7 million).

Implications for Public Health

Examining global mortality trends is critical for identifying needs, public health programs, and for the allocation of public health resources and personnel to address various health challenges in both developed and developing regions of the world. These findings suggest that public health efforts should be targeted towards low- and middle-income countries to further reduce mortality. Moreover, the researchers caution that there is a potential to underestimate achievement in reference to the Millennium Development Goal 4 due to limitations of available demographic data on child mortality for the most recent decades. Improvements of civil registration system worldwide are crucial for better tracking of global mortality rates and trends.

Source: Wang et al. (2012).

mechanisms such as the WHO (2014c) *Framework Convention on Tobacco Control* (see link http://www.who.int/fctc/en/) are required with increasing urgency as international markets merge and accelerate the circulation and access to health damaging commodities such as tobacco and certain processed foods high in sodium, fat, and sugar.

The current global economic recession, which surfaced in 2008, has resulted in negative ripple effects in terms of the availability of healthcare finances and government-funded research initiatives in various countries and regions of this world (e.g., Africa, Australia, European Union, North America). For example, Strully (2009) reports that unemployment in the United States was associated with a 54% chance of reporting fair or poor health; and for individuals with no pre-existing health conditions, the chances of reporting a new state of ill increased by 83%.

Bartfay et al. (2013) employed a phenomenological investigation to examine the effects of the recent global economic recession on the health of unemployed blue-collar autoworkers in the Durham Region of Ontario, Canada. Subjects reported high levels of stress, anxiety, and depression; increased physical pain and discomfort; changes in weight and sexual function; and financial hardships including the inability to pay for required prescription drugs and loss of housing.

Stuckler et al. (2011) examined the negative health effects associated with the recent global recession in 2008–2009 in 26 countries in the European Union. The researchers found that every 1% increase in unemployment was associated with a 0.79% rise in the rates of suicide and homicide. Moreover, it is now estimated that 55–90 million people are living in extreme poverty conditions, as a consequence of the 2008 global financial crisis and this includes high-income countries of the G8 attempting to reduce public expenditures (UNDP 2009). *Extreme poverty* is defined as individuals who live on less than $1.75 Canadian per day (or approximately $2.00 U.S.) and includes the costs of food, water, shelter, medicines, and other necessities of life (Deviney 2013). Deviney (2013) reports that currently approximately 1.4 billion individuals are living in extreme poverty globally. Food prices have also been increasing globally resulting in increased states of hunger. An estimated 1.02 billion

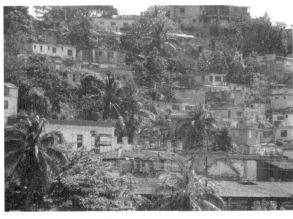

Source: Wally J. Bartfay

Photo 9.9 The slums of Casa Blanca, Cuba. Extreme poverty remains a major public health concern globally. The average minimum wage for a worker in Cuba in 2016 was approximately 11 cents per hour or a monthly income of $20.00 (US).

people who are malnourished, including an estimated 642 million in Asia, 265 million in sub-Saharan Africa, and 15 million undernourished people, are now living in high-income countries which represent an alarming increase of 50% in comparison to 2003 levels (Food and Agriculture Organization [FAO] 2009).

The year 2015 marked the 30th anniversary of the so-called Big Mac Index, which was first published by Pam Woodall in the September edition of *The Economists* as an informal and light-hearted guide for assessing the "Purchasing Power Parity" between two different currencies, and provides a guide to test the extent to which market exchange rates result in goods costing the same in different countries (Jacobsen 2008; Tough and Preece 2015). The name for this index is derived from the "Big-Mac," a hamburger sold at McDonald's restaurants in approximately 120 countries around the world. For example, if a Big Mac burger costs $4.00 in one country and $8.50 in another, it is likely that the cost of living is much higher in the $8.50-per-burger country. In addition, workers in the higher priced country will have to earn a much higher salary to stay above the poverty line, in comparison to the $4.00-per-burger country. It may be argued that the Big Mac Index may provide a more representative and realistic view of the actual purchasing power of the average individual in various countries, since it takes into account factors such as local wages. For example, the average price of a Big Mac in the United States in July 2015 was $4.79, while in China it was only $2.74 at market exchange rates. Hence, this "raw" Big Mac Index suggests that the yuan was undervalued by approximately 43% during this time period (The Statistical Portal 2015).

The *Gini Index (or coefficient)* is a measure of the inequality in the distribution of incomes within a given country (Armartya 1977; Guillermina 1979; Jacobsen 2008). A country with a Gini Index of zero (0 or perfect equality) means that everyone in that country has the same income, whereas an index of 100 would indicate perfect inequality. For example, Namibia has a Gini Index score of 70.7 and a very unequal distribution in terms of income earned by its residents. Hence, the richest 10% of the population makes 128.8 times more than the poorest 10% of wage earners in Namibia. By comparison, Denmark has a Gini Index of 24.7 and a very equal distribution of income where the wealthiest 10% of the population make only 8.1 times more than the poorest 10% of wage earners.

In India, as much as 40% of all fruits, vegetables, and food grains produced never make it to market due to a variety of issues such as inefficient harvesting, inadequate local transportation networks, and poor infrastructures. In Niagara, apples are often shipped 100 km away to a distribution centre, and then sent back to Niagara to be sold in markets. Moreover, it is estimated that 7 million tonnes of food, worth an estimated $16 billion (U.S.), are discarded each year globally by consumers before the "best before" date is reached, which costs the average household an estimated $763 per year (Westhead 2013). Buying discounted items in bulk in North America and "two-for-the-price-of-one" offers also encourages individuals to buy in excess of what they can often consume. Given that the current world population of approximately 7 billion individuals is expected to grow to 9.5 billion by 2075, we

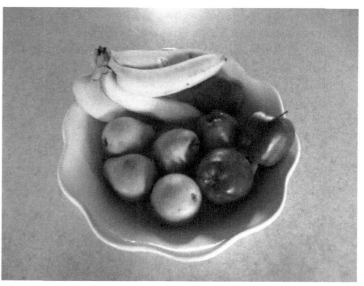

Source: Wally J. Bartfay

Photo 9.10 Westhead (2013) reports that in Canada and other developed nations in the world, approximately one-third of vegetable crops and fruits are rejected and discarded simply because they do not look appealing enough for large supermarket grocery chains.

must address these issues related to food supplies, how they are harvested and distributed, and the prevention of edible foods going to waste (Bartfay and Bartfay 2015).

There is also an increase in the reported incidence of type 2 diabetes in children and adolescents in countries as diverse as Canada, the United States, England, France, Germany, Japan, Hong Kong, Singapore, Bangladesh, and Libya (Lee, Yach, and Kamradt-Scott 2012; Wild et al. 2004). It is notable that until recently, most children and adolescence diagnosed with diabetes had the type 1 disease (insulin dependent). The rise in the incidence of type 2 diabetes has been linked to the effects of globalization which includes the adaption of increasingly sedentary lifestyles and obesity attributed to diets and processed food products high in fat, sugar, salt, and calories (Bartfay and Bartfay 2015; O'Dea and Piers 2002; Thomas and Bartfay 2010).

Table 9.2 provides the reader with a comparison of the top 10 leading causes of mortality globally for low- versus high-income countries (WHO 2011). It is notable that the top 10 leading causes of death for low-income countries are lower respiratory infections, diarrheal diseases, HIV/AIDS, ischaemic heart disease, malaria, stroke and other cerebrovascular disease, TB, prematurity and low birth weight, birth asphyxia and birth trauma, and neonatal infections.

Table 9.2 The Top 10 Leading Causes of Death Globally in Low-Income Countries in 2008

Reported causes of death	Death in millions	Percentage (%) of deaths
(i) Lower respiratory infections	1.05	11.3
(ii) Diarrheal diseases	0.76	8.2
(iii) HIV/AIDS	0.72	7.8
(iv) Ischaemic heart disease	0.57	6.1
(v) Malaria	0.48	5.2

Reported causes of death	Death in millions	Percentage (%) of deaths
(vi) Stroke and other cerebrovascular disease	0.45	4.9
(vii) Tuberculosis	0.40	4.3
(viii) Prematurity and low birth weight	0.30	3.2
(ix) Birth asphyxia and birth trauma	0.27	2.9
(x) Neonatal infections	0.24	2.6

Source: Adapted from the World Health Organization (2011). http://www.who.int/mediacentre/factsheets/fs310/en/index.html.

The next two decades will see major changes in the healthcare needs of all the world's regions. For example, by the year 2020 non-communicable diseases are expected to account for 7 out of every 10 deaths in the developing nations of the world, compared with less than half in the latter part of the twentieth century. These changes are expected because of the rapid aging of the populations in developing countries worldwide (Thomas and Bartfay 2010). Figure 9.2 provides a comparison of the 10 leading causes of burden of disease for the year 2004 with those predicted for the year 2030. We observe a dramatic increase in unipolar depressive disorders and chronic non-communicable diseases such as ischaemic heart disease, cerebrovascular disease, Chronic obstructive pulmonary disease (COPD), and diabetes mellitus.

Table 9.3 shows the top 10 reported leading causes of death globally for high-income countries. By contrast, the leading causes of death in high-income developed countries globally are ischaemic heart disease; stroke and other cerebrovascular disease; trachea, bronchitis, lung cancers; Alzheimer and other dementias; lower respiratory infections; chronic obstructive pulmonary disease; colon and rectum cancers; diabetes mellitus; hypertensive heart disease; and breast cancer.

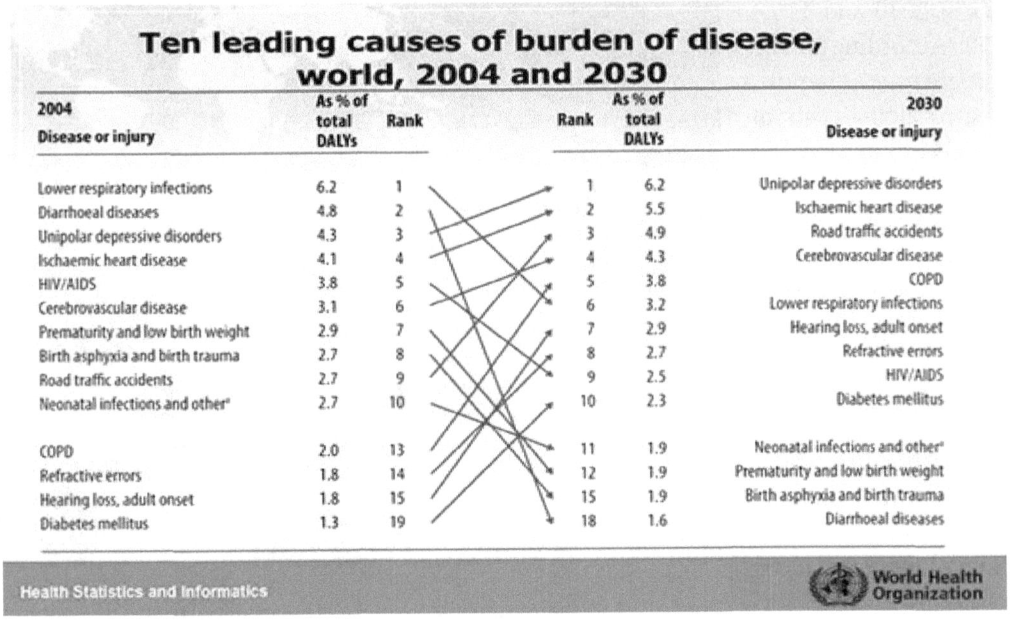

Figure 9.2 Ten leading causes of burden of disease, world, 2004 and 2030.

Reprinted from *The Global Burden of Disease, 2004 Update*. Part 4 Burden of disease: DALYs, figure 27, pg. 51, 2004.

Table 9.3 The Top 10 Leading Causes of Death Globally in High-Income Countries in 2008

Reported causes of death	Death in millions	Percentage (%) of deaths
(i) Ischaemic heart disease	1.42	15.6
(ii) Stroke and other cerebrovascular disease	0.79	8.7
(iii) Trachea, bronchus, lung cancers	0.37	4.1
(iv) Alzheimer and other dementias	0.57	6.1
(v) Lower respiratory infections	0.35	3.8
(vi) Chronic obstructive pulmonary disease	0.32	3.5
(vii) Colon and rectum cancers	0.30	3.3
(viii) Diabetes mellitus	0.24	2.6
(ix) Hypertensive heart disease	0.21	2.3
(x) Breast cancer	0.17	1.9

Source: Adapted from the World Health Organization (2011). Available at http://www.who.int/mediacentre/factsheets/fs310/en/index.html.

Prince et al. (2013) report that the global prevalence of dementia worldwide was 35.6 million in 2010, with numbers expected to almost double every 20 years to 65.7 million in 2030 and 115.4 million in 2050. According to the 2010 World Alzheimer's Report, the total estimated global costs of dementia was $604 billion (U.S.) in 2010 alone, and it is estimated that the associated costs will increase 85% by 2030 based on predicted increases in the number of people with dementia globally (Wimo and Prince 2010).

If we examine this trend from the Canadian perspective, we currently know that the life expectancy in Canada is more than 80 years, and the number of senior aged 65 years or older is expected to reach 6.7 million in 2020 and 9.2 million in 2041 (CIHI 2015; PHAC 2008). In 2015, life expectancy for a male and a female born

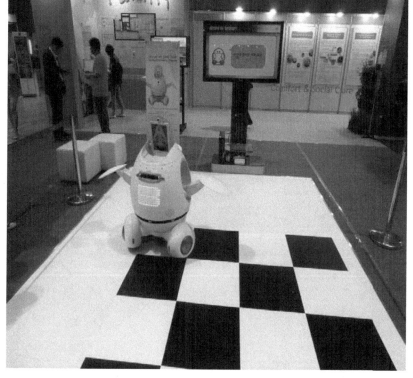

Source: Wally J. Bartfay

Photo 9.11 The robot called "Silbot" (meaning a "friend of senior citizens") is a cognitive rehabilitation robot developed in Seoul, Korea for clients with dementia and Alzheimer's disease to carry out daily cognitive brain-training games and exercises.

in 2012 was 80 and 84, respectively (Canadian Broadcasting Corporation [CBC] 2015). By comparison, the top three countries for life expectancies for males born in 2012 were Iceland at 81.2 years, Switzerland at 80.7 years, and Australia at 80.5 years. For females born in 2012, the top three countries were Japan at 87.0 years, Spain at 85.1 years, and Switzerland at 85.1 years (CBC 2015). In Canada, individuals aged 65 years or older account for approximately 15% of the total population, but consume more than 45% of all public sector healthcare costs (CIHI 2015). In 2015, healthcare costs rose to $219.1 billion (10.9% of GDP), or an average cost of $6105 per person. However, that cost of health care rose to $8383 for a person aged 70–74 years; $11,557 for a person aged 75–79 years, and $20,917 for a person aged 80 years or older (CIHI 2015).

Given that age is a primary and unchangeable risk factor associated with the development of various chronic non-communicable diseases (e.g., heart disease, stroke, Alzheimer's disease), the incidence of these diseases is predicted to increase as our population continues to age in the next few decades. For example, Alzheimer Society of Canada (2010) reports that in 2008 alone, 103,700 new dementia cases per year (or one new case every 5 minutes) were diagnosed, and this number is projected to increase to 257,800 new diagnosed cases in 2038 (or one new case every 2 minutes) with an associated cumulative economic burden of $872 billion and the total informal caregiver opportunity costs are projected to exceed $301 billion annually.

Table 9.4 shows the top 10 leading causes of mortality globally for all combined income level countries (WHO 2011). The top 10 leading causes of mortality globally are ischaemic heart disease; stroke and other cerebrovascular disease; lower respiratory infections; chronic obstructive pulmonary disease; diarrheal diseases; HIV/AIDS; trachea, bronchus, lung cancers; tuberculosis; diabetes mellitus; and road traffic accidents.

Table 9.4 The Top 10 Leading Causes Globally in 2008 for All Combined Income Level Countries

Reported causes of death	Death in millions	Percentage (%) of deaths
(i) Ischaemic heart disease	7.25	12.8
(ii) Stroke and other cerebrovascular disease	6.15	10.8
(iii) Lower respiratory infections	3.46	6.1
(iv) Chronic obstructive pulmonary disease	3.28	5.8
(v) Diarrheal disease	2.46	4.3
(vi) HIV/AIDS	1.78	3.1
(vii) Trachea, bronchus, lung cancers	1.39	2.4
(viii) Tuberculosis	1.34	2.4
(ix) Diabetes mellitus	1.26	2.2
(x) Road traffic accidents	1.21	2.1

Source: Adapted from the World Health Organization (2011). http://www.who.int/mediacentre/factsheets/fs310/en/index.html.

Common Global Burden of Disease Measures

Traditionally, life expectancy and mortality measures have been employed as indicators of population health. The reader is referred to Chapter 6 for a detailed discussion of life expectancy and the various types of mortality measures commonly employed by epidemiologist and public healthcare professionals. In the year 2009, the global life expectancy was 68 years (WHO 2012a). For comparison purposes, the average life expectancy was 83 in Australia, Japan, Norway, and the Netherlands, 82 in Singapore, Switzerland, and the United Kingdom, 81 in France and the United States, 79 years in Canada, 74 in the Czech Republic, Thailand, and Viet Nam, 72 in China, 70 in Brazil, 60 in Kenya, 53 in Congo, 50 in Swaziland, Zimbabwe, and Zambia, and 47 in Afghanistan, Chad, and Malawi (WHO 2011). The life expectancy for both males and females born in 2012 is still less than 55 years in nine sub-Saharan African countries: Angola, Central African Republic, Chad, Ivory Coast, Democratic Republic of Congo, Lesotho, Mozambique, Nigeria, and Sierra Leanne (CBC 2015).

The WHO (2012a) reports that globally approximately 57 million individuals die each year; almost 15% of these deaths occur in children under the age of 5 years, and 74% of these child-related deaths occur in Africa and South-East Asia. During the past two decades, increased international effort has been put into the development of global summary measures of population health that integrate information related to mortality and non-fatal outcomes and indicators such as morbidity measures and health-related quality of life (Mathers 2006; Thomas and Bartfay 2010). The reader is referred to Chapter 6 for a more detailed discussion of mortality and morbidity measures.

The *global burden of disease (GBD)* is defined as measures to quantitatively express, examine, and compare the societal impact of a particular disease, condition, and/or altered state of health and includes measures of societal burden caused by death and morbidity including injuries and disabilities in different regions or countries around the world (Bartfay and Bartfay 2015). Use of indicators that integrate the societal burden caused by both mortality and morbidity allows for the comparison of the burden due to various risk factors, SDH or diseases (Porta 2008). Sophisticated methodologies enable the combined measurement of mortality and non-fatal health outcomes, and provide comparable and comprehensive measures of population health across countries and different regions of the world. They are also critical for the investigation of healthcare costs, efficacy, effectiveness, and other health outcome measures (Porta 2008). In this section, we shall examine four of the most commonly employed and reported composite measures of population health for determining and assessing the GBD impact: (a) The *disability-adjusted life years* (DALYs), (b) the *healthy life years* (HeaLY) lost measure, (c) the *health-adjusted life expectancy* (HALE) measure, and (d) the *quality-adjusted life year* (QALY) (Hyder, Puvanachandra, and Morrow 2012; Jamison et al. 2006; Lopez et al. 2006).

The term GBD was first coined by Murray and Lopez (1996) in their landmark publication *The Global Burden of Disease and Injury Series*. This work was the result of a major collaborative 5-year study that involved the WHO, World Bank, and the Harvard School of Public Health. This work provided projections of disease and injury to 2020, and the researchers not only quantified the number of deaths, but also the effects of premature death and disability on populations due to certain risk factors such as tobacco use, consumption of alcohol, unsafe sex practices, and sanitation. The researchers then combined these various measures into a single measure referred to as the GBD. The use of GBD measures has been expanding worldwide and several countries have completed or are in the process of undertaking national burden of disease assessments. The WHO publishes GBD results and promotes its development and application as a global measure of health. According to Murray and Lopez (1996), the GBD has three major aims:

i. To include both mortality and non-fatal conditions for assessing health status. In certain countries of the world, statistics on the health status of their population are limited and age- and death-specific mortality rates are difficult to obtain and may be based on estimates only. Even in developed nations such as Canada, the United States, and the United Kingdom, where these statistics are more readily available often fail to identify the impact of non-fatal outcomes of disease or injuries (e.g., dementia, blindness, immobility) on population health.

ii. To produce objective, independent, and demographically plausible assessments of the burdens of particular conditions and diseases (p. 6).

iii. To measure disease and injury burden that permit objective comparisons for the relative cost-effectiveness of different healthcare interventions in terms of cost per unit of disease burden averted. For example, the cost of long-term care for mental health issues such as schizophrenia versus ischaemic heart disease. Policy-makers can utilize this data to help make rational decisions related to healthcare priorities and for the allocation of scare resources, which requires this information.

According to Murray and Lopez (1996), one death in three in 1990 was present in the Group I series of GBDs, which include communicable, maternal, perinatal, and nutritional conditions, and the majority of these deaths were in developing regions of the world. Over half of the deaths were from Group II causes (noncommunicable diseases) and approximately 1 death in 10 was from Group III causes (injuries). Table 9.5 shows the GBD and injury series categories as first described by Murray and Lopez (1996). Over the past few decades, we have observed a shift in the GBDs from communicable (infectious) diseases (e.g., TB, smallpox) to non-communicable (noninfectious) diseases (e.g., diabetes, heart disease, depression). A study commissioned by the World Economic Forum estimates that mental illness, heart disease, cancer, diabetes, and respiratory illnesses would cost the global economy more than $47 trillion (U.S.) due to lost productivity due to illness and disease over the next 20 years (Bloom et al. 2011). The reader is referred to Chapter 7 for a detailed discussion of acute, chronic, communicable, and non-communicable diseases.

Table 9.5 Global Burden of Disease and Injury Series Categories

Group I	Group II	Group III
Communicable diseases Maternal conditions Perinatal conditions Nutritional conditions	Noncommunicable diseases	Injuries

Source: Adapted from Murray and Lopez (1996).

Disability-Adjusted Life Year

The **DALY** is defined as a standardized international measure that expresses the number of years lost due to premature death and years lived with a disability of specified duration and severity (Bartfay and Bartfay 2015). Hence, one DALY refers to the loss of 1 year of healthy life. Burden of disease calculations in DALY's may help to determine priorities among disease and disorders for policy-making, available interventions, and research (Melse et al. 2000). The DALY was first introduced as an estimate of the GBD in the 1993 *World Development Report* (World Bank 1993). DALY is the best-known health gap measure and quantifies the gap between a population's actual health and a normative health goal which is based on a global standard life table which specifies the healthy years of life lost (YLL) due to mortality at any given age (Hyder, Puvanachandra, and Morrow 2012; Jamison et al. 2006; Mathers 2006). DALYs are calculated as two separate components for the measurement of life lost due to disease: (a) YLL, which refers to the loss of healthy life due to mortality, and (b) the total number of years of life lived with a disability (YLD), which refers to the loss of healthy life from disability. Hence,

$$DALY = YLL + YLD$$

Three social value choices may also be included in the calculation of DALYs including life expectation values, discount rates for future life, and weighing for life lived at different ages (Hyder, Puvanachandra, and Morrow 2012; Jamison et al. 2006; Lopez et al. 2006). DALYs are calculated using a *disability weight* (a proportion less than 1) multiplied by the chronological age to reflect the burden of the disability. Hence, DALYs' measures can produce estimates that accord greater value to fit for disabled persons and to the middle years of life rather than to youth or to seniors (Porta 2008).

Table 9.6 shows the estimated cost to prevent one DALY from being lost, and the large number of DALYS averted indicates a highly cost-effective intervention for reducing mortality in children under 5 years of age in developing countries (Jamison et al. 2006).

Table 9.6 The Estimated Cost per DALY ($U.S.) to Reduce Mortality in Children Under the Age of 5 Years in Developing Countries

Public health intervention or service	Cost per DALY ($U.S.)	Estimated number of DALYs averted per $1,000,000 spent
Improving the care of children under 28 days old (including resuscitation of newborns when required)	10–400	2500–100,000
Expanding immunization coverage with standard child vaccines	2–20	50,000–500,000
Adding Hib and Hepatitis B vaccines to the standard child immunization program	40–250	4000–24,000
Switching to the use of combination drugs for malaria where there is a noted drug resistance in sub-Saharan Africa	8–20	50,000–125,000

Source: Adapted from Jamison et al. (2006).

Chronic conditions (e.g., mental health disorders) that limit the individual's productivity for long periods and childhood diseases associated with mortality are given additional weight in DALY estimates (Jacobsen 2008; WHO 2006a). For example, while neuropsychiatric conditions are estimated to account for approximately 2.0% of deaths annually, they are estimated to contribute 13.5% of the DALY measure. When self-inflicted injuries are also considered in reference to neuropsychiatric conditions, the adjusted estimates are 3.6% and 14.9% for deaths and DALY estimates, respectively.

According to Jacobsen (2008), it will never be possible to assign an accurate rank order to the decrease in the quality of life caused by blindness, loss of a limb, depression, a brain tumour, or asthma, because the experience of illness and disability varies based on the individual, the level of community support, living conditions, and other factors. Nonetheless, the DALY remains the best tool to date for estimating the GBD and disability. Furthermore, the DALY helps to underscore the global burden resulting from mental health conditions and disorders, which were not even considered a few decades ago. Indeed, an estimated 450 million people worldwide have a psychiatric disorder, which includes 121 million with depression, 70 million with alcohol dependence, 37 million with dementia, and 24 million with schizophrenia (The WHO World Mental Health Survey Consortium 2004; WHO 2004b). Moreover, the WHO (2004b) reports that 5 of the 10 leading causes of disability worldwide in individuals aged 15–44 years are psychiatric conditions including unipolar depression, alcohol abuse, self-inflicted injuries, schizophrenia, and bipolar disorder (formally known as manic depression) (World Health Organization (WHO) World Mental Health Survey Consortium 2004). Mental and behavioural disorders account for approximately 12% of the GBD and contribute to as many days of lost work as physical ailments and disease. Similarly, the *Global Burden of Disease Study* conducted by the WHO, World Bank, and the Harvard School of Public Health found that psychiatric (e.g., depression, bipolar disorder, schizophrenia) and neurological conditions (e.g., dementia, Parkinson's disease, multiple sclerosis) accounted for 38.2% of the DALYs globally (WHO 2006b).

Healthy Life Years (HeaLY) Lost Measure

The *HeaLY* is defined as a composite measure that combines the total amount of health life lost due to morbidity with that lost to disease, and therefore provides an estimate of the loss of life expected had the disease or condition not occurred (Bartfay and Bartfay 2015). In other words, the HeaLY measure is based on the total number of years of life that would have been lived had the disease or condition not occurred, and is often employed as tool for the planning of health services and priorities in different countries and regions (Hyder, Puvanachandra, and Morrow 2012; Last 2000; Morrow and Bryant 1995; Murray and Lopez 1994).

The specific information needed to calculate HeaLY includes the incidence rate and case fatality ratio for the age of disease onset, the age of death, and the expectation of life at these ages. Hence, HeaLY incorporates three components for determining disability: (a) case disability (compared to the case fatality ratio), (b) extent of disability, and (c) the duration of the specific disability measured. The HeaLYs lost from death and from the noted disability are added up and expressed as the total YLL per 1,000 populations per year. The duration of the disability may be temporary or permanent (lifelong) in nature. For example, a cohort that comprised 1,000 newborns with a life expectation of 75.0 years has the potential of 75,000 years of healthy life. Each year this cohort would experience events which result in the 1,000 years of healthy life lost attributable to mortality, with a distribution of age at death equivalent to that which lead to the life expectancy of 75.0 years. Any disease or condition that leads to mortality or disability earlier than that set for this *age-at-death* distribution would increase the amount of HeaLY beyond this minimum.

The onset of a disease condition typically involves the date from the onset of overt clinical signs and symptoms as determined by an individual and/or diagnosed by a laboratory or healthcare professional. The reader is referred to Chapter 7 for a more detailed discussion of disease nomenclature, classifications, and clinical signs and symptoms. Each disease or condition will have a typical distribution of ages at which onset or death may occur, but for most the average is employed as a proxy measure for a defined population. In the case of recurrent diseases or conditions with multiple episodes (e.g., diarrhea), the age of onset denotes the average age for the first episode experienced. Malaria present in a country in Africa, for example, may be considered for each individual as a single, lifelong disease with chronic, usually asymptomatic, parasitemia but with intermittent severe clinical attacks (which result in high mortality in late infancy and early childhood while immunity is being acquired), followed by recurring, non-fatal clinical episodes after age 10 (Hyder, Puvanachandra, and Morrow 2012).

Moreover, taking into consideration the natural history of a disease or condition, or how one may response to different primary health interventions based on different age cohorts, the disease or condition is often classified by age cohorts (e.g., child versus adult pneumonia, neonatal versus adult tetanus). Public health interventions may be directed at reducing identifiable risk factors, such as tobacco smoking and the development of health disease; or engaging in unprotected sex, and the development of sexually transmitted infections such as HIV/AIDS. For example, every $1.00 spent on tobacco prevention campaigns results in a health care saving of $20.00, or a return on investment (ROI) of 1900%.

Health-Adjusted Life Expectancy Measure

The *HALE* is defined as a composite measure of a population health status that belongs to a defined family of health expectancies, and summarizes the expected number of year's equivalent to a state of so-called full-health and well-being (Bartfay and Bartfay 2015). This can also be envisioned as the number of years of full-health and well-being a newborn can expect to live, based on current rates of ill-health and mortality. The HALE estimate is considered to be the best available summary estimate for measuring the overall level of health for populations and is employed by the WHO for their annual global health reports (Mathers et al. 2001; Skolnik 2012; WHO 2000). To calculate HALE, the years of ill-health are weighed in accordance with its severity and then subtracted from the overall life expectancy at birth. The HALE is calculated using the prevalence of disability at each age, and then divides the years of life expected at each age (according to a life table cohort) into years with and without disability. Mortality is captured by using a life table method, while the disability component is expressed by additions of prevalence of various disabilities within the life table (Hyder, Puvanachandra, and Morrow 2012).

When compared with the total life expectancy at birth, HALE translates into an estimate of the total disability burden in a defined population. It is important to note that HALE does not relate to specific diseases, but is a measure of the average extent of disability among the proportion for each age cohort that is disabled. Hence, the lack of correlation between a specific condition or disease and the HALE estimate makes it less valuable in terms of resource allocation and for cost-effectiveness calculations (Hyder, Puvanachandra, and Morrow 2012). Table 9.7 shows the life expectancy and the HALE for males and females for selected low-, middle-, and high-income countries (WHO 2004a).

Table 9.7 Life Expectancy and HALE for Males and Females in Select Low-, Middle-, and High-Income Countries

Select countries	Life expectancy at birth (males)	HALE (males)	Life expectancy at birth (females)	HALE (females)
Afghanistan	42	35.3	42	25.8
Bangladesh	62	55.3	63	53.3
Bolivia	63	53.6	66	55.2
Brazil	67	57.2	74	62.4
Cambodia	51	45.6	58	49.5
Cameroon	50	41.1	51	41.8
China	70	63.1	74	65.2
Costa Rica	75	65.2	80	69.3
Cuba	75	67/1	80	69.5
Denmark	75	68.6	80	71.1
Ethiopia	49	40.7	51	41.7
Ghana	56	49.2	58	50.3
India	61	53.3	63	53.6
Indonesia	65	57.4	68	58.9
Jordan	69	59.7	73	62.3
Malaysia	69	61.6	74	64.8
Nepal	61	52.5	61	51.1
Niger	42	35.8	41	35.2
Nigeria	45	41.3	46	41.8

Select countries	Life expectancy at birth (males)	HALE (males)	Life expectancy at birth (females)	HALE (females)
Peru	69	59.6	73	62.4
Philippines	65	57.1	72	61.5
Sri Lanka	68	59.2	75	64.0
Turkey	69	61.2	73	62.8
The United States	75	67.2	80	71.3
Vietnam	69	59.8	74	62.9

Source: Adapted from the World Health Organization (2004c).

Quality-Adjusted Life Year

The QALY was first introduced in 1976 as a guiding measure for selecting among alternative tertiary healthcare interventions in defined populations (Zeckhauser and Shepard 1976). There is a popular contention that low quality of health is primarily a reflection of inadequate financial resources (Skolnik 2012). However, there is a growing body of evidence to show that quality can be enhanced in a variety of ways even in the absence of additional financial resources.

This generic measure sums time spent in different health states using weights on a scale which ranges from 0.00 (dead) to 1.00 (perfectly healthy) (see Figure 9.3) for each health state, and is regarded as an arithmetic product of duration of life and a global measure of quality of life also (health state weight) (Hyder, Puvanachandra, and Morrow 2012; Kaplan 1990; Morrow and Bryant 1995). For examples, 5 years of so-called perfect health = 5 QALYs, whereas 2 years in a state measured as 0.5 of perfect health followed by 5 years of perfect health = 4 QALYs. Since its conception, a variety of QALY measures and survey instruments have been developed and tested over the years such as the *European Quality of Life with Five Domains and Five Domains* (EQ-5D, see www. eruoqol.org), which has three defined levels for each of the five domains. The QALY estimate, which typically comprises a large family of measures, has been employed as a common denominator to measure utility in cost-utility analysis and for cost-effectiveness analysis to assist healthcare policy-makers and health-care public professionals with healthcare resource allocation among alternative health interventions by ranking the interventions in terms of costs per QALY (Hyder, Puvanachandra, and Morrow 2012; Kaplan 1990; Morrow and Bryant 1995).

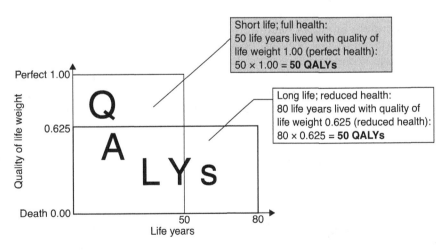

Figure 9.3 Understanding quality-adjusted life years (QALYs) estimates.

The **QALY** is defined as a measure that provides an estimate for the adjustment of life expectancy that reduces the overall life expectancy of populations by numerical amounts that reflect the existence of chronic conditions that result in impairments, disability and/or handicaps based on a specified chronological age which is multiplied by a so-called utility-weight for each health state or condition.

Source: http://holisticpracticedevelopment.com/wp-content/uploads/2011/01/QALYs2.jpg.

Research Focus Box 9.2

Measuring Global Health Inequality

Study Aim/Rationale

The researchers argue that the notion of equity is a major cornerstone for achieving and assessing global health initiatives. Health inequality refers to the uneven distribution of health in or between populations and includes measures such as population attributable risk, rate ratios, rate differences, and the concentration index. Health inequity is typically measured by using these measures of health inequality as a proxy, implicitly conflating the terms equity and equality. Moreover, measure of global inequality does not take into account the health inequity associated with the additional, and unfair, encumbrances associated with poor health status in poorer and less developing nations. Accordingly, this study seeks to address this disparity by proposing a new measure of global health inequality.

Methodology/Design

The researchers employed global health data from the WHO's 14 mortality sub-regions. The analysis was based on the decomposition of an index of inequality known as the Robin Hood Index (Pietra ratio), which in effect represents the share of wealth that has been "robbed from the rich and given to the poor." This inequity measure weights the inequality data by regional economic capacity (GNP per capita). The GNP for each of the mortality sub-regions was derived from the World Bank "World Development Indicators-1999" CD-ROM, following and adjustment for the purchasing power of a so-called international dollar in each of the WHO sub-regions. When GNP figures were not available for a specific country in a respected sub-region, the researchers employed the medium GNP per capita for the available countries as the missing value.

Major Findings

Based on the statistical analysis performed by the researchers, the results suggest that the least healthy sub-regions of the world are approximately four times worse off when we consider a health inequity analysis, when compared to the traditional straight health inequality analysis. By contrast, the wealthiest sub-regions of the world are approximately four times better off. These findings suggest that an analysis based on the inequality of health substantially underestimates the magnitude of the health inequity in sub-regions of the world.

Implications for Public Health

These findings provide further quantitative evidence that exists between wealthy and poor WHO sub-regions of the world in terms of health disparities. Lastly, it is important to note that measures of inequity do not necessarily encompass current health policy initiatives being carried out in certain regions (e.g., immunization programs) which require additional time (e.g., decades) to assess their true impact on reducing the global burden of disease. Nonetheless, by measuring the inequity and simply the inequality in various regions of the world, the magnitude of health disparities can be better understood when planning for and assessing the impact of various economic and health policy planning decisions.

Source: Reidpath and Allotey (2007).

What Are Neglected Tropical Diseases (NTDs)?

NTDs are defined as those diseases that no longer attract world headlines and are ignored in reference to research development efforts for new interventions or drugs, yet still pose a significant health burden on individuals affected by these diseases who typically reside in poor and mainly tropical and subtropical regions of the world (Bartfay and Bartfay 2015). The term "neglected" is often employed because most countries are not required to report the prevalence of these diseases, they occur below the threshold of surveillance and detection methods available in that country or region, and usually do not develop into an immediate global health crisis per se.

When people find out someone has leprosy, they typically say "get out," says Ghosh, an official with the aid organization Calcutta Rescue, which treats leprosy patients. Ghosh estimates there could be more than 200,000 lepers in the state of West Bengal [India] alone. In the Middle Ages, lepers were given a bell and ordered to ring it whenever they went as warning to others of their presence. Even today, lepers are shunned . . . Backing up his claim that cases are overlooked, a study funded by the Indian Council of Medical Research found leprosy prevalence in the city of Agra was 40 times higher than official government statistics. (Westhead 2011, A11).

The WHO (2012) reports that an estimated 1 billion people (or 1:7 individuals worldwide) suffer from NTDs. This includes lymphatic filariasis which in 2009 was endemic in 81 countries. There were over 220,000 cases of cholera reported in 2009, an increase over the previous year, and 244,617 cases of leprosy were reported, down from 5.2 million in 1985. Birn et al. (2009) report that individuals who are affected by NTDs are typically the poorest and most vulnerable populations including indigenous groups, infants, the elderly, migrant workers, and slum dwellers. In fact, NTDs are among the most common infections in an estimated 2.7 billion people who live on less than $2 (U.S.) per day.

For example, pneumonia kills more children than any other illness including HIV/AIDS, malaria, and measles combined and respiratory infections claim nearly 2 million children under the age of 5 annually (Birn, Pillay, and Holtz 2009). The global prevalence for soil-transmitted helminthiasis (worms) is an estimated 573 million people, Schistosomiasis (freshwater parasite) affects 207 million, lymphatic filariasis (parasitic infection transmitted via bites from mosquitoes) affects 120 million, river blindness or onchocerciasis (parasitic worm disease transmitted through blackfly bites) affects 37 million, human leishmaniasis (parasitic infection through sandfly bites) affects 12 million, Chagas disease (caused by infection via Triatominae insects, transfusions of infected blood or mother-to-child transmission) affects 8–9 million, leprosy (transmitted through human-to-human contact) affects 0.4 million, African trypanosomiasis (sleeping sickness caused by parasitic protozoa infection via bit of a tsetse fly) affects 0.3 million, and Dracunculiasis (parasitic infection caused by ingesting water containing guinea worm larvae) affects 0.01 million (Birn, Pillay, and Holtz 2009; WHO 2007).

Malaria is perhaps the best-known example of a vector-borne diseases spread via mosquitoes that are present in temperate regions of the world (e.g., sub-Saharan Africa, Caribbean island of Hispaniola, Middle East, Indian continent, Southeast Asia, Oceania, and South America) (Centers for Disease Control and Prevention 2012; Kachur, de Oliveria, and Bloland 2008). Malaria is present in 107 countries of the world and affects between 300 and 500 million individuals each year globally (WHO and UNICEF 2005).

More recently, public health officials and researchers have been monitoring the Zika virus which has been linked to a 20-fold increase in miscarriages and birth defects including over 4400 cases of microcephaly in Brazil from October 2015 to February 2016 alone (Ferguson 2016; PHAC 2016; WHO 2016b). Similarly, Martinique and French Guiana had reported 2500 potential cases of Zika virus and 100 confirmed cases for a period ranging from December 2015 to February 2016, which included 20 pregnant women and 2 victims suffering from temporary paralysis resulting from Guillain–Barre Syndrome (Nebehay 2016). Honduras declared a state of emergency on February 2, 2016, after having 3469 suspected cases of the Zika virus in less than three months (Chai 2016). On February 1, 2016, the WHO Director-General Margaret Chan declared the Zika virus to be an "international emergency" in Geneva, Switzerland (Ferguson 2016; Keaten and Cheng 2016).

Typical symptoms of exposure include fever, headaches, conjunctivitis, rash, and joint and muscle pain and last for a duration of 2–7 days. The Zika virus is spread by the Aedes mosquitoe and was first detected in rhesus monkeys in Uganda, Africa, in 1947 (Gallagher 2016; Rod 2016; WHO 2016b). This mosquitoe is also responsible for transmitting three other vector-borne diseases—dengue, chikungunya, and yellow fever. The WHO and other public health agencies indicated that the Zika virus could be spread via sexual contact (Lunau 2016; Nebehay 2016). For example, one confirmed case of Zika virus transmission via semen was confirmed by public health officials in the United States for a male traveller in Dallas, Texas, who fell ill after visiting Venezuela. There was also one report of an American male who returned from Senegal in 2008, and was suspected of having infected his wife.

The Zika virus is believed to be first introduced to Brazil during the 2015 FIFA World Cup tournament for soccer held there. Currently, public health officials warn that it has the potential to spread throughout South and Central America's, Mexico, the Caribbean, Oceanic Pacific regions, and parts of the United States (Mulholland 2016; PHAC 2016; WHO 2016b). As of February 20, 2016, 24 countries reported to have cases of Zika virus present, including 31 cases in the United States and 7 Canadians who travelled to high-risk areas (Aljazeera American 2016; CBC News 2016b; Ferguson 2016; Rod 2016). Up to 1.5 million cases could be present in Brazil alone, and the WHO predicted in January 2016 that the Zika virus could potentially affect 4 million people worldwide (Aljazeera American 2016; Lunau 2016). By comparison, a total of only 8098 people worldwide became sick during the 2003 pandemic of SARS. The six Canadians infected were from British Columbia (two cases), Alberta (one case), Ontario (one case), and Québec (three cases) (Ferguson 2016; Lunau 2016). On February 3, 2016, the Canadian Blood Services had moved to ban blood donations from individuals who travelled to affected areas for a period of 21 days, to help ensure that enough time has elapsed for the virus to be eliminated from the bloodstream (Chai 2016). However, the Canadian Blood Services asked individuals to postpone donating blood for at least one month after returning from travel to high-risk-affected areas. The 21-day ban also applied to cord blood and stem cell donations. Héma-Québec, the provinces blood operator, also implemented similar protocols (Chai 2016). There is currently no vaccine or antiviral medication to treat victims infected with the Zika virus (Gallagher 2016; PHAC 2016; WHO 2016b). The best and currently only available public health interventions include fumigation, use of insect repellents with DEET, covering-up exposed skin as much as possible with light, loose-fitting bright-coloured clothing, emptying, cleaning and covering-up kiddy swimming pools, puddles, ponds, and/or other containers or sources that can hold water, and sleeping under mosquitoe nets.

Many global public health efforts are currently underway to control and manage NTDs and decrease associated mortalities. For example, although boiling the water will often kill copepods such as the Guinea (Dracunculiasis) worm larvae, most individuals in developing regions of the world are often too poor to afford the fuel necessary to boil their drinking water supplies. However, the application of temephos (Abate larvicide at 1 part per million) to ponds, wells, and other drinking water supplies at 4-week intervals during the transmission season has been shown to be a safe and effective public health means of vector control, which does not harm humans, fish, plants, or other aquatic species. These collective public health efforts are making a major contribution to decreasing the incidence of Guinea worm infestations, and the *World Health Organization International Commission for the Certification of Dracunculiasis Eradication* has already certified 180 countries as free of Guinea worm (Hopkins 2008). For example, only 3190 cases of Dracunculiasis were reported in 2009, compared to the 1989 estimate of almost 900,000 confirmed cases (World Health Association 2012). The reader is referred to Chapter 7 for a future discussion on select NTDs (e.g., malaria, parasitic infections, TB) and associated public health efforts to manage and control them.

The main determinants of NTDs are non-portable water sources and poor sanitation practices, and a lack of access to public primary healthcare services or healthcare professionals. Table 9.8 shows the total global research and development (R&D) funding by disease in 2008 in U.S. dollars (Moran et al. 2009). *Platform technologies* are defined as technologies that can be applied to a range of diseases and products (e.g., a slow-release technology that could be used to deliver different drugs) (Bartfay and Bartfay 2015). Core funding refers to the organizational grants that are not tied to specific disease projects per se. For example, *schistosomiasis* is a major endemic NTD that affects millions of individuals in rural areas of Africa, Asia, and Latin America through use of contaminated water, and is clinically characterized by infection and gradual destruction of the tissues of the kidneys, liver, and other organs. Currently, the only available drug for the treatment of this NTD is praziquantel. Hence, it is imperative to develop new and cost-effective

Table 9.8 Total Global Research and Development Funding by Select Diseases in 2008 in U.S. Dollars.

Disease	Nominal (U.S. dollars)	Percentage
HIV/AIDS	1,215,841,708	39.4
Malaria	565,985,827	18.3
Tuberculosis (TB)	467,538,635	15.1
Kinetoplastids	145,676,517	4.7
Diarrheal diseases	138,159,527	4.5
Dengue	132,470,770	4.3
Core funding of a multi-disease R&D organization	110,403,053	3.4
Bacterial pneumonia and meningitis	96,071,934	3.1
Unspecified disease	78,179,894	2.5
Helminth infections (worms and flukes)	69,518,274	2.3
Salmonella infections	41,079,293	1.3
Leprosy	10,073,184	0.3
Rheumatic fever	2,268,099	0.1
Trachoma	2,225,330	0.1
Buruli ulcer	2,140,303	0.1
Plateform technologies	16,569,978	0.1
Totals	**3,094,202,328**	**100**

Source: Adapted from Moran et al. (2009).

drugs. *Phytol* is a diterpene alcohol derived from chlorophyll that is widely employed as a food additive and is non-mutagenic. There is preliminary evidence to suggest that phytol possesses antischistosomal properties *in vitro* and offers promise as a potential new drug for the treatment of schistosomiasis (De Moraes et al. 2014).

Effective drugs for the treatment and/or prevention of a variety of NTDs are currently available, but they are infrequently used clinically because large pharmaceutical companies see no profit in their marketing and distribution in the poorer affected regions of the world where affected individuals cannot afford to purchase them. Developing countries continue to face challenges in respect to the availability and high costs associated with essential medicines. Surveys by the World Health Association (2011) in over 40 low- and middle-income countries indicate that selected generic medicines were available in approximately 42% of healthcare facilities in the public sector. The WHO (2011) reports that a lack of available medicines in the public sector forces individuals to purchase medicines from the private sector, where generic medicines costs on average 630% more than their international reference price with originator brands being generally even more expensive. Figure 9.4 shows the geographical distribution of confirmed counterfeiting incidents for the year 2011 alone in selected regions of the world. This is a growing global public health challenge, especially in developing regions of the world due to the growing volume of counterfeit drugs being produced and the required resources for policing and monitoring their illicit distribution, uses, and associated negative ripple effects.

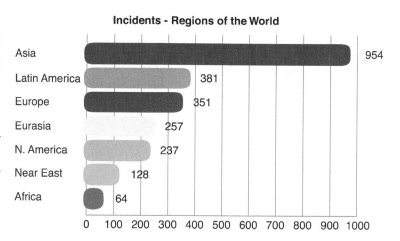

Figure 9.4 Geographical distribution of confirmed counterfeit drugs in 2011 by regions of the world.

Source: http://globalvoicesonline.org/wp-content/uploads/2012/08/Total-counterfeit-drugs-incidents-by-year-375x291.jpg.

The lack of availability of certain drugs in different regions of the world has also resulted in the growth of counterfeit medications (Cockburn et al. 2005; Deisingh 2005). In response to this, the WHO (1999) has published global guidelines directed at combating the manufacturing and distribution of counterfeit drugs. In Nigeria, for example, counterfeit drugs and adulterated drugs in circulation decreased from a high of 70% to 16%, whereas in India the share of counterfeit medications has increased from 10% to 20% (International Medical Products Anti-Counterfeiting Taskforce [IMPACT] 2006).

Funding for the total global investment in NTD R&D amounted to $2.9 billion in 2009 (Hanson et al. 2012; Moran et al. 2009). It is important to consider that the relative risk–benefit tradeoff for NTD research may be viewed dramatically different in highly developed and wealthy industrialized regions of the world such as Canada, the United States, and England versus those that are poor and developing such as sub-Saharan Africa or Bangladesh.

For example, Hanson et al. (2012) report that the *RotaShield*, the first vaccine against the rotavirus, was registered in the United States in 1998 but was subsequently withdrawn in 1999 due to an 1:10,000 risk of intussusceptions in children. An *intussusception* is defined as a potentially serious disorder in which part of the intestine slides or telescopes into an adjacent part of the intestine, which results in the blockage of food, fluid, and/or blood supply to that affected region of the intestine (Bartfay and Bartfay 2015). In the United States, where the rotavirus results in less than 60 childhood deaths per year, the risk–benefit ratio was deemed unacceptable. Conversely, the same risk–benefit calculations could result in different outcomes in poorer nations where mortality attributed to the rotavirus are as high as 5% in children under the age of five years (i.e., mortality rates of 183 per 100,000 population). Hence, the likelihood of dying from the rotavirus in poor and developing nations is 18 times greater than the risk of intussusceptions associated with the vaccine. Unfortunately, since the 2008 global economic crisis, several key public funders have substantially scaled back on their R&D efforts in regard to NTDs, while demand continues to increase annually. Hanson et al. (2012) note that R&D funding for global health issues relies on a handful of donors, with 10 organizations providing 75% of global funds for research into NTDs in 2008. Two notable organizations include the U.S.-based National Institutes of Health (NIH) and the Bill and Melinda Gates Foundation, which collectively provides a striking 60% of the global total. The remaining 25% come from the pharmaceutical industry (12% of global investments), the general public (12%), and philanthropic donors (1%). The reader is referred to the Web-Based Resource Box 9.2 for additional information related to various global health organizations.

Web-Based Resource Box 9.2 Global Health Organizations

Learning resource	Website
Canadian Nurses Association's (CNA's) Global Health and Equity Position Statement This website describes the CNA's position on global health which endorses a primary health-care approach whereby essential health care aimed at prevention and promoting health is universally accessible to all.	http://www.can-aiic.ca/cna/ international/resources/ publications/default_e.aspx
Doctors Without Borders This website describes the history of this voluntary non-profit organization and aims which includes providing independent, impartial assistance in more than 60 countries to people whose survival is threatened by violence, neglect, or catastrophe, primarily due to armed conflict, epidemics, malnutrition, exclusion from health care, or natural disasters.	http://msf.org

Global Spread of Infections

Despite ongoing global efforts to enhance disease surveillance and response, many poorer and developing countries and regions of the world face challenges with respect to accurately diagnosing, identifying, and reporting infectious diseases which is often attributed to the remoteness of villages and communities, a lack of reliable transportation and communication infrastructures, lack of public health and laboratory facilities, and a shortage of trained and skilled public healthcare professionals and workers (Bartfay and Bartfay 2015; Seear 2007). To correctly track and interpret global epidemiological patterns of disease, mortality and morbidity, data collection, and reporting efforts must be taken into consideration. Although some diseases are reported under the International Health Regulations, others are simply monitored by the respected countries or by the WHO in the context of specific control programs (e.g., vaccine-preventable diseases).

The WHO (2011) argues that these diseases are best managed through preventative measures such as vaccinations and mass drug treatment programs. The reporting of the number of cases should have a lower priority than estimating the populations at most risk. Indeed, diseases such as the H5N1 influenza, Japanese encephalitis, and malaria are difficult to clinically diagnosis without specialized laboratory tests that are often not available in developing countries. For vaccine-preventable diseases, the number of cases is directly affected by immunization rates. Notably, every $1.00 spent on an immunization campaign results in a healthcare cost saving of $16.00, or an ROI of 1,500%. In many settings, cases of some diseases (such as malaria, pneumonia) are identified only via presenting clinical signs and symptoms, and opposed to imaging (e.g., x-rays) or laboratory confirmed diagnosis (e.g., blood samples, sputum cultures) (WHO 2011).

Heymann (2008) reports that infectious (communicable) diseases (e.g., HIV/AIDS, TB, malaria, measles) kill more than 14 million people annually and these deaths are primarily in developing and poorer nations. The revised *International Health Regulations* (IHR) issued by WHO (2005b) was updated in an attempt to help prevent, protect from, and control the spread of communicable disease globally. Although these regulations provide a public health response mechanism when a disease becomes pandemic, the effectiveness of the regulation per se is dependent on the country's pandemic preparedness and their overall public primary health systems to effectively identify, monitor, and manage disease outbreaks. Accordingly, public healthcare professionals need to be cognizant of infectious disease prevention, monitoring, control, and management and have an understanding of how best to forestall negative health ripple effects both locally and globally. According to the WHO (2010), an influenza pandemic may occur when a new influenza virus appears against which the human population has no current immunity. With the increase in global travel and trade, as well as urbanization and overcrowded conditions in some areas, epidemics due to a new influenza virus are likely to take hold around the world, and become a pandemic faster than before. Pandemics can be either mild or severe for the illness resulting in death, and the severity of a pandemic can change over the course of the pandemic (WHO 2010). The reader is referred to Chapters 6 and 7 for a more detailed discussion on pandemics and communicable disease, respectively.

The successfully control, prevention, management, and treatment of communicable disease require both national and international efforts. Public healthcare professionals and workers play major roles in health promotion and education, direct care, community mobilization and development, liaison with stakeholders, research, advocacy, program planning and evaluation, and policy formulation. All of these skills are essential for the successful prevention, control, treatment, and management of communicable diseases in Canada and abroad. Figure 9.5 shows the global distribution of influenza A (H1N1) infections as of May 29, 2009, in 53 countries globally.

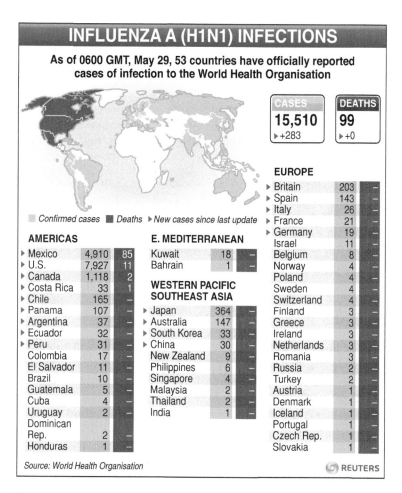

Figure 9.5 Global spread of Influenza A (H1N1) in May 29, 2009.

Reprinted by permission of Thompson Reuters.

For example, in April 2009, the first deaths from the H1N1 influenza virus (swine flu) were reported in Mexico and the United States. This virus quickly spread to other countries around the world including Canada due to travel, trade, and commerce. As of July 2009, the WHO reported that approximately 100,000 confirmed cases of human infections globally and approximately 500 deaths, including 25 Canadians. During this pandemic, there were 428 deaths and 8,678 hospitalizations in Canada due to influenza A/H1N1 (Public Health Agency of Canada [PHAC] 2010). Public healthcare professions and policy-makers were under tremendous public pressure to make informed healthcare decisions based on the best available scientific evidence available. To facilitate this process, the Canadian Institutes of Health Research, Rx&D Health Research Foundation, and Canadian Food Inspection Agency (2009) sponsored a one-day research meeting in Toronto, Ontario, on July 8, 2009, that consisted of approximately 180 influenza and pandemic experts from across Canada. This meeting had three primary goals: (a) to facilitate information sharing among researchers and other influenza expects in Canada, (b) to network and develop collaborations in order to focus the Canadian research response to the pandemic, and (c) to discuss gaps in the research knowledge about the pandemic H1N1/09 virus.

In addition to the above, recommendations made by the PHAC were followed by all public healthcare professionals and workers working in acute and chronic healthcare facilities and in communities during the H1N1 pandemic. As a result, the infection resulted in minimal deaths in Canada in comparison to other nations and societal disruption was kept to a minimum. Hence, pandemic preparedness is critical to mitigate the negative health ripple effects felt in a single country and beyond its borders. In fact, Canada was one of the few countries that had a pandemic plan in place due to the lessons learned from the previous SARS and the Avian Flu pandemics known as the *Canadian Pandemic Influenza Plan for the Health Sector*, which was first published in 2004 and is updated regularly.

Future Directions and Challenges

In order to significantly address current and emerging global health issues and challenges, there must be strong international collaboration. Given that there is no single governing authority for addressing global health issues and challenges that transcend national boundaries by their nature and scale, nations, governments, NGOs, faith-based organizations, citizens, and other stakeholders must work collaboratively to achieve common goals. The September 2012 *E. coli* outbreak from the XL beef processing plant in Alberta is a recent example of how human error, the failure to follow government protocols and the many challenges industry and the Canadian Food Inspection Agency (CFIA) face in assuring that our food supplies are safe in Canada. This outbreak not only affected Canadians, but alerts and recalls were extended beyond our bounders to the United States and Hong Kong in October 2012. Hence, contamination at a single meat processing plant can have negative ripple effects that span international borders and threaten the health and well-being of citizens abroad. One of the major challenges for the public health of nations in this new millennium will be to envision and incorporate health from a global perspective in terms of research involving primary healthcare initiatives and education. Indeed, we are living in an increasingly global society where knowledge is becoming easier to access due to technology and greater opportunities for sharing public health expertise and resources to meet global health challenges.

Research into current and emerging global health issues is affected by the availability of public healthcare professionals, researchers, and academics; access to graduate programs and training; and the availability of funding initiatives (Carlton et al. 2007; Drager and Sunderland 2007; Skolnik 2008; Walraven 2010). For example, if we consider that the majority of researchers in the health sciences are from higher income and developed countries such as Canada, the United States, and Western Europe, who have been primarily educated, trained, and funded to study emerging issues. This phenomenon has been referred to as the "90/10 divide." which refers to the fact that only 10% of all international health research is dedicated to studying problems associated with 90% of the world's GBD (Resnik 2004). Moreover, we must also consider that fact that healthcare researchers from these affluent countries frequently publish their findings in English, which has been referred to as the "21st-century language of science" (Gennaro 2009; Mancia and Gastaldo 2004). This, of course, constitutes a significant barrier in reference to both accessing and utilizing research for evidence-based practice in poorer developing countries where English may not be the prominent language spoken.

In Canada, the establishment of a growing number of federal and provincial initiatives in recent years has helped to address the need to both investigate and teach future generations of public healthcare professionals and workers about global health issues and perspectives. The *Global Health Research Initiative* (GHRI) of the Canadian Institute of Health Research (CIHR) and other federal partners, and the not-for-profit *Canadian Coalition for Global Health Research* (CCGHR), are examples of funding agencies which encourages Canadian researchers to partake in global health research projects and initiatives. According to Riddle et al. (2008), the key to promoting and maintaining this enthusiasm for global health research at the provincial and national levels is the role that students and new researchers will play, and a variety of strategies should be pursued to ensure that new researchers are genuine partners in this endeavour.

There is also a growing need to train and educate future generations of public healthcare professionals and workers to be prepared for global health issues that may emerge and affect Canadians (e.g., HIV/AIDS, SARS, Avian Flu, H1N1, bioterrorism) (Johnson, Donovan, and Parboosingh 2008; Moloughney and Skinner 2006; Mowat and Moloughney 2004; Spasoff 2005; The Joint Task Group on Public Health Human Resources 2005; Tulchinsky and Bickford 2006). Indeed, if we take into account the rapid and growing ripple effects of globalization, public healthcare professionals need to be educated as global citizens who have both a moral responsibility and the professional competencies necessary to provide primary healthcare services beyond their local communities or national institutions (Friedman 2000; Herdman 2004; WHO 2005a, 2005b). During the 1970s, only two schools of public health/hygiene existed in Canada at the University of Toronto (1927–1975) and the University of Montréal (1945–1975) (Defries 1957; Desrosiers, Gaumer, and Keel 1994; Massé and Moloughney 2011). Graduate training in the public health sciences has grown from 5 programs during the 1990s to 15 programs as of September 2011, and the involvement of more than 20 different academic institutions has resulted in a strong interest to create a network of programs and schools of public health across Canada (Massé and Moloughney 2011). Various graduate programs in community, public, and global health have emerged over the past decade due to increased need and demand for specialists in these noted fields (PHAC 2013a).

In March 2009, the Public Health Agency of Canada's Centre for Food-borne, Environmental and Zoonotic Infectious Diseases (CFEZID) hosted the *One World One Health*™ (OWOH) Expert Consultation in Winnipeg, Manitoba, at the Fort Garry Hotel (PHAC 2013b). The OWOH approach is primarily preventive in nature and seeks to address public health issues and threats the source of the problem and is consistent with various surveillance and disease monitoring programs for currently in place for both animals and humans in Canada, such as the *Canadian Integrated Program for Antimicrobial Resistance Surveillance* (CIPARS) (PHAC 2013b). At this 3-day conference, experts from 23 countries shared knowledge and expertise related to best practices, challenges, and barriers towards implementation of the OWOH approach. Experts included individuals from academia, government and NGOs, United Nations organizations, and the private sector. A number of delegates provided presentations and case studies on a variety of key issues including surveillance data gathering and management, interdisciplinary training, and maintaining political will. The key recommendations of these experts included creating transdisciplinary networks for information sharing; engaging grass roots involvement in animal, human, and ecosystem health initiatives; supporting partnerships and collaboration; building capacity (infrastructure and skills); and developing a global health university curriculum (PHAC 2013b).

A group of Canadian researchers reviewed the global health focus being carried out in university-based public health programs at five universities in Québec (Ridde, Mohindra, and LaBossiere 2008). The researchers surveyed and interviewed both students and professors and a total of 36 researchers who have worked on a total of 76 global health projects or initiatives over the past 5 years. The majority of these projects were undertaken in sub-Saharan Africa and Asia and the dominant themes included infectious/parasitic diseases, health services, and health policy initiatives. The authors note that there is a strong and growing presence of global health in Québec universities—although the situation varies according to specific institutions across Canada (Ridde, Mohindra, and LaBossiere 2008).

Many of these new and emerging graduate programs are offering courses or a focus concentration in global health. In addition, there are also a limited number of Canadian universities offering public health-focused undergraduate degree programs (e.g., Ryerson University, Brock University, University of Lethbridge), while others are developing specialized streams for BHSc programs where courses in global health are currently being offered or developed (e.g., University of Ontario Institute of Technology). The future development of these schools and programs will be highly dependent on close collaborations with all the stakeholders and actors involved. A detailed enumeration to ascertain the actual capacity of the public system is required as is an assessment of current and future educational needs, which should be regarded as major priorities in our highly decentralized system (Massé and Moloughney 2011).

Group Review Exercise "Half the Sky: Turning Oppression Into Opportunity for Women Worldwide"

About This Global Health Documentary

This two-part Public Broadcasting Station documentary film entitled "Half the Sky: Turning Oppression into Opportunity for Women Worldwide" is based on the acclaimed book of the same name written by Nicholas Kristof and Sheryl WuDunn. This documentary film was filmed in 10 developing countries around the world and the series follows Nicholas Kristof and various celebrities and activists including Meg Ryan, Gabrielle Union, Olivia Wilde, America Ferera, Diane Lane, and Eva Mendes on their journey to document inspiring stories of courageous women and girls. This film highlights how the oppression of women and girls is being confronted through various public healthcare interventions, education, and economic empowerment. The issues confronted include forced prostitution of young girls and women and sex trafficking, gender-based mutilations and violence, and maternal mortality which claims the life of one woman every 90 seconds in certain regions of the world.

Instructions

This assignment may be done alone, in pairs or in groups of up to 5 people (note: if you are doing this assignment in pairs or groups, please only submit one hard or electronic copy to your instructor). The assignment should be type-written and no more than 4–6 pages maximum in length (double-spaced please). View the two-part documentary film entitled *"Half the Sky: Turning Oppression into Opportunity for Women Worldwide"* See links: http://www.pbs.org/independentlens/half-the-sky/ and http://www.pbs.org/independentlens/half-the-sky/video/Take notes during the viewing of this documentary film.

   i. Provide a brief overview of the salient issues highlighted in this documentary film.

   ii. Describe which MDGs were addressed in the documentary and the current barriers and challenges in meeting these goals.

   iii. Describe some of the SDH described in this two-part documentary.

   iv. Discuss the positive "ripple effects" that public health, education, and economic freedom are having on the lives of girls and young women in these developing nations.

Summary

- Global health embraces a wide range of health-promoting and health-preserving activities and challenges that span international borders and boundaries.
- Global health is defined as an area of research and practice that seeks to improve health via the SDH by promoting social justice and equity, human rights, and sustainable development both on the national and on the international scale, and by fostering and promoting the availability and access to healthcare professionals; healthcare financing, and delivery of primary healthcare services to all citizens of this planet.
- Developing an understanding and need to examine health and public healthcare challenges from an international perspective is critical for all public healthcare professionals and workers in Canada.
- SARS, H1N1, and the West Nile Virus are recent examples of how quickly diseases can spread and the global challenges faced by public healthcare professionals and officials in terms of their surveillance, tracking, and management.

- There is also a need to be cognizant of the negative ripple effects associated with climate change, global warming, and natural disasters (e.g., tsunamis, hurricanes) which often extends beyond borders.
- The 2009 United Nations Millennium Declaration consists of the following eight specific goals with targets set for the year 2015: (a) eliminate extreme poverty and hunger, (b) achieve universal education for all, (c) empower women and promote gender equality, (d) decrease mortality in children, (e) improve maternal health, (f) combat major diseases such as malaria, HIV/AIDS, TB, and malaria, (g) ensure and maintain environmental sustainability, and (h) develop a global partnership for development.
- We defined globalization as a fundamental and relatively accelerated change to human societies and social–cultural–political and geographical environments around the world due to a variety of processes by which individuals, groups, and entire nations or regions are becoming increasingly more connected and interdependent via commerce and trade; information technology, knowledge and communication exchanges, migration and cultural diffusion, and healthcare issues.
- NTDs are those diseases that no longer attract world headlines and are ignored in reference to research development efforts for new interventions or drugs, yet still pose a significant health burden on individuals affected by these diseases.
- NTDs currently affect a staggering 1 billion people globally or 1:7 individuals worldwide, primarily in the poorer tropical and subtropical regions of the world.
- Despite ongoing international efforts to enhance disease surveillance and management, many poorer regions of the world face challenges with respect to accurately diagnosing, identifying, and reporting infectious diseases.
- These challenges include a lack of reliable communication and transportation networks, lack of public health and laboratory facilities, and a critical shortage of trained and skilled healthcare professionals and workers.

Critical Thinking Questions

1. Why is it important to assess the relationship between culture and health in specific societies by the extent to which cultural practices, expectations, and norms promote and hinder good health? Name two cultural practices that are health promoting and two cultural practices that hinder health.
2. How do multinational organizations enhance and impede global health in developing regions of the world?
3. How does the health of infants and young children in low- versus high-income countries vary with the mother's level of education?
4. Why are psychiatric disorders so critical to the burden of disease in both developed and developing countries if so few individuals die from them annually?
5. What are some of the key differences in the burden of disease between men and women in developed versus developing countries? Identify and discuss three associated SDH.

References

Aljazeera American. *Zika Virus Could See "Explosive" Spread to 4 Million People: UN Agency*. Doha, Qatar: Author, January 28, 2016. Retrieved January 30, 2016. http://america.aljazeera.com/articles/2016/1/28/zika-virus-to-affect-up-to-4-million-people.html.

Alzheimer Society of Canada. *Rising Tide: The Impact of Dementia on Canadian Society. (A Study Commissioned by the Alzheimer's Society). Executive Summary*. Toronto, ON: Author, 2010. ISBN:978-0-9733522-2-1.

Armartya, S. *On Economic Inequality*, 2nd ed. London, England: Oxford University Press, 1977.

Bartfay, W. J., and E. Bartfay. *Public Health in Canada*. Boston, MA: Pearson Learning Solutions, 2015. ISBN:13:978-1-323-01471-4.

Bartfay, W. J., Bartfay, E., and T. Wu. "Impact of the Global Economic Crisis on the Health of Unemployed Autoworkers." *Canadian Journal of Nursing Research* 45, no. 3 (2013): 66–79.

Birn, A. M., Y. Pillay, and T. H. Holtz, eds. *Textbook of International Health: Global Health in a Dynamic World*. New York: Oxford University Press, 2009.

Bloom, D., E. Cafiero, E. Jane-Llopis, S. Abraham-Gessel, L. Bloom, S. Fathima, et al., *The Global Economic Burden of Noncommunicable Diseases*. Geneva, Switzerland: World Economic Forum, 2011. Retrieved January 10, 2014. http://www.weforum.org/reports/global-economic-burden-non-communicalbe-diseases.

Branigan, T. "Chinese Figures How Fivefold Rise in Babies Sick Form Contaminated Milk." *The Guardian (London)*, December 2, 2008. Retrieved January 8, 2014. http://www.guardian.co.uk/world/2008/dec/02/china.

Campbell, A. *The SARS Commission. Spring of Fear: Final Report. Ontario Ministry of Health and Long-Term Care (MOHLTC)*. Toronto, ON: MOHLTC, December, 2006. Retrieved January 6, 2012. http://www.health.gov.ca/english/public/pub/ministry_reports/campbell06/oinlinerep/index.html.

Canadian Broadcasting Services. *Life Expectancy in Canada Hits 80 for Men and 84 for Women. For Both Sexes Life Expectancy Is Up at Birth*. Toronto, ON: CBC, May 15, 2014. Retrieved November 10, 2015. http://www.cbc.ca/news/health/life-expectancy-in-canada-hits-80-for-men-84-for-women-1.2644355.

Canadian Broadcasting News Services. "WWF Reports Criticizes Canada's Ecological Footprint." *CBC News*, 2016a. Totonto, ON. Retrieved January 25, 2016. http://www.cbc.ca/news/technology/wwf-report-criticizes-canada-s-ecological-footprint-1.1263041.

———. "Zika Virus Confirmed Among 4 Canadian Travelers: Human Tests on Vaccine Could Start as Early as September, Says Scientists Gary Kobinger." *CBC News*, 2016b. Toronto, ON. Retrieved January 30, 2016. http://www.cbc.ca/news/health/canadian-us-zika-vaccine-1.3425647.

Canadian Institute for Health Information. National Health Expenditure Trends, 1975 to 2015. Ottawa, ON: CIHI, 2015. ISBN:978-1-77-109-413-9 (PDF). Retrieved November 10, 2015. https://www.cihi.ca/en/spending-and-health-workforce/spending/canadas-slow-health-spending-growth-continues.

Canadian Institutes of Health Research, Rx & D Health Research Foundation, and Canadian Food Inspection Agency. *Canadian Pandemic Preparedness Meeting: H1N1 Outbreak Research Response*. Toronto, ON: Canadian Institutes of Health Research, July 8, 2009. Retrieved December 9, 2011. http://www.chir-irsc.gc.ca/e/documents/iii_cppm_report_2009.e.pdf.

Carlton, K. H., M. Ryan, N. S. Ali, and B. Kelsy. "Integration of Global Health Concepts in Nursing Curricula: A National Study." *Nursing Education Perspectives* 28, no. 3 (2007): 124–29.

Centers for Disease Control and Prevention. *Climate Effects on Health*. Atlanta, GA: CDC, 2015. Retrieved January 7, 2016. http://www.cec.gov/climateandhealth/effects.

———. *Malaria Parasites*. Atlanta, GA: Author, November 9, 2012. Retrieved December 16, 2013. http://www.cdc.gov/malaria/about/biology/parasites.html.

Chai, C. "Zika Virus: Don't Donate Blood for 3 Weeks After Returning Home from Travel." *Global News*, February 3, 2016. Toronto, ON. Retrieved February 4, 2016. http://globalnews.ca/news/2495745/zika-virus-dont-donate-blood-for-3-weeks-after-returning-home-from-travels/.

Chen, S. "Melamine—An Industry Staple." *South China Morning Post*, September 18, 2008: A2. Hong Kong.

Cockburn, R., P. N. Newton, E. K. Agyarko, D. Akunyili, and N. J. White. The Global Threat of Counterfeit Drugs: Why Industry and Governments Must Communicate the Dangers. *Public Library of Science Medicine* 2, no. 4 (2005): e100. doi:10.1371/journal.pmed.0020100.

Commission on the Social Determinants of Health. *Closing the Gap in a Generation. Health Equity through Action on the Social Determinants of Health*. Geneva, Switzerland: World Health Organization, 2008. ISBN:978-92-4-156370-3.

Defries, R. D. "Postgraduate Teaching in Public Health in the University of Toronto, 1913–1955." *Canadian Journal of Public Health* 48 (1957): 285–94.

Deisingh, A. K. "Pharmaceutical Counterfeiting." *Analyst* 130 (2005): 271–79.

de Moraes, J., R. N. de Oliveiria, J. P. Costa, A. L. Junior, D. P. de Sousa, R. M. Freitas, S. M. Allegretti, and P. L. Pinto. "Phytol, A Diterpene Alcohol from Chlorophyll, as a Drug Against Neglected Tropical Disease Schistosomiasis Mansoni." *PLoS Neglected Tropical Disease* 8, no. 1 (January 2, 2014): e26217. doi:10.1371/journal/pntd.0002617.

Desrosiers, G., Gaumer, B., and Keel, O. (1994). "Contribution de l'École d'Hygiéne de l'Université á un enseignement francophone de santé publique, 1946–1970." *Revue d'histoire de l'Amérique française* 47 (1994): 323–47.

Deviney, E. "Could You Live on $1.75 a Day?." *The Huntington Post*, July, 2013. Retrieved January 9, 2014. http://www.huntingtonpost.ca/tag/extreme-poverty-canada.

Drager, N., and L. Sunderland. "Public Health in a Globalizing World: The Perspective From the World Health Organization." In *Governing Global Health: Challenge, Response, Innovation*, edited by A. F. Cooper, J. J. Kirton, and T. Schrecker, 67–78. Aldershot, UK: Ashgate, 2007.

Ehrenberg, J. P., and S. K. Ault. "Neglected Diseases of Neglected Populations: Thinking to Reshape the Determinants of Health in Latin America and the Caribbean." *BioMed Central Public Health* 5, no. 1 (2005): 119–31.

Etches, V., J. Frank, E. Di Ruggiero, and D. Manuel. "Measuring Population Health: A Review of Indicators." *Annual Review of Public Health* 27 (2006): 29–55.

Ferguson, R. "Ontario Has First Confirmed Case of Zika." Toronto, ON: *The Star.com.* (Queen's Park Bureau), February 19, 2016. Retrieved February 20, 2016. http://www.thestar.com/news/canada/2016/02/19/ontario-has-first-case-of-zika-virus-in-person-who-travelled-to-colombia.html.

Friedman, M. "Educating for World Citizenship." *Ethics*, 110, no. 3 (2000): 586–601.

Food and Agriculture Organization. *The State of Agricultural Commodity Markets: High Food Prices and the Food Crisis-Experiences and Lessons Learned.* Rome: FAO, 2009.

Food Banks Canada. *Hungercount 2012. A Comprehensive Report on Hunger and Food Bank Use in Canada, and Recommendations for Change.* Toronto, ON: Author, 2012. ISBN: 978-0-9813632-8-8.

Gallagher, J. "*Zika Virus: Outbreak 'Likely to Spread Across Americas' Say WHO.*" *BBC News*, 2016. London, UK. Retrieved January 25, 2016. http://www.bbc.com/news/health-35399403.

Gates, B., and M. Gates. "About Us, Our Values (Letter)." *Gates Foundation*, June 27, 2006. Retrieved January 7, 2012. http://www.gatesfoundation.com/About/Us/OurValues/GalesLetter.htm.

Gennaro, S. "Searching for Knowledge." *Journal of Nursing Scholarship* 41 no. 1 (2009): 1–2.

Hanson, K., B. Palafox, S. Anderson, J. Guzman, M. Moran, R. Shretta, and T. Wuliji. "Pharmaceuticals." In *Global Health: Diseases, Programs, Systems and Policies.* 3rd ed., edited by M. H. Michael, R. E. Black, and A. J. Mills, 707–55. Toronto, ON: Jones & Bartlett Learning, 2012.

Guillermina, J. "On Gini's Mean Difference and Gini's Index of Concentration." *American Sociological Review* 44, no. 5 (1979): 867–70.

Herdman, E. "Globalization, Internationalism and Nursing." *Nursing and Health Sciences* 6 (2004): 237–38.

Heymann, D. L. *Control of Communicable Diseases Manual: An Official Report of the American Public Health Association*, 19th ed. Washington, DC: American Public Health Association, 2008.

Hopkins, D. R. "Dracunculiasis." In *Public Health and Preventative Medicine.* 15th ed., edited by R. B. Wallace, 320–22. Toronto, ON: McGraw Medical, 2008.

Hyder, A. A., Puvanachandra, P., and Morrow, R. H. "Measures of Health and Disease in Populations." In *Global Health: Diseases, Programs, Systems and Policies*, 3rd ed., edited by M. H. Michael, R. E. Black, and A. J. Mills, 1–42. Toronto, ON: Jones & Bartlett Learning, 2012.

International Medical Products Anti-Counterfeiting Taskforce [IMPACT]. *Counterfeit Medicines: An Update on Estimates.* Geneva, Switzerland: IMPACT, WHO, 2006.

Jacobsen, K. H. *Introduction to Global Health.* Toronto, ON: Jones and Bartlett Publishers, 2008.

Jamison, D. T., J. G. Breman, A. R. Measham, G. Alleyne, M. Claeson, D. B. Evans, P. Jha, A. Mills, and P. Musgrove. *Disease Control Priorities in Developing Countries*, 2nd ed. Washington, DC: Oxford University Press, 2006, 25.

Johnson, I., D. Donovan, J. Parboosingh. "Steps to Improve the Teaching of Public Health to Undergraduate Medical Students in Canada." *Academic Medicine* 83 (2008): 414–18.

Kachur, S. P., A. M. de Oliveria, and P. B. Bloland. In *Public Health and Preventive Medicine.* 5th ed., edited by R. B. Wallace, N. Kohatsu, and J. M. Last, 373–86. Toronto, ON: McGraw Hill Medical, 2008.

Kaplan, R. M. "The General Health Policy Model: An Integrated Approach." In *Quality of Life Assessment in Clinical Trials*, edited by B. Spiker. New York: Raven Press, 1990, 156.

Keaten, J., and M. Cheng, M. "WHO Declares Zika Virus an International Emergency." *CTV News and The Associated Press*, February 1, 2016. Toronto, ON. Retrieved February 4, 2016. http://www.ctvnews.ca/health/who-declares-zika-virus-an-international-emergency-1.2759788.

Landsman, I. Y. *Public Health Management of Disasters: The Practice Guide*. 2nd ed. Washington, DC: American Public Health Association, 2005.

Last, J. M., ed. *A Dictionary of Epidemiology*, 4th ed. New York: Oxford University Press, 2000.

Lee, K., D. Yach, and A. Kamradt-Scott. "Globalization and Health." In *Global Health: Diseases, Programs, Systems and Policies*. 3rd ed., edited by M. H. Merson, R. E. Black, and A. J. Mills, 885–913. Mississauga, ON: Jones & Bartlett Learning, 2012.

Lenton, R., Wright, A. M., Lewis, K., and the UN Millennium Project Task Force on Water and Sanitation. *Health, Dignity, and Development: What Will It Take?* Sterling, VA: United Nations Development Programme, 2005.

Lopez, A., C. Mathers, M. Ezzati, D. Jamison, and C. Murray, eds. *Global Burden of Disease and Risk Factors*. New York: The World Bank and Oxford University Press, 2006.

Lunau, K. "Zika: The New Global Health Terror." *Maclean's*, February 4, 2016, Toronto, ON: Rogers Media Inc. Retrieved February 4, 2016. http://www.msn.com/en-ca/health/medical/zika-the-new-global-health-terror/ar-BBp5LZs?li=AAggNb9.

Lunn, S. "Ebola Outbreak: No New Medical Personnel for Now, Rona Ambrose Says. Drills Underway to Prepare for Potential Cases in Canada." *Canadian Broadcasting Corporation (CBC)*, October 20, 2014. Toronto, ON: CBC. Retrieved January 29, 2016. http://www.cbc.ca/news/health/ebola-outbreak-no-new-medical-personnel-for-now-rona-ambrose-says-1.2805765.

Mackenbach, J. P., A. E. Junst, F. Groenhof, J. Borgan, G. Costa, F. Faggiano, P. l. Jozan, et al. "Socioeconomic Inequalities in Mortality Among Women and Among Men: An International Study." *American Journal of Public Health* 89, no. 12 (1999): 1800–13.

Mancia, J. R., and D. Gastaldo. "Production and Consumption of Science in a Global Context." *Nursing Inquiry* 11, no. 2 (2004): 65–66.

Massé, R., and B. Moloughney. "New Era for Schools and Programs of Public Health in Canada." *Public Health Reviews* 33, no. 1 (2011): 1–11.

Mathers, C. D. "Measuring the Health of Populations: The Conceptual and Analytic Approach of the Global Burden of Disease Study." *Proceedings of Statistics Canada Symposium 2006: Methodological Issues in Measuring Population Health. Statistics Canada International Symposium Series (Abstract Proceedings)*. Ottawa, ON: Statistics Canada, 2006 (Cat. No. 11-522-XIE).

———, T. Vos, A. Lopez, J. Salomon, R. Lozano, and M. Ezzati, eds. *National Burden of Disease Studies: A Practical Guide*, Edition 2.0. Geneva, Switzerland: WHO, 2001.

McDonald, S. "Nearly 53,000 Chinese Children Sick From Milk." Last modified September 22, 2008. Retrieved January 8, 2014. http://web.archive.org/web/20110521092518/http://ap.goggle.com/article/ALeqM5iCL58EMBN1tqq6xujZlsalTAFpCQD93BHE880.

McGuinn, D. *How Much in Food Do Canadian Waste a Year? Think Billions*. Toronto, ON: The Globe and Mail, October 1, 2012. Retrieved January 25, 2016. http://www.theglobeandmail.com/life/the-hot-button/how-much-in-food-do-canadians-waste-a-year-think-billions/article4580509/.

Medicines for Malaria Venture. "How Cost Effective Is MMV?" . Retrieved January 9, 2012. http://www.mmv.org/article.php3?id_article=131.

Melse, J. M., M. Essink-Bot, P. G. Kramers, and N. Hoeymans. "A National Burden of Disease Calculation: Dutch Disability-Adjusted Life Years." *American Journal of Public Health* 90, no. 8 (2000): 1241–47.

Messias, D. K. H. "Globalization, Nursing and Health for All." *Journal of Nursing Scholarship* 33, no. 1 (2001): 9–11.

Moloughney, B. W., and H. A. Skinner. "Rethinking Schools of Public Health: A Strategic Alliance Model." *Canadian Journal of Public Health* 97 (2006): 251–56.

Moran, M., J. Guzman, K. Henderson, A. L. Ropars, A. McDonald, L. McSherry, G. Finder. *Neglected Disease Research and Development: New Times, New Trends*. London, UK: George Institute for International Health, 2009.

Morrow, R. H., and J. H. Bryant. "Health Policy Approaches to Measuring and Valuing Human Life: Conceptual and Ethical Issues." *American Journal of Public Health* 85 (1995): 1356–60.

Mowat, D. L., and B. W. Moloughney. "Developing the Public Health Workforce in Canada: A Summary of Regional Workshops on Workforce Education and Training." *Canadian Journal of Public Health* 95 (2004), 186–87.

Mulholland, A. "Zika Virus Could Spread to North America, Researchers Say." *CTV News*, January 14, 2016. Toronto, ON. Retrieved January 25, 2016. http://www.ctvnews.ca/health/zika-virus-could-spread-to-north-america-researchers-say-1.2738002.

Murray, C. J., and Lopez, A. D. *Global Comparative Assessments in the Health Sector.* Geneva, Switzerland: WHO, 1994.

Murray, C. J., and A. D. Lopez. *Summary: The Global Burden of Disease. Global Burden of Disease and Injury Series.* Cambridge, MA: Harvard School of Public Health on Behalf of the World's Health Organization and the World Bank: Harvard University Press, 1996.

Nebehay, S. "WHO Concerned by Report of Sexual Spread of Zika Virus." *The Globe and Mail*, February 3, 2016. Toronto, ON. Retrieved February 4, 2016. http://www.theglobeandmail.com/news/world/who-concerned-by-report-of-sexual-spread-of-zika-virus/article28531722/.

Neibergall, C. *Most of Canada's Wasted Food Dumped from Homes. 37B Worth of Food Wasted Across the Country Every Year, Research Group Says.* Toronto, ON: CBC News and Associated Press, October 1, 2012. Retrieved January 26, 2016. http://www.cbc.ca/news/canada/most-of-canada-s-wasted-food-dumped-from-homes-1.1132998.

O'Dea, K., and L. S. Piers. "Diabetes." In *The Nutrition Transition: Diet and Disease in the Developing World*, edited by B. Caballero and B. M. Popkins, 165–90. London, UK: Academic Press, 2002.

Ontario Association of Food Banks. *The Costs of Poverty: An Analysis of the Economic Costs.* Toronto, ON: Author, June 5, 2008.

Paris, R., F. Lavigne, P. Wassimer, and J. Sartohadi. "Coastal Sedimentation Associated with the December 26, 2004 Tsunami in Lhok Nga, West Banda Aceh (Sumatra, Indonesia)." *Marine Geology* 238, nos. 1–4 (2007): 93–106. doi:10.1016/j.margeo.2006.12.009.

Poladian, C. "Ebola in the United States: Nina Pharm Update, Calls for Hospital Response Reform and New Policies." *International Business Times*, October 19, 2014. Retrieved January 26. http://www.ibtimes.com/ebola-us-nina-pham-update-calls-hospital-response-reform-new-policies-1707547.

Porta, M. *A Dictionary of Epidemiology.* 5th ed. Toronto, ON: Oxford University Press, 2008.

Prince, M., R. Bryce, E. Albanese, A. Wimo, W. Riberiro, and C. P. Ferri. "The Global Prevalence of Dementia: A Systemic Review and Metaanalysis." *Alzheimers and Dementia* 9, no. 1 (2013): 63–75. doi:10.1016/j.jalz.2012.11.007.

Public Health Agency of Canada. *Core Competencies for Public Health in Canada: Release 1.1.* Ottawa, ON: Author, September, 2007. http://www.phac-aspc.gc.ca/core_competencies or http://www.phac-aspc.gc.ca/php-psp/ccph-cesp/pdfs/cc-manual-eng090407.pdf.

———. *Canada's Aging Population. Division of Aging Seniors.* Ottawa, ON: PHAC, 2008. Retrieved January 10, 2014. http://www.phac-aspc.gc/ca/seniors-aines/publications/public/various-varies/papier-fed-paper/index-eng.php.

———. *Surveillance: Deaths Associated with H1N1 Flu Virus in Canada.* Ottawa, ON: PHAC, 2010. Retrieved December 9, 2011. http://www.phac-aspc.gc.ca/alert-alerte/h1n1/surveillance-archieve/201000128-eng.php.

———. *Master's Programs in Public Health.* Ottawa, ON: Author, October 23, 2013a. Retrieved January 8, 2014. http://www.phac-aspc.gc.ca/php-psp/master_of_php-eng.php.

———. *One World, One Health Conference: From Ideas to Action.* Ottawa, ON: Author, March 28, 2013b. Retrieved January 7, 2014. http://www.phac-aspc.gc.ca/owoh-umus/index-eng.php.

———. *Zika Virus Infection in the Americas. Travel Health Notice.* Ottawa, ON: Author, January, 15, 2016. Retrieved January 25, 2016. http://www.phac-aspc.gc.ca/tmp-pmv/notices-avis/notices-avis-eng.php?id=143.

Quinlan, E., and Dickinson, H. D. "The Emerging Public Health System in Canada." In *Health, Illness, and Health Care in Canada.* 4th ed., edited by B. Singh Bolaria and H. D. Dickinson, 42–55. Toronto, ON: Nelson Education, 2009.

Ramzy, A., and L. Yang. "Tainted-Baby-Milk Scandal in China." *Time*, September 16, 2008. Retrieved January 8, 2014. http://www.time.com/time/world/article/0,85999,1841535,00.html.

Reidpath, D. D., and P. Allotey. "Measuring Global Inequity." *International Journal for Equity in Health* 6 (2007): 16. doi:10.1186/1475-9276-6-16.

Resnik, D. B. "The Distribution of Biomedical Research, Resources and International Justice." *Developing World Bioethics* 4, no. 1 (2004): 42–57.

Ridde, V., Mohindra, K. S., LaBossiere, F. "Driving the Global Public Health Research Agenda Forward by Promoting the Participation of Students and New Researchers." *Canadian Journal of Public Health* 99, no. 6 (2008): 460–65.

Rod, N. *Gov't Says Four Canadians Infected With Zika Virus after Travel.* Winnipeg, MB: Reuters, January 24, 2016. Retrieved January 30, 2016. http://www.reuters.com/article/us-health-zika-canada-idUSKCN0V722S.

Ruckert, A., and R. Labonté. "The Global Financial Crisis and Health Equity: Early Experiences From Canada." *Global Health* 10, no. 1 (January 6, 2014): 2.

Salvation Army. *Canada Speaks. Exposing Myths About the 150,000 Canadians Living on the Street.* Toronto, ON: Author, May, 2011. ISBN:978-88-8912-965-4.

Seear, M. *An Introduction to International Health.* 2nd ed. Toronto, ON: Canadian Scholars' Press Inc., 2007.

Skolnik, R. *Essentials of Global Health.* Sudbury, MA: Jones and Bartlett, 2008.

Spasoff, R. *A Pan-Canadian Strategy for Public Health Workforce Education 2005. Pan-Canadian Public Health Human Resources Committee (PPHHRC).* Ottawa, ON: Public Health Agency of Canada, 2005. Retrieved December 8, 2011. http://www.phac-aspc.gc.ca/php-psp/pan_canadian_strategy_for_public_health_workforce_education_e.pdf.

———. *Global Health 101.* 2nd ed. Mississauga, ON: Jones & Bartlett Learning Canada, 2012.

Strully, K. W. "Job Loss and Health in the US Labor Market." *Demography* 46 (2009): 221–46.

Stuckler, D., S. Basu, M. Suhrcke, A. Coutts, and M. McKee. "Effects of the 2008 Recession on Health: A First Look at European Data." *Lancet* 378, no. 9786 (2011): 124–25.

Taylor, S. "Wealth, Health and Equity: Convergence to Divergence in Late 20th Century Globalization." *British Medical Bulletin* 91, no. 1 (2009): 29–48.

The Joint Task Group on Public Health Human Resources. *Advisory Committee on Health Delivery and Human Services. Advisory Committee on Population Health and Health Security. Building the Public Health Workforce for the 21st Century. A Pan-Canadian Framework for Public Health Human Resources Planning.* Ottawa, ON: Public Health Agency of Canada, 2005. Retrieved December 8, 2011. http://www.phac-aspc.gc.ca/php-psp/pdf/building_the_public_health_workforce_fo_%20the-21stc_e.pdf.

The Statistical Portal. "Global Prices for a Big Mac in July 2015, by Country (in U.S. Dollars): Statistics and Studies From More Than 18,000 Sources." *The Statistical Portal,* 2015. Retrieved January 27, 2016. http://www.statista.com/statistics/274326/big-mac-index-global-princes-for-a-big-mac/.

Thomas, S. A., and W. J. Bartfay. "Global Health Perspectives for Community Health Nurses." In *Community Health Nursing: Caring in Action,* edited by J. E. Hitchcock, P. E. Schubert, S. A. Thomas, and W. J. Bartfay, 143–72. Toronto, ON: Nelson Education, 2010.

Tough, J., and W. Preece. *Return on Investment.* Toronto, ON: TD Wealth, August, 2015.

Tulchinsky, T. H., and M. J. Bickford. "Are Schools of Public Health Needed to Address Public Health Workforce Development in Canada for the 21st Century?" *Canadian Journal of Public Health* 97 (2006): 248–50.

UNICEF. *Innocenti Research Centre. Innocenti Report Card 10: Measuring Child Poverty. New League Tables on Child Poverty in the Worlds Rich Countries.* Florence, Italy: Author, 2012.

UNICEF Canada. *UNICEF Report Card 11: Child Well-Being in Rich Countries.* Toronto, ON: Author, 2013. Retrieved January 8, 2014. http://www.unicef.ca/en/discover/article/child-well-being-in-rich-countries-a-comprehensive-overview.

United Nations. *General Assembly August 12, 2014: Report of the Open Working Group of the General Assembly on Sustainable Development Goals.* New York: United Nations, 2014. Retrieved January 21, 2016. http://www.un.org.ga/search/view_doc.asp?symbol=A/68/970&Lang-E.

———. *Millennium Development Goals Indicator.* New York: United Nations, 2008. Retrieved December 8, 2011. http://unstats.un.org/unsd/mdg/Host.aspx?Content=Indicators/OfficialList.htm.

———. *We Can End Poverty: Millennium Development Goals and Beyond 2015.* New York: United Nations, 2013. Retrieved January 3, 2014. http://www.un.org/millenniumgoals/.

United Nations Food and Agricultural Organization. *Global Food Losses and Food Waste: Extent, Causes and Prevention.* Rome, Italy: Author, 2011. ISBN:978-92-5-107205-9. Retrieved January 25, 2016. http://www.fao.org/docrep/014/mb060e/mb060e00.pdf.

United Nations Development Program. *Sustainable Development Goals (SDGs)*. New York: United Nations, 2015. Retrieved January 21, 2016. http://www.undp.org/content/undp/en/home/mdgoverview/post-2015-development-agenda.

———. *The Millennium Development Goals Report 2009*. New York: United Nations, 2009.

United Nations Secretary-General. *Keeping the Promise: A Forward-Looking Review to Promote an Agreed Action Agenda to Achieve the Millennium Development Goals by 2015*. New York: United Nations, 2010. Retrieved January 16, 2016. http://www.un.org/en/mdg/summit2010.

United States Bureau of the Census. *Statistics for Industry Groups and Industries: 2005. Annual Survey of Manufacturers*. Washington, DC: Author, 2006.

Vidal, J. "Global Warming Causes 300,000 Deaths a Year, Says Kofi Annan thinktank." *The Guardian,* May 29, 2009. Retrieved January 3, 2014. http://www.theguardian.com/environment/2009/may/29/1.

Walraven, G. *Health and Poverty: Global Health Problems and Solutions*. Sterling, VA: Stylus, 2010.

Wang, H., L. Dwyer-Lindgren, K. T. Lofgren, J. K. Rajaratnam, J. R. Marcus, A. Levin-Rector, C. E. Levitz, A. D. Lopez, and C. J. Murray. "Age-Specific and Sex Sex-Specific Mortality in 187 Countries, 1970–2010: A Systematic Analysis for the Global Burden of Disease Study 2010." *Lancet* 380, no. 9859 (December 15, 2012): 2071–94. doi:10.1016/S0140-6736(12)61719-X.

West, L. "Global Warming Leads to 150,000 Deaths Every Year. Infectious Diseases and Death Rates Rise Along Global Temperatures." *About News,* 2015. Retrieved December 8, 2015. http://environment.about.com/od/global warmingandhealth/a/gw_deaths.htm.

Westhead, R. *Half of World's Food Wasted, Report Finds. Global Effort Needed to End Harmful Trend*, A1 and A4. Toronto, ON: The Toronto Star, January 11, 2013.

———. *Leprosy Making a Quiet Comeback*, A11. Toronto, ON: Toronto Star, May 30, 2011.

Wild, S., G. Roglie, A. Green, R. Sicree, and H. King. "Global Prevalence of Diabetes Estimates for 2000 and Projections for 2003." *Diabetes Care* 27 (2004): 1047–53.

Wilson, J. "Facing an Uncertain Climate." *Annuals of Internal Medicine* 146, no. 2 (January, 2007): 153–56.

Wimo, A., and M. Prince. *Alzheimer's Disease International World Alzheimer's Report 2010: The Global Impact of Dementia*. London: Alzheimer's Disease International, September, 2010.

Wolfensohn, J. D. "A Partnership for Development and Peace." An Address at the Woodrow Wilson International Center on March 6, 2002. Washington, DC, March 6, 2002.

Wong, G. "China's Dairy Farmers Fret as Milk Scandal Grows." *International Herald Tribune,* September 22, 2008. Associated Press. Retrieved January 8, 2014. http:www.iht.com/articles/ap/2008/09/21/asia/AS-China-Dairy-Farmersphp.

Woodward, D., N. Drager, R. Beaglehold, and D. Lipson. "Globalization and Health: A Framework for Analysis and Action." *Bulletin of the World Health Organization* 79 (2001): 875–81.

World Bank. *World Development Report 1993: Investing in Health*. New York: Oxford University Press, 1993.

World Health Organization. *Declaration of Alma Alta: International Conference on Primary Health Care, Alma-Ata, USSR, 6-12*. Europe: WHO, 1978. Retrieved December 8, 2011. http://www.who.int/topics/primary_health_care/en/.

———. *Guidelines for the Development of Measures to Combat Counterfeit Drugs*. Geneva, Switzerland: Author, 1999.

———. *The World Health Report 2000*. Geneva, Switzerland: Author, 2000.

———. *Core Health Indicators*. Geneva, Switzerland: WHO, 2004a. http://www3.who.int/whosis/core/core_select_process.cfm.

———. *World Health Organization, World Health Report 2001: Mental Health: New Understanding, New Hope*. Geneva, Switzerland: WHO, 2004b.

———. *Bangkok Charter of Health Promotion. From the 6th Global Conference on Health Promotion, Bangkok, Thailand, August 11, 2005*. Geneva, Switzerland: WHO, 2005a. Retrieved December 8, 2011. http://www.who.int/health promotion/conferences/6gchp/hpr_050829_%20BCHP.pdf.

———. *International Health Regulations 2005*. 2nd ed. Geneva, Switzerland: WHO, 2005b. Retrieved December 8, 2011. http://www.who.int/ihr/9789241596664/en/index.html.

———. *Global Burden of Disease Database*. Geneva, Switzerland: WHO, 2006a.

———. *Neurological Disorders: Public Health Challenges*. Geneva, Switzerland. Author, 2006b. Retrieved January 10, 2014. http://www.who.int/mental_health/neurology/nurodiso/en/.

_____. *World Health Organization, Global Tuberculosis Control: Surveillance, Planning, Financing.* WHO Report. Geneva, Switzerland: WHO, 2006c.

_____. *Control of Neglected Tropical Diseases (NTD).* Geneva, Switzerland: Author, 2007. http:www.who.int/neglected_diseases/en/.

_____. *Promoting Health and Development: Closing the Implementation Gap. The 7th Global Conference on Health Promotion.* Geneva, Switzerland: WHO, 2009. Retrieved December 8, 2011. http://www.who.int/mediacentre/events/meetings/7gchp/en/index.html.

_____. *Pandemic Preparedness.* Geneva, Switzerland: WHO, 2010. Retrieved December 9, 2011. http://www.who.int/csr/disease/influenza/pandemic.

_____. *World Health Statistics 2011.* Geneva, Switzerland: Author, June, 2011. ISBN:978-92-4-156419-9.

_____. *Global Health Observatory (GHO): Mortality and Global Burden of Disease (GBD).* Geneva, Switzerland: Author, 2012a. Retrieved January 12, 2012. http://www.who.intohlo/mortality_burden_disease/en/.

_____. *Millennium Development Goals: Progress Towards the Health-Related Millennium Development Goals* (Fact Sheet No. 20). Geneva, Switzerland: Author, May, 2012b.

_____. *2014 Ebola Virus Disease (EVD) Outbreak in West Africa.* Geneva, Switzerland: WHO, 2014a. Retrieved January 29, 2016. http://www.who.int/update/20140421/en/.

_____. *Ebola Virus Disease Fact Sheet No. 103.* Geneva, Switzerland: WHO, 2014b. Retrieved January 29, 2016. http://www.who.int/mediacentre/factsheets/fs103/en/.

_____. *Framework Convention on Tobacco Control (FCTC).* Geneva, Switzerland: Author, 2014c. Retrieved January 8, 2014. http://www.who.int/fctc/en/.

_____. *The Ottawa Charter for Health Promotion. First International Conference on Health Promotion. November 21, 1986. Ottawa.* Geneva, Switzerland: Author, 2014d. Retrieved January 4, 2014. http://www.who.int/healthpromotion/conferences/previous/ottawa/en/index4.html.

_____. *Ebola Virus Outbreak: Guidance for Survivors.* Geneva, Switzerland: WHO, 2016a. Retrieved February 1, 2016. http://www.who.int/scr.disease/ebola/en.

_____. *Health Topics: Zika Virus.* Geneva, Switzerland: WHO, 2016b. Retrieved February 1, 2016. http://www.who.int/topics/zika.en.

World Health Organization and UNICEF. *World Malaria Report, 2005.* Geneva, Switzerland: Author, 2005.

World Health Organization (WHO) World Mental Health Survey Consortium. "Prevalence, Severity, and Unmet Need for Treatment of Mental Disorders in the World Health Organization World Mental Health Survey." *JAMA* 291 (2004): 2581–90.

Zeckhauser, R., and D. Shepard. "Where Now for Saving Lives?" *Law and Contemporary Problems* 40, no. b (1976): 5–45.

Zhu, C. "2 Executed Over Baby Formula Scandal." *China Daily*, November 25, 2009. Retrieved January 8, 2014. http://www.chinadaily.com.cn/bizchina/2009-11/25/content_9046968.htm.

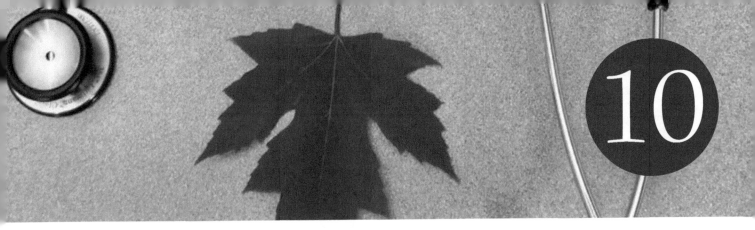

Program Planning and Evaluation in Public Health

This is a story of four people named Everybody, Somebody, Anybody, and Nobody. There was an important job to be done and Everybody was sure that Somebody would do it. Anybody could have done it, but Nobody did it. Somebody got angry about that because it was Everybody's job. Everybody thought Anybody could do it, but Nobody realized that Everybody wouldn't do it. It ended up that Everybody blamed Somebody when actually Nobody accused Anybody.

—Anonymous

Learning Objectives

After completion of this chapter, the student will be able to:

- Explain the importance of evidence-informed health-related information for program planning and evaluation;
- Discuss the growing importance and use of web-based technologies and platforms to plan for, develop, implement, and disseminate information related to a variety of primary health care programs in Canada and globally;
- Define and differentiate between the terms program planning, strategic (allocative) planning, operational (activity) planning, program evaluation, formative evaluation, process evaluation, and summative evaluation;
- Recognize and describe the importance of including key stakeholders in program planning and evaluation processes;
- Describe the significance of program planning and evaluation by health care professionals, workers, and policy makers in Canada and internationally;
- Describe how program logic models may be utilized by health care professionals and workers to assess the impact of public health programs in Canada and abroad;
- Describe and differentiate between the eight critical steps of the program planning and evaluation process;

(Continued)

(Continued)

- List and describe how health services research (HSR) and outcomes research can be utilized by public health care professionals, workers, and policy makers to monitor, evaluate and/or improve primary health care services and initiatives in diverse populations across the lifespan; and
- List and discuss ethical considerations and principles related to program planning and evaluation for public health professionals and workers.

Core Competencies for public health addressed in Chapter 10

Core Competencies	Competency Statements
1.0 Public Health Sciences	1.1, 1.2, 1.3, 1.4, 1.5
2.0 Assessment and Analysis	2.2, 2.3, 2.4, 2.5, 2.6
3.0 Policy and Program Planning, Implementation, and Evaluation	3.1, 3.2, 3.3, 3.4, 3.5, 3.6, 3.7
4.0 Partnerships, Collaboration, and Advocacy	4.1, 4.2, 4.3, 4.4
5.0 Diversity and Inclusiveness	5.2
6.0 Communication	6.2, 6.3
7.0 Leadership	7.1, 7.2, 7.3, 7.4

Note: Please see the following document or web-based link for a detailed description of these specific competencies (Public Health Agency of Canada 2007a, http://www.phac-aspc.gc.ca/core_competencies or http://www.phac-aspc.gc.ca/php-psp/ccph-cesp/pdfs/cc-manual-eng090407.pdf).

Introduction

In all health care organizations and systems in Canada and globally, decisions are made as to how resources, health care personnel and technologies will be utilized to address projected health care needs in the future. With increasing scrutiny, demands for transparency and accountability of how public funds in Canada are being utilized, program planning, and evaluation are critical components to address current and emerging public health issues and challenges (Health Canada 2001; Public Health Agency of Canada 2008; Senate Subcommittee on Population Health 2009). Unfortunately, public health systems in Canada and internationally are under pressure "to do more with less," or "to do better with the same," and are increasingly being swayed to employ industrial or corporate models to guide health care reforms (Bartfay and Bartfay 2015). Public health professionals and workers must work in partnership with other health care providers, citizens, organizations, families, community stakeholders, and various levels of government during the program planning and evaluation process.

   Program planning and evaluation mirrors and complements the research process. Refer Chapter 5 for a detailed discussion of the critical nine steps of the research process. This chapter provides an overview of program planning and evaluation in public health. A framework for program planning and evaluation is presented to highlight the critical steps involved in this process which can be utilized to address a variety of current or emerging health issues and/or underlying social determinants of health. We shall begin with a discussion of how to access and develop web-based health programs and sites in our evolving technologically driven society in Canada. We shall then detail the formal processes involved in program planning and evaluation. We shall provide the reader with an overview of

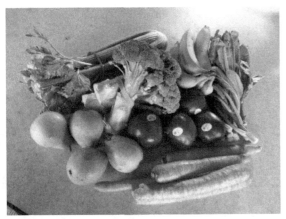
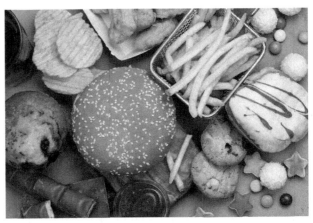

Source: Wally J. Bartfay

© Ekaterina Markelova/Shutterstock.com

Photo 10.1a and Photo 10.1b There is a strong body of empirical evidence which demonstrates that eating a variety of natural occurring fruits and vegetables (Photo 10.1a), as opposed to a variety of highly processed and nutritionally compromised foods (e.g., candy-bars), helps to maintain and promote good health across the lifespan in diverse cultures and societies globally.

health services research (HSR) and outcomes research. Lastly, we shall examine ethical principles and considerations when engaging in program planning and evaluation by public health professionals and workers.

Accessing and Developing Web-Based Health Programs and Sites

Evidence-informed public health (EIPH) is defined as "the process of distilling and disseminating the best available evidence from research, practice and experience and using that evidence to inform and improve public health policy and practice" (National Collaborating Centres for Public Health [NCCPH] 2011, 1). The **evidence** may include, but is not limited to, published research reports from a variety of disciplines; current best practice guidelines; existing legislations and policies; observations and experiences; and both expert and lay opinions and perspectives for all stakeholders concerned (Bartfay and Bartfay 2015). For example, it is critical to take into account the ability and willingness of all stakeholders to mutually agree that the evidence being accessed, graded, and employed is, in fact, relevant to their unique health situation, goal or need when planning and implementing various public health interventions, programs or when formulating policies. Similarly, it is critical to recognize cultural, moral, ethical, spiritual, financial, and political issues and values that may impact practice or public health policy decisions. Refer Chapter 1 for a detailed discussion on EIPH, types of evidence that may be employed by public health professionals and workers, and guidelines related to determining their significance, suitability and applicable.

The retrieval of EIPH-related knowledge and its pursuit is taking place within an ever widening network of both online and offline resources. Indeed, the availability, use, and access to the *world wide web* (WWW) and online resources and materials (e.g., peer-reviewed journals, conference proceedings, World Health Organization reports) have expanded exponentially during the past few decades globally (Bowen and Zwi 2005; Ciliska, Thomas, and Buffet 2008; Oxman, Lavis, and Fretheim 2007; Pach 2008). Web-based health-related sites are increasingly being accessed by health care professionals and workers and by the lay public (Rycroft-Malone 2008; Statistics Canada 2007, 2010a, 2010b). Indeed, 95% of youth are online every day, and in July 2010 Canada had the world's greatest number of Facebook users in proportion to its population; the United Kingdom was in second place; and the United States in third (CEFRIO 2010; Robinson and Robertson 2010).

The International Telecommunications Union (ICT 2011) reports that one-third of the world's population is online and 45% of Internet users are below the age 25. From the years 2006 to 2011, developing countries have increased their share of the world's total number of Internet users from 44% to 62%, respectively. By mid-2011, 90% of countries had 2G services available and a total of 159 countries have launched 3G commercial Internet services with the total number of active mobile broadband subscriptions of almost 1.2 billion individuals (ICT 2011). According to Internet World Stats (IWS 2012), 44.8% of Internet users were from Asia; 21.5% for Europe; 11.4% for North America; 10.4% from Latin America and the Caribbean; 7% from Africa; 3.7% from the Middle East; and 1.0% for Oceania and Australia. In comparison to December 31, 2000 figures (N = 360,985,492), this represents a global growth of 566.4% (N = 2,405,518,376) in Internet usage for the year 2012 (IWS 2012).

Primary public health services and their delivery can be enhanced through the use of innovative and interactive telehealth or e-health interventions that are specifically tailored to meet the client's health care needs. **Telehealth** or **e-health** is defined as "the use of telecommunications technologies and electronic information to exchange health care information and to provide and support services such as long distance clinical healthcare to clients" (Hebda and Czar 2013, 505). The online world has the empowering potential for lay individuals and public health professionals and workers alike in regards to finding health information that is contextually relevant; to identify peers or experts in various health-related fields; to locate support groups online;

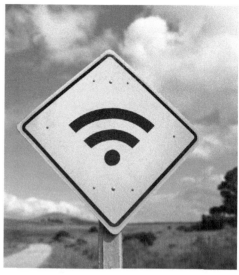

Source: Wally J. Bartfay

Photo 10.2 Access to and use of available hotspot WIFI hubs has been growing exponentially even in remote areas of the world. According to the Internet World Stats Usage and Population Statistics (2017), 49.6% of the population of the world had internet penetration (% total population), and the internet penetration was 88.1% for North America; 77.4% for Europe; 59.6% for Latin America and the Caribbean; 56.7% for the Middle East; 45.2% for Asia, and 27.7% for Africa.

and to plan for and engage in preventative actions for change and health promotion (Eysenbach 2008; Flicker, Maley, and Ridgley 2008; Kreps and Neuhasuer 2010; Robinson and Robertson 2010). For example, the Public Health Agency of Canada (2006) has developed a portal for knowledge exchange entitled the "Canadian Best Practices Portal for Health Promotion and Chronic Disease Prevention" (see link: http://cbpp-pcpe.phac-aspc.gc.ca or http://www.phac.gc.ca/cbpp). The aims of this portal include the enhancement of knowledge exchange between public health care professionals, and it also serves as a central access point for EIPH. This portal serves as a convenient and single point of quick access to EIPH practices for a variety of public health care professionals in Canada. The portal consists of a searchable database of community-level interventions, resources to help with public health planning, chronic disease prevention and health promotion goals, and a user-friendly catalogue of best practice systematic reviews of the scientific literature. The portal is constantly being updated and consists of over 255 interventions and resources. This portal is increasingly being accessed and utilized by various public health care professionals for program planning and evaluation. Janis Letterman, for example, is a member of a national team for the *Victoria Order of Nurses* (VON) for the management of chronic disease prevention and its management who described her experience with the portal as follows:

Having a centralized, credible source of information was very helpful in developing our overarching chronic disease prevention and management program," Janis notes. Now she tends to refer to the Portal at the beginning of planning for a project and in responding to requests for proposals for project funding. "I find the (population health approach) organizing frame-work very helpful. It's a comprehensive, but simply place to start, helping me identify what I may be missing in program planning.

—Ontario Health Promotion E-Bulletin 2010, 2

Public health care professionals can also register to complete skills enhancement modules online (see http://www.phac-aspc.gc.ca/sehs-acss/index-eng.phpl).

The *NurseONE/INF-Fusion* portal was developed by the Canadian Nurses Association (2006), and is an interactive Web 2.0 resource designed to assist nurses to connect with their colleagues nationally, assist in their professional development, and as a central access point to access credible and current informational resources and tools to support evidence-informed nursing practice in Canada (see link: http://www.cna-nurses.ca/CNA/ nursing/portal/about/default_easpx). The *Effective Public Health Practice Program* provides numerous links to systematic reviews and summaries of health research and practice outcomes (see link: http://www.ephpp.ca/). In addition, the *National Collaborating Centre of Methods and Tools* (NCCMT) provides resources and information about a variety of knowledge translation approaches and tools relevant to the practice of public health in Canada and globally for both practitioners and students (see link: http://www.nccmt.ca).

The development and use of mobile information and communication technologies (ICTs) have had considerable effects on our daily lives affecting how we work, communicate and socially interact. The term "ICTs" includes a variety of computer-based technology systems and applications for collecting, sending, retrieving and processing information, data and communications. Mobile ICTs are widespread and prevalent in a variety of setting including public schools, universities and colleges, businesses, restaurants, hospitals, retirement homes, community and sporting centres, shopping malls, airports and private homes (Petrič, Petrovčič, and Vehovar 2011; Pew Research Centre 2014; Thomée 2012). Most individuals use mobile technologies as functional tools in everyday life and many cannot imagine living in a world without daily access to the Internet for work, play, shopping, banking, entertainment or educational purposes. Canadians on average have 4.5 connected devices in their households; 52% watch television while using their mobile devices, and 51% sleep with their mobile devices next to their bed, based on a national online survey conducted by Harris/Deima involving 1,009 individuals aged 16 and over who owned a smartphone or tablet device (Christensen 2013; Rogers Communication 2013).

The availability and use of the Internet has without doubt brought about a variety of conveniences to our modern life including doing university courses online, online banking and shopping, accessing information related to a variety of topics, and as a means of socializing to name but a few applications. Canadians are amongst the most active Internet users globally, and spend on average approximately 43.5 hours per week online, compared to the global average of 23.1 hours (Canadian Broadcasting Corporation [CBC] 2011). Hence, public health care professionals and workers need to be aware of these trends and develop public health promotion programs and campaigns with these in mind. Comparatively, the United States ranked second with 35.5 hours online (CBC 2011). The percentage of individuals using the Internet in Canada has grown from 51.3% in 2000 to 85.8% in 2013 (ICT Data and Statistics Division 2014). Similarly, the number of fixed (wired) broadband subscriptions has increased from 1,410,932 in 2000 to 11,709,900 in 2013 (ICT Data and Statistics Division 2014). Kende (2014) reports that there were over 1 billion Internet hosts in 2013 and by 2015 there will be over 3 billion regular Internet uses globally.

According to the *Internet Use Survey*, 69% of individuals in Canada searched for medical or health-related information using the Internet (Statistics Canada 2010a, 2010b). Similarly, results from the US-based *Pew Internet Survey* conducted between 2002 and 2008 revealed that between 75% and 83% of Internet users searched for health information online (Fox and Jones 2009). Bennett and Glasgow (2009) conducted a review of the Internet as a delivery platform for public health interventions, and their review showed potential and positive results for the dissemination of primary and secondary interventions for diverse populations. Lüchtenberg et al. (2008) reported that 82% of the 139 Internet-based health information sites evaluated were not fully accessible to the visually impaired.

A random survey of 2038 adults in the Pew Internet Project found that adults who were sick or disabled were more likely to use the Internet, and searched for more online health information in comparison to healthy adults surveyed (Goldner 2006). Hesse et al. (2005) found that although study participants viewed physicians as the most credible source for obtaining health information, 48.6% of respondents reported using the Internet first, while only 10.9% consulted with a physician first. Underhill and McKeown (2008) found that higher-educated women and those with higher incomes were more likely to search for health-related information online, while young adult men were the least likely to perform Internet-based searches for health-related information.

The Internet and newer Web 2.0 platforms (e.g., social networking sites, video sharing and mobile e-technologies, wikis, blogs) are slowly changing public health practice settings and scope, as well as the public's expectations and capabilities to make evidence-informed decisions related to their health and well-being. In fact, more than 83% of Canadians regularly use the Internet and approximately 70% of users search online for health-related information (Statistics Canada 2010a, 2010b). The challenges for employing online web-based prevention and health promotion in virtual settings are to provide a balanced and targeted communication; provide information to diverse populations and interests across the lifespan; and ensure quality control checks related to content with collaborative filtering of links towards high-quality EIPH. Hence, the key public health challenge in these virtual settings is to actively engage individuals and public health professionals and workers, and to offer empowering health information, resources and networks. With this in mind, there is little doubt that the online world is increasing becoming a major setting in Canada and globally where *people live, love, work and play.* Access to and the availability of high-quality and reputable health information on the Internet provides individuals, families and health care professionals and workers with valuable information to make informed decisions about their health (Kivits 2009; Korp 2006; Mehra, Merkel, and Bishop 2004; Public Health Agency of Canada 2006). However, a growing number of Internet users have expressed concern about the claims made and credibility of health information obtained from certain Internet sites. Moreover, comfort and familiarity with the Internet does not necessarily guarantee the ability to obtain credible online evidence-informed health-related information (Eysenbach and Kohler 2002; Goldner 2006; Hess et al. 2005; Rice 2006). For example, Changrani and Gany (2005) investigated the Internet behaviour and use of sixty English-speaking Caribbean women in New York City, and findings from this study revealed that Internet users did not know the differences among cancer websites with domain names such as .edu, .gov, .com or .net.

Health care professionals and workers and the individuals, families or communities they serve can help to determine the credibility of online web-based sites by accessing the health-related information provided based on the *Health on the Net Foundation (HON) Code* (2009). Table 10.1 shows the eight principles of the HON Code (2009). Individuals may also submit a URL to the *Worldwide Online Reliable Advice to Patients*

Table 10.1 The Health on the Net Foundation (HON) Code of Conduct for Medical and Health Websites (2009)

Specific Principles	Criteria and Comments
1. Authority	Any medical or health advice provided and hosted on this site will only be given by medically trained and qualified health professionals unless a clear statement is made that a piece of advice is from a non-medically qualified individual or organization.
2. Complementarity	The information provided on this site is designed to support, not replace, the relationship that exists between a patient/site visitor and his or her existing physician.
3. Privacy	Confidentiality of data relating to individual clients and visitors to a medical/health website, including their identity is respected by this website. The website owners undertake to honour or exceed the legal requirements of medical/health information privacy that apply in the country and state where the website and mirror sites are located.
4. Attribution	Where appropriate, information contained on this site will be supported by clear references to source data and, where possible, have specific HTML links to that data. The date when a clinical page was last modified will be clearly displayed (e.g., at the bottom of the page).

Specific Principles	Criteria and Comments
5. Justifiability	Any claims relating to the benefits/performance of a specific treatment, commercial product or service will be supported by appropriate balanced evidence in the manner outlined in Principle 4.
6. Transparency	The designers of this website will be clearly identified, including the identities of commercial and non-commercial organizations that have contributed funding, services or material for the site.
7. Financial disclosure	Support for this website will be clearly identified, including the identities of commercial and non-commercial organizations that have contributed funding, services or material for this site.
8. Honesty in advertising and editorial policy	If advertising is a source of funding, it will be clearly stated. A brief description of the advertising policy adopted by the website owners will be displayed on the site. Advertising and other promotional material will be presented to viewers in a manner and context that facilitates differentiation between it and the original material created by the institution operating the site.

Source: Adapted from the Health on the Net Foundation (HON 2009).

and Individuals (WRAPIN 2007) service (http://www.wrapin.org) to determine if the health-related website is accredited or trustworthy in nature.

The *World Wide Web Consortium* (W3C 2009) is an international organization that provides the standardization and operation for the web and helps to ensure the universal and equitable access to information for all, including individuals with disabilities (see W3C—http://www.w3.org). The W3C has created accessibility standards for web content designers and developers, including the *Web Content Accessibility Guidelines* (WCAG), which was last updated in 2008 (Caldwell, Slating, and Vanderheiden 2008). Similarly, the Treasury Board of Canada Secretariat (2007) has also developed guidelines to ensure accessibility to all Canadian government websites known as the *Common Look and Feel for the Internet* document. Refer Web-Based Resource Box 10.1 for further information related to how to access and evaluate the quality of online health-related information and resources for program planning and evaluation in public health.

The development, usability and easy access to web-based health information by health care professionals and workers and consumers of health information often relates to more than just the credibility and accuracy of the health information provided (Canadian Public Health Association 1999, 2010; Health Summit Working Group 2010). Indeed, readability of the text and materials provided on the website is a critical design aspect to convey health-related information to all potential users and health consumers. In fact, 7% of Anglophones and 18% of Francophones in Canada have not completed Grade 9, and 42% of the working-age population scored below the functional level on international prose literacy scales (Statistics Canada 2006, 2008). Reading experts suggest that the majority of the population prefers that written materials provided be at least three grades below the last grade completed, which is typically at the grade 5–6 level (Gottlieb and Rogers 2004; McLaughlin 1969). However, a study by Ache and Wallace (2009) found that health-related web-based materials were on average written at the grade 11 level with a range between grades 7 and 12.

Public health care professionals and workers who are either developing or recommending Internet-based websites for their clients can determine the readability of the site by using the *Simple Measure of Gobbledygook (SMOG) Readability Test,* (Gottlieb and Rogers 2004; McLaughlin 1969). Table 10.2 shows an adapted SMOG readability assessment tool which can be utilized by public health care professionals and workers to assess the readability of a website they are developing or one they may be recommending to their clients.

Web-Based Resource Box 10.1 How to access and evaluate the quality of online health related information and resources

Learning Resource	Website
Canadian Nurses Association, (2006). NurseONE, the Canadian Nurses portal This web-based resource box provides nurses with credible and reliable information to support their evidence-informed practice, managing their careers and connecting with colleagues and health care experts	http://www.cna-nurses.ca/ CNA/nursing/portal/about/ default_e.aspx
Canadian Public Health Association (2010). Plain language service and Canadian Public Health Association (1999). Directory of plain health information These websites by the PHAC provides public health care professionals and workers with so-called "user-friendly" hints related to health terms, conditions and how to write clear health goals and outcomes.	http://www.cpha.ca/en/ portals/h-l/resources http://www.cpha.ca/en/pls. aspx
Health on the Net Foundation. (2009). HON code of conduct (HOHcode) for medical and health Websites. Health on the Net Foundation This website describes how the HON seeks to promote and guide the deployment of useful and reliable online health information, and its appropriate and efficient uses.	http://www.hon.ch/HONcode/ Guidelines/guidelines.html
Public Health Agency of Canada (2006). The Canadian Best Practices Portal for health promotion and chronic disease prevention: About the portal This portal provides public health professionals and workers with resources and solutions to plan programs for promoting health and preventing diseases in their community.	http://cbpp-pcpe.phac-aspc-gc.ca
WRAPIN (2007). WRAPIN Project-IST-2001-33260 This website helps to determine the reliability of health-related documents by checking the ideas contained against established benchmarks, and enables users to determine the relevance of a given document from a page of search results.	http://www.wrapin.org

Table 10.2 The *Simple Measure of Gobbledygook (SMOG) Readability Assessment Tool*: Adapted for the Assessment for the Approximate Grade Level of Reading Skill for Health-Related Websites

Step 1: Sample selection	Select 30 sentences from the text material of the health-related Website: 10 consecutive sentences from the start, the middle, and the end of the material. A sentence is a complete idea with a period, question mark, a bulleted point, or both parts of a sentence with a colon included.
Step 2: Word count	Count the number of words with more than three syllables (polysyllabic) in the 30-sentence sample. Include all repetitions of a word, proper nouns, the full text of abbreviations and hyphenated words as one word.

Step 3: Short text conversion	For web-related documents of fewer than 30 sentences, multiply the number of polysyllabic words by a factor to simulate a sample of 30 sentences. For example, if the web document contained 15 sentences, the factor would be 30 divided by 15 to equal a factor of 2. For web documents of 24 sentences, the factor would be 30 divided by 24 to equal 1.25.
Step 4: Calculate	Determine the nearest square root of the number of words in the sample. A square root is a number multiplied by itself to equal a perfect square. For example, 8 multiplied by 8 (square root) equals 64 (perfect square). The number that is square root is usually between 3 and 15.
Add the constant "3" to the square root obtained in step 4	Example: A sample is assessed as having 86 polysyllabic words in 30 sentences. The nearest square root is 9 (9 times 9 equals 81). The constant of 3 is added to give an approximate reading level of 12, or more appropriately described as a reading level requiring the reading skills approximately at the grade 12 reading level.

Source: Adapted from McLaughlin (1969).

Similarly, Norman and Skinner (2006) have developed a reliable and valid scale to assess an individual's e-health literary based on their comfort level, knowledge and perceived skills at finding, evaluating and applying health information obtained. The reader can review this scale at http://www.jmir .org/2006/4/e27.

In addition to the above, the Canadian Public Health Association (PHAC 1999, 2010) has published the *Directory of Plain Language Health Information* to assist public health care professionals and workers to produce and publish clear and easily understood written materials for the public. These include the use of an active voice by stating the action first and by writing directly to the reader (i.e., you). For example: *You should eat five to ten fruits and vegetables per day* instead of *five to ten fruits and vegetables should be eaten every day*. The PHAC also recommends the use of short words and sentences and the replacement of technical or difficult words with simpler words (e.g., heart in place of cardiac); the use of bullets and boxes to highlight important points or information; to write instructions in the order in which you want them to be carried out; and to evaluate/test whatever you write with learners before you formalize them.

Interactivity is defined as a process where a user is an active participant in utilizing technology and for acquiring and engaging in the exchange of information (Bartfay and Bartfay 2015). When designing health-related websites, the use of graphics, diagrams, short video clips or props to illustrate concepts (e.g., what a serving of meat is in comparison to a deck of cards) will often help to clarify or reinforce text and to have a more professional and pleasing appearance in nature. Lastly, health-related websites that are interactive in nature may help to attract users and to monitor their progress (e.g., calculations of body mass index, calorie counters or self-report charts and graphs, and chat rooms) (Ferney and Marshall 2006; Stout, Villegas, and Kim 2001; Suggs and McIntyre 2009; Yasnoff et al. 2000). Research Focus Box 10.1 provides an example of how Canadian youth in Ontario are accessing and employing online health-related resources and information, and some of their major concerns related to issues of privacy.

What Is Program Planning?

Planning is a critical component of public health which seeks to make informed decisions today based on the best available evidence to influence future health outcomes and directives based on competing resources and/or priorities (Bartfay and Bartfay 2015). Indeed, decisions on resource usage and allocation need to take into account the possibility of future changes to the health needs of your target population or community, the availability of qualified public health care professionals and workers, required financial and resource forecasts and technologies. Program planning and eval-

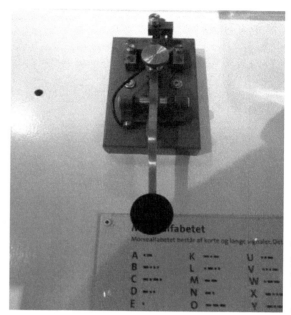

Photo 10.3 An early nineteenth century keypad receiver and sender for Morse code. The availability and means of communicating and sharing information globally has dramatically changed in the past few decades.

Source: Wally J. Bartfay

uation in public health are also critical components which ultimately seek to promote community development and health partnerships, build community capacity based on the available resources on hand, and to promote social justice for all residents of Canada. The Public Health Agency of Canada (2007a, p. 14) defines

---

Research Focus Box 10.1

How adolescents use technology for health information: Implications for health professionals from focus group studies

Study Aim/Rationale
Although the use of the Internet and web-based resources has increased exponentially during the past decade, little is known about the use and forms of health-related information accessed by adolescent youth in Ontario, Canada. Accordingly, the aim of this present study was to assess how youth access and utilize Internet-based health resources.

Methodology/Design
Convenience sampling was employed to determine what forms of health-related information were being accessed by 210 youth. The youths were from a variety of socioeconomic and cultural and geographical backgrounds including Indigenous youth and street teens. Results from a total of twenty-seven focus groups in different locations in the province of Ontario, Canada, were examined by the researchers.

Major Findings
Based on the findings from the focus groups, the most common health-related topics searched were specific diseases or medical conditions (67%); body image and nutrition (63%); violence and personal safety (59%); sexual health and sexually transmitted infections (STIs) (56%) and mental health issues (22%).

Implications for Public Health

These findings suggest that youth (teens) in Ontario are concerned about privacy issues when accessing Internet-based health resources. Youth also expressed concern about the difficulty in locating specific health-related information or answers to specific questions they had. Public health care professionals and workers should encourage privacy when youth are accessing Internet-based health resources, and teach youth various search strategies that will help them to locate and access specific health-related information in a more effective manner employing credible websites. The use of technology may provide an effective vehicle for building collaborative partnerships between youth in Ontario and various health care professionals and workers through the identification of common concerns and issues.

Source: Skinner, Biscope, and Goldberg (2003).

the concept of **social justice** as a society that gives individuals and groups fair treatment and an equitable share of the benefits of society. In this context, social justice is based on the concepts of human rights and equity where all groups and individuals are entitled to important rights such as health protection and minimal standards of income. One of the major goals of public health is to minimize preventable death and disability for all residents in Canada, and this goal is integral to social justice. The specific objectives of Health Canada are as follows:

- Prevent and reduce risks to individual health and the overall environments;
- Promote healthier lifestyles;
- Ensure high-quality health services that are efficient and accessible;
- Integrate renewal of the health care system with longer term plans in the areas of prevention, health promotion, and protection;
- Reduce health inequalities in Canadian society; and
- Provide health information to help Canadians make informed decisions (Public Health Agency of Canada 2007a, 3–4).

Program planning is defined as an organized and structured systemic decision-making process which attempts to meet specific primary health care aims or objectives through the application of currently available, and competing or needed resources in the future based on identified priorities or projected needs (Bartfay and Bartfay 2015). The growth of multidrug-resistant strains of tuberculosis (TB) seen in certain immigrant populations, and the potential spread of diseases carried by mosquitoes (e.g., West Nile Virus) in Canada due to climate change, are salient examples. Budgen, Cameron, and Bartfay (2010) note that an analogy can be made between planning a public health program and creating an architectural design for a building. Indeed, the more carefully the architect consults with the stakeholders for whom the building is being constructed, the greater the likelihood that the building will be satisfactory to all. The more clearly specified the vision of that which is wanted, the more likely the vision will be realized. The more attention the architect pays to the physical and social environments where the building will to be located, the more likely the building will be appreciated and compatible with the environment, and viewed as an overall positive addition to the neighbourhood. This analogy is much the same in regards to program planning and evaluation in public health (Bartfay and Bartfay 2015; Budgen, Cameron, and Bartfay 2010).

Strategic or Allocative Planning

Strategic or **allocative planning** is defined as an open and transparent formalized decision-making process which seeks to determine which health care needs should be addressed in accordance with the available resources and closely resembles policy making (Bartfay and Bartfay 2015). The establishment of health care needs or priorities may be situational (e.g., aging population) or reactive in nature (e.g., SARS, Avian flu pandemic).

For example, in April of 2009, a novel strain of influenza (H1N1) was recognized in Mexico, which resulted in a cluster of illness with the potential to become a deadly pandemic (Public Health Agency of Canada 2009). On June 11, 2009, the World Health Organization (WHO) raised the pandemic alert level to 6, which indicated that the H1N1 virus was rapidly spreading from human to human globally. The WHO reported that as of July 2009, there were almost 100,000 confirmed cases worldwide and

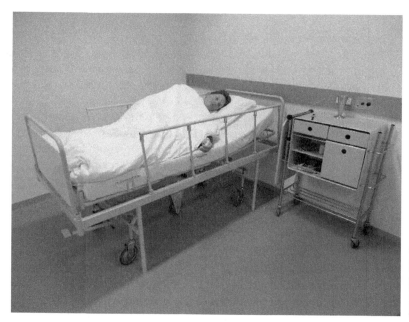

Source: Wally J. Bartfay

Photo 10.4 During the 2009 A/H1N1 pandemic, there were 428 deaths and 8,678 hospitalizations in Canada (PHAC 2010).

500 deaths, including twenty five in Canada (Canadian Institutes of Health Research, Rx & D Health Research Foundation, and Canadian Food Inspection Agency 2009). Consequently, many nations declared this to be a global pandemic and various public health initiatives were quickly considered and implemented (e.g., tracking and surveillance, primary prevention measures such proper handwashing and the development of vaccines). The overall goals of the *Canadian Pandemic Influenza Plan* were to minimize serious illness, overall deaths and social disruption associated with this pandemic. We must also be cognizant of the fact that all the decisions regarding how public health priorities are identified and set often entail ethical, sociopolitical or value-laden aspects and tensions (Bartfay and Bartfay 2015). Indeed, health care systems in Canada often reflect each of the provinces' and territories' unique political and social conditions, health challenges and aspirations and willingness to address these current or emerging issues and concerns.

Operational or Activity Planning

Operational or **activity planning** is defined as a formalized decision-making process which focuses on the implementation of plans based on detailed time frames (Bartfay and Bartfay 2015). For many planning systems, both short- and long-term planning outcomes may be identified. Short periods are typically a few months to a year, whereas a period of five years is employed as the standard time frame for long-term planning (Green 2007; Green, Collins, and Mirzoev 2012). Short-term planning outcomes are the immediately apparent results of the program, such as a community-based immunization campaign to prevent the spread of a potentially life-threatening virus. The long-term planning outcomes reflect the ultimate goals of the program. For example, building the clinical knowledge base of health care professionals (e.g., public health nurses, nurse practitioners, family physicians) and youth workers in remote First Nations communities related to suicide over a period of 12–18 months would be an example of a short-term planning outcome. Reducing the incidence of attempted and successful suicides in this target population over a five-year period would be an example of a long-term planning outcome.

Unfortunately, planning in public health often does not have a good reputation due to a lack of implementation of plans or the failure of ineffective or insufficient plans. The reasons for these failures vary, but frequently include a failure to involve and consult key stakeholders such as community members who will access these proposed services; rigid top-down bureaucratic centralist processes; a failure to do a needs assessment; access issues; budgetary constraints; a variety of sociopolitical reasons; and the lack of formalized program outcome or impact evaluations (Green 2007; Green, Collins, and Mirzoev 2012; Victora et al. 2012). Another criticism of planning in public health involves the feasible issue in periods of social, environmental, economic or political uncertainty or instability (e.g., minority governments, growing provincial/territorial health care deficits, global recession, climate changes and extreme weather, bioterrorism). Nonetheless, it may also be argued that planning is a mechanism for dealing with these noted uncertainties by highlighting priorities or groups with needs (e.g., Indigenous with diabetes) and/ or trends (e.g., aging population), and for developing a strategic plan to address these projected gaps or needs.

What Is Program Evaluation?

Program evaluation is defined as a formalized ongoing and dynamic process to monitor, assess and refine public health program activities and interventions and to identify gaps or actual or potential flaws in the original program design and implementation (Bartfay and Bartfay 2015). Although governments and non-governmental organizations in Canada and abroad spend literally billions of dollars annually on health programs which seek to restore, maintain and/or improve health outcomes in diverse populations across the lifespan, there is a growing realization that few of these initiatives have been formally evaluated (Evaluation Gap Working Group 2006; Oxman et al. 2010). Moreover, current interests in so called "results-based financing" for health outcomes is increasing the pressure on public and private health funders and implementers to carry out formal program impact evaluations (Victora et al. 2012; World Bank 2010).

Evaluation is best understood as a process ultimately intended to determine the worth of something new, presumably in comparison with some current norm or standard of *goodness* (Bartfay and Bartfay 2015; Budgen, Cameron, and Bartfay 2011). For example, comparisons for evaluation purposes may be conducted (Brinkerhoff et al. 1983; Herman, Morris, and Fitz-Gibbon 1987; Horne 1995; Hudson, Mayne, and Thomlison 1992; McKenzie and Jurs 1993; Van Marris and King 2007):

- To make comparisons with similar programs (e.g., comparing one Indigenous diabetes community health centre with another);
- To make comparisons with different programs (e.g., comparing weight gains of infants whose parents participated in community-based maternal health classes versus infants whose parents did not participate in these classes);
- To confirm and establish new clinical practice and outcome standards of care (e.g., best practice guidelines for stroke care by health care professionals such as nurses, physicians and rehabilitation therapists);
- To determine the impact of a public health program (e.g., the effectiveness of school-based safe-sex primary prevention programs in terms of condom use and sexually transmitted infections (STIs) rates in a region);
- To establish baselines and monitor trends associated with the delivery of various health programs and services and their associated costs (e.g., diagnostic imaging and laboratory tests);
- To justify a change in public health policy or legislation (e.g., legislation to ban smoking in public places such as workplaces, restaurants and shopping centres and its impact on mortality rates of lung cancer associated with chronic exposure to second-hand smoke);

- To evaluate access to health care services and programs (e.g., wait times for hip and knee replacement surgeries in rural versus urban communities in Newfoundland);
- To test a hypothesis related to the outcomes or delivery of a health program;
- To monitor and determine what needs to be changed to improve the overall effectiveness of a program and to ensure continuous quality improvement of program delivery and outcomes;
- To determine the efficiency and cost benefit of a public health program; and
- To determine what public health programs work for certain target groups, communities or entire populations, what doesn't work and why.

The United Nations Committee on Economic, Social and Cultural Rights (2002) suggests using four basic criteria to evaluate access to health: (a) availability (of functioning, staffed and stocked with supplies health care facilities); (b) accessibility (all individuals have affordable access to health care and health information and are not discriminated against in reference to their sex, age, marital status, physical ability or other characteristics); (c) acceptability (health care interventions and practices adhere to current standards of care and ethical practices that are confidential and respectful of cultural, gender and life cycle requirements); and (d) quality (of health facilities, goods and services utilized are scientifically appropriate and of good overall quality).

Appropriate comparisons can sometimes be a challenge in terms of comparing one public health program with another due to a variety of complex physical and socopolitical issues (e.g., transportation issues, availability of required infrastructures, access in remote communities, unemployment, availability of health professionals and specialists required to carried out the program). When comparisons cannot be made in a straightforward nature, creativity is required. For example, a so-called "tracer method" may be employed to evaluate the effectiveness of a health program (Bartfay and Bartfay 2015; Budgen, Cameron, and Bartfay 2010; Kaluzney and Veney 1999). This method is analogous to the use of a radioactive tracer used for clinical diagnostic purposes. The radioactive tracer is introduced into a vein via an intravenous device and is literally traced throughout the patient's body to assess the health of vessels, glands and/or entire organ systems. With this method, a health problem or issue is literally traced through a community or defined population, and variables such as the socioeconomic conditions present, changing demographics, health care access, availability of health care professionals and required infrastructures, and the like are examined.

Group Activity-Based Learning 10.1

Program planning and evaluation: What are the first steps to consider?
This Group Activity-Based Learning Box 10.1 highlights the importance of EIPH and decision-making for program planning and evaluation. Working in small groups of three to five students, discuss and answer the following questions:

1. What resources would you employ to find out about a current health challenge or issue in your community or region?

2. What information would you need to gather to address this health challenge or issue and why?

3. Which health care professionals and workers would you include on your program planning and evaluation team?

4. Which community partners and stakeholders would you involve in this process and why?

What Are the Types of Program Evaluations Conducted?

There are a variety of program evaluation types that can be broadly classified into the following three main categories, which are typically based on when the evaluations are being conducted and the type of information being collected (Bartfay and Bartfay 2015; Budgen, Cameron, and Bartfay 2010; Van Marris and King 2007): (a) formative, (b) process, and (c) summative. **Formative evaluations** focus on public health programs that are being planned and developed to help ensure that the stakeholder's needs are being addressed and that the program uses effective and appropriate structures, resources, facilities, procedures and/or materials (Bartfay and Bartfay 2015). Formative evaluations include such things as needs assessments; program logic models (detailed below); pretesting or piloting of program materials or educational resources; and a preliminary analysis to determine if your program's intended aims, goals or outcomes can be achieved, measured and evaluated. The term **structure** is often employed to describe all the resources and personnel required to support the health process. A **structural evaluation** is a common component of formative evaluations and involves the assessment of resources used in the program (Bartfay and Bartfay 2015).

Process evaluations focus on programs that have gone through the formal planning stages and have been implemented or are already underway and seek to answer the question "What health services are actually being delivered and to whom?" In reality, public health programs are rarely implemented exactly according to plans. Hence, a process evaluation focuses on the specific tasks and procedures necessary to carry out the program and includes a variety of activities, including (Bartfay and Bartfay 2015):

- implementation evaluations;
- quantity and quality of public primary health care services rendered and to whom;
- providing descriptions of what actually transpired while providing health services; and
- descriptions of the users who access the public primary health program.

Summative evaluations are carried out for health programs that are well underway or have been completed and can be used to asses short-, medium- or long-term aims, goals or desired outcomes of the program both intended and unintended. Summative evaluations seek to answer the questions "Did the health program make a difference?" and "Did the health program meet all of its aims and goals?"

The terms *outcome measures* and *impact measures* are often used interchangeably to describe the effects of a health program during summative evaluations; however, they are distinct

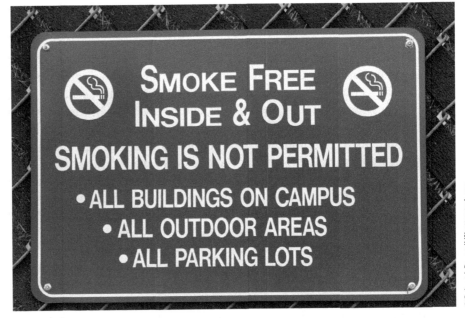

Photo 10.5 A sign prohibiting smoking near entrances and exits on a university campus. Signs such as this one and legislation banning smoking in workplaces, theaters, shopping centres, bars and restaurants in Canada are examples of a positive outcome measure which helps to protect non-smokers from the harmful effects associated with exposure to second-hand smoke in their environment.

entities (Borus, Buntz, and Tash 1982; Lorig et al. 1996; Van Marris and King 2007). An **outcome measure** evaluates what specifically occurred as the result of the health program being implemented in reference to its noted aims or goals (Bartfay and Bartfay 2015). Conversely, **impact measures** are used to evaluate the effect of the implemented health program on the users, stakeholders and implementers and specifically measure what changes (positive, negative or neutral) occurred as a result of the program (Bartfay and Bartfay 2015). Both outcome and impact measures require quantifiable indicators or measures. Indicators might be, for examples, public safety, behavioural changes, health-related quality of life measures, health-related policies, public participation, individual health status, population health status, use of resources and the like (Budgen, Cameron, and Bartfay 2010).

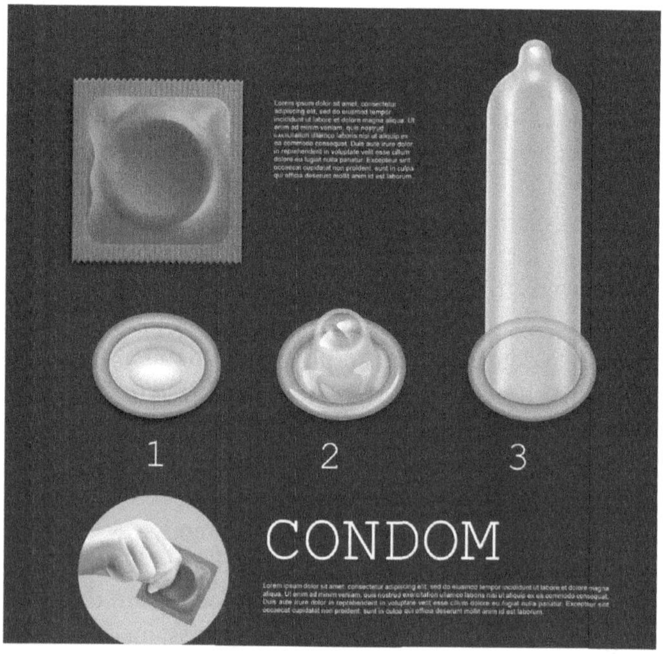

What Is the Program Planning and Evaluation Process?

There are a variety of program planning and evaluation process models that have been described in the literature and are beyond the purpose and scope of this chapter. We present here a simple, easy to understand and implement eight-step process, which is based on several of these process models. The reader is cautioned that the terminology or concepts used in this process often

Photo 10.6 Satisfaction of stakeholders may or may not also be a good indicator of program success per se. For example, parents of teens may not be "satisfied" about the availability of condom machines in school washrooms or their open display and availability in community pharmacies, although they have been shown to help to prevent the contraction and spread of STIs and unwanted pregnancies (Budgen, Cameron, and Bartfay 2010).

varies depending on the specific program planning and evaluation model employed (Bartfay and Bartfay 2015; Budgen, Cameron, and Bartfay 2010). We shall also describe in a section below the program logic model, which is currently being utilized by various public health agencies and departments in Canada (Mullet 1995; Porteous, Sheldrick, and Stewart 1997, 2002; Public Health Agency of Canada 2008).

The process involved in program planning and evaluation is similar to the research process. Indeed, there is often a fine line between formal program planning and evaluation and research in the health sciences. Hence, it is imperative to protect the stakeholders involved in terms of the principles of autonomy, confidentiality, beneficence and social justice every time your program planning and evaluation involves the collection or documentation of opinions, observations, interviews, surveys or the collection of personal health-related data or outcomes. Both require a review of the best available evidence, critical thinking and formal planning and evaluation or assessment techniques for EIPH. When you plan and design a public health program for evaluation, it is important to consider whether you will need to get ethical approval from all stakeholders involved and/or a formal review of your program proposal from one or more institutional review boards (IRBs). IRBs are found at most universities, health care centres and hospitals, public health departments and other governmental and non-governmental organizations. Figure 10.1 shows the eight critical steps involved in the program planning and evaluation process (Bartfay and Bartfay 2015).

Step I

The first step consists of a **needs assessment** which helps to formulate a clear understanding by all stakeholders and implementers as to what the actual or potential needs, problems or health-related issues are that need to be addressed to positively influence health and well-being in a defined community or region. Figure 10.2 provides some factors that are often considered during a typical needs assessment.

Actual problems are those that currently exist in a defined group or community (e.g., high incidence of STI's in teens in a community). Potential problems are those that may occur at some later time or date (e.g., development of heart disease or diabetes in adults who were obese as children). **Stakeholders** are defined as all individuals or groups (both internal and external) who have an interest in the program or those who may be affected by the program either directly or indirectly, including community volunteers, potential program participants, policy makers, governmental agencies, non-governmental agencies or industry (Bartfay and Bartfay 2015).

This first step is critical in crystallizing what the program's intent is (e.g., decrease the incidence of type 2 diabetes); for whom (e.g., young adults aged 18–40 living on First Nations reserves); and who will implement the program (e.g., public health care professionals in concert with volunteers and community leaders). The program's

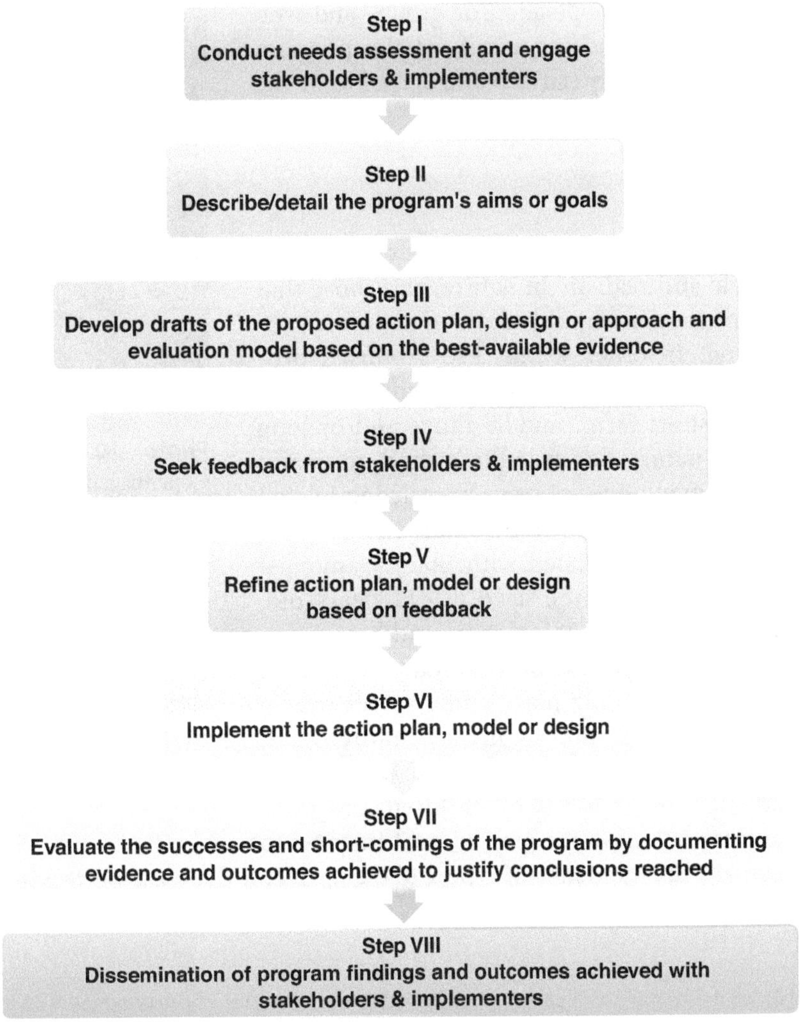

Step I
Conduct needs assessment and engage stakeholders & implementers

Step II
Describe/detail the program's aims or goals

Step III
Develop drafts of the proposed action plan, design or approach and evaluation model based on the best-available evidence

Step IV
Seek feedback from stakeholders & implementers

Step V
Refine action plan, model or design based on feedback

Step VI
Implement the action plan, model or design

Step VII
Evaluate the successes and short-comings of the program by documenting evidence and outcomes achieved to justify conclusions reached

Step VIII
Dissemination of program findings and outcomes achieved with stakeholders & implementers

Courtesy of Wally J. Bartfay

Figure 10.1 Critical steps in the program planning and evaluation process.

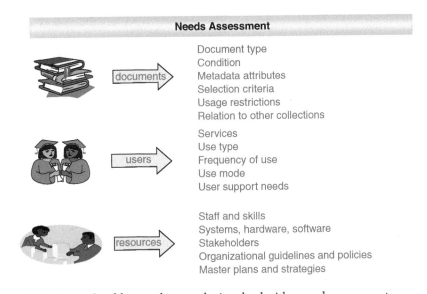

Needs Assessment

documents
Document type
Condition
Metadata attributes
Selection criteria
Usage restrictions
Relation to other collections

users
Services
Use type
Frequency of use
Use mode
User support needs

resources
Staff and skills
Systems, hardware, software
Stakeholders
Organizational guidelines and policies
Master plans and strategies

Figure 10.2 Example of factors that may be involved with a needs assessment.

intended target population or groups and who will ultimately deliver and fund the program needs to be clearly clarified and agreed to by the stakeholders and implementers.

Step II

Program aims or goals should be clear, measureable and realistic in nature, and those that are not specific should be clarified before proceeding. In other words, the proposed program should have measurable indicators that can be short term, middle range and/or long term in nature. For example, a short-term aim or goal may be to increase knowledge related to inactivity, poor nutritional choices and the hazards associated with obesity amongst school-aged children aged 10–12 years old, parents or guardians, teachers and caregivers. A middle-term aim or goal may be related to improving body mass index scores over a period of 8–12 months in the children, and a decrease in the consumption of high fat and high sugar foods by children and their parents. A long-term aim or goal may be to decrease the incidence of type 2 diabetes over a five-year period in high-risk school-aged children.

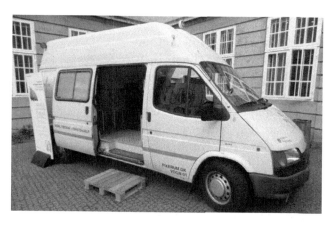

Source: Wally J. Bartfay

Photo 10.7 Community stakeholders were consulted in Copenhagen, Denmark to deal with health-related concerns associated with intravenous (IV) drug use (e.g., STIs, hepatitis B). This converted ambulance is known as the "Fixulance" and was the first safe drug consumption room (DCR) in Denmark. This unique DCR provides public health care professionals such as nurses to supervise clients during IV drug injections, provide them with sterile supplies (e.g., syringes and needles), dispose of used supplies safely, and also to provide health education, counselling and referrals to other community-based health services and professionals. The first DCR began operations in September, 2011 and there are currently four DCRs total due to the success of this pilot project.

Step III

The third step of the program planning and evaluation process is to develop a draft program plan based on a critical review of the best available evidence and the current state of knowledge related to the actual or potential problem(s) or issue(s) identified. For example, what is the current state of knowledge related to cosmetic pesticides and the development of skin rashes, neurological disorders and cancer? A variety of portals may be consulted, as noted above. In addition, there are a variety of reputable websites and search engines that can be accessed by public health care professionals and workers (e.g., MEDLINE, CINAHL, PUBMED). It is also critical to review the outcomes of similar programs and determine what worked and what did not work and why at this point in time.

This plan of action is like a blueprint for the construction of a home which shows where all the support beams will go, the electrical wiring and plumbing, the size of each room, timelines for completion, and so on. This action plan should be evidence informed and each proposed intervention of the program plan needs to be carefully detailed. Many kinds of action strategies can be considered or created, and imagination is an essential ingredient for success. Resources should be sought from both within and outside the community or group. Plans of action, for example, may involve a specific research methodology, approach or design (e.g., pretest–posttest experimental design, prospective cohort study, cross-sectional design study). It is critical that public health care professionals and workers clearly understand the stakeholders' interests and expectations. Successful program planning must be linked with time estimates and task specifications (e.g., Gantt charts described below). Timelines indicate tasks or activities that must be done and by whom and when.

A **task development timeline** specifies the specific tasks or activities that need to be completed and the time frame in which the tasks are estimated to be completed by (McKenzie, Neiger, Thackeray 2009). Making an optimistic and an alternative timeline (if things take longer) may be wise. As with all aspects of

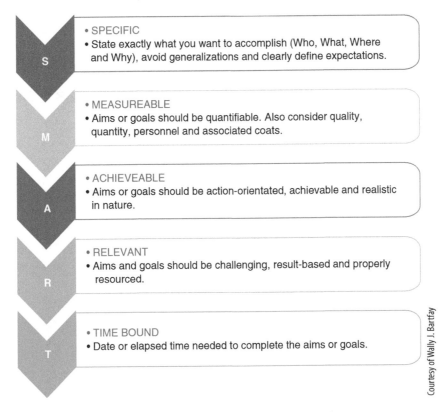

Figure 10.3 The "SMART" method for writing aims or goals.

Note: "SMART" is a mnemonic acronym that can be utilized to guide public health professionals, workers and stakeholders to write clear, realistic, measureable, and attainable aims or goals (Bogue 2013; Doran 1981).

program planning and evaluation, flexibility is needed in combination with goal directedness (Bartfay and Bartfay 2015; Budgen, Cameron, and Bartfay 2010). For example, if students in a public high school are involved, note when the students must have their tasks completed; if seniors in a community need immunizations prior to flu season, note when the immunizations should be finished; or if an agency or institution has provided funding for a project or primary health care intervention, note when a final report is expected. The Gantt chart was first developed by Henry Gantt in 1971 as a production tool and provides a list of tasks to be completed and associated timelines; monitors the progress made towards completing the noted tasks; and uses a marker (e.g., *) above the columns to indicate the current date or time period (TechTarget 2007; Timmreck 2003). **Gantt charts** are typically depicted in a tabular format and are a commonly employed visual tool to present the sequence and timing of tasks or activities that must take place in order to accomplish the specific objectives of the program or project (Bartfay and Bartfay 2015). Hence, a Gantt chart provides stakeholders and planners with a visual aid to monitor tasks completed and progress made on a regular basis. Table 10.3 presents an example of a fictitious Gantt chart for a pilot community-based health promotion program.

It is also critical to determine the availability of funding or potential funding sources for the program at this point in time; the availability of community-based resources and facilities, staff, volunteers, and how potential users will learn about your program and how it will be accessed. One needs to also determine and articulate how you will formally evaluate the effectiveness, outcomes and/or impact factor of the program based on its intended aims or goals. You should select the type of evaluation that shall take place; an evaluation framework or tools for evaluation (e.g., survey, clinical data, mortality and morbidity rates); determine when it will be conducted; and how qualitative and quantitative data will be analyzed. The action plan, design or approach and evaluation model should use easy-to-understand terms and health-related jargon or technical terms

Table 10.3 Sample Gantt Chart of a Pilot Community-Based Health Promotion Program

Major Tasks	JAN	FEB	MARCH	APRIL*	MAY	JUNE	JULY	AUG	SEPT	OCT	NOV	DEC
1. Develop pilot program rationale	XO	XO	XO									
2. Conduct needs assessment for all stakeholders concerned	XO	XO	XO									
3. Develop program goals and objectives		XO	XO									
4. Detail health promotion interventions			XO	XO								
5. Assemble necessary resources and train program facilitators				XO	X	X						
6. Promote and pilot test program						X	X	X				
7. Collect and analyze data and evaluate program outcomes							X	X	X			
8. Write report									X	X	X	
9. Present findings to key stakeholders											X	X

X—planned time frame; XO—completed.

*—marker for current date or time frame.

should be avoided. It is often helpful to show each step of your plan of action using flowcharts, diagrammatic models, conceptual maps, symbols or even photos or pictures.

These can also be utilized to help guide the formal evaluation process once the program has been implemented. Although the primary intent of diagrammatic models is to make clear the connections between values, goals, program activities, and outcomes, other relevant program dimensions may be included for practical purposes (Bartfay and Bartfay 2015; Budgen, Cameron, and Bartfay 2010). Diagrams such as program logic models and conceptual maps may be created in a variety of forms for planning purposes, updated regularly and used finally to help guide the evaluation process. Cartoonlike sketches, for example, may be helpful in depicting the human experiences represented within the diagrams. Of importance is not the form of the diagrams per se, but that they effectively depict in the visual sense that which is planned, is happening or has happened. Constructing diagrams in conjunction with community stakeholders helps to promote clarity, a shared vision and ownership for the process and outcomes achieved (Bartfay and Bartfay 2015; Budgen, Cameron, and Bartfay 2010).

Step IV

The fourth step of this process is seeking feedback and suggestions from all stakeholder's and implementer's. It is critical to determine that you have identified all the program aims or goals, how the program will be implemented and by whom, the target dates for completion and so on. In other words, have you done a good job communicating what the proposed program is all about and what it wants to accomplish? Communities and groups work from their own values, experiences and definitions of situations, and public health care professionals and workers need to be supportive of these. Effective communication emphasizes the need to find a common language and ground which recognizes the interdependence between stakeholders and public health care professionals and workers.

Step V

The feedback and suggestions received by the stakeholders and implementers above should be carefully recorded and considered. This information may be utilized to help clarify program aims or goals, target populations or users, resources available or needed, definitions of actual or potential health-related issues or concerns, action plans and timelines, and/or evaluation tools or methods. Feedback may occur in a variety of formats (e.g., town hall meetings, focus group sessions, e-mails). For example, programs involving the use of community volunteers as resources are becoming increasingly popular as a way to help contain costs and, hopefully, encourage community partnerships and empowerment in term. This is an example of the so-called "art of effective program planning and evaluation" where the feedback and inputs from volunteers are actively sought. Furthermore, this helps to solidify their active involvement and the success of the proposed program under review.

Step VI

Once the program is implemented, it is critical to carefully monitor and assess the program on an ongoing basis for unforeseen events or circumstances that may negatively impact on the overall success of the program. For example, suppose a rural community-based dialysis program is implemented and the clinic was initially planned to run between the hours of 9 am and 4 pm. The rationale for the clinic was to decrease travel times for dialysis patients so they wouldn't have to engage in long commutes to urban-based dialysis clinics. Based on feedback from users of the rural dialysis program, you learn that these proposed program hours conflict with school and work schedules and that users would prefer the clinic to run after 5 pm. Changing the dialysis clinic hours in response to user feedback would help to facilitate access to the clinic for more users and likely increase the success of this rural community-based dialysis program.

Step VII

This step involves the formal evaluation of the program aims or goals. The evaluation is based on the documented outcomes achieved and an analysis of the qualitative and/ or quantitative data collected. Evaluation approaches must be flexible and holistic in nature; whenever possible, to permit a better understanding of the outcomes of the program and its true impact on the target group or community. A variety of questions may be addressed during this stage. It is important to remember that different questions may be important to different stakeholders and implementers of the program. As much as possible, evaluations must be designed to answer pertinent questions for all stakeholders and implementers involved with the program. Standardized tools may be employed or tools may be developed specifically for the program to answer these critical questions. For example: *Were the aims of the program met, partially met, or not met at all? What contributed to the program's overall success and/or shortcomings? Was the program carried out as planned within the timelines? Were the outcomes or results of the program worth the effort and associated costs? What has changed as a result of the program being implemented?*

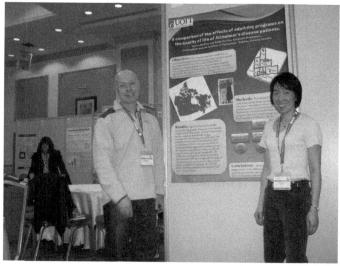

Photo 10.8 A research poster presented at an international research conference related to Alzheimer's disease. The last step of the program planning and evaluation process is dissemination and communication of the findings observed in a timely, unbiased and consistent fashion. Bartfay, E, and W.J. Bartfay: A Comparison of the Effect of Adult Day Programs on the Quality of Life of Alzheimer's Disease Patients. *The 25th International Conference on Alzheimer's Disease International*, March, 2010, Thessaloniki, Greece (Poster: P043).

Source: Wally J. Bartfay

Step VIII

This step serves as a vehicle for providing feedback related to the program findings and outcomes achieved to all stakeholders and implementers in reference to the program aims or goals. Although formal documentation of the evaluation is often a requirement for various health programs, informal mechanisms may also be employed. Regardless of how communications are delivered or their format, the goal of dissemination is to achieve full and impartial reporting and disclosure of the program outcomes in reference to its intended aims or goals. A checklist to consider during this stage may include tailoring the content of your report to the specific intended audience(s) (e.g., lay public, public health care professionals, governmental agencies, non-governmental agencies [NGOs]); explaining the focus of the evaluation; and listing both the strengths and limitations of the evaluation methods or tools employed. **SWOT** (see Figure 10.4) is an acronym for Strengths, Weaknesses, Opportunities and Threats (Fraser and Stupak 2002; Helms and Nixon 2010). A SWOT analysis can be employed to identify both internal and external strengths and analysis of the proposed program along with potential barriers, gaps, challenges and opportunities.

A variety of forums can be employed to provide feedback to stakeholders and implementers of the program including the publication of the results (e.g., public health reports or bulletins, peer-reviewed journals, conference proceedings); online forums (e.g., e-mails, a website developed for the program); social media (e.g., Facebook, Twitter, YouTube); town hall meetings or public lectures; and the mass media (e.g., local newspapers, television, radio).

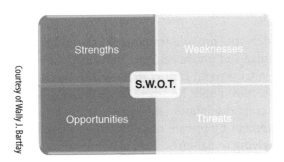

Courtesy of Wally J. Bartfay

Figure 10.4 The SWOT method.

Note: Users of the SWOT method need to ask and answer questions that generate meaningful information for each of the categories (strengths, weaknesses, opportunities, and threats) in order to generate meaningful analysis.

A cost analysis of the program may also be provided at this stage, and which evaluates the total costs of the program in relation to actual health outcomes (e.g., program total accounting costs; cost benefit and effectiveness analysis). Conclusions reached can be strengthened by providing stakeholders and implementers with plausible mechanisms that resulted in noted health outcomes achieved; delineating a temporal order between the sequence of program interventions or activities and outcomes achieved; searching for possible alternative explanations based on similar findings from the empirical literature; and demonstrating the desired outcomes were replicable in users of the program.

Lastly, recommendations are actions for future consideration that result from the evaluation process. For example, knowing that a specific community-based fitness program for young adults may reduce the risk of developing heart disease or stroke does not necessarily translate into a recommendation to continue the effort, especially when competing priorities or other effective alternatives exists. Hence, recommendations for continuing, expanding, redesigning or terminating a specific program should be viewed as separate judgments regarding a program's overall effectiveness or impact factor. Refer Web-Based Resource Box 10.2 for additional resources related to program planning and evaluation.

Web-Based Resource Box 10.2 Program planning and evaluation

Learning Resource	Website
Canadian Journal of Program Evaluation This journal deals exclusively with the field of program planning and evaluating and includes reviews of the literature and research investigations.	http://www.ucalgary.ca/UofC/departments/UP/UCP/CJPE.html
Centers for Disease Control (CDC) Introduction to program evaluation for public health programs and CDC Evaluation Brief This website provides the reader with a brief introduction to program planning and evaluation though a public health lens.	http://www.cdc.glov/eval/evalguide.pdf and www.cdc.gov/healthyyouth/evaluation/pdf/brief18.pdf
Chronic Disease Prevention Program Planning and Evaluation (Toronto Public Health) This website provides public health care professionals and workers with numerous guides and resources related to program planning and evaluation for the prevention and management of communicable and non-communicable diseases.	http://www.toronto.ca/health/chronicdisease-prevent.htm or http://www1.toronto.ca/wps/portal/contentonly?vgnextoid=a253ba2ae8b1e310VgnVCM10000071d60f89RCRD

What Are Program Logic Models?

There are numerous program planning and evaluation models that provide frameworks or guides to assist public health care professionals and workers to collect, organize and utilize evidence-informed data to form coherent action plans for public health. However, there are often several factors that need to be considered when choosing a particular framework or guide. For example, most public health agencies utilize a standardized planning framework or guide that is often employed across disciplines and departments. A particular framework or guide may also be a funding program requirement by private or government organizations, NGOs and institutions (e.g., to define and examine the underlying social-environmental determinants of the health problem). In addition, the selection of a particular framework or guide may be influenced by a set of underlying principles or social values deemed critical for the specific public health program in Canada or abroad internationally (e.g., participatory decision-making or social justice).

Although a discussion of all the available frameworks and guides available to health care professionals and workers is beyond the scope of this chapter, we shall provide an overview of the program logic model that is used extensively in many municipal, regional, provincial and federal governmental public health agencies in Canada (Mullet 1995; National Collaborating Centre for Methods and Tools 2010; Porteous, Sheldrick, and Stewart 1997, 2002; Public Health Agency of Canada 2008; Wooten et al. 2014) (see Figure 10.5).

Program logic models are often employed by public health agencies and institutions in Canada because of their simplicity for use and ability to clearly reveal program interrelationships and linkages (Cooksy, Gill, and Kelly 2001; Porteous, Sheldrick, and Stewart 1997, 2002). The logic model provides a diagram of *what the program is supposed to do, with whom and why* (Porteous, Sheldrick, and Stewart 2002). Development of a logic model consists of two main planning stages: (a) *Components, Activities and Target groups (CAT)* and (b) the *Short-term Outcomes and Long-term Outcomes (SOLO)*. During the CAT stage, activities are typically clustered thematically into components for the public health program under consideration or review.

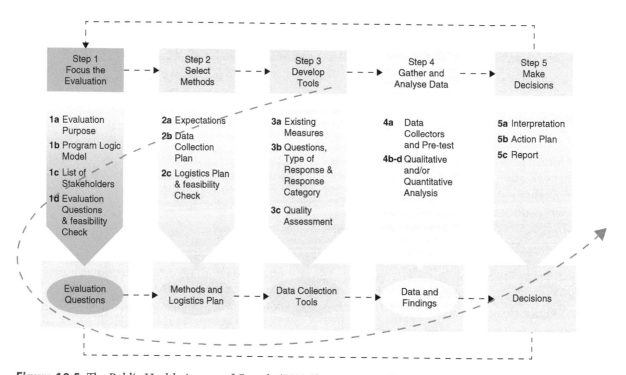

Figure 10.5 The Public Health Agency of Canada (PHAC) program evaluation toolkit.

For example, a program to address the prevention of sexually transmitted infections (STIs) on a First Nations reserve may include the components of risk assessment, targeted face-to-face and web-based health education in schools and/or community centres, and support for community workers and teachers. The activities are the specific intervention strategies that are employed as a primary health care intervention (e.g., development of a website targeting Indigenous youth; providing information and resources to community workers, teachers and parents). The target groups are the intended recipients of the specific community-based primary prevention program (e.g., Indigenous youth).

During the SOLO stage, short- and long-term health-related outcomes of the community-based STI primary prevention program are identified. The short-term outcomes are the immediate effects of the program. For example, increasing knowledge related to the types of STIs, their possible clinical manifestations and outcomes and primary prevention strategies that can be employed to prevent their occurrence (e.g., latex condoms, abstinence). Building the knowledge base of parents related to STIs, community workers and teachers may also be a short-term goal that can be assessed. The long-term outcomes may involve the achievement of goals related to decreasing incidence rates of STIs, clinical interventions (e.g., prescription of antibiotics to treat bacterial STIs such as syphilis, chlamydia and gonorrhoea) and associated clinical complications for this targeted First Nations Reserve over the course of a five-year plan.

Figure 10.5 shows the *Program Evaluation Toolkit* employed by the Public Health Agency of Canada (2008). This toolkit is based on a program logic model and highlights which specific evaluation processes can be employed to inform and assist with the decision-making process during program planning and implementation. It is based on a relatively inexpensive *do-it-yourself approach* and is designed to be user friendly and free of technical jargon. The toolkit has been developed specifically to evaluate public health programs based on five basic steps: (a) focus the evaluation; (b) select methods; (c) develop tools; (d) gather and analyze data; and (e) make decisions (see Figure 10.6). The toolkit is presented as a series of short learning modules with simply explanations and specific tools, and worksheets are provided to assist individuals through the process (Public Health Agency of Canada 2008). The toolkit is tailored specifically to the decision-making needs of managers of public health programs, public health officials, and frontline field staff plus anyone assisting with evaluation, such as health unit program evaluation specialists, epidemiologists, public health nurses, health planners and educators, information analysts, or outside consultants. The toolkit presents a decision-orientated model of program evaluation and has been specifically designed as a concise in-house guide to the necessary steps and processes involved (Public Health Agency of Canada 2008).

The evaluation component is a dynamic and ongoing process that helps to support and guide programs, their refinements, along with previously unknown gaps, deficiencies, and/or flaws in the original design of the public health program. This toolkit can be used in conjunction with community stakeholders and groups to help build partnerships when engaging in program planning and evaluation. Indeed, involvement of all community stakeholders, public health professionals and workers, agencies, and organizations will help to build and foster commitment to the public health program and aid in its design, implementation, and evaluation of outcomes achieved.

What Is Health Services Research?

A brief overview of health services and outcomes research shall be highlighted in this section to familiarize the reader with these associated terms. A **health service** is simply any primary health care service provided by a public health care professional or worker for the purpose of maintaining, promoting, protecting, and/or restoring the health of diverse populations across the lifespan (Bartfay and Bartfay 2015). **Health services research (HSR)** is defined as an integrative and multidisciplinary scientific field that involves the integration of knowledge, the study and evaluation of the organization, and functioning and performance of health services (Bartfay and Bartfay 2015). Health services research does not involve a specific research design or methodological approach per se, but is a field of scientific inquiry that seeks to better understand organizational influences, functions and the performance of various health services provided. According to Porta (2008, 113), HSR requires the formal evaluation of four critical components:

1. **Structure**—which is concerned with resources, facilities, and human resources available.
2. **Process**—which seeks to evaluate matters related to the where, by whom and how health care services are provided.
3. **Output**—which is concerned with the amount and the exact nature of health services provided.
4. **Outcome**—which is ultimately concerned with the results of the health services provided based on measureable benefits (e.g., improved survival rates, decreased mortality rates, improvements related to DALYs).

HSR investigations seek to determine how various personal behaviours, economic and sociopolitical factors, financing systems, organizational structures and processes, the availability of various laboratory and diagnostic imaging technologies, and geography affect access to public primary health care services, their overall costs and quality and their health impact in terms of quantity and quality of life measures. The primary aims of HSR is to improve the overall quality of primary health care services provided to diverse populations across the lifespan; determine the most effective and cost-efficient ways of managing and delivering these health care services; reduce errors by health care personnel; and to improve overall client safety and satisfaction (Agency for Healthcare Research and Quality 2002).

What Is Outcomes Research?

An **outcome** for a public health service provided includes all possible results (negative, positive or neutral) that may stem from exposure to a known causal factor (e.g., H1N1), determinant of health and/or from a primary health care intervention (Bartfay and Bartfay 2015). End results may include such things as mortality, survival, disability, individual's experience with the public health services provided and morbidity measures such as their overall health-related quality of life (Black and Gruen 2005; Clancy and Eisenberg 1998). **Outcomes research** is designed to critically and objectively examine and document the effectiveness of health-care policies and services and the end results of care provided to clients (Bartfay and Bartfay 2015).

Outcomes research examines the specific outcomes of primary health care interventions and seeks to understand why these end results were obtained or not. Outcomes research seeks to provide important insights about making public health services efforts more effective, equitable, timely and client focused by filling in the gaps in evidence needed by health care professionals and workers and the individuals they serve to make informed decisions in concert. Outcomes research, in other words, seeks to provide evidence about which primary health care interventions work best for each client and under what specific circumstances. The urgent need for outcomes research was highlighted in the early 1980s, when researchers discovered that *geography is destiny* (Agency for Healthcare Research and Quality 2000). Time and again, studies documented that certain routine medical procedures (e.g., hysterectomy, hernia repairs, cardiac bypass surgeries) were performed much more frequently in some areas than in others, even if there were no differences in the underlying rates of disease. Furthermore, there was often no information about the end results for the individuals who received a particular procedure, and few comparative studies were undertaken to show which interventions were most effective or had the most beneficial health-related outcomes (Agency for Healthcare Research and Quality 2000).

The Research Focus Box 10.2 highlights the results from a two-generation program designed to address the link between the lack of school readiness in children and parenting stress and the social determinants of health involving poverty, unemployment and inadequate housing. The researchers employed outcomes research to determine the effectiveness of this community-based program.

Research Focus Box 10.2

What are the short-term effects of a two-generation preschool program on parenting stress, self-esteem, life skills, and children's receptive language?

Study Aim/Rationale

Poverty and its associated sequelae is a critical determinant of health, especially for young children and their families. There is a proposed link between the lack of school readiness in children and parenting stress associated with poverty, unemployment and inadequate housing. The aim of this two-generation program was to determine if early interventions addressing the needs of parents and their preschool children could offset negative associated health effects.

Methodology/Design

Outcomes research was utilized to determine the effectiveness of a two-generation program which consisted of early childhood education (20 hours per week provided by the Centre), parenting life skills education (designed and implemented by off-site program staff members), and family support administered by social workers in the home setting. This multi-intervention program was offered to interested parents and children at no costs and a pretest–posttest experimental design study was employed to evaluate changes to outcomes. Specifically, caregivers were asked to complete a parenting stress index, community life skills scale, and a self-esteem scale at the onset of the program and upon its completion. Fifty-five caregivers of seventy-six preschool-aged children partook in the portion of the study examining the impact of the program and 112 children participated in the child outcomes portion.

Major Findings

In comparison to pretest measures, parents who attended the program reported significantly decreased parental stress and defensive responding, decreased total stress, increased levels of self-esteem and an increase in daily management skill scores. Preschool-aged children demonstrated a statistically significant improvement in receptive langue skills. Interestingly, for Indigenous children who partook in the program, a longer duration of time in the program was associated with increased gains in language skills.

Implications for Public Health

These findings suggest that the program had a positive effective on both parents and children who partook in the program. Moreover, appropriate and timely supports and services for low-income families may help to reduce the negative impacts of their financial status.

Source: Benzies et al. (2009).

In the formal appraisal of health care outcomes, various factors need to be considered. Donabedian (1987), whose pioneering efforts in this field of scientific inquiry, created a simply framework for conducting outcomes research that consists of the following three factors:

1. *Structure of care*—which refers to the broad organizational and administrative features (e.g., type of facilities, technologies employed, range of services provided, size, location, organizational climate);
2. *Processes*—which include the various aspects of clinical care provided, clinical management, decision-making processes and health care interventions; and
3. *Outcomes*—which refer to the specific outcomes achieved as a result of a given primary health care intervention carried out.

By providing a critical link between the health services individuals access and those that are offered or provided with and the actual outcomes they experience, outcomes research has become a critical component to develop better ways to monitor and improve the quality of care (Agency for Healthcare

Research and Quality 2000; Black and Gruen 2005). Moreover, governments, NGOs, public health institutions and departments, and policy makers are all interested in identifying ways to improve the quality and value of health care services while decreasing their associated costs. Mitchell, Ferketich, and Jennings (1988) argue that the emphasis on evaluating quality of care has shifted from structures (having the rights things) to processes (doing the right things) to outcomes (having the right things happen).

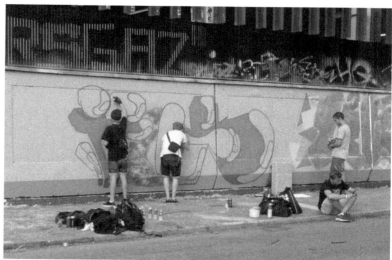

Source: Wally J. Bartfay

Photo 10.9 Youth engaged in "tagging their territory" via graffiti. Ethics deals with the study of human nature, behaviours, and decisions surrounding ethical or moral issues in society.

Ethical Considerations for Public Health Professionals and Workers

Ethics is defined as a branch of philosophy which deals with the study of nature and justification of principles that guide human behaviours and decisions and are applied when moral issues or dilemmas arise (Bartfay and Bartfay 2015). **Public health ethics** is defined as a practical means of collaboratively determining a moral course of action with all stakeholders concerned and their impacts and consequences (Bartfay and Bartfay 2015). It may be argued that public health ethics focuses more on issues related to the interaction of individuals, families, communities and entire populations, reflecting on collective responsibilities, and common goals or desires. The right to health care includes the right to goods and services to maintain and promote health across the lifespan (Commission on the Social Determinants of Health 2008).

Hardly anyone would question the many positive contributions and ripple effects achieved via public health programs, activities, and policies in regards to improving the health and well-being of various groups, communities and entire populations across the lifespan. At first glance, public health policies (e.g., tobacco legislation, compulsory seat belt use) and programs (e.g., immunization, promoting active lifestyles, and healthy eating) may appear sufficient to ethically justify their need and impact for preserving and promoting health and for prevention disease and illness. But a moment of critical reflection makes it apparent that there are several ethical issues and challenging questions that need to be considered throughout the program planning and evaluation process in public health (Arah 2009; Baylis, Kenny, and Sherwin 2008; Buchanan 2008; Gostin and Gostin 2009).

Recent public health events, such as SARS, H5N1, and the Walkerton *E coli* outbreak, along with the growing recognition of the disparities present for certain populations (e.g., Indigenous peoples, immigrants, elderly) in terms of the social determinants of health (SDH), have reinforced the need for ethical reflection in practice (Dawson and Verweij 2007; Holland 2007; University of Toronto Joint Centre for Bioethics 2012). For example, when a particular communicable disease begins to affect a larger than usual number of people, or to circulate globally among populations that have little or no immunity against it (e.g., SARS, AH1N1), the specific program aims of public health interventions, programs, policies or legislations and how they should be prioritized requires that difficult decisions be made for the "collective good" of society. Indeed, during a global pandemic, the area of communicable disease control in public health has no shortage of ethical issues related to mandatory reporting requirements, trade and travel restrictions, quarantines, school closers, bans on public gatherings, staffing management and workplace safety assurances, contact tracing and the use of public health powers and legislation to alter behaviour, to name but a few public health actions that may be required (Barry 2009; McDougal 2010; Paranthaman et al. 2009).

The PHAC (2012) reports that there is a growing need to consider the ethical foundations for and implications of our work in public health, and to need to reflect upon the values underlying public health practice in Canada. The *Chief Public Health Officer's Ethics Advisory Committee* assists with integrating ethical thinking into the development of public health policies, programs, and services (PHAC 2012). The PHAC (2013) has released a set of thirty-six core competencies deemed essential for all public health professionals and workers in Canada. Refer Chapter 1 for a detailed discussion of these thirty-six core competencies. Unfortunately, specific competencies related to ethical decision-making or practice per se for public health professionals and workers are not clearly identified in the document, but inferred or implied as highlighted by the following quote:

All public health professionals share a core set of attitudes and values. These attitudes and values have not been listed as specific core competencies for public health because they are difficult to teach and even harder to assess. However, they form the context within which the competencies are practiced . . . If the core competencies are considered as the notes to a musical score, the values and attitudes that practitioners bring to their work provide the tempo and emotional component of the music. One may be a technically brilliant musician but without the correct temp, rhythm and emotion, the music will not have the desired effect.

—PHAC 2013, 3

Rapid advances in the allied health sciences and health care technologies have precipitated a dramatic rise in ethical dilemmas for public health care professionals and workers. Ethical questions often arise when sociocultural values, norms or expectations are infringed upon. For examples, *what if the aims or goals of the proposed program infringes on individual civil liberties or shared values of minority groups or vulnerable populations or communities (e.g., immigrants, Indigenous peoples, homeless, unemployed)? How far should public health programs go in presenting health information campaigns for protecting the health of the majority without unduly stigmatizing individuals or groups by making them feel guilty for their non-compliance (e.g., smokers, individuals who are obese)? Should society stigmatize women who choose to feed their new born infants with infant formula as opposed to breast feeding, despite the many noted health benefits for both mother (e.g., decreased incidence of breast cancer) and child (e.g., passive immunity)?* Hence, we argue that program planning and evaluation is an inherently value-laden process that also requires ethical reflection and consideration in order to comprehend and negotiate the potentially conflicting fundamental values of public health professionals and workers and stakeholders who will ultimately be affected. Table 10.4 provides a list of some basic ethical principles relevant to the practice of public health, what they entail and examples of each (Dawson 2007; Holland 2007; McDougal 2010; Nuffield Council on Bioethics 2007; University of Toronto Joint Centre for Bioethics 2012).

We argue that public health is, by its very nature, both a normative and acculturative practice. It is normative because it recommends or makes inferences about what is "good health" and how to preserve, maintain, and promote it; what are acceptable versus unacceptable risks and environments. Given that many health-related behaviours, practices, lifestyles, and/or environments are contextually bound in social and cultural values, public health is therefore also an acculturative enterprise. Ethics in public health, therefore, involves applying a critical, analytical, and value-laden lens to address a particular need, program or policy. Refer Chapter 1 for a detailed discussion on how health, disease, illness, and sickness are influenced by various social, cultural, and environmental factors.

Understanding ethical principles and theories are helpful to address ethical issues and moral planning and decision-making related to ethical practices, policies and programs for all stakeholders concerned (Dawson and Verweij 2007; Holland 2007; Nuffield Council of Bioethics 2007; Thompson 2010). Ethical decisions in health care are guided primarily by two classical ethical theories: (a) deontology and (b) teleology, especially the utilitarianism form. **Deontology** is defined as the classical ethical theory based on moral obligations and duties that require individuals to act in certain ways in response to moral, cultural and social norms, and expectations or motivations (Bartfay and Bartfay 2015). **Teleology** is defined as a classical theory that

Table 10.4 Basic Ethical Principles

Ethical Principle	What the Principle Entails	Example
Autonomy	Deals with respect for persons and the right to self-determination and destiny. (Note: Informed consent, confidentiality, fidelity, and veracity all rely on the acceptance and exercise of this principle).	Allowing a client in their home the right to refuse a treatment or intervention (e.g., IV medication, dressing change, insertion of a Foley catheter).
Active collaboration	Requires formalized input from public health professionals and workers and all stakeholders considered in order to ensure active discussions, decision-making, prioritization of needs, education, and communication.	Holding a community-based meeting to discuss a proposal related to fluoridation of drinking water supplies on a First Nations reserve with several boil water advisories.
Beneficence	Deals with doing or promoting good that requires abstention from injuring others, and the promotion of the opinions or interests of others primarily by decreasing, preventing or limiting possible harms.	Installing hand-rails and other safety equipment in an elderly client's bathroom to prevent falls.
Equitable processes	Requires that specific protocols, plans, and/or standards be collective made by all stakeholders concerned via an open, transparent, and accountable process, as well as the formal application of the decisions made in a consistent manner without discrimination and in proportion to the identified need, degree of scarcity, and/or scale of the public health emergency identified.	During a global pandemic when there may be a scarcity of vaccines available, priority will be given to high-risk individuals (e.g., elderly, children, individuals with chronic diseases and those immunocompromised) in community-based immunization clinics.
Fairness	Requires that decisions and public health interventions be based on the best available evidence and be responsive to the needs of those affected, acceptable to all, while respecting professional obligations and duties related to care, compassion, resource stewardship, and maintenance of public trust.	Setting up a mandatory screening station outside all public health facilities to screen all health professionals and workers and the general public prior to entrance (e.g., temperature check, screening survey related to travel abroad, fever, coughing) during a global pandemic (e.g., SARS).
Fidelity	Deals with keeping/honouring one's promise made to others.	A public health nurse makes a follow-up home visit to a client in the community at the agreed-upon date and time.
Following the Rule of Law	Requires that appropriate public health legislations, actions, standards, and/or incentives are only made by the proper designated public authorities (e.g., Minister of Health) or agencies (e.g., Health Canada, PHAC) via appropriate processes and laws.	A decision by the federal government to increase taxes on tobacco products sold in Canada as a means to discourage smoking by individuals and associated negative health outcomes.

(Continued)

Table 10.4 Basic Ethical Principles(*Continued*)

Ethical Principle	What the Principle Entails	Example
Non-maleficence	Deals with doing no harm to the client.	A public health nurse helps a homeless man in distress to a community clinic for follow-up diagnostic services.
Social Justice	Deals with the issue of fairness that an individual is entitled to, deserves or has a legitimate claim to.	A client is placed upon the provincial waiting list for cardiac surgery based on priority needs.
Veracity	Deals with telling the truth to clients.	A public health professional informs a teen that they have contracted a STI based on laboratory findings.

determines rightness or wrongness based solely on the basis of an estimate, likelihood or probably outcomes (Bartfay and Bartfay 2015). **Utilitarianism** is one form of teleology which is based on usefulness or utility of the outcomes achieved. The utility of action is decided on the basis of whether the action would bring about the greatest number of beneficial outcomes or consequence, and has a long association with public health. Some argue that public health may be envisioned as the practical implementation of a utilitarian ethic (Dawson 2007; Holland 2007; Nuffield Council on Bioethics 2007; University of Toronto Joint Centre for Bioethics 2012). To assist the reader in distinguishing between the two theoretical positions, consider the issue of an abortion resulting from severe trauma following a motor vehicle accident (MVA). To the deontologist, abortion remains unjustifiable even if it may save the life of the mother due to complications (e.g., serious internal injuries sustained and bleeding) because the action would violate the moral duty to preserve life and avoid killing at all cost. On the other hand, a utilitarian may argue that preserving the life of the woman is justified by aborting the foetus in utero, which will allow her to recover, return to her family or to contribute to society in general. Although the abortion of the foetus is viewed as tragic by the utilitarian, this action represents the potential for greater good than allowing both the foetus and mother to die as a result of the MVA.

In the past decade, considerable attention has been devoted to the existence of inequities leading to disparities in reference to access to public health care services and health outcomes, which are rooted in our greater understanding of the SDH (Commission on the Social Determinants of Health 2008; Raphael 2009). Refer Chapter 1 for a detailed discussion on the fifteen SDH. The existence of these marked disparities has led to the analysis of the relationship between social justice and public health (Commission on the Social Determinants of Health 2008; Powers and Faden 2006; University of Toronto Joint Centre for Bioethics 2012). For example, Powers and Faden (2006) argue that a social justice lens addresses the twin moral impulses that bring to life the practice of public health:

. . . to improve human well-being by improving health and to do so in particular by focusing on the needs of those who are the most disadvantaged. A commitment to social justice . . . attaches a special moral urgency to remediating the conditions of those whose life prospects are poor across multiple dimensions of well-being. Placing a priority on those so situated is a hallmark of social justice.

—Powers and Faden 2006, 82

We argue that for public health ethics to contribute to effective program planning and evaluation, policy and practice, it must be understood in the context of an applied ethics that is relevant to all public health professionals, workers, and stakeholders concerned (Bartfay and Bartfay 2015). No one ethical principle, theory or framework will be appropriate for all situations, needs or decisions ultimately reached based on some magical algorithm that always provides the right moral solution. These are simply meant to assist with the systematic and transparent examination of the issues, including consideration of the interests of all stakeholders concerned. A discussion of all professional ethical codes of practice, principles, and frameworks for decision-making in public health is beyond the scope of this chapter. The Web-Based Resource Box 10.3 provides various ethical codes for health care professionals in Canada, frameworks, guides, and aids to assist with formal training, skills, and professional competencies related to ethical analysis and practices in the public health context.

Web-Based Resource Box 10.3 Ethical codes and guides

Learning Resource	Website
Community Health Nurses of Canada (2013). Canadian Community Health Professional Practice Model This document provides the reader with codes of ethical practice and standards for community health nurses in Canada.	http://chnc.ca/documents/ CanadianCommunityHealthNursing ProfessionalPracticeCompoments-E.pdf
Canadian Nurses Association (2008 Centennial edition). Code of Ethics for Registered Nurses Provides a statement of the ethical values of nurses and of nurses' commitments to persons with health care needs and persons receiving care. It is intended for nurses in all contexts and domains of nursing practice and at all levels of decision-making.	http://www.cna-aiic.ca/en/on-the-issues/best-nursing/ nursing-ethics **and/or** http://www.cna-aiic.ca/~/media/cna/page%20content/ pdf%20fr/2013/09/05/18/05/code_of_ethics_ 2008_e.pdf
Canadian Medical Association (Update 2004, last reviewed March 2012) Code of Ethics Provides ethical guidelines for physicians, including residents, and medical students. Its focus is the core activities of medicine—such as health promotion, advocacy, disease prevention, diagnosis, treatment, rehabilitation, palliation, education, and research. It is based on the fundamental principles and values of medical ethics, especially compassion, beneficence, non-maleficence, respect for persons, justice, and accountability.	http://policybase.cma.ca/dbtw-wpd/PolicyPDF/ PD04-06.pdf
Public Health Ontario (April 2012). A framework for the ethical conduct of public health initiatives This document presents a framework to assist public health professionals and workers employing an evidence-informed lens.	http://www.publichealthontario.ca/en/eRepository/ PHO%20%20Framework%20for%20Ethical%20 Conduct%20of%20Public%20Health%20Initiatives%20 April%202012.pdf
University of Toronto Joint Centre for Bioethics (2012). Population and public health ethics. Cases from research, policy, and practice. Toronto, ON: University of Toronto. ISBN 978-1-261-00001-5 This document provides the reader with an excellent resource related to public health ethics, theory, frameworks and various cases related to public health research, policy making, and practice.	http://www.jointcentreforbioethics.ca/publications/documents/Population-and-Public-Health-Ethics-Casebook-ENGLISH.pdf

Future Directions and Challenges

Primary health care is an integral part of the Canadian health care system and provides a set of guiding principles for public health care professionals and workers to help empower citizens to make informed decisions about their health and well-being, build community capacity, and promote harmony with our environments (Bartfay and Bartfay 2015; Budgen, Cameron, and Bartfay 2010; English 2000; McKnight 2001). To reach this aim in public health, we must devote our knowledge, clinical skills and will to planning for effective primary health care services and also formally evaluating the impact of these public health actions.

Program planning and evaluation are also critical components for project management. In October 1969, the *Project Management Institute* (PMI) was founded as a global non-profit professional organization for professionals in this noted field (Sliger and Broderick 2008; PMI 2013). The objectives of the PMI are to foster professionalism in the field of project management; provide a forum for the exchange of problems, solutions, and applications; coordinate both industrial and academic research efforts in this field; develop common techniques and terminology; provide interface between users and suppliers of software and hardware products for project management activities; and provide guidelines in reference to career development (see link: http://www.pmi.org/). The PMI offers a range of services including the development of standards, research, education, publications, networking opportunities in local chapters, conferences and training seminars and for obtaining additional training and credentials related to project management. Currently, there are PMI chapters in various cities across Canada including Victoria, Vancouver, Calgary, Edmonton, Saskatoon, Region, Winnipeg, Kitchener, London, Mississauga, Toronto, Oshawa, Ottawa, Montréal, Québec City, Fredericton, Saint John, Moncton, Halifax, and St. John's.

As the primary targets of public health interventions have greatly expanded over the past few decades in Canada beyond the management and prevention of communicable diseases to include non-communicable and chronic diseases, domestic violence, an aging population, emerging pathogens (e.g., H1N1, West Nile Virus), threats of bioterrorism, climate change and the social determinants of health, and so on, the task of program planning and evaluation for public health has become more complex and fluid in nature. As these public health challenges expand, so do the associated costs. For example, it is generally agreed upon that health care costs tend to increase with age in Canada due to a growing number of associated disabilities and the higher incidence of chronic disease. For example, in 2015 health care costs exceeded $219.1 billion or $6,105 per Canadian under the age of 65; compared to $11,557 for those 70–74 years, and $20,917 for those 80 years and older (CIHI 2015).

Program planning and evaluation in public health should not occur in isolation from the setting or situation, but should consist of an interdisciplinary team of health care professionals, community stakeholders, governmental and NGOs, and institutions in order for the program to be ultimately successful in achieving its short and long-term goals. Budgen, Cameron, and Bartfay (2010) note that thoughtful consideration of the context within which a health program will be developed and implemented contributes directly to the program's overall success. Local contexts are nested with regional, national and international contexts. Although these contexts may vary considerably, important factors and trends relevant to health usually can be identified if the public health care professional or worker is open minded, observant and questioning and works in partnership with the community or target population.

Regional, national or international health programs often consist of a web of complex and interacting determinants of health. Poverty and its associated outcomes (e.g., inadequate housing, malnutrition), for example, is an important SDH across the lifespan in Canada and globally (Commission of Social Determinants of Health 2008; Raphael 2008). The challenge is to acknowledge and identify the often complex web of relationships and associated outcomes during the program planning and evaluation process for these determinants of health.

Dramatically changing and/or evolving technologies have created an unprecedented flow of health-related information, screening, and diagnostic tools as well as advancements in how various health-associated conditions are managed. For example, until the 1960s, all health care professionals could offer an individual with kidney failure was supportive and/or palliative care until they finally succumbed to their condition. Shortly after, the available options greatly increased with the introduction of dialysis to clinically manage the condition, followed by kidney transplantation. All of these had to be formally evaluated in terms of their effectiveness and impact on the clients receiving these treatment options (Dieppe 2007). Although new treatment regimens often result in limited gains in terms of the total years of survival or cure per se, it could be deemed preferable if the individual's perceptions of their broader health-related quality of life were improved by adopting these.

The increasing emphasis on the individual's perspective of primary health care services received during the past few decades in Canada has created a paradigm shift in the approach to the operationalization and measurement of the impact of health outcomes achieved. Making an overall judgment about the quality of primary health care services received requires, therefore, a complex assessment of the individual's experiences and health care priorities. These health care priorities are often fluid in nature and change and evolve due to a variety of health events and challenges. National and international social-political, economic and environmental forces and trends (e.g., 2009 global recession, climate change, bioterrorism) are driving health care reforms and a multitude of proposed healthcare approaches with ethical, legal, social, cultural and economic implications, as well as negative iatrogenic health effects (Armstrong et al. 2000; Budgen, Cameron, and Bartfay 2010; Canadian Public Health Association 2000). Public health care professionals and workers should anticipate encountering these forces and dilemmas in their practice. Societal trends are significant to program planning and evaluation because they are directly linked to the community and the types of programs that would be most useful.

For example, unemployment in the auto sector in the Durham Region of Ontario during the recent global economic recession in 2009 had significant negative social-psychological, economic and physical health effects on unemployed autoworkers and their families (Bartfay, Bartfay, and Wu 2011, 2013). Programs directed at supporting laid-off autoworkers and their families are imperative during economic downfalls resulting in unemployment. These programs may include community-based support groups and resources, housing, medication and dental assistant programs, food banks, and job retaining. Health care professionals and workers who consider current and emerging health care challenges and societal trends can use this knowledge to avoid pitfalls, realize opportunities and increase the likelihood that the program will be successful (Bartfay and Bartfay 2015). Indeed, opportunities for program planning and evaluation in Canada and globally have never been greater.

Group Review Exercise Child family health program planning in public health: What's the evidence?

About this public health webinar

This ninty-minute webinar first aired on February 2, 2012, and was hosted by Maureen Dobbins, the Scientific Director of Health Evidence. This webinar focused on child and family health program planning in public health and examined the evidence presented on the following four systematic reviews of the scientific literature. The first systematic review in this webinar focused on Internet-based innovations for the prevention of eating disorders (also see Newton 2006 at http://www.health-evidence.ca/articles/show/16914). The second examined alternatives to inpatient mental health care for children and young people (also see Shepperd 2009 at http://www.health-evidence.ca/articles/show/19286). The third systematic review consisted of internet-based self-management interventions for youth with health conditions (also see Stinson 2009 at http://www.health-evidence.ca/articles/show/20114). The last systematic review in this webinar examined the literature related to supplementation with calcium to improving bone mineral density in children (also see Winzenberg 2006 at http://www.health-evidence.ca/articles/show/17768). This webinar also hosted an online discussion which allowed participants to further discuss these presentations, pose additional questions and comments and also share information with other public health care professionals and workers. This webinar helps to highlight the importance of program planning in evaluation in public health and the importance of critically evaluating the scientific literature to help guide evidence-based practice related to child and family health programs in the community.

Instructions

This assignment may be done alone, in pairs or in groups of up to five people (note: if you are doing this assignment in pairs or groups, please only submit one hard or electronic copy to your instructor). The assignment should be typewritten and no more than 4–6 pages maximum in length (double-spaced please). View the ninty-minute webinar and take notes during the presentations. See link http://www.youtube.com/watch?v=TtrErDdz9g (and links noted above for specific topic systematic reviews).

1. Provide a brief overview of the importance of examining the empirical evidence in reference to program planning and evaluation in public health.

2. Provide a brief summary of the salient findings highlighted in the four systematic reviews.

3. Describe some of the social determinants of health described in these four systematic reviews of the literature and their implications for public health practice.

Summary

- Program planning is defined as an organized and structured systemic decision-making process which attempts to meet specific primary health care aims or objectives through the application of currently available, competing or needed resources in the future based on identified priorities or projected needs.
- Strategic or allocative planning is defined as an open and transparent formalized decision-making process which seeks to determine which health care needs should be addressed in accordance with the available resources and closely resembles policy making.
- Operational or activity planning is defined as a formalized decision-making process which focuses on the implementation of plans based on detailed time frames.
- Program evaluation is defined as a formalized ongoing and dynamic process which seeks to monitor, assess and refine health program activities and interventions and to identify gaps or actual or potential flaws in the original program design and implementation.
- Evaluation in public health may be viewed as a process that is ultimately intended to determine the worth of something, presumably in comparison with some norm or standard of goodness.
- There are a variety of program evaluation types that can be broadly classified into the following three main categories based on when the evaluations are being conducted and the type of information being collected: (a) formative, (b) process, and (c) summative.
- Outcome measure evaluates what specifically occurred as the result of the health program being implemented in terms of its noted aims or goals.
- Impact measures are used to evaluate the effect of the implemented health program on the users, stakeholders and implementers and specifically measures what changes (positive, negative or neutral) occurred as a result of the program.
- There are eight critical steps in the program planning and evaluation process:
- Step I includes the need to conduct a needs assessment and the active engagement of stakeholders and implementers (e.g., public health nurses).
- Stakeholders are defined as all individuals or groups (both internal and external) who have an interest in the program or those who may be affected by the program either directly or indirectly including community volunteers, potential program participants, policy makers, governmental agencies, NGOs or industry.
- Step II requires that the stakeholders and implementers collectively describe and detail the program's aims or goals.
- Step III involves the development of a draft proposed action plan, design, or approach and a proposed evaluation model based on the best available evidence.

- Step IV consists of seeking feedback from the stakeholders and implementers regarding the draft proposed action plan, design or approach and proposed evaluation model.
- During Step V, the action plan, model or design is formally refined based on the feedback and suggestions received.
- Step VI consists of the formal implementation of the action plan, model or design.
- Step VII consists of the evaluation the successes and outcomes of the program via the formal documentation of the evidence and outcomes achieved to justify the conclusions reached.
- Step VIII involves the dissemination of the program findings and outcomes achieved with the stakeholders and implementers.
- The program logic model is used extensively in many municipal, regional, provincial and federal governmental public health agencies in Canada.
- The development of a logic model consists of two main planning stages: (a) CAT and (b) SOLO.
- During the CAT stage, activities are typically clustered thematically into components for the public health program under construction or review.
- During the SOLO stage, short- and long-term health-related outcomes are identified. An example of the program logic model.
- HSR is defined as an integrative and multidisciplinary scientific field that involves the integration of knowledge, and the study and evaluation of the organization, functioning and performance of health services.
- HSR requires the evaluation of the following four critical components: (a) structure, (b) process, (c) output, and (d) outcome.
- Outcomes research seeks to study the specific outcomes of primary health care interventions and seeks to determine why these end results were obtained or not and is designed to critically and objectively examine and document the effectiveness of health care policies and services and the results of care provided to clients.
- The emphasis on evaluating the quality of primary health care interventions has shifted from structures to an understanding of the critical processes involved.
- Public health care professionals and workers need to be cognizant of various ethical principles and dilemmas that may arise during the process of program planning and evaluation.

Critical Thinking Questions

1. Your health care agency is collaborating with a senior's advocacy group in your community to address the issue of elder abuse. What are some of the underlying SDH that may put seniors at risk? How would you conduct a needs assessment to address these issues?
2. Based on the elder abuse issue above, what types of evidence would you need to collect or assemble to support the need for the development of an elder abuse prevention program in your community? What specific levels of prevention do you believe need to include and how would you prioritize them?
3. What would the specific aims or goals of your community-based elder prevention program be, and how would you determine its impact factor or success?

References

Agency for Healthcare Research and Quality (AHRQ). *Outcomes Research Fact Sheet*. Rockville, MD: AHQ Publication No. 00-P011, March, 2000. Accessed May 22, 2012. http://www.ahrq.gov.clinic/outfact.htm.

———. *Health Services Research*. Rockville, MD: AHQ Publication No. 00-P011, February, 2002. Accessed May 22, 2012. http://www.ahrq.gov/.

Arah, O. A. "On the Relationship between Individual and Population Health." *Medicine Health Care and Philosophy* 12, no. 3 (2009): 235–44.

Armstrong, P., H. Armstrong, I. Bourgeault, J. Choiniere, E. Mykhalovsky, and J. White. *Health Thyself: Managing Health Care Reform*. Aurora, ON: Garamond, 2000.

Barry, J. M. *White Paper on Novel N1N1. Prepared for the MIT Center for Engineering Systems Fundamentals*. Massachusetts: Massachusetts Institute of Technology, 2009. Accessed January 26, 2014. http://.esd.mit.edu/WPS/2009/esd-wp-2009-07-072709.pdf.

Bartfay, W. J., and E. Bartfay. *Public Health in Canada*. Boston, MA: Pearson Learning Solutions, 2015. (ISBN:13:978-1-323-01471-4).

Bartfay, W. J., E. Bartfay, and T. Wu. "Impact of the Global Economic Crisis on the Health of Unemployed Autoworkers." *Canadian Journal of Nursing Research* 45, no. 10 (September 2013): 66–79.

Bartfay, E., W. J. Bartfay, and T. Wu. "The Health and Well-being of Laid-off Automobile Industry Workers in Durham, Canada." *Journal of Epidemiology and Community Health* 65 (August 2011): A458. IEA World Congress of Epidemiology, August 7–11, 2011. Edinburgh International Conference Centre Edinburgh, Scotland: SPg-12. doi:10.1136/jech.2011.14296p.83.

Baylis, F., N. P. Kenny, and S. Sherwin. "A Relational Account of Public Health Ethics." *Public Health Ethics* 1, no. 3 (2008): 196–209.

Bowen, S., and A. B. Zwi. "Pathways to 'Evidence-informed' Policy and Practice: A Framework for Action." *PLoS Medicine* 2, no. 7 (May 31, 2005): 1–6. doi:10.1371/journal.pmed.0020166.

Bennett, G. G., and R. E. Glasgow. "The Delivery of Public Health Interventions via the Internet: Actualizing Their Potential." *Annual Review of Public Health* 30 (2009): 273–92.

Benzies, K., S. Tough, N. Edwards, K. Nagan, B. Nowicki, R. Bychasiuk, and C. Donnelly. "Effects of a Two-generation Canadian Preschool Program on Parenting Stress, Self-esteem, and Life skills." *Early Childhood Services: An Interdisciplinary Journal of Effectiveness* 3, no. 1 (2009): 19–32.

Black, N., and R. Gruen. *Understanding Health Services*. New York: London School of Hygiene and Tropical Medicine, 2005.

Bogue, R. "Use S.M.A.R.T. Goals to Launch Management by Objectives Plan". *TechRepublic*, 2013. Accessed January 7, 2016. http://www.techrepublic.com/article/use-smart-goals-to-launch-management-by-objectives-plan/.

Borus, M., C. Buntz, and W. Tash. *Evaluating the Impact of Health Programs: A Primer*. Cambridge, MA: MIT Press, 1982.

Brinkerhoff, R. O., D. M. Brethower, T. Hluchyj, and J. R. Nowakowski. *Program Evaluation: A Practitioner's Guide for Trainers and Educators*. Boston: Kluwer-Nijhoff Publishing, 1983.

Buchanan, D. R. "Autonomy, Paternalism, and Justice: Ethical Priorities in Public Health." *American Journal of Public Health* 98, no. 1 (2008): 15–21.

Budgen, C., G. Cameron, and W. J. Bartfay. "Program Planning, Implementation, and Evaluation." In *Community Health Nursing: Caring in Action*, 1st Canadian edition, edited by J. E. Hitchcock, P. E. Schubert, S. A. Thomas, and W. J. Bartfay, 284–24. Toronto, ON: Nelson Education, 2010.

Caldwell, B., J. Slatin, and G. Vanderheiden. "Web Content Accessibility Guidelines 2.0." *World Wide Web Consortium W3C*, 2008. Accessed April 03, 2012. http://www.w3.org/TR/WCAG20/.

Canadian Broadcasting Corporation (CBC). *Canadians Lead World in Internet Use: A Report*. Toronto, ON: CBC, March 9, 2011. Accessed January 16, 2016. http://www.cbc.ca/news/technology/canadians-lead-world-in-Internet-use-report-1.1063588.

Canadian Institute for Health Information. *National Health Expenditure Trends, 1975 to 2015*. Ottawa, ON: CIHI, 2015. ISBN 978-1-77-109-413-9 (PDF). Accessed November 10, 2015. https://www.cihi.ca/en/spending-and-health-workforce/spending/canadas-slow-health-spending-growth-continues.

Canadian Institutes of Health Research, Rx & D Health Research Foundation, and Canadian Food Inspection Agency. *Canadian Pandemic Preparedness Meeting: H1N1 Outbreak Research Response*. Toronto, ON: CIHR, July 8, 2009. Accessed April 24, 2012. http://www.cihr-irc.gc.ca/e/documents/iii_cppm_report_2009_e.pdf.

Canadian Nurses Association. *NurseOne, the Canadian Nurses Portal*. Ottawa, ON: Author, 2006. Accessed April 10, 2012. http://www.cnanurses.ca/CNA/nursing/portal/about/default_easpx.

Canadian Public Health Association. *Directory of Plain Language Health Information.* Ottawa, ON: Author, 1999. Accessed April 10, 2012. http://www.cpha.ca/en/portals/h-l/resources.aspx.

———. *An Ounce of Prevention: Strengthening the Balance in Health Care Reform.* Ottawa, ON: Author, 2000.

———. *Plain Language Service.* Ottawa, ON: Author, 2010. Accessed April 10, 2012. http://www.cpha.ca/en/pls.aspx.

CEFRIO. "L'explosion des media sociaux au Québec." *Netendances 2010,* 14, 2010. Accessed January 25, 2014. http://www.cefrio.qc.ca/fileadmin/documents/Publication/NETendances-Vol1-1.pdf.

Changrani, J., and F. Gany. "Online Cancer Education and Immigrants: Effecting Culturally Appropriate Websites." *Journal of Cancer Education* 20 (2005): 183–86.

Chistensen, S. "20 Million Canadians Suffer from Nomophobia Rogers Says, and This is Just the Beginning." *Techvibes,* January 2, 2013. Accessed April 10, 2015. http://www.techvibes.com/blog/canadians-suffer-from-nomophobia-2013-01-02.

Ciliska, C., H. Thomas, and C. Buffet. *An Introduction to Evidence-informed Public Health and a Compendium of Critical Appraisal Tools for Public Health Practice.* 2008. Accessed October 8, 2013. http://www.nccmt.ca/pubs/eiph_backgrounder.pdf.

Clancy, C. M., and J. M. Eisenberg. "Outcomes Research: Measuring the End Results of Health Care." *Science* 282, no. 5387 (October, 1998): 245–46. doi:10.1126/science/282.5387.245.

Commission of Social Determinants of Health (CSDH). *Closing the Gap in a Generation: Health Equity through Action on the Social Determinants of Health. Final Report of the Commission on Social Determinants of Health.* Geneva, Switzerland: World Health Organization, 2008.

Cooksy, L. J., P. Gill, and P. A. Kelly. "The Program Logic Model as an Integrative Framework for a Multimethod Evaluation." *Evaluation and Program Planning* 24 (2001): 119–28.

Daniel, M., L. Green, S. Marion, D. Gamble, C. Herbert, C. Hertzman, and S. Sheps. "Effectiveness of Community-directed Diabetes Prevention and Control in a Rural Population in British Columbia, Canada." *Social Science and Medicine* 48 (1999): 815–32.

Dawson, A., and M. Verweij. *Ethics, Prevention, and Public Health.* New York: Oxford University Press, 2007.

Dieppe, P. "Research on Health and Health Care." In *Handbook of Health Research Methods,* edited by A. Bowling and S. Ebrahim, 3–11. Berkshire, England: Open University Press, 2007.

Dickerson, S. S. "Women's Use of the Internet: What Nurses Need to Know." *Journal of Obstetric Gynecologic and Neonatal Nursing* 35 (2006): 151–56.

Donabedian, A. "Some Basic Issues in Evaluating the Quality of Health Care." In Vol. 1 of the *Outcomes Measures in Home Care,* edited by L. T. Rinke, 3–28. New York: National League for Nursing, 1987.

Doran, G. T. "There's a S.M.A.R.T. Way to Write Management's Goals and Objectives." *Management Review (AMA FORUM)* 70, no. 11. (1981): 35–36.

English, J. "Community Development." In *Community Nursing: Promoting Canadians' Health,* 2nd ed., edited by M. Stewart, 403–19. Toronto, ON: W. B. Saunders, 2000.

Evaluation Gap Working Group. *When Will We Learn? Improving Lives Through Impact Evaluations.* Washington, DC: Center for Global Development, 2006. Accessed May 18, 2012. http://www.cgdev.org/content/publications/detail/973.

Eysenbach, G. "Medicine 2.0: Social Networking, Collaboration, Participation, Apomediation, and Openness." *Journal of Medical Internet Research* 10, no. 3 (2008): e22. Accessed January 25, 2014. http://www.jmir.org/2008/3/e22.

Eysenbach, G., and C. Kohler. "How Do Consumers Search for and Appraise Health Information on the World Wide Web? Quality Study Using Focus Groups, Usability Tests, and in-depth Interviews." *British Medical Journal* 324 (2002): 573–77.

Ferney, S. L., and A. L. Marshall. "Website Physical Activity Interventions: Preferences of Potential Users." *Health Education Research: Theory and Practice* 21 (2006): 560–66.

Flicker, S., O. Maley, and A. Ridgley. "Using Technology and Participatory Action Research to Engage Youth in Health Promotion." *Action Research* 6 (2008): 285–303.

Fox, S., and S. Jones. *The Social Life of Health Information: Americans' Pursuit of Health Takes Place with a Widening Network of Both Online and Offline Resources* (Rep. No. 202-149-4500). Washington, DC: Pew Internet and American Life Project, 2009.

Fraser, D. L., and R. J. Stupak. "A Synthesis of the Strategic Learning Process with the Principles of Andragogy: Learning, Leading and Linking." *International Journal of Public Administration* 25, no. 9 2002: 1199–20.

Goldner, M. "Using the Internet and Email for Health Purposes: The Impact of Health Status." *Social Science Quarterly* 87 (2006): 690–710.

Gosselin, P., and P. Poitras. "Use of an Internet 'Viral' Marketing Software Platform in Health Promotion." *Journal of Medical Internet Research* 10 (2008): e47.

Gostin, L. O., and K. G. Gostin. "A Broader Liberty: J. S. Mill, Paternalism and the Public's Health." *Public Health* 123, no. 3 (2009): 214–21.

Gottlieb, R., and J. L. Rogers. "Readability of Health Sites on the Internet." *International Electronic Journal of Health Education* 7 (2004): 38–42.

Green, A. *An Introduction to Health Planning in Developing Health Systems*, 3rd ed. Oxford, UK: Oxford University Press, 2007.

Green, A., C. Collins, and T. Mirzoev. "Management and Planning for Global Health." In *Global Health: Diseases, Programs, Systems, and Policies*, 3rd ed., edited by M. H. Merson, R. E. Black, and A. J. Mills, 653–706. Mississauga, ON: Jones & Bartlett Learning, 2012.

Health Canada. *The Population Health Template: Key Elements and Actions that Define a Population Health Approach.* Ottawa, ON: Strategic Policy Directorate of the Population and Public Health Branch, Health Canada, 2001. Accessed May 01, 2012. http://www-phac.aspc.gc.ca/ph-sp/pdf/discussion-eng.pdf.

Health on the Net Foundation. "HON Code of Conduct (HONcode) for Medical and Health Web Sites." *Health on the Net Foundation*, 2009. Accessed April 10, 2012. http://www.hon.ch/HON.code/Guidelines/guidelines.html.

Health Summit Working Group. *Information Quality Tool. Mitretek Systems.* 2010. Accessed April 10, 2012. http://www. ieee.org/organizations/pubs/newsletter/npss/march2000/health.htm.

Hebda, T., and P. Czar. *Handbook of Informatics for Nurses & Healthcare Professionals*, 5th ed. Boston, MA: Pearson, 2013.

Helms, M. M., and J. Nixon. "Exploring SWOT Analysis—Where Are We Now? A Review of Academic Research from the Last Decade." *Journal of Strategy Management* 3, no. 3 (2010): 215–51.

Herman, J., L. L. Morris, and C. Fitz-Gibbon. *Evaluator's Handbook.* Newbury Part, CA: SAGE Publications, 1987.

Hesse, B. W., D. E. Nelson, G. L. Kreps, R. T. Croyle, N. K. Arora, B. K. Rimer, and K. Viswanath. "Trust and Sources of Health Information." *Archives of Internal Medicine* 165 (2005): 2618–24.

Holland, S. *Public Health Ethics.* Cambridge: Polity Press, 2007.

Horne, T. *Making a Difference: Program Evaluation for Health Promotion.* WellQuest Consulting, 1995.

Hudson, J., J. Mayne, and R. Thomlison, eds. *Action-oriented Evaluation in Organizations: Canadian Practices.* Toronto, ON: Wall & Emerson Inc, 1992.

ICT Data and Statistics Division. *World Telecommunications/ICT Indicators Database 2014*, 18th ed. Geneva, Switzerland: ICT Data and Statistics Division, 2014. Accessed April 02, 2015. www.itu.int/ict.

International Telecommunications Union. *ICT Facts and Figures: The World in 2011.* Geneva, Switzerland: ICT Data and Statistics Division Telecommunications Development Bureau, ICT, 2011.

Internet World Stats. "Usage and Population Statistics." *Miniwatts Marketing Groups*, June 30, 2012. Accessed January 16, 2014. http://www.internet worldstats.com/stats/htm.

Internet World Stats. "Usage and Population Statistics" (March 25, 2017). *World Internet Penetration.* Miniwatts Marketing Group. Retrieved April 14, 2017, http://www.internetworldstats.com/stats.htm.

Kaluzney, A., and J. Veney. "Evaluating Health Care Programs and Services." In *Introduction to Health Services*, edited by S. Williams and P. Torrens. New York: Wiley, 1999.

Kende, M. *Internet Society Global Internet Report 2014. Open and Sustainable Access for All.* Geneva, Switzerland: Internet Society, 2014. Accessed April 02, 2014. http://www.Internetsociety.org/doc/ global-Internet-report?gclid=CPLOx4yj1cQCFQsAaQodIqoAnA.

Kivits, J. "Everyday Health and the Internet: A Mediated Health Perspective on Health Information Seeking." *Sociology of Health and Illness* 31, no. 5 (2009): 673–87.

Korp, P. "Health on the Internet: Implications for Health Promotion." *Health Education Research* 21 (2006): 78–86.

Kreps, G. L., and L. Neuhauser. "New Directions in eHealth Communication: Opportunities and Challenges." *Patient Education and Counseling* 78 (2010): 329–36.

Lorig, K., A. Stewart, P. Ritter, V. Gonzalez, D. Laurent, and J. Lynch. *Outcome Measures for Health Education and Other Health Care Interventions*. Thousand Oaks, CA: SAGE Publications, 1996.

Lüchtenberg, M., C. Kuhli-Hattenbach, Y. Sinangin, C. Ohrloff, and R. Schalnus. "Accessibility of Health Information on the Internet to the Visually Impaired User." *Ophthalmologica* 222, no. 3 (2008): 187–93.

McDougal, C. W. *Public Health Ethics-selected Resources: Ethics in a Pandemic*. Montréal, QC: National Collaborating Centre for Healthy Public Policy, May 2010. Accessed January 26, 2014. http://www.ncchpp.ca/43/Contact_Us.ccnpps.

McKenzie, J. F., and J. L. Jurs. *Planning, Implementing and Evaluating Health Promotion Programs*. New York: MacMillian Publishing Company, 1993.

McKenzie, J. F., B. L. Neiger, and R. Thackeray. *Planning, Implementing, and Evaluating Health Promotion Programs: A Primer*, 5th ed. Toronto, ON: Pearson Benjamin Cummings, 2009. ISBN-10:0-3214-9511-X.

McKnight, J. *Community Capacity: People, Place, Technology*. Workshop on Community Development at Vernon, BC: Vernon School District, 2001.

McLaughlin, G. H. "SMOG-grading: A New Readability Formula." *Journal of Reading* 12 (1969): 639–49.

Mehra, B., C. Merkel, and A. P. Bishop. "The Internet for Empowerment of Minority and Marginalized Users." *New Media and Society* 66 (2004): 781–802.

Mitchell, P. H., S. Ferketich, and B. M. Jennings. "Quality Health Outcomes Model." *Image: The Journal of Nursing Scholarship* 20 (1998): 43–46.

Mullet, J. *Program Performance Evaluation Framework for Regional Health Boards and Community Health Councils*. Unpublished paper. Victoria, BC: Ministry of Health, 1995.

National Collaborating Centre for Methods and Tools. *Program Evaluation Toolkit*. Hamilton, ON: McMaster University, 2010. Accessed January 13, 2016. http://www.nccmt.cas/registry/view/eng/68.html.

National Collaborating Centres for Public Health (NCCPH). *What Is Evidence-informed Public Health? Fact Sheet*. Last modified November, 2011. Accessed October 12, 2013. http://www.nccmt.ca/eiph/.

Norman, C. D., and H. A. Skinner. "eHealth Literacy: Essential Skills for Consumer Health in a Networked World." *Journal of Internet Research* 8, no. 2 (2006):e9. doi:10.2196/jmir.8.2.e9.

Nuffield Council on Bioethics. *Public Health: Ethical Issues*. Cambridge: Cambridge Publishers, 2007.

Ontario Health Promotion E-Bulletin (OHPE). "Canadian Best Practice Portal Makes Program Planning Easier for Public Health Practitioners." *OHPE Bulletin* 2010 no. 658 (April 16, 2010). Accessed May 12, 2012. http://www.ohpe.ca/node/11256.

Oxman, A. D., A. Bjorndal, F. Becerra-Possada, M. Gibson, M. A. Block, A. Haines, M. Hamid, C. H. Odom, H. Lei, B. Levin, M. W. Lipsey, J. H. Littell, H. Mshinda, P. Ongolo-Zogo, T. Pang, N. Sewankambo, F. Songane, H. Soydan, C. Torgerson, D. Weisburd, J. Whitworth, S. Wibulpolprasert. "A Framework for Mandatory Impact Evaluations to Ensure Well Informed Public Policy Decisions." *Lancet* 375, no. 9012 (2010): 427–31.

Oxman, A. D., J. N. Lavis, and A. Fretheim. "Use of Evidence in WHO Recommendations." *The Lancet* 369, no. 9576–78 (June 2007): 1883–89.

Pach, B. *What Is the "Evidence" in Evidence-based Public Health? Pathways to Evidence Informed Public Health Policy and Practice*. Toronto, ON: Ontario Public Health Libraries Association (OPHL) Foundation Standard Workshop, November 14, 2008.

Paranthaman, K., C. P. Conlon, C. Parker, and N McCarthy. "Resource Allocation during an Influenza Pandemic." *Emerging Infectious Diseases* 14, no. 3 (2008). Accessed January 26, 2014. http://www.cdc.gov/EID/content/13/3/520.htm.

Petrič, G., A. Petrovčič, and V. Vehovar. "Social Uses of Interpersonal Communication Technologies in a Complex Media Environment." *Communication Technology* 11, no. 5 (2011): 339–48. doi:10.1007/s00779-0060078-3.

Pew Research Centre. *Mobile Technology Use*. Washington, DC: Pew Research Centre, October, 2014. Accessed April 8, 2015. http://www.pewInternet.org/fact-sheets/mobile-technology-fact-sheet/.

Porta, M. *A Dictionary of Epidemiology*, 5th ed. New York: Oxford University Press, 2008.

Porteous, N., B. Sheldrick, and P Stewart. "Introducing Program Teams to Logic Models: Facilitating the Learning Process." *The Canadian Journal of Program Evaluation* 17, no. 3 (2002): 113–14.

——. *Program Evaluation Tool Kit: A Blueprint for Public Health Management*. Ottawa, ON: Ottawa-Carleton Health Department, 1997.

Powers, M., and R. Faden. *Social Justice. The Moral Foundations of Public Health and Public Health Policy*. New York: NY: Oxford University Press, 2006.

Project Management Institute. *A Guide to the Project Management Body of Knowledge* (PMBOK® Guide), 5th ed. Newtown, Pennsylvania: Author, 2013 (BSR/PMI 99-001-2013).

Public Health Agency of Canada. *The Canadian Best Practices Portal for Health Promotion and Chronic Disease Prevention: About the Portal*. Ottawa, ON: Author, 2006. Accessed April 02, 2012. http://cbpp-pcpe.phac-aspc.gc.ca/.

——. *Core Competencies for Public Health in Canada: Release 1.1*. Ottawa, ON: Author, September, 2007a.

——. *A Framework for Strategic Risk Communications with the Context of Health Canada and the PHAC's Integrated Risk Management*. Ottawa, ON: Author, March, 2007b. Accessed May 01, 2012. http://www.phac-aspc.gc.ca/publicat/2007/risk-com/index-eng.php.

——. *Program Evaluation Tool Kit*. Ottawa, ON: Author, 2008. Accessed May 01, 2012. http://www.phac-aspc.gc.ca/php-psp/toolkit-eng.php.

——. *Influenza*. Ottawa, ON: Author, 2009. Accessed April 23, 2012. http://wwwphac-aspc.gc.ca/influenza/index-eng.php.

——. *Surveillance: Deaths Associated with H1N1 Flu Virus in Canada*. Ottawa, ON: Author, 2010. Accessed April 24, 2012. http://www.phac-aspc/gc/ca/alert-alerte/h1n1/surveillance-archive/20100128-eng.php.

——. *Public Health Ethics and Ethical Research*. Ottawa, ON: Author, November 14, 2012. Accessed January 26, 2014. http://www.phac-aspc.gc.ca/php-psp/phe-esp.eng.php.

——. *Core Competencies for Public Health in Canada*. Ottawa, ON: Author, 2013. Accessed January 26, 2014. http://www.phac-aspc.gc.ca/php-psp/ccph-cesp/stmts-enon-eng.php.

Purcell, K., J. Brenner, and L. Rainie. "Search Engine Use 2012." *Pew Research Center*, March 9, 2012. Accessed January 16, 2016. http://www.pewinternet.org/2012/03/09/search-engine-use-2012/.

Rainie, L., K. Purcell, and A. Smith. "The Social Side of the Internet." *Pew Research Center*, June 18, 2011. Accessed January 16, 2014. http://www.pewinternet.org/Reports/2011/The-Social-Side-of-the-Internet.aspx.

Raphael, D, ed. *Social Determinants of Health*, 2nd ed. Toronto, ON: Canadian Scholars Press, Inc, 2009.

Rice, R. E. "Influences, Usage, and Outcomes of Internet Health Information Searching: Multivariate Results from the Pew surveys." *International Journal of Medical Informatics* 75 (2006): 8–28.

Rieger, O. Y. http://www.dlib.org/dlib/july07/rieger/rieger-fig2-rev.png.

Robinson, M., and S. Robertson. "Young Men's Health Promotion and New Information Communication Technologies: Illuminating the Issues and Research Agenda." *Health Promotion International* 25 (2010): 363–70.

Rogers Communication. *Rogers Innovation Report Infographic 2013*. Toronto, ON: Author, 2013. Accessed April 10, 2015. http://redboard.rogers.com/rogers-innovation-report-infographic-2013/.

Rycroft-Malone, J. "Evidence-informed Practice: From Individual to Context." *Journal of Nursing Management* 16, no. 4 (May, 2008). 404–08. doi:10.111/j.1365-2834.2008.00859.x.

Senate Subcommittee on Population Health. *A Healthy, Productive Canada: A Determinants of Health Approach*. Ottawa, ON: The Standing Senate Committee on Social Affairs, Science and Technology, 2009. Accessed May 01, 2012. http://www-parl.gc.ca/40/2/parlbus/commbus/senate/com-e/popu-e/rep-e/rephealth1jun09-e.pdf.

Skinner, H., S. Biscope, and E. Goldberg. "How Adolescents Use Technology for Health Information: Implications for Health Professionals from Focus Group Studies." *Journal of Medical Internet Research* 5, no. 4 (2003): 32.

Sliger, M., and S. Broderick. *The Software Project Manager's Bridge to Agility*. New York: Addison-Wesley, 2008. ISBN 0321502752.

Statistics Canada. *Literacy and the Official Languages Minority*. Ottawa, ON: Author, 2006. Accessed April 10, 2012. http://www.statcan.gc.ca/daily/quotidian/080612/dq080612b-eng.htm.

——. *Canadian Internet Use Survey*. Ottawa, ON: Author, 2007. Accessed April 10, 2012. http://www.statcan.gc.ca/daily-quotidein/080612/dq080109/dqa-eng.htm.

————. *International Survey of Reading Skills*. Ottawa, ON: Author, 2008. Accessed April 10, 2012. http://www.statcan. gc.ca/daily-quotidien/080109/dq080109a-eng.htm.

————. *Internet Use by Individuals, By Type of Activity*. (CANSIM Table 358-0130). Ottawa, ON: Author, 2010a. Accessed April 02, 2012. http://www40.statcan.gc.ca/01;cst01/comm29a-eng.htm?sdi=internet.

————. *Canadian Internet Use Survey*. Ottawa, ON: Author, 2010b. Accessed January 25, 2014. http://www.statcan/gc/ ca/daily/quotidian/100510/dq100510a-eng.htm.

Stout, P. A., J. Villegas, and H. Kim. Enhancing Learning through the Use of Interactive Tools on Health-related Websites. *Health Education Research* 16 (2001): 721–33.

Suggs, L. S., and McIntyre, C. "Are We There Yet? An Examination of Online Tailored Health Communication." *Health Education and Behavior* 36 (2009): 278–88.

TechTarget. "Gantt chart." *TechTarget*, 2007. Accessed January 16, 2014. http://searchsoftwarequality.techtarget.com/ sDefinition/0,,sid92_gci331391,00.html.

Thompson, V. D. *Health and Health Care Delivery in Canada*. Toronto, ON: Mosby Elsevier, 2010.

Timmreck, T. C. *Planning, Program Development, and Evaluation*, 2nd ed. Boston, MA: Jones and Bartlett Publishers, 2003.

Tomée, S. "ICT Use and Mental Health in Young Adults. Effects of Computer and Mobile Phone Use on Stress, Sleep Disturbances, and Symptoms of Depression." PhD thesis. Gotehnburg, Sweden, Sahlgrenska Academy, Institute of Medicine, 2012. ISBN: 978-91-628-8432-1. Accessed April 15, 2015 from https://gupea.ub.gu.se/ bitstream/2077/28245/1/gupea_2077_28245_1.pdf.

Treasury Board of Canada Secretariat. *Common Look and Feel Standards for the Internet (CLF 2.0)*. *Treasury Board of Canada Secretariat*. Ottawa, ON: Author, 2007. Accessed April 03, 2012. http://www.tbs-sct.gc.ca/clf-nsi/index-eng.asp.

Underhill, C., and L. McKeown. "Getting a Second Opinion: Health Information and the Internet." *Health Report* 19 (2008): 65–69.

United Nations (UN) Committee on Economic, Social and Cultural Rights. *Twenty-Five Questions and Answers on Health and Human Rights*. Health and Human Rights Publication Series, Issue No.1. New York: UN, July, 2002.

University of Toronto Joint Centre for Bioethics. *Population and Public Health Ethics: Cases from Research, Policy, and Practice*. Toronto, ON: Joint Centre for Bioethics, University of Toronto, 2012. ISBN: 978-1-261-99991-5.

Van Marris, B., and B. King. *Evaluating Health Promotion Programs (version 3.6)*. Toronto, ON: Health Communication Unit at the Centre for Health Promotion Department of Public Health Sciences, University of Toronto, August 15, 2007. hc.unit@utoronto.ca or http://www.thcu.ca.

Victora, C. G., D. Walker, B. Jones, and J. Bryce. "Evaluations of Large-scale Health Programs." In *Global Health: Diseases, Programs, Systems, and Policies*, 3rd ed., edited by M. H. Merson, R. E. Black, and A. J. Mills, 815–51. Mississauga, ON: Jones & Bartlett Learning, 2012.

Wooten, K. C., R. M. Rose, G. V. Ostir, W. J. Calhoun, B. T. Ameredes, and A. R. Briaser. "Assessing and Evaluating Multidisciplinary Translational Teams: A Mixed Methods Approach." *Evaluation & Health Professions* 37, no. 1 (2014): 33–49. doi:10.1177/0163278713504433.

World Bank. *Results-based Financing*, 2010. Accessed May 18, 2012. http://web.worldbank.org/ WBSITE/EXTERNAL/TOPICS/EXTHEALTHNUTRITIONALANDPOPULATION?EXTHSD/0,,menu PK:376799~pagePK:149018~piPK:149093~theSitePK:376793,00.html.

Worldwide online Reliable Advice to Patients and Individuals (WRAPIN). *Worldwide Online Reliable Advice to Patients and Individuals*. *European Project-IST-2001-33260*. 2007. Accessed April 10, 2012. http://www/wrapin.org.

World Wide Web Consortium W3C. "Web Accessibility Initiative (WAI)." *World Wide Web Consortium W3C*, 2009. Accessed April 02, 2012. http://www/w3.org/WAI/.

Yasnoff, W., P. O'Carroll, D. Koo, R. Linkins, and E. Kilbourne. "Public Health Informatics: Improving and Transforming Public Health in the Information Age." *Journal of Public Health Management Practice* 6 (2000): 67–75.

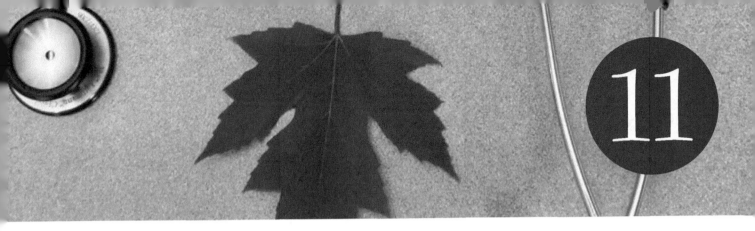

Current and Emerging Mental Health Issues in Canada

When inspiration does not come to me, I go halfway to meet it.

(Sigmund Freud 1856–1939)

Learning Objectives

After completion of this chapter, the student will be able to

- Define mental health and list three major mental illnesses and disorders along with their clinical manifestations.
- Critically examine the role of stress and how it affects individuals from various social, psychological, and biological perspectives.
- Explain the role and objectives of the Mental Health Commission of Canada (MHCC), the Pan-Canadian Joint Consortium for School Health (JCSH), and the Mental Health First Aid (MHFA) Canada program in maintaining, promoting, and/or decreasing stigma associated with mental health issues and challenges faced by Canadians.
- Describe and critically examine theories associated with the development of mental illness and their associated treatment regimens.
- Describe the role of public healthcare professionals and workers in helping individuals' families, entire communities, and populations regain, maintain, and promote their mental health and well-being.
- Critically examine and discuss current and emerging mental health issues and challenges facing Canadians across the lifespan.

Core Competencies for Public Health Addressed in Chapter 11

Core Competencies	Competency Statements
1.0 Public Health Sciences	1.1, 1.2, 1.3, 1.4
2.0 Assessment and Analysis	2.1, 2.3, 2.5, 2.6
3.0 Policy and Program Planning, Implementation, and Evaluation	3.1, 3.2, 3.6, 3.7
4.0 Partnerships, Collaboration, and Advocacy	4.1, 4.2, 4.3, 4.4
5.0 Diversity and Inclusiveness	5.1, 5.2, 5.3
6.0 Communication	6.2
7.0 Leadership	7.1, 7.2

Note: Please see the following document or web-based link for a detailed description of these specific competencies. Public Health Agency of Canada (2007).

Introduction

Simply stated, "There can be no health without mental health." In fact, mental health is intrinsically indispensable and a critical component of health and well-being of individuals, families, and entire communities. Mental health promotion from the public health context focuses on enhancing the social, structural, environmental, spiritual, and psychological resources that enable Canadians to cope, and experience positive quality of life. It is also a necessary component required to enable individuals to contribute to the social, economic, and environmental dimensions of our society (Canadian Mental Health Association [CMHA], 2017; PHAC, 2012).

Hence, promoting mental health provides the capacity of individuals to realize abilities; develop effective coping skills to manage a variety of daily and unexpected stressors; take control of one's life, and make positive contributions to society at large. Most of us feel "down-and-out" on the occasional basis, but we are able to cope and our resiliency is strong enough to carry-out our required various activities of daily living rather than being trapped in a state of despondency. However, for some individuals, these "down-and-out" times become persistent and chronic in nature, and coping mechanisms and strategies are excessively taxed or insufficient in nature resulting in alterations to one's mental health and well-being.

This chapter examines the role of public healthcare professionals and workers in helping individuals, families, entire communities, and populations regain, maintain, and promote their mental health across the lifespan. Current and emerging major mental health issues are highlighted and critically examined from the public health perspective. A realization by public healthcare professionals and workers that community-based services requires

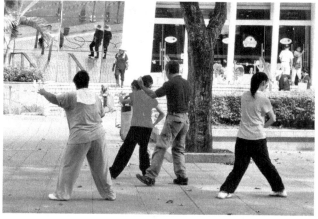

Source: Photo by Wally J. Barfay (2017), Hong Kong.

Photo 11.1 Tai Chi (Qigong or Chi Kung) is an ancient form of martial arts which dates back to over 700 years and consists of slow breathing and movements, visualizations, and relaxation of the entire body and mind. An increasing amount of scientific evidence suggests that Tai Chi is an effective means to decrease stress and blood pressure, improve mental and physical health and well-being, and improve self-reported sleep duration in diverse populations across the lifespan (e.g., McCain, Gray, & Elswick, 2008; Zhang, Layre, Lawder, & Liu, 2012).

timely diagnosis, evidence-informed treatment and care, health promotion and prevention, and rehabilitation and/or supportive services for clients and their families afflicted with specific mental health disorders, is critical to the art and science of public health. In addition, a growing voice of Canadians are demanding and expecting active collaboration and decision making with their healthcare providers, as opposed to being passive recipients of healthcare services. Recognition of the social determinants of health (SDH) and how they contribute or impact mental health; the need for clients to be involved in policy development and implementation; the value of self-help groups and peer consultations, and the importance of the recovery model of rehabilitation which goes far beyond the conventional symptom management approach, are critical to public health. For example, according to the Canada census count, 20,170 individuals were homeless and living in a shelter in 2011 alone (MHCC, 2015). Homelessness is a national public health concern and many homeless individuals suffer from mental illness and addictions. The reader is referred to Chapter 1 for a detailed discussion of the SDH.

What Is Mental Health?

Mental health is a critical component of public health and holistic health and well-being in Canada and globally. Each year, one in every five Canadians experiences one or more mental health problems, creating a significant cost to the health system of over $50 billion annually (Canadian Mental Health Association [CMHA], 2016a; George, Thomson, Chaze, & Guruge, 2015; Smetanin et al., 2011). The PHAC (2006, 2012) defines **mental health** as the capacity of each and all of us to feel, think, and act in ways that enhance our ability to enjoy life and deal with the challenges we face, and a positive sense of emotional and spiritual well-being that respects the importance of culture, equity, social justice, interconnections, and personal dignity.

The World Health Organization (WHO, 2014a) defines **mental health** "as a state of well-being in which every individual realizes his or her own potential, can cope with the normal stresses of life, can work productively and fruitfully, and is able to make a contribution to her or his community." The WHO concept of mental health embraces promotion of mental well-being, the prevention and treatment, as well as rehabilitation of individuals affected with mental illness and disorders (George et al., 2015; WHO, 2014a). Hence, mental health may be perceived as a necessary resource for living a healthy life and a critical factor in overall health and well-being that involves striking a balance in all aspects of one's self including social, physical, spiritual, cultural, environmental, occupational, economic, and psychological components. Reaching this balance involves a continuous learning process and journey that requires employing and/or learning new coping skills, being flexible, and willing to adapt to changing situations, developing resilience, and managing the many stressors Canadians face.

The MHCC (2015) reports that 72.1% of Canadians aged 20 to 64 years reported their mental health as very good or excellent in 2011/2012. Moreover, 77.2% of Canadians aged 12 to 19 years reported their mental health as very good or excellent during this assessment period. Good mental health in adolescence is associated with good mental health and quality of life in adulthood. Poor mental health in youth can signal a lack of resilience, the presence of stressors and/or other vulnerabilities.

Mental Health Commission of Canada

The MHCC was created by the federal government in its budget of March 2007, with the goal of creating an integrated mental health system that places individuals living with mental illness at its centre or core. Since the March 2007 announcement, a board of directors and eight advisory committees have been established to guide the work of MHCC. The MHCC mandate is to encourage cooperation and collaboration among various levels of government, mental health service providers and healthcare professors, employers, the scientific and research communities, as well as Canadians living with mental illness, their families and caregivers in their community. The MHCC's strategy calls for promoting the health and well-being of all Canadians and to improve mental health outcomes (Goldbloom & Bradley, 2012; MHCC, 2012).

The MHCC (2012, p. 11) identified the following six priority strategic directions for Canadians across the lifespan, which are summarized below:

1. Promote mental health across the lifespan in homes, schools, and workplaces, and prevent mental illness and suicide wherever possible.
2. Foster recovery and well-being for people of all ages living with mental health problems and illnesses, and uphold their rights.
3. Provide access to the right combination of services, treatments, and supports, when and where people need them.
4. Reduce disparities in risk factors and access to mental health services, and strengthen the response to the needs of diverse communities and Northerners.
5. Work with First Nations, Inuit, and Métis to address their mental health needs, acknowledging their distinct circumstances, rights, and cultures.
6. Mobilize leadership, improve knowledge, and fosters collaboration at all levels.

The MHCC (2013) reports that approximately 6.7 million people in Canada are living with a mental health condition or illness today. For comparative purposes, approximately 2.2 million individuals in Canada have type 2 diabetes and only 1.4 million have heart disease. Approximately 28% of Canadians aged 20 to 29 years experience a mental illness in a given year. By the time people reach 40 years of age, one in two people in Canada will have had or currently have a mental illness. Moreover, mental health problems and illnesses account for approximately 30% of short- and long-term disability claims and are rated amongst the top three of claims reported by more than 80% of Canadian employers. It is notable that the predictive cumulative cost of providing treatment, care, and supportive services is projected to reach $625 billion in the year 2021; $1.42 trillion in the year 2031, and $2.5 trillion in the year 2041 (MHCC, 2013). Hence, one may clearly argue that mental health illness is a major public health issue in Canada and one that is predicted to continue to be a major challenge in the next 30 years to come. We shall examine some of the major current and emerging mental health issues in great detail later.

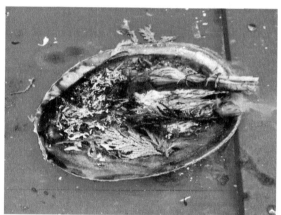

Source: Photo by Wally J. Bartfay (2017), St. Catharine's, Ontario.

Photo 11.2 Smudging ceremonies or rituals are carried-out by First Nations people and often involve the burning of sage, cedar, sweet grass, juniper, and other herbs. Negative energies, feelings, and emotions are believed to be carried-away by the smoke, and it is often employed to promote healing and cleansing of the mind, body, and soul of First Nation's people. The MHCC (2012) has identified the need to work with indigenous people in Canada to address their current and emerging mental health needs, while acknowledging their distinct circumstances, rights, and cultures.

School-Based Mental Health Promotion

Schools are an effective means to provide developmentally specific targeted mental health promotion to children, with the specific aim of encouraging children to remain active during and after school in their communities (Bartfay & Bartfay, 1994, 2015; Lavin, Shapiro, & Weills, 1992; Vander-Ploeg, McGavock, Maximova, & Vengelers, 2013). For example, Vander-Ploeg et al. (2013) examined the change in physical activity during and after school among students (*N* = 1157) participating in a *Comprehensive School Health* (CSH) intervention in Edmonton, Alberta over a period of two years. The investigators conducted a quasi-experimental, pre–post trial with a parallel, non-equivalent control group. Pedometer recordings (seven full days) and demographic data were collected from cross-sectional samples of fifth grade students from 10 intervention schools and 20 comparison schools. Intervention schools were targeted in socioeconomically disadvantaged neighbourhoods. Compared to baseline data taken in 2009, children were more active on schools days (1172 steps per day; $p = .001$) and on weekends (1450 steps per day; $p = .001$) in 2011. This study highlights the effectiveness of school-based health promotion programs to affect children's physical activity during and outside of the school environment.

A growing global movement of community-based health-promoting initiatives recognizes "the direct influence schools can have on positive student health" (WHO, 2006). JCSH, a partnership of Canadian provincial, territorial, and federal health and education ministries, has been formed to support this movement in Canada. To support the advancement of healthy school communities across Canada, the JCSH has developed the *Healthy School Planner*, which is a free, web-based tool that elementary and secondary schools can employ to assess their school's current health environment. The Healthy School Planner also helps to develop program plans to address gaps in identified priority areas, and was developed for the JCSH by the Propel Centre for Population Health Impact at the University of Waterloo (see link: http://hsp.uwaterloo. ca/). First launched in 2009, the purpose of this initiative is to help individual schools **EVOLVE**, which is an acronym for: (i) **E**valuate current conditions; (ii) **V**alidate untapped resources in the community; (iii) **O**rganize increased support for change; (iv) **L**ead the decision-making process to determine action steps; (v) **V**isualize outcomes through shared success stories; and (vi) **E**valuate progress over time. The reader is referred to the Web-based Resources Box 11.1 for more information related to the Health School Planner initiative in Canada.

In Canada this movement is known as "Comprehensive School Health" (CSH). The MHCC (2015) reports that there are over 14,000 schools in Canada and only 7% (or $N = 1012$) of Canadian schools that have completed the Foundational Module of the Healthy School Planner (HSP-FM) developed by the Pan-Canadian Joint Consortium for School Health (PCJCSH, 2010). Schools are a logical setting to promote the health and well-being of children and youth. The number of schools that use a comprehensive school health approach in planning for a healthier school environment is one measure of the extent to which schools are interested, and involved, in creating healthy school communities. The PCJCSH (2010) includes a focus on the school's social environment which addresses factors and noted SDH closely linked to mental health promotion.

Web-Based Resources Box 11.1: Healthy School Planner Initiative in Canada

Learning Resource	Website
JCSH Healthy School Planner Video. -This video provides an overview of the Healthy School Planner: a free online tool that schools can use to assess the current health environment and build a plan to make improvements.	https://www.youtube.com/ watch?v=4GQ77goWzdY
Zummach, D., & Craig, J. E. (2014, November 25). *Highlights of the healthy school planner.* **Pan Canadian Joint Commission for School Health. Propel Centre for Population Health Impact.** -This is a 26.53-min webinar that provides an overview of the Healthy School Planner initiative and is intended for healthcare professionals and workers, educators, and other school officials.	https://www.youtube.com/ watch?v=Coh3liLel4I&list=UU_ 42JlLmmkFVo0XFMQzGthA

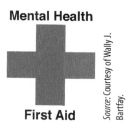

Mental Health

First Aid

Source: Courtesy of Wally J. Bartfay.

Figure 11.1 The Mental Health First Aid (MHFA) Canada program seeks to address the issue of stigma associated with mental health illness and disorders through the development of mental health literacy and by equipping individuals with the necessary knowledge and skill sets to address and respond to mental health issues themselves, for a family member, friend, colleague or individual in their community (MHCC, 2015, 2017a).

Mental Health First Aid Training in Canada

The MHFA program was developed and designed with the goal of responding promptly to a person developing a mental health problem or issue and/or experiencing a mental health crisis. MHFA participants receive a training manual while attending a training session (see link: http://www.mentalhealthcommission.ca/English/focus-areas/mental-health-first-aid). The idea is similar to someone providing physical first aid to an injured person before professional treatment can be obtained by a healthcare professional. MHFA is an international program that is currently active in over 20 countries including Canada (MHCC, 2017a). Research has shown that this evidence-informed course offers significant positive impacts including greater recognition of common mental health conditions; decreased social distance from individuals living with mental health issues in their workplaces and community; increased confidence in helping others, and improved mental health of the MHFA participant themselves. The MHCC (2017a) reports that more than 200,000 individuals have already participated in MHFA training programs across Canada.

Major Theories Related to the Origins of Mental Illness and Disorders

Throughout history there have been three general theories related to the aetiology of mental illness and disorders: (i) Supernatural; (ii) psychogenic; and (iii) somatogenic (Burton, 2012, 2015; Viney & Zorich, 1982). We shall examine these from a historical context below and highlight the implications for public health for each of the three aforementioned major theories.

i. *Supernatural theory*
   Supernatural theories of mental illness and disorders attribute these conditions to possession and/or punishment by evil or demonic spirits, displeasure of gods or deities, solar or lunar eclipses, comets, curses, and/or sin. For example, the First Book of Samuel describes how King Saul became "mad" after neglecting his religious duties and angering God as a consequence (Burton, 2012, 2015).

   But the Spirit of the Lord departed from Saul, and an evil spirit from the Lord troubled him... And it came to pass, when the evil spirit from God was upon Saul, that David took an harp, and played with his hand: so Saul was refreshed, and was well, and the evil spirit departed from him. (1 Samuel 16:14, 23-Old Testament, Holy Bible)

   Even today, many cultures around the world still believe that unusual behaviours and mental illness and disorders are caused by spirit possession or supernatural causes, especially in some less developed regions of the world (Davey, 2014; Hanwella, deSilva, Yoosuf, Karunoratre, & de Silva, 2012; Levack, 1992; Neuner et al., 2012). Hence, public healthcare professionals and workers need to be cognizant of these beliefs and practices, especially given that Canada is a land of increasing diversity and immigration since Confederation. Indeed, Statistics Canada (2016a) reports that since 2011, the estimated foreign-born population was 6,775,700, which represented 20.6% (or approximately 1:5) of the total population in Canada (see Figure 11.2). Since the early 1990s, the number of landed immigrants has remained relatively high, with an average of approximately 235,000 new immigrants per year.

Migration is one of the noted SDH since migrants often face social isolation, poverty, unemployment and/or under-employment, and other social inequities in their new host country (Davis, Basten, & Frattini, 2009; Fuller-Thomson, Noack, & George, 2011; George et al., 2015; Kennedy, McDonald, & Biddle, 2006). It is notable that the majority of immigrants to Canada are so-called "economic immigrants" who are accepted on the basis of their potential to contribute to the Canadian labour market through a points system based on language skills (i.e., proficiency in English and/or French), professional qualifications, and work experiences. However, research indicates that these new immigrants are more likely to be underemployed, in comparison to native-born Canadians. Moreover, although new immigrants tend to have overall better health in comparison to their native-born counterparts, a phenomenon termed the "healthy immigrant effect" occurs where their physical and mental health tends to decrease over the subsequent decade following immigration (Davis et al., 2009; Fuller-Thomson et al., 2011; George et al., 2015; Kennedy et al., 2006). For example, **acculturative stress** is defined as difficulties faced by new immigrants in adapting to their new host country and society. Acculturations to Western lifestyles and society often holds significant consequences for the mental health of diverse immigrant groups including increased rates of depression and other mental health issues and challenges (George et al., 2015; Kuo, Chong, & Joseph, 2008; Lou & Beaujot, 2005).

For example, Neuner et al. (2012) investigated the prevalence of "cen," a local variant of spirit possession among 1113 former child soldiers and war-affected civilians from Northern Uganda, Africa aged between 12 and 25 years. Cen is widely believed to be a form of spirit possession where the "ghost of a deceased person visits the affected individual and replaces his or her identity" in this region of Africa. The researchers reported that spirit possession was significantly higher in former abducted child soldiers than in non-abductees. They also found that reports of spirit possession were

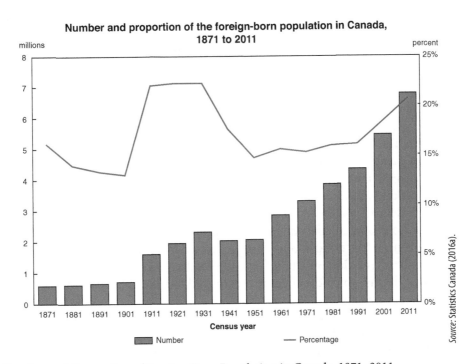

Figure 11.2 Number and Proportion of Foreign-Born Population in Canada, 1871–2011

related to trauma exposure (e.g., sexual assault or being forced to kill), psychological distress, and to higher rates of suicide and post-traumatic stress disorder (PTSD; Neuner et al., 2012).

In Western societies demonology survived as an explanation of mental illness until the 18th century, when witchcraft and demonic possession were common explanations for socially undesirable behaviours or thought processes (i.e., suicide, schizophrenia) (Davey, 2014; Hanwella et al., 2012; Levack, 1992). Treatment often entailed exorcism, voodoo, and physical attacks on the individual's body (e.g., flogging, starvation), or trephination in an attempt to force out the evil spirits or demon causing the possession. **Trephination** (a.k.a., trepanning or burr holing) is a surgical intervention where a hole is drilled, incised, or scraped into the skull using simple tools, and is an example of one of the earliest treatments and supernatural explanation for mental illness (i.e., madness or insanity) and epilepsy. Evidence of this practice has been found in prehistoric human remains from Neolithic times (6500 BCE) and onwards (Faria, 2013; Restak, 2000). Trephination is still employed today to relieve pressure in the cranial cavity often resulting from traumatic head injuries that result in bleeding and/or severe inflammation of the brain (Mondorf, Abu-Owaimer, Gaab, & Oertel, 2009; Lu, Guan, & An, 2015).

ii. *Psychogenic theories*
Psychogenic theories of mental illness or disorders focus on traumatic or stressful experiences, maladaptive learned associations and cognitions, or distorted perceptions. Sigmund Freud (1856–1939), Alfred

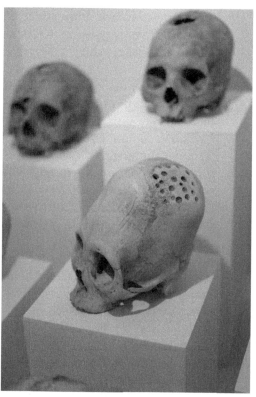

Source: Photo by Wally J. Bartfay.

Photo 11.3 Trephination of a skull. Trepanned skull of a male who survived the surgery, at least for a period of time, as evidenced by bone healing at the edges of the two holes drilled. In ancient times, holes were surgically drilled or scraped into a person's skull who was believed to be behaving abnormally or was deemed "possessed and insane" to let out or release what they believed were evil spirits or demons.

Adler (1870–1937), Carl Gustav Jung (1875–1961), and their disciples, influenced much of 20th century treatment of clients with mental illness and disorders via psychotherapy and psychoanalysis (Caplan, 2011; Cushman, 1996). **Psychotherapy**, also known as "talk therapy," is defined as a process whereby mental health issues and concerns are treated through communication and relationship factors between a client and a trained mental health professional. Modern psychotherapy is often time-limited (e.g., 45–50 min per session weekly) and consists of focused sessions where clients learn about their specific conditions, moods, feelings, thoughts, and behaviours (Herkov, 2016). **Psychoanalysis** is defined as a theory first developed by Freud during the 1890s, and is a form of therapy that seeks to treat mental health disorders by analyzing the interaction of conscious and unconscious elements in the mind and bringing repressed fears and conflicts into the conscious mind. **Psychoanalytic techniques** include the interpretations of dreams and free association treatment sessions during which the client is encouraged to talk freely about personal experiences, and especially about early childhood conflicts.

Adler was a physician by training and psychotherapist, and is credited as being the founder of *Adlerian psychology*, which is also known as "individual psychology" (Anbacher & Anbacher, 1959; Sharp, 1899). It is notable that Alder is regarded as the first community-based psychologist, because his work pioneered attention to community life, prevention, and population-based mental health issues based on the SDH. He was also one of the first healthcare professionals to provide family and group counselling sessions, and to use public education as a way to address community-based mental health issues. In fact, by the second half of the 20th century a majority of psychiatrists in the United States (although not in the United Kingdom) believed that mental disorders such as schizophrenia and depression, resulted from unconscious conflicts originating in early childhood (Burton, 2012, 2015; Faria, 2013).

Frontal lobotomy, the sectioning of the prefrontal cortex, and leucotomy, the severing of the underlying white matter, for the treatment of mental disorders, reached a peak of popularity after World War II. This surgical treatment helped address the pressing problem of overcrowding in mental institutions in an era when no other forms of effective treatment were available (Faria, 2013; Kucharski, 1984). It is notable that Dr Egas Moniz received the Nobel Prize in 1949 for his pioneering work on frontal leucotomy in which, specifically, the white matter connections between the prefrontal cortex and the thalamus were sectioned to alleviate severe mental illness, including depression and schizophrenia in the long-term hospitalized patients (Faria, 2013; Kucharski, 1984). The reader is referred to the Web-based Resources Box 11.2 below for documentary on Dr Walter Freeman who popularized the treatment of the mentally ill via frontal lobectomies in the United States during the 1940s and performed this procedure on over 4000 mentally ill clients. Freeman had used alcohol injections initially, but subsequently adapted his procedure by using a modified "ice-pick" instrument to traverse the roof of the orbit and enter the base of the skull.

It must be remembered that this movement toward surgical interventions for the treatment of mental disorders and illnesses did not occur in a vacuum. It was engendered at a time when drug therapy was not available, and it involved mostly severely incapacitated hospitalized patients for whom psychotherapy was ineffective or unavailable. Psychotropic drugs were not available until the 1950s, and in their absence, the only treatment options used in conjunction with long-term hospitalization were physical restraint with the feared strait jackets, isolation in padded cells, and other inhumane treatment regimes. During the 1960s, a philosophical shift proposed that clients could be more effectively and humanely managed and treated in their respective communities, which resulted in a gradual deinstitutionalization of long-term mental health hospitals and asylums which also resulted in associated cost saving measures (Davis, 2006).

iii. *Somatogenic theories*
Somatogenic theories of mental illness or disorders identify disturbances in physical functioning resulting either from illness, genetic inheritance, brain damage, or chemical or force of nature imbalances. For example, around 2700 B.C.E., Chinese medicine's concept of complementary positive and negative bodily forces ("yin and yang") attributed both mental and physical illnesses to an imbalance

Web-Based Resource Box 11.2

The Lobotomist: Dr Walter J. Freeman

Learning Resource	Website
Public Broadcasting Station (PBS). The American Experience—*The Lobotomist, Walter J. Freeman.* (2008, January 21). -This video documentary highlights the psychosurgical practice of performing frontal lobotomies that was popularized by Dr Walter Freeman in the United States, and reached a zenith in the 1940s, only to come into disrepute in the late 1950s.	https://www.youtube.com/watch?v=0nOnUQ0qOd8. Or http://www.pbs.org/wgbh/americanexperience/lobotomist/program/

between these forces. As such, a harmonious life that allowed for the proper balance of yin and yang and movement of vital air was essential (Donahue, 1996; Porter, 1997; Tseng, 1973).

It was around 400 B.C.E. that the Greek physician Hippocrates of Cos (460–370 B.C.E.) attempted to separate superstition and religion from the concept of health by systematizing the belief that a deficiency in or especially an excess of one of the four essential bodily humours (i.e., blood, yellow bile, black bile, and phlegm) was the root cause for both physical and mental illness (see Figure 2.1, Chapter 2). The first classifications of mental disorders proposed by Hippocrates were mania, melancholy, phrenitis, insanity, disobedience, paranoia, panic, epilepsy and hysteria (Burton, 2012,

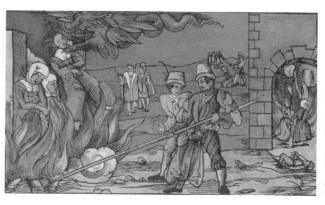

Photo 11.4 Burning of Suspected Witches. Three women executed because they were accused of being witches by being burnt alive while tied to a wooden stake in Derneburg, Germany in 1555. It is notable that during the 14th through 16th centuries, the mentally ill and especially women were often persecuted as witches who were alleged to be possessed by the devil.

2015; Kleisioris, Sfakianakis, & Papathonosiou, 2014). It is interesting to note that several of these disorders described are still relevant today, although the exact terms have been replaced (e.g., melancholy is now depression and panic is panic disorder). We shall examine these conditions in greater detail below.

By the Middle Ages (11th and 15th centuries A.D.), however, attempts to explain mental illness through rational mechanisms were quickly replaced by theories of demonology and witchcraft on the European continent fueled by the Roman Catholic Church (Laden, 2012; Levack, 1992; Stephens, 2000). For example, in 1326, The Holy Catholic Church in Rome authorized the "Inquisition to Investigate Witchcraft," which subsequently led to the development of demonology (Laden, 2012; Levack, 1992; Stephens, 2000). Indeed, supernatural theories of mental illnesses and disorders were fueled by natural disasters like plagues and famines that common- and laypeople believed were linked to evil spirits and/or the devil. Consequently, superstition, astrology, and alchemy took hold with common treatments and interventions including prayer rites, relic touching, confessions, and atonement became commonplace on the European continent.

During the 17th century and onwards, mental illness began to be viewed somatogenically once again, so treatments were similar to those for physical illnesses during the period (e.g., purges, blood-letting, application of leeches, emetics) (Donahue, 1996; Porter, 1997). During the 18th century, individuals with mental illness were often restrained using a variety of devices (e.g., shackles, chains). In 1785, the Italian physician Vincenzo Chiarughi (1759–1820) removed the chains of patients at his St. Boniface hospital in Florence, Italy. By contrast, his treatment regime consisted of encouraging good hygiene, physical and recreational activities, and occupational training for patients.

French physician Philippe Pinel (1745–1826) and his former patient Jean-Baptiste Pussin created a "traitement moral" at La Bicêtre and the Salpêtrière in 1793 and 1795 that also included unshackling patients, moving them to well-aired, well-lit rooms, and encouraging purposeful activity and freedom to move about the grounds freely (Micale, 1985). In fact, Philippe Pinel (1745–1826) has been described as the father of modern psychiatry. (Rahman, 2011). A landmark in the history of psychiatry, Pinel's Traité Médico-philosophique sur l'aliénation mentale ou la manie (*A Treatise on Insanity*) called for a more humane approach to the treatment of mental disorder.

The patient's in Bicêtre in Paris had led very different lives from ourselves; most striking is Pinel's writing is the shadow of violence of the French Revolution and Terror which lay over the patient's and frequently had drastic effects on life inside the hospital…[He] believed so much in the effect of environmental disasters in precipitating insanity. (Cited in Smith, 1967, p. 85).

It was published in France in 1801, and a popular translation (*A Treatise on Insanity*) was published in England in 1806 (Pinel, 1806; Rahman, 2011; Smith, 1967). This book had an enormous influence on French and Anglo-American psychiatrists during the 19th century and beyond (Rahman, 2011; Smith, 1967). This "moral treatment," as it had already been dubbed, included respect for the patient, a trusting and confiding doctor–patient relationship, decreased stimuli, routine activity and occupation, and the abandonment of old-fashioned Hippocratic treatments (Burton, 2012, 2015).

When retired school teacher Dorothea Dix discovered the negligence that resulted from such conditions, she advocated for the establishment of state hospitals. Between 1840 and 1880, she helped establish over 30 mental institutions in the United States and Canada (Viney & Zorich, 1982). During the mid-19th century, specialized mental health hospitals or asylums were built in several provinces across Canada to provide care to individuals with mental illnesses. Psychiatry first began as a specialized branch or field of medicine in 1846, which emphasized finding cures for mental illness based on the medical model of health (Nolan, 1993; Sussman, 1998). When clinical and societal expectations of having clients return to their respective communities proved to be unrealistic, mental health hospitals and asylums quickly became overcrowded and understaffed by nurses and physicians, and basically became warehouses to house these clients.

During the past few decades, the "*chemical imbalance theory*" of mental illness and disorders has been propagated by psychiatrist and by the pharmaceutical industry. For example, in 1965 Joseph Schidkraut was the first to propose the theory

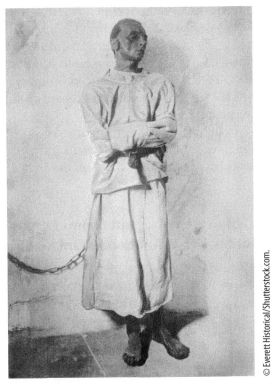

© Everett Historical/Shutterstock.com.

Photo 11.5 A Hospitalized Patient in a Straight-Jacket. Most inmates in asylums were inhumanely treated, institutionalized against their will, lived in filth and were often malnourished, shackled, or chained to walls and/or put into strait jackets or other restraining devices, and were commonly exhibited to the public for a fee.

that depression was associated with low levels of norepinephrine (Schidkraut, 1965). It is still currently argued and promulgated that depression is "caused" by simple chemical imbalances of serotonin (5-hydroxytryptamine, 5-HT), norepinephrine, and/or cortisol in the brain by the medical establishment and big pharma (e.g., Deakin, 1988; Dinan, 1994; Lacasse & Leo, 2005; Moncrieff, 2007, 2014). It is noteworthy that this laboratory-based unicausal model of disease causation is in concert with the medical model of health. The reader is referred to Chapter 2 for a detailed description of the medical model of health and its noted limitations.

In fact, the powerful and influential American Psychological Association (APA) continues to support and propagate the unicausal chemical imbalance theory for depression. For example, the APA's online public information brochure entitled *Let's Talk Facts About Depression* makes the following claims regarding the origins and treatment of depression:

Abnormalities in two chemicals in the brain, serotonin and norepinephrine, might contribute to symptoms of depression, including anxiety, irritability and fatigue…[AND] Anti-depressants may be prescribed to correct imbalances in the levels of chemicals in the brain (APA, 2005, p. 2).

However, published scientific peer-reviewed studies of serotonin 1A receptors in living human subjects remain contradictory and inconsistent in nature with some finding lowered levels of receptors in individuals with depression compared to those without; some finding elevated levels by contrast, and some finding no differences at all (e.g., Drevets et al., 1999; Lacasse & Leo, 2005). It may be argued that propaganda from the APA and the pharmaceutical industry, which targets healthcare consumers, psychiatrists, and physicians directly, has led the way in advocating this chemical imbalance theory for depression (e.g., Cowen, 2002; Lacasse & Leo, 2005; Moncrieff, 2007, 2014). In fact, it has been reported that approximately 70% of the task force members for the updated *DSM-V* (American Psychological Association [APA], 2013) had direct financial ties to the pharmaceutical industry, which represents an increase of 57% in comparison to the *DSM-IV* task force membership (Cosgrove & Drimsky, 2012; Nemeroff et al., 2013). The reader is referred to Chapter 7 for a detailed discussion on current criticism related to the *DSM-V* and corporate influences by big pharma.

Hence, it is not surprising that selective serotonin reuptake inhibitor (SSRI) anti-depressants are among the most profitable and best-selling drugs on the market globally. For example, sertraline (Zoloft) was the sixth best-selling medication in the United States, with over $3 billion in sales in 2004 alone (International

Table 11.1.   Content Claims Propagating the Chemical Imbalance Theory for Depression for Sselected Antidepressant Medications

Medication	Selected Content from Consumer Advertisement
Citalopram	"Celexa helps to restore the brain's chemical balance by increasing the supply of a chemical messenger in the brain called serotonin. Although the brain chemistry of depression is not fully understood, there does exist a growing body of evidence to support the view that people with depression have an imbalance of the brain's neurotransmitters" [57].
Escitalopram	"LEXAPRO appears to work by increasing the available supply of serotonin. Here's how: The naturally occurring chemical serotonin is sent from one nerve cell to the next. The nerve cell picks up the serotonin and sends some of it back to the first nerve cell, similar to a conversation between two people. In people with depression and anxiety, there is an imbalance of serotonin–too much serotonin is reabsorbed by the first nerve cell, so the next cell does not have enough; as in a conversation, one person might do all the taking and the other person does not get to comment, leading to a communication imbalance. LEXAPRO blocks the serotonin from going back into the first nerve cell. This increases the amount of serotonin available for the next nerve cell, like a conversation moderator. The blocking action helps balance the supply of serotonin, and communication returns to normal. In this way, LEXAPRO improves symptoms of depression" [58].
Fluoxetine	"When you're clinically depressed, one thing that can happen is the level of serotonin (a chemical in your body) may drop. So you may have trouble sleeping. Feel unusually sad or irritable. Find it hard to concentrate. Lose your appetite. Lack energy. Or have trouble feeling pleasure... to help bring serotonin levels closer to normal, the medicine doctors now prescribe most often is Prozac®" [59]
Paroxetine	"Chronic anxiety can be overwhelming. But it can also be overcome... Paxil, the most prescribed medication of its kind for generalized anxiety, works to correct the chemical imbalance believed to cause the disorder" [60].
Sertraline	"While the cause is unknown, depression may be related to an imbalance of natural chemicals between nerve cells in the brain. Prescription Zoloft works to correct this imbalance. You just cshouldn't have to feel this way anymore" [5].

Source: Seratonin and Depression: A Disconnect Between the Advertisements and the Scientific Literature" by Jeffrey R. Lacasse and Jonathan Leo, in PLOS Medicine, 2005, 2(12): E392.

Marketing Services Health, 2004; Lacasse & Leo, 2005). Tencer (2013) reports that a survey conducted by the OECD found that consumption of anti-depressants in Canada was the third-highest among 23 developed countries, with 86 doses consumed daily per 1000 people. Only Australia (89 doses per 1000 people) and Iceland (106 doses per 1000 people) ranked higher. Similarly, Statistics Canada (2015a) reports that anti-depressants are among the top five prescription medications taken by adults aged 24 to 79 years, and are among the top two prescription medications taken by individuals aged 6 to 24 years.

Table 11.1 above shows content claims being propagated by the pharmaceutical industry in mass and social media related to the chemical imbalance theory for depression and selected anti-depressant medications, which target the general health consumer. For example, one of Pfizer's television advertisement campaigns for the anti-depressant sertraline (Zoloft), which featured a little cartoon blob that was sad, stated that depression is a "*serious medical condition*" that may be due to a "chemical imbalance," and that "Zoloft works to correct this imbalance" (Pfizer, 2004- see link: https://www.youtube.com/watch?v=twhvtzd6gXA). Although so-called "direct-to-consumer" television and print advertising of anti-depressants has been a controversial practice since its introduction in 1997, and its prohibition in all countries except for the United States and New Zealand, the introduction of YouTube in 2005 and other social media sites makes this difficult to police and enforce on both the national and international levels (Greenslit, 2012).

It is noteworthy that in January 2013 a class-action lawsuit was filed against Pfizer regarding its marketing of Zoloft (*Plumlee v. Pfizer, Inc.*, Case No. 13-cv-00414, N.D. Cal.). The allegation is that the drug label and marketing materials do not make mention of the numerous clinical trials in which Zoloft was shown to be no more effective in treating depression than placebo (e.g., Ioannidis, 2008). By contrast, Pfizer's consumers are given the impression that Zoloft has been clinically proven to be very effective for treating depression. Furthermore, there are various clinical trials which have not only reported that certain anti-depressants are no more "statistically effective" (e.g., $p \leq .05$) when compared to placebos, but may have serious life threatening side effects and complications (e.g., suicide, cardiovascular events) (e.g., Fergusson et al., 2005; Ioannidis, 2008; Jakobsen et al., 2017; Lacasse & Leo, 2005; Nezafati, Eshraghi, Vojdanparast, Abtahi, & Nezafati, 2016). For example, a recent meta-analysis involving 131 placebo-controlled trials with anti-depressants that involved 27,422 participants total concluded that SSRIs, when compared to placebos alone:

... seem to have statistically significant effects on depressive symptoms, but the clinical significance of these effects seems questionable and all trials were at high risk of bias. Furthermore, SSRIs versus placebo significantly increase the risk of both serious and non-serious adverse events. Our results show that the harmful effects of SSRIs versus placebo for major depressive disorder seem to outweigh any potentially small beneficial effects. (Jakobsen et al., 2017, doi:10.1186/s12888-016-1173)

The reader is referred to the Group Review Exercise Box 11.1 below near the end of this chapter for more insights into the current dominance of the chemical imbalance theory for mental illness and disorders, and how the pharmaceutical industry has influenced the development of previous and the current 5th edition of *Diagnostic and Statistical Manual of Psychological Disorders* (APA, 2013).

What Is Stress?

Stress is **a** fact of daily living and when it is intense or chronic in nature, it can lead to a variety of health issues and conditions. **Stress** is defined as a unique and subjective perception or reaction to a specific current existing or imminent situation or condition that results in emotional and physiological responses resulting from various demands, expectations, and/or unpredictable circumstances experienced in our daily lives. Moreover, stress can also be defined as any physical, social, political, economic, or cultural force which creates an imbalance, and which can have either negative or positive influence on an individual or group (Bartfay & Bartfay, 2015).

Group Activity-Based Learning Box 11.1

How Do You Respond to Stress?
This group activity seeks to examine how individuals identify and cope with stress in their daily lives. Working in small groups of three to five students, discuss and answer the following questions:

1. Make a list of current stressors affecting individuals in your group. Label them as everyday minor stressors (e.g., traffic jams, upcoming quizzes) and major stressors (e.g., not being able to pay the rent, death in the family, chronic pain).

2. Make a separate list of coping mechanisms employed by members of your group. Identify any short-comings and potential community resources to assist individuals in managing their stressors.

Certain levels of stress related to one's family, going to school, work or life in general is expected and normal. Indeed, it may be argued that a certain level of stress is often what provides us with the motivation and energy to meet our daily challenges at home, at school, or in the workplace. However, when stress turns into unwanted feelings, pressure, anxiety, frustration, unmet needs, or dissatisfaction, it can manifest itself as a negative ripple effect (Bartfay & Bartfay, 2015; Statistics Canada, 2014, 2001).

In 2014, 23.0% of Canadians aged 15 years and older (6.7 million people) reported that most days were "quite a bit" or "extremely stressful" (Statistics Canada, 2014) (See Figure 11.3). In addition, since 2003, females were more likely than males to report that most days were "quite a bit" or "extremely stressful." The rate for females was 23.7%, compared to 22.3% for their male counterparts. The rate of daily stress was found to be higher for females than males in all age groups except for those aged 35 to 64 years. Similarly, 22% of immigrants to Canada aged 15 years or older reported that most days are quite a bit stressful or extremely stressful in 2011/2012 (MHCC, 2015). Moreover, approximately one in five (19.6%) residents of Northern communities report very high levels of stress (MHCC, 2015). Unemployment, low income, housing difficulties, transportation challenges, and under-servicing are among the issues faced by residents of Northern communities. These factors may increase the level of stress experienced by individuals who reside in these

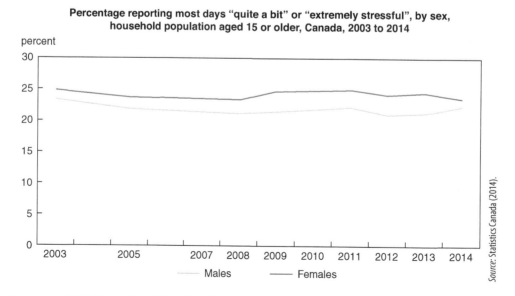

Figure 11.3 Perceived Life Stress Levels for Canadians Aged 15 Years and Older 2003–2014.

communities. The reader is referred to Chapter 4 for a detailed discussion of several challenges and health issues facing indigenous people in Canada.

Daily reported stress rates appear to be highest in the core working age groups (i.e., 35–54 years), peaking at approximately 30% in the 35 to 44 years and 45 to 54 years age groups (Statistics Canada, 2014). Individuals in these age groups are most likely to be managing multiple responsibilities, which includes career and family obligations (Statistics Canada, 2014). The reader is referred to Chapter 8 for a detailed discussion of work-related stress and the associated implications for public health.

For example, on May 1, 2016 a forest fire began southwest of Fort McMurray, and on May 3rd it required the evacuation of the entire community which forced the largest wildfire evacuation in Alberta's history to date (Barkto, 2016; Pruden, 2016). The direct and indirect costs of this major disaster was estimated to be $9.5 billion which included the expense of replacing buildings and infrastructure as well as lost income, profits, and royalties in the oil sands and forestry industries (Weber, 2017). The wildfire destroyed approximately 2400 homes and buildings and another 2000 residents in three communities were displaced after their homes were declared unsafe for reoccupation due to contamination. Firefighters from across Alberta and other Canadian provinces responded to the massive fire along with personnel from the Canadian Armed Forces, RCMP and other Canadian and provincial agencies. Aid for evacuees was provided by various governments and via donations through the Canadian Red Cross and other local and national charitable organizations for stress management, medical issues, childcare, pet rescues, emergency food, shelter and gas, and assistance with insurance claims and financial aid (Postmedia News, 2016). This example highlights how a single natural disaster can result in negative ripple effects across an entire community and region and result in high levels of chronic negative stress.

Web-Based Resources Box 11.3 Recognizing, Coping, and Managing Stress

Learning Resource	Website
Canadian Mental Health Association (CMHA) -This website provides current statistics related to the incidence of mental illness in Canada and associated healthcare costs, and current national policies and reports.	http://www.cmha.ca/media/fast-facts-about-mental-illness/#.WSLoh-vyupo.
Canadian Mental Health Association & Heart and Stroke Foundation of Canada. *Coping with stress.* -This website provides the reader with information on the negative effects of stress on health, how to recognize it, stress management, and coping skills (e.g., meditation, counselling services available), and additional mental health resources available by province and territory.	https://www.heartandstroke.ca/-/media/pdf-files/canada/other/coping-with-stress-en.ashx
Health Canada (2008). *Mental Health: Coping with Stress.* **Ottawa, ON: Her Majesty the Queen in Right of Canada.** -This website provides helpful information to health consumers and health-care professionals about the signs and symptoms of stress, the negative associated health risks, how to cope with stress, and the federal government's role in dealing with this important public health issue.	http://www.hc-sc.gc.ca/hl-vs/iyh-vsv/life-vie/stress-eng.php
Mental Health Commission of Canada. (2012). *Changing directions. Changing lives: The mental health strategy for Canada.* **Calgary, AB: Author.** -This report and strategic directions paper outlines various mental health challenges facing diverse Canadian populations (e.g., immigrants and refugees, First Nations) across the lifespan.	http://strategy.mentalhealth-commission.ca/pdf/strategy-images-en.pdf

Stress is an individual's unique reaction and emotional and physiological response to a specific situation or condition, as opposed to the actual situation or condition. Stress in itself is neither negative nor positive (Canadian Mental Health Association [CMHA], 2016a, 2016b). Rather, it is our reactions to stress that can be described as being negative or positive. Hence, the term "stress" really refers to two different things: (i) Situations that trigger physical and emotional reactions, and (ii) the reactions to stressors themselves (Conversano et al., 2010; Donatelle, Munroe, Munroe, & Thompson, 2008; Hahn, Payne, Gallant, & Fletcher, 2006; Insel, Roth, Irwin, & Burke, 2016; Kleiman et al., 2017). What is perceived as being stressful varies greatly among individuals due to a variety of factors including coping mechanisms, genetic makeup, life experiences, environmental influences, ethnicity, and culture. We usually feel stressed when we think that the demands of the situation or condition are greater than our resources, resilience, and coping skills to deal with that situation. For example, someone who feels comfortable speaking in public in front of a large crowd of individuals may not worry about giving a public presentation, while someone who isn't confident in their skills may feel a lot of stress about an upcoming presentation.

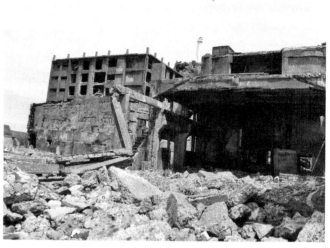

Source: Wally J. Bartfay. Nagasaki, Japan.

Photo 11.6 Coping Mechanisms and Stress Overload. Conflicts, war and natural disasters that include earth quakes, tsunamis, hurricanes, floods, and fire can result in stress "overload" when traditional coping mechanisms are overwhelmed or are insufficient to meet current or emerging demands. Public healthcare professionals and workers play a vital role in helping individuals, families, and entire communities to manage and cope with the stressor and the potential negative physical and emotional health effects associated with it.

Seyle (1974, 1983) argued that stress was a subjective condition such as pain or grief. For example, a client may react with a smile and chuckle when she is told by a public health nurse that she has type 2 diabetes. Indeed, for weeks this client has been suffering from anxiety and insomnia due to fear that her signs and symptoms were related to cancer. A **stressor** is defined as any situation or event that triggers an emotional or physiological response by an individual (Donatelle et al., 2008; Insel et al., 2016; Hahn et al., 2006; Seyle, 1974). Examples of *physiological stressors* include inadequate nutrition, chronic pain and discomfort, a burn, excessive heat or noise, and having an infectious disease. Examples of *emotional stressors* include losing one's job or source of income, death of a spouse or family member, being a victim of child abuse or rape, and being diagnosed with a life threatening disease such as cancer.

Work-related stress is a growing occupational health concern in Canada and internationally. In fact, one in four adult workers (27% or 3.7 million workers) described their lives as being highly stressful in nature, and mental health issues are estimated to cost employers in excess of $20 billion annually and account for 3-out-of-4 short-term work-related disability claims in Canada (Crompton, 2014). It is notable that healthcare expenditures are also approximately 50% greater for workers who report high degrees of stress, and stress-related absences cost employers in excess of $3.5 billion annually in Canada (Druxbury & Higgins, 2001; Williams, 2003). The reader is referred to Chapter 8 for a discussion on work-related stress, and Table 8.6 for a list of potential stressors that can contribute to increased workplace stress and alterations to health.

The **stress response** is defined as the individual's reaction to a specific stressor. Seyle (1974, 1983) coined the terms "eustress" and "distress" which are defined in Figure 11.4.

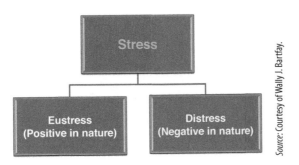

Source: Courtesy of Wally J. Bartfay.

Figure 11.4 Positive and Negative Stress. **Eustress** is regarded as positive stress that presents the opportunity for personal growth, satisfaction, and new and desirable life experiences (e.g., getting married, starting university, learning a new language or musical instrument, beginning a new career). **Distress** is regarded as negative stress that consists of unpleasant situations or experiences (e.g., death of a loved one, job loss, loss of a home due to fire or a natural disaster, being diagnosed with a life-threatening health condition). If distress is not controlled and managed, it can result in physical and/or mental health issues, illness, or even death.

General Adaption Syndrome Model

Seyle (1974, 1983) developed the **general adaptation syndrome (GAS) model**, which describes how the human body moves through three stages when confronted by stressors: (i) Alarm reaction; (ii) resistance; and (iii) exhaustion. The alarm stage consists of involuntary changes controlled by hormonal and nervous system responses that trigger the "fight-flight- freeze" response, which is detailed below (Donatelle et al., 2008; Hahn et al., 2006; Insel et al., 2016; Seyle, 1974). This stage requires high amounts of energy. The resistance stage reflects the body's attempt to reestablish homeostasis by decreasing or reducing the intensity of the initial stress response to a more manageable level by decreasing the production of adrenocorticotropic hormone (ACTH). During this stage, a person can typically cope with normal activities of daily living and the added stressor. However, if the resistance stage is prolonged or chronic in nature and the individual in not able to reestablish homeostasis via their coping mechanisms, the person may begin to develop mind-induced psychogenic and/or psychosomatic disorders associated with chronic stress. During the exhaustion stage, bodily adjustments resulting from chronic stress can result in depletion of adaptation energy stores and systems overload resulting in increased stress-inducing hormone levels again. In extreme cases of stress, this state may be life threatening in nature (Donatelle et al., 2008; Hahn et al., 2006; Insel et al., 2016; Seyle, 1974). Although the GAS model is regarded as a key conceptual model for understanding how individuals react to stress and stressors, some of its components are currently viewed as being outdated or incorrect in nature.

Allostatic load is defined as the "wear and tear on the body" which accumulates as a function of time due to chronic or repeated episodes of stress that result in fluctuating or heightened neural or neuroendocrine responses. An individual's allostatic load is dependent on several factors including previous life experiences and coping mechanisms, resilience levels, genetics, and behavioural responses to stressors (Crimmins, Johnston, Hayward, & Seeman, 2003; McEwen, 2000; Szanton, Gill, & Allen, 2005). **Allostasis** is defined as the process by which the body responds to stressors in order to regain stability or homeostasis (Bechie, 2012; McEwen, 2017). High stress levels and allostatic loads have been linked to an increased risk of developing heart disease, hypertension, obesity, diabetes, certain cancers, sleep disorders, depression, recurrent seizures, and impaired immune system responses to name but a few (e.g., Bocke, Seidle, Latza, Rossnagel, & Schumann, 2012; Baldin, Hauser, Pack, & Hesdorffer, 2017; Bechie, 2012; Chiang & Chang, 2012; Li et al., 2013; McEwen, 2017; Seeman, Singer, Rowe, Horwitz, & McEwen, 1997; Zota, Shenassa, & Morello-Frosch, 2013).

Although excessive or chronic stress can lead to a variety of negative health problems (e.g., increased incidence of heart disease, stroke, certain cancers, mental health issues, sexual dysfunction), a certain moderate

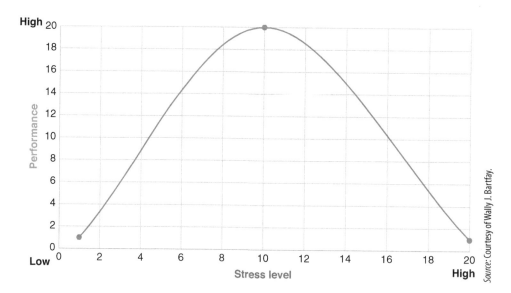

Source: Courtesy of Wally J. Bartfay.

Figure 11.5 Yerkes–Dodson Law. Yerkes–Dodson Law is often illustrated graphically as a bell-shaped curve which increases and then decreases with higher levels of stress and arousal.

and manageable level of stress may be beneficial in nature. Indeed, stress can also be seen as very motivating and energizing and without some degree of stress in our daily lives, we would accomplish little. Recognizing the appropriate level of stress for your ideal performance level is critical in reaching your personal potential. Figure 11.5 shows a bell-shaped curve known as the **Yerkes–Dodson Law**, which demonstrates graphically the theoretical association between optimal levels of stress and peak performance for an individual (Andreassi, 1998; Calabrese, 2008; Hanoch & Vitouse, 2004). Too little or too much stress is not helpful; however, a moderate level of stress encourages or helps to foster peak performance. This law was originally developed by the psychologists Robert M. Yerkes and John Dillingham Dodson in 1908 who argued that performance increases with physiological or mental arousal, but only up to a certain point.

Physiological Responses to Stressors

Imagine for a minute that you step-off a curb to cross a quiet street and suddenly a truck beeps its horn and within a split second of colliding you leap away to safety. Your heart is racing, your breathing is rapid and your body is physically shaking after the experience. This is an example of a physiological response to a potential lethal stressor (i.e., a truck about to collide with you). There are three major systems in your body that control your physiological responses to stress: (i) Central nervous system (CNS); (ii) endocrine system; and (iii) immune system (Donatelle et al., 2008; Hahn et al., 2006; Insel et al., 2016). Figure 11.6 illustrates the neurochemical links among these three aforementioned systems. The CNS consists of your brain, spinal cord which controls your reflexes, and nerves.

1. *Central Nervous System*

    The **autonomic nervous system** (ANS) is the part or component of the nervous system that controls basic body processes such as your heart rate, breathing, blood pressure, and hundreds of other involuntary process, and consists of the sympathetic and parasympathetic divisions (Donatelle et al., 2008; Hahn et al., 2006; Insel et al., 2016). The sympathetic division of the ANS reacts to the perceived stressor or danger by instantly accelerating body processes through the use of the neurotransmitter norepinephrine. **Norepinephrine**, which is also known as noradrenaline, is a neurotransmitter released by the sympathetic division and targets specific tissues (e.g., muscles) and organs (e.g., heart) to enable the individual to quickly handle the stress situation, and it also increases alertness, awareness, and attention. In general, the sympathetic division of the ANS hinders or stops the storage of energy in the body and uses it to handle the stressor or threat. The cerebral cortex evaluates the stressor based on past life experiences and the perception of future consequences in relation to that stressor, and plans a course of action (Hoehn & Marieb, 2010; McCance & Heuther, 2010).

The hypothalamus sits at the base of the brain just above the pituitary gland and it plays a critical role by serving as the central connection between the nervous and endocrine systems during the stress event (Hoehn & Marieb, 2010; McCance & Heuther, 2010). The hypothalamus sends signals via nerve fibres to activate the sympathetic nervous system, and also releases hormones that regulate the secretion of ACTH by the pituitary gland (Donatelle et al., 2008; Hahn et al., 2006; Insel et al., 2016). The limbic system is located in the inner mid-portions of the brain and when it is stimulated by a stressor, emotions, feelings, and behaviours that help to ensure the survival of the individual may be aroused. A stressor may also stimulate the reticular activating system (RAS) located between the lower end of the brainstem and thalamus. During such an event, the RAS may be activated to increase arousal, alertness, and certain emotional responses to the stressor at hand. However, chronic stimulation of the RAS has been linked to stress-induced insomnia and sleep disturbances (e.g., Basta, Chrousas, Vela-Bueno, & Vgontzos, 2007; Riemann et al., 2010).

2. *Endocrine System*

Once the hypothalamus is activated in response to a stressor perceived as harmful or threatening in nature, the endocrine system becomes activated via the sympathetic nervous system to release hormones and other chemical messengers into the bloodstream to increase metabolism and other bodily functions (Hoehn & Marieb, 2010; McCance & Heuther, 2010). Walter Bradford Cannon (1929) was the first to describe the so-called "fight or flight response" where an animal (e.g., seal) reacts to a threat stressor (e.g., polar bear) with a general discharge of the sympathetic nervous system, which prepares it for either fighting or fleeing. This response is also recognized as the first stage of the GAS that regulates the stress response among vertebrates including humans. Stress experts around the world are now adding the word "freeze" to this response in deference to the fact that instead of fighting or fleeing, sometimes we tend to freeze (e.g., like a deer caught in the headlights of a car on the

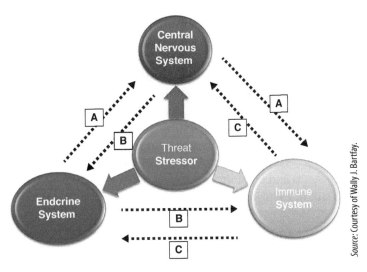

Figure 11.6 Neurochemical Links Among the Central Nervous System, Endocrine System and Immune System. The communication among these three major systems is regarded as being bidirectional in nature. It is important to note that stress activation of these systems may also affect other body systems such as the cardiovascular (e.g., increased heart rate, stroke volume, and cardiac output); blood vessels (e.g., peripheral vasoconstriction, redistribution of blood to vital organs); respiratory (e.g., increased respiration rate), and gastrointestinal systems (e.g., increased glycogenosis, decreased digestion). *Note:* A = neuropeptides; B = endocrine hormones, and C = cytokines.

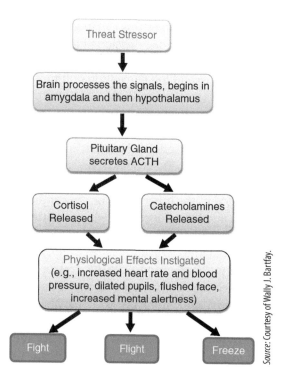

Source: Courtesy of Wally J. Bartfay.

Figure 11.7 Physiological Effects of the "Fight-Flight-Freeze" Response. A simplified flowchart showing the major physiological responses experienced by an individual following a threat stressor and the "fight-flight-freeze" response. *Note:* Catecholamines include norepinephrine and epinephrine, and ACTH = adrenocorticotropic hormone.

highway) in traumatic situations (e.g., Bracha, 2004; Schmidt, Richery, Zvolensky, & Moner, 2015; Seltzer, 2015). Hence, the **fight-flight-freeze response** describes how an individual ultimately reacts to a threat stressor, and its major physiological effects are summarized in Figure 11.7.

During the fight, flight, or freeze response, the adrenal medulla releases a hormonal cascade that results in the secretion of catecholamines such as norepinephrine and epinephrine known as the *sympathoadrenal response* (Donatelle et al., 2008; Hahn et al., 2006; Insel et al., 2016). The hormones testosterone, estrogen, and cortisol, and the neurotransmitters dopamine and serotonin also affect how the animal reacts to the treat stressor. **Cortisol**, also called hydrocortisone, is a primary corticosteroid secreted by the cortex of the adrenal gland that produces a number of physiological responses to the threat stressor such as increasing blood glucose levels, potentiating the action of epinephrine and norepinephrine on blood vessels and inhibiting inflammatory responses *in-vivo*. This reaction, for examples, results in the dilation of blood vessels supplying skeletal muscles necessary for quick movements, and increases cerebral blood flow which enhances mental alertness. Cortisol also "turns-off" inflammatory processes and cytokines (e.g., tumour necrosis factor & interleukin-1), which if left uncontrolled could result in cellular injury and/or destruction (Hoehn & Marieb, 2010; McCance & Heuther, 2010).

3.   *Immune System*

Psychoneuroimmunology (PNI) is an interdisciplinary science and field of investigation that seeks to examine the relationships and interactions between psychological, neurological, and immune responses to stressors. For example, current evidence shows that high levels of stress can predispose individuals to the development of colds and compromise the functioning of the immune system to fight-off infections (Donatelle et al., 2008; Insel et al., 2016; Segerstrom & Miller, 2004, 2010). The interaction or communication between the immune system and the brain is largely medicated via cytokines, which play a critical role in the coordination of the immune response. For example, interleukin-1 is a specific kind of cytokine produced by monocytes which act on the temperature control centre of the hypothalamus that initiates the "febrile response" (i.e., increase in body temperature) to help combat various infectious agents in the body.

Both acute and chronic forms of stress can affect the immune system differently and how the individual is ultimately able to cope and manage threat stressor in play. For example, during an acute stress period resulting from a trauma, burn, or injury to the skin, white blood cells (i.e., neutrophils, natural killer T cells) migrate into the skin where they enhance the immune response during the stressful event sequence (Donatelle et al., 2008; Segerstrom & Miller, 2004). Acute stress events (e.g., being in a car accident, missing your train for work, writing a quiz) typically last between five and 100 min (Insel et al., 2016). By contrast, chronic forms of stress (e.g., unemployment, poverty, war) appear to have negative outcomes on both cellular and humoral (i.e., antibody) components of the immune system (Segerstrom & Miller, 2004). Chronic stress, for example, may result in the chronic secretion of cortisol which may accelerate and/or predispose individuals to a variety of diseases that have been associated with inflammation (e.g., multiple sclerosis, type 2 diabetes, cardiovascular disease) (Bechie, 2012; McEwen, 2017; Zota et al., 2013). In addition, immune responses may be ineffective and/or suboptimal in nature with chronic forms of stress.

In short, acute stress often results in beneficial physiological changes that are important to human adaptation and survival. Conversely, chronic stress that is excessive in nature and prolonged may result in maladaptive physiological responses that can result in harm, injury to vital organs, and disease. For example, chronic stress may have profound effects on both brain structure and function such as the hippocampus, which plays a critical role in long-term memory, spatial learning, and other vital cognitive functions. In fact, studies reveal that individuals who have experienced chronic forms of stress (e.g., domestic violence, childhood neglect, war) have decreased hippocampal volumes and activity (Bechie, 2012; McEwen, 2017; Weiss, 2007).

Several questions about the effects of stress on immune responses remain to be answered. For example, it is currently not known if stress is required to initiate these aforementioned changes *in-vivo* or how much of an alteration in the immune system is required before an individual becomes susceptible to disease processes. Moreover, it is important to acknowledge that there are conflicting findings that have found no association between prolonged arousal by stressors and negative health outcomes (Donatelle et al., 2008; Insel et al., 2016). Indeed, the relationship between stressors and negative health outcomes such as disease is affected by the nature, number, and persistence of stressors, and by the individual's biological vulnerability (i.e., genetics, constitutional factors), psychosocial resources, and learned patterns of coping and individual coping mechanisms (Alkadhi, 2013; Scheiderman, Ironside, & Siegel, 2005). We shall explore these coping mechanisms in greater detail later.

Personality-types and stress

Personality is defined as the sum of all cognitive, behavioural, and emotional tendencies of a specific individual that are formed and developed over-time due to personal memories, social relationships, interactions with one's environment (i.e., physical, social, environmental, occupational), values, attitudes, habits, and skill sets. Various personality theorists present their particular definitions of the word "personality" based on their own unique theoretical positions and constructs. The term **personality trait** refers to enduring personal characteristics that are revealed in particular patterns of behaviour in a variety of social situations and interactions. Some individuals are generally less irritable and easygoing and not easily upset by minor annoyances (e.g., being caught in a traffic jam or being tailgated by another car), while others get highly emotional, upset, and are prone to verbal or physical outbursts (e.g., road rage) by similar minor annoyances. Table 11.2 shows the four basic personality types, a brief description of each and how they tend to respond to stressors.

Table 11.2　Four Major Personality Types

Personality Type	Description	Response to Stressors
Type A	Individuals are highly controlling in nature, ultracompetitive in nature, impatient, aggressive, cynical, confrontational, verbally, emotionally and/or physically hostile or abusive.	Tend to have higher perceived stress levels and more problems coping with stress. This personality type was first described as a potential risk factor for **heart disease** during the 1950s by cardiologists Meyer Friedman and Ray Rosenman (Fisher, 1963; Friedman & Rosenman, 1959).
Type B	Individuals are generally relaxed, laid-back, easy going, and contemplative. These individuals tend to be better at relaxing without feeling guilty and working without becoming overly anxious or agitated.	Tend to have lower perceived stress levels in comparison to type A. They may enjoy achievement, although they have a greater tendency to disregard physical or mental stress when they do not achieve.
Type C	Individuals with this personality type tend to be introverts are characterized by the suppression of anger and feelings. These individuals prefer to be alone, appear to lack emotions, are often perfectionist in nature, often have feelings of hopelessness, suppress their wants, needs or desires, do not usually assert themselves, and prefer to pacify others. They often find it hard to work with others, so prefer to work on their own.	Tend to have exaggerated responses to minor stressors, and these heightened responses may impair immune functions. Over the long term, this can bring about high degrees of frustration, anger, and stress which can lead to the development of depression. Lydia Temoshok was the first to propose the "cancer prone" personality hypothesis during the late 1980s (Temoshok, 1987; Temoshok et al., 1985).
Type D	This is a relatively new personality construct where individuals tend to have a joint tendency toward negative affectivity (e.g., anger, contempt, disgust, guilt, and fear, and nervousness) and social inhibition (e.g., reticence and a lack of self-assurance). These individuals often possess a negative outlook on life, are gloomy, socially inept, and anxious worriers who live with a constraint fear of rejection by others. These individuals tend to be pessimistic and overall negative in nature, and often expect the worse to happen.	The letter D stands for "distressed" with this personality type. These individuals tend to have an overall negative outlook on life, live with a constraint fear of rejection by others resulting in chronic levels of stress which may make them more prone to the development of coronary heart disease, diabetes, and major depressive disorder (Al-Quezweny et al., 2016; Denollet & Conraads, 2011; Park, Ko, Lee, Lee, & Kim, 2014; Sher, 2005).

Note: Not all individuals will fit perfectly or wholly into a specific personality type category per se, but may possess characteristics, traits, and/or behaviours that are present in other personality type descriptions as well (i.e., mixed types).

Studies on types A, C, and D personality types suggest that expressing one's emotions, desires, and feelings tends to be beneficial, whereas suppressing in general may have negative health outcomes in general and decreased health-related quality of life (Donatella et al., 2008; Huang et al., 2017; Insel et al., 2016; Roberts, Kuncel, Shiner, Caspi, & Goldberg, 2007). Researchers have examined personality traits that enable individuals to deal more successfully with stressors in life, such as "hardiness" which can be described as a particular form of optimism (e.g., Conversano et al., 2010; Kleiman et al., 2017). It is important to note from a public health perspective that personality is not an inherited trait per se. Hence, it doesn't matter whether the individual happens to be Type A, B, C, or D, because all clients have the power to make changes to positively affect their health and well-being. For example, modification of Type A personality to decrease the risk of developing cardiovascular disease (CVD) is possible when certain "learned behaviours" or habits are modified (e.g., hurried-rush behaviours, becoming more tolerant, calm, and better-humoured in nature). In fact, although approximately 80% of Canadian's know that prolonged stress can increase their risk of developing CVD, only one in four knows that associated lifestyle and/or personality changes can reduce their risk by up to 80% as well (Canadian Mental Health Association and Heart and Stroke Foundation of Canada; Health Canada, 2008).

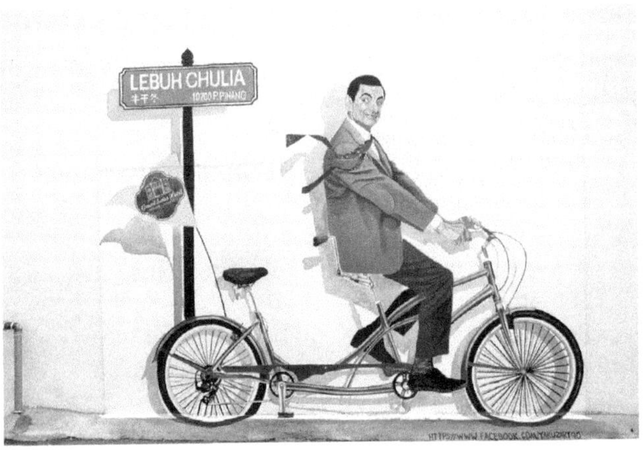

Coping and Managing Stressors

Coping is defined as an individual's cognitive and/ or behavioural attempts and resources to manage specific physiological or emotional/psychological

Photo 11.7 A comical street mural in Georgetown, Malaysia. When it comes to stress, "Laughter is perhaps the best and oldest medicine." Laughter can boost your spirits by producing changes in the autonomic nervous system; decreasing stress hormones, and stimulating immune function and the production of infection-fighting antibodies. Laughter also triggers the release of *endorphins*, the body's natural feel-good biological opiate peptides, which also provide temporarily relief of pain and discomfort.

stressors that they are confronted with. Forty-one Canadian post-secondary institutions participated in the ACHA National College Health Assessment II (NCHA II) Canadian Reference Group survey, and a total of 43,780 surveys were completed by students on these campuses nationwide (American College Health Association National College Health Assessment ACHA NCHA II, 2016). Notably, 49.2% of survey respondents reported that they were experiencing "more than average stress" in their lives, and 14.4% reported experiencing "tremendous stress" levels. In addition, 67.8% of survey respondents indicated that they have not received any information related to how to help others in distress. Nonetheless, 74.7% of these respondents reported that they would be interested in receiving information on how to help others in distress. Moreover, 67.6% of respondents indicated that they had received information from their college or university on the topic of "stress reduction." The reader is referred to the Web-Based Resources Box below for the full 63-page ACHA NCHA II Canadian Reference Group II Group report.

Coping resources are defined as internal and external assets, characteristics, behaviours, problem solving skills, and/or actions that can be employed by an individual to manage a stress response. Table 11.3 provides the reader with some examples of internal and external coping resources. It is critical to be flexible in terms of assessing the nature of the stressor, the client's perception of control over it, and the ability to adapt coping resources and strategies overtime as needed (Zong et al., 2010).

Web-Based Resources Box ACHA NCHA Canadian Reference Group II Report

Learning Resource	Website
ACHA NCHA **II): Canadian Reference Group (Spring, 2016). Data Report**	http://www.acha-ncha.org/docs/NCHA-II%20 SPRING%202016%20CANADIAN%20REFERENCE%20 GROUP%20DATA%20REPORT.pdf

Table 11.3   Examples of Internal and External Coping Resources

Internal Resources	External Resources
• Effective communication skills • Ability to identify problem & collection of appropriate information • Flexibility and ability to propose or generate alternative courses of action to solve problems • Self-efficacy • Positive outlook on life and beliefs • Generally positive health-related quality of life • High moral standards • Spirituality • High energy levels • Effective social skills	• Strong social network of friends, family, and co-workers • Social contracts • Positive financial resources • Knowledge and willingness to access social agencies in workplace or community • Knowledge and application/use of stress-management resources (e.g., spa, massage therapist, gym) • Access and use of self-help websites, books, community-based workshops, and/or seminars

Positive coping and stress management techniques

Emotion-focused coping involves positively managing and dealing with the emotions that arise when a stressful life event occurs. For example, an individual diagnosed with a terminal form of cancer may seek spiritual guidance and comfort from their place of worship in the community. Although this form of coping may not appear to be working toward a solution or resolution of the stressor per se, it is nonetheless an essential and valid mechanism to deal with the stressor. In this context, spirituality deals with the individual's ability to remain connected to the world around them and their unique spiritual quality of life beliefs and associated meanings, be it religious or not in nature. For example, Desbiens and Fillion (2007) investigated the associations between coping strategies, emotional outcomes (distress and vigor), and spiritual quality of life in 120 palliative care nurses in Québec. The researchers found that whether through religious beliefs or the ability to reinterpret life experiences and assign positive meaning to them, were shown to positively mediate bereavement-related stress.

Problem-focused coping is a type of cognitive approach in which the individual attempts to deal with and find effective workable solutions to the stressor in question. For instance, an older individual who has renal failure that requires frequent travel to a dialysis clinic may sign-up and arrange for volunteer driver services in their community. Emotion- and problem-focused types of coping may be employed as individual strategies or in combination by the individual experiencing the stressor. For example, a client diagnosed with heart failure and chronic obstructive pulmonary disease (COPD) may engage in problem-focused coping by deciding to quit smoking and partake in an integrated community exercise program. This same client may decide to seek support from their healthcare provider and also join a smoking cessation support group in their community. Desveaux (2017) reported that group-based integrated community exercise programs tailored to the participant's functional ability help to facilitate adherence and sustainability. In addition, participant support for group-based integrated community exercise programs; which included the benefit of sharing multiple perspectives, helped to increase accountability.

Benson (1975) was the first to describe the **relaxation response**, which is defined as the counterpart to the fight-flight-freeze response where the body is no longer in perceived danger, and the ANS functioning returns to a normal state. Benson (1975) characterized this response as a state of physiological and psychological deep rest that helps clients deal with their stressors by increasing control over them and also decreasing tension. The relaxation process does not involve sleeping or lying on the couch and being lazy. By contrast, it is a mentally active process that is trainable and which becomes more profound and effective with practice overtime, which leaves both the body and mind more relaxed in concert. For example,

Papathanassoglou (2010) conducted a systematic review of 14 studies which highlighted the benefits of the relaxation response among patients in critical care units in terms of psychological support, use of imagery, and other relaxation techniques. Table 11.4 provides examples of various positive coping and stress management techniques.

Table 11.4 Examples of Various Coping and Stress Management Techniques

Technique	Brief Description
Animal assisted therapy (AAT)	• Involves the use of specially trained animals (e.g., dogs, horses) to assist in the attainment of motivational, educational, recreational, or other therapeutic health-related goals that seek to help individuals deal and manage actual or perceived stressors in their daily lives. The goal of AAT is to improve a client's social, emotional, or cognitive functioning.
Art therapy	• Involves the creative expression of one's self through artistic mediums (e.g., drawing, painting, sculpting) to help decrease stress, facilitate healing from current stressors or past trauma.
Biofeedback	• Involves the use of an electronic monitoring device of a normally automatic bodily response (e.g., heart rate, brain activity, muscle tension, skin temperature, or conductance), which helps train an individual to acquire voluntary control of that function.
Community-based social or self-help support groups	• Involve professional and/or non-professional groups and organizations (e.g., Alcoholics Anonymous, support groups for parents with autism, women undergoing mastectomies due to breast cancer) formed by individuals with a common problem or life situation, for the purpose of pooling resources, gathering and sharing information or experiences, and offering mutual support, services, or care.
Exercise and physical activity	• Moderate- and vigorous -intensity forms of movement-related activities (e.g., jogging, boxing, lap swimming, cycling, rope skipping, aerobic dancing) help to reduce stress, expand energy in a positive outlet, provide social contact, promote relaxation, and promote the release of endorphins (mood-enhancing natural opiate peptide pain killers) into the bloodstream.
Guided imagery	• Involves the use of relaxation and mental visualization to improve mood and/or physical well-being. May involve the use of vision, sounds, smells, or taste, as well as the senses of touch, movement, and position which help to produce a calming effect on the mind and body including decreased stress and anxiety, enhanced immune responses, and positive hormonal responses.
Hypnosis and hypnotherapy	• Is employed to create subconscious change in a client in the form of new responses, thoughts, attitudes, behaviours, or feelings to certain stressors or life events and is undertaken with a subject in hypnosis, and which may help to increase motivation, alleviate stressors, and/or alter behaviours.
Journal keeping	• The individual expresses their self in a written format, which helps to increase self-awareness and coping. May describe thoughts, feelings, behaviours, memories, and perceptions of events or stressors.
Massage therapy	• Involves the manipulation of soft tissues and joints to improve circulation to the area, improve health, and promote health and healing via relaxation, reduced muscle tension, improve immune function, increased flexibility and range of motion, and pain management.

(Continued)

Table 11.4   Examples of Various Coping and Stress Management Techniques (*Continued*)

Technique	Brief Description
Mindfulness	• A therapeutic technique involving a mental state achieved by focusing one's awareness on the present moment, while calmly acknowledging and accepting one's feelings, thoughts, and bodily sensations which can be achieved through the practice of yoga or other techniques.
Music therapy	• Includes creating and/or listening to various forms of music chosen by the individual to promote relaxation, alter moods, decrease anxiety and stress, and to manage pain and discomfort.
Relaxation breathing	• Involves slow and/or deep breathing techniques and exercises to induce the relaxation response in clients.
Yoga	• Regarded as a Hindu-based spiritual and ascetic discipline and part of Ayurvedic medicine, which involves controlled breathing techniques, simple meditation, and the adoption of specific bodily postures to promote overall health and relaxation and decrease stress.

Negative coping and stress management techniques

Negative coping strategies include the use of tobacco products, alcohol, and other drugs (e.g., cocaine, methamphetamines, cannabis). The ACHA National College Health Assessment II (NCHA II) Canadian Reference Group survey (ACHA NCHA II, 2016) reported that 52.3% of college and university students have not received any health-related information related to alcohol or other drug use on their campus, although 63.1% reported that they were interested in receiving information on this topic. It is notable that 21.5% of respondents surveyed reported consuming alcohol in the past one to two days, and 19.8% in the past three to five days of the survey. Moreover, 23.7% reported consuming marijuana (pot, hashish, hash oil); 8.8% MDMA (Ecstasy); 5.5% cocaine (crack, rock, freebase); 3.6% hallucinogens (LSD, PCP), and 1.3% methamphetamine (crystal, meth, ice, crank) in the past.

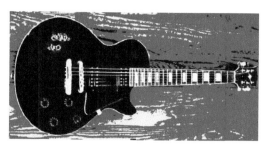

Source: Photo by Wally J. Bartfay.

Photo 11.8 Music Therapy. Music therapy includes creating and/or listening to various forms of music chosen by the client. It has been documented to be an effective means to promote relaxation, alter moods, decrease anxiety, stress, and blood pressure, and to help manage pain and discomfort.

For instance, alcohol (e.g., beer, liquor, spirits, wine and wine coolers) is classified as a "depressant," which means that it slows down and alters physical and cognitive functions resulting in slurred speech, unsteady and coordinated bodily movements, disturbed perceptions, decreased reflex times, distorted judgment and decreased ability to think and reason rationally. Under the *Food and Drugs Act* in Canada (see link http://laws-lois.justice.gc.ca/eng/regulations/C.R.C.%2C_c._870/), alcohol is identified/classified as a "food." However, alcohol contains psychoactive chemicals, which also makes it technically a psychoactive drug or substance in terms of its impacts on health (WHO, n.d.). Between April 2013 and March 2014, over $20.5 billion worth of alcohol was sold to Canadians (Statistics Canada, 2015b). The PHAC (2015) reports that an estimated 22 million Canadians (approximately 80%), drank alcohol in the previous year. Moreover, 3.1 million Canadians 15 years or older drank enough alcohol to be at risk for immediate injury and harm, and 4.4 million individuals were at risk for developing health disorders associated with its chronic consumption (e.g., liver cirrhosis, various forms of cancer) (PHAC, 2015b). In fact, more recent data show that the associated cost of hospitalizations for substance use disorders from psychoactive drugs has been steadily increasing overtime, reaching $267 million in 2011 alone, over half of which was due to alcohol (Young & Jesseman, 2014). From a global public health perspective, alcohol has been linked to over 3 million deaths per year, slightly more than lung cancer and HIV/AIDS combined (WHO, 2014b, 2015b).

Public health caution related to natural health products and stress

Public healthcare professionals and workers should be cognizant of the fact that individuals with life-threatening conditions (e.g., cancer, heart or liver failure) and older adults are more likely to employ complementary and alternative therapies to help manage their stress responses. In fact, a 2010 Ipsos-Reid survey reported that 73% of Canadians regularly take natural health products (NHPs) like vitamins and minerals, herbal products, and homeopathic medicines (Health Canada, 2016a). Older adults, for example, may use a variety of over-the-counter (OTC) supplements, herbs and/or natural remedies that rises safety concerns and possible toxicities from polypharmacological interactions with prescriptions medications or age-related pharmacokinetics changes (e.g., decreased renal or liver function) (Gujjariamudi, 2016; Scholz, Holmes, & Marcus, 2008; Trappman, 2012; Johns & Gray-Donald, 2002).

For example, St. John's wort (*Hypericum perforatum)* is a common plant-derived herbal product taken orally in the form of a pill or capsule, and it is widely sold in healthcare stores and pharmacies throughout Canada. St. John's wort is often taken by Canadians as a non-prescription-based "natural health product" for the short-term treatment of mild-to-moderate anxiety and depression. However, this herbal supplement can have serious interactions with other OTC drugs and prescription medications, which include interference with the metabolism of prescription-based drugs through the cytochrome P450 enzyme system, and may lead to potentially harmful interactions when taken in combination with other anti-depressants. In fact, St. John's wort when taken in combination with other drugs may elevate 5-HT (serotonin) levels in the CNS, which could result in "serotonin syndrome," a potentially life-threatening adverse drug reaction (Borrelli & Izzo, 2009; Kober, Pohl, & Efferth, 2008; Whorry, 2000). Moreover, it decreases the levels of estrogens, such as estradiol, by speeding up its metabolism, and should therefore not be taken by women prescribed contraceptive pills (Health Canada, 2016b).

As part of the Health Products and Food Branch of Health Canada, the Natural and Non-prescription Health Products Directorate (NNHPD) is the federal authority for regulating the sale of natural health products in Canada (Health Canada, 2016a, 2016b). The mandated role of the NNHPD is to ensure that Canadians have ready access to natural health products that are deemed safe, effective, and of high quality, while also respecting freedom of choice and philosophical and cultural diversity surrounding healthcare choices (Health Canada, 2016b).

For example, the herb "Kava" (*Piper methysticum)* is a plant native to the western Pacific islands and may be taken by some individuals to decrease stress and anxiety levels, and to treat restlessness and insomnia (Pittler & Ernest, 2000; Singh & Singh, 2002). Kava has been banned for sale or import in Canada and many European countries including Britain, France, and Germany due to reports of liver damage/failure and associated mortalities as of August 2002 (Health Canada, 2002a, 2002b; Mills, Singh, Ross, Ernst, & Ray, 2003). The reader is referred to the study by Mills et al. (2003) in the research focus box below. This study highlights the public health concern that despite a ban on specific natural herbal health products by Health Canada, certain restricted products continue to be recommended and sold to unknowing Canadian consumers, which could result in serious and even life-threatening health consequences.

Research Focus Box 11.1

Sale of Kava Extract in Some Health Food Stores

Study Aim/Rationale

To examine the availability and sale of Kava (*Piper methysticum*), a herbal plant-derived so called "natural health product" used to treat anxiety, stress, insomnia and ADHD, in Canadian health food stores following the 2002 ban of this product by Health Canada.

Methodology/Design

The researchers employed a "participant-as-observer" method to best simulate the real-life interactions between a customer and a natural health store employee. The interactions between a total of 33 health food stores employees was documented in regards to whether or not they recommended Kava to their customers after the reported ban of this natural herbal product by Health Canada.

Major Findings

Even though the herbal product kava had been the subject of a Health Canada advisory, employees in 22 (67%) of the 33 health food stores recommended kava to their simulated customers. The simulated customers returned to the same stores two months after Health Canada issued a stop-sale order for products containing kava, but found that 17 (57%) of the 30 stores still in business continued to stock kava on their selves and sell it to unknowing consumers.

Implications for Public Health

These findings are of major concern to Canadian healthcare professionals and workers and consumers alike. The study raises the questions of how Health Canada can actually enforce a nationwide ban on a specific natural health product, and the potential negative health on Canadians might be if stop-sale orders are, in fact, ignored. The sale of Kava represents an important test case with respect to Health Canada's approach to informing Canadian consumers about the potential negative or potentially lethal health outcomes associated with consuming certain natural health products. Indeed, the sale of kava in health food stores two months after a stop-sale order was issued by Health Canada reflects the confusion surrounding the regulation and enforcement of herbs and other natural health products. This study highlights the critical need for regulation not only of the natural products themselves, but also at various points of sale. Informing consumers of the potential risks of non-prescription pharmaceuticals through product labelling would be a prudent public health intervention.

Source: Mills et al. (2003).

Major Mental Illnesses

Mental illness arises from a complex interaction of genetic, biological, social, personality, and environmental factors, and affects people of all ages, education levels, income levels, and cultures. **Mental illnesses** are defined as alterations in thinking, mood, or behaviour—or some combination thereof—associated with significant distress and impaired functioning (APA, 2013; PHAC, 2015a). The symptoms of mental illness vary from mild to severe, depending on the type of mental illness, the individual, the family and the socio-economic environment. Mental illnesses take many forms, including mood disorders, schizophrenia, anxiety disorders, personality disorders, eating disorders, and addictions such as substance dependence and gambling (PHAC, 2006, 2012). Although a detailed discussion of each mental illness and disorder is beyond the scope and purpose of this chapter, we shall highlight some of the major mental illnesses and disorders affecting Canadians.

The laboratory-based medical model of disease causation has historically focused on the identification of chemical imbalances in the brain and/or genome studies to identify specific regions of chromosomes that have been linked to specific mental illness (e.g., schizophrenia, bipolar disorder, depression, attention deficit disorder) (e.g., MacIntyre et al., 2003; National Institute of Mental Health, 2013; Pies, 2014). The reader is referred to Chapter 2 for a detailed discussion of the evolution of the medical model of health and its noted limitations in dealing with complex and multi-faceted health conditions. For example, despite the passage of decades of research, the "chemical imbalance hypothesis" for the development of mental illness and disorders has failed to be proven. Nonetheless, the "magic bullet" approach to finding a cure for mental illness and its associated treatment remains a clinical staple in Canada and abroad.

In the narrative of the antipsychiatry movement, a monolithic entity called "Psychiatry" has deliberately misled the public as to the causes of mental illness, by failing to debunk the chemical imbalance hypothesis. Indeed, this narrative insists that by promoting this simplistic notion, psychiatry betrayed the public trust and made it seem as if psychiatrists had "magic bullets" for psychiatric disorders (Pies, 2014).

Moreover, traditional notions of mental health and mental illness tend to describe their relationship on a single continuum. Mental illness is represented at one end of the continuum while mental health is at the other end. However, mental health is more than the absence of overt signs and symptoms of mental illness and distress. In fact, for people with mental illness, promoting mental health as we previously defined earlier, is a powerful force in aiding the recovery process (CMHA, 2017; PHAC, 2006, 2012). Hence, there is a growing acknowledgement and recognition that mental illness and disorders need to be viewed beyond the laboratory-based unicausal medical model of health, and the need to investigate and address the influence of various SDH (e.g., safety and shelter, domestic violence, income levels, racism, homophobia, oppression) (CMHA, 2017; McGibbon, 2012; MHCC, 2015).

For instance, different communities or populations have different experiences with the SDMH. The impact of these differences can lead to health inequities, where entire communities have poorer health or mental health outcomes than the general population. For example, a 2016 Statistics Canada report again confirmed that SDH, specifically food security and housing, were significant factors for the mental health of First Nations people living off-reserves (Statistics Canada, 2016b). The reader is referred to Chapter 4 for a detailed discussion of mental health challenges faced by indigenous people in Canada.

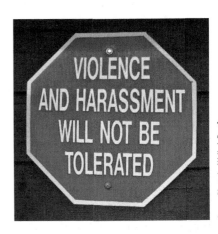

Source: Photo by Wally J. Bartfay.

Photo 11.9 The Canadian Mental Health Association (2017) reports that the following three social determinants of mental health (SDMH) are especially important from the Canadian context and experience: (i) Freedom from discrimination and violence; (ii) social inclusion; and (iii) access to economic resources.

Anxiety disorders

The MHCC (2015) notes that 7% of Canadians aged 12 to 19 years reported in 2011/2012 that they had an anxiety disorder which had been diagnosed by a healthcare professional. The rate of 7.0% in the most recent survey was higher, when compared to 2003 (4.6%) and 2005 (4.7%) rates (MHCC, 2015). Clients with anxiety disorders are plagued by chronic and persistent feelings of threat and anxiety about everyday problems associated with living. Common symptoms include chronic fatigue, lower back pain, headaches, feelings of unreality, sleep disturbances, perceptions of generalized weakness in the lower extremities, and fear of losing control. Anxiety disocrders include generalized anxiety disorder (GAD), obsessive compulsive disorder (OCD), PTSD, panic disorders and social phobias. Anxiety disorders affect approximately 12% of Canadians of which 16% are females and 9% are males (Insel et al., 2016; MHCC, 2015). The former *DSM-IV* category of "Anxiety Disorders" has been expanded into the following three separate categories in the updated and revised *DSM-V* (APA, 2013; Zupanick, 2014):

1. **Anxiety Disorders** (i.e., separation anxiety disorder, selective mutism, specific phobia, social phobia, panic disorder, agoraphobia, and generalized anxiety disorder).
2. **Obsessive–Compulsive Disorders** (i.e., obsessive–compulsive disorder, body dysmorphic disorder, hoarding disorder, trichotillomania, and excoriation disorder).
3. **Trauma and Stressor-Related Disorders** (i.e., reactive attachment disorder, disinhibited social engagement disorder, PTSD, acute stress disorder, and adjustment disorder).

Improved detection of anxiety disorders could result in improved self-management and treatment outcomes. Anxiety disorders are among the most common mental health conditions in children and youth, which can also negatively affect social and academic functioning. Early identification and treatment can prevent the development of more severe problems and improve long-term health outcomes (MHCC, 2015).

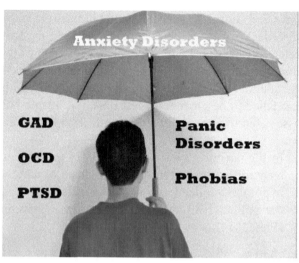

Source: Photo by Wally J. Bartfay.

Photo 11.10 Major mental health disorders falling under the umbrella of anxiety disorders. Anxiety disorders are amongst the most common mental health conditions in adults and contribute to significant distress and impairment. Examples under this "umbrella-term" classification include Generalized Anxiety Disorder (GAD), Obsessive Compulsive Disorders (OCD), Post-Traumatic Stress Disorder (PTSD), panic disorders, and phobias.

According to the MHCC (2015), 6.8% of immigrants aged 12 years or older reported in 2011/2012 that they had an anxiety disorder, which has been diagnosed by a healthcare professional. Immigrants to Canada may be vulnerable to mental health problems because of the difficulties associated with resettlement in a new country. While the lower rate of anxiety disorders among immigrants may be a promising finding, it could also be attributed to an under-reporting or detection. The rate of reported anxiety disorders and/or mood disorders among people living in Canadian territories aged 12 years or older in 2011/2012 (9.6%) was higher than in 2003 (6.5%) (MHCC, 2015). Limited access to mental health professionals and language/ cultural barriers may result in fewer diagnoses. People in Northern communities may be more vulnerable to mental health conditions, including anxiety, than people in non-Northern regions of Canada. This may result from social and economic disparities, access and transportation issues and, in many communities, limited healthcare resources and mental health professional and workers.

Generalized Anxiety Disorder

Generalized anxiety disorder (GAD) is defined as a psychological disorder that can affect both children and adults and is characterized by a chronic and exaggerated anxiety, tension and/or worry about an impending disaster related to some aspect of life or daily living; which may include work or career matters, social relationships, and/or financial matters even when, in fact, nothing seems to be provoking it (APA, 2013; Statistics Canada, 2015c). At least three of the following symptoms must accompany the worry:

- Restlessness or feeling on edge
- Being easily fatigued
- Difficulty concentrating
- Irritability; muscle tension
- Sleep disturbances, which occur more often than not for at least a six months duration

Individuals with GAD find it difficult to control their worry and anxiety. The persistent anxiety that they feel is much more severe than the normal anxiety experienced by the average individual, and clients with GAD tend to anticipate an impending disaster. Clients with GAD are always thinking about the "what ifs" in life and activities of daily living, and fear the worst in every situation. GAD affects approximately 2.5% to 3% of the general Canadian population in a given year, and the lifetime prevalence is approximately 5% globally (Insel et al., 2016; Statistics Canada, 2015c).

The two most common treatments for GAD are anti-anxiety medications (e.g., benzodiazepines, Buspirone) and psychotherapy, which can be administered alone or in combination (Mayo Clinic, 2017; Statistics Canada, 2015c). Benzodiazepines are clinically effective for symptom reduction only. Hence, they should only be taken for short periods of time since they are highly addictive in nature. Cognitive-behavioural therapy can help clients identify negative thoughts, stressors, or behaviours and replace them with positive ones. Exposure therapy may also be employed to narrow down the anxiety-causing stimuli and help individuals to cope with their anxieties and fears.

Obsessive Compulsive Disorder

Obsessive compulsive disorder (OCD) is characterized by obsessions or compulsions that are recurrent and persistent in nature, and thoughts that are intrusive and inappropriate often result in high levels of anxiety and/or distress (APA, 2013; Statistics Canada, 2015c). **Obsessions** are defined as unwanted thoughts or impulses. **Compulsions** are defined as repetitive actions, behaviours, or mental acts that are difficult to resist or control by the individual, and which are often performed rigidly in response to an obsession in an attempt to prevent or reduce anxiety and stress. In the classic play *Macbeth,* for example, William Shakespeare employed compulsive handwashing ritual as a literary device to reveal the guilt pangs that Lady Macbeth felt at having goaded her husband, Macbeth, to kill the King. The most common obsession is concern with contamination by dirt or germs or "misophobia." Hence, individuals with misophobia consequently attempt to avoid all sources of contamination (e.g., handshakes, doorknobs, elevator buttons, shopping cart handles) and often wash and/or disinfect their hands frequently or take frequent baths or showers.

To be clinically diagnosed with OCD, the person must self-recognize that their behaviour is excessive and unreasonable in nature, are time consuming (at least 1 hour per day), results in marked distress, and interferes with their normal, occupational, or social functions. OCD affects approximately 2% of Canadians, and clients with this disorder often feel anxious, out of control and embarrassed about their condition (Insel et al., 2016). Behavioural therapy is often employed to teach the affected individual techniques to avoid their compulsive ritual, and to deal with their anxiety and stress (Statistics Canada, 2015c). In addition, serotonin reuptake inhibitors (anti-depressants) are often clinically prescribed to decrease symptoms (Bloch et al., 2013; Pittenger, Kelmendi, Bloch, Krystal, & Coric, 2005).

Post-Traumatic Stress Disorder

Post-Traumatic Stress Disorder (PTSD) is a disorder caused by a traumatic event that is outside the normal realm of human experience, such as rape, assault, torture, being kidnapped or held captive, military combat, being in severe motor vehicle accident, bioterrorism, and natural or man-made disaster that results in emotional and/or social impairments due to anxiety, depression hypervigilance, guilt, memory impairments, recurrent flashbacks, difficulty sleeping and concentrating, and feelings of guilt of having survived when others may not have (APA, 2013; Donatelle et al., 2008; Statistics Canada, 2015c). According to the National Centre for PTSD about seven or eight out of every 100 people will experience PTSD at some point in their lives and it affects almost twice as many women, in comparison to men (Canadian Broadcasting Corporation CBC-TV, 2017). In general, the traumatic event involves real or threatened physical harm to oneself or to others, and causes intense fear, hopelessness, and/or horror. PTSD symptoms typically subside or decrease within three months following the traumatic event, and approximately half of individuals' recovery within six months. Unfortunately, certain individuals can experience symptoms for years after the traumatic event.

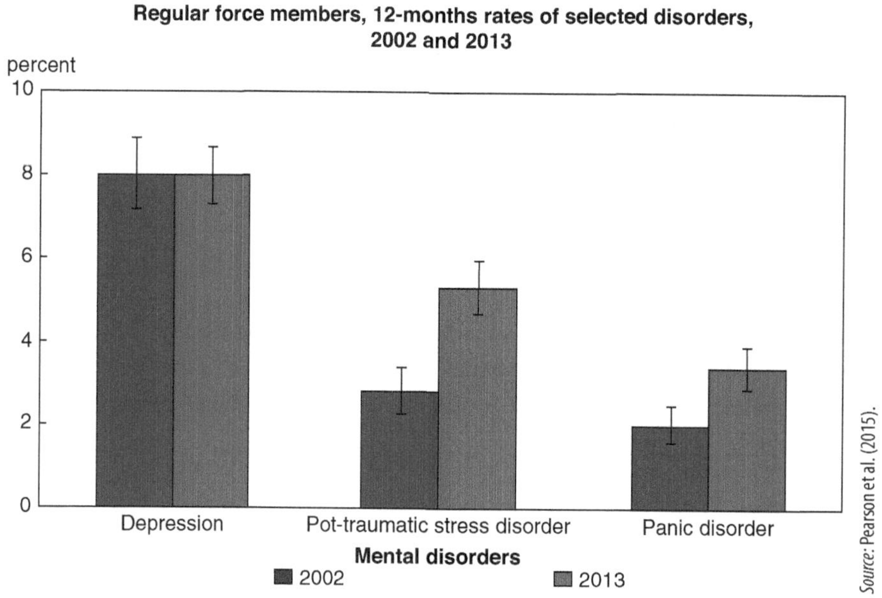

Regular force members, 12-months rates of selected disorders, 2002 and 2013

percent

Source: Pearson et al. (2015).

Depression   Pot-traumatic stress disorder   Panic disorder

Mental disorders

■ 2002   ■ 2013

Figure 11.8 Regular Force Members, 12-Month Rates of Selected Disorders, 2002 and 2013

Member of the Canadian Armed have increased rates of mental health issues, including depression, PTSD, and panic disorders as shown in Figure 11.8. It is noteworthy that PTSD was reported to be twice as high in 2013 (5.3%), in comparison to 2002 figures (2.8%) (Pearson, Zamorski, & Janz, 2015).

Pharmacological interventions include the prescription of SSRIs and/or tricyclic anti-depressants and benzodiazepines. Psychotherapy, including cognitive-behavioural therapy, is critical for the effective treatment and management of PTSD, where individuals learn how to change their thought patterns to overcome their noted anxieties. NSD's Service Dog for PTSD Program was launched in 2011 in Canada and is currently offering this service to Veterans and First Responders in Ontario, British Columbia, and Alberta (see link: http://www.nsd.on.ca/programs/skilled-companion-dogs-for-veterans/). These service dogs are employed to assist individuals suffering from long-term PTSD. Like all assistance dogs, a psychiatric service dog is individually trained to do work or perform tasks that mitigate their handler's disability, and are permitted in all work places and public establishments (e.g., shopping malls, hotels, restaurants) and modes of transport (e.g., taxi's, buses, planes, ferries) by national and provincial laws.

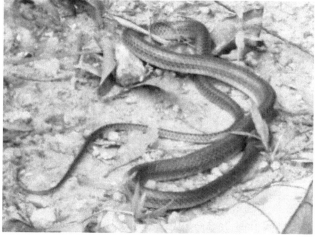

Source: Photo by Wally J. Bartfay, Malaysia.

Photo 11.11 Do you Suffer from Ophidiophobia or Herpetophobia? A venomous brown snake (*Pseudonaja textilis*) in Malaysia. **Ophidiophobia** (or ophiophobia) is a specific phobia associated with the abnormal fear of both venomous and non-venomous snakes. Fear of snakes is sometimes called by a more general term, **herpetophobia**, or the general fear of reptiles and/or amphibians.

Panic Disorders

A **panic disorder** is defined as a syndrome of severe surges in anxiety, accompanied by physical symptoms such as tachycardia, shortness of breath, loss of physical balance or equilibrium, and a feeling of losing mental control. Approximately 2% of Canadians suffer from a panic disorder, and 4% will experience it at some point in their lifetime (Donatelle et al., 2008). A **panic attack** is defined as a sudden and intense acute form of anxiety that often results in intense disabling physical reactions and feeling of dread or terror.

Phobias

A **phobia** is a profound and persistent fear of a specific object, event, activity, or situation that results in a compelling desire to avoid that specific source of fear. Phobias are reported to be more prevalent in women than in men. Simple phobias (e.g., fear of flying, spiders) are often successfully treated with behavioural therapy. Social phobias (e.g., fear of public speaking, eating in public, fear of inadequate sexual performance) require more extensive therapies (Donatelle et al., 2008; Insel et al., 2016).

Mood Disorders, Depression, and Suicide

Mood disorders are one of the most common mental illnesses and conditions present in the general population. A **mood disorder** is defined as an emotional disturbance that is intense and persistent enough in nature to affect normal daily functions and routines. It is noteworthy that the number of categories and specifiers for mood disorders has increased with each successive edition of the *Diagnostic and Statistical Manual for Mental Disorders (DSM)*. In addition, there has been a shift from conceptualizing these disorders as episodic/remitting conditions to viewing them as chronic/intermittent conditions (Klein, 2008; Malhi et al., 2015). Examples of mood disorders include depression, bipolar disorder, and seasonal affective disorder. We shall examine these in greater detail later.

Depression

Depression is a common type of mood disorder characterized by the loss of interest, feelings of sadness, melancholy, dejection, worthlessness, emptiness, hopelessness, changes to libido, appetite, sleep disturbances and other physical symptoms that are inappropriate and out of proportion to reality. Some of the common signs and symptoms of depression are highlighted in Table 11.6. At any given time in Canada, approximately 3 million Canadians suffer from depression, but less than one-third actually seek treatment or counselling for it. The Mood Disorders Society of Canada (2009) estimates that depression affects approximately 11% of Canadians aged 15 years and older at some point during their lifespan. Moreover, twice as many women are likely to experience depression in comparison to their male counterparts, at 14.1% and 8.5%, respectively.

Despite considerable work on the aetiology of depression, which has included neurobiological, genetic, and psycho-sociological investigations, there remains no reliable classificatory system which conclusively links to either the proposed underlying aetiology or has a proven strongly predictive response to the prescribed treatment regime(s) to date (APA, 2013; Kanter, Busch, & Weeks, 2008; Malhi et al., 2015; National Center for Biotechnology Information [NCBI], 2017; Smith & Craddock, 2011). Hence, a number of clinical classification systems and subgroupings have been employed over the past few decades, including reactive and endogenous depression, melancholia, atypical depression, depression with a seasonal pattern/seasonal affective disorder and dysthymia (APA, 2013; NCBI, 2017; Kanter et al., 2008; Malhi et al., 2015; Smith & Craddock, 2011).

For instance, when a depression develops after a period of difficulty (e.g., divorce, loss of a job or loved one), it may be classified as a *reactive-*, *secondary-*, or *exogenous*-type of depression (Donatelle et al., 2008; Hahn et al., 2006; Kanter et al., 2008). Similarly, a depression may be classified as being *endogenous* in nature or a *primary depression*, which is alleged to be caused by biochemical imbalances of various neurotransmitters in the brain. When considered in combination, these two major types of depression noted may be incapacitating enough to be further classified as a *major depression*. When one also considers the depth and duration of an underlying major depression, it may be in contrast to another clinical condition characterized by chronic periods of "feeling blue" that is clinically defined as *dysthymia*.

As one can see from these examples above, the clinical classification of depression remains a challenge. Nonetheless, there are common signs and symptoms which often manifest and can be easily recognized by the general population at large. It is important to note that depression takes on different forms for each individual and any of the following indicators highlighted in Table 11.6 may be indicators of depression. For example, although some individuals may experience poor appetite, others may experience weight gain due to a stimulated appetite.

Table 11.6   Common Signs and Symptoms of Depression

Signs and Symptoms
• Persistent feelings of sadness or melancholy
• Sleep disturbances and insomnia
• Changes to energy levels and libido
• Restlessness, or alternatively, fatigue
• Problems concentrating, remembering, and/or making decisions
• Changes to appetite and/or eating disorders
• Marked and sudden weight loss or gain
• Persistent physical symptoms of pain or discomfort that do not respond to treatment or pain medications
• Thoughts of suicide and death

Depression affects all ethnic groups in Canada, although not equally. For example, only 3.1% of Inuit have experienced a major depressive episode, compared to 16% of First Nations people (Insel et al., 2016). According to Statistics Canada's (2012) Canadian Community Health Survey (CCHS) on Mental Health, 5.4% of the Canadian population aged 15 years and over reported symptoms that met the criteria for a mood disorder in the previous 12 months, including 4.7% for major depression and 1.5% for bipolar disorder (Findlay, 2017). Furthermore, almost one in 8 adults (12.6%) identified symptoms that met the criteria for a mood disorder at some point during their lifetime, including 11.3% for depression and 2.6% for bipolar disorder. It is notable that 15- to 24-year olds had the highest rates of mood and anxiety disorders of all age groups. About 7% of them were identified as having had depression in the past 12 months, compared with 5% of people aged 25 to 64 years and 2% of those aged 65 or older (Findlay, 2017).

Depression is a major risk factor for suicide across the lifespan, and programs that seek to increase public awareness and recognition of this disorder are critical. For example, *Partners for Life* is a depression awareness program which targets youth in Québec secondary schools by the Mental Illness Foundation (MHCC, 2012). This program employs classroom-based sessions that are interactive in nature to help students recognize the signs and symptoms of depression, substance abuse, and suicidal thoughts and behaviours. In addition, the program provides valuable knowledge about what they can do to get help for themselves or a friend in need. The Partners for Life program has reached over 750,000 secondary school students in Québec (approximately 60%); 8000 parents and guardians, and 22,000 care providers (MHCC, 2012). This school-based program has helped to raise awareness of depression as a risk factor for suicide, and has empowered and aided many youth to be referred and treated for depression.

Bipolar Disorder

Bipolar disorder, which was previously known as manic depressive illness, is characterized by altering and unusual periods or cycles of depression and elevated mood that can last for days, weeks, or even months in duration (APA, 2013). It is notable that almost nine out of 10 Canadians who reported symptoms that met the 12-month criteria for bipolar disorder (86. 9%) reported that the condition interfered with their lives. The elevated mood component is known as *mania* or *hypomania*, depending on its severity, and/or whether or not symptoms of psychosis are present. Statistics Canada (2009) reports that approximately 1% of Canadians aged

15 years and over reported symptoms that met the criteria for a bipolar disorder in the previous 12 months. Moreover, approximately one in 50 adults aged 25 to 44 years or 45 to 64 years reported symptoms consistent with bipolar disorder at some point in their lifetime (Statistics Canada, 2009).

Seasonal Affective Disorder

Seasonal affective disorder (SAD) is a type of depression which affects approximately 2% to 6% of Canadians, especially during the fall and winter months; and is characterized by irritability, apathy, carbohydrate cravings, weight gain, sleep disturbances of prolonged duration, apathy, fatigue, and general feelings of sadness (Greaves, 2016; Mood Disorders Association of Canada, n.d.). Women are up to eight times as likely as men to report having SAD, and individuals residing in more northern communities in Canada are at increased risk attributed in part to decreases in total exposure to natural sunlight which disrupt natural circadian rhythms (our natural biological clock), depletion of vitamin D and tryptophan (natural precursor of serotonin) levels (Centre for Addictions & Mental Health [CAMH], 2012; Kwong, 2015; Mood Disorders Association of Canada, n.d.). Non-pharmaceutical treatments include light therapy (a.k.a., phototherapy) which has been found to have an anti-depressant effect in over 70% of people with SAD treated within two weeks. Light therapy is delivered through special full-spectrum lights or through a light visor. Daily treatment sessions usually last between 15 and 30 min.

Suicide: A Canadian Context

What separates the potentially suicidal individual from the non-suicidal one is the extent and degree of depression and despair the person feels, their coping mechanisms, social support network, and awareness of the presenting signs and symptoms. A large number of individuals with thoughts of committing suicide have depressive orders and/or other mental health disorders. There are a number of warning signs and symptoms that the general public at large should be aware of and brought to the immediate attention of authorities (e.g., teacher, parent, guidance worker) and/or healthcare professionals, and include

- Individuals who openly talk about wanting to die and/or the revealing of contemplated methods
- Sudden social withdrawal and isolation of self
- A sudden and inexplicable lightening of mood, which may indicate that the person has decided on the means and date to commit suicide
- Changes in sleep patterns, appetite, concentration, increased agitation, feeling of self-reproach and guilt
- A history of previous unsuccessful attempts
- A history of substance abuse, depression, and/or other mental health issues
- A suicide by a family member or friend
- A person who is giving away or donating their prized personal possessions
- A person who has experienced an extreme loss (e.g., family member or loved one)
- A person who is being bullied and/or is experiencing extreme humiliation or public ridicule

Suicide is a preventable cause of death, but rates in Canada remain unacceptably high. An examination of suicide rates over time in relation to demographic, social, and clinical factors can help identify which youth and adults are at higher risk. The MHCC (2015) reported that 6.6% of Canadian college and university students in 2013 reported having intentionally cut, burned, bruised, or otherwise injured themselves over the past 12 months. The ACHA NCHA II (2016) reports that only 39.7% of college and university students have received information about suicide prevention on their respected campuses; 70.8% reported that they have never seriously considered suicide, and 9.1% have not seriously considered suicide in the past 12 months.

The MCHH (2015) reports that 6.4% of Canadian youth aged 15 to 19 years reported having "seriously thought about suicide" or "taking their own life" in the last 12 months, which appears to be consistent with statistics over the past decade. The actual rate of suicide was nine per 100,000 Canadians aged 15 to 19 years in 2011 (MHCC, 2015). Youth who disclose thoughts of suicide are regarded as being at a higher risk for suicidal behaviours. While the majority of youth with these thoughts will not make an attempt to end their life, serious consideration of suicide is associated with emotional distress and more severe forms of depression, warranting immediate attention by a health professional.

The MHCC (2015) noted that 3.5% of adults reported having serious suicidal thoughts over the past 12 months, and the actual rate for suicide per 100,000 Canadians aged 20 to 64 years was 13.8%. The highest rates were observed among males aged 45 to 49 and 50 to 54 (26.6 per 100,000 and 25.7 per 100,000, respectively) (MHCC, 2015). Overall rates have declined only slightly since the year 2000 (15.6 per 100,000) with some year-to-year variability over the last decade.

The rate of suicide in older adults aged 55 years and older, which is 10.4 per 100,000 has been very stable over the past decade. Rates are considerably higher for males in comparison to their female counterparts, with men over 85 years having the highest suicide rate (29 per 100,000) (MHCC, 2015). Several factors may contribute to this noted increased risk of depression and suicide with ageing. These include potential deterioration in health, loss of independence, income reduction, loss of significant others (e.g., spouse) and social isolation. In addition, there is some evidence to suggest that suicide rates tend to increase during major holidays and celebrations (e.g., New Years, Christmas) when the individual is isolated and alone.

Suicide rates in the territories differ dramatically from rates for the rest of Canada. The rate of 30.9 suicide deaths per 100,000 is nearly three times that for the general population (10.8) (MHCC, 2015). People in Northern and rural communities tend to have poorer overall health and lower life expectancy than people in more densely populated and serviced urban centres (Kirby & Keon, 2006; Ryan-Nichollis & Haggarty, 2007). In fact, higher mortality rates are evident for all causes including suicide.

Indigenous people have a suicide rate that is approximately twice the national average, and shows little change since 1979. It is notable that the suicide rate for Inuit is among the highest in the world, which is also 11 times the national average (Health Canada, First Nations and Inuit Health, 2015). For example, Bell (2013) reports that 120 suicides occurred in Nunavut between the years 2003 and 2006, and that depression and borderline personality disorders were major associated factors. Risk factors for Indigenous people include historical oppression, the legacy of colonization by Europeans, overcrowding, poverty, chronic unemployment, community demoralization, and the lack of culturally appropriate mental health services and professionals in the region (Bell, 2013; Chacahamovich & Tomlinson, 2013). Suicide prevention efforts targeting Indigenous people need to be better coordinated, culturally appropriate and holistic in nature (Health Canada, First Nations and Inuit Health, 2015). Canada is currently leading an international study to address ways to prevent suicide in eight countries with Indigenous people living in the Artic regions of the world (Weber, 2014). The reader is referred to Chapter 4 for a detailed discussion of health issues and challenges faced by Indigenous people in Canada.

Schizophrenia

Schizophrenia is defined as a mental disorder characterized by abnormal social behaviour(s), marked disturbances in thinking and cognition, and perceptions of reality. The clinical definition and criteria for making a diagnosis of schizophrenia has changed and evolved through the six editions of the *DSM* to date (Grohol, 2014; Tandon et al., 2013). Most notable is the removal of different subtypes of schizophrenia (e.g., paranoid, disorganized, catatonic, undifferentiated, residual) from the *DSM-5* because of their apparent "limited diagnostic stability, low reliability, and poor validity" (APA, 2013; Grohol, 2014). Instead, schizophrenia is now clinically viewed as a single mental disorder with an array of different presenting symptoms.

The five characteristic symptoms for the diagnosis of schizophrenia with the requirement that at least two of the following five symptoms be present for a month is retained in the current *DSM-5* (APA, 2013; Grohol, 2014; Tandon et al., 2013): (i) Delusions; (ii) hallucinations; (iii) disorganized speech; (iv) grossly disorganized or catatonic; and (v) negative symptoms (i.e., diminished emotional expression or avolition).

Positive symptoms include delusions, thought withdrawal, erratic behaviours, and paranoia. Irrational thought patterns are also common. Positive symptoms make it difficult for clients to connect with reality. Indeed, clients often report feeling overwhelmed, hearing voices and seeing and/or feeling things that do not exist. *Negative symptoms* tend to be long-lasting and persistent in nature and include alogia (difficulty in speaking), absence of motivation, flattened mood, volition, and motivation (apathy), lack of pleasure in life, social isolation, and/or withdrawal, decreased level of functioning, and poor social interactions with others. Of the four symptom domains highlighted above, negative symptoms appear to have the greatest impact on individual functioning and recovery, and hence our society and economy, and several of the current medications developed to mitigate negative symptoms have fallen short (Kirkpatrick, Fenton, Carpenter, & Marder, 2016; Public Policy Forum, 2013).

The prevalence rate of schizophrenia in Canada is approximately 1.5%, and we are only one of five countries with a lifetime prevalence greater than 1% based on a 2015 systematic review of published estimates from 65 countries between the years 1990 and 2013 (Simeone, Ward, Rotella, Collins, & Windisch, 2015). There are approximately 26 new cases per 100,000 individuals diagnosed with schizophrenia in Canada, which is more than twice the global incidence rate of approximately 12 cases per 100,000 individuals (Dealberto, 2013; Public Policy Forum, 2013).

The Canadian Institute of Health Research (Canadian Institute for Health Information CIHI, 2015) reports that youth aged 15 to 17 years with a diagnosis of schizophrenia had increased rates of emergency room visits (up by 53%) and inpatient rates (up by 74%) since 2006 to 2007. In fact, one in 12 acute care hospital beds in Canada is reported to be taken-up by a client with schizophrenia, which represents 1.7% of Canada's national health expenditure and a cost of over $2 billion to our economy each year (Ledwell, McLean, & Griller, 2013). Moreover, it is critical to note that 72% of primary caregivers of individuals with schizophrenia are typically family members, and 15% of these caregivers spend on average 12.5 work days/ year looking after the loved one in need (Awad & Varuganti, 2016). Suicide remains a major cause of death amongst clients diagnosed with schizophrenia, although the death rates have been decreasing from 102 total in 2008 to 79 total in 2013 (Statistics Canada, 2013).

In Canada, upward of 96% of individuals who have been diagnosed with schizophrenia reported that they have been victims of discrimination (Public Policy Forum, 2013).

Stigma is one of the most prominent social challenges affecting people with schizophrenia. For decades, patients have been portrayed in film and television as unstable, dangerous and unable to participate in society. Pejorative terms, stereotypes and other discriminatory behaviour are also common despite campaigns to bring greater global awareness to mental health issues. (Public Policy Forum, 2013, p. 8).

Hence, one may argue that from a public health practice and policy standpoint, the case for developing multi-stakeholder frameworks to address the health, social, and economic effects of schizophrenia is needed. For example, in Ontario, the provincial government embraced early intervention programs in 1999 when it partnered with the Ontario Working Group on Early Intervention in Psychosis. Clients and families received enhanced assistance through coordination of counselling, information-sharing and support networks with documented positive outcomes (Public Policy Forum, 2013).

Major Eating Disorders

Eating disorders are characterized by severe disturbances in perceptions of one's body shape, negative body image, unhealthy eating patterns and behaviours, and unhealthy efforts to control one's body weight and/or fat. These altered perceptions of weight and body image results in dysfunctional attitudes toward eating, preoccupation with food, restrictive dieting, and weight control measures. The three main eating disorders that we will examine in this section are anorexia nervosa, bulimia nervosa, and binge eating. It is critical to note that obesity is neither a mental health illness nor an eating disorder per se. The National Eating Disorder Information

Centre (NEDIC) is a non-profit organization providing critical information and resources on eating disorders and weight preoccupation for Canadians (see www.nedic.ca). The reader is referred to Chapter 14 for a detailed discussion on the origins of obesity and the implications for public health in Canada and globally.

At any given time in Canada, as many as 600,000 to 990,000 Canadians may meet the diagnostic criteria for an eating disorder, and approximately 80% of these are females (LeBlanc, 2014; McVey, 2014). In general, these disorders often begin during early adolescent, although cases may occur at any age and affect women and girls 10 times more frequently than men and boys (Smink, Hocken, & Hock, 2012; Statistics Canada, 2015d; Surgenor & Maguire, 2013). Although eating disorders span all social classes and ethnic groups, they tend to be predominately present in industrialized, affluent, and developed nations such as Canada.

Individuals with an eating disorder often have a perfectionistic attitude toward school or work, low self-esteem, and a distorted body image of themselves (Donatelle et al., 2008; Insel et al., 2016; Smink, Hocken, & Hock, 2012). Female athletes (e.g., gymnasts, swimmers) and dancers (e.g., ballet) that are constantly under pressure to be highly fit and thin are especially vulnerable. Moreover, individuals with other emotional or psychological disorders, particularly substance abuse, personality disorders, or affective disorders (depression), are at higher risk of developing an eating disorder (Statistics Canada, 2015d; Surgenor & Maguire, 2013). It is notable that anorexia nervosa has the highest overall mortality rate of any mental illness in Canada, which is estimated to be between 10% and 15% of individuals with the illness; and the mortality rate for individuals with bulimia nervosa is about 5% (LeBlanc, 2014; McVey, 2014). Combined, these two disorders alone kill an estimated 1000 to 1500 Canadians annually, and this number is likely higher as death certificates often fail to record eating disorders as the cause of death.

Anorexia Nervosa

Anorexia nervosa is a mental health disorder characterized by a refusal to maintain a body weight at a minimal health level; a distorted view of one's body shape or weight; intense pathological fear of getting fat or gaining weight; unnecessary influence on self-evaluation; denial of the seriousness of their low body weight, and amenorrhea in female clients of childbearing age (for at least three consecutive mental cycles) (APA, 2013; LeBlanc, 2014; MHCC, 2015). Clients with this eating disorder view weight loss and control as an impressive achievement and a sign of extraordinary self-control and discipline. Conversely, any weight gain is perceived as an unacceptable failure of self-control and discipline. Self-imposed starvation often results in damage to the bones, muscles, and vital organs (e.g., kidneys, liver, heart), and also affects various body systems including the digestive, nervous, and immune systems. Individuals often lose hair or develop excessively fine facial and body hair due to associated malnutrition. In comparison to their peers without this eating disorder, the risk of premature death is approximately 10-fold greater in a person with anorexia nervosa (Smink, Hocken, & Hock, 2012; Surgenor & Marguire, 2013).

There are currently two clinically recognized subtypes of anorexia nervosa: (i) Restricting type and (ii) binge-eating or purging type (APA, 2013). The **restricting type of anorexia nervosa** is the most common form whereby an individual severely restricts their food intake via dieting and/or fasting (APA, 2013; Eating Disorders Victoria, 2017; Statistics Canada, 2015d).

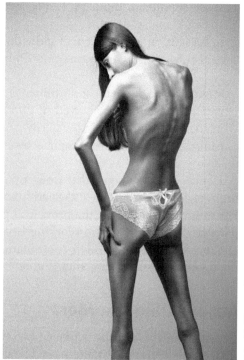

© Den Rise/Shutterstock.com.

Photo 11.12 Female Client with Anorexia Nervosa. The diagnosis of anorexia nervosa occurs when clients weigh less than 85% of their normal weight.

Restriction may take many forms (e.g., maintaining very low calorie count; restricting types of food eaten; eating only one meal a day), and may follow obsessive and rigid rules (e.g., only eating food of one specific colour, raw foods). Individuals with restricting type of anorexia nervosa do not regularly engage in binge-eating or purging behaviours (e.g., self-induced vomiting or misuse of laxatives, diuretics, or enemas). **Binge-eating/purging type of anorexia nervosa** is less recognized and common in nature where an individual restricts their caloric intake of food items, but also regularly engage in binge-eating and/or purging behaviours (at least weekly) (APA, 2013; Eating Disorders Victoria, 2017; Statistics Canada, 2015d). **Purging behaviours** include self-induced vomiting, misuse of laxatives or diet pills, diuretics and/or enemas, and excessive amounts of exercise to combat weight gain.

Bulimia Nervosa

Bulimia nervosa is a mental disorder characterized by recurrent episodes of binge eating followed by purging (APA, 2013; Statistics Canada, 2015d). Although bulimia nervosa typically presents during adolescence or young adulthood, it has begun to emerge as early as 11 and 12 years of age, and also in adults aged 40 to 60 years. Approximately 90% of clients diagnosed with bulimia nervosa are females. Binge eating consists of eating large amount of food in a short period of time and typically occurs in secret during periods of increased stress. It is difficult for the client to control or stop the binging episode once it has started (Donatelle et al., 2008; Insel et al., 2016). For example, clients may gorge themselves with up to 10,000 calories in a single session. Clients with bulimia nervosa may maintain or present within normal weight categories for their height and weight, although fluctuation of 5 to 10 kg is not uncommon.

Binge-Eating Disorder

Binge-Eating Disorder (BED) is characterized by uncontrollable binge-eating sessions, usually followed by feelings of guilt and shame and associated weight gain (APA, 2013). BED is also known by the popular term "compulsive eating," and approximately 2% of Canadians are estimated to suffer from this disorder. Unlike bulimia nervosa, clients with BED do not engage in measures to rid themselves of the excess calories consumed during the binge sessions (i.e., no purging rituals or excessive exercise) or report abnormal attitudes toward dieting or body image (Donatelle et al., 2008; Insel et al., 2016).

Public Health Challenges Related to Eating Disorders

The current obstacles to address eating disorders from a public health perceptive among Canadians are numerous. They include entrenched stereotypes and stigma associated with eating disorders; a general lack of public awareness; a need for greater community-based supports; bias in the healthcare field against clients with these disorders; financial constraints; the challenges of concurrent disorders, and the lack of community-based research examining the extent of these disorders; and/or the effectiveness of public health interventions (Austin, 2011; Gauvin & Steiger, 2012; LeBlanc, 2014; McVey, 2014). Although the exact causes or aetiology for developing a specific eating disorder remains unknown, a variety of factors are likely involved. These factors include a family history, presence of a recent traumatic event or loss (e.g., death of a loved one), and the presence of other mental health issues or disorders (e.g., depression) (Statistics Canada, 2015d; Surgenor & Maguire, 2013).

Societal mindsets and convictions, and the mass and social media tend to portray the message that individuals who are thin are successful, popular, attractive, and more "healthy" than individuals who are overweight. Thin models, actresses, and celebrities appear to be a common standard in the mass and social media who are ever-present on television, and in magazines, movies, and Internet sites. Advertisements targeting young women often feature thin models portrayed in desirable circumstances and/or locations in order to sell cosmetics, clothing, accessories, and other products. These portrayals may, in part, collectively contribute to a creation of a distorted body image.

Reversing the rising tide of eating disorders needs to be a public health priority (Austin, 2011; Gauvin & Steiger, 2012; LeBlanc, 2014; McVey, 2014). These include disorders characterized by the pathological pursuit of thinness (e.g., anorexia nervosa and bulimia nervosa). A growing body of research shows that greater exposure to images in the mass and social media which promote excessively thin body ideals can elicit maladaptive weight-control practices and disordered eating behaviours, especially when viewers are female adolescents (e.g., Durkin, Paxton & Sorbello, 2007; Hogan & Strasburger, 2008; van den Berg et al., 2007; van Vonderer & Kinnally, 2012). Such images are markedly prevalent in Western cultures and industrialized and developed nations such as Canada.

In the province of Québec, the Ministry of Culture, Communications, and the Status of Women spearheaded an initiative in 2009 to create a health promotion tool to challenge the "thin-is-in" message propagated by the fashion industry via mass and social medias (Bondareff, 2009; Meney, 2015). The *Québec Charter for a Healthy and Diverse Body Image* (a.k.a. "La Chic" for short) outlines consensual actions and principles that can be undertaken by organizations and citizens to reduce media pressures and influences, which predominately display thin females. The development of this Charter was based on a collaborative, educational, and a non-coercive inducement toward voluntary engagement on the part of actors in the fashion and media industries and in the health, social services, and education networks.

Six months after the Charter's launch, Gauvin and Steiger (2012) surveyed 1003 Québec residents aged 18 years or older about their knowledge of the Charter (La Chic), their willingness to adhere to it, and their perceptions of its potential in overcoming the unhealthy pursuit of thinness. The study showed that approximately one-third of respondents recognized La Chic health promotion program, and approximately two-thirds expressed a willingness to personally adhere to the Charter. The researchers concluded that public health promotion campaigns such as La Chi have a great potential to make individuals aware of the negative consequences of disordered eating and excessive thinness. Moreover, this study provides preliminary evidence to demonstrate that such public health initiatives aimed at encouraging healthy and diverse body images in the mass and social media, created through consensus building and disseminated through accessible media events can reach a key segment of the adult population (Gauvin & Steiger, 2012).

Future Directions and Challenges

Canada urgently requires a multifaceted public health approach to address mental health issues and concerns facing Canadians across the lifespan and high risk groups including indigenous people, homeless individuals, immigrants, inmates in correctional facilities, and individuals residing in rural and remote areas. This approach should include assessment, treatment, universal health promotion, mental health triage, and access to mental healthcare facilities and healthcare professionals and workers in both urban and rural and remote areas across Canada.

For instance, there are a number of inmates in correctional facilities in Canada that have mental health issues and/or serious addictions (Canadian Medical Association, 2013; Government of Canada, 2014). We argue that this often overcrowded environment is simply not conducive to meet the healthcare needs of inmates with mental illness who are often dealt with via solitary confinement, being pepper sprayed or other means of force and punishment. There are over 40,000 inmates in Federal and Provincial prisons in Canada, and 13% of male and 29% of female offenders are identified on admission as presenting with a mental health issue or disorder (Government of Canada, 2014), For example, the 2007 death of Ashley Smith who committed suicide in solitary confinement in prison while being watched by prison guards highlights the failure of both the healthcare and correctional systems in Canada to effectively recognize and help individuals with mental health challenges (Bromwich, 2015; Canadian Broadcasting Corporation, 2013). In December 2013, an all-woman inquest jury shocked Canadians by rendering a bold verdict of homicide in the inquest to determine Smith's cause of death. This was the first time a death in custody had been found to be the fault of someone other than an inmate. The jury made 104 recommendations to improve conditions in Canadian correctional facilities; however, conditions remain abhorrent to date (Bromwich, 2015).

The Canadian Institutes of Health Research (CIHR) has responded in part by identifying mental health issues and services as one of its research priorities. Nonetheless, preventative programs remain both a low research and health policy priority in Canada. Furthermore, if professional healthcare training schools (e.g., medicine, nursing) in Canada continue to emphasize the recognition of predominately physical health signs and symptoms, there is a danger that actual or potential mental health issues or disorders may not be revealed.

Based on recommendations outlined in the Kirby Commission Report (Kirby, 2008; Kirby & Keon, 2006), the federal government established the MHCC in 2007 to help facilitate a national approach to mental health issues in Canada with a mandate to reform mental health policies and improve healthcare services, decrease the stigma and associated discrimination associated with mental illness, and disseminate evidence-informed research to all levels of government, community stakeholders and the general public at large. In 2012, a national mental health strategy for Canada was developed in an attempt to both improve mental health outcomes and to address inadequacies within the current mental health systems (MHCC, 2012). For example, some clients with depression tend not to seek treatment or support from a healthcare professional, and believe that the most effective strategy is to "self-manage" their depression on their own (Griffiths, Crisp, Jorm, & Christensen, 2011).

Sixty percent of people with a mental health problem or illness won't seek help for fear of being labelled and one in seven (15.4%) Canadians aged 15 years or older reported feelings of being discriminated in the past five years (MHCC, 2017b). This perception has been linked to feelings of increased vulnerability and poor physical and mental health outcomes in general (MHCC, 2015). Perceived discrimination increases the likelihood of both physical and mental health problems. Research evidence suggests that the experience of unfair treatment, rather than the reason for discrimination, is responsible for psychological distress. The occurrence of perceived discrimination across individuals with diverse sociodemographic characteristics suggests that it represents an important vulnerability factor in population health. Higher rates of discrimination are evident among people with mental health conditions than among those without such difficulties. Indeed, nearly 40% of people affected by mental health conditions reported some form of discrimination or unfair treatment, while only 14.2% of those without mental health problems reported this experience (MHCC, 2015).

Opening Minds is the largest systematic effort in Canadian history to date to focus on reducing stigma related to mental illness (MHCC, 2017b). Established by the MHCC in 2009, it seeks to change Canadians' behaviours and attitudes toward people living with mental illness to ensure they are treated fairly and as full citizens with opportunities to contribute to society like anyone else. Opening Minds is addressing stigma within four main target groups: healthcare providers, youth, the workforce, and the media. As such, the initiative has multiple goals, ranging from improving healthcare providers' understanding of the needs of people with mental health problems, to encouraging youth to talk openly and positively about mental illness. Ultimately, the goal of Opening Minds is to cultivate an environment in which those living with mental illness feel comfortable seeking help, treatment, and support on their journey toward recovery.

According to the MHCC (2015), 26.3% of Canadians aged 15 years or older with mental disorders self-reported that during specific times they were in need of mental healthcare services, but did not receive the sought after care required. Receipt of mental healthcare in their respected communities when needed is critical to support improvement and recovery and to prevent worsening of mental health conditions that could lead to increased disability or to other harms. Moreover, 22.6% of Canadians were hospitalized for a mental illness for more than 30 consecutive days in 2012/2013, and 11.5% of these were readmitted within 30 days. Often readmission for clients previously hospitalized for a mental illness indicates relapse or complications. However rapid readmission may reflect lack of stabilization during the previous hospitalization, poor discharge planning, or inadequate community support. Multiple hospital admissions in the same year may be warranted in people with serious mental health disorders, but may also reflect poor discharge planning or shortcomings in community care supports available.

The MHCC (2015) reports that there are over 4 million family caregivers in Canada. Among these, 7.6% (or 322,556 individuals) provide care to a family member with a mental illness or disorder. This large population of caregivers should be monitored and supported. The extent of family caregiving to support individuals with mental illness reflects the degree of disability associated with mental illness and their impact on families. Caregivers may experience enduring stress associated with caregiving responsibilities themselves. This stress has been linked to poor outcomes such as depression. Very high levels of stress are reported by 16.5% of the population in family caregiving roles (MHCC, 2015). Canada's ageing population means higher projected numbers of people with dementia and other chronic illnesses. This may result in an increase in the number of family caregivers and consequently, a rise in those subject to excessive stress.

Accreditation of both hospital- and community-based mental health services is in its early stages in Canada. Accreditation Canada has developed accreditation standards for mental health programs in both the hospital and, since 2011, community-based settings (MHCC, 2015). The most recent standards put greater emphasis on the recovery aspects of mental healthcare. An increase in mental health program accreditation would suggest increasing availability of recovery-based services for people with mental disorders. Only 250 Canadian programs have reported meeting the current standards for mental health programs developed by Accreditation Canada as of 2013 (MHCC, 2015).

Group Review Exercise Box 11.1 "The DSM: Psychiatric's deadliest scam"

Overview of this Investigative Documentary
The *Diagnostic and Statistical Manual of Mental Disorders, Fifth Edition (DSM-5)* is the standard classification system for mental disorders employed by various mental health professionals (e.g., psychiatrics, physicians, nurses, psychologists, social workers, and counsellors) in Canada and globally. The *DSM* consists of three major components: (i) The diagnostic classification; (ii) diagnostic criteria sets; and (iii) a descriptive text. It is intended to be used in all clinical settings by clinicians of different theoretical orientations. The *DSM*-5 claims that it can also be used for research in both clinical and community-based populations, and that it is a necessary tool for collecting and communicating accurate public-health statistics.

Instructions
This assignment may be done alone, in pairs, or in groups of up to 5 people (note: if you are doing this assignment in pairs or groups, please submit only one hard or electronic copy as requested by your instructor). The assignment should be type-written and between 4 and 6 pages maximum in length (double-spaced please). View and take notes on the documentary entitled "The DSM: Psychiatric's deadliest scam." You may choose to watch the documentary on YouTube, BBC, or elsewhere on the World Wide Web (www). For examples, see: https://www.youtube.com/watch?v=mTzTgJLwSeo or http://www.cchr.org/videos/diagnostic-statistical-manual.html or https://www.youtube.com/watch?v=XEg7UNphRgQ or https://www.youtube.com/watch?v=Qn0mgisVhgM), and answer the following 5 questions below:

i. Briefly highlight the evolution and social stimuli for the development of the *DSM-1* to the current *DSM-5*. Provide a time line highlighting major changes between each new version of this manual and "growth trends" detailing the number of diagnostic disorders listed.

ii. What is the "best available scientific evidence," if any, utilized to support the current 374 disorders listed in the *DSM-5*? Provide specific examples from the video and how "psychiatry" has attempted to justify/validate itself as a legitimate medical specialty.

iii. Discuss the merits of how current diagnosis is added by the *DSM* committee to new editions or recategorized. Highlight/debate the role of "big pharma" (pharmaceutical industry) for influencing the addition of new disorders to the *DSM*.

iv. Discuss/highlight how the *DSM* has been employed as a means of "social control" mechanism for the behaviour of children. Provide specific examples from the video. As a public health professional/ worker, how would you convey this information to parents or guardians?

v. Given that over 90% of individuals who undergo screening will have a subsequent mental health disorder diagnosed, what would be the repercussions or negative effects of proposed mass population-based mental health screening programs? What would be the implications for public health in Canada in terms of sustainability of our current healthcare system, associated costs to treat and manage clients diagnosed with mental health disorders, and/or the general health and well-being of vulnerable groups (e.g., elderly, Aboriginal, new immigrants to Canada)?

Summary

- Mental health is defined as the capacity of each and all of us to feel, think, and act in ways that enhance our ability to enjoy life and deal with the challenges we face, and a positive sense of emotional and spiritual well-being that respects the importance of culture, equity, social justice, interconnections, and personal dignity.
- The WHO concept of mental health embraces promotion of mental well-being, the prevention and treatment, as well as rehabilitation of individuals affected with mental illness and disorders.
- MHCC (2013) reports that approximately 6.7 million people in Canada are living with a mental health condition or illness today.
- MHFA Canada program seeks to address the issue of stigma associated with mental health illness and disorders through the development of mental health literacy and by equipping individuals with the necessary knowledge and skill sets to address and respond to mental health issues themselves, for a family member, friend, colleague, or individual in their community.
- Throughout history there have been three general theories related to the aetiology of mental illness and disorders: (i) Supernatural; (ii) psychogenic; and (iii) somatogenic.
- Supernatural theories of mental illness and disorders attribute these conditions to possession and/or punishment by evil or demonic spirits, displeasure of gods or deities, solar or lunar eclipses, comets, curses, and sin.
- Psychogenic theories of mental illness or disorders focus on traumatic or stressful experiences, maladaptive learned associations and cognitions, or distorted perceptions.
- Somatogenic theories of mental illness or disorders identify disturbances in physical functioning resulting from either illness, genetic inheritance, brain damage, or chemical or force of nature imbalance.
- Stress is defined as a unique and subjective perception or reaction to a specific current existing or imminent situation or condition that results in emotional and physiological responses resulting from various demands, expectations and/or unpredictable circumstances experienced in our daily lives.
- Allostatic load is defined as the "wear and tear on the body" which accumulates as a function of time due to chronic or repeated episodes of stress that result in fluctuating or heightened neural or neuroendocrine responses.
- Allostasis is defined as the process by which the body responds to stressors in order to regain stability or homeostasis.
- Fight-flight-freeze response describes how an individual ultimately reacts to a threat stressor.
- Coping is defined as an individual's cognitive and/or behavioural attempts and resources to manage specific physiological or emotional/psychological stressors they are confronted with.

- Mental illnesses are defined as alterations in thinking, mood, or behaviour—or some combination thereof—associated with significant distress and impaired functioning.
- Schizophrenia is defined as a mental disorder characterized by abnormal social behaviour(s), marked disturbances in thinking and cognition, and perceptions of reality.
- Anxiety disorders include generalized anxiety disorder (GAD), obsessive compulsive disorder (OCD), post-traumatic stress disorder (PTSD), panic disorders and social phobias.
- A mood disorder is defined as an emotional disturbance that is intense and persistent enough in nature to affect normal daily functions and routines.
- Depression is a common type of mood disorder characterized by the loss of interest, feelings of sadness, melancholy, dejection, worthlessness, emptiness, hopelessness, changes to libido, appetite, sleep disturbances and other physical symptoms that are inappropriate and out of proportion to reality.
- Bipolar disorder is characterized by altering and unusual periods or cycles of depression and elevated mood that can last for days, weeks, or even months in duration.
- Eating disorders are characterized by severe disturbances in perceptions of one's body shape, negative body image, unhealthy eating patterns and behaviours, and unhealthy efforts to control one's body weight and/or fat.
- Canada urgently requires a multifaceted public health approach to address mental health issues and concerns facing Canadians across the lifespan and high risk groups including indigenous people, homeless individuals, immigrants, inmates in correctional facilities, and individuals residing in rural and remote areas.

Critical Thinking Questions

1. Depression is the single most frequently occurring mental health condition in the general population in Canada. Depressive signs and symptoms are often missed or incorrectly attributed to organic disorders in older Canadians aged 65 years and older. As a public healthcare professional or worker, how would you assess for the presence of depression?
2. What community-based resources are currently present in your region to assist older adults with a clinical diagnosis of depression? What are the noted gaps related to access to care for these vulnerable or at-risk older adults in your community?

References

Alkadhi, K. (2013). Brain physiology and pathophysiology in mental stress. *ISRN Physiology*, 2013. Article ID 806104. Retrieved from http://dx.doi.org/co.1155/2013/806014

American College Health Association National College Health Assessment II (ACHA NCHA II): Canadian Reference Group (2016, Spring). *Data report*. Author. Retrieved from http://www.acha-ncha.org/docs/NCHA-II%20SPRING%20 2016%20CANADIAN%20REFERENCE%20GROUP%20DATA%20REPORT.pdf

American Psychological Association. (2005). *Let's talk facts about depression*. Washington, DC. Author. Retrieved from http://www.fcphp.usf.edu/courses/content/rfast/Resources/depression.pdf

American Psychological Association. (2013, May). *Diagnostic and statistical manual of psychological disorders* (5th ed.). Washington, DC: Author. Retrieved from https://www.psychiatry.org/psychiatrists/practice/dsm

Anbacher, H. L., & Anbacher, R. R. (1959). *Individual psychology of Alfred Adler*. Oxford, England: Basic Books, Inc.

Andreassi, J. L. (1998). Psychophysiological interpretations of Yerkes-Dodson. *International Journal of Psychophysiology, 30*, 9–10.

Austin, S. B. (2011). The blind spot in the drive for childhood obesity prevention: Bringing eating disorders prevention into focus as a public health priority. *American Journal of Public Health, 101*(6), e1–e4. doi:10.2105/AJPH.2011.300182. Retrieved from http://ajph.aphapublications.org/doi/10.2105/AJPH.2011.300182

Awad, A., & Varuganti, L. (2016). *Quality of life and health costs: The feasibility of cost-utility analysis in schizophrenia. Beyond assessment of quality of life in schizophrenia.* Springer Link: 175–183. Retrieved from https://link.springer.com/chapter/10.1007/978-3-319-30061-0_12?no-access=true

Bocke, E. M., Seidle, A., Latza, U., Rossnagel, K., & Schumann, B. (2012). The role of psychosocial stress at work for the development of cardiovascular diseases: A systematic review. *International Archives of Occupational and Environmental Health, 85,* 67–79.

Baldin, E., Hauser, W. A., Pack, A., & Hesdorffer, D. C. (2017, April 18). Stress is associated with an increased risk of recurrent seizures in adults. *Epilepsia, 58*(6), 1037–1046. doi:10:1111/epi.13741 (Epub ahead of print).

Barkto, C. (2016, May 4). *Fort McMurray wildfire update: Roughly 1600 building destroyed in 'catastrophic' fire.* Toronto, Ontario: Global News. Retrieved from http://globalnews.ca/news/2679178/fort-mcmurray-wildfire-how-many-homes-have-been-lost-in-the-fire/

Bartfay, W. J., & Bartfay, E. (1994, August). Promoting health in schools through a board game. *Western Journal of Nursing Research, 16*(4), 438–446. doi:10.1177/019394599401600408. Retrieved from https://www.ncbi.nlm.nih.gov/pubmed/7941489

Bartfay, W. J., & Bartfay, E. (2015). *Public health in Canada.* Boston, MA: Pearson Learning Solutions. ISBN: 13978-1-323-01471-4.

Basta, M., Chrousas, G. P., Vela-Bueno, A., & Vgontzos, A. N. (2007, June). Chronic insomnia and stress. *Sleep Medicine Clinics, 2*(2), 279–291. doi:10.1016/j.jsmc.2007.04.002

Bechie, T. M. (2012, September 23). A systematic review of allostatic load, health, and health Disparities. *Biological Research for Nursing,* 1–39. Retrieved from http://journals.sagepub.com/doi/full/10.1177/1099800412455688

Bell, J. (2013, June 6). Suicide in Nunavut: Child abuse, pot smoking, mental disorders the biggest factors. *Iqaluit: Nunatsiaq On-line (News).* Retrieved from http://www.nunatsiaqonline.ca/stories/article/65674suicide_in_nunavut_child_abuse_pot_smoking_mental_disorders_the_bigges/

Benson, H. (1975). *The relaxation response.* New York, NY: Avon.

Bloch, M. H., Green, C., Kichuk, S. A., Dombrowski, P. A., Wasylink, S., Billingslea, E., … Pittenger, C. (2013, August). Long-term outcomes in adults with obsessive-compulsive disorder. *Depression and Anxiety, 30*(8), 716–722. doi:10.1002/da.22103

Bondareff, D. (2009, October 16). *Québec 'charter' fights use of skinny models: Aims to promote healthier image of women.* Toronto, ON: Associated Press and CBC News. Retrieved from http://www.cbc.ca/news/canada/montreal/Québec-charter-fights-use-of-skinny-models-1.864408

Borrelli, F., & Izzo, A. A. (2009, December). Herb-drug interactions with St. John's wort (Hypericum perforatum): An update on clinical observations. *The AAPS Journal, 11*(4), 710–27. doi:10.1208/s12248-009-9146-8

Bracha, H. S. (2004). Freeze, flight, fight, fright, faint: Adaptionist perspectives on the acute stress response spectrum. *CNS Spectrums, 9,* 679–685.

Bromwich, R. (2015, October 13). Eight years after Ashley Smith's death, prison conditions remain abhorrent. *Ottawa Citizen,* Ottawa, ON: Retrieved from http://ottawacitizen.com/news/politics/bromwich-eight-years-after-smiths-death-prison-conditions-remain-abhorrent

Burton, N. (2012, June 2). A brief history of psychiatry. *Psychology Today.* Retrieved from https://www.psychologytoday.com/blog/hide-and-seek/201206/brief-history-psychiatry

Burton, N. (2015, October 30). *The meaning of madness* (2nd ed.). Oxford: Acheron Press.

Calabrese, E. J. (2008, January). Converging concepts: Adaptive response, preconditioning, and the YERKES-DODSON Law are manifestations of hormesis. *Ageing Research Reviews, 7*(1), 8–20.

Canadian Broadcasting Corporation (CBC). (2013, December 19). *Ashley's coroner's jury rules prison death a homicide.* Toronto, ON: CBC. Retrieved from http://www.cbc.ca/news/canada/new-brunswick/ashley-smith-coroner-s-jury-rules-prison-death-a-homicide-1.2469527

Canadian Broadcasting Corporation (CBC) TV. (2017, January 19). *PTSD: Beyond trauma—The healing process. The Nature of Things.* Toronto, ON: CBC. Retrieved from http://www.cbc.ca/natureofthings/features/ptsd-canada-has-the-highest-rate-and-other-surprising-things

Canadian Institute for Health Information [CIHI]. (2015). *Many more young Canadians using health services for mental disorders.* Ottawa, ON: CIHI. Retrieved from https://www.cihi.ca/en/many-more-young-canadians-using-health

Canadian Medical Association. (2013). Imprisoning the mentally ill. *Canadian Medical Association Journal, 19, 185*(3), 201–202.

Canadian Mental Health Association (CMHA). (2016a). *Fast facts about mental illness.* Toronto, ON: CMHA. Retrieved from http://www.cmha.ca/media/fast-facts-about-mental-illness/#.WSLoh-vyupo

Canadian Mental Health Association (CMHA). (2016b). *Your mental health: Stress.* Toronto, ON: CMHA. Retrieved from http://www.cmha.ca/mental_health/stress/#.WP9NE_nyupo

Canadian Mental Health Association (CMHA). (2017). *Social determinants of health.* Toronto, ON: CMHA. Retrieved from https://ontario.cmha.ca/provincial-policy/social-determinants/

Cannon, W. B. (1929). *Bodily changes in pain, hunger, fear and rage.* New York, NY: Appleton-Century-Crofts.

Caplan, E. (2001). *Mind Games: American Culture and the birth of psychotherapy.* Berkeley: University of California Press.

Centre for Addictions and Mental Health [CAMH]. (2012). *Seasonal depression, winter blues and seasonal affective disorder: CAMH expert available for interview.* Toronto, ON: CAMH. Retrieved from http://www.camh.ca/en/hospital/about_camh/newsroom/news_releases_media_advisories_and_backgrounders/current_year/Pages/Seasonal-depression,-winter-blues-and-seasonal-affective-disorder--CAMH-expert-available-for-interview-.aspx

Chacahamovich, E., & Tomlinson, M. (2013). *Nunavut suicide follow-back study: Identifying the risk factors for Inuit suicide in Nunavut. Learning from lives that have been lived.* Toronto: ON: Toronto Distress Centre. Retrieved from http://torontodistresscentre.com/sites/torontodistresscentre.com/files/Learning%20from%20lives%20that%20have%20been%20lived.pdf

Chiang, Y. M., & Chang, Y. (2012) Stress, depression, and intention to leave among nurses in different medical units: Implications for healthcare management/nursing practice. *Health Policy, 108,* 149–157.

Conversano, C., Rotondo, A., Lensi, E., Della Vista, D., Arpone, F., & Reda, M. A. (2010, May 14). Optimism and its impact on mental and physical well-being. *Clinical Practice Epidemiology & Mental Health, 6,* 25–29. doi:10.2174117 4501790.1006010025

Cosgrove, L., & Drimsky, L. (2012, March). A comparison of DSM-IV and DSM-V panel member's financial association with industry: A pernicious problem persists. *PLoS Medicine, 9*(3), 1–5.

Cowen, P. J. (2002, February). Cortisol, serotonin and depression: All stressed out? *The British Journal of Psychiatry, 180*(2), 99–100. doi:10.1192/bjp.180.2.99. Retrieved from http://bjp.rcpsych.org/content/180/2/99

Crimmins, E. M., Johnston, M., Hayward, M., & Seeman, T. (2003). Age differences in allostatic load: An index of physiological dysregulation. *Experimental Gerontology, 38*(7), 731–734.

Crompton, S. (2014). What's stressing the stressed? Main sources of stress among workers. *Statistics Canada.* Ottawa, ON: Retrieved from http://www.statcan.gc.ca/pub/11-008-x/20111002/article/11562-eng.htm

Cushman, P. (1996). *Constructing the self, constructing America: A cultural history of psychotherapy.* Boston, MA: Da Capo Press.

Davey, G. C. C. (2014, December 31). "Spirit possession" and mental health. *Psychology Today,* Retrieved from https://www.psychologytoday.com/blog/why-we-worry/201412/spirit-possession-and-mental-health

Davis, A. A., Basten, A., & Frattini, C. (2009). *A social determinant of health of migrants. International Organization for Migration (IOM) back paper.* Geneva, Switzerland: IOM. Retrieved from http://www.migrant-health-europe.org/files/Migration%20a%20Determinant%20of%20Health_Background%20Paper(1).pdf

Davis, S. (2006). *Community mental health in Canada: Policy, theory, and practice.* Vancouver, BC: UBC Press.

Deakin, J. F. (1988, April). 5-HT$_2$ receptors, depression and anxiety. *Pharmacology, Biochemistry and Behavior, 29* (4), 819–820. Retrieved from http://www.sciencedirect.com/science/article/pii/0091305788902158

Dealberto, M. J. (2013). Are the rates of schizophrenia unusually high in Canada? A comparison of Canadian and international data. *Psychiatry Research, 209*(3), 259–265. Retrieved from http://www.sciencedirect.com/science/article/pii/S0165178113000061

Denollet, J., & Conraads, V. M. (2011, August). Type D personality and vulnerability to adverse outcomes in heart disease. *Cleveland Clinic Journal of Medicine,* (Suppl. 1), S13–S19. doi:10.3949/ccjm.78.s1.02

Desbiens, J., & Fillion, L. (2007). Coping strategies, emotional outcomes and spirituality quality of life in palliative care nurses. *International Journal of Palliative Nursing, 13*(6), 291–300. doi:10.12968/ijpn.2007.13.6.23746

Desveaux, L., Harrison, S., Lee, A., Mathur, S., Goldstein, R., & Brooks, D. (2017, May). "We are all there for the same purpose": Support for an integrated community exercise program for older adults with heart failure and COPD. *Heart Lung.* Retrieved from https://www.ncbi.nlm.nih.gov/pubmed/28527832. doi:10.1016/j.hrtlng.2017.04.00

Dinan, T. G. (1994, March). Glucocorticoids and the genesis of depressive illness. A psychobiological model. *British Journal of Psychiatry, 164* (3), 365–371. Retrieved from https://www.ncbi.nlm.nih.gov/pubmed/7832833

Donahue, P. (1996). *Nursing: The finest art.* Toronto, ON: Mosby Company.

Donatelle, R. J., Munroe, A. J., Munroe, A., & Thompson, A. M. (2008). *Health the basics* (4th Canadian ed.). Toronto, ON: Pearson Benjamin Cummings.

Drevets, W. C., Frank, E., Price, J. C., Kupfer, D. J., Holt, D., & Greer P. J. (1999, November). PET imaging of serotonin 1A receptor binding in depression. *Biological Psychiatry, 46*(10):1375–1387. Retrieved from https://www.ncbi.nlm.nih.gov/pubmed/10578452

Druxbury, L., & Higgins, C. (2001). *Work-life balance in the new millennium: Where are we? Where do we need to go?* Canadian Policy Research Networks (CPRN), Discussion type paper No. W/12. Ottawa, ON: Author.

Durkin, S. J., Paxton, S. J., & Sorbello, M. (2007). An integrative model of the impact of exposure to idealized female images on adolescent girls' body satisfaction. *Journal of Applied Social Psychology, 37*(5):1092–1117.

Eating Disorders Victoria. (2017). *What is anorexia nervosa?* Victoria, BC: Author. Retrieved from https://www.eatingdisorders.org.au/eating-disorders/anorexia-nervosa

Faria, M. A. Jr. (2013, April 5). Violence, mental illness, and the brain. A brief history of psychosurgery. Part 1-From trephination to lobotomy. *Surgical Neurology, 4*(49). doi:10.4103/2152-7806.110146. Retrieved from https://www.ncbi.nlm.nih.gov/pmc/articles/PMC3640229/

Fergusson, D., Doucette, S., Glass, K. C., Shapiro, S., Healy, D., Hebert, P., & Hutton, B. (2005). Association between suicide attempts and selective serotonin reuptake inhibitors: Systematic review of randomized controlled trials. *British Medical Journal, 330*(7488), 396 10.1136/bmj.330.7488.396

Findlay, L. (2017, January 18). *Health reports: Depression and suicide ideation among Canadian aged 15-24.* Ottawa, ON: Statistics Canada. Cat. No. 82-003. Retrieved from http://www.statcan.gc.ca/pub/82-003-x/2017001/article/14697-eng.htm

Fisher, S. H. (1963, January 1). Psychological factors and heart disease. *Circulation, XXVII,* 113–117. doi:10.1161/01.CIR.27.1.113

Friedman, M., & Rosenman, R. (1959). Association of a specific overt behavior pattern with increases in blood cholesterol, blood clotting time, incidence of arcus senilis and clinical coronary artery disease. *JAMA, 169,* 1286–1296.

Fuller-Thomson, E., Noack, A. M., & George, U. (2011). Health decline among recent immigrants to Canada: Findings from a national-representative longitudinal survey. *Canadian Journal of Public Health, 102,* 237–280. Retrieved from http://journal.cpha.ca/index.php/cjph/article/view/2423

Gauvin, L., & Steiger, H. (2012, August). Overcoming the unhealthy pursuit of thinness: Reaction to the Québec Charter for A Healthy and Diverse Body Image. *American Journal of Public Health, 102*(8). doi:10.2105/AJPH.2011.300479. Retrieved from https://www.ncbi.nlm.nih.gov/pmc/articles/PMC3464821/

George, U., Thomson, M. S., Chaze, F., & Guruge, S. (2015). Immigrant mental health, a public health issue: Looking back and moving forward. *International Journal of Environmental Research and Public Health, 12,* 13624–13648. doi:10.3390/ijerph121013624

Goldbloom, D., & Bradley, L. (2012). The Mental Health Commission of Canada: The first 5 years. *Mental Health Review Journal, 17*(4), 221–228. doi:10.1108/13619321211289290

Government of Canada. (2014). *Annual report of the office of the correctional investigator 2013-2014.* Ottawa, ON: Office of the correctional investigator. Retrieved from http://www.oci-bec.gc.ca/cnt/rpt/annrpt/annrpt20132014-eng.aspx

Greaves, K. (2016, November 11). Seasonal affective disorder affects many Canadians, but it's treatable. Toronto, ON: *The Huffington Post Canada.* Retrieved from http://www.huffingtonpost.ca/2016/11/14/seasonal-affective-disorder_n_12965660.html

Greenslit, N. (2012). Op-ED: *Why YouTube matters to the science of depression.* Wired.com. Retrieved from https://www.wired.com/2012/02/zoloft-video-parodies/

Griffiths, K. M., Crisp, D. A., Jorm, A. E., & Cristensen, H. (2011). Does stigma predict a belief in dealing with depression alone? *Journal of Affective Disorders, 132,* 413–417.

Grohol, J. M. (2014, May 29). *DSM-5 changes: Schizophrenia & psychotic disorders.* Newsburyport, MA: Psych Central Professional. Retrieved from https://pro.psychcentral.com/dsm-5-changes-schizophrenia-psychotic-disorders/004336.html

Gujjariamudi, H. B. (2016, July/September). Polytherapy and drug interactions in elderly. *Journal of Midlife Health, 7*(3), 105–107. doi:10.4103/0976-7800.191021

Hahn, D. B., Payne, W. A., Gallant, M., & Fletcher, P.C. (2006). *Focus on health* (2nd Canadian ed.). Toronto, ON: McGraw-Hill Ryerson.

Hanoch, Y., & Vitouse, O. (2004, August 1). When less is more: Information, emotional arousal and the ecological reframing of the Yerkes-Dodson Law. *Theory and Psychology, 14*(4), 64–71.

Hanwella, R., deSilva, V., Yoosuf, A., Karunoratre, S., & de Silva, P. (2012). Religious beliefs, possession states, and spirits: Three case studies from Sri Lanka. *Case Report Psychiatry*, 232740. doi:10.1155/2012/232740. Epub 2012, August 30. Retrieved from https://www.ncbi.nlm.nih.gov/pubmed/22970398

Health Canada. (2002a, January 16). *Health Canada is advising consumers not to use any products containing kava*. Ottawa, ON: Author. Retrieved from www.hc-sc.gc.ca/english/protection/warnings/2002/2002_02e.htm3

Health Canada. (2002b, August 21). *Health Canada issues a stop-sale order for all products containing kava*. Ottawa, ON: Author. Retrieved from www.hc-sc.gc.ca/english/protection/warnings/2002/2002_56e.htm

Health Canada. (2008). *Mental health: Coping with stress*. Ottawa, ON: Her Majesty the Queen in Right of Canada. Retrieved from http://www.hc-sc.gc.ca/hl-vs/iyh-vsv/life-vie/stress-eng.php

Health Canada. (2016a). *Natural and non-prescription health products*. Ottawa, ON: Author. Retrieved from http://hc-sc.gc .ca/dhp-mps/prodnatur/index-eng.php

Health Canada. (2016b). *Natural and health products directorate*. Ottawa, ON: Author. Retrieved from http://hc-sc.gc.ca/ ahc-asc/branch-dirgen/hpfb-dgpsa/nhpd-dpsn/index-eng.php

Health Canada, First Nations and Inuit Health. (2015). *Mental health and wellness*. Ottawa, ON: Government of Canada. Retrieved from http://www.hc-sc.gc/fniah-spnia/promtion/mental/index-eng.php

Herkov, B. (2016, September). What is psychotherapy? *Psych Central*. Retrieved from https://psychcentral.com/lib/ what-is-psychotherapy/

Hogan, M. J., & Strasburger, V. C.(2008). Body image, eating disorders, and the media. *Adolescent Medical State Art Review, 19*(3), 521–546.

Hoehn, K., & Marieb, E. N. (2010). *Human anatomy & physiology*. San Francisco, CA: Benjamin Cummings. ISBN: 0-321-60261-7.

Huang, I. C., Lee, J. L., Ketheeswaran, P., Jones, C. M., Revicki, D. A., & Wu, A. W. (2017, March 21). Does personality affect health-related quality of life? A systematic review. *PLoS ONE, 12*(3), e0173806. doi:10.1371/journal.pone.0173806

Insel, P. M., Roth, W. T., Irwin, J. D., & Burke, S. M. (2016). *Core concepts in health*. Toronto, ON: McGraw Hill Education.

International Marketing Services Health. (2004). *Year-end U.S. Prescription and sales information and commentary. (Connecticut): Fairfield. International Marketing Services Health Year-end U.S. Prescription and sales information and commentary 2004*. Connecticut: Fairfield International Marketing Services Health. Available at: http://www.imshealth .com/ims/portal/front/articleC/0,2777,6599_3665_69890098,00.html

Ioannidis, J. P. A. (2008). Effectiveness of antidepressants: An evidence myth constructed from a thousand randomized trials? *Philosophy, Ethics, and Humanities in Medicine, 3*, 14. doi:10.1186/1747-5341-3-14. Retrieved from https:// peh-med.biomedcentral.com/articles/10.1186/1747-5341-3-14

Jakobsen, J. C., Katakam, K. K., Schou, A., Hellmuth S. G., Stallknecht, S. E., Leth-Møller, K … Gluud, C. (2017). Selective serotonin reuptake inhibitors versus placebo in patients with major depressive disorder. A systematic review with meta-analysis and Trial Sequential Analysis. *BMC Psychiatry, 17*(58). doi:10.1186/s12888-016-1173

Kanter, J. W., Busch, A. M., Weeks, C. E., & Landes, S. J. (2008, Spring). The nature of clinical depression: Symptoms, syndromes, and behavior analysis. *Behavioral Analysis, 31*(1), 1–21. Retrieved from https://www.ncbi.nlm.nih.gov/ pmc/articles/PMC2395346/

Kennedy, S., McDonald, J. T., & Biddle, N. (2006). *The healthy immigrant effect and immigrant selection: Evidence from four countries*. Retrieved from https://ideas.repec.org/p/mcm/sedapp/164.html

Kirby, M. J. (2008). Mental health in Canada: Out of the shadows forever. *Canadian Medical Association Journal, 178*(10), 1320–1322.

Kirby, M. J., & Keon, W. J. (2006). *Out of the shadows at last: Transforming mental health, mental illness and addiction services in Canada*. Ottawa, ON: Standing Committee on Social Affairs, Science and Technology.

Kirkpatrick, B., Fenton, W. S., Carpenter, W. T., & Marder, S. R. (2016, April). The NIMH MATRICS consensus statement on negative symptoms. *Schizophrenia Bulletin, 32*(2), 214–219. Retrieved from https://academic.oup.com/schizophreniabulletin/article/32/2/214/1901232

Kleisioris, C. F., Sfakianakis, D., & Papathonosiou, I. V. (2014, March 15). Healthcare practices in ancient Greece: The Hippocratic ideal. *Journal of Medical Ethics, History and Medicine, 7,* 6. (PMCID: PMC4263393) Retrieved from https://www.ncbi.nlm.nih.gov/pmc/articles/PMC4263393/

Kleiman, E. M., Chiara, A. M., Liu, R. T., Jager-Hyman, S. G., Choi, J. Y., & Allay, L. B. (2017, February). Optimism and well-being: A prospective multi-method and multi-dimensional examination of optimism as a resilience factor following occurrence of stressful life events. *Cognition & Emotions, 31*(2), 269–283. doi:10.108010269993.2015.1108284

Klein, D. N. (2008, August). Classification of depressive disorders in DSM-V: Proposal for a two-dimensional system. *Journal of Abnormal Psychology, 117*(3), 552–560. doi:10.1037/0021=843X.117.3.552. Retrieved from https://www.ncbi.nlm.nih.gov/pmc/articles/PMC3057920/

Kober, M., Pohl, K., & Efferth, T. (2008). Molecular mechanisms underlying St. John's wort drug interactions. *Current Drug Metabolism, 9*(10), 1027–1037. doi:10.2174/138920008786927767

Kucharski, N. (1984). A History of frontal lobotomy in the United States, 1935–1955. *Neurosurgery, 14,* 765–772. Retrieved from https://www.ncbi.nlm.nih.gov/pubmed/6379496

Kuo, B. C. H., Chong, V., & Joseph, J. (2008). Depression and its psychosocial correlates among older Asian immigrants in North America: A critical review of two decades' research. *Journal of Aging and Health, 20,* 615–652.

Kwong, M. (2015, March 5). SAD science. Why winter brings us down, but won't for long. Severe seasonal affective disorder affects up to 1 in 20 Canadians. Toronto, ON: *CBC News.* Retrieved from http://www.cbc.ca/news/health/sad-science-why-winter-brings-us-down-but-won-t-for-long-1.2981920

Lacasse, J. R., & Leo, J. (2005). Serotonin and depression: A disconnect between the advertisements and the scientific literature. *PLoS Med, 2*(12), e392. doi:10.1371/journal.pmed.0020392

Laden, G. (2012). How many people were killed as witches in Europe from 1200 to present? *ScienceBlogs.* Retrieved from http://scienceblogs.com/gregladen/2012/12/02/how-many-people-were-killed-as-witches-in-europe-from-1200-to-the-present/

Lavin, A. T., Shapiro, G. R., & Weill, K. S. (1992, August). Creating an agenda for school-based health promotion: A review of 25 selected reports. *Journal of School Health, 62*(6), 212–228. Retrieved from http://onlinelibrary.wiley.com/doi/10.1111/j.1746-1561.1992.tb01231.x/full

LeBlanc, H. (Chair). (2014, November). *Eating disorder among girls and women in Canada.* Ottawa, ON: House of Commons (FEWO Committee Report), 41st Parliament, 2nd session. Retrieved from http://www.ourcommons.ca/DocumentViewer/en/41-2/FEWO/report-4/page-18

Ledwell, P., McLean, J., & Griller, D. (2013). *Schizophrenia in Canada* (1st ed.). Ottawa, ON: Public Policy Forum.

Levack, B. P. (Ed.). (1992). *Articles on witchcraft, magic, and demonology: A twelve volume anthology of scholarly articles.* New York, NY: Garland Publications. Retrieved from http://www.worldcat.org/title/articles-on-witchcraft-magic-and-demonology-a-twelve-volume-anthology-of-scholarly-articles/oclc/58587899/editions?referer=di&editionsView=true

Li, J., Jarczok, M. N., Loerbroks, A., Schöllgen, I., Siegrist, J., Bosch, J. A., … Fischer, J. E. (2013). Work stress is associated with diabetes and prediabetes: Cross-sectional results from the MIPH Industrial Cohort Studies. *International Journal of Behavioral Medicine, 20,* 495–503.

Lou, Y., & Beaujot, R. (2005). *What happens to the healthy immigrant effect: The mental health of immigrants to Canada.* Discussion paper No. 05-15. Population Studies Centre, University of Western Ontario, London, ON, Volume 7 (Issue 15). Retrieved from http://ir.lib.uwo.ca/cgi/viewcontent.cgi?article=1031&context=pscpapers

Lu, T., Guan, J., & An. C. (2015, July). Preoperative trepanation and drainage for acute subdural hematoma: Two case reports. *Experimental Therapies and Medicine, 10*(1), 225–230. Retrieved from https://www.ncbi.nlm.nih.gov/pmc/articles/PMC4487041/

MacIntyre, D. J., Blackwood, D. H. R., Porteous, D. J., Pickard, B. S., & Muir, W. J. (2003). Chromosomal abnormalities and mental illness. *Molecular Psychiatry, 8,* 275–287.

Malhi, G. S., Basset, D. I., Boyce, P., Bryant, R., Fitzgerald, P. B…Singh, A. B. (2015). The Royal Australian and New Zealand College of Psychiatrists Clinical Practice Guidelines for Mood Disorders. *Australian and New Zealand Journal of Psychiatry, 49*(12), 1–185. Retrieved from https://www.ranzcp.org/Files/Resources/Publications/CPG/Clinician/Mood-Disorders-CPG.aspx

Mayo Clinic. (2017). *Diseases and conditions: Generalized anxiety disorder.* Retrieved from http://www.mayoclinic.org/diseases-conditions/generalized-anxiety-disorder/basics/treatment/con-20024562

McCance, K. L., & Huether, S. E. (2010). *Pathophysiology: The biologic basis for disease in adults and children* (6th ed.) St, Louis, MO: Elsevier Mosby.

McCain, N. L., Gray, D. P., & Elswick, R. K. Jr. (2008). A randomized clinical trial of alternative stress management interventions in persons with HIV infection. *Journal of Consulting & Clinical Psychology, 7*(3), 431–441. doi:10.1037/0022-006X.76.3.431

McEwen, B. S. (2000). Allostasis and allostatic load: Implications for neuropsychopharmacology. *Neuropsychopharmacology, 22*(2), 108–124. doi:10.1016/S0893-133X(99)00129-3

McEwen, B. S. (2017, April). Allostasis and the epigenetics of brain and body health over the life course. *JAMA Psychiatry.* doi:10.1001/jamapsychiatry.2017.0270

McGibbon, E. (2012). *Oppression: A social determinant of health.* Winnipeg, MB: Fernwood.

McVey, G. (2014, March 4). Existing gaps in eating disorder services and recommendations. Ontario Community Outreach Program for Eating Disorders, *Brief submitted to the House of Commons Standing Committee on the Status of Women*, March 4, 2014. Community Health Systems Resource Group, Ontario, Community Outreach Program for Eating Disorders, The Hospital for Sick Children of Toronto, ON.

Meney, F. (2015, July 5). The Québec Charter for A Health and Diverse Body Image still relevant. Montreal, QC: The Douglas Mental Health University Institute. Retrieved from http://www.douglas.qc.ca/news/1142?locale=en

Mental Health Commission of Canada. (2012). *Changing directions. Changing lives: The mental health strategy for Canada.* Calgary, AB: Author. Retrieved from http://strategy.mentalhealthcommission.ca/pdf/strategy-images-en.pdf

Mental Health Commission of Canada. (2013a). *Making the case for investing in mental health in Canada.* Ottawa, ON: MHSC. Retrieved from http://www.mentalhealthcommission.ca/sites/default/files/2017-03/Making%20the%20Case%20for%20Investing%20in%20Mental%20Health%20in%20Canada.pdf

Mental Health Commission of Canada. (2015). *Informing the future: Mental health indicators for Canada.* Ottawa, ON: Author. Retrieved from http://www.mentalhealthcommission.ca/sites/default/files/Informing%252520the%252520Future%252520-%252520Mental%252520Health%252520Indicators%252520for%252520Canada_0.pdf

Mental Health Commission of Canada. (2017a). *Mental health first aid.* Ottawa, ON: Author. Retrieved from (see link: http://www.mentalhealthcommission.ca/English/focus-areas/mental-health-first-aid

Mental Health Commission of Canada. (2017b). *Opening minds.* Ottawa, ON: Author. Retrieved from http://www.mentalhealthcommission.ca/English/initiatives/11874/opening-minds

Micale, M. S. (1985). The Salpêtrière in the age of Charcot: An institutional perspective on medical history in the late nineteenth century. *Journal of Contemporary History, 20*, 703–731.

Mills, E., Singh, R., Ross, C., Ernst, E., & Ray, J. G. (2003). Sale of kava extract in some health food stores. *CMAJ, 169*(11), 1158–1159.

Moncrieff, J. (2007). Rebuttal: Depression is not a brain disease. *Canadian Journal of Psychiatry, 52*, 100–101. Retrieved from http://journals.sagepub.com/doi/pdf/10.1177/070674370705200206

Moncrieff, J. (2014). The chemical imbalance theory of depression: Still promoted but still unfounded. *Critical Psychiatry.* Retrieved from https://joannamoncrieff.com/2014/05/01/the-chemical-imbalance-theory-of-depression-still-promoted-but-still-unfounded/

Mondorf, Y., Abu-Owaimer, M., Gaab, M. R., & Oertel, J. M. (2009). Chronic subdural hematoma—craniotomy versus burr hole trepanation. *British Journal of Neurosurgery, 23*, 612–616. doi:10.3109/0268869090337029. Retrieved from https://www.ncbi.nlm.nih.gov/pmc/articles/PMC4487041/

Mood Disorders Association of Canada. (n.d.). *Frequently asked questions: Seasonal Affective Disorder (S.A.D.).* Retrieved from https://www.mooddisorders.ca/faq/seasonal-affective-disorder-sad

Mood Disorders Society of Canada. (2009, October). *Quick facts: Mental illness and addictions in Canada* (3rd ed.). Guelph, ON: Author. Retrieved from https://mdsc.ca/documents/Media%20Room/Quick%20Facts%203rd%20Edition%20Eng%20Nov%2012%202009.pdf

National Center for Biotechnology Information (NCBI). (2017). *Depression: The treatment and management of depression in adults (updated edition).* Betheseda, MD: U.S. National Library of Medicine and NCBI. Retrieved from https://www.ncbi.nlm.nih.gov/books/NBK63740/

National Institute of Mental Health. (2013, March 1). *Five major mental disorders share genetic roots.* Bethesador, MD: Author. Retrieved from https://www.nimh.nih.gov/news/science-news/2013/five-major-mental-disorders-share-genetic-roots.shtml

Nemeroff, C. B. D., Wienberger, M., Rutter, H. L., Macmillan, R. A., Bryant, S., … Lysaker, P. (2013, September 12). DSM-5: A collection of psychiatrist views on changes, controversies, and future directions. *BMC Medicine, 12*(11), 202. doi:10.1186/1741-7015-11-202.

Neuner, F., Pfeiffer, A., Schauer-Kaiser, E., Adenwald, M., Elbert, T., & Erti, V. (2012, August). Prevalence, predictors and outcomes of spirit possession experiences among former child soldiers and war-affected civilians in Northern Uganda. *Social Science and Medicine, 75*(3), 548–554. Retrieved from http://www.sciencedirect.com/science/article/pii/S027795361200295X

Nezafati, M. H., Eshraghi, A., Vojdanparast, M., Abtahi, S., & Nezafati, P. (2016). Selective serotonin reuptake inhibitors and cardiovascular events: A systematic review. *Journal of Research, Medicine and Science, 21,* 66. Retrieved from http://www.jmsjournal.net/article.asp?issn=1735-1995;year=2016;volume=21;issue=1;spage=66;epage=66;aulast=Nezafati

Nolan, P. W. (1993). A history of the training of asylum nurses. *Journal of Advanced Nursing, 18*(8), 1193–1201.

Papathanassoglou, E. (2010). Psychological support and outcomes of ICU patients. *Nursing in Critical Care, 15*(3), 118–128. doi:10.111/j.1478-5153.2009.00383x

Pan-Canadian Joint Consortium for School Health (PCJCSH). (2010). *Schools as a setting for promoting positive mental health: Better practices and perspectives.* Ottawa, ON: PCJCSH. Retrieved from http://www.jcshpositivementalhealth-toolkit.com

Park, Y. M., Ko, Y. H., Lee, M. S., Lee, H. J., & Kim, L. C. (2014, July). Type D personality can predict suicidality in patients with major depressive disorder. *Psychiatric Investigations, 11*(3), 232–236. doi:10.4306/pi.2014.11.3.232

Pearson, C., Zamorski, M., & Janz, T. (2015). *Health at a glance. Mental health of Canadian Armed Forces.* Ottawa, ON: Statistics Canada (Catalogue No. 82-624X). Retrieved from http://www.statcan.gc.ca/pub/82-624-x/2014001/article/14121-eng.htm

Pies, R. W. (2014, April 11). Nuances, narratives, and the "chemical imbalance" debate. *Psychiatric Times,* Retrieved from http://www.psychiatrictimes.com/blogs/nuances-narratives-chemical-imbalance-debate

Pittenger, C., Kelmendi, B., Bloch, M., Krystal, J. H., & Coric, V. (2005, November). Clinical treatment of obsessive compulsive disorder. *Psychiatry (Edgmont), 2*(11), 34–43. Retrieved from https://www.ncbi.nlm.nih.gov/pmc/articles/PMC2993523/

Pittler, M., & Ernst, E. (2000). Efficacy of kava extract for treating anxiety: Systematic review and meta-analysis. *Journal of Clinical Psychopharmacology, 20*(1), 83–89

Pinel, P. H. (1806). *A treatise of insanity.* Sheffield, England: Printed by W. Todd for Cadell and Davis.

Porter, R. (1997). *The greatest benefit to mankind: A medical history of humanity form antiquity to the present.* New York, NY: Harper Collins.

Postmedia News. (2016, May 11). Here's our list of resources for Fort McMurray wildfire evacuees and how you can help. *Edmonton Journal.* Edmonton, Alberta. Retrieved from http://edmontonjournal.com/storyline/heres-our-list-of-resources-for-fort-mcmurray-wildfire-evacuees-and-how-you-can-help

Pruden, J. G. (2016, May 10). A week in hell: How Fort McMurray burned. *Globe and Mail.* Toronto, ON. Retrieved from http://www.theglobeandmail.com/news/a-week-in-hell-how-fort-mcmurrayburned/article29932799/

Public Health Agency of Canada (PHAC). (2006 & 2012 [updated]). *The human face of mental health and mental illness in Canada 2006.* Ottawa, ON: Author. Retrieved from http://www.phac-aspc.gc.ca/publicat/human-humain06/index-eng.php

Public Health Agency of Canada. (2007, September). *Core competencies for public health in Canada: Release 1.1.* Ottawa, ON: Author. Web-based link: http://www.phac-aspc.gc.ca/core_competencies or http://www.phac-aspc.gc.ca/php-psp/ccph-cesp/pdfs/cc-manual-eng090407.pdf

Public Health Agency of Canada (PHAC). (2015a). *Mental illness*. Ottawa, ON: Author. Retrieved from http://www.phac-aspc.gc.ca/cd-mc/mi-mm/index-eng.php

Public Health Agency of Canada (PHAC). (2015b). *The Chief Public Health Officer's Report on the State of Public Health in Canada 2015: Alcohol Consumption in Canada*. Ottawa, ON: Author. Cat. No. HP2-10E-PDF. Retrieved from http://healthycanadians.gc.ca/publications/department-ministere/state-public-health-alcohol-2015-etat-sante-publique-alcool/alt/state-phac-alcohol-2015-etat-aspc-alcool-eng.pdf

Public Policy Forum. (2013). *Schizophrenia in Canada. The social and economic case for a collaborative model of care*. Ottawa, ON: Author. ISBN: 978-1-927009-51-2. Retrieved from http://www.ppforum.ca/sites/default/files/Schizophrenia%20in%20Canada%20-%20Final%20report_0.pdf

Pfizer. (2004, March). *Zoloft advertisement*. Burbank (California): NBC. Pfizer Zoloft advertisement 2004. March, Burbank (California): NBC Retrieved from https://www.youtube.com/watch?v=twhvtzd6gXA

Rahman, S. (2011, May 11). A treatise on insanity. *British Medical Journal, 342*, d2953. doi:10.1136/bmj.d2953. Retrieved from http://www.bmj.com/content/342/bmj.d2953

Restak, R. (2000). *Mysteries of the mind*. Washington, DC: National Geographic Society.

Riemann, D., Spiegelholder, K., Feige, B., Vaderhalzer, U., Berger, M, Perlis, M., & Nissen, C. (2010, February). The hyperarousal model of insomnia: A review of the concept and its evidence. *Sleep Medicine Reviews, 14*(1), 19–31.

Roberts, B. W., Kuncel, N. R., Shiner, R., Caspi, A., & Goldberg, L. R. (2007). The power of personality: The comparative validity of personality traits, socioeconomic status, and cognitive ability for predicting important life outcomes. *Perspectives on Psychological Science, 2*(4), 313–345. pmid:26151971.

Ryan-Nichollis, K. D., & Haggarty, J. M. (2007). Collaborative mental healthcare in rural and isolated Canada: Stakeholder feedback. *Journal of Psychosocial Nursing, 45*(12), 37–45.

Schmidt, N. B., Richery, J. A., Zvolensky, M. J., & Moner, J, K. (2008, September). Exploring human freeze response to a threat stressor. *Journal of Behavioral Therapy and Experimental Psychiatry, 39*(3), 292–304. doi: 10.1016/j.jbtep.2007.08.002

Scheiderman, N., Ironside, G., & Siegel, S. D. (2005, October 16). Stress and health: Psychological, behavioral and biological determinants. *Annual Review of Clinical Psychology, 1*, 607–628. doi:10.1146/annurev.clinpsy.1.102803.144141

Schidkraut, J. J. (1965). The catecholamine hypothesis of affective disorders: A review of supporting evidence. *Journal of Neuropsychiatry and Clinical Neuroscience, 7*, 524–533. Retrieved from https://www.ncbi.nlm.nih.gov/pubmed/8555758

Scholz, B. A., Holmes, H. M., & Marcus, D. M. (2008). Use of herbal medications in elderly patients. *Annals of Long-Term Care, 16*(12), 24–28.

Seeman, T. E., Singer, B. H., Rowe, J. W., Horwitz, R. I., & McEwen, B S. (1997). Price of adaptation—Allostatic load and its health consequences. MacArthur studies of successful aging. *Archives of Internal Medicine, 157*, 2259–2268.

Segerstrom, S. C., & Miller, G. E. (2004). Psychological stress and the human immune system: A meta-analytic study of 30 years of inquiry. *Psychological Bulletin, 130*(4), 601–630.

Segerstrom, S. C. (2010). Resources, stress, and immunity: An ecological perspective on human psychoneuroimmunology. *Annals of Behavioral Medicine, 40*(1), 114–135. doi:10.1007/s12160-010-9155-3

Seltzer, L. F. (2015, July 8). Trauma and the freeze response: Good, bad or both? *Psychology Today*. Retrieved from https://www.psychologytoday.com/blog/evolution-the-self/201507/trauma-and-the-freeze-response-good-bad-or-both

Seyle, H. (1974). *Stress without distress*. New York, NY: Lippincott.

Seyle, H. (1983). The stress concept: Past, present, and future. In C. L. Cooper (Ed.), *Stress research: Issues for the eighties*. New York, NY: Wiley.

Sharp, S. E. (1899, April). Individual psychology: A study in psychological method. *The American Journal of Psychological Method, 10*(3), 329–391. doi:10.23071/1412140. Retrieved from http://www.jstor.org/stable/1412140?seq=1#page_scan_tab_contents

Sher, L. (2005, May). Type D personality: The heart, stress and cortisol. *Quarterly Journal of Medicine, 98*(5): Epub. doi:10.1093/qimed/hciO64

Simeone, J. C., Ward, A. J., Rotella, P., Collins, J., & Windisch. R. (2015). An evaluation of variation in published estimates of schizophrenia prevalence from 1990 to 2013: A systematic review. *BMC Psychiatry, 15*(1). doi:10.1186/s

12888-015-0578-7. Retrieved from https://www.semanticscholar.org/paper/An-evaluation-of-variation-in-published-estimates-Simeone-Ward/8376cd23446c426c0a179ef9c7f2cefab2585792

Singh, Y. N., & Singh, N. N. (2002). Therapeutic potential of kava in the treatment of anxiety disorders. *CNS Drugs,* *16*(11), 731–743.

Smetanin, P., Stiff, D., Briante, C., Adair, C., Ahmad, S., & Khan, M. (2011). *The life and economic impact of major mental illnesses in Canada: 2011 to 2041. Risk Analytica, on behalf of the Mental Health Commission of Canada.* Calgary, AB: Author.

Smink, F. R. E., Hocken, D. V., Hock, H. W. (2012, May 27). Epidemiology of eating disorders: Incidence, prevalence and mortality rates. *Current Psychiatry Reports, 144,* 406–414. doi:10.1007/s11920-0121-0282-y. Retrieved from https://link.springer.com/content/pdf/10.1007%2Fs11920-012-0282-y.pdf

Smith, A. C. (1967, March). Clinical notes on Pinel's Treatise of Insanity. *British Medical Journal, 40*(1), 85–100. doi:10.1111/j.2044-8341.1967.tb00558.x. Retrieved from http://onlinelibrary.wiley.com/doi/10.1111/j.2044-8341.1967.tb00558.x/abstract

Smith, D. J., & Craddock, N. (2011, September). Unipolar and bipolar depression: Different or the same? *The British Journal of Psychiatry, 199*(4), 272–294. doi:10.1192/bjp.111.092726. Retrieved from http://bjp.rcpsych.org/content/199/4/272

Statistics Canada. (2001). Stress and well–being. *Health Reports, 12*(3). Statistics Canada Catalogue no. 82-003. 22. http://www.statcan.gc.ca/studies-etudes/82-003/archive/2001/5626-eng.pdf

Statistics Canada. (2009). *What should I know about bipolar disorder (manic-depression)?* Ottawa, ON: Author. Retrieved from https://www.canada.ca/en/public-health/services/chronic-diseases/mental-illness/what-should-know-about-bipolar-disorder-manic-depression.html

Statistics Canada. (2012). *Canadian Community Health Survey Report.* Ottawa, ON: Author. Retrieved from https://www.statcan.gc.ca/eng/survey/household/3226

Statistics Canada. (2013). *Deaths by cause. Chapter V: Mental and behavioural disorders (F00 to F99), age group and sex, Canada.* Ottawa, ON: Author. Retrieved from http://www5.statcan.gc.ca/cansim/a26?lang=eng&id=1020525

Statistics Canada. (2014). *Perceived life stress.* Ottawa, ON: Author. Cat. No. 82-625X. Retrieved from http://www.statcan.gc.ca/pub/82-625-x/2015001/article/14188-eng.htm

Statistics Canada. (2015a). *Prescription medication use by Canadians aged 6 to 79.* Ottawa, ON: Author. Cat. No. 82-003-X, Vol. 25, No. 6. Retrieved from http://www.statcan.gc.ca/pub/82-003-x/2014006/article/14032-eng.htm

Statistics Canada. (2015b). *Control and sales of alcoholic beverages, for the year ending March 31, 2014.* Ottawa ON: Statistics Canada. 8. Retrieved from http://vghtrauma.vch.ca/control-sale-alcoholic-beverages-year-ending-march-31-2015/

Statistics Canada. (2015c). *Section B: Anxiety disorders.* Ottawa, ON: Author. Cat. No. 82-619-M. Retrieved from http://www.statcan.gc.ca/pub/82-619-m/2012004/sections/sectionb-eng.htm

Statistics Canada. (2015d). *Section D: Eating disorders.* Ottawa, ON: Author. Cat. No. 82-619M. Retrieved from http://www.statcan.gc.ca/pub/82-619-m/2012004/sections/sectiond-eng.htm

Statistics Canada. (2016a). *150 years of immigration in Canada.* Ottawa, ON: Author. Retrieved from http://www.statcan.gc.ca/pub/11-630-x/11-630-x2016006-eng.htm

Statistics Canada. (2016b). *Study: Social determinants of health for the off-reserve First Nations population aged 15 years and older, 2012.* Ottawa, ON: Author. Cat. No. 89-653-X. Retrieved from http://www.statcan.gc.ca/daily-quotidien/160412/dq160412a-eng.htm?cmp=mstatcan

Stephens, W. (2000). *Demon lovers: Witchcraft, sex and belief.* Chicago: University of Chicago Press.

Surgenor, L. J., & Maguire, S. (2013). Assessment of anorexia nervosa: An overview of universal issues and contextual challenges. *Journal of Eating Disorders, 1*(2), 29. Retrieved from https://jeatdisord.biomedcentral.com/articles/10.1186/2050-2974-1-29

Sussman, S. (1998). The first asylums in Canada: A response to neglectful community care and current trends. *Canadian Journal of Psychiatry, 43,* 260–264.

Szanton, S., Gill, J. M., & Allen, J. K. (2005, July). Allostatic load: A mechanism of socioeconomic health disparities? *Biological Research for Nursing, 7*(1), 7–15. doi: 10.1177/1099800405278216

Tandon, R., Gaebel, W., Barch, D. M., Bustillo, J., Gur, R. E., … Carpenter, W. (2013). Definition and description of schizophrenia in the DSM-5. *Schizophrenia Research,* 1–8. Retrieved from http://ccpweb.wustl.edu/pdfs/2013_defdes.pdf

Temoshok, L., Hellen, B. W., Sagebiel, R. W, Sweet, D. M., DiClemente, R. J., & Gold, M. L (1985). The relationship of psychosocial factors to prognostic indicators in cutaneous malignant melanoma. *Journal of Psychosomatic Research, 29*, 139–154.

Temoshok, L. (1987). Personality, coping style, emotion and cancer: Towards an integrative model. *Cancer Survey, 6*, 545–567.

Tencer, D. (2013, November 22). Antidepressant use in Canada among highest in the world: OECD. *The Huffingston Post*. Retrieved from http://www.huffingtonpost.ca/2013/11/22/antidepressant-use-world-canada_n_4320429.html

Tseng, W. (1973). The development of psychiatric concepts in traditional Chinese medicine. *Archives of General Psychiatry, 29*, 569–575.

Troppmann, L., Johns, T., & Gray-Donald, K. (2002). Natural health product use in Canada. *Canadian Journal of Public Health, 93*, 426–430.

Vander-Ploeg, K. A., McGavock, J., Maximova, K., & Vengelers, P. J. (2013, November 14). School-based health promotion and physical activity during and after school. *Pediatrics*. doi:10.1542peds.2013-2383. Retrieved from http://www.appleschools.ca/files/PA-DuringAfterSchool.pdf

van den Berg, P., Paxton, S. J., Keery, H., Wall, M., Guo, J., & Neumark-Sztainer, D. A. (2007). Body dissatisfaction and body comparison with media images in males and females. *Body Image, 4*(3):257–268.

van Vonderer, K. E., & Kinnally, W. (2012, Spring). Media effects on body image: Examining exposure in the broader context on internal and other social factors. *American Communications Journal, 14*(2), 41–57. Retrieved from http://www.ac-journal.org/journal/pubs/2012/SPRING%202012/McKinnally3.pdf

Viney, W., & Zorich, S. (1982). Contributions to the history of psychology: XXIX. Dorothea Dix and the history of psychology. *Psychological Reports, 50*, 211–218.

Weber, B. (2014, November 12). Canada leading global effort to curb high Inuit suicide rate. Toronto, ON: *The Canadian Press*. Retrieved from https://beta.theglobeandmail.com/news/national/canada-leading-global-effort-to-curb-high-rate-of-inuit-suicide/article21419168/?ref=http://www.theglobeandmail.com&

Weber, B. (2017, January 17). Costs of Alberta Wildfire reach $9.5 billion: Study. Ottawa, ON. The Canadian Press. Retrieved from http://www.bnn.ca/costs-of-alberta-wildfire-reach-9-5-billion-study-1.652292

Weiss, S. (2007). Neurobiological alterations associated with traumatic stress. *Perspectives in Psychiatric Care, 43*(3), 114–122. doi:10.1111/j.1744-6163.2007.00120.x

Whorry, S. (2000, June 13). Health Canada sounds warning over St. John's wort. *CMAJ, 162*(12). Retrieved from http://www.cmaj.ca/content/162/12/1723.3.full

Williams, C. (2003, June). Sources of workplace stress. *Perspectives on Labour and Income, 4*(6), 1–11 (on-line). Statistics Canada, Ottawa, ON. Retrieved from http://www.statcan.gc.ca/pub/82-003-x/2006007/article/10191-eng.htm

World Health Organization. (2006, March). *What is the evidence on school health promotion in improving health or preventing disease and, specifically what is the effectiveness of the health promoting schools approach?* Geneva, Switzerland: WHO. Retrieved from www.euro.who.int/document/e88185.pdf

World Health Organization. (2014a, August). *Mental health: A state of well-being*. Geneva, Switzerland. WHO. Retrieved from http://www.who.int/features/factfiles/mental_health/en/

World Health Organization. (2014b). *Global status report of alcohol and health—2014 edition*. Geneva, Switzerland: WHO, Press. 49. Retrieved from http://www.who.int/substance_abuse/publications/global_alcohol_report/en/

World Health Organization. (2015). *Alcohol: Fact sheet*. Geneva, Switzerland, WHO. Available at http://www.who.int/mediacentre/factsheets/fs349/en/50

World Health Organization. (n.d.). *World Health Organization: Definition of psychoactive substances*. Geneva, Switzerland: WHO. Retrieved from http://www.who.int/substance_abuse/terminology/psychoactive_substances/en/4

Young, M.M., Jesseman, R. (2014, November). *The impact of substance use disorders on hospital use*. Ottawa, ON: Canadian Centre on Substance Abuse. Retrieved from http://www.ccsa.ca/Resource%20Library/CCSA-Substance-Use-Hospital-Impact-Report-2014-en.pdf

Zhang, L., Layre, C., Lawder T., & Liu, J. (2012). A review focused on the psychological effectiveness of tai chi on different populations. *Evidence-based Complementary & Alternative Medicine*. (2012). Article ID 678107. Retrieved from https://www.hindawi.com/journals/ecam/2012/678107/

Zong, J., Cao, X., Cao, Y., Shi, Y., Wang, Y., Yan, C., … Chan, R. (2010). Coping flexibility in college students with depressive symptoms. *Health & Quality of Life Outcomes, 8,* 66. doi:10.1186/1477-7525-8-66

Zota, A. R., Shenassa, E. D., & Morello-Frosch, R. (2013, August). Allostatic load amplifies the effect of blood levels on elevated blood pressure among middle-aged U.S. adults: A cross-sectional study. *Environmental Health, 12,* 64. doi:10.1186/1476-069X-12-64

Zupanick, C. E. (2014, February 23). *The new DSM-5 anxiety disorders and obsessive-compulsive disorders.* MentalHealth.net. Retrieved from https://www.mentalhelp.net/articles/the-new-dsm-5-anxiety-disorders-and-obsessive-compulsive-disorders/

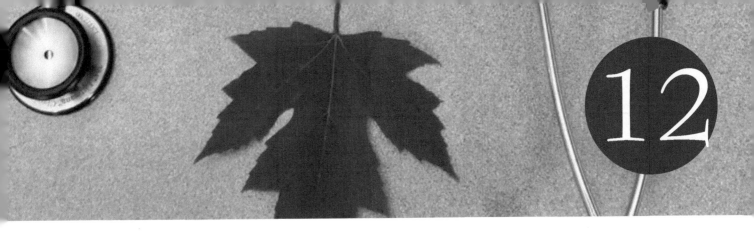

Neurological Disorders: A Growing Public Health Challenge

In all our studies of the brain, no mechanism has been discovered that can force the mind to think, or the individual to believe anything.
The mind continues free ...

—*(Wilder Penfield, 1891–1976)*

Learning Objectives

After completion of this chapter, the student will be able to
- Describe the major structural components of the central nervous system and their primary functions.
- Compare and contrast the costs and benefits of prevention versus treatment and management of traumatic head injuries and concussions in Canada
- Describe current and emerging neurological conditions and diseases in Canada and globally.
- Discuss the direct and indirect healthcare costs and impact associated with caring for clients diagnosed with a neurological condition and their implications from a public health perspective.
- List and describe various non-pharmaceutical or non-invasive interventions to help clients with neurological disorders improve and/or maintain their quality of life.

Core Competencies for Public Health addressed in this Chapter

Core Competencies	Competency Statements
1.0 Public Health Sciences	1.1, 1.2, 1.3, 1.4, 1.5
2.0 Assessment and Analysis	2.1, 2.2, 2.3, 2.4, 2.5, 2.6
3.0 Policy and Program Planning, Implementation, and Evaluation	3.1, 3.2, 3.6, 3.7
4.0 Partnerships, Collaboration, and Advocacy	4.1, 4.2, 4.3, 4.4
5.0 Diversity and Inclusiveness	5.1, 5.2
6.0 Communication	6.2
7.0 Leadership	7.1, 7.2

Note: Please see the following document or web-based link for a detailed description of these specific competencies. Public Health Agency of Canada (2007).

Introduction

During the 19th and early 20th centuries, laboratory-based research into the human brain and neurological systems concentrated primarily on their associated morphological, physiological, and psychological functions. However, in the new millennium a much deeper and holistic interdisciplinary understanding of the brain and nervous systems and associated neurological disorders is required from a public health perspective (World Health Organization, 2017b). Indeed, many distinctions can be made between the practice of public health and that of clinical neurology per se. For example, public health professionals and workers:

> ...approach neurology more broadly than neurologists by monitoring neurological disorders and related health concerns of entire communities and promoting healthy practices and behaviours among them to ensure that populations stay healthy ... [and] focus on health and disease of entire populations rather than on individual patients (WHO, 2017b, p. 7).

Hence, neurological disorder from a public health context is concerned with actual and potential threats to the overall health of Canadians across the lifespan from a holistic perspective. Evidence-informed interventions and public health policy initiatives are therefore concerned with the monitoring of health at the community and population levels through surveillance; the identification of aetiological factors including the social determinants of health, and the promotion of healthy lifestyles, behaviours, and environments.

For example, one's environment or location of where care is provided to a client with a neurological disorder or disease may affect the timing of one's diagnosis, treatment regime, and overall quality of life. The reader is referred to Research Focus Box 12.1. This population-based study suggests that clients with dementia who reside in residual care facilities in Ontario, Canada are diagnosed significantly later in comparison to clients in home-care settings, and are only clinically diagnosed when their cognitive and functional statuses have already significantly deteriorated (Bartfay, Bartfay, & Gorey, 2016).

Neurological disorders are defined as diseases of the central and peripheral nervous system, which include the brain, spinal cord, cranial nerves, peripheral nerves, nerve roots, autonomic nervous system (ANS), neuromuscular junction, and muscles (World Health Organization, 2016, 2017b). These disorders include but are not limited to: Alzheimer disease and other dementias, stroke, multiple sclerosis (MS), Parkinson's disease

Research Focus Box 12.1

Dementia Care in Ontario, Canada: Evidence of More Timely Diagnosis Among Persons With Dementia Receiving Care at Home Compared With Residential Facilities

Study Aim/Rationale

Home care in Canada has been promoted as a cost-effective alternative to long-term residential care. Currently, little is known about the welfare of persons who receive home versus residential care. This study examined cognitive and functional status of persons with dementia receiving home care (HC) or residential care (RC) at their time of diagnosis in Ontario, Canada.

Methodology/Design

The researchers employed a population-based secondary data analysis study to compare cognitive and functional statuses of persons with dementia. Data from the Canadian Institute for Health Information's Continuing Care Reporting System and the Home care Reporting System for the years 2009 to 2011 were employed. Representative populations of 39,604 and 21,153 persons with dementia who received either RC or HC were included, respectively. It was hypothesized that persons with dementia receiving RC would have declined further, both cognitively and functionally. Cognitive and functional statuses were assessed via a cognitive performance scale (CPS) and an activities of daily living (ADL) scale, respectively.

Major Findings

The proportion of individuals diagnosed when impairment was moderate to very severe was higher in the RC group (32% vs. 13.3%). The mean CPS score was also higher (3.2 vs. 2.5) for the RC group and also for the ADL score (3.5 vs. 1.6), in comparison to the HC group. The proportion of individuals diagnosed when they required extensive assistance or where deemed totally dependent (ADL > 3) were significantly higher in the RC group, when compared to the HC group (72.3% vs. 27.3%). All reported findings were statistically significant ($p < .0001$). Subsequent multivariable analysis suggested that RC clients were approximately four times more likely than HC clients to be diagnosed at a later state of dementia (odds ratio [OR] = 3.74, 95% confidence interval [CI]: 3.54–3.95).

Implications for Public Health

These findings suggest that clients with dementia who reside in RC facilities in Ontario, Canada are diagnosed significantly later in comparison to clients in HC situations. Moreover, clients in RC facilities tend to be diagnosed only when their cognitive (CPS) and functional (ADL) statuses have markedly declined, in comparison to HC clients. There is a growing need for community-based support mechanisms to support primary caregivers looking after persons with dementia in their homes. Furthermore, clients with already advanced dementia residing in RC facilities may be at a risk of not receiving proper individual evidence-informed treatment or care regimes for their dementia due to missed or delayed diagnosis.

Source: Bartfay et al. (2016).

(PD), epilepsy, meningitis, Japanese encephalitis, tetanus, and traumatic disorders of the nervous system. We shall examine some of these major disorders in greater detail later. Public health professionals and workers approach these disorders by monitoring neurological disorders and related health concerns of individuals, families, entire communities, and populations; and by promoting healthy practices and behaviours among them to ensure the health of all Canadians across the lifespan. The reader is referred to Web-Based Resources Box 12.1 for additional information on current and emerging neurological disorders, diseases, and injuries in Canada and globally.

The *Global Burden of Disease Study*, which is an ongoing international collaborative project between the WHO, the World Bank, and the Harvard School of Public Health has produced a significant body of data since 1990 that pinpoints neurological disorders as one of the greatest threats to public health facing various nations in the new millennium (World Health Organization, 2017a, 2017b, 2017c). This global collaborative

Web-Based Resources Box 12.1 Current and Emerging Neurological Disorders, Diseases, and Injuries

Learning Resource	Website
Canadian Institute for Health Information. (CIHI, 2007). *The burden of neurological diseases, disorders and injuries in Canada.* **Ottawa, ON: CIHI (ISBN: 978-1-55465-025-5).** - Provides an overview of major neurological disorders and injuries in Canada, risk factors, and associated costs.	https://secure.cihi.ca/free_products/BND_e.pdf
World Health Organization. (2017b). *Neurological disorders: Public health challenges.* **Geneva, Switzerland: WHO.** - Provides an international perspective on current and emerging major neurological disorders and the critical role of public health in providing treatment, care, and support services.	http://www.who.int/mental_health/neurology/neurological_disorders_report_web.pdf.

initiative has revealed the current lack of information regarding the burden of neurological disorders (e.g., cerebrovascular disorders, epilepsy, Alzheimer's disease and other dementias, PD, multiple sclerosis, meningitis, Japanese encephalitis, tetanus), and an alarming lack of policies, programs and resources for their identification and management. For example, mortalities due to dementias alone have more than doubled between 2000 and 2015, making it the seventh leading cause of deaths globally in 2015 (WHO, 2017c). Moreover, deaths directly attributed to neurological diseases globally were 11.67% in 2005; 11.84% in 2015, and are predicted to increase to 12.22% by 2030 (WHO, 2017a).

A growing burden of neurological disorders is reaching a significant proportion of countries now with a growing percentage of older individuals affected who are aged 65 years and older (WHO, 2017b). In fact, the number of Canadians aged 65 years and older is expected to reach 6.7 million in 2020 and 9.2 million in 2041 (CIHI, 2015; Public Health Agency of Canada, 2008). It is noteworthy from a public health context that in 2015, Canadians aged 65 years or older comprised 15% of the total population, but consumed more than 45% of all public health sector care costs (CIHI, 2015).

Indeed, several parts of the nervous system are directly affected by ageing processes. For example, in the CNS, neurons are slowly lost in certain areas of the brainstem, cerebellum, and cerebral cortex, ventricles widen and brain weight may decrease by 10% to 15% (Porter & Kaplan, 2011). This loss is a gradual process which first begins during the second and ninth decades of life. In fact, older adults are more prone to sensory changes, including decreased perception of taste and smell, which may result in dietary alterations and weight changes (Donatelle, Munroe, Munroe, & Thompson, 2008; Hahn, Payne, Gallant, & Flectcher, 2006). Similarly, declines in visual and auditory acuity can result in perceptual challenges, and problems with balance and coordination can put them at increased risk for falls and injury. Figure 12.1 provides estimates for the projected prevalence rates of select neurological conditions in Canada for the years 2011 and 2031.

This chapter examines the role of public healthcare professionals and workers in helping individuals, families, entire communities, and populations regain, maintain, and promote their neurological health across the lifespan. Current and emerging neurological disorders and issues are highlighted and critically examined from the public health perspective.

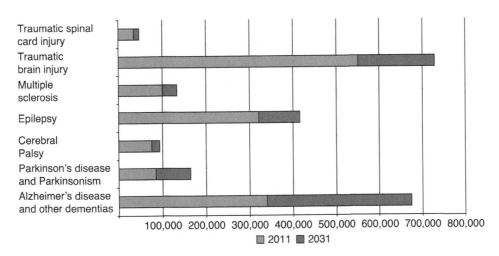

Figure 12.1 Projected prevalence rates with select neurological conditions in canada during 2031 (e.g., wife, daughters).

Source: Fines (2010, May 28).

A Brief Overview of the Human Brain and Nervous System

The weight of a newborn's brain is approximately 350 to 400 g; whereas an adult's brain weighs between 1300 and 1400 g (or approximately 3 pounds) on average (Rosenbluth, 2003). Brain growth that occurs in humans is typically completed by 5 to 6 years of age. By comparison, the sperm whale is believed to have the largest brain known of all species on Earth, weighing approximately 7820 g (or approximately 17 pounds) (Mink Blumenschine, & Adams, 1981; Rehkamper, Frahm, & Zilles, 1991).

Interesting, approximately 60% of our brain is composed of fat (i.e., essential fatty acids; EFAs), and we have learned in recent decades that fatty acids are, in fact, among the most crucial molecules that determine your brain's integrity and ability to perform (Chang, Ke, & Chen, 2009). EFAs are required for maintenance of optimal health, but they cannot be synthesized by the body and must therefore be obtained from dietary sources. A growing body of evidence has linked an imbalance of dietary EFAs to impaired brain performance, cognition, memory, and certain diseases in humans (e.g., Kidd, 2007; McCann & Ames, 2005; Wainwright, 2002; Witte et al., 2014). Figure 12.2 shows the major anatomical regions of the human brain.

The **gray matter** component of the brain contains the cells bodies that are responsible for voluntary motor neurons and preganglionic autonomic motor neurons, along with cells bodies for association neurons (interneurons). The **white matter** component of the brain contains the axons of the ascending sensory and descending (suprasegmental) motor fibres, and the myelin surrounding these fibres gives them the characteristic white appearance. The gray matter is made up of about 100 billion neurons that gather and transmit signals, whereas the white matter is made of dendrites and axons that the neurons use to transmit signals (Rosenbluth, 2003).

The human **nervous system** is a highly complex and specialized system responsible for the control and integration of the body's many functions and activities, and consists of two main divisions: (i) central nervous system (CNS), and (ii) peripheral nervous system (PNS). Major structural components of the CNS are the cerebrum (cerebral hemispheres), telencephalon and diencephalons, brainstem, cerebellum, and spinal cord. The **PNS** consists of cranial nerves III through XII, the spinal nerves, their associated ganglia (groupings of cell bodies) and the peripheral components of the ANS. Although the ANS is typically considered a part of the PNS by convention, components of the ANS are found in both the CNS and the PNS anatomically. The **ANS** is divided into sympathetic and parasympathetic components, which control various body functions and responses highlighted in Table 12.1.

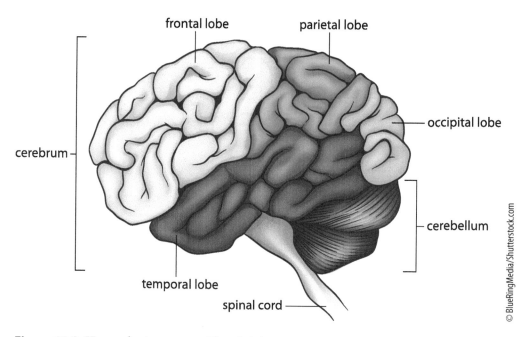

© BlueRingMedia/Shutterstock.com

Figure 12.2 Human brain anatomy. The adult brain is composed of approximately 40% gray matter and 60% white matter, and weights between 1300 and 1400 g total on average.

Table 12.1 Select Organs or Glands Controlled by the Sympathetic and Parasympathetic Components of the ANS. The ANS governs involuntary functions of both cardiac and smooth (involuntary) muscles and glands.

Organ or Gland	Parasympathetic ANS	Sympathetic ANS
Eye	• Constricts pupils	• Dilates pupils
Salivary and parotid glands	• Stimulates saliva production	• Inhibits saliva production
Blood vessels	• Causes constriction in skeletal muscles	• Causes dilation in skeletal muscles
Sweat glands	• Inhibits sweat production	• Stimulates sweat production
Lungs	• Constricts bronchi	• Dilates bronchi
Heart	• Slows/decreases heart rate	• Increases/accelerates heart rate
Liver	• Inhibits the release of glucose (glycogen)	• Stimulates the release the glucose (glycogen)
Gallbladder	• Stimulates production of bile	• Inhibits production of bile
Intestines	• Stimulates intestinal motility	• Inhibits intestinal motility
Kidneys and adrenal gland	• Stimulates adrenal gland & inhibits production of renin	• Inhibits adrenal glands and stimulates renin production

Traumatic Brain Injuries and Concussions

A **traumatic brain injury (TBI)** is defined as any insult or injury to the brain which is not of a degenerative or congenital nature, but caused by an external physical force that may produce a diminished or altered state of consciousness resulting in an impairment of cognitive abilities and/or physical functioning. A **concussion** is a type of brain injury caused by the brain moving inside of the skull which often causes damage and/or results in changes of how brain cells function, leading to symptoms that can be physical (headaches, dizziness); cognitive (problems remembering or concentrating), and/or emotional (feeling depressed) in nature. A concussion can result from any impact to the head, face, or neck or by a blow to the body that results in a sudden jolting of the head.

Profound disturbances of cognitive, emotional, and behavioural functioning after a TBI may produce permanent impairments that result in partial or total functional disability and psychosocial maladjustment (Belanger, Vanderploeg, & McAllister, 2016; Dismore, 2013; O'Neil-Pirazzi, Kennedy, & Sohlberg, McKay 2016). Brain damage can occur along the path where an object (e.g., bullet, knife, nail, rock, or other projectile) enters the brain. TBIs can also occur as a result of a sudden acceleration/deceleration of the structures of the brain within the cranium. For example, if a hockey player receives a slap shot to the head with a hockey puck, or as the result of a fall to the hard ice surface. Currently, no effective TBI therapy exists, with clients treated through a combination of surgery (i.e., if bleeding is present in the brain); rehabilitation, and pharmacological agents to manage posttraumatic conditions such as depression (Dismore, 2013; Haddad & Arabi, 2012; Tabish & Syed, 2014).

TBI is a heterogeneous condition in terms of its aetiology, severity, and outcomes. There are three generally acknowledged levels of severity for TBIs that is assessed via the *Glasgow Coma Scale* (GCS) as being: (i) Mild (GCS = 13–15); (ii) moderate (GCS = 9–12), or (iii) severe (GCS = 3–8) in nature. The clinical components that make up the GCS assessment scores are detailed in Figure 12.3.

A mild TBI typically results in a confused state or a loss of consciousness of less than 30 min, and posttraumatic amnesia typically lasts less than 24 hours. A moderate TBI often results in a loss of consciousness of 30 min to 24 hours, and posttraumatic amnesia can last 24 hours to seven days in duration. Lastly, a severe TBI often results in a loss of consciousness of greater than 24 hours, with a typical posttraumatic amnesia period of greater than seven days. However, factors such as hypoxia, hypotension, and/or intoxication via alcohol or narcotics can all affect GCS scores, resulting in potential diagnostic confusion. Moreover, clinical management algorithms based on GCS scores alone often ignore individual client variability and associated injury-specific factors (Dismore, 2013; Haddad & Arabi, 2012; National Institute for Health and Clinical Excellence, 2007).

Glasgow Coma Scale

The Glasgow Coma Scale (GCS) is widely employed internationally to assess acute head and brain injuries and/or trauma by emergency medical [service] (EMS) responders in community settings, and by other health care professionals (e.g., nurses, physicians) to monitor neurological changes in clients in acute care neurological trauma centres and intensive care hospital settings. The GCS was originally published by Graham Teasdale and Jennett (1974) who were professors of neurosurgery at the University of Glasgow's Institute of Neurological Sciences in Scotland. The GCS is currently employed in over 80 countries around the world; has been transcribed into various languages, and it is the most widely quoted scale in published neuroscientific journals. The original scale consisted of 14 points maximum (Teasdale & Jennett, 1974), and the more updated and modified scale consists of 15 points maximum (Teasdale et al., 2014). The GCS has three main components: (i) eye (E), (ii) verbal (V), and (iii) motor (M) response to external stimuli. The best or highest responses are recorded (see Figure 12.3). The client is assessed against the criteria of the scale, and the resulting points give a score between 3 (indicating deep unconsciousness) and either 14 (original scale) or 15 (the more widely used modified or revised scale). Hence, the higher the score obtained, the higher the level of brain functioning present at assessment.

Table 12.2 The Glasgow Coma Scale (GCS). The GCS is a relatively quick, practical, and standardized neurological scale widely employed around the world for assessing the degree to which consciousness is impaired via three main clinical indicators: (i) Best eye opening response, (ii) best verbal response, and (iii) best motor response.

Appropriate Stimulus	Response Obtained by Client	Score
i. Best eye opening response	• Spontaneous response • Opens eyes to name or command • No opening of eyes to previous stimuli, but opening to painful stimuli • No opening of eyes to any stimuli • Untestable (e.g., periorbital edema, trauma to eyes or orbital socket)	4 3 2 1 *U
ii. Best verbal response	• Orientated X 3 spheres (person, place, and time) • Confusion, conversant, but disoriented to one or more spheres • Disorganized or confused conversation or lack of sustained conversation • Incomplete or inaudible words or sounds (e.g., moaning) • No sound, even with painful stimuli • Untestable (e.g., endotracheal tube)	5 4 3 2 1 *U
iii. Best motor response	• Obeys/follows verbal commands (e.g., squeeze my hands, raise your hands) • Does not obey/follow verbal commands, localization of pain, reacts, or attempts to remove stimuli (purposeful movement) • Has flexion withdrawal of arm in response to painful stimuli without abnormal flexion position (non-purposeful movement) • Abnormal flexion present, flexing of arm at elbow and pronation, clenched fist • Abnormal extension present, extension of arm at elbow usually with adduction and internal rotation of arm at shoulder • No or lack of response noted • Untestable (e.g., injury to extremities, traction, amputation)	6 5 4 3 2 1 *U
	Total score obtained =	_____

Note: *Added to the original scale by many health institutions and centres. Grading = Severe head injury/trauma, GCS < 8–9; Moderate head injury/trauma, GCS 8 or 9–12, and Minor head injury or trauma, GCS ≥ 13. Modified 15-point scale adapted from Teasdale and Jennett (1974) and Teasdale et al. (2014).

TBIs: A Growing Public Health Concern

TBIs are a growing public health concern in Canada and globally, and are leading causes of death and disability. In fact, it is estimated than 1 million Canadians are currently living with a TBI, and over 10 million people experience a TBI every year (Brain Injury Canada, 2017a, 2017b; Hyder, Wunderlich, Puvanachandra, & Kobusingye, 2007; Tabish & Syed, 2014). It is estimated that 452 people suffer from a serious brain injury every day in Canada, which amounts to one person injured with a TBI every 3 min (Northern Brain Injury Association [NBIA], 2017). The annual incidence of acquired brain injury in Canada is 44 times more common than spinal cord injuries; 30 times more common than breast cancer, and 400 times more common than HIV/AIDS (NBIA, 2017). In fact, brain injury occurs at a rate greater than that of all known cases of MS, spinal cord injuries, HIV/AIDS, and breast cancer cases per year. It is noteworthy that the WHO predicts that TBIs and road traffic accidents will be the third leading cause of death and injury worldwide by 2020 (Tabish & Syed, 2014).

TBIs are also a leading cause of death and disability for Canadians under the age of 40 years. Of those, tens of thousands of individuals will become partially or permanently disabled, and more than 11,000 Canadians will die due to complications (NBIA, 2017). Deaths attributed to head trauma tend to occur at three specific intervals or time points after injury: (i) Immediately after the injury; (ii) within 2 hours following the injury, and (iii) three weeks or longer after the initial injury often resulting from multisystem failure. It is estimated that 30% of all TBIs in Canada are suffered by children and youth, with acquired brain injury being the leading cause of death and disability among children (McGauron, 2017; NBIA, 2017). For example, in one Canadian study, hockey was linked to nearly half (44.3%) of TBIs in children aged 11 years and older due to body checking, followed by football and rugby at 13% and 5.6%, respectively (Cusimano, 2003; Ubelacher, 2013).

Individuals between the ages of 15 and 24 years experience the highest number of TBIs. Males have twice the risk of sustaining a TBI compared to females, and fourfold the chance of associated resultant death. Estimates put the brain injury rate among indigenous people at four to five times the rate of the general non-indigenous population in Canada (NBIA, 2017). Research also shows that TBIs usually requires long-term care and management, which therefore incurs high economic cost to health systems across Canada. In fact, the economic burden of acquired brain injuries and treatment, when combined, is estimated to be in excess of $12.7 billion per year in Canada alone (NBIA, 2017).

Recognition and prevention of TBIs and concussions remain a major public health challenge in Canada and internationally (Bell, Taylor, & Breiding, 2015; Hyder et al., 2007; Tabish & Syed, 2014; WHO, 2017d). Indeed, there is an old adage that "an ouch of public health prevention is worth a pound of cure" resonates loudly in regards to TBIs and concussions. Countries such as Canada need to develop public health surveillance systems and conduct epidemiologic studies to measure the impact of neurotraumas, including TBIs and concussions across the lifespan to help guide the development of more effective preventive methods (WHO, 2004, 2017b). A number of methods have already proven effective, such as the use of motorcycle helmets, head supports in vehicles and on sports equipment, and the padding of goal posts for various sports such as soccer, hockey, and football. Nonetheless, individuals who engage in certain types of contact sports (e.g., boxing, mixed martial arts, hockey, tackle football, and rugby) are at increased risk of sustaining a TBI and concussion.

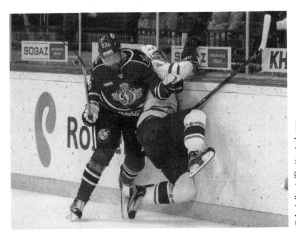

Photo 12.1: Hazards of contact sports One video-based study found that 88% of clinically diagnosed concussions in the National Hockey League (NHL) involved player-to-opponent contact (Hurtchinson, Comper, Meeuwisse, & Echemendia, 2013).

For example, a Canadian study by Goodman, Gaetz, and Meichenbaum (2001) documented various aspects of concussion in Canadian Amateur hockey including demographics, causes, treatment, and prevention. The researchers obtained detailed prospective and retrospective concussion history from British Columbia Junior Hockey League players over the course of two seasons (1998–2000). Higher rates of concussions occurred during competitive games versus practice sessions, and there was an overrepresentation of forwards injured versus defensemen or goaltenders. There was between 4.63 and 5.95 concussions per 1000 player/game hours with the average age of the first hockey-related concussion in the 15th year (Goodman et al., 2001).

Hutchinson and coworkers (2013) conducted a systematic video analysis of how concussion occurs in the National Hockey League (NHL). The researchers found that 88% ($n = 174/197$) of concussions involved player-to-opponent contact, and 16 clinically diagnosed concussions resulted from fighting. Of the 158 concussions that involved player-to-opponent body contact, the most common mechanisms were direct contact to the head initiated by the shoulder 42% ($n = 66/158$); followed by the elbow 15% ($n = 24/158$)

and by gloves in 5% of cases (*n* = 8/158). As a result of growing public concern and recognition of TBI and concussions in hockey, Hockey Canada in partnership with Parachute Canada Education (2017) has developed a *concussion card* which includes information on what a concussion is; signs and symptoms; how to respond when there is an initial loss of consciousness; concussion management, and prevention strategies.

It is noteworthy that none of the current recommendations emphasizes the importance of counselling and educating children, youth, or adults and their families who play contact sports (e.g., hockey, football, rugby) about the associated risks of returning to play and/or the option of not playing in a non–body-contact league. In our opinion, too much emphasis is placed on "when" to return to play and not enough on "whether" to return to play after a suspected TBI or concussion.

Helmets for the Prevention of TBI's and Concussions Example

The WHO (2004) recommends that member countries set an enforce helmet wearing law, and WHO data shows that almost a quarter of the victims of road traffic collisions who require admission to a hospital facility have sustained a TBI. With the emergence and growing popularity of off-road all-terrain vehicles (ATVs) and skidoos in Canada that can be driven at higher speeds, it is predicted that both injury and mortalities resulting from these motorized accidents will also increase in the years to come. Laws and legislation which mandate the use of helmets as a form of primordial prevention are effective public health strategies to significantly reduce associated fatalities and injuries. For examples, in Malaysia, the introduction of a helmet law led to a 30% reduction in motorcycle deaths; and in Italy the introduction and implementation of a law on helmet use resulted in helmet use increasing from 20% in 1999, to more than 96% in 2001 (WHO, 2004). There was also a dramatic decrease in the number of associated TBIs.

Wearing a helmet is the single most cost-effective method to reduce severe head injuries and fatalities resulting from motorcycle, ATVs, skidoo, skiing, and bicycle accidents. In fact, wearing a helmet as a primordial (e.g., mandatory legislations) and/or primary level of prevention intervention has been shown to decrease the risk and severity of injuries among motorcyclists by approximately 70%, and mortality by approximately 40% (Safe Kids Canada, 2007; Thompson, Rivara, & Thompson, 2000; WHO, 2017b).

If all cyclists wore a Canadian Safety Association (CSA)-approved helmet, it is estimated that half of deaths and numerous head injuries could be averted. For example, systematic reviews of the literature (e.g., Korkhaneh, Kalenga, Hagel, & Rowe, 2006; Macpherson & Spinks, 2008; Thompson et al., 2000) and meta-analysis (e.g., Attewell, Glase, & McFadden, 2001; Elrick, 2011) have demonstrated that helmets dramatically reduce the risk and incidence of head injuries associated with cycling. In a Cochrane-based systematic review, helmets were estimated to reduce the risk of head and brain injuries by 69%; severe brain injuries by 74%, and facial injuries by 65% with similar effects for cyclists in collisions with motor vehicles and across all age groups investigated (Attewell et al., 2011). Similarly, a meta-analysis-based study found that helmets reduced head injury risk by 60%, brain injury risk by 58%, facial injuries by 47% and fatal injury by 73% (Thompson et al., 2000).

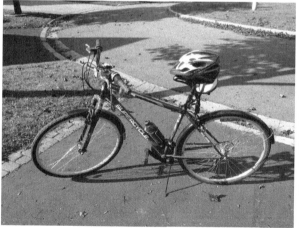

Source: Photo by Wally J. Bartfay.

Photo 12.2 Helmets help prevent serious head injuries and associated mortalities across the lifespan. Between 30% and 53% of cycling fatalities occur in children and youth, with most resulting from collisions with motor vehicles (Hagel & Yanchar, 2013). According to a Canadian study, cyclists who died of a head injury were three times as likely to not be wearing a helmet compared with those who died of other injuries (Persaud, Coleman, Zwolakowski, Lauwers, & Cass, 2012).

Based on the best available evidence and the critical importance of preventing head injuries in children and youth, the Canadian Paediatric Society has made the following recommendations (Hagel & Yanchor, 2013):

- All jurisdictions across Canada should legislate and enforce mandatory bicycle helmet use for all ages of users (children, youth, and adults).
- Legislation should be introduced via social marketing and public education campaigns related to bicycle helmet efficacy, accessibility and importance for the prevention of head injuries.
- Multi- and varied public health prevention strategies that seeks to prevent bicycling injuries should be implemented concurrently along with mandatory helmet use (e.g., separating cyclists from motor traffic with designated cycle lanes, pathways for commuting and recreational cycling, community-based safety programs).
- Healthcare professionals (e.g., physicians, nurses) should counsel families about the importance of wearing bicycle helmets.
- Where mandatory all-age legislation does not exist, parents should wear a bicycle helmet to model good behaviour and protect themselves and their children.
- Sales tax exemptions and rebates and/or federal tax credits to make the purchase of bicycle helmets less expensive should be implemented.

Parkinson's Disease

PD is the second most common neurological disease after Alzheimer's disease (detailed later) (Parkinson's Society of Canada, 2012; Wong, Gilmour, & Ramage-Morin, 2015). PD is defined as a progressive neurodegenerative disease of the CNS (basal ganglia) characterized by a constellation of clinical manifestations; which includes a slowing down in the initiation and execution of movement (akinesia and bradykinesia), increase muscle tone rigidity, mild tremors at rest, slowness of movement, and impaired and decreased balance, muscle coordination, and postural reflexes. PD is more common in men than women by a ratio of 3:2. As the disease progresses, body movements such as walking and talking are affected that was first described in a classic essay on "shaking palsy" by James Parkinson in 1817.

PD develops when there is a loss of nerve cells in the brain which produce the chemical neurotransmitter *dopamine* that transmits impulses between nerve cells in the brain to control body movements (Hickey, 2003; UBC Canada, 2017). Without enough dopamine, nerves in the brain which control muscle action do not work properly. When the loss of nerve cells reaches 80%, clinical symptoms of PD begin to manifest themselves over time as dopamine levels gradually decline. The onset of PD is insidious in nature and usually manifests unilaterally with mild symptoms, eventually progressing bilaterally.

The classic triad of symptoms of PD includes: (i) *Tremor* which is often the first symptom and is present in 70% to 100% of clients, and is often more prominent at rest and which can also be aggravated by emotional stress; (ii) *rigidity* occurs in over 90% of clients and is characterized by slow jerky movements (a.k.a., cogwheel rigidity) caused by sustained muscle contraction; and (iii) *bradykinesia* that is present in 80% to 100% of clients and involves the loss of automatic movements that become involuntary (e.g., blinking of eyelids, swinging of arms while walking, short and shuffling gait, difficulty in speaking, has difficulty with swallowing of saliva, stooped posture and masklike appearance of face, sleeping disorders) (Hickey, 2003; Tugwell, 2008; UBC Canada, 2017; Victor & Ropper, 2001; Wong et al., 2015).

Hand tremors can affect handwriting of clients with PD making it to be small and irregular in appearance. These hand tremors are often exaggerated by the resting posture; is often relieved by movements, and typically disappears during periods of sleep. Hand tremors are often described as "pill-rolling" in nature because the thumb and forefinger appear to move in a rotary fashion as if rolling a pill, coin, or other small object in the hand. In addition to the motor symptoms described above, clients often suffer from depression, anxiety, fatigue, pain, constipation, impotence, and short-term memory impairments (Aminoff, 2001; Hickey, 2003; Tugwell, 2008; Victor & Ropper, 2001). The reader is referred to the Web-Based Resource Box 12.2 for current

Web-Based Resource Box 12.2: Canadian Guidelines on Parkinson's Disease

Learning Resource	Website
Parkinson's Society of Canada (2012). Canadian guidelines on Parkinson's disease. *Canadian Journal of Neurological Sciences, 39*(Suppl. 4), S1–S30. This guide provides best-practice clinical guidelines for the diagnosis and treatment of PD in Canada.	http://www.parkinsonclinicalguidelines.ca/sites/default/files/PD_Guidelines_2012.pdf

Canadian guidelines for the management of PD that were developed with input from movement disorder specialists, functional surgery specialists, family physicians, nurses, methodologists, physiotherapists, and the Parkinson's Society Canada, as well as clients living and affected with PD.

Prevalence of PD

PD affects approximately one in every 500 people and more than 25 individuals will be diagnosed with this neurological disease each day in Canada (Parkinson's Society of Canada, 2012; UBC Canada, 2017; Wong et al., 2015). Currently, over 100,000 Canadians are living with PD, and approximately 6600 new cases are diagnosed annually (based on annual incidence of 20 new cases per 100,000 people). Most clients are diagnosed over the age of 60; however, at least 10% of the Parkinson's population develops symptoms before the age of 50. Moreover, there are an estimated 10 million people worldwide currently living with PD (Parkinson's Association of Carolinas, 2013; WHO, 2017b).

Impact of PD and Implications for Public Health

Wong et al. (2015) report that in the previous 12 months, 56% of people with PD received formal and/or informal assistance at home, work, or school because of their condition. The types of assistance most frequently reported were help with activities such as housework, home maintenance, or outdoor work (80%); emotional support (77%); transportation including trips to the doctor or for shopping (70%); and meal preparation or delivery (64%). Among those who received assistance because of PD, 84% relied at least in part on family, friends, or neighbours (Wong et al., 2015). Referred to as "informal" assistance, or caregiving, this is distinguished from "formal" assistance provided by organizations with paid or volunteer workers. Sources of assistance may be influenced by the availability of caregivers and volunteers and paid services, as well as financial resources. More than half (56%) of PD clients relied solely on informal assistance. Figure 12.3 shows the prevalence of out-of-pocket expenses in the past 12 months for individuals caring for family members with PD in Canada aged 18 years and older.

According to a study by Statistics Canada (Wong et al., 2015), main or primary caregivers looking after a client diagnosed with PD were typically females (62%) who lived in the same household (72%), and provided unpaid assistance on a daily basis (76%). For the most part, the client's spouse was the main caregiver (64%). Main caregivers who were not family members included friends and/or neighbours that tended to be younger on average (mean = 52 years, $p < .05$), and 66% of them were employed full or part-time (Wong et al., 2015). Although caregiver burden and indirect healthcare costs were not assessed in this investigation, these findings suggest that a significant amount of unpaid primary caregiving is provided by spouses, neighbours, and friends.

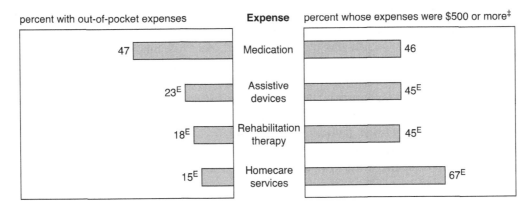

Figure 12.3 Prevalence of out-of-pocket expenses in past 12 months because of parkinson's disease, household population aged 18 or older, canada, excluding territories, 2011 Almost two-thirds (61%) of clients with PD reported out-of-pocket expenses during the past 12 months in 2011 resulting from their condition that was not reimbursed via provincial or territorial health programs (Medicare). In addition, close to half (46%) of clients who reported out-of-pocket required drug expenses indicated that these costs amounted to $500 or more.

Source: Wong et al. (2015).

Multiple Sclerosis

MS is defined as a chronic and progressive degenerative autoimmune disorder of the CNS characterized by disseminated and demyelination of nerve fibres of the brain, spinal cord, and optic nerves and inflammation and gliosis (scarring) in the CNS. The onset of MS is often insidious with vague signs and symptoms that occur intermittently over a period of months or years, and the clinical manifestations vary according to the areas of the CNS involved (Aminoff, 2001; Hickey, 2003; Multiple Sclerosis Society of Canada-National Executive Committee, 2017b; Victor & Ropper, 2001). While it is most often diagnosed in young adults aged 15 to 40 years, younger children and older adults may also be diagnosed with the disease (Multiple Sclerosis Society of Canada, 2017a). Remission or improvement in symptoms may occur with MS as a consequence of the healing process or in response to the conclusion of an acute inflammatory episode. Nonetheless, eventually the axis cylinder of the neuron may be affected, so that associated disabilities increase and become permanent in nature.

The most common diagnostic criterion for MS is the *McDonald Criteria* that makes use of recent advances in MRI techniques (Lancaster, 2010; Multiple Sclerosis International Federation [MSIF], 2013; Polman et al., 2011). Specifically, the updated 2010 McDonald Criteria calls for at least one year of demonstrated progression (done prospectively or retrospectively), plus two of the following three clinical findings on a MRI:

- Evidence of DIS in the brain, seen in at last T2 lesion in the three key brain regions (periventricular, juxtacortical or infratentorial).
- Evidence of DIS in the spinal cord, based on at least two T2 lesions DIS (≥ 2 T2 damage).
- Positive CSF involvement, again as seen in the presence of oligoclonal bands and/or a high IgG index.

However, it is critical to note that access to radiologists who can read MRI scans and/or neurologists remains a challenge in many rural and remote areas of Canada, and also in several developed and developing nations globally.

The 2013 *Atlas of MS* remains the most comprehensive compilation of MS resources for clients and healthcare professionals around the world (Browne et al., 2014).

The estimated number of people with MS has increased from 2.1 million in 2008 to 2.3 million in 2013, and the 2:1 ratio of women to men with this neurological disease has not changed significantly since 2008 (Browne et al., 2014; MSIF, 2013). The ratio of women to men with MS varies, and is considerably higher in some regions, such as East Asia where the female-to-male ratio is 3.0, and the Americas where it is 2.6. The reason for this difference in MS risk between men and women is not fully understood, and neither is the cause of the apparent increase in the ratio in many countries over recent decades, though it is likely to be caused by the interaction of changes in a range of social and environmental factors with underlying genetic differences.

Multiple Sclerosis Society of Canada has recently branded MS as "Canada's disease" based on data that the country is home to the world's highest incidence of this incurable degenerative neurological condition (Kingston, 2015). The direct cost of caring for and treating Canadians with MS is estimated at $139 million annually, with drugs accounting for approximately half of these direct costs (Kingston, 2015). Ernstsson et al. (2016) conducted a systematic review of the costs of illness associated with MS and examined 1326 peer-reviewed publications published between January 1969 and January 2014. Drugs were the main cost drivers for MS clients with low disease severity, representing 29% to 82% of all direct costs, while the main cost components for clients with more advanced MS symptoms were production (i.e., work related) losses and informal care, together representing 17% to 67% of the costs, respectively.

In many countries, MS is the leading cause of non-traumatic disability in young adults. While some people with MS experience little disability during their lifetime, as many as 60% may be unable to walk without assistance 20 years after onset (Browne et al., 2014; MSIF, 2013). This has major implications for the quality of life of clients with MS and their families and friends, and for the cost to society if their condition is not managed adequately. Despite our awareness of the considerable impact of MS, information and research related to its impact on clients' quality of life is limited. In 2005 the MSIF published *Principles to promote the quality of life of people with multiple sclerosis* (MSIF, 2005) and in 2008 the United Nations (UN) *Convention on the Rights of Persons with Disabilities* (United Nations, 2008) reaffirmed that people with disabilities have human rights and that they should enjoy them on an equal basis with other people (e.g., work settings, school, access to primary healthcare services). During the past decade, there have been initiatives across Europe, North America, and Australia/New Zealand to identify the needs of people with MS and the services and expertise required to meet those needs (Browne et al., 2014). Nonetheless, awareness and education regarding MS to combat discrimination and equity remains a global public health challenge.

The MS Society of Canada (2017b) has released a report entitled *The costs of caring: Implications for family members*, which highlights some of the challenges faced by family members in providing indirect and unpaid care to a loved one diagnosed with MS. In fact, an estimated 3 million Canadians are informal caregivers who provide care and assistance for their family members and friends who are ill, injured or have a disability (Canadian Caregiver Coalition, 2014).

> They prepare meals, do cleaning, transport and accompany loved ones to medical appointments, manage financial matters and provide both personal and specialized medical care. Caregivers contribute more than $5 billion of unpaid labour annually to the health care system and save governments millions of dollars in annual costs for hospitalization, long-term institutional care and home care (MS Society of Canada, 2017b, p. 3).

Family members, public health professionals, non-governmental organizations and all levels of governments need to work in concert to address the growing burden of neurological disorders in Canada and globally. Many Canadian family caregivers (41%) use their personal savings to weather financial hardships associated with looking after a family member at home, and spend between $100 to $300 extra per month on expenses directly related to their caregiver responsibilities (The Canadian Caregiver Coalition, 2014). The Canadian Caregiver Coalition (2014) released a pan-Canadian strategy with the following five essential actions and recommendations to support family caregivers:

1. Safeguard the health and well-being of family caregivers.
2. Minimize the financial burden placed on family caregivers.
3. Enable access to user friendly information and education.
4. Create flexible workplace/educational environments that respect caregiving obligations.
5. Invest in research on family caregiving as a foundation for evidence-informed decision making.

These recommendations not only apply to caregivers looking after family members with neurological disorders, but all disorders, injuries, and disabilities facing Canadians across the lifespan.

Web-Based Resource Box 12.3: Additional Resources Related to MS

Learning Resources	Web-Based Links
Multiple Sclerosis International Federation (MSIF) (2005). *Principles to promote the quality of life of people with multiple sclerosis. London, UK: Author.* - This document provides the reader with an overview of current issues and challenges faced by clients with MS in terms of discrimination, equity, and quality of life issues from an international perspective.	http://www.msif.org/about-ms/publications-and-resources/
Multiple Sclerosis International Federation (MSIF). (2013). *Atlas of multiple sclerosis 2013: Mapping multiple sclerosis around the world.* **London, UK: Author.** - This report provides information about current diagnostic challenges, quality of life issues, and the prevalence of MS from a global perspective.	http://www.msif.org/wp-content/uploads/2014/09/Atlas-of-MS.pdf
Multiple Sclerosis Society of Canada. **Resources for clients.** - This website provides various links to support services across Canada including telephone and Internet-based peer support programs, access to MS drug reimbursement programs, day away programs, and various advocacy and educational programs.	https://mssociety.ca/support-services/programs-and-services
Multiple Sclerosis Society of Canada-National Executive Committee. (2017b, October 23). *The costs of caring: Implications for family caregivers.* **Quebec: Author.** - This report provides an overview of the indirect costs of looking after an individual with MS by a family member or friend, and makes several recommendations and how to improve healthcare services and information.	https://mssociety.ca/en/pdf/socact_caregiver-pospaper-feb08-EN.pdf

Amyotrophic Lateral Sclerosis

Amyotrophic lateral sclerosis (ALS), also known as *Lou Gehrig's disease,* is defined as a progressive motor neuron disease that involves both the upper and lower motor neurons and is characterized by wasting of the muscles of the body resulting from the destruction of motor neurons in the brain stem and anterior gray horns of the spinal cord and degeneration of the pyramidal tracts. ALS is a progressive disease that eventually leads to death resulting from respiratory arrest for the affected client. Sensory changes are not part of the disease and intellect may remain unaffected, although muscles become progressively weaker and atrophy; whereas spasticity and hyperreflexia are common in other clients (Aminoff, 2001; Hickey, 2003; Victor & Ropper, 2001). The exact aetiology of the disease is not known (90% to 95%) and most cases are therefore "sporadic in nature" with no known specific cause. Approximately 5% to 10% of cases are inherited as an autosomal dominant trait termed "familial ALS." Regardless of whether a client has the sporadic- or familial-type ALS, 30% of all clients have a form referred to as "Bulbar ALS" (ALS Canada, 2017). In the early stages of Bulbar ALS, the motor neurons in the corticobulbar area of the brainstem are the first affected. This means that the muscles of the head, face, and neck become paralyzed before muscles in other parts of the body. Men tend to be more affected than women and the typical onset is between 40 and 80 years of age.

There is no cure for this fatal disease, and the lifetime risk of developing ALS is approximately 1:1000 (ALS Canada, 2017; Aminoff, 2001; Hickey, 2003; Victor & Ropper, 2001). ALS became a household name in North America during the 20th century when it affected the professional baseball player Lou Gehrig, and later internationally in 1963 when it affected Stephen Hawkins. In 2014, videos of the "Ice Bucket Challenge" went viral on the Internet and also helped to increased public awareness of this disease globally. Approximately 80%

of clients with ALS die within 3 to 5 years after being diagnosed; however, there are notable exceptions including the renowned theoretical physicists Professor Stephen Hawkins who continued his work on black holes and cosmology at Cambridge University in England, until his death at age 76 on March 14, 2018. Hawking spent 30 years as a full professor of mathematics at the University of Cambridge, and was director of research at the school's Centre for Theoretical Cosmology. Professor Hawkins' ashes were buried in "*Scientists Corner*" located in Westminster Abbey in London, England on March 31, 2018.

Currently, approximately 3000 Canadians are living with ALS, and more than 200,000 people around the world are living with motor neuron disease (ALS Canada, 2017). Chio and coworkers conducted a systematic review of peer-reviewed articles that examined quantitative data from population-based studies on ALS incidence and prevalence rates for the years 1995 to 2014 inclusive. The median (IQR) incidence rate (per 100,000 population) was 2.08 (1.47–2.43), corresponding to an estimated 15,355 (10,852–17,938) cases. Median (IQR) prevalence (per 100,000 population) was 5.40 (4.06–7.89), or 39,863 (29,971–58,244) prevalent cases (Chio et al., 2013).

The number of ALS cases across the globe will increase from 222,801 in 2015 to 376,674 in 2040, representing an alarming increase of 69% (Arthur et al., 2016). This predicted increase is predominantly due to ageing populations internationally, particularly among developing nations, and is likely an underestimate. This ageing pattern is especially significant in developing countries, where the proportion of older individuals will increase from about 9% in 2015 to 16% by 2040 (Arthur et al., 2016; United Nations, 2013).

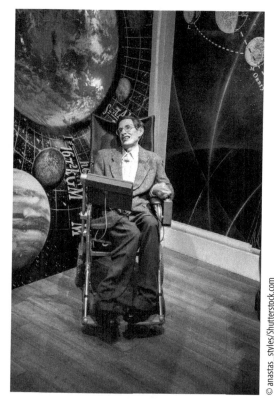

Photo 12.3 Wax figure of Professor Stephen Hawkins in Madame Tussard's Wax Museum in London, England. Professor Hawkins was diagnosed with ALS at the age of 21 and has defined all odds for his prognosis made by his neurologists living until his death at the age of 76 years (Harmon, 2012; McCoy, 2015). Available at https://www .Shutterstock.com/image-photo/london-england-april-2017-stephen-hawking-723919972?src=W4 YfotHJuCI1LXmpRqtlhw-1-36

Myasthenia Gravis

Myasthenia gravis (MG) is defined as a chronic disease of the neuromuscular junction in which an autoimmune process slowly destroys acetylcholine (ACh) receptors at the postsynaptic muscle, and is characterized by fatigability and fluctuating muscle weakness of selected voluntary muscle distribution, especially those innervated by motor nuclei of the brain stem (e.g., extraocular, mastication, facial, swallowing, and speech). Weakness in clients with MG tends to increase with repeated activity, but improves somewhat with rest (Myasthenia Gravis Society of Canada, 2017).

Carr and coworkers conducted a systemic review comprised of 55 peer-reviewed population-based MG epidemiological studies performed between 1950 and 2007, representing 1.7 billion population-years. The estimated pooled incidence rate was 5.3 per million person-years (CI: 4.4, 6.1), with a range of 1.7 to 21.3; and the estimated pooled prevalence rate was 77.7 per million persons (CI: 64.0, 94.3), with a range of 15 to 179. Early clinical findings upon assessment include ptosis and diplopia involving the levator palpebrae and extraocular muscles (Aminoff, 2001; Hickey, 2003; Victor & Ropper, 2001). The next muscles that tend to be affected include the facial, masticator, speech and neck muscles of affected clients. Hence, clients may be at increased risk of aspiration due to problems in managing saliva and/or difficulty with swallowing. There is no cure for MG currently available. The onset of MG is typically gradual in nature, although rapid onsets have been reported in concert with respiratory infections and/or emotional stress.

Huntington's Disease

Huntington's disease (HD) is defined as a genetically transmitted autosomal dominant disorder that affects both men and women equally, and is characterized by chronic, devastating loss of all neurological functions resulting in dementia. We shall examine the various forms of dementia in greater detail later. HD causes cells in parts of the brain to die including the caudate, putamen, and cerebral cortex as the disease progresses. As the brain cells die, a client with HD becomes less able to control movements, recall events, make decisions, and control their emotions (Huntington's Society of Canada, 2016).

In fact, the offspring of a parent diagnosed with HD has a 50% risk of inheriting this genetic disorder (Aminoff, 2001; Victor & Ropper, 2013). Since 1986, genetic testing for HD has been available in Canada; however, a direct test for the disease was developed in 1993. This means individuals who are at-risk for developing HD, or who believe they have the symptoms, can take a simple blood test to determine whether they have the gene that causes HD. The onset of HD typically occurs between the ages of 30 to 50 years, yet the range can be from two to 80 years. Approximately one in every 10,000 Canadians has HD; approximately five in every 10,000 individuals are at risk of developing HD, and individuals with European ancestry tend to have a higher incidence of the disease (Huntington's Disease Society of Canada, 2016). Fisher and Hayden (2014) estimated the prevalence of HD at 13.7 per 100,000 (95% CI: 12.6–14.8 per 100,000) in the general Canadian population, and 17.2 per 100,000 (95% CI: 15.8–18.6 per 100,000) in the Caucasian population.

Dementia and Alzheimer's Disease

Dementia is defined as a chronic and often progressive neurological disorder that results in a deterioration of mental processes; and is clinically characterized by memory disorders, personality and behavioural changes, emotional and mood disturbances, and impaired cognition, concentration, judgment, and/or reasoning. Dementia is caused by a variety of diseases and injuries that affect the brain (Alzheimer's Society of Canada, 2010, 2017a, 2017b; Chapman, Marshale Williams, Strine, Andra, & Moore, 2006; Wong, Gilmour, & Ramage-Morin, 2016). In addition to impaired memory, dementia often affects the client's ability to effectively communicate, carryout purposeful movements and other ADL. It is critical to note that there is currently no cure for dementia and that it is not part of the normal ageing process per se (Alzheimer's Society of Canada, 2010, 2017a, 2017b; Smetanin et al., 2011). Dementia is irreversible when caused by degenerative disease or trauma, but might be reversible in some cases when caused by drugs, alcohol, metabolic conditions, hormone or vitamin imbalances, and/or depression. Nonetheless, potentially reversible dementias are extremely rare, accounting for less than 1% of clients presenting with dementia-related signs and symptoms (Chapman et al., 2006; Clarfield, 2003; Hejl, Hogh, & Waldermar, 2002; Walstra, Teunisse, van Gool, & van Crevel, 2002). Table 12.3 provides a brief overview of the major types of dementia, a brief description of their aetiology and pathology, and prevalence rate estimates (Aminoff, 2001; Chapman et al., 2006; Hickey, 2003; Victor & Ropper, 2001; Zekry, Hauw & Gold, 2002).

Dementia is the most common type of neurodegenerative disorder globally. In 2010, an estimated 35.6 million people worldwide were living with dementia, and that number is expected to double in 20 years (Chambers, Bancej, & McDowell, 2016; WHO, 2017b). In fact, it is estimated that there are globally 47.5 million people with dementia with 7.7 million new cases diagnosed every year, and Alzheimer's disease is the most common cause of dementia and may contribute to 60% to 70% of cases (WHO, 2016). The Alzheimer's Society of Canada (2010) report entitled "Rising tide: The impact of dementia in Canada" notes that approximately 500,000 individuals have dementia; every year about 104,000 acquire dementia, and Alzheimer's disease accounts for approximately 50% of new cases of dementia diagnosed for Canadians aged 65 years and older. Moreover, by 2038, over 1.1 million Canadians will have dementia, and more than 257 new cases of dementia will be diagnosed each year.

Current demographic ageing trends in Canada and globally suggest that the costs associated with caring for clients living with dementia and their caregivers will increase rapidly unless there are significant reductions in the incidence of dementia (Alzheimer's Society of Canada, 2017a, 2017b; Chambers et al., 2016; WHO, 2016, 2017b).

Table 12.3 Major Types of Dementia

Major Types	Brief Description	Prevalence Estimates
Alzheimer's Disease (AD)	The most common form of dementia that was first described by the German psychiatrist Alois Alzheimer in 1907 while treating a 55-year-old female client. AD is a chronic and progressive degenerative disease of the brain. Characteristic findings are related to brain structure and function and include: (i) Amyloid plaques; (ii) neurofibrillary tangles, and (iii) loss of connections between cells and cells death. Age is the most critical risk factor as only a small percentage of clients develop AD prior to the age of 60 years.	50%–80% of all cases
Vascular Dementia (VD)	VD is the second most common form of dementia. Results from ischemic, ischemic-hypoxic, or hemorrhagic brain damage caused by cardiovascular disease, which results in reduced blood and oxygen supply to the brain or via a blockage. May result from a single stroke (infarct) or multiple strokes.	20%
Dementia with Lewy Bodies (DLB)	DLB has features of both AD and Parkinson's disease (PD) and there are no known risk factors. Associated with the presence of Lewy Bodies (i.e., deposits of alpha-synuclein protein) in the brain which are abnormal brainstem, amygdala, and/or cortex.	15%
Parkinson's Disease related Dementia (PdD)	The key brain changes linked to PD and PdD are abnormal microscopic deposits composed chiefly of alpha-synuclein, a protein that is found widely in the brain but whose normal function is not yet known. These deposits are called Lewy bodies. The average time from onset of Parkinson's to developing PdD is approximately 10 years, and it is estimated that 50%–80% of clients with PD eventually experience and develop PdD.	2%–5%
Frontotemporal Dementia or Pick's disease	Characterized by degeneration of the frontal lobe, temporal lobe, or both where nerve cells die due to abnormal accumulation of proteins in the neurons including tau proteins, TDP-43 and ubiquitin. Tends to strike at a younger age typically between the ages of 50 and 60 years.	2%–5%
Creutzfeldt-Jakob Disease (CJD) related Dementia	A rare but fatal infectious brain disorder though to be caused by the accumulation of abnormally folded proteins called "prions." More than 50 variations of CJD have been identified, and all of these mutations can have very different symptoms. There are three major types of CJD are: (i) Sporadic; (ii) hereditary; and (iii) acquired. No diagnostic test or treatment for CJD is currently available and only autopsy and examination of brain tissue can confirm diagnosis.	Extremely rare (1 per 1 million people per year globally)
Mixed or multifactorial dementias	Mixed dementia is a condition in which abnormalities characteristic of more than one type of dementia occur simultaneously in the brain. In the most common form of mixed dementia, the abnormal protein deposits associated with AD coexist with blood vessel problems linked to VD. Alzheimer's brain changes also often coexist with Lewy bodies, the abnormal protein deposits characteristic of dementia with Lewy bodies and PdD.	Unknown

Note: Prevalence rates are approximations based on commonly reported published ranges, and therefore may not add up to 100% (Aminoff, 2001; Chapman et al., 2006; Hickey, 2003; Victor & Ropper, 2001; Zekry et al., 2002).

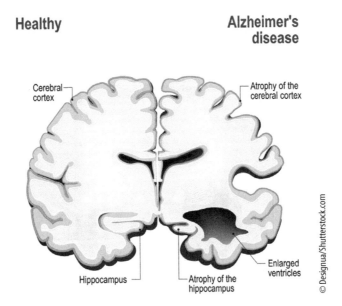

Healthy   Alzheimer's
                                           disease

Cerebral cortex   Atrophy of the cerebral cortex

Hippocampus   Atrophy of the hippocampus
                                           Enlarged ventricles

© Designua/Shutterstock.com

Figure 12.4 Cross-section comparisons of a healthy brain versus a client with alzheimer's disease Alzheimer's disease is an incurable and progressive neurological disorder and the leading type of dementia which affects approximately 500,000 Canadians. Every year about 104,000 new cases of dementia will be diagnosed in Canada (Alzheimer's Society of Canada, 2010).

The Alzheimer's Society of Canada (2010) *Rising Tide* report makes the following recommendations to address this growing public health issue:

1. Accelerated investment in all areas of dementia research.
2. A clear recognition of the important role played by informal caregivers.
3. Increased recognition of the importance of prevention and early intervention.
4. Greater integration of care and increased use of chronic disease prevention, and management.
5. Strengthening of Canada's dementia workforce.

Direct and Indirect Health Care Costs Associated With Dementia

Dementia is a disease that disrupts all aspects of personal, social, and family life. Individuals caring for loved ones with dementia frequently describe this as being very disruptive and distressful in nature. Indeed, caregivers are affected on various dimensions including reversed family roles (e.g., child caring for parent), have personal health deterioration themselves, work and/or career disruptions, financial constraints (e.g., hiring a personal care worker), and social disruptions. Support groups for caregivers and family members help to provide critical emotional support and information about dementia and related topics (e.g., safety concerns, legal issues such as power of attorney), and are often facilitated by nurses, social workers, and/or occupational therapists in community settings. The Alzheimer's Society of Canada, for example, has many educational and support systems available to help caregivers look after loved ones in their communities.

Figure 12.5 shows the estimated and projected direct costs associated with caring for clients diagnosed with Alzheimer's disease and other dementias of both sexes combined for years 2011, 2021, and 2031 (Fines, 2010). It is predicted that the direct healthcare costs associated with Alzheimer's disease and other dementias will reach $10.9 billion by the years 2021 to 2022, and will reach a staggering $15.8 billion by the years 2031 to 2032, which suggests an impending public health crisis on the horizon especially given ageing population trends in Canada.

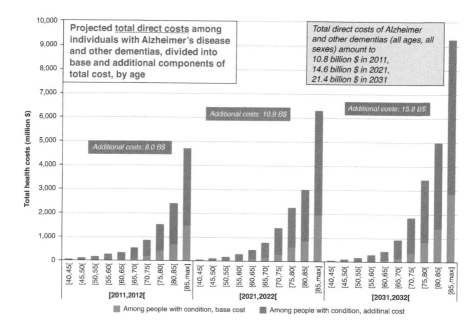

Figure 12.5 Estimated and projected costs of caring for clients diagnosed with alzheimer's disease and other dementias, both sexes combined for years 2011, 2021, and 2031 Note the estimated costs are for publicly funded (i.e., tax-based) healthcare (Medicare) systems in Canada only, and do not include out-of-pocket costs and/or informal caregiver costs often provided by family members of clients with AD and other dementias.

Source: Fines (2010, May 28).

The Alzheimer's Society of Canada (2017a, 2017b) reports that there are 25,000 new cases of dementia diagnosed each year; 564,000 are currently living with dementia and this number is predicted to increase to over 937,000 in the next 15 years, and the associated indirect costs to care for individuals with dementia is $10.4 billion annually or five and one-half times greater than for those who are dementia-free. In Canada, the total healthcare system costs and out-of-pocket costs of caring for people with dementia were $10.4 billion in 2016, and is projected to double by 2031 (Alzheimer's Society of Canada, 2010, 2017a, 2017b; Chambers et al., 2016). By 2038, the Alzheimer's Society of Canada (2010) predicts that total direct healthcare costs associated with managing dementia will surpass $152 billion annually.

Figure 12.6 shows the percentage of individuals in Canada with dementia receiving informal assistance, by type of care, for household populations aged 45 years or older in 2011 (Wong et al., 2016). It is important to note that clients living with dementia often have other health conditions that could increase their need for assistance and make caring for them more complex. For example, in 2011, 6% of the general population without dementia reported having incontinence; whereas the likelihood of a client with dementia having incontinence was 10-fold higher. Age also contributes to these noted differences. As noted in Figure 12.6, the burden of care provided by informal caregivers in Canada in 2011 alone were quite substantial, and as our population continues to age, so will the associated burden of informal caregiving.

In addition to the above, the estimated 19.2 million hours of informal unpaid caregiver time occurred in 2011 (conservatively valued at $1.2 billion), and this number is projected to double by 2031 due largely to our ageing population in Canada (Chambers et al., 2016). Indeed, the costs for caring for clients with dementia are estimated to be 5.5 times greater than those who are dementia free. *Formal* assistance to individuals with dementia is provided by organizations with paid or volunteer workers; whereas *informal* assistance, or caregiving, is provided by family (typically a daughter), friends, or neighbours (Chambers et al., 2016).

Statistics Canada reports that among clients diagnosed with dementia nationally, 85% relied, at least in part, on family, friends, or neighbours for assistance of which 43% also received some formal assistance, and the remaining 41% relied solely on informal assistance to manage their ADL (Wong et al., 2016). An additional 15% of clients in need received neither formal nor informal assistance.

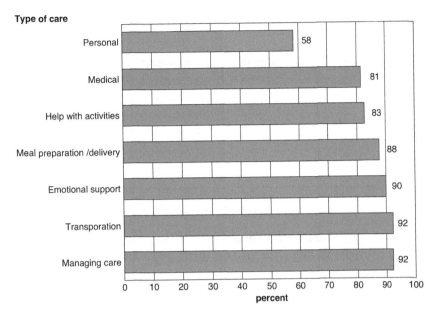

Figure 12.6 Percentage with dementia receiving informal assistance, by type of care, household population aged 45 years or older, Canada excluding territories, 2011 Among people with at least one of the chronic conditions, those with dementia were, on average, almost 15 years older than those without dementia (i.e., 79 vs. 65). When age was taken into account, clients with dementia were significantly more likely to also have heart disease, a mood disorder, or incontinence (data not shown) (Wong et al., 2016).

Source: Wong et al. (2016).

The Alzheimer's Society of Canada (2010) *Rising Tide* report predicts that by 2038, 1,125,200 Canadians will have some form of dementia; the cumulative economic burden will be in excess of $872 billion, and the need and demand for long-term care for these clients will increase 10-fold. The reader is also referred to Chapter 6, Table 6.4 which details the predicted annual total economic burden attributed to dementia for the years 2008, 2018, 2028, and 2038 in terms of: (i) direct costs (e.g., includes costs of prescription medications, hospital and physician costs, and long-term care); (ii) total unpaid caregiver opportunity costs (i.e., lost wages that could have been earned by informal caregivers in the labour force); (iii) total indirect costs (e.g., lost wages and corporate profits); and (iv) total economic burden estimates (Alzheimer's Society of Canada, 2010).

Providing community-based interventions for clients with dementia and their caregivers is imperative to maintaining one's quality of life (QOL), and for decreasing associated burden of care and direct and indirect healthcare costs (Bartfay & Bartfay, 2015). For example, Bartfay and Bartfay (2013) employed a cross-sectional comparative design study to examine how community-based adult day programs for family members were benefiting QOL measures in 62 female self-identified primary caregivers with family members diagnosed with Alzheimer's disease. The study was comparative in nature because a control group comprised of individuals without Alzheimer's disease or dementia was used to assess QOL measures, in comparison to primary caregivers looking after loved ones with Alzheimer's disease. Caregivers were recruited at 5 community-based adult day programs in the Durham Region of Ontario, and primary data collection consisted of a self-report questionnaire administered to both primary caregivers and controls along with a 13-item QOL scale. The findings suggest that primary caregivers of clients with Alzheimer's disease who utilize and access community-based adult day programs enjoy similar QOL levels, in comparison to controls. Hence, community-based interventions such as adult day programs and caregiver support groups may be beneficial in maintaining and promoting the QOL of primary caregivers of clients with dementia (Bartfay & Bartfay, 2013, 2015). The reader is also referred to the Research Focus Box 12.2 that describes the development of a novel telehealth videoconferencing approach to provide critically needed support for rural caregivers of spouses with atypical early-onset forms of dementia.

Web-Based Resources Box 12.4 ACHA NCHA Canadian Reference Group II Report

Learning Resource	Website
ACHA NCHA II): Canadian Reference Group (2016 Spring). Data Report	http://www.acha-ncha.org/docs/NCHA-II%20 SPRING%202016%20CANADIAN%20REFERENCE%20 GROUP%20DATA%20REPORT.pdf

---

Research Focus Box 12.2

Development and Evaluation of a Telehealth Videoconferenced Support Group for Rural Spouses of Individuals Diagnosed with Atypical Early-Onset Dementias

Study Aim/Rationale

To describe the development and examine the effectiveness of a telehealth videoconferencing support system to provide support for a group of rural primary caregivers of spouses with atypical and early-onset form of dementia, with specific emphasis on frontotemporal dementia (FTD) during mid-life. Clients with FTD often present with several behavioural challenges including aggression, impulsiveness, disinhibition and other forms of socially inappropriate behaviours. Primary caregivers of these clients often experience high degrees of stress resulting from these behaviours. In addition, rural clients are often faced with additional stressors including geographical isolation with little or no formal mental health services and financial hardships.

Methodology/Design

The researchers employed a qualitative methodology to evaluate the effectiveness of a telehealth videoconferencing support system for primary caregivers in Saskatchewan. All participants in this investigation were family members who were referred to a Rural and Remote Memory Clinic (RRMC) at the University of Saskatchewan for dementia diagnosis and follow-up care. The specific intervention consisted of monthly telehealth videoconferenced support group sessions of 90 min each. These support group sessions were co-facilitated by two members of neuropsychological team at the urban centre of the RRMC in Saskatchewan. Qualitative data collection occurred after a time period of 18 months at an in-person retreat comprised of nine group members. The qualitative data was subsequently coded and thematically analyzed.

Major Findings

Although the sample size was limited in nature, this qualitative study provides preliminary evidence in support of the use of telehealth videoconferenced sessions for spouses who were primary caregivers of clients living with atypical forms of dementia in rural and remote areas of Saskatchewan. The RRMC effectively provided access to mental health support services across a large geographical area through the use of telehealth services, and decreased needed travel for group members by 262 to 532 km per session.

Implications for Public Health

These findings support the use of telehealth videoconferencing sessions to provide cost-effective mental health services to clients living in rural and remote regions of Canada. Telehealth also appears to be an effective means to decrease the costs associated with travel to these rural and remote areas in Canada. Additional noted benefits included the open structure of the group, flexibility due to the lack of preplanned artificial agenda, and sharing of similar experiences between group members and what worked for them in providing care.

Source: O'Connell et al. (2013).

Future Directions and Challenges

We have attempted to highlight some of the most common neurological injuries and diseases encountered in Canada and globally; however, we acknowledge that there are many other disorders that are too numerous to cover within the limits of a single chapter. Nonetheless, a common thread for all conditions discussed is that client and family education and community-based supports are critical for the navigation and management of their conditions, and to prevent caregiver stress and burnout. It is critical to note that although there may be no cures available for many of the disorders highlighted, public healthcare professionals and workers play a critical role in helping to maintain and preserve independence and quality of life for the affected client and their family at each stage of the illness journey.

To increase the awareness of public health professionals and workers about the public health aspects of caring for individuals with neurological disorders, and to emphasize the need for the prevention of these disorders and the necessity to provide neurological care at all levels of the primary healthcare model, WHO launched a number of international public health projects in 1993, including the *Global Initiative on Neurology and Public Health* (Janca, Pricipko, & Costa e-Silva, 1997; WHO, 2017b). The outcome of this global collaborative endeavor revealed a paucity of information about the prevalence and burden of neurological disorders and a lack of policies, programs, and resources for their associated treatments and management (Janca et al., 1997; WHO, 2017b).

In Canada, a 2007 report released by the Canadian Institute for Health Information (CIHI); the Canadian Neurological Sciences Federation (CNSF), and the Canadian Brain and Nerve Health Coalition (CBANHC) entitled *The burden of neurological diseases, disorders and injuries in Canada* echoed the call by the WHO for collective public health action and initiatives on neurological conditions (CIHI, 2007). In Canada, neurological disorders are currently estimated to affect 3.6 million Canadians living in their respective communities and a further 170,000 Canadians living in long-term care facilities (Public Health Agency of Canada, 2014). A four-year study conducted by the PHAC (2014) entitled *Mapping connections: On understanding of neurological conditions in Canada* highlighted the fact that prevalence and incidence of some of the most common neurological conditions tend to increase with age, and that both the number of individuals facing these challenges and the healthcare cost are expected to rise dramatically as the Canadian population ages. Indeed, over a 20-year period from 2011 to 2031, the Canadian population is projected to grow by an estimated 40 million people. Along with this growth in population, it is predicted that both the prevalence and associated healthcare costs for managing neurological disorders in Canada will also increase dramatically as highlighted in Figure 12.7.

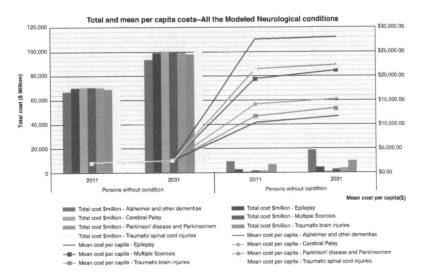

Figure 12.7 Projected health care costs associated with neurological conditions in Canada for 2011 and 2031 Note the estimated costs are for publicly funded (i.e., tax-based) healthcare (Medicare) systems in Canada only, and do not include out-of-pocket costs and/or informal caregiver costs often provided by family members of clients with neurological disorders.

Source: Fines (2010, May 28).

Group Review Exercise Box

Alive Inside: A Story of Music and Memory

Overview of This Investigative Documentary

This documentary won the Audience Award at the 2014 Sundance Film Festival and chronicles the power of personalized music therapy with various clients in long-term nursing homes with various forms of advanced dementia and Alzheimer's disease. Dan Cohen is a social worker by profession and the founder of the non-profit organization *Music & Memory*. Mr. Cohen seeks to challenge a so-called "broken health-care system" in the United States by demonstrating music's ability to combat memory loss and restore a deep sense of self to clients suffering from it. In this documentary, Rossato-Bennett visits family members in long-term care facilities and records the immediate and positive effects of personalized music on clients diagnosed with various forms of advanced dementia. Since music is stored in many areas of the brain and is a basic part of several human life experiences (e.g., weddings, first loves, various holiday events), employing music therapy via an iPod that consists a personalized playlist may help reach and engage clients with dementia even as memory continues to fail. This documentary highlights how music therapy may help to improve communication and increase overall quality of life for clients with dementia residing in long-term care facilities in their community.

Instructions

This assignment may be done alone, in pairs, or in groups of up to five people (note: if you are doing this assignment in pairs or groups, please submit only one hard or electronic copy as requested by your instructor). The assignment should be type-written and between four and six pages maximum in length (double-spaced please). View and take notes on the documentary entitled "Alive Inside: A Story of Music and Memory." See links: https://www.youtube.com/watch?v=8HLEr-zP3fc or https://www.youtube.com/watch?v=Hlm0Qd-4mP-I or http://www.aliveinside.us/

1. Briefly highlight the benefits of music therapy described by recreational therapists Yvonne Russel and neurologists Oliver Sacks in this documentary.

2. Henry is one of the clients in a long-term nursing home highlighted in the documentary. Briefly describe Henry's typical demeanor prior to receiving personalized music therapy via an IPod device, during music therapy and immediately after.

3. Based on the results highlighted in this documentary, how can personalized music therapy be utilized to benefit clients with dementia in both home settings and residential care facilities in your community?

The distribution of risk factors in a population has major implications for public health strategies related to the various levels of prevention. The reader is referred to Chapter 1 for a detailed discussion on the five levels of prevention. Indeed, a large number of individuals exposed to a small risk may generate several more cases of a specific neurological disorder or disease than a small number exposed to a known high-risk factor. Consequently, a public health preventative strategy or campaign that focuses only on high-risk individuals will deal only with the surface or "tip-of-the-iceberg" for the problem, and will not have any impact on major amounts of the neurological disorder or disease occurring in the large proportion of people who are at low-to-moderate risk. In contrast, we argue that population and community-based strategies and policies that seek to shift the whole distribution of identified risk factors have the potential to control the incidence of a neurological disorder on a macro-level (e.g., wearing bicycle helmets, banning body checking for youth in hockey).

We further argue that simple prevalence estimates derived from health administrative, hospital, and/or other chart-based or electronic data sources are often not based on standardized clinical neurological assessments and may therefore underestimate the true prevalence of neurological disorders in population-based studies.

Furthermore, autopsies on suspected cases with neurological disorders are seldom performed although this is often a superior method for confirming a clinical diagnosis. There is a need to provide robust benchmarks against which future trends and needs assessments can be conducted for both formal and informal healthcare services planning in Canada. Current demographic ageing trends in Canada and globally suggest that the costs associated with caring for clients living with neurological disorders and their caregivers will increase rapidly unless there are significant reductions in their incidence (Chapman et al., 2006; PHAC, 2014; WHO, 2017b). While there is unavoidable uncertainty in estimating and projecting these direct and indirect costs, we argue that informal caregiving should also be formally documented and counted as part of the robust public healthcare costs and burden associated with managing neurological disorders in Canada. Lastly, efforts to foster increased public recognition and decreased stigma associated with neurological disorders and disease, along with their prevention and management where possible, are emerging as increasingly important facets of public health in Canada and globally (Chapman et al., 2006; PHAC, 2016; WHO, 2017b).

Summary

- Neurological disorders of the central and peripheral nervous system include the brain, spinal cord, cranial nerves, peripheral nerves, nerve roots, ANS, neuromuscular junction, and muscles.
- A growing burden of neurological disorders is reaching a significant proportion of countries now with a growing percentage of older individuals affected who are aged 65 years and older.
- Mortalities due to dementias alone have more than doubled between 2000 and 2015, making it the seventh leading cause of death globally in 2015.
- The human nervous system is a highly complex and specialized system responsible for the control and integration of the body's many functions and activities, and consists of the CNS and PNS.
- Adult brain is composed of approximately 40% gray matter and 60% white matter, and weighs between 1300 and 1400 g on average.
- PNS consists of cranial nerves III through XII, the spinal nerves, their associated ganglia (groupings of cell bodies) and the peripheral components of the ANS.
- ANS is divided into sympathetic and parasympathetic components, which control various body functions and responses.
- TBI is a heterogeneous condition in terms of its aetiology, severity, and outcomes.
- There are three generally acknowledged levels of severity for TBIs that is assessed via the Glascow Coma Scale (GCS): (i) Mild (GCS = 13–15); (ii) moderate (GCS = 9–12); and (iii) severe (GCS = 3–8).
- PD is the second most common neurological disease after AD and affects approximately one in every 500 people and more than 25 individuals will be diagnosed with this neurological disease each day in Canada.
- Canada has the highest rates of MS in the world at 291 cases per 100,000 people.
- Direct cost of caring for and treating Canadians with MS is estimated at $139 million annually, with drugs accounting for approximately half of these costs.
- ALS is a progressive disease that leads to death resulting from respiratory arrest.
- Approximately 3000 Canadians are living with ALS, and more than 200,000 people around the world are living with motor neuron disease.
- MG is a chronic disease of the neuromuscular junction in which an autoimmune process slowly destroys ACh receptors at the postsynaptic muscle, and is characterized by fatigability and fluctuating muscle weakness of selected voluntary muscle distribution.
- HD is a genetically transmitted autosomal dominant disorder that affects both men and women equally, and is characterized by chronic, devastating loss of all neurological functions resulting in dementia.

- Dementia is the most common type of neurodegenerative disorder globally, and is caused by a variety of diseases and injuries that affect the brain.
- The Alzheimer's Society of Canada (2010) *Rising Tide* report predicts that by 2038, 1,125,200 Canadians will have some form of dementia; the cumulative economic burden will be in excess of $872 billion, and the need and demand for long-term care for these clients will increase 10-fold.
- Providing community-based interventions for clients with neurological disorders and diseases and their caregivers is imperative to maintaining one's QOL and decreasing associated burden of care and healthcare costs.

Critical Thinking Questions

Mrs Hickell is a 65-year old recently retired school teacher who reports increased difficulty with speech and swallowing and has lost 10 kg in the past year. She has developed a "pill rolling" motion and tremor in her both hands that are present at rest and has been suffering from constipation over the past week. Moreover, Mrs Hickell encounters "cogwheel rigidity" during passive range of motion exercises performed by a visiting public health nurse. Her husband informs the nurse that a neurologist has recently diagnosed Mrs Hickell with PD, and that he is worried that she may fall while climbing stairs in their home.

1. What is the pathogenesis of PD?
2. Based on the presenting signs and symptoms and concerns expressed by Mrs Hickell's husband, what are the major priorities and why? What would you suggest that Mr Hickell do to help make his home safer and help manage her constipation? Justify your answers.
3. What community-based services and/or resources are available in your community to help clients and their loved ones diagnosed with PD?

References

ALS Canada. (2017). *What is ALS?* Toronto, ON: Author. Retrieved from https://www.als.ca/about-als/what-is-als/

Alzheimer's Society of Canada. (2010). *Rising tide: The impact of dementia on Canadian society.* Toronto, ON: Author. ISBN: 978-0-9733522-21. Retrieved from http://www.alzheimer.ca/sites/default/files/files/national/advocacy/asc_rising_tide_full_report_e.pdf; http://www.alzheimer.ca/en/suroit/Get-involved/Advocacy/Latest-info-stats/Rising-Tide

Alzheimer's Society of Canada. (2017a). *Dementia numbers in Canada.* Toronto, ON: Author. Retrieved from http://www.alzheimer.ca/en/about-dementia/what-is-dementia/dementia-numbers

Alzheimer's Society of Canada. (2017b). *What is dementia?* Toronto, ON: Author. Retrieved from http://www.alzheimer.ca/en/Home/About-dementia/What-is-dementia

Aminoff, M. J. (2001). *Neurology and general medicine* (3rd ed.). New York, NY: Churchill Livingstone.

Arthur, K. C., Caluo, A., Price, T. R., Geiger, J. T., Chio, A., & Traynor, B. J. (2016). Projected increased in amyotrophic lateral sclerosis from 2015 to 2040. *Nature Communications, 7* (article No. 12408). Retrieved from https://www.nature.com/articles/ncomms12408

Attewell, R. G., Glase, K., & McFadden, M. (2001, May). Bicycle helmet efficacy: A meta-analysis. *Accident Analysis and Prevention, 33*(3), 345–352. Retrieved from https://www.ncbi.nlm.nih.gov/pubmed/11235796

Bartfay, E., & Bartfay, W. J. (2013, January). Quality of life outcomes among Alzheimer's disease family caregivers following community-based interventions. *Western Journal of Nursing Research, 35*(1), 98–116. doi:10.1177/0103945911400763

Bartfay, E., Bartfay, W. J., & Gorey, K. M. (2016, January). Dementia care in Ontario, Canada: Evidence of more timely diagnosis among persons with dementia receiving care at home compared with residential facilities. *Public Health, 130*, 6–12. doi:10.1016/j.puhe.2015.10.992

Bartfay, W. J., & Bartfay, E. (2015). *Public health in Canada.* Boston, MA: Pearson Learning Solutions. ISBN: 13978-1-323-01471-4.

Belanger, G., Vanderploeg, R. D., & McAllister, T. (2016, May/June). Subconcussive blows to the head: A formative review of short-term clinical outcomes. Journal of Head Trauma Rehabilitation, *31*(3), 159–166.

Bell, J. M., Taylor, C. A., & Breiding, M. J. (2015, May/June). The public health approach to TBI. Journal of Head Trauma Rehabilitation, *30*(3), 148–149.

Brain Injury Canada. (2017a). *Brain injury Canada ABI fact sheet with TBI incidence pie chart*. Ottawa, ON: Brain Association of Canada. Retrieved from https://braininjurycanada.ca/wp-content/uploads/2014/07/ABI-Fact-Sheet-with-TBI-Incidence-Pie-Chart.pdf

Brain Injury Canada. (2017b). *June is brain injury awareness month #BIAM17*. Ottawa, ON: Brain Association of Canada. Retrieved from https://www.braininjurycanada.ca/2017/06/05/june-brain-injury-awareness-month/

Browne, P., Chandraratna, D., Angood, C., Tremlette, H., Baker, C., Taylor, B. V., & Thompson, A. T. (2014, September 9). Atlas of multiple sclerosis 2013: A growing global problem with widespread inequity. *Neurology, 83*(11), 1022–1024. Retrieved from https://www.ncbi.nlm.nih.gov/pmc/articles/PMC4162299/

Canadian Caregiver Coalition. (2014, February). *Canadian caregiver strategy: Are we making progress?* Mississauga, ON: Author. Retrieved from http://www.carerscanada.ca/wp-content/uploads/2015/09/Pan-Canadian-Family-Caregiver-2013_WEB-PAGES-2.pdf

Canadian Institute for Health Information (CIHI). (2007). *The burden of neurological diseases, disorders and injuries in Canada*. Ottawa, ON: CIHI (ISBN: 978-1-55465-025-5). Retrieved from https://secure.cihi.ca/free_products/BND_e.pdf

Canadian Institute for Health Information (CIHI). (2015). *National health expenditure trends, 1975 to 2015*. Ottawa, ON: CIHI. ISBN 978-1-77-109-413-9 (PDF). Retrieved from https://www.cihi.ca/en/national-health-expenditure-trends

Carr, A. S., Cardwell, C. R., McCorron, P. O., & McConville, J. (2010, June 18). A systematic review of population-based epidemiological studies in myasthenia gravis. *BMC Neurology, 10*, 46, PMC 2905354. doi:10.1186/1471-2377-10-46

Chambers, L. W., Bancej, C., & McDowell, I. (Eds.) (2016). *Prevalence and monetary costs of dementia in Canada*. Toronto, ON: Alzheimer's Society of Canada & The Public Health Agency of Canada. Retrieved from http://www.alzheimer.ca/~/media/Files/national/Statistics/PrevalenceandCostsofDementia_EN.pdf

Chang, C. Y., Ke, D. S., & Chen, J. Y. (2009, December). Essential fatty acids and human brain. *ACTA Neurology Taiwan, 18*(4), 231–241. Retrieved from https://www.ncbi.nlm.nih.gov/pubmed/20329590

Chapman, D. P., Marshale Williams, S., Strine, T., Andra, R. F., & Moore, M. (2006, April). Dementia and its implications for public health. *Preventing Chronic Disease, 3*(2), A34. Retrieved from https://www.ncbi.nlm.nih.gov/pmc/articles/PMC1563968/

Chio, A., Logroslino, G., Traynor, B. J., Collins, J., Simeone, J. C., Goldstein, L. A., & White, L. A. (2013). Global epidemiology of amyotrophic lateral sclerosis: A systematic review of the published literature. *Neuroepidemiology, 41*(2), 118–130.

Clarfield, A. M. (2003). The decreasing prevalence of reversible dementias: An updated meta-analysis. *Archives of Internal Medicine, 163*, 2219–2229. doi:10.1001/archinte.163.18. 2219

Cusimano, M. A. (2003). Bodychecking and concussions in ice hockey: Should our youth pay the price? *Canadian Medical Association Journal, 169*(2), 124–128. Retrieved from http://www.cmaj.ca/content/169/2/124.full?ijkey=b0062e904532ed2771f0dc5419a727550ad75844&keytype2=tf_ipsecsha

Dismore, J. (2013, February 24). Traumatic brain injury: An evidence-based review of management. *Continuing Education in Anaesthesia, Critical Care & Pain, 13*(6), 189–195. doi:10.1093/bjaceaccp/mkt010

Donatelle, R. J., Munroe, A. J., Munroe, A., & Thompson, A. M. (2008). *Health the basics* (4th ed.). Toronto, ON: Pearson Benjamin Cummings.

Elrick, R. (2011). Publication bias and time-trend bias in meta-analysis of bicycle helmet efficacy: A re-analysis of Attewell, Glase and McFadden, 2001. *Accident Analysis and Prevention, 43*(3), 1245–1251. Retrieved from https://www.ncbi.nlm.nih.gov/pubmed/21376924

Ernstsson, O., Gyllensten, H., Alexanderson, K., Tinghög, P., Friberg, E., & Norlund, A. (2016, July 13) Cost of illness of multiple sclerosis—A systematic review. *PLoS ONE, 11*(7), e0159129. doi:10.1371/journal.pone.0159129

Fines, P. (2010, May 28). *Estimating costs of health care for neurological conditions in Canada in 2031*. Ottawa, ON: Statistics Canada. Retrieved from https://www.cahspr.ca/en/presentation/5574e17837dee87418501956

Fisher, E. R., & Hayden, M. R. (2014, January). Multisource ascertainment of Huntington's disease in Canada: Prevalence and population at risk. *Movement Disorders, 29*(1), 105–114. Retrieved from https://www.ncbi.nlm.nih.gov/pubmed/24151181

Goodman, D., Gaetz, M., & Meichenbaum, D. (2001, December 1). Concussions in hockey: There is a cause for concern. *Medicine & Science in Sports & Exercise, 33*(12), 2004–2005. Retrieved from http://europepmc.org/abstract/med/11740291

Haddad, S. H., & Arabi, Y. M. (2012, February 3). Critical care management of severe traumatic brain injuries in adults. *Scandinavian Journal of Trauma, Resuscitation and Emergency Medicine, 20*, 12. Retrieved from https://www.ncbi.nlm.nih.gov/pmc/articles/PMC3298793/

Hagel, B. E., & Yanchar, N. L. (2013, November 1). Bicycle helmet use in Canada: The need for legislation to reduce the risk of head injury. *Paediatric Child Health, 18*(9), 475–480. Retrieved from https://www.cps.ca/en/documents/position/bike-helmets-to-reduce-risk-of-head-injury

Hahn, D. B., Payne, W. A., Gallant, M., & Flectcher, P. C. (2006). *Focus on health* (2nd ed.). Toronto, ON: McGraw-Hill Ryerson.

Harmon, K. (2012, January). How has Stephen Hawkins lived past 70 with ALS? *Scientific American.* Retrieved from https://www.scientificamerican.com/article/stephen-hawking-als/

Hejl, A., Hogh, P., & Waldemar, G. (2002). Potentially reversible conditions in 1000 consecutive memory clinic patients. *Journal of Neurology Neurosurgery and Psychiatry, 73*, 390–394.

Hickey, J. V. (2003). *The clinical practice of neurological and neurosurgical nursing* (5th ed.). New York, NY: Lippincott Williams & Wilkins.

Huntington's Disease Society of Canada. (2016). *What is Huntington's disease?* Kitchener, ON: Author. Retrieved from https://www.huntingtonsociety.ca/learn-about-hd/what-is-huntingtons/

Hurtchinson, R. G., Comper, P., Meeuwisse, W. H., & Echemendia, R. J. (2013, June 13). A systematic video analysis of National Hockey League (NHL) concussions, part II: How concussions occur. *British Journal of Science and Medicine, 49*, 547–551. Retrieved from https://www.researchgate.net/profile/Michael_Hutchison4/publication/236603534_A_systematic_video_analysis_of_National_Hockey_League_NHL_concussions_part_II_How_concussions_occur_in_the_NHL/links/54e5fb080cf277664ff1cf9c/A-systematic-video-analysis-of-National-Hockey-League-NHL-concussions-part-II-How-concussions-occur-in-the-NHL.pdf

Hyder, A. A., Wunderlich, C. A., Puvanachandra, P., Gururaj, G., & Kobusingye, O. C. (2007, December 7). The impact of traumatic brain injuries: A global perspective. *Neurorehabilitation, 22*(5), 341.

Janca, A., Pricipko, C., & Costa e-Silva, J. A. (1997). The WHO global initiative on neurology and public health. *Journal of Neurological Sciences, 145*(1), 1–2.

Korkhaneh, M., Kalenga, J. C., Hagel, B. E., & Rowe, B. H. (2006, April). Effectiveness of bicycle helmet legislation to increase helmet use: A systematic review. *Injury Prevention, 12*(2), 76–82. Retrieved from https://www.ncbi.nlm.nih.gov/pmc/articles/PMC2564454/

Kidd, P. M. (2007). Omega-3 DHA and EPA for cognition, behavior and mood: Clinical findings and structural–functional synergies with cell membrane phospholipids. *Alternative Medicine Review, 12*(3), 207–227.

Kingston, A. (2015, April 20). *Could Canada cause MS?* Toronto, ON: Macleans Magazine. Retrieved from http://www.macleans.ca/society/health/could-canada-cause-multiple-sclerosis/

Lancaster, J. (2010). *Guidelines for the MS diagnosis: McDonald criteria.* Dallas, TX: BioNews Services. Retrieved from https://multiplesclerosisnewstoday.com/multiple-sclerosis-diagnosis/mcdonald-criteria/

Macpherson, A., & Spinks, A. (2008). Bicycle helmet legislation for the uptake of helmet use and prevention of head injuries. *Cochrane Database Systematic Review,* (3), CD005401. doi:10.1002/14651858.CD005401.pub3

McCann, J. C., & Ame, B. N. (2005). Is docosahexaenoic acid, an n-3 long-chain polyunsaturated fatty acid, required for development of normal brain function? An overview of evidence from cognitive and behavioral tests in humans and animals. *American Journal of Clinical Nutrition, 82*, 281–295.

McCoy, T. (2015, February 24). *How Stephen Hawkins, diagnosed with ALS decades ago, is still alive.* Washington, DC: The Washington Post. Retrieved from https://www.washingtonpost.com/news/morning-mix/wp/2015/02/24/how-stephen-hawking-survived-longer-than-possibly-any-other-als-patient/?utm_term=.1de5fa443c27

McGauron, D. (2017, August 10). Let's talk about traumatic brain injuries. *Active Beat*. Retrieved from http://www .activebeat.co/your-health/lets-talk-about-traumatic-brain-injury/?utm_medium=cpc&utm_source=- google&utm_campaign=AB_GGL_CA_DESK-SearchMarketing&utm_content=g_c_164099518300&cus_widget= kwd-529677050&utm_term=traumatic%20brain%20injury%20cases&cus_teaser=

Mink, J. W., Blumenschine, R. J., & Adams, D. B. (1981). Ratio of central nervous system to body metabolism in verte-brates: Its constancy and functional basis. *American Journal of Physiology, 241*, R203–R212.

Multiple Sclerosis International Federation (MSIF). (2005). *Principles to promote the quality of life of people with multiple sclerosis*. London, UK: Author. Retrieved from http://www.msif.org/about-ms/publications-and-resources/

Multiple Sclerosis International Federation (MSIF). (2013). *Atlas of multiple sclerosis 2013: Mapping multiple sclerosis around the world*. London, UK: Author. Retrieved from http://www.msif.org/wp-content/uploads/2014/09/Atlas-of-MS.pdf

Multiple Sclerosis Society of Canada. (2017a). *What is multiple sclerosis?* Quebec: Author. Retrieved from https://mssociety.ca/about-ms/what-is-ms

Multiple Sclerosis Society of Canada-National Executive Committee. (2017b, October 23). *The costs of caring: Implications for family caregivers*. Quebec: Author. Retrieved from https://mssociety.ca/en/pdf/socact_caregiver-pos-paper-feb08-EN.pdf

Myasthenia Gravis Society of Canada. (2017). *What is myasthenia gravis?* Stouffville, ON: Author. Retrieved from http:// www.mgcanada.org/pages/about-mg/

National Institute for Health and Clinical Excellence. (2007). *Head injury: Triage, assessment, investigation and early management of head injury in infants, children and adults*. London, England: Author (NICE Clinical Guideline 56). Retrieved from https://www.nice.org.uk/guidance/CG176/documents/head-injury-draft-scope2

Northern Brain Injury Association. (2017). *Brain injury statistics*. Prince George, BC: Author. Retrieved from http://nbia .ca/brain-injury-statistics/

O'Neil-Pirozzi, T. M., Kennedy, M. R. T., & Sohlberg, McKay M. (2016, July/August). Evidence-based practice for the use of internal strategies as a memory compensation technique after brain injury: A systematic review. *Journal of Head Trauma Rehabilitation, 31*(4), E1–E11.

Parkinson's Association of the Carolinas. (2013). *Statistics on Parkinson's disease*. Charlotte, NC. Retrieved from http:// www.parkinsonassociation.org/facts-about-parkinsons-disease/.

Parkinson's Society of Canada. (2012). Canadian guidelines on Parkinson's disease. *Canadian Journal of Neurological Sciences, 39*(Suppl. 4), S1–S30. Retrieved from http://www.parkinsonclinicalguidelines.ca/guidelines

Persaud, N., Coleman, E., Zwolakowski, D., Lauwers, B., & Cass, D. (2012). Nonuse of bicycle helmets and risk of fatal head injury: A proportional mortality, case–control study. *Canadian Medical Association Journal, 184*(12), E921–E923. doi:10.1503/cmaj.120988. Retrieved from https://www.safetylit.org/citations/index.php?fuseaction=citations. viewdetails&citationIds%5b%5d=citjournalarticle_379077_37

Polman, C. H., Reingold, S. C., Banwell, B., Clanet, M., Cohen, J. A., Filippi M., … Wolinsky, J. S. (2011, February). Diagnostic criteria for multiple sclerosis: 2010 revisions to the McDonald criteria. *Annals of Neurology, 69*(2), 292–302. doi:10.1002/ana.22366

Porter, R. S., & Kaplan, J. L. (2011). *Merck manual of diagnosis and therapy* (19th ed.). West Point, PA: Merck & Company.

Public Health Agency of Canada (2007, September). *Core competencies for public health in Canada: Release 1.1*. Ottawa, ON: Author. Web-based link: http://www.phac-aspc.gc.ca/core_competencies or http://www.phac-aspc.gc.ca/php-psp/ccph-cesp/pdfs/cc-manual-eng090407.pdf

Public Health Agency of Canada (PHAC). (2008). *Canada's aging population. Division of seniors*. Ottawa, ON: PHAC. Retrieved from https://www.canada.ca/en/public-health/services/health-promotion/aging-seniors/aging-seniors-publications.html

Public Health Agency of Canada (PHAC). (2014). *Mapping connections: On understanding of neurological conditions in Canada*. Ottawa, ON: Author (Cat. No. HP 35-45/2014E-PDF). Retrieved from http://www.phac-aspc.gc.ca/publicat/ cd-mc/mc-ec/assets/pdf/mc-ec-eng.pdf

Rehkamper, G., Frahm, H. D., & Zilles, K. (1991). Quantitative development of brain and brain structures in birds (Galliformes and Passeriformes) compared to that in mammals (Insectivores and Primates). *Brain Behavior and Evolution, 37*, 125–143.

Rosenbluth, R. S. (2003). *The physics fact book. An encyclopedia of scientific essays (Mass of the human brain)*. High North Alliance. Retrieved from https://hypertextbook.com/facts/2003/RachelScottRosenbluth.shtml

Safe Kids Canada. (2007). *Child and youth unintentional injury: 10 years in review; 1994–2003*. Retrieved from https://prevention/skc_injuries.pdf

Tabish, S. A., & Syed, N. (2014, December). Recent advances and emerging medicine. *Emergency Medicine-Open Access, 5*, 229. doi:10.4172/2165-7548.1000229. Retrieved from https://www.omicsonline.org/open-access/recent_advances_and_future_trends_in_traumatic_brain_injury-2165-7548.1000229.php?aid=36101

Teasdale, G., & Jennett, B. (1974, July 13). Assessment of coma and impaired consciousness: A practical scale. *The Lancet, 304*(7872), 81–84. Retrieved from http://www.sciencedirect.com/science/article/pii/S0140673674916390

Teasdale, G., Maas, A., Lecky, F., Manley, G., Stocchetti, N., & Murray, G. (2014, August). The Glasgow Coma Scale at 40 years: Standing the test of time. *The Lancet Neurology, 13*(8), 844–854. Retrieved from http://www.thelancet.com/journals/laneur/article/PIIS1474-4422%2814%2970120-6/fulltext

Thompson, D. C., Rivara, F. P., & Thompson, R. (2000). Helmets for preventing head and facial injuries in bicyclists. *Cochrane Database Systematic Reviews, (2)*, CD001855.

Tugwell, C. (2008). *Parkinson's disease in focus*. London, UK: Pharmaceutical Press.

UBC Canada. (2017). *Parkinson's disease*. Oakville, ON: Author. Retrieved from https://www.ucb-canada.ca/en/Patients/Conditions/Parkinson-s-Disease

Ubelacher, S. (2013, March 29). *Hockey linked to half of brain injuries in Canada's kids, teen athletes*. Toronto, ON: CTV News and The Canadian Press. Retrieved from http://www.ctvnews.ca/?cid=ie9_taskbar_ctvnews

United Nations. (2008). *Convention on the rights of persons with disabilities*. New York, NY: Author. Retrieved from http://www.un.org/disabilities/convention/conventionfull.shtml

United Nations. (2013). *World population ageing 2013*. New York, NY: Department of Economic and Social Affairs-Population Division. Retrieved from http://www.un.org/en/development/desa/population/publications/pdf/ageing/WorldPopulationAgeing2013.pdf

Victor, M., & Ropper, A. H. (2001). *Adams and victor's principles of neurology* (7th ed.). Toronto, ON: McGraw-Hill Companies, Inc.

Walstra, G. J. M., Teunisse, S., van Gool, W. A., & van Crevel, H. (1997). Reversible dementia in elderly patients referred to a memory clinic. *Journal of Neurology, 244*, 17–22.

Wainwright, P. E. (2002, February 28). Dietary essential fatty acids and brain function: A developmental perceptive on mechanisms. *Proceedings of the Nutrition Society, 61*(1), 61–69. Retrieved from https://www.cambridge.org/core/journals/proceedings-of-the-nutrition-society/article/dietary-essential-fatty-acids-and-brain-function-a-developmental-perspective-on-mechanisms/3B7745C313EE695E5DF881A711A19490

Witte, A. V., Kerti, L., Hermannstadter, H. M., Fiebach, J. B., Schrieber, S. J., Schuchardt, J. P., … Hahn, A. (2014, November). Long-chain omega-3 fatty acids improves brain function and structure in older adults. *Cerebral Cortex, 24*(11), 3059–3068. Retrieved from https://academic.oup.com/cercor/article/24/11/3059/304487

Wong, S. L., Gilmour, H., & Ramage-Morin, P. L. (2015). *Parkinson's disease: Prevalence, diagnosis and impact*. Ottawa, ON: Statistics Canada (82-003). Retrieved from https://www.statcan.gc.ca/pub/82-003-x/2014011/article/14112-eng.htm

Wong, S. L., Gilmour, H., & Ramage-Morin, P. L. (2016, May 18). *Health reports: Alzheimer's disease and other dementias in Canada*. Ottawa, ON: Statistics Canada (82-003-x). Retrieved from https://www.statcan.gc.ca/pub/82-003-x/2016005/article/14613-eng.htm

World Health Organization. (2004). *Facts: Road safety helmets*. Geneva, Switzerland: WHO. Retrieved from http://www.who.int/violence_injury_prevention/publications/road_traffic/world_report/helmets_en.pdf?ua=1

World Health Organization. (2016). *What are neurological disorders?* Geneva, Switzerland: WHO. Retrieved from http://www.who.int/features/qa/55/en/

World Health Organization. (2017a). *Chapter 2: Global burden of neurological disorders estimates and projections* (pp. 27–39). Geneva, Switzerland: WHO. Retrieved October 9, 2017 from http://www.who.int/mental_health/neurology/chapter_2_neuro_disorders_public_health_challenges.pdf

World Health Organization. (2017b). *Neurological disorders: Public health challenges*. Geneva, Switzerland: WHO. Retrieved from http:www.file:///C:/Users/100241938/Desktop/Neurology%20WHO%202017.pdf

World Health Organization. (2017c). *The top 10 leading causes of death: Fact sheet*. Geneva, Switzerland: WHO. Retrieved from http://www.who.int/mediacentre/factsheets/fs310/en/

World Health Organization. (2017d). *Violence and injury prevention and disability (VIP): Neurotrauma*. Geneva, Switzerland: WHO. Retrieved from http://www.who.int/violence_injury_prevention/road_traffic/activities/neurotrauma/en/

Zekry, D., Hauw, J. J., & Gold, G. (2002). Mixed dementia: Epidemiology, diagnosis and treatment. *Journal of the American Geriatric Society, 50*, 1431–1438. Retrieved from https://s3.amazonaws.com/academia.edu.documents/45125887/Mixed_dementia_Epidemiology_diagnosis_an20160427-14145-1520zqc.pdf?AWSAccessKeyId=AKIAIWOWYYGZ2Y53UL3A&Expires=1511202443&Signature=bn5UY1srNXVDR2S3RLAXPcfx03g%3D&response-content-disposition=inline%3B%20filename%3DMixed_Dementia_Epidemiology_Diagnosis_an.pdf

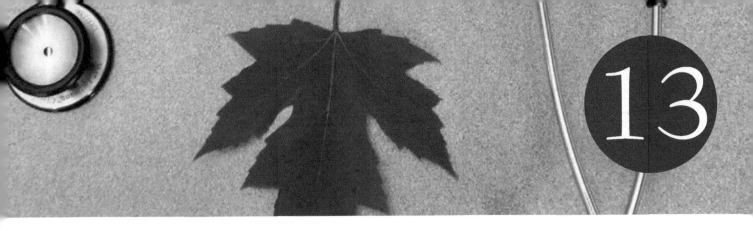

Major Emerging and Reemerging Infectious Diseases: A Canadian Perspective

Germ theory which secularized infectious disease, had a side effect: It sacralized epidemiology.
—(Jill Lepore, Professor of American History at Harvard University)

Learning Objectives

After completion of this chapter, the student will be able to:
- Describe and summarize the function of the immune system and the step-by-step process by which infectious diseases are transmitted.
- List and describe common risk factors, pathogens, and routes of invasion associated with infectious diseases.
- Recognize and critically examine various environmental and social determinants of health associated with infectious disease in Canada and globally.
- List and describe five emerging infectious diseases (EIDs) or reemerging infectious diseases (REIDs) of growing concern to public health in Canada; their zoonotic nature, and public health prevention strategies.
- Critically examine and explain the public health impact of EIDs and REIDs.
- List and discuss the importance of various public health plans and approaches for outbreak management in Canada; including tracking and surveillance, pandemic emergency preparedness, and vector control.

Core Competencies for Public Health addressed in Chapter 13

Core Competencies	Competency Statements
1.0 Public Health Sciences	1.1, 1.2, 1.3, 1.4
2.0 Assessment and Analysis	2.1, 2.2, 2.4, 2.5, 2.6
3.0 Policy and Program Planning, Implementation, and Evaluation	3.1, 3.2, 3.6, 3.7
4.0 Partnerships, Collaboration, and Advocacy	4.1, 4.4
5.0 Diversity and Inclusiveness	5.1, 5.2, 5.3
6.0 Communication	6.2, 6.4
7.0 Leadership	7.1, 7.2

Note: Please see the following document or web-based link for a detailed description of these specific competencies. Public Health Agency of Canada (PHAC, 2007).

Introduction

Every moment of every day of your life, you are in contact with literally billions of microscopic organisms which are found in the air you breathe, in the foods you eat, and on nearly every inanimate surface (e.g., door knobs, elevator buttons, smartphones, computer keyboards) or living person or animal(s) (e.g., family pet, livestock) you come into contact with. It may surprise you to learn that many of these are microorganisms; which include bacteria, are, in fact, beneficial to humans. For example, gram-positive probiotic bacteria such as *Lactobacillus acidophilus* present in over-the-counter probiotic capsules, yogurt, miso, and tempeh help aid with digestion of lactose, treat traveler's diarrhea, and irritable bowel syndrome (IBS), combat vaginal infections, lower LDL cholesterol levels and boost your immune system; and there are more than 80 strains of this bacteria alone (Begtrup, Muckadell, Kjeldsen, Christensen, & Jarbol, 2013; de Vrese & Marteau, 2007; Goldin & Gorbach, 2008; McFarland, 2007; Rerksuppaphol & Rerksuppaphol, 2012). **Probiotics** are defined as living microorganisms (e.g., bacteria), which when administered in adequate amounts confer a positive health benefit to the host.

The "normal flora" of humans is remarkably diverse and complex consisting of more than 200 species of bacteria alone. The normal flora of bacteria present on or within us usually develops in an orderly sequence after birth, resulting in relatively stable populations of bacteria. *In utero*, fetal skin is sterile; however, colonization quickly occurs immediately after birth following vaginal delivery or in the minutes following birth by caesarian section (Dominguez-Bello et al., 2010; Grice & Segre, 2011). In fact, the average person has more bacterial cells than human cells combined residing on their skin, nose, and ears and within them in their respiratory or intestinal tracts. It is notable that the human body contains about 10^{13} eukaryotic cells in all the tissues and organs combined, and also routinely harbours approximately 10^{14} bacteria in the gastrointestinal tract alone (Davis, 1996; Todor, 2012).

However, when bacteria leave their normal site of residence, they may cause illness or disease. For example, *Staphylococcus aureus* bacteria live harmlessly on your skin and inside your nose. However, a break in your skin barrier (e.g., open cut or wound on your leg), could quickly lead to contamination and a subsequent localized infection. Furthermore, it is important to note that unnecessary antibiotic prescriptions (e.g., to treat viral infections), and improper or clinically incorrect use of antibiotics regimes (e.g., using broad spectrum or a combination of agents instead of first-line agents) allows for the survival of bacteria with antibiotic resistance genes. Biochemically, bacteria counteract antibiotics by enzymes that destroy or are inactive to these drugs. Indeed, methicillin-resistant *Staphylococcus aureus* (MRSA), vancomycin-resistant enterococci (VREs), and penicillin-resistant *Streptococcus pneumonia* are three of the most problematic resistant bacteria,

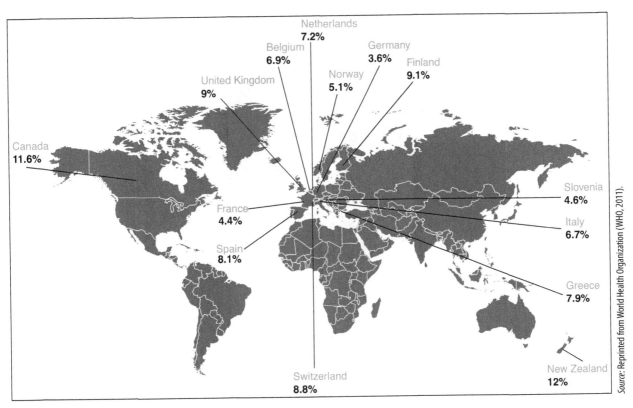

Figure 13.1 Prevalence of healthcare-associated infections (HAIs) in high income countries, 1995–2010. It is noteworthy that Canada was ranked second in the world for HAIs at 11.6% (just behind New Zealand at 12%) as a high-income and developed country.

and have been flagged as major public health challenges in Canada and internationally (Cunhn, 2006; Tortora, Funke, & Case, 2016; World Health Organization [WHO], 2017c).

Figure 13.1 for shows the global prevalence of HAI's in high income countries between the years 1995 and 2010.

The *Canadian Nosocomial Infection Surveillance Program* (CNISP) was established in 1994, and monitors healthcare associated infections at 54 sentinel hospitals located across 10 provinces (PHAC, 2012a). The CNISP provides a mechanism to compare provincial infection rates (benchmarks), and also to develop national guidelines on clinical issues related to HAIs. It is estimated that one in nine hospitalized clients will develop a HAI, and there are over 220,000 infections that occur each year in Canada; between 8000 and 12,000 Canadians die as a result of HAIs each year, and it costs our healthcare systems in excess of $1,000,000,000 annually (Canadian Patient Safety Institute [CPSI], 2018; Government of Canada, 2013; PHAC, 2013). The reader is referred to Chapter 7 for a detailed discussion on community-and-hospital acquired nosocomial infections, and the growing public health concern related to antibiotic resistance.

This chapter examines current major EIDs and REIDs that are of growing public health concern in Canada and internationally. We begin with a brief overview of what infectious diseases are. We examine the functioning of the human immune system and how various public health interventions help break the chain of infection. We also examine select major EIDs and REIDs from a Canadian perspective. Lastly, we examine current public health challenges related to infection control in various environments and individuals across the lifespan.

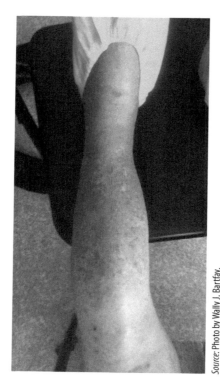

Source: Photo by Wally J. Bartfay.

Photo 13.1 A severely infected left leg (cellulitis) acquired during hospitalization. It is estimated that approximately one in nine patients will develop a HAI in Canada, and the increasing incidence of antibiotic resistant strains of bacteria is a major public health concern in Canada and internationally.

What Are Infectious Diseases?

An **infectious disease** is defined as a communicable disease caused by a specific pathogen (e.g., bacteria, viruses, fungi, protozoa, prion) or its toxic products that results through its transmission from an agent to a susceptible host. An **infection** is defined as an invasion of the body caused by a pathogen that results in specific signs and symptoms that develop in response to the pathogen which may be localized or systemic in nature. *Localized infections* are limited in scope and nature to a small area (e.g., eye, tooth, specific finger); whereas, *systemic infections* are broader in scope and widespread throughout the body, and are often spread via the circulatory system (Cooke, 2008; Heymann, 2015; Webber, 2016). You may also *autoinoculate* yourself, or transmit a pathogen from one part of your body to another. For example, you may touch a sore on your lip teeming with herpes simplex virus-1 (HSV-1), and then transmit this virus to your eye when you rub it resulting in conjunctivitis (aka, "pink eye").

For several centuries, infectious diseases such as smallpox, tuberculosis, syphilis, pertussis (a.k.a., whooping cough), and the plague have resulted in millions of casualties and threatened the survival of our species on Earth (Cooke, 2008; Tortora et al., 2016; Webber, 2016). For example, during the 14th century in Euroasia, an estimated 75 to 200 million people died as a consequence of Bubonic plague (a.k.a., "Black Death") alone (Heymann, 2015; WHO, 2017h). During medieval times, people believed that the plague resulted from punishment from God for sins committed; linked it to the movement of planets; comets; solar or lunar eclipses; and noxious unhealthy vapours or smells termed "miasma" to name but a few suspected causes.

We currently know that the plague is caused by the zoonotic bacteria *Yersinia pestis* that may be present on some rodents (e.g., rats, squirrels), and which can be transmitted to humans via bites from infected fleas. There are two types of plague: (i) *Bubonic*, which accounts for 30% to 60% of all associated mortalities when contracted; and (ii) *pneumonic*, which results in almost 100% mortality if not treated with antibiotics. Plague has not been eradicated and continues to result in deaths to this very day. For example, the WHO (2017h) reports that during the years 2010 through 2015 there were 3248 cases of plague reported worldwide; including 584 deaths, and the most endemic areas include the Democratic Republic of Congo, Madagascar and Peru.

By convention and tradition since the turn of the 19th century, when an organism was transmittable, it was deemed *infectious* (or communicable) in nature; otherwise the disease was labelled *non-infectious* (or non-communicable). However, this simple distinction is becoming less clear-cut and defined as we continue to learn about the nature and evolution of various diseases. For examples, the links between hepatitis B virus and the development of hepatocellular cancer, and human papilloma virus (HPV) and cervical cancer are well established and documented; whereas both can now be prevented via routine vaccinations (Cooke, 2008; Webber, 2016). Hence, we argue that the key to understanding the difference from a public health context, is to examine the manifestation and presence, or not, of a necessitated and requisite "chain of infection."

What Is the Chain of Infection?

Infectious (a.k.a., communicable) diseases are transmitted from one host to another through a series of steps known as the "chain of infection" (Hahn, Payne, Gallant, & Fletcher, 2006; Heymann, 2015; Insel, Roth, Irwin, & Burke, 2016; Tortora et al., 2016). Figure 13.2 shows the various links in the chain of infection, which forms the basis for an understanding of how certain communicable diseases are transmitted. Fortuitously for humans, there are only a limited number of microscopic organisms known as "pathogens" that can make us sick or cause disease. A **systemic infection** is defined as an invasion by a microorganism that spreads through the blood or lymphatic system to large portions of the host's body or tissues.

Pathogens are defined as any microorganism (e.g., virus, bacteria, fungi) or other matter (e.g., prion) that can cause disease in humans or animals and/or result in a morbid process or state. Through mutation, some pathogenic agents, particularly viruses and certain bacteria, become virulent in nature over time. The reader is referred to Chapter 7 for a detailed discussion on the communicability of a disease and the various modes of disease transmission.

The environment forms the second necessary link in the chain of infection and is referred to as the "reservoir." A **reservoir** is defined as the natural environment in which a pathogen typically resides, and may be a person, animal, or environment (e.g., soil, water, unpasteurized milk product). For example, spores of the tetanus bacterium (*Clostridium tetani*) can survive in non-living environments such as soil or dust for up to 50 years, and infect individuals via a puncture wound, cut, or laceration (e.g., during gardening). When the tetanus bacterium enters via a wound, cut, or laceration; spores quickly grow into bacteria that can produce a powerful neurotoxin known as *tetanospasmin*, which impairs the nerves that control your facial, neck, and/ or

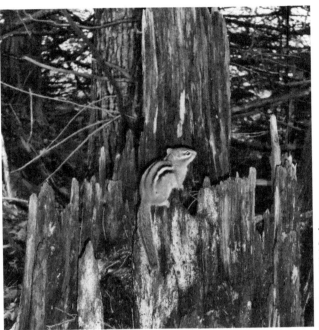
Source: Photo by Wally J. Bartfay.

Photo 13.2 Small Rodents: Carriers of the Plague. Over 200 species of animals can carry and transmit the plague via infected fleas. The bacteria (*Yersinia pestis*) is maintained in nature by wild rodents, such as chipmunks, ground squirrels, prairie dogs, deer mice, voles, and household pets such as cats and dogs. On average seven cases occur every year in the southwestern regions of the United States. A small number of human deaths have also been observed in recent years including four cases 2015 and one case in 2013. Human cases of plague are very rare in Canada with the last documented case reported in 1939 (PHAC, 2017c).

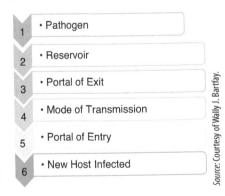
Source: Courtesy of Wally J. Bartfay.

1. • Pathogen
2. • Reservoir
3. • Portal of Exit
4. • Mode of Transmission
5. • Portal of Entry
6. • New Host Infected

Figure 13.2 The Chain of Infection

skeletal muscles (motor neurons). In fact, "lock jaw" is a term and clinical symptom commonly associated with tetanus and refers to spasms of the jaw, neck, and/or facial muscles which cause them to remain tightly closed. Tetanus can be a potentially life-threatening condition if left untreated, and approximately 10% to 20% of infections are fatal (Centers for Disease Control and Prevention [CDC], 2017b).

The **host** refers to the animal and/or human on which the pathogen or agent acts to create disease or altered states of health and well-being. The reader is referred to Chapter 6 for a detailed discussion on the *epidemiological triangle* of communicable disease involving the host, agent, environment, and time (see Figure 6.3). However, a person who is a reservoir for a pathogen (e.g., HIV, hepatitis B) may be an asymptomatic carrier who can spread the infection to another person (e.g., unprotected sex, sharing IV needles, contaminated dental equipment) (Hahn et al., 2006; Heymann, 2015; Insel et al., 2016; Tortora et al., 2016).

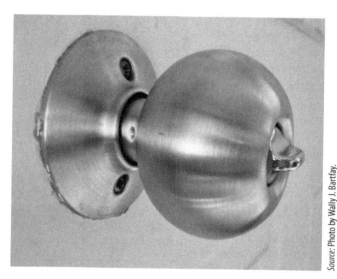

Source: Photo by Wally J. Bartfay.

Photo 13.3   How Many Doorknobs Have You Touched Today? Doorknobs in your home, or in public and work places, are the most commonly touched surfaces by several individuals during a typical day where pathogens (e.g., viruses, bacteria, fungi) can easily be transferred from person-to-person. One germy doorknob can infect up to half of your workplace, building of residence, hotel, airline flight, university campus, daycare, or healthcare facility within a manner of hours (Blaszczak, 2014). For example, one single bacteria cell can become more than 8 million cells in less than 24 hours (Manning, 2017). Most flu viruses can survive 24 to 48 hours on non-porous surfaces (e.g., steel doorknobs), and 8 to 12 hours on porous surfaces (e.g., wooden doorknobs); whereas, avian influenza may survive for as long as six days on certain surfaces (O'Connor, 2009). Be sure to use an alcohol-based (e.g., ethanol 60% or higher) hand sanitizer and wash your hands frequently as a form of primary prevention.

Research Focus Box 13.1: Elevator Buttons as Unrecognized Sources of Bacterial Colonization in Hospitals

Study Aim/Rationale
Although many inanimate objects harbour bacteria (e.g., keyboards, smartphones, door knobs), hospital elevator buttons represent a frequently encountered fomite because of their frequency of use, and they are considered commonplace technologies in Canadian society. The aim of this study was to estimate the prevalence of bacterial colonization present on elevator buttons in three large urban teaching hospitals located in Toronto, Ontario. These hospitals collectively represent a total of 1490 acute inpatient hospital beds (range of 353–677 beds per hospital).

(Continued)

(Continued)

Methodology/Design

At each acute care teaching hospital located in Toronto, Ontario, four separate elevator buttons were swabbed for the presence of bacteria on 10 separate days. Swabs for the elevators were taken from two interior buttons (i.e., ground floor and one randomly selected upper-level floor) and two exterior buttons (i.e., the "up" and "down" buttons) due to their frequency of use. Toilet surface swabs were taken from the exterior and interior handles of the entry door, the privacy latch, and the toilet flusher. Four toilet surfaces were swabbed over eight separate days. Hence, a total of 120 elevator buttons and 96 toilet surfaces were swabbed over separate intervals at three separate acute care teaching hospitals. Samples were obtained using standard bacterial collection techniques, which were subsequently plated and cultured in the laboratory. Species identification was done by a laboratory technician who was blinded to the sample source.

Major Findings

In brief, elevator buttons had higher colonization rates than toilet surfaces in the same hospitals sampled (61% vs. 43%, $p = .008$). Specifically, a total of 73 elevator samples from 120 cultures showed the presence of microbiological growth, which is a prevalence rate of 61% (95% confidence interval [CI]: 52%–70%). The most common organisms cultured were coagulase-negative *staphylococci*, followed by *Streptococcus*; whereas, *Enterococcus* and *Pseudomonas* species were deemed to be infrequent in the colonies. For toilets, a total of 41 samples showed microbiological growth, which is a prevalence rate of 43% (95% CI: 33%–53%).

Implications for Public Health

Hospital-acquired infections (HAIs) are a substantial cause of morbidity and mortality in Canada, and a growing public health concern. Hospital elevator buttons appear to be a frequently colonized site for bacteria in this study, although most pathogens identified were not deemed to be clinically relevant. Nonetheless, surface contamination of bacteria that can persist for days in various hospital and community settings, has been implicated in the propagation of drug-resistant bacteria. The risk of pathogen transmission to patients, staff, and healthcare personnel might be reduced by simple infection control countermeasures; such as the use of alcohol-based hand sanitizers (e.g., ethanol 60% or higher) strategically placed inside and/or outside elevators, and frequent handwashing. Additional ergometric countermeasures could include redesigning and enlarging elevator buttons to allow for activation by elbows, and/or installing touchless proximity or voice-activated sensors. Lastly, increased public education about proper hand hygiene targeted to individuals exiting elevators and visitors and staff who tend to exhibit poor hand hygiene should be implemented. Ultimately, an increased awareness of risk of contamination might spur greater attention throughout the hospital environment and into the surrounding community.

Source: Kandel, Simor, and Redelmier (2014).

The environment plays a key role in the chain of infection. For example, before the introduction of proper sanitation practices during the 18th century in Europe, rubbish and bodily waste (e.g., urine, faeces) were often tossed into narrow streets and allowed to rot or be washed away by rain. These were ideal breeding grounds for rats which carried the fleas associated with plague and other diseases. Today, if there is a breakdown in the collection of trash by the city's or town's sanitation department (e.g., war, earthquake, tsunamis, labour dispute or strike), this could provide a fertile breeding ground for rats which could spread infectious diseases into the community (Cooke, 2008; Webber, 2016).

The third required link in the chain of infection is the **portal of exit**, where pathogenic agents leave their reservoirs; and include the circulatory, urinary, respiratory, reproductive, and/or digestive systems. In the case of human reservoirs, portal of exit may include discharges from the mouth (e.g., certain HPV's, saliva for mumps); nose or throat (e.g., sneeze, sputum for influenza); genitalia and mucous membranes (e.g., STI transmission, sperm); faeces (e.g., for parasitic infections), and blood (e.g., HIV or hepatitis B).

The **mode of transmission** is the fourth required link in the chain of infection and refers to the way the pathogen is passed from a reservoir to a susceptible host; which involves two principle methods: (i) Direct transmission and (ii) indirect transmission (Hahn et al., 2006; Heymann, 2015; Insel et al., 2016; Tortora et al.,

2016). There are three types of *direct transmission* involved for human-to-human transmission: (i) Contact between body surfaces (e.g., touching, sexual intercourse, kissing); (ii) inhalation of contaminated air droplets (e.g., influenza virus via sneeze), and (iii) fecal–oral route. *Indirect transmission* includes travel by non-human or innate objects or materials (e.g., food items, soil, kitchen sponges and towels, clothing, doorknobs, elevator buttons). Indirect transmission of a pathogen or infectious agent may also occur via vectors such as insects, birds, or other animals. For example, Lyme disease (or Lyme borreliosis) in humans is an infectious disease caused by the spirochete *Borrelia burgdorferi*. Lyme disease is spread by ticks present on infected animals including mice, squirrels, other small rodents, birds, and deer during the spring and summer seasons in Canada. We shall examine Lyme disease in greater detail later. The reader is referred to Chapter 7 for a detailed discussion on vector-borne diseases and other common modes of disease transmission (i.e., horizontal and vertical modes, fecal/oral, airborne, waterborne, parasitic mode, vector-borne, zoonotic mode).

The fifth link in the chain of infection is the **portal of entry**, where pathogenic agents enter the body of a susceptible host. For several infections, the portal of entry are within the same system as the portal of exit. However, cross-system contamination can also occur. For example, oral, vaginal, and anal sex allows for HIV (infectious agent) to pass between warm, moist mucous membranes and tissues of the reproductive and digestive systems. Pathogens tend to enter via one of the following four common ways: (i) Via direct contact with the pathogen or penetration of the skin, or contact with mucous membrane; (ii) inhalation of droplets via the respiratory tract (i.e., mouth or nose); (iii) via ingestion of contaminated food or water; and/or (iv) contact with blood (e.g., vector such as mosquitoe for transmission of malaria parasite).

One single bacteria cell can become more than 8 million cells in less than 24 hours. The number of bacteria it takes to make an individual sick can range from as few as 10 up to several millions (Manning, 2017). Infections can easily spread when germs are transferred from a contaminated item, (e.g., door handle, elevator button, kitchen

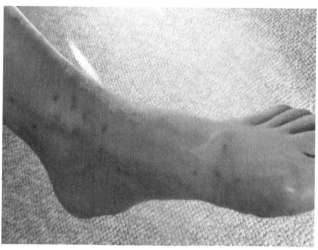

Source: Photo by Wally J. Bartfay.

Photo 13.4   Bedbug Bites Present on the Foot and Ankle Region. Bedbugs (*Cimex lectularius*) are readily transported via luggage, clothing, bedding, and furniture, and have undergone a dramatic resurgence worldwide. Chagas disease is a vector-borne disease caused by a parasitic protozoan called *Trypanosoma cruzi* that slowly attacks internal organs like the heart. According to a recent laboratory-based study, bedbugs may be just as dangerous as its sinister cousin, the "kissing bug" (*triatomine*), which can transmit the parasite that causes Chagus disease (Salazar et al., 2015). Chagus disease affects between 6 and 8 million people worldwide, and approximately 50,000 die annually from the disease, mostly in Latin America.

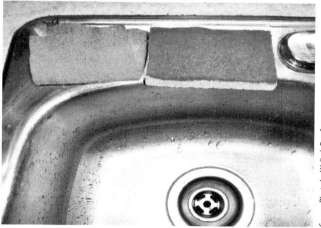

Source: Photo by Wally J. Bartfay.

Photo 13.5   What's Growing on Your Kitchen Sponge? A study by Cordinale, Kaiser, Lueders, Schnell, and Egert (2017) on used kitchen sponges revealed the presence of 362 different species of bacteria including *Acinetobacter*, *Moraxella*, and *Chryseobacterium*. In fact, one square centimeter of sponge could contain up to 45 billion bacteria. Microwaving sponges on a high setting for 1 min kills 99.99% of bacteria present, and do not forget to replace your kitchen sponges every week or so.

Group Activity-Based Learning 13.1 Thinking About the Chain of Infection

This group activity-based learning box highlights and reinforces critical links in the chain of infection in community-based settings. Working in small groups of three to five students, discuss and answer the following questions:

1. Identify the last time you had the flu, the cold, or an intestinal infection. What was the potential reservoir for this infection?

2. What was the mode of infection?

3. List and describe actions or behaviours you could have taken in hind-site to break the chain of infection?

---

sponge, cutting board, hand towel, smartphone, computer keyboard), to an individual's hand. Once a pathogen enters a potential new host, a variety of factors determine whether the pathogen will be able to establish itself and cause an infection. In theory, all people are at risk for contracting infectious diseases, and so can be considered *susceptible hosts*. In public health practice, however, we know that a variety of factors can affect the chain of infection including the clients' overall health, age, acquired immunity, access to healthcare services, nutritional status, and health-related practices and behaviours (e.g., handwashing, wearing a mask). For example, people with compromised immune systems (e.g., transplant clients, HIV/AIDS, clients receiving chemotherapy or radiation, diabetics, elderly) may be more likely to contract the disease (Hahn et al., 2006; Insel et al., 2016). The number of pathogens that enter the body of the new host is also an important factor. Interrupting the chain of infection at any point can prevent disease and include practices such as quarantining infecting individuals, public sanitation practices including chlorination of drinking water, rodent and vector control, and routine immunization against known infectious diseases (e.g., MMR, hepatitis, tetanus), to name but a few.

For example, immunization is a proven and cost-effective primary prevention public health strategy for controlling and even eradicating known infectious diseases. In fact, a global immunization campaign carried out by WHO from 1967 to 1977 resulted in the eradication of smallpox. When the smallpox immunization program first began, the disease threatened approximately 60% of the world's population, and 1:4 infected individuals died as a result of the disease (WHO, 2017g). More recently, the *Global Vaccine Action Plan* (GVAP) was a framework adopted at the 65th World Health Assembly held in May 2012; with the goal of attaining "a world in which all individuals and communities enjoy lives free from vaccine-preventable diseases" (WHO, 2015). By 2010, an estimated 85% of children under 1 year of age had received at least three doses of DTP vaccine (DTP3) globally. Additional vaccines (e.g., hepatitis B, Hemophilus influenzae type b) have now been added also to this list (WHO, 2017g).

A Brief Overview of the Human Immune System

Although a detailed review of the human immune system is beyond the purpose and scope of this chapter, we shall highlight some of the critical basic components that all public health professionals and workers should be cognizant of. One potential outcome of the adaptive coevolution of humans and bacteria is the development of commensal relationships in nature; where neither partner nor collaborator is harmed. These unique partnerships and collaborations in nature are commonly referred to as a "symbiotic relationships" where unique metabolic traits or other mutual benefits happily and opportunely coexist. For example, we should think of our gastrointestinal tract as a vast community of colonized symbionts and commensals that have important effects on our immune function, nutrient processing, and a broad range of other host activities (Hooper & Gorden, 2001; Tortora et al., 2016). In fact, our gastrointestinal system plays a central role in immune system homeostasis. It is the main route of contact with the external environment and is overloaded every day with external stimuli, which include dangerous pathogens (bacteria, protozoa, fungi, viruses) or toxic substances on occasion. In other cases, the gastrointestinal system plays a key role in the breakdown of food items for nutrition, and is also a source of commensal flora (Oregon State University, 2013). In fact, it is estimated that 70% to 80% of your total immune system responses reside in your intestinal tract or "gut" (Furness, Wolfgang, & Kunze, 1999; Hooper & Gorden, 2001; Vighi, Marcucci, Sensi, Di Cara, & Fratti, 2008). The crucial position of the gastrointestinal system is demonstrated and affirmed by the huge amount of immune cells that reside within it. Indeed, gut-associated lymphoid tissue (GALT) is the prominent part of mucosal-associated lymphoid tissue (MALT), representing almost 70% of the entire immune system. Moreover, about 80% of plasma cells, which are mainly immunoglobulin A (IgA)-bearing cells, reside in GALT (Furness et al., 1999; Hooper & Gorden, 2001; Vighi et al., 2008). Hence, our gut plays a critical and central role in our immune system, and any disruption will affect our ability to effectively respond to potentially harmful pathogens in our environment.

The **immune system** is defined as a complex system that is responsible for distinguishing a host from everything foreign, and for protecting the body against a host of infectious agents and foreign substances. The immune system also has two types of responses for invading pathogens: (i) Natural or innate and (ii) acquired or adaptive (Hahn et al., 2006; Insel et al., 2016; Tortora et al., 2016). Without a normal immune system which employs both cellular and humoral elements, we would quickly fall victim to serious life-threatening infections and/or malignancies. **Immunological competence** is defined as the body's ability to defend itself against pathogens and includes factors such as age, heredity, temperature, nutritional status, presence of other diseases (e.g., diabetes, AIDS, Cooley's anemia), and environmental factors. The reader is referred to Chapter 7 for a detailed discussion related to the various types of immunity (e.g., acquired or passive, natural, active, herd), and a discussion on the antigenicity of various infectious agents.

Once a host has been invaded by a foreign organism or substance, an elaborate system of responses is activated, which includes both inflammatory and immune responses (Donatelle, Johnson-Munroe, Munroe, & Thompson, 2008; Hahn et al., 2006; Insel et al., 2016). The **inflammatory response** occurs when the body in injured or infected resulting in the release of *histamine* and other substances that cause blood vessels to dilate and fluid to flow-out of capillaries into the surrounding tissue. This results in localized heat, swelling, and redness. Moreover, white blood cells including *neutrophils*, *dendritic cells*, and *macrophages* are drawn into the area and attack invading pathogens, and are regarded as components of the natural response. *Natural killer cells* also destroy infected body cells by breaking the chain of reproduction of the pathogen. In brief, they recognize pathogens as being "foreign" in nature, but have no previous innate memory of a similar past infection. Hence, they respond identical to each subsequent invasion of the foreign substance no matter how many times the pathogen invades the body.

T cells (or T-lymphocytes) and *B cells* (or B-lymphocytes) are part of the acquired responses developed from stem cells in the bone marrow, and are altered or changed after initial contact with the pathogen via the development of a "memory for the antigen" (Hahn et al., 2006; Insel et al., 2016; Tortora et al., 2016). Both T- and B cells are found primarily in blood and lymphoid organs and their responses of cellular immunity focus on attacking antigens that make their way inside cells. In brief, T cells do not bind to antigens directly, but recognize antigenic peptides after they have been processed by phagocytic cells such as macrophages. T cells respond to antigens by means of a receptor on the surface termed "T-cell receptors" (TCRs). B cells help remove bacteria, viruses and other toxins from body tissue fluids and blood by recognizing antigens, and by making antibodies against them. Hence, the immune response requires a series of coordinated and complex biochemical actions between different cells in the body.

Cytokines are soluble proteins or glycoprotein chemical messengers secreted by lymphocytes that help to regulate and coordinate immune responses. In fact, there are over 200 different types of cytokines that have been identified to date, and *interleukins* and *interferons* are two key examples. Cytokines play a critical role in stimulating the production of B cells and T cells along with antibodies; promote the activities of natural killer cells, and produce fever and other anti-pathogenic responses in the human body. Dead cells, destroyed

---

Group Activity-Based Learning 13.2 Thinking About the Spread of Infectious Disease

This group activity-based learning box highlights and examines EIDs and REIDs in Canada and globally. Working in small groups of three to five students, discuss, and answer the following questions:

1. Why do you think there has been an increase in both community- and hospital-acquired infectious diseases in Canada and internationally?

2. List and describe current clinical practices and/or treatment regimens that result in increased antibacterial resistance?

3. List and describe practices individuals can do to reduce their own risk of contracting an infectious disease?

---

pathogens, and other debris that result from the immune response are typically filtered-out by the liver and spleen, and excreted by the kidneys. Hence, this is why it is important to inform clients to "drink plenty of fluids" to help clear the body of waste byproducts associated with the immune response. *Pus* is simply a local collection of dead white cells and cellular debris at the site of an infection, and may be required to be drained via lancing and/or surgical debridement.

What Are EIDs and REIDs?

The WHO (2017d) defines an **emerging infectious disease (EID)** as one that has appeared in a population for the first time, or that may have existed previously; but is rapidly increasing in incidence or geographic range. Recent examples of EIDs that have appeared in the mass and social media include Zika, Ebola, chikungunya, West Nile virus (WNV), severe acute respiratory syndrome (SARS), avian influenza (Type A H5N1), Middle East respiratory syndrome coronavirus (MERS-CoV), and Lyme disease. A particular feature of many EIDs is their capacity to spread internationally due to travel, trade, and/or migration of species (e.g., birds), and consequently impact health from a global perspective.

Re-emerging infectious diseases (REIDs) are defined as diseases that were once regarded as major public health problems globally or in a particular country, and then declined dramatically; but have subsequently reemerged as a public health concern for a significant proportion of the population. Examples include malaria, tuberculosis, measles, cholera, typhoid, and Rift Valley fever. Malaria, for example, is endemic in 91 countries, and approximately 40% of the world's population is at risk. Up to 500 million cases occur every year; 90% of them in Africa, and there are up to 2.7 million associated deaths annually (WHO, 2018k). Figure 13.3 shows a map of examples of major EIDs and REIDs from a global health perspective.

The National Institute of Allergy and Infectious Disease (NIAID) classifies EIDs and REIDs into three major groups (Bowman, 2008; National Institutes of Health [NIH], 2012; NIAID, 2018). Group I pathogens are agents which are new or have been recognized within the past two decades (e.g., Acanthamebiasis, *Helicobacter pylori*, Hepatitis E, Human herpesvirus 8, Parvovirus B19). Group II pathogens are regarded as agents that have previously been recognized, but are now reemerging (e.g., Enterovirus 71, *Clostridium difficile*, Mumps virus, Streptococcus Group A).

Group III are regarded as agents with bioterrorism potential and are further classified into three subcategories (Bowman, 2008; NIAID, 2018; NIH, 2012). Category A pathogens are those organisms/biological agents that pose the highest risk to national security and public health because they are: (i) Easily disseminated and/or transmitted from person-to-person; (ii) have the potential to result in high mortality rates and have major impact on public health; (iii) have potential to result in social disruption and/or panic by public at large; and (iv) requires special plans of action and public health preparedness. Examples of Category A

Global Examples of Emerging and Re-Emerging Infectious Diseases

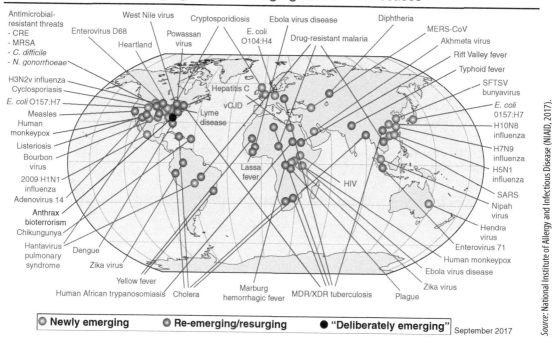

Figure 13.3   Global Examples of Emerging and Reemerging Infectious Diseases. It is noteworthy that approximately 75% of all emerging and reemerging infectious diseases are zoonotic in nature (CDC, 2017d; Ogden, Abdel-Malik, & Pulliam, 2017; Wang & Cramer, 2014). Drivers of change include the modernization of agricultural practices (e.g., large scale single animal farm factories)—particularly in developing regions of the world, habitat destruction (e.g., clear cutting rain forests, open pit mining), human encroachment, increasing global trade and travel, and climate change.

pathogens include *Bacillus anthracis* (Anthrax), *Clostridium botulinum* (botulism), *Y. pestis* (plague), *Variola major* (smallpox), *Francisella tularensis* (tularemia), and various viral hemorrhagic fevers including Lassa fever, Ebola, and Marburg.

Category B pathogens are the second highest priority organisms/biological agents because they are: (i) Regarded as moderately easy to disseminate; (ii) result in low mortality rates and/or moderate morbidity rates; and (iii) require specific diagnostic capacities and enhanced disease surveillance systems (Bowman, 2008; NIAID, 2018; NIH, 2012). Examples of Category B pathogens include Ricin toxin, *Staphylococcus* enterotoxin B, Typhus fever (*Rickettsia prowazekii*), Pathogenic vibrios, *Shigella* species, *Salmonella*, and *Campylobacter jejuni*. Category C agents consist of EID treats such as Nipah virus and additional hantaviruses (e.g., tick-borne hemorrhagic fever viruses, yellow fever, multidrug-resistant TB, rabies, prions, chikungunya virus, SARC-CoV, *Coccidioides immitis*, and posadosil) (Bowman, 2008; NIAID, 2018; NIH, 2012). The reader is referred to Chapter 7 for a detailed discussion on bioterrorism and emergency preparedness in Canada.

Adaptive emergence is defined as a genetic change in a microorganism that results in a phenotype that is capable of invading a new ecosystem, particularly via jumping to a new host species including humans. The emergence of SARS and MERS-CoV in humans, for examples, is believed to be facilitated by genetic changes enhancing transmissibility and pathogenicity between different species (WHO, 2018q). Notably, it is estimated that over 75% of EIDs and EIDs affecting humans are, or were originally *zoonotic* in nature (CDC, 2017d; Ogden, Abdel-Malik, & Pulliam, 2017; Wang & Cramer, 2014). That is to say, infectious diseases transmitted from animals to humans. Some zoonoses are intrinsically highly transmissible from human-to-human once infected. Hence, an epidemic can occur in the human population as evidenced during the outbreak of Ebola in West Africa in 2013 to 2016 (Ogden, Abdel-Malik, & Pulliam, 2017). We shall examine Ebola in greater detail later. Consequently, the capacity to predict, identify, and respond to infectious diseases in Canada and internationally is a major preoccupation of public health. The reader is referred to Chapter 7 for a detailed discussion of zoonotic mode infections.

There are two main ways by which infectious diseases can emerge or reemerge: (i) By changes in their geographical regions and ranges, or (ii) by adaptive emergence that results from a genetic change in a microorganism (Ogden, Abdel-Malik, & Pulliam, 2017). That latter makes the microorganism potentially capable of jumping to a new host species including humans. Management of EID events is a key challenge facing public health professionals, workers, and agencies. Increasingly, emphasis is being placed on predicting EID and REID occurrences, or to "get ahead of the curve"— that is, allowing health systems to be poised to respond to them, and public health to be ready to prevent them. Predictive models estimate where and when EIDs and REIDs may occur and the levels of risk they pose. Evaluation of the internal and external drivers that trigger emergence events is increasingly considered in predicting EID and REIDS events. For example, it is critical to mon-

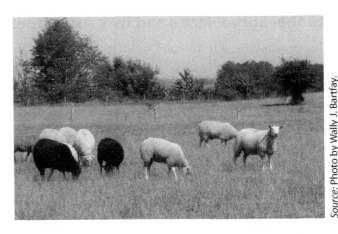

Photo 13.6   Zoonotic Infections are Major Drivers of EIDs and REIDs Globally. The zoonotic mode of transmission involves transmission of pathogens from animals to humans. Examples of zoonotic infections associated with sheep or goats include: Ringworm, Q-fever, chlamydiosis, leptospirosis, campylobacteriosis, salmonellosis, listeriosis, cryptosporidiosis, and giardiasis.

itor climate change and extreme weather events as actual or potential future drivers for the emergence of climate-sensitive diseases in Canada (e.g., Lyme disease, which typically occurs during the late spring and summer seasons) (Gasmi et al., 2017; Ogden, Abdel-Malik, & Pulliam, 2017). We shall examine Lyme disease in greater detail later.

Climatic factors also influence the emergence and reemergence of infectious diseases, in addition to multiple human, biological, and ecological determinants of health (Bartfay & Bartfay, 2015). The reader is referred to Chapter 8 for a detailed discussion on how climate change affects health, and Chapter 9 for discussion on global warming and its influence on the spread of infectious diseases. For example, climatologists in recent decades have identified upward trends in global temperatures and now estimate an unprecedented rise of 2.0+°C by the year 2100 (Epstein, 2001; Liang & Gong, 2017; Patz, Epstein, Burke, & Balbus, 1995; Wu, Lu, Zhou, Chen, & Xu, 2016). Of major concern is that these climatic changes can affect the introduction and dissemination of many serious and potentially lethal infectious diseases. The incidence of mosquitoe-borne diseases, including malaria, dengue, and viral encephalitis are among those diseases most sensitive to climate change. Climate change would directly affect disease transmission by shifting the vector's geographic range and increasing reproductive and biting rates, and by shortening the pathogen's required incubation period. Moreover, climate-related increases in sea surface temperature and sea level can lead to higher incidence of water-borne infectious and toxin-related illnesses, such as cholera and shellfish poisoning. Human migration and damage to health infrastructures from the projected increase in climate variability could also indirectly contribute to disease transmission.

Currently, global changes are driving an increased occurrence of EIDs and REIDs, but our capacity to prevent and deal with them is also increasing concurrently. For example, web-based scanning and analysis methods are increasingly allowing us to detect EIDs and REIDs outbreaks, modern genomics, and bioinformatics are increasing our ability to identify their genetic and geographical origins; while developments in geomatics and earth observation enable more real-time tracking of outbreaks. EIDs and REIDs will, however, remain a major public health challenge in our globalized world where demographic, climatic, and other environmental changes are altering the interactions between hosts and pathogen; in ways that increase spillover from animals to humans and global spread (Ogden, Abdel-Malik, & Pulliam, 2017). The reader is referred to Chapter 8 for a detailed discussion on how the environment and climate change is affecting the incidence of infectious diseases from a global context.

Global Surveillance and Risk Assessments of EIDs and REIDs

The growing need to respond to EIDs and REIDs has served as a catalyst for the creation and/or design of many international (e.g., WHO) and national (e.g., Public Health Agency of Canada [PHAC]) public health organizations and agencies; and the development of management plans for local, national, and international outbreaks (PHAC, 2017a; WHO, 2018q). Risk assessment is critical to decide, clarify, and justify public health preparedness, response, and recovery actions (Bartfay & Bartfay, 2015). To further facilitate the detection, communication, and management of global health threats the international community partnered with the WHO to create the *International Health Regulations* (IHR) in June 2017 (WHO, 2017b, 2017e). The IHR is regarded as a legally binding instrument on 196 countries across the globe, including Canada and other member states of WHO, and provides action plans to help prevent and respond to acute public health risks that have the potential to cross borders and threaten people worldwide.

For example, human influenza or the "common flu," is a respiratory infection caused by the influenza virus. While there are three types of influenza virus (A, B, and C), only influenza A and B cause seasonal outbreaks in humans (Government of Canada, 2017b; PHAC, 2017a). Influenza typically begins with a headache, chills, and cough, followed rapidly by fever, loss of appetite, muscle aches and fatigue, running nose, sneezing, watery eyes, and throat irritation. Nausea, vomiting, and diarrhea may also occur, especially in children. Most individuals will recover from influenza within a week or ten days. However, some individuals are at greater risk of complications (e.g., pneumonia) and mortality including those over 65 years of age; children less than 60 months of age; adults and children with chronic conditions (e.g., COPD, diabetes, heart disease); clients who underwent organ transplants, and immune-compromised clients (e.g., HIV/AIDS, cancer patients receiving chemotherapy or radiation). Notably, it is estimated that 12,200 hospitalizations and 3500 deaths linked to the flu occur annually in Canada alone (Government of Canada, 2017b). Globally, there are an estimated 1 billion cases of which 3 to 5 million results in severe illness or complications; and between 250,000 and 500,000 deaths occur annually due to the flu (Government of Canada, 2017b).

In 1947, WHO's Interim Committee recognized the importance of influenza and instigated a global coordinated effort for its surveillance, study, and control (WHO, 2018a). This subsequently resulted in the establishment of the *Global Influenza Programme* (GIP) and the *Global Influenza Surveillance and Response System* (GISRS). GISRS is an unique international disease surveillance network built on voluntary collaboration and real-time reporting, and includes 143 institutions in 113 member states. Similarly, "FluNet" is a web-based global surveillance, reporting, and analysis platform of GISRS that was first launched in 1997 (WHO, 2018a, 2018l). The virological data entered into FluNet (e.g., number of influenza viruses detected by subtype), are critical for real-time tracking of the movement of viruses globally, and for the interpretation of epidemiological data (WHO, 2018a, 2018l).

Surveillance entails the systematic collection and analysis of health-related data and timely communication of these health events to public health agencies, professionals, and workers. The reader is referred to Chapter 7 for a detailed discussion of active and passive surveillance activities in Canada. Surveillance for EIDs and REIDs is an ongoing regional, national, and international public health activity and priority that takes on many forms. One of the core requirements of the IHR is that all WHO member states are duty-bound to have the capacity for both indicator- and event-based surveillance, and are required to report "unusual or unexpected" events to WHO in a timely manner (Ogden, Abdel-Malik, & Pulliam, 2017; WHO, 2017d).

In addition to the IHR, there are a number of other global surveillance systems currently in play. For example, the *Global Early Warning System* (GLEWS) tracks zoonotic-based EIDS and REIDs, and recognizes the risks of human–animal–ecosystems interfaces (WHO, 2018t). Accordingly, GLEWS is run jointly by the following three sister organizations: (i) Food and Agriculture Organization (FAO); (ii) World Organization for Animal Health (OIE), and (iii) WHO. Similarly, the *GeoSentinel Surveillance Network* is a voluntarily international network of participating clinics and laboratories that engage in passive surveillance and communication of travel-related morbidity (International Society of Travel Medicine [ISTM], 2018; Torresi &

Leder, 2009). GeoSentinel was first initiated in 1995 by the ISTM with support from the CDC. Collectively, these surveillance systems and programs described above allow for a large numbers of individual members in several countries to be rapidly linked together to share observations and data, and to facilitate direct interaction with public health agencies and authorities.

Examining Major EIDs and REIDs From a Canadian Context

The global spread of communicable diseases is a growing concern largely as a result of increased international travel and global trade. In Canada, the provinces and territories have the primary responsibility to prepare for and respond to health threats within their borders (Bjatia et al., 2015; Lior & Njoo, 2015). This mandated responsibility covers the spectrum of clinical care and treatment; to the development and implementation of policies and programs that seek to prevent and/or mitigate the consequences of an outbreak. Although most public health management of ICDs occurs at the front line, the federal government also takes actions to prevent and mitigate their importation. The PHAC plays a central role in collaboration with its provincial/territorial partners to advance preparedness for emerging and reemerging high-consequence infectious diseases (Bartfay & Bartfay, 2015; Lior & Njoo, 2015).

For example, PHAC plays a key role in providing evidence-informed travel health notices and advice to help reduce associated risks when travelling abroad for pleasure or business; works closely with Canadian Border Services (CBS) to screen for infectious diseases, and closely regulates the entry of pathogens and toxins into Canada (Bhatia et al., 2015). The PHAC has also developed "Rapid Response Teams" to help contain an EID outbreak, and this team idea was first conceptualized and developed during the 2014 Ebola outbreak in Africa (Lior & Njoo, 2015). We shall examine the Ebola outbreak in greater detail later. The reader is referred to Chapter 7 for a detailed discussion of active and passive surveillance systems; notifiable/reportable infectious diseases in Canada, and bioterrorism. The reader is referred to Chapter 8 for a detailed discussion on public health preparedness and response and emergency management systems, and how climate change and global warming affect the distribution and prevalence of various infectious diseases. Although a discussion of all major EIDs and REIDs is beyond the scope and purpose of this chapter, we shall examine select key EIDs and REIDs that are also impacting or have impacted Canadians across the lifespan.

Avian Influenza (Avian Flu or Bird Flu)

Avian influenza, often called "Avian flu" or "Bird flu" in the mass and social media, is a contagious viral infection that can affect several species of food producing birds (e.g., chickens, turkeys, quails, guinea fowl) as well as pet birds and wild birds. Avian influenza viruses are broadly classified into the following two types; which is based on the severity of the illness they cause in birds: (i) Low pathogenic avian influenza (LPAI) and (ii) highly pathogenic avian influenza (HPAI) (Canadian Food Inspection Agency [CFIA], 2017a). Avian influenza viruses are further divided by subtypes based on the following two proteins found in the viruses: (i) Hemagglutinin (HA or "H" protein) and (ii) neuraminidase (NA or "N" protein). To date, there are 16 H types and 9 N types that have been identified, which creates a total 144 possible combinations (CFIA, 2017a).

There are four main kinds of influenza viruses, which are categorized as types A, B, C, and D (WHO, 2018o). Aquatic birds are the primary natural reservoir for most subtypes of influenza A viruses, and are of most concern to public health professionals and officials due to their potential to cause a pandemic in humans populations, Type A influenza viruses are classified into subtypes according to the combinations of two different virus surface proteins HA and NA. To date, there have been 18 different HA subtypes and 11 different NA subtypes identified (WHO, 2018n). Influenza B viruses may also circulate among human populations and cause seasonal epidemics. Influenza C viruses can infect both humans and pigs (swine), but these infections are typically mild in nature and are rarely reported. Influenza D viruses primarily affect cattle and are not known to infect or cause illness in humans (WHO, 2018n, 2018o).

Avian influenza viruses, such as the highly pathogenic H5N1 virus present in Asia, can, on rare occasions, cause disease in humans through close contact with infected birds or heavily contaminated environments. It is notable that the H5N1 Asian strain of avian influenza virus has been confirmed in poultry and wild birds in several countries in the following regions: Asia, Europe, Africa, and the Middle East (Government of Canada, 2008; WHO, 2018n, 2018o). This example highlights how a virus can quickly spread over wide geographical regions. Table 13.1 shows the number of confirmed human cases and deaths for avian influenza A (H5N1) reported to WHO between the years 2003 and 2017 (WHO, 2017a). There were a total of 860 confirmed cases and 454 associated deaths. The greatest risk to humans appears to occur when the virus becomes established in small backyard poultry flocks, which allows for close human contact, exposures, and infections to occur (Government of Canada, 2008; WHO, 2018n, 2018o).

The first outbreak of avian influenza A (H5N1) virus in humans arose in 1997 in Hong Kong, and consisted of 18 confirmed cases and six associated deaths (Chan, 2002; Snacken, Kendal, Haaheim, & Wood, 1999). Infections were acquired by humans directly from interactions with chickens; without the involvement of an intermediate host. The clinical spectrum of avian H5N1 infection ranged from asymptomatic

Table 13.1   Cumulative Number of Confirmed Human Cases for Avian Influenza A (H5N1) Reported to WHO, 2003–2017

Country	Confirmed Cases	Deaths
Azerbaijan	8	5
Bangladesh	8	1
Cambodia	56	1
Canada	1	1
China	53	31
Djibouti	1	0
Egypt	359	120
Indonesia	200	168
Iraq	3	2
Lao People's Democratic Republic	2	2
Myanmar	1	0
Nigeria	1	1
Pakistan	3	1
Thailand	25	17
Turkey	12	4
Viet Nam	127	64
Totals	860	454

Source: Adapted from WHO (2017a).

infections to fatal pneumonitis and multiple organ failure. Reactive hemophagocytic syndrome was the most distinguishing pathologic finding, which may have contributed to other complications including lymphopenia, liver dysfunction, and abnormal clotting profiles observed in hospitalized clients. In fact, this outbreak raised worldwide concern on the possibilities that such an influenza virus may become the next global influenza pandemic. In fact, it has killed nearly 60% of the clients who have been infected. This outbreak was halted by a territory-wide slaughter in Hong Kong of more than 1.5 million chickens by the end of December, 1997 (Chan, 2002; Snacken et al., 1999).

Certain avian H7 viruses (e.g., H7N2, H7N3, and H7N7) are also a growing public health concern in Canada and globally, because they have occasionally been found to infect humans as well (WHO, 2018o). From 1996 to 2012, for example, human infections with H7 avian influenza viruses (e.g., H7N2, H7N3, and H7N7) have been reported in Canada, Italy, Mexico, the Netherlands, the United Kingdom, and the United States (WHO, 2018o). Between February 24 and March 7, 2017, a total of 58 additional laboratory-confirmed cases of human infection have also been reported to WHO from mainland China and Hong Kong's Special Administrative Region (WHO, 2018m).

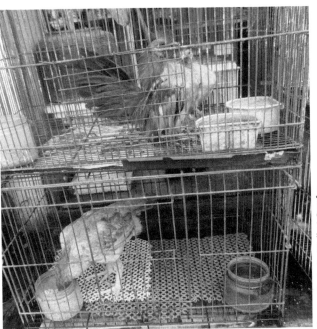

Source: Photo by Wally J. Bartfay.

Photo 13.7 Chickens Being Sold in a Wet Market in Hong Kong. The available epidemiological and virological information strongly suggests that most known human H7N9 infections result from direct contact (e.g., animal husbandry, farming practices) with infected poultry, or indirect contact with infected poultry (e.g., faeces, blood). For example, by visiting wet markets and having contact with environments where infected poultry have been kept or slaughtered.

More recently, avian influenza A (H7N9) is a subtype of influenza viruses that have been detected in birds in the past, but has not previously been seen in either animals or humans until it was found in March 2013 in China (WHO, 2018b, 2018n, 2018o). The H7N9 strain is a growing public health concern because most clients who become infected become severely ill. Nonetheless, this virus does not appear to transmit easily from person-to-person, and sustained human-to-human transmission has not yet been reported (WHO, 2018b). The WHO (2018m) advises that individuals travelling to regions with known outbreaks of avian influenza avoid visiting poultry farms, having contact with animals in live poultry markets, entering areas where poultry may be slaughtered, or come into contact with any surfaces that appear to be contaminated with faeces from poultry or other animals. Individuals should also follow good food safety and hygiene practices, including washing their hands often with soap and water.

The emergence of the 2009 influenza pandemic virus, animal-to-human transmission of A (H5N1), A (H7N9); and other animal influenza viruses highlight the importance of monitoring and assessing the potential risks of emerging influenza viruses to cause future pandemics (WHO, 2016a, 2016b). Advanced emergency planning and preparedness are critical to help mitigate the impact of an influenza pandemic. Accordingly, the WHO (2016b) has developed a document entitled a "Tool for Influenza Pandemic Risk Assessment (TIPRA)" (see Web-Based Resource Box 13.1) with the aim of harmonizing national and international preparedness and response. TIPRA also enables the identification of gaps in knowledge so that attention and resources can be dedicated to address these shortcomings.

Web-Based Resource Box 13.1: Tool for Influenza Pandemic Risk Assessment (TIPRA)

Learning Resource	Website
World Health Organization (May, 2016b). *Tool for influenza pandemic risk assessment (TIPRA) Version I.* Geneva, Switzerland: Author. -Tool developed to monitor and assess the potential risks of emerging influenza viruses to cause future pandemics.	http://www.who.int/influenza/publications/TIPRA_manual_v1/en/ **or** http://apps.who.int/iris/bitstream/10665/250130/1/WHO-OHE-PED-GIP-2016.2-eng.pdf?ua=1

Blastomycosis (Gilchrist's Disease)

Blastomycosis, which is also known as "Gilchrist's disease," is defined as an invasive fungal disease caused by the organism *Blastomyces dermatitidis;* and whose natural reservoir is found in decaying wood, leaves, and soil. It is estimated that 70% of human cases can be attributed to pulmonary blastomycosis, which usually presents as a flulike illness. Dogs, and more rarely cats, can also be infected. Blastomycosis infection occurs primarily through the inhalation of airborne spores. It can also rarely occur via a puncture in the skin and via sexual contact. Exposure to potential fungal spores may increase during excavation and construction operations, as well as during recreational activities that involve contact with soil near waterways. Hence, individuals with weakened immune systems (e.g., HIV/AIDS, clients receiving chemotherapy or radiation therapy) should avoid hiking in forested and wooded areas in Canada where the fungus is present (Government of Canada, 2016c; Manitoba Health Communicable Disease Control Unit, 2015).

Common clinical signs and symptoms may take 21 to 45 days to manifest post-exposure; and include fever and night sweats, cough, brown or bloody mucus, pneumonia, fatigue, general discomfort, malaise, open sores, or ulcers on the skin that can develop into abscesses, bone and joint pain, and unintentional weight loss (Government of Canada, 2016c; PHAC, 2010). Antifungal treatments with Amphotericin B and itraconazole continue to be the main drugs employed to treat blastomycosis.

The annual incidence rate of blastomycosis is 0.62 cases per 100,000 people in the provinces of Québec, Ontario, Manitoba, and Saskatchewan; and the mortality rate ranges from 0% to 2% in treated clients, and 42% in untreated clients (Government of Canada, 2016c; PHAC, 2010). Cases of blastomycosis have been reported in eastern areas of North America, including the Great Lakes Basin (i.e., Ontario, Michigan, Wisconsin, Minnesota) and the St. Lawrence Valley, and in the Midwestern United States and Central Canada (Litvinjenko & Lunny, 2017; Manitoba Health Communicable Disease Control Unit, 2015; Seitz, Adjemian, Steiner, & Prevots, 2015). Blastomycosis is spread via the inhalation of small particles of the fungus into the lungs where they develop into yeast and cause swelling. The yeast can subsequently spread through your blood to other parts of the body. Although the lungs are the primary site of infection; it may also spread to the kidneys, brain and spinal cord, bones, stomach and intestines (Government of Canada, 2016c; PHAC, 2010).

Research Focus Box 13.2 describes an epidemiological investigation which examined hospitalized cases of blastomycosis in Ontario between the years 2006 and 2010.

Research Focus Box 13.2 Blastomycosis Hospitalizations in Northwestern Ontario: 2006–2015

Study Aim/Rationale

Blastomycosis is a fungal disease caused by the organism *B. dermatitidis*, which is an invasive species found in soil in Central Canada and Central and Midwestern United States. The aim of this investigation was to examine

---

(Continued)

(Continued)

and describe trends in reported cases of blastomycosis requiring hospitalization among Northwestern Ontario residents between the years 2006 and 2015, inclusive.

Methodology/Design

An epidemiological investigation was undertaken to examine documented cases of blastomycosis. Specifically, hospital-based data were extracted from the Discharge Abstract Database (DAD) that was accessed through IntelliHEALTH Ontario. The DAD includes administrative (e.g., time of admission and discharge); clinical (e.g., diagnosis, treatment, medications), and demographic information (e.g., client's age, sex) on hospital discharges provided by the Canadian Institute for Health Information (CIHI). Confirmation of a blastomycosis diagnosis in the records were identified using ICD-10 codes B40.0 to B40.9. Hospitalization rates were calculated as well as age-specific hospitalization rates by local health regions. Moreover, data pertaining to time, seasonality, and presenting clinical signs and symptoms were analyzed.

Major Findings

There were a total of 581 cases of blastomycosis in Ontario over the 10-year assessment period. It is noteworthy that 245 cases (i.e., 42%) were from Northwestern Ontario, although this region accounts for only 0.6% of the entire population in this province. The average hospitalization rate was 35.0 per 100,000 per year, with a range from 1.7 in the Red Lake region to 57.9 in the Kenora region of the province. Pulmonary symptoms (e.g., flulike) were the most common clinical presentation on admission to the hospital. Males were 1.36 times more likely to be hospitalized for blastomycosis, in comparison to their female counterparts (95% CI: 1.06–1.75, $p < .05$).

Implications for Public Health

Based on data which spans a 10-year period, this study suggests that areas of Northwestern Ontario are at increased risk of contracting blastomycosis. It is interesting to note that most hospitalized cases were registered in the late fall months, which suggests prior blastomycosis exposure in the spring/summer seasons followed by a lengthy incubation period. Interregional differences may warrant prioritizing public health strategies for the prevention and control of blastomycosis. In addition, epidemiological research, tracking, and surveillance of this fungal infection are warranted in Ontario.

Source: Litvinjenko and Lunny (2017).

Chikungunya

Chikungunya is a reemerging infectious mosquitoe-borne RNA viral disease that was first described during an outbreak in Southern Tanzania in 1952 (Chhabra, Mittal, Bhattacharya, Rana, & Lal, 2008; Powers & Lague, 2007; WHO, 2018c, 2018d). Specifically, this RNA virus belongs to the alphavirus genus of the family *Togaviridae*. The name "Chikungunya" is derived from a word in the Kimakonde language, meaning "to become contorted," and is employed to describe the stooped appearance of sufferers afflicted with severe joint pain (arthralgia) (Weaver, 2006; WHO, 2018c, 2018d). The virus is transmitted from human-to-human via bites from infected female mosquitoes, which include the *Aedes aegypti* and *Aedes albopictus* species (Chhabra et al., 2008; Powers & Lague, 2007; Weaver, 2006; WHO, 2018c, 2018d).

Clinical signs and symptoms typically appear between 4 and 7 days after the client has been bitten by an infected mosquitoe, and include very high fever (39+°C), severe joint pain, and swelling that is often debilitating in nature (e.g., lower back, ankle, knees, wrists, or phalanges), skin rashes, headache, muscle pain, nausea, and fatigue (Chhabra et al., 2008; Powers & Lague, 2007; Weaver, 2006). Chikungunya does not often result in death per se, but the severe disabling joint pain may last for months or years; which often becomes a cause of chronic pain and disability (Pan American Health Organization [PAHO], 2017). There is no specific antiviral drug treatment or commercial vaccine currently available for Chikungunya. Treatment is directed primarily at relieving the symptoms, which include analgesics for pain management (e.g., for relieving severe joint pain), use of anti-pyretics, and maintaining hydration via fluids.

Chikungunya has been identified in over 60 countries in Asia, Africa, Europe, Mexico, Caribbean, and the Americas. In 2015 alone, 693,489 suspected cases and 37,480 confirmed cases of Chikungunya were reported in the Americas; and Colombia had the greatest burden with 356,079 suspected cases (PAHO, 2017). Nonetheless, this number was less in comparison to 2014 figures when more than 1 million suspected cases were reported in the same region. In 2016, there was a total of 349,936 suspected and 146,914 laboratory confirmed cases reported to the PAHO. The countries reporting the highest number of cases were Brazil with 265,000 cases; and Bolivia and Colombia had 19,000 cases, respectively (PAHO, 2017; WHO, 2018d).

As of December 9, 2014, there were 320 confirmed cases and 159 probable cases of Chikungunya infections in Canada associated with travel to Caribbean countries, Mexico and the Americas, and Asia–Pacific regions (CTV News, 2015; PAHO, 2017; The Canadian Press, 2017). Protecting travelers going abroad is a major public health concern because Canadians make an estimated 2.5 million visits to Caribbean countries each year, and are therefore at increased risk for infection (CTV News, 2015). In fact, almost 800,000 people have been reported infected in the Caribbean in 2014,

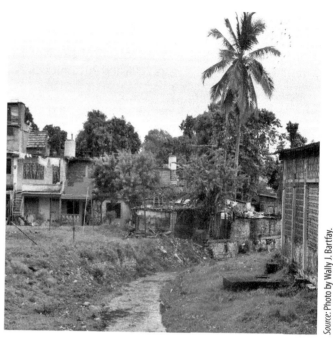

Source: Photo by Wally J. Bartfay.

Photo 13.8   Slums of Santa Clara, Cuba. Vector-control is a major public health challenge in developing nations such as Cuba, Dominican Republic, Haiti, Puerto Rico, and the U.S. Virgin Islands. The PAHO (2014) reports that between 2013 and 2014, there were 5000 confirmed cases of Chikungunya fever and as many as 160,000 suspected cases in the Caribbean, which are often visited by Canadian tourists.

and the majority where from the Dominican Republic (The Canadian Press, 2017). Moreover, most provinces in Canada had at least one confirmed case with the majority diagnosed in Ontario ($N = 165$) and Québec ($N = 114$) (CTV News, 2015).

Prevention and control relies heavily on reducing the number of natural and artificial water-filled container habitats that support breeding of the mosquitoes (e.g., flower pots, bird baths, kiddy pools). This requires mobilization of affected communities. During outbreaks, insecticides may be sprayed to kill flying mosquitoes, applied to surfaces in and around containers where the mosquitoes land, and used to treat water in containers to kill the immature larvae. For protection during outbreaks of Chikungunya, clothing which minimizes skin exposure to day-biting vectors is advised. Mosquitoe repellents should also be applied to exposed skin and/or clothing in strict accordance with product label instructions. Repellents should contain DEET (N,N-diethyl-3-methylbenzamide), IR3535 (3-[N-acetyl-N-butyl]-aminopropionic acid ethyl ester) or icaridin (1-piperidinecarboxylic acid, 2-(2-hydroxyethyl)-1-methylpropylester) (WHO, 2018d). For those who sleep or take naps during the daylight hours; which include particularly young children and infants or sick or older people, and insecticide-treated mosquitoe nets may be employed.

Ebola Virus Disease

Ebola virus disease (EVD), formally known as "Ebola hemorrhagic fever," is a rare yet potentially deadly viral disease which can affect humans and primates alike (e.g., monkeys, gorillas, and chimpanzees), and was first recognized in 1976 in Nzara, South Sudan, and in Yambuku, the Democratic Republic of Congo (formerly Zaire) (Government of Canada, 2017a; Payne, 2016a; WHO, 2018g). This disease is named after the Ebola River located in the Democratic Republic of Congo in Africa. During the 1976 outbreak, 284 cases and 151 deaths were present in Sudan with a case fatality rate of 55%. In the Democratic Republic of Congo, 318 cases were identified with 280 deaths or a case fatality rate of 88% (see Table 13.2). In both cases, this zoonotic disease—meaning it can be transmitted from animals to humans—was primarily spread through close personal contact within hospitals, and through contaminated needles and syringes. Ebola resurfaced three years later in Zaire, Africa when 34 people became infected in 1979. Case fatality rates have varied from 25% to 90% during past outbreaks, and the average rate is approximately 50% for those who contract the disease (Infection Control and Prevention Canada [IPAC], 2018; WHO, 2018g).

Table 13.2   Chronology of Previous Ebola Virus Disease Outbreaks, Species, Human cases, Deaths and Case Fatalities

Year	Country	Ebolavirus species	Cases	Deaths	Case fatality
2015	Italy	Zaire	1	0	0%
2014	DRC	Zaire	66	49	74%
2014	Spain	Zaire	1	0	0%
2014	UK	Zaire	1	0	0%
2014	USA	Zaire	4	1	25%
2014	Senegal	Zaire	1	0	0%
2014	Mali	Zaire	8	6	75%
2014	Nigeria	Zaire	20	8	40%
2014–2016	Sierra Leone	Zaire	14,124[a]	3956[a]	28%
2014–2016	Liberia	Zaire	10,675[a]	4809[a]	45%
2014–2016	Guinea	Zaire	3811[a]	2543[a]	67%
2012	Democratic Republic of Congo	Bundibugyo	57	29	51%
2012	Uganda	Sudan	7	4	57%
2012	Uganda	Sudan	24	17	71%
2011	Uganda	Sudan	1	1	100%
2008	Democratic Republic of Congo	Zaire	32	14	44%
2007	Uganda	Bundibugyo	149	37	25%
2007	Democratic Republic of Congo	Zaire	264	187	71%
2005	Congo	Zaire	12	10	83%

(Continued)

Table 13.2   Chronology of Previous Ebola Virus Disease Outbreaks, Species, Human cases, Deaths and Case Fatalities (*Continued*)

Year	Country	Ebolavirus species	Cases	Deaths	Case fatality
2004	Sudan	Sudan	17	7	41%
2003 (Nov–Dec)	Congo	Zaire	35	29	83%
2003 (Jan–Apr)	Congo	Zaire	143	128	90%
2001–2002	Congo	Zaire	59	44	75%
2001–2002	Gabon	Zaire	65	53	82%
2000	Uganda	Sudan	425	224	53%
1996	South Africa (ex-Gabon)	Zaire	1	1	100%
1996 (Jul–Dec)	Gabon	Zaire	60	45	75%
1996 (Jan–Apr)	Gabon	Zaire	31	21	68%
1995	Democratic Republic of Congo	Zaire	315	254	81%
1994	Côte d'Ivoire	Taï Forest	1	0	0%
1994	Gabon	Zaire	52	31	60%
1979	Sudan	Sudan	34	22	65%
1977	Democratic Republic of Congo	Zaire	1	1	100%
1976	Sudan	Sudan	284	151	53%
1976	Democratic Republic of Congo	Zaire	318	280	88%

[a] Includes suspect, probable, and confirmed Ebola virus disease (EVD) cases.
Source: Adapted from the WHO (2018g).

The West African Ebola outbreak that occurred between 2013 and 2016 garnered international headlines in the mass and social media. The *Public Health Emergency of International Concern* (PHEI) declaration related to Ebola outbreak in West Africa issued by WHO was finally lifted on March 29, 2016. The outbreak was considered to be over when 42 days (double the 21-day incubation period of the ebolavirus) had elapsed since the last identified case in isolation was laboratory confirmed negative for the EVD virus (IPAC, 2018). By the time the outbreak was over, a total of 28,616 confirmed, probable, and suspected cases had been reported to WHO, and 11,310 individuals died as a consequence of EVD (CDC, 2016; Payne, 2016a; WHO, 2016c, 2018f, 2018g; Figure 13.4).

The incubation period of EVD varies from 2 to 21 days, with an average onset of 10 days postexposure (CDC, 2014; IPAC, 2018). Clinical signs and symptoms of EVD include sudden onset of high fever (39+°C), myalgia, unexplained bruising or bleeding, pharyngitis, sore throat, skin rash, muscle aches and pain, severe headache, malaise, fatigue, nausea and vomiting, diarrhea, abdominal pain, and decreased and impaired liver and kidney function. Death is usually attributed to low blood pressure and severe loss of body fluids or blood. These are often accompanied by a maculopapular or petechial rash that may progress to purpura. Bleeding (hemorrhaging) may also occur in approximately 50% of cases from the gums, nasal cavity, injection sites or wounds, and the gastrointestinal tract (Government of Canada, 2017a; WHO, 2018g).

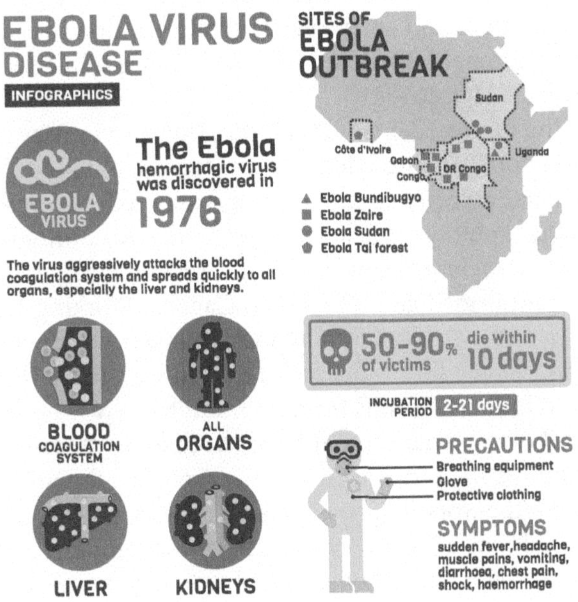

Within the genus *Ebolavirus* (family = *Filoviridae*), five species of EVD have been identi-

Figure 13.4 Understanding Ebola Virus Infection

fied to date: (i) Zaire; (ii) Bundibugyo; (iii) Sudan; (iv) Reston; and (v) Taï Forest (CDC, 2016; Heymann, 2015; WHO, 2018g). The first three (i.e., Bundibugyo ebolavirus, Zaire ebolavirus, and Sudan ebolavirus) have been responsible for large outbreaks in humans in Africa and are regarded as being endemic in nature. The virus which caused the 2014 to 2016 West African outbreak belonged to the Zaire ebolavirus species. It is notable that four of the five virus strains that occur in an animal host is native to the African continent (CDC, 2016; WHO, 2018g).

The exact natural reservoir host for the Ebola virus remains unknown. Nonetheless, on the basis of epidemiological evidence and the nature of similar viruses, researchers believe that EVD is animal-borne in origin, and that bats are the most likely reservoir. Specifically, it is hypothesized that fruit bats of the *Pteropodidae* family are natural Ebola virus hosts (CDC, 2016; Heymann, 2015; Wang & Cramer, 2014; WHO, 2018g). The Ebola virus can be introduced into the human population via close contact with the blood, secretions, organs or other bodily fluids or discharges of infected animals including fruit bats, chimpanzees, gorillas, monkeys, forest antelope, and porcupines found ill or dead in the rainforest.

Human-to-human transmission of the EVD can occur via contact with blood, body fluids (e.g., semen, urine, saliva, breast milk) or tissue from an infected person or corpse, contaminated medical equipment (e.g., syringes, needles, surgical equipment) and/or sexual intercourse (e.g., oral, vaginal, anal). Ebola may also spread in healthcare settings if staff do not wear proper protective equipment, such as masks, gowns, and gloves (CDC, 2016; Government of Canada, 2017a; IPAC, 2018; WHO, 2018g). Hence, EVD can spread through human-to-human transmission via direct contact with the blood, secretions, organs, or other bodily fluids of infected people (e.g., through broken skin or mucous membranes); and/or with surfaces and materials (e.g., bedding, clothing) contaminated with these fluid (WHO, 2018g). The WHO (2018g) cautions that the Ebola virus is reported to persist in immune-privileged sites in certain clients who have recovered from EVD (e.g., testicles, inside of the eye, CNS). In women who have been infected while pregnant, the virus can persist in the placenta, amniotic fluid, and fetus. In women who have been infected while breastfeeding, the virus may also persist in breast milk and be passed on to their infants.

Community engagement is key to successfully controlling outbreaks. Suitable and proper outbreak control relies on applying a package or set of interventions; which includes case management, infection prevention and control practices, surveillance and contact tracing, adequate laboratory services, safe burial practices, public education, and social mobilization (Bartfay & Bartfay, 2015; WHO, 2018g). Early supportive care with rehydration, and symptomatic treatment improves survival rates. Currently there is no licensed treatment proven to neutralize the virus; but a range of blood, immunological, and drug therapies are under development (WHO, 2018g).

The unprecedented extent, duration and impact of the EVD outbreak in West Africa which began in the spring of 2014; provided worldwide recognition of the importance for a multidisciplinary, international and national capacity to initiate and sustain effective public health responses over an extended period of time for such outbreaks (Lior & Njoo, 2015). Accordingly, the PHAC has established *Ebola Virus Disease (EVD) Rapid Response Teams* that were available to any requesting provincial/territorial jurisdiction with a laboratory confirmed case of EVD in Canada. Working with provincial and territorial officials, a *Rapid Response Team Concept of Operations* was developed, which outlined the process for Rapid Response Team engagement as well as the suite of technical expertise available (Lior & Njoo, 2015).

Preliminary results from a clinical trial ($N = 11,841$) in Guinea conducted by WHO in 2015 suggests that an Ebola vaccine created by researchers in Winnipeg, Manitoba was effective against the so-called "Zaire strain" of the virus; which was responsible for more than 11,300 deaths in Western Africa starting in late 2013—the worst Ebola outbreak in history (Payne, 2016b; Semeniuk, 2017; WHO, 2018f, 2018p). During this clinical trial, a "ring vaccine strategy" was employed by WHO; where only those individuals who were in close contact with a new Ebola case (e.g., family members, neighbours), as well as contacts of those contacts, were vaccinated. Whereas members of a randomly chosen West African cohort might only have a minute chance of contracting Ebola, those in the ring of contacts around a new case would have a significant risk. This translated into a higher confidence level obtained with results of the trial. A total of 117 rings (or "clusters") were identified, each made up of an average of 80 individuals. Amongst the 5837 people who received the vaccine, no Ebola cases were recorded 10 days or more post-vaccination. In comparison, there were 23 cases 10 days or more post-vaccination among those who did not receive the vaccine (WHO, 2018f, 2018p). Interestingly, the trial also revealed that unvaccinated individuals in the rings were indirectly protected from Ebola virus via the ring vaccination approach due to herd immunity. Researchers report that the vaccine, called rVSV-ZEBOV, is likely to be more than 80% effective when deployed across an entire population, as a form of herd immunity. In brief, the rVSV-ZEBOV vaccine is an altered form of vesicular stomatitis virus (VSV), which affects animals but not human. Due to a genetic modification, it carries a surface protein that is identical to one found on the human Ebola virus. Hence, this protein serves to prime the body's immune system so that it recognizes and attacks any real Ebola it encounters. A parallel vaccine is still required for the Sudan strain, which is more prevalent in Eastern Africa (Semeniuk, 2017; WHO, 2018p).

Lyme Disease (Lyme Borreliosis)

The disease received its name from town of Old Lyme, Connecticut, in 1975 where it was first reported, but has since spread to over 80 countries in the world including Canada, Australia, European continent, and Asia (Lyme Disease Association, Inc. 2018; Steere, Coburn, & Glickstein, 2004; WHO, 2018s). **Lyme disease**, is a multisystem infection that is manifested by progressive stages and is caused by the spirochete *B. burgdorferi* sensu stricto transmitted by blacklegged deer ticks (Ixodes species) (Gasmi et al., 2017; Hatchette, Davis, & Johnson, 2014; Ogden, Koffi, Pelcat, & Lindsay, 2014; PHAC, 2017b). Many species of mammals (e.g., dogs, humans) can be infected, and rodents and deer act as primary reservoirs. Immature ticks are called nymphs, and they are about the size of a pinhead. Nymphs pickup bacteria when they feed on small rodents, such as mice, that are infected with *B. burgdorferi*.

Lyme disease is diagnosed through a combination of clinical signs and symptoms, history of exposure or potential exposure to infected ticks (e.g., hiking in tick infected woods), and via validated laboratory test results. Early signs and symptoms of Lyme disease include fever, chills, headache, fatigue, muscle and joint pain. The development of a red circular rash (i.e., erythema migrans) that resembles a "bull's eye" mark may develop in certain clients; which typically begins as a small erythematous papule or macule that appears at the site of the tick bite one to two weeks post-infection (range, 3–32 days) (Canadian Lyme Disease Foundation,

2018; Hahn et al., 2006; Shapiro, 2014). However, approximately 25% to 50% of infected clients never develop an erythema migrans rash, and it may be more difficult to detect in clients with dark coloured skin tones. Based on Canadian data, the most common presenting symptom reported between the years 2009 and 2015 was a single erythema migrans rash (74.2%), and arthritis (35.7%) (Gasmi et al., 2017).

If left untreated, Lyme disease symptoms could progress to cardiac symptoms (e.g., heart palpitations), arthritic symptoms, extreme fatigue and general weakness, and central and peripheral nervous system disorders (e.g., paralysis) (Shapiro, 2014; Steere et al., 2004; WHO, 2018s). Arthritis, which typically affects the knee joints of infected clients, is a late sign of disseminated Lyme disease, occurring weeks to months after initial infection; but occurs in less than 10% of all cases (Shapiro, 2014). Progression through the stages of Lyme disease in humans can take a number of months and in some cases years to manifest. Symptoms tend to worsen during each stage of infection; ranging from flu-like symptoms to cardiac complications, and neurological illnesses which may include paralysis. It is important to note that as time passes, both treatment options and client relief become more difficult to manage. Nonetheless, most cases of Lyme disease

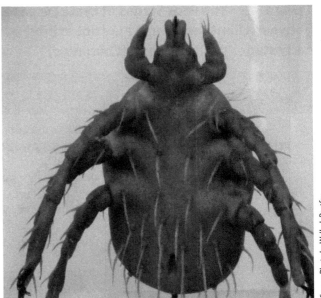

Source: Photo by Wally J. Bartfay.

Photo 13.9 Lyme Disease Is Transmitted by Blacklegged Ticks in Canada. Lyme disease is the most commonly reported vector-borne disease in North America transmitted by blacklegged ticks, *Ixodes scapularis*, in Central and Eastern Canada and *Ixodes pacificus* in Western Canada. The increase in geographic distribution of Lyme disease cases is associated, in part, with effects of climate change and global warming on range spread of these tick vectors in Canada (PHAC, 2017b).

can be treated successfully with a course of antibiotics. Table 13.3 provides an overview of the four stages of Lyme disease; common signs and symptoms, and treatment options currently available (Canadian Lyme Disease Foundation, 2018; Lind, 2018; Lyme Disease Association of Australia, 2018; Shapiro, 2014; Steere et al., 2004; WHO, 2018s).

Table 13.3   The Four Stages of Lyme Disease. Clinical signs and symptoms may vary between clients and some may not exhibit overt signs and symptoms, especially in the early stages of the disease.

Stage and Description	Common Signs and Symptoms	Treatment Options
Stage I: Early localized Lyme Disease (one to a few days after infection) -Bacteria have not yet spread throughout the body or organ systems.	Initial flu-like symptoms, chills, headaches, muscle and joint pain, low-grade fever, nausea, jaw pain, light sensitivity, red eyes, muscle aches and neck stiffness, circular red-rash described as being "bull's-eye" (erythema migraines) in shape and appearance.	Oral course of antibiotics such as doxycycline, cefuroxime, and amoxicillin may be prescribed.

(Continued)

Table 13.3   The Four Stages of Lyme Disease. Clinical signs and symptoms may vary between clients and some may not exhibit overt signs and symptoms, especially in the early stages of the disease. (*Continued*)

Stage and Description	Common Signs and Symptoms	Treatment Options
Stage II: Disseminated Lyme disease (several days to weeks following infection) -Bacteria have begun to spread throughout the body and organ systems.	Flu-like symptoms that are often similar to or worse than those noted in Stage 1, fever, sore throat, chills, joint and muscle pain, fatigue, visual disturbances, including blurry vision, stiffness of neck, headache, swollen lymph nodes or glands, pain or numbness in the jaw area, and disorders of the nervous system and heart (e.g., palpitations).	Oral course of antibiotics such as azithromycin, doxycycline, amoxicillin, or cefuroxime may be prescribed. Note: doxycycline should not be given to children under eight years of age or to nursing or pregnant women. For more severely ill clients, a 10- to 30-day course of intravenous antibiotics such as ceftriaxone may be prescribed.
Stage III: Late disseminated Lyme disease (days to weeks after infection if left untreated, or not properly treated) -Bacteria have now spread throughout the body and organ systems.	Arthritis of major large joints (e.g., knees, hips, elbow), extreme fatigue, temporary paralysis of facial muscles, numbness or tingling in extremities (arms, legs, feet or hands), severe migraines or headaches, heart arrhythmias or palpitations, memory loss (short term), difficulty concentrating, mental fogginess or sluggishness, sleep and mood disturbances.	Treatment at this stage is typically the same as in the first two stages, which involves a course of oral or intravenous antibiotics.
Stage IV: Chronic Lyme disease a.k.a. Chronic Lyme Arthritis (several months or years after initial infection)	Symptoms may include episodes lasting 6 months or more and include: chronic arthritis, joint inflammation (especially the knee), redness and fluid build-up in joints, pain and discomfort in extremities, alterations to short-term memory, confusion, and disorientation at times.	As above.

Lyme disease became a nationally notifiable disease on the *Canadian Notifiable Disease Surveillance System* (CNDSS) in 2009; with provincial and territorial health departments reporting clinician-diagnosed cases to the PHAC (2017b). Subsequently, the *Lyme Disease Enhanced Surveillance* (LDES) system, which was designed by a working group of the Pan-Canadian Public Health Network, was implemented in 2010. Since Lyme disease became a nationally notifiable disease in Canada in 2009, the number of reported confirmed cases has continued to increase from 0.4 to 2.6 per 100,000 population; and most cases were reported from Ontario, Québec and Nova Scotia. The number of reported Lyme disease cases increased more than sixfold, from 144 in 2009 to 917 in 2015, mainly due to an increase in infections acquired in Canada (Gasmi et al., 2017).

Ongoing surveillance, preventive strategies as well as early disease recognition and treatment will continue to abate and combat the impact of Lyme disease in Canada (Gasmi et al., 2017; Ogden et al., 2014). The best way to prevent Lyme disease is to avoid tick bites by using insect repellents when outdoors or in tick-infected regions, wearing proper clothing (e.g., tucking pants into socks worn over shoes or hiking boots), protecting family pets including cats and dogs from bites and infestations, removing ticks from the body as soon as they are detected, and removing tick habitats from around the home.

Sudden Acute Respiratory Syndrome (SARS)

Sudden Acute Respiratory Syndrome (SARS) is defined as a potentially life-threatening coronavirus (SARS-CoV) infection that affects the respiratory system with an average incubation period of six days, and which is spread by close person-to-person contact by infected individuals; most often via droplets expelled into the air during coughing or sneezing episodes. SARS is listed as a severe emerging viral disease due to its noted high fatality rates (WHO, 2018i). Initial symptoms of SARS are typically flu-like in nature and include fever (38+°C), myalgia, malaise, lethargy and generalized weakness, dry cough, sore throat, diarrhea (in approximately 10%–20% of cases), along with other non-specific symptoms. SARS may eventually lead to severe shortness of breath (at rest); respiratory failure, and/or pneumonia resulting from either direct viral pneumonia or due to secondary bacterial pneumonia (CDC, 2017a; Peiris, Guan, & Yuen, 2004; Zhong, Zheng, Li, Poon Xie, & Chan, 2003).

SARS-CoV was first identified in 2003, and is believed to be derived from an animal reservoir reported to be horseshoe bats; which was tracked and isolated to a remote damp cave located in Yunnan Province, China (Cyranoski, 2017; Hu et al., 2017). The SARS-CoV subsequently spread to other exotic animals (e.g., civet cats, raccoon dog, red fox, Chinese ferret badger); which are often sold as protein sources in Chinese markets, and then to humans (Cyranoski, 2017; Hu et al., 2017; Li et al., 2006). The first human case appeared in November 2002, and was speculated to be a farmer from the Foshan County located in the Guangdong province of Southern China (WHO, 2018i, 2018j, 2018r). This area is currently considered as a potential zone for the reemergence of SARS-CoV.

After SARS first emerged in Southern China in 2002, it rapidly initiated a global pandemic in 2003. On February 21, 2002 Liu Jianlun, a 64-year-old physician who had treated suspected cases in Guangdong, China checked into the ninth floor of Metropole Hotel in Hong Kong to attend an upcoming wedding (WHO, 2018j). By February 22, he required admission to the intensive care unit at Kwong Wah Hospital in Hong Kong, but subsequently died on March 4 of acute respiratory failure. Interestingly, approximately 80% of all initial Hong Kong cases have been traced back to this physician from China, including the first Canadian case who was also a guest at this hotel in Hong Kong (WHO, 2018j). The reader is referred to Chapter 7 for a detailed discussion on contact tracing, and for passive and active surveillance done by public health professionals and workers.

The WHO (2018i, 2018j) reports that between November 2002 and July 2003, the SARS pandemic caused an eventual 8098 cases, resulting in 774 deaths (9.6% fatality rate) in 37 countries; which included 251 cases (151 females and 100 males) and 44 deaths (18% fatality rate) in Canada (mostly in the greater Toronto area). The first human case in Canada was identified in March, 2003 in a client who returned from a trip to Hong Kong. All subsequent cases in Canada were traced to individuals who were in close contact with this female (e.g., family members, healthcare providers), and/or to travelers who had been in Asia. Indeed, by April 10 in Canada, there were already 253 suspected and probable cases, and 206 were in the greater Toronto area (GTA, Health Canada, 2003; Maunder et al., 2003). It is noteworthy that most cases of human-to-human transmission in Canada first occurred in acute healthcare settings due to the absence of adequate infection control precautions and procedures (Health Canada, 2003; Maunder et al., 2003; PHAC, 2012b). Other countries and regions of significance in which chains of human-to-human transmission occurred included: Hong Kong Special Administrative Region of China, Chinese Taipei, Singapore, Hanoi in Viet Nam, and Canada.

The WHO (2003) declared that the SARS outbreak "was contained" on July 5, 2003 when it removed Taiwan as the last country on its list based on two consecutive 10-day incubation periods (or 20 days total), since its last reported case on June 15, 2003. By this time, the global pandemic of SARS had affected 26 countries, claimed the lives of 916 individuals, 8422 were infected, and it cost the world economy in excess of $60 billion (U.S.) (Payne,

2006; WHO, 2018h, 2018r). Hence, SARS has been pronounced as one of the most significant global public health threats of the 21st century (Peiris, Guan, & Yuen, 2004; WHO, 2018i, 2018j; Zhong et al., 2003).

During the SARS pandemic, WHO coordinated an international investigation with the assistance of the Global Outbreak Alert and Response Network, and worked closely with health authorities and agencies in the affected countries to provide epidemiological, clinical, and logistical support (WHO, 2018h). In Canada, public health efforts to contain the spread of SARS included infection control measures in hospitals; and community-based quarantine measures mainly throughout the GTA in the province of Ontario. Specifically, the instigated provincial public health measures included restricted access to hospitals, screening of all employees and personnel entering hospitals, strict isolation precautions for cases, and restrictions on transfers of patients between institutions (Health Canada, 2003; Maunder et al., 2003).

It is noteworthy that the PHAC was established by Parliament in September, 2004 in response to the 2003 SARS outbreak in the GTA; which highlighted several deficiencies in our capacity and readiness to both anticipate and respond to such global health treats. In fact, the PHAC was confirmed as a legal entity in December 2006 by the Public Health Agency of Canada Act (Act 2006-12-12) (Government of Canada, 2006; PHAC, 2012b). The PHAC is currently responsible for emergency preparedness, and response; and infectious and chronic disease control and prevention in Canada. The PHAC works closely in collaboration with all levels of government (provincial, territorial, and municipal) to build on each other's skills and strengths, as well as with non-government organizations (NGOs), including civil society and business, other countries (e.g., CDC; European Centre for Prevention and Control) and international organizations (e.g., Global Security Action Group, WHO) to share knowledge, expertise, and experiences. The reader is referred to Chapter 1 for a detailed discussion on the establishment of the PHAC, and Chapter 2 for the evolution of public health in Canada.

West Nile Virus

WNV is a mosquitoe-borne arbovirus and a member of the flavivirus genus (Family *Flaviviridae*) that was first discovered in 1927 and isolated in 1937 from the blood of a febrile client in the West Nile province of Uganda, Africa. The first serious human outbreaks of WNV occurred in the mid-1990s in Algeria and Romania (Calistri et al., 2010; Drebot et al., 2003; Murgue, Zeller, & Duebel, 2002). It is believed that migratory birds, which may have been infected in their African wintering regions, carried the virus northward to European sites during their spring migrations. Species of *Culex* found amongst mosquitoes and magpies (*Pica pica*); carrion crows (*Corvus corone*); rock pigeons (*Columba livia*), and similar resident birds are believed to be the most probable species involved (Calistri et al., 2010; Murgue et al., 2001).

Serological assays are commonly employed for monitoring MNV disease in human cases, and for undertaking case investigations. Conversely, genomic amplification procedures are typically employed for testing animal (e.g., horses, birds) and mosquitoe specimens collected as part of ongoing surveillance efforts (BC Centre for Disease Control, 2018; Drebot et al., 2003; Government of Canada, 2017e; PHAC, 2017d).

The unexpected intrusion and spread of WNV into North America occurred during the summer of 1999 when an outbreak of neurological illness among humans, birds, and horses was identified in the metropolitan area of New York City in the United States (Asnis, Conetta, Teixeira, Waldman, & Sampson, 2000; Drebot et al., 2003; Vector Disease Control International, 2013). Notably, 62 human cases were identified in the New York City metropolitan area in 1999 alone. This unexpected and dramatic outbreak underscores the ability of viruses to appear suddenly, often without prior warning, in unanticipated or predicted areas. WNV is typically transmitted to humans by mosquitoes that have previously fed upon an infected bird. While over 150 species of mosquitoes have been known to carry the WNV, the main vector species in the United States are Culex pipiens, Culex tarsalis, and *Culex quinquefasciatus* (Vector Disease Control International, 2013).

The incubation period for WNV disease is typically 2 to 6 days, but may range from 2 to 14 days; and can be several weeks in duration for immunocompromised clients (e.g., clients receiving chemo- or radiation-therapy for cancer, organ transplant recipients, HIV/AIDS) (CDC, 2015; Public Health Ontario, 2017; Vector Disease Control International, 2013). An estimated 70% to 80% of human WNV infections are subclinical or asymptomatic in nature. Approximately 20% (1:5) of clients will experience flu-like symptoms including fever, headache, nausea, muscle pain or discomfort, and swollen lymph glands. Some infected clients may also experience sleep disturbances, disorientation, or confusion, a skin rash and/or complain of a stiff neck. Less than 1% (1:150) of infected clients will develop West Nile encephalitis or meningitis, which can lead to coma, tremors, convulsions, paralysis, and even death (CDC, 2015; Public Health Ontario, 2017; Vector Disease Control International, 2013).

The WNV was first detected in Windsor, Ontario on August 8, 2001; and public health officials responded by including surveillance of mosquitoes, horses, and birds (e.g., blue jays, crows, raven, magpies) (PHAC, 2017d; Public Health Ontario, 2017). By 2002, public health officials documented the presence of the WNV in Saskatchewan, Manitoba, Ontario, Québec, and Nova Scotia and the first human case was also confirmed this year (Drebot et al., 2003; PHAC, 2017d). WNV disease has been a nationally notifiable disease in Canada since 2003, and all human and animal cases need to be reported to local public health authorities in a timely manner (CFIA, 2017b; Government of Canada, 2016a, 2016d). The total number of human cases of WNV in Canada for the years 2002 to 2016 was 5414 (see Table 13.4) (PHAC, 2017d).

There are currently no vaccines to prevent or medications to cure WNV (BC Centre for Disease Control, 2018; CDC, 2015; Public Health Ontario, 2013, 2017). Public health professionals and workers need to

Table 13.4   Number of Human Cases of West Nile Virus in Canada, 2002–2016

Year	Number of Cases
2002	414
2003	1481
2004	25
2005	225
2006	151
2007	2215
2008	36
2009	13
2010	5
2011	101
2012	428
2013	115
2014	21
2015	80
2016	104
Total number of confirmed cases in Canada from 2002 to 2016	5414

Source: Data adapted from PHAC (2017d).

educate the general public about the importance of vector-control and prevention in their communities (BC Centre for Disease Control, 2018; Public Health Ontario, 2013, 2017). Individuals, for examples, should be encouraged to ensure that all windows and doors have screens and any holes present are promptly repaired. Individuals should also be encouraged to sleep under a mosquitoe bed net if air conditioning is not available during the late spring or summer seasons; when sleeping outdoors (e.g., camping under the stars), or when air conditioning units are not available. It is critical to empty, turn-over, cover, and/or throw-out items that hold water necessary for mosquitoes to breed (e.g., old tires, buckets, planters, discarded bottles or cans, toys, kiddy pools, birdbaths, flowerpots, garbage containers). Individuals should also avoid going outside when mosquitoes are most active, including dust and dawn; wear long protective clothing (e.g., long sleeves), and apply a topical insect repellent containing DEET or similar product (BC Centre for Disease Control, 2018; Public Health Ontario, 2013, 2017; Scutti, 2013). Icaridin, formerly known as "Picaridin," is a new topical insect repellent that first entered the U.S. market in 2005, and was approved by Health Canada in 2012 (HealthLinks, 2017; Government of Canada, 2012). Icaridin is considered to be as effective as DEET for offering protection for both mosquitoe and tick bites alike. IR3535 is currently not available as an insect repellent in Canada, but can be purchased and employed in other parts of the world (including the United States) to prevent insect bites by Canadian tourists (HealthLinks, 2017; Scutti, 2013). Figure 13.5 shows the 5 Ds of West Nile prevention that are easy to remember, and which could be employed for public health promotion purposes.

The reader is referred to Web-Based Resource Box 13.2 for additional information on the surveillance, control, and management of WMN in Canada.

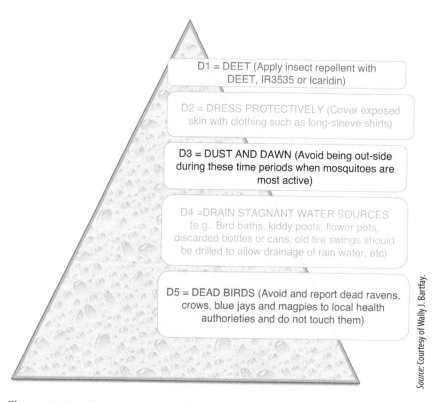

Figure 13.5 The 5 Ds of West Nile Prevention

Web-Based Resource Box 13.2: Resources for the Surveillance, Control, and Management of West-Nile Virus in Canada

Learning Resource	Website
BC (British Columbia) Centre for Disease Control. (2018). *West Nile virus.* **Vancouver, BC: Provincial Health Services Authority.** -Provides current information for healthcare professionals related to case identification, clinical signs and symptoms, laboratory testing, and available treatment regimens and medications.	http://www.bccdc.ca/health-info/diseases-conditions/west-nile-virus-wnv
Government of Canada. (2017e, December 4). *Surveillance of West Nile virus.* **Ottawa, ON: Author.** -Provides current information about national surveillance efforts in Canada for the WNV for animals, birds, and human cases, and also surveillance being done in First Nations communities.	https://www.canada.ca/en/public-health/services/diseases/west-nile-virus/surveillance-west-nile-virus.html
Public Health Ontario. (2013, August). *Guide for public health units: Considerations for adult mosquitoe control.* **Toronto, ON: Queen's Printer for Ontario.** -This resource provides helpful guidelines for public healthcare professionals and workers responsible for vector-control in communities.	https://www.publichealthontario.ca/en/eRepository/Guide_Considerations_Mosquitoe_Control_2013.pdf

Zika Virus Infections

Zika virus is a mosquitoe-borne flavivirus transmitted primarily via the *Aedes* mosquitoe (CDC, 2017c; Government of Canada, 2016e; WHO, 2017j, 2017l). The Zika virus can also be transmitted through sexual intercourse and can persist for an extended period of time in the semen of infected males. Moreover, the virus can also be transmitted from an infected pregnant women to her developing fetus *in-utero*. Clinical signs and symptoms of Zika virus infection include mild fever, headache, malaise, conjunctivitis, skin rash, joint and/or muscle pain. Illness is typically mild in nature and lasts for only two to seven days in duration; whilst the majority of infected individuals may not exhibit any signs or symptoms.

Zika virus was first detected in 1947 in rhesus monkeys residing in the Zika forests of Uganda (see Figure 13.6) through a surveillance network of scientists that were monitoring yellow fever. It was later identified in humans in 1952 in Uganda and also the United Republic of Tanzania (WHO, 2017l). Outbreaks of Zika virus disease have subsequently been recorded on African continent, the Americas, Asia and the Pacific. In fact,

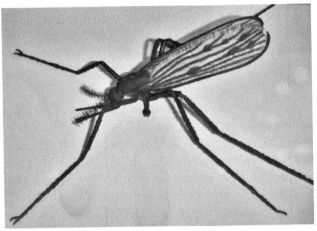

Source: Photo by Wally J. Bartfay.

Photo 13.10 What Is the Deadliest Animal in the World? It might seem impossible that something so small can be the most deadly animal in the world, but it's true. Of all disease-transmitting insects, the mosquitoe is the greatest menace, responsible for spreading Zika virus, malaria, dengue and yellow fever, lymphatic filariasis, and Japanese encephalitis; which together are responsible for several million deaths and hundreds of millions of cases every year (WHO, 2018k). By undermining the health and working capacity of hundreds of millions of people globally, the mosquitoe is also closely linked to poverty and negatively affects social and economic development.

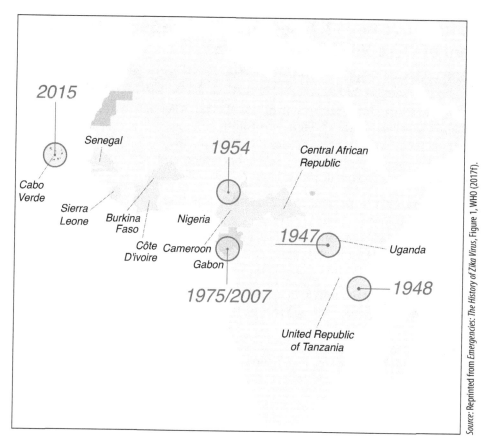

Source: Reprinted from Emergencies: The History of Zika Virus, Figure 1, WHO (2017f).

Figure 13.6   Zika Virus Was First Isolated in 1947 and Quickly Spread to Humans. In 1947, scientists conducting routine surveillance of yellow fever in the Zika forest of Uganda, Africa isolate the newly discovered "Zika virus" from a captive sentinel rhesus monkey. By 1952, the first human cases of Zika are detected in Uganda and the United Republic of Tanzania (WHO, 2017f).

from the 1960s to 1980s, human infections of Zika were found across Africa and Asia; which were typically accompanied by mild illness.

The first large outbreak of disease caused by Zika infection was reported from the Island of Yap (Federated States of Micronesia) in 2007. In July 2015 Brazil reported an association between Zika virus infection and Guillain–Barré syndrome. In October 2015 Brazil also reported an association between Zika virus infection and microcephaly in newborn infants (WHO, 2017j, 2017l). Between December 2015 and February 2016, public health officials reported a 20-fold increase in miscarriages and birth defects linked to the Zika virus, which included 4400 cases of microcephaly in Brazil (Ferguson, 2016; PHAC, 2016; WHO, 2016a).

Similarly, 2500 cases of Zika virus and 100 confirmed cases suffering from associated Guillain–Barré syndrome were reported in French Guiana and Martinique between December 2015 and February 2016 (Nebehay, 2016). On February 1, 2016 the WHO Director-General Dr Margaret Chan declared the Zika virus pandemic as an "international emergency," and the province of Ontario had its first confirmed case of Zika (Ferguson, 2016; Keaton & Chang, 2016). Honduras subsequently declared a state of emergency on February 2, 2016 after having 3469 suspected cases of the Zika virus in their country in less than three months (Nebehay, 2016). The Government of Canada (2017c, 2017d) notes that as of December 1, 2017, 544 travel-related cases of Zika and four sexually transmitted cases have been reported in Canada; and a total of 37 cases have been reported amongst pregnant women, along with two newborn cases with Zika-related anomalies.

March 10, 2017 *Zika Situation Report* released by the WHO (2017k) noted that as of February 1, 2017 there were no countries reporting new cases of vector-borne Zika virus. However, 84 countries, territories, or subnational areas have evidence of vector-borne Zika virus transmission. This included a total of 31 countries or territories who reported microcephaly and other central nervous system (CNS) malformations potentially associated with the Zika virus, and 23 have also reported an increased incidence of Guillain–Barré syndrome (GBS). Moreover, there were 64 countries, territories, or subnational areas where the competent vector is established; but have no documented past or current transmission. Since February, 2016, 13 countries have reported evidence of person-to-person transmission; which included Argentia, Canada, Chile, Peru, the United States, France, Germany, Italy, the Netherlands, Portugal, Spain, the United Kingdom, Northern Ireland, and New Zealand (CDC, 2017c; WHO, 2017k). Figure 13.7 shows a map of high risks countries and regions for Zika virus transmission (CDC, 2017c).

In September of 2016, *A. albopictus* mosquitoes (a.k.a., Asian Tiger mosquitoes), were caught and identified in Windsor, Ontario (Brockman, 2016). The Asian Tiger mosquitoe is found in the Southern United States, but it typically only reached the State of Michigan.

Though these particular mosquitoes tested negative for Zika, the insects are a known carrier of the disease. The species is uncommon in Canada, but is an invasive species that has been reported in the Niagara Region. It's believed the four mosquitoes were brought to Ontario by a cross-border traveler from the United States

(Brockman, 2016)

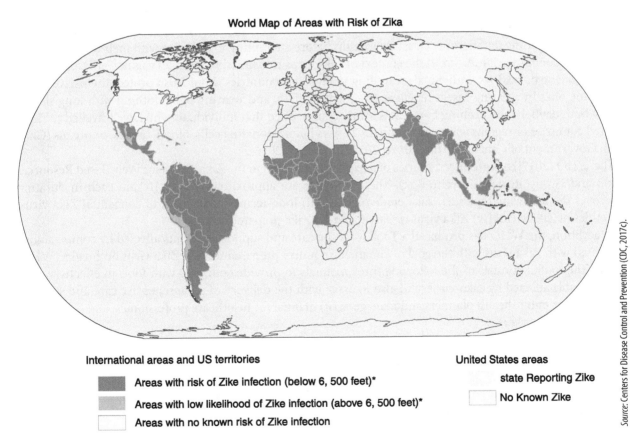

Figure 13.7   World Map of Areas With Risk of Zika Virus Transmission. On February 1, 2016 the WHO (2017f) declared that the confirmed association of Zika virus infection with clusters of microcephaly and other neurological disorders constituted a "Public health emergency of international concern."

Web-Based Resources Box 3: Zika Virus

Learning Resource	Website
WHO. (2017j). *WHO Zika podcast episodes—Evidence in action.* **Geneva, Switzerland: Author.** -Consists of the following five podcasts on the Zika virus of approximately 9 to 10 min each.	http://www.who.int/mediacentre/multimedia/podcasts/2017/en/
WHO. (2017i). *WHO toolkit for the care and support of people affected by complications associated with Zika virus.* **Geneva, Switzerland: Author. (ISBN: 978-92-4-151271-8).** -262-page toolkit is intended to provide a system approach involving public health planners and managers so that the necessary infrastructure, personnel, and resources can be identified.	http://www.who.int/mental_health/neurology/zika_toolkit/en/

The Government of Canada (2016e, 2017c, 2017d) reports that there have been travel-related cases of Zika virus reported in Canada in returned travelers from countries with ongoing Zika virus outbreaks. Hence, travel advisors which include recommendations that pregnant women and those planning a pregnancy avoid travel to high-risk countries. This includes the states of Texas and Florida in the United States. It is also recommended that women planning a pregnancy wait at least two months before trying to conceive to ensure that any possible Zika virus infection has cleared the body. Similarly, for male travelers, the Zika virus can persist for extended periods of time in the semen and they are therefore strongly advised to avoid having sexual intercourse for the duration of at least six months before attempting to conceive with their female partner, and to use a condom prior to. Sex in the context of Zika virus transmission includes vaginal, anal, or oral sex, and the sharing of sex toys. Individuals travelling to high risk countries should also protect themselves from mosquitoe bites by wearing insect repellent (e.g., with DEET), and wearing light clothing with long sleeves during both daylight and evening hours. It is also recommended that individuals who have travelled to Zika-affected countries or regions wait a minimum of 21 days before donating cells, blood, tissues, or organs (Chai, 2016; Government of Canada, 2016e, 2017c, 2017d; Nebehay, 2016).

The WHO (2017j) has produced a series of five podcasts related to the Zika virus (see Web-Based Resources Box 3 and Group Review Exercise Box). These podcasts are approximately 9 to 10 min each in duration and cover the following topics: (i) Zika epidemiology; (ii) long-term management of congenital Zika virus; (iii) ethics of Zika virus; (iv) Zika virus research; and (v) Zika preparedness.

In addition, the WHO has produced a Toolkit for the care and support of clients affected by complications associated with Zika virus with the goal of enhancing country preparedness for Zika virus outbreaks (WHO, 2017i). The toolkit consists of the following three manuals to provide countries with tools to effectively recognize people affected by Zika virus, and also to assist with the delivery of comprehensive care and support: (i) Manual for public health planners and managers; (ii) manual for healthcare professionals; and (iii) manual for community workers.

Future Directions and Challenges

Recent outbreaks, and the emergence and establishment of diseases new to human populations (e.g., avian flu, *blastomycosis*, chikungunya, Ebola, SARS, WNV, and Zika), illustrate how intimately associated and linked human health is with the health and welfare of animals globally. In fact, approximately 75% of currently known EIDs and REIDs originate from animal sources (CDC, 2017d; Ogden, Abdel-Malik, & Pulliam, 2017; Wang & Cramer, 2014). Canadians can never be certain that they will be completely safe from infectious diseases. Nonetheless, we can certainly be prepared from a public health perspective. This includes tracking and surveillance, establishing protocols and mechanisms to monitor outbreaks, training of healthcare personnel, and ensuring that we have the necessary resources and structures in place to respond to an outbreak in a coordinated, rehearsed, and effective fashion (Government of Canada, 2006; PHAC, 2012b). Indeed, the Director General of WHO, Dr Tedros Adhanom remarked during an address to delegates at the G20 summit held on July 8, 2017 in Hamburg, Germany that pandemic health emergencies represent some of the greatest risks to the global economy and our security as a species (WHO, 2018e). Furthermore, Dr Adhanom cautioned that

We do not know where the next global pandemic will occur, we don't know when it will occur, but it will be costly in lives and dollars. With airline travel (3 billion travellers every year) global spread of any new pathogen would occur in hours. As well as untold human suffering, the economic losses would be measured in trillions, including the losses of tourism, trade, consumer confidence and also including political problems and challenges. There will be 2 epidemics—one caused by the virus, and the other one caused by fear.

(WHO, 2018e).

The prevention and control of EIDs and REIDs, along with other public health emergencies, requires both national and international coordinated efforts (Ogden, Adel-Malik, & Pulliam, 2017; PHAC, 2012b; WHO, 2017d). For example, the PHAC participates in a number of international networks to facilitate information sharing and collaboration (e.g., risk communication networks). Similarly, the development of the *North American Pandemic and Avian Influenza Plan* is an example of a successful collaboration with the United States and Mexico through the *Security and Prosperity Partnership* (SPP).

We argue that our provincial/territorial, national, and global public health agencies and communities must replenish and increase capacity that has been depleted during years of inadequate funding; while simultaneously incorporating new health technologies and planning for emergency preparedness in the new millennium (Bartfay & Bartfay, 2015). Among these public health challenges is the need for coordinated, national and global, multi-sectoral approaches to identifying, tracking, preventing, and controlling complex EIDs and REIDs. Indeed, this is in a world where increased trade and globalization, travel, demographic changes, climatic and other environmental changes are collectively enhancing the emergence of new pathogens; their transmission from animals to humans, and their global prevalence and spread (Binder, Levitt, Sacks, & Hughes, 1999; Ogden, Adel-Malik, & Pulliam, 2017; WHO, 2017d).

Specifically, public health must continue to focus and develop their capacity to conduct upstream risk assessments of EIDS and REIDS; build capacity for tracking and surveillance, and engage in emergency response and preparedness exercises and training in order to effectively respond to outbreaks in a coordinated manner. Further efforts to identify and link different approaches into comprehensive globalized network systems that capitalize on available historical and contextual data would further strengthen the ability to detect, prepare for, and respond to EIDs and REIDs.

Group Review Exercise "WHO Zika Podcast-Evidence in Action Episode I: Zika Epidemiology"

About this podcast

This podcast is the first in a series of five podcasts produced by WHO (2017j) examining the Zika virus pandemic and challenges faced by public health professionals, workers, researchers, and agencies in combating this EID. The podcast is approximately 10 min in duration and examines the role of

(Continued)

(Continued)

epidemiology surrounding the transmission of Zika virus to humans; and rare but serious neurological disorders associated with it, in particular Guillain–Barré syndrome and microcephaly.

Instructions

This assignment may be done alone, in pairs, or in groups of up to five people (note: if you are doing this assignment in pairs or groups, please submit only one hard or electronic copy to your instructor). The assignment should be typewritten and no more than four to six pages maximum in length (double-spaced please). View the 10-min podcast and take notes during the presentations. See links http://www.who.int/mediacentre/multimedia/podcasts/2017/en/ and/ or http://www.who.int/mediacentre/multimedia/podcasts/2017/en/

1. Provide a brief overview of what epidemiology is and its role in the aetiology, surveillance, and tracking of the Zika virus pandemic?

2. How was epidemiology employed to identify a causal link between the Zika virus and Guillain–Barré syndrome and microcephaly? What was the importance of "time" and "place" in making these causal links?

3. What action did the WHO take on February 1, 2016 in regards to the Zika virus? Describe public health strategies associated with combating the spread and transmission of Zika virus in humans.

Summary

- Normal flora of humans is remarkably diverse and complex consisting of more than 200 species of bacteria alone.
- Probiotics are living microorganisms (e.g., bacteria), which when administered in adequate amounts confer a positive health benefit to the host.
- *Canadian Nosocomial Infection Surveillance Program* (CNISP) was established in 1994, and monitors healthcare associated infections at 54 sentinel hospitals located across 10 provinces.
- An infectious disease is a communicable disease caused by a specific pathogen (e.g., bacteria, viruses, fungi, protozoa, prion) or its toxic products that results through its transmission from an agent to a susceptible host.
- An infection is an invasion of the body caused by a pathogen that results in specific signs and symptoms that develop in response to the pathogen, which may be localized or systemic in nature.
- Infectious (a.k.a., communicable) diseases are transmitted from one host to another through a series of steps known as the "chain of infection"; which consists of the reservoir, portal of exit, mode of transmission, portal of entry and infection of a new host.
- Immune system is a complex system that is responsible for distinguishing a host from everything foreign, and for protecting the body against a host of infectious agents and foreign substances.
- Immune system also has two types of responses for invading pathogens: (i) natural or innate and (ii) acquired or adaptive.
- EID is as one that has appeared in a population for the first time, or that may have existed previously but is rapidly increasing in incidence or geographic range.
- REIDs are diseases that were once regarded as major public health problems globally or in a particular country, and then declined dramatically; but have subsequently reemerged as a public health concern for a significant proportion of the population.
- Adaptive emergence is a genetic change in a microorganism that results in a phenotype that is capable of invading a new ecosystem, particularly via jumping to a new host species including humans.

- Approximately 75% of all EIDs and REIDS that affect humans are of zoonotic origin.
- Avian influenza is a contagious viral infection that can affect several species of food producing birds (e.g., chickens, turkeys, quails, guinea fowl) as well as pet birds and wild birds.
- Blastomycosis (a.k.a., "Gilchrist's disease") is as an invasive fungal disease caused by the organism *B. dermatitidis*, and whose natural reservoir is found in decaying wood, leaves, and soil.
- Chikungunya is a reemerging infectious mosquitoe-borne RNA viral disease that was first described during an outbreak in Southern Tanzania in 1952.
- EVD is a rare yet potentially deadly viral disease which can affect humans and primates alike (e.g., monkeys, gorillas, and chimpanzees), and was first recognized in 1976 in Africa.
- Lyme disease, is a multisystem infection that is manifested by progressive stages and is caused by the spirochete *B. burgdorferi* sensu stricto transmitted by blacklegged deer ticks.
- Sudden Acute Respiratory Syndrome (SARS) is a potentially life-threatening coronavirus (SARS-CoV) infection that affects the respiratory system with an average incubation period of six days; and which is spread by close person-to-person contact by infected individuals, most often via droplets expelled into the air during coughing or sneezing episodes.
- WNV is a mosquitoe-borne arbovirus that was first discovered in 1927 and isolated in 1937 from the blood of a febrile client in the West Nile province of Uganda, Africa, and is a member of the flavivirus genus (Family *Flaviviridae*).
- Zika virus is a mosquitoe-borne flavivirus transmitted primarily via the *Aedes* mosquitoe.
- The prevention and control of EIDs and REIDs, along with other public health emergencies, requires both national and international coordinated efforts.

Critical Thinking Questions

You work in health department for Immigration Canada located in a busy port that is a major centre for both national and international passenger traffic, shipping, and freight cargo. There is a general concern about how your department ought to respond to situations where an individual (e.g., tourist on a cruise ship, crew member of a cargo chip) is deemed ill upon arrival to Canada. This is especially true when there is a strong suspicion, but no certainty based on a laboratory confirmed diagnosis, that the unidentified disease is potentially deadly and highly contagious in nature (e.g., Ebola, measles). You have been asked to help develop a new set of national guidelines to help guide staff respond to such situations.

1. What ethical issues are relevant to removing a suspected individual from a ship or halting their legal entry into Canada? What are the factors (e.g., evidence of risk of exposure, clinical signs, symptoms, etc.) that should be taken into account in developing guidelines and/or action plans?
2. If the number of healthcare officers is limited in a specific port of entry, how should priorities about the use of staff time be set? For example, is it acceptable for staff to be asked to work beyond their contacted hours to ensure that individuals are not detained on a ship longer than a few hours? Justify your answer.
3. What details, if any, of a specific suspected case should be disclosed to the mass and/or social media to protect the health and safety of Canadian residents? What details, if any, should be disclosed to fellow passengers, crew members, or family members? Justify your answers.

References

Asnis, D. S., Conetta, R., Teixeira, A. A., Waldman, G., & Sampson, B. A. (2000). The West Nile virus outbreak of 1999 in New York: The Flushing Hospital experience. *Clinical Infectious Diseases, 30,* 413–418.

Bartfay, W. J., & Bartfay, E. (2015). *Public health in Canada.* Boston, MA: Pearson Learning Solutions (ISBN: 13:978-1-323-01471-4).

BC (British Colombia) Centre for Disease Control. (2018). *West Nile virus.* Vancouver, BC: Provincial Health Services Authority. Retrieved from http://www.bccdc.ca/health-info/diseases-conditions/west-nile-virus-wnv

Begtrup, L. M., de Muckadell, O. B., Kjeldsen, J., Christensen, R. D., & Jarbol, D. E. (2013). Long-term treatment with probiotics in primary care patients with irritable bowel syndrome—A randomized, double-blind, placebo controlled trial. *Scandinavian Journal of Gastroenterology, 48*(10), 1127–1235.

Bhatia, N., Sarwal, S., Robinson, H., Geduld, J., Huneault, F., Schreiner, H., Collins, S., ... Hickey, R. (2015, December 17). Federal public health strategies to minimize the importation of communicable diseases into Canada. *Canada Communicable Disease Report (CCDR),* S15–S16. Retrieved from http://publications.gc.ca/collections/collection_2015/aspc-phac/HP3-1-41S6-eng.pdf

Binder, S., Levitt, A. M., Sacks, J. J., & Hughes, J. M. (1999, May). Emerging infectious diseases: Public health issues for the 21st century. *Science, 284*(5418), 1311–1313. doi:10.1126/science/284.5418.1311. Retrieved from http://science.sciencemag.org/content/284/5418/1311

Blaszczak, A. (2014, September 8). *One germy doorknob can infect half your office within hours.* New York, NY: CBS News. Retrieved from https://www.cbsnews.com/news/one-germy-doorknob-can-infect-half-your-office-within-hours/

Bowman, D. (2008, October 30). *List of NIAID emerging and re-emerging diseases.* Newton, MA: FierceHealthcare-A Division of Questex. Retrieved from https://www.fiercehealthcare.com/healthcare/list-niaid-emerging-and-re-emerging-diseases

Brockman, A. (2016, October 6). *Zika mosquitoe in Windsor.* Toronto, ON: Canadian Broadcasting Corporation (CBC). Retrieved from http://www.cbc.ca/news/canada/windsor/potential-zika-carrying-mosquitoes-windsor-1.3793683

Calistri, P., Giovannini, A., Hubalek, Z., Ionescu, S., Monaco, F., Sarini, G., & Lelli, R. (2010, April 22). Epidemiology of west Nile in Europe and in the Mediterranean basin. *Open Virology Journal, 4,* 29–37. Retrieved from https://www.ncbi.nlm.nih.gov/pmc/articles/PMC2878979/

Canadian Food Inspection Agency. (2017a). *Fact sheet: Avian influenza.* Ottawa, ON: Author. Retrieved from http://www.inspection.gc.ca/animals/terrestrial-animals/diseases/reportable/ai/fact-sheet/eng/1356193731667/1356193918453#a3

Canadian Food Inspection Agency. (2017b). *Fact sheet: West Nile virus.* Ottawa, ON: Author. Retrieved from http://www.inspection.gc.ca/animals/terrestrial-animals/diseases/immediately-notifiable/west-nile-virus/fact-sheet/eng/1305853043399/1305853235540

Canadian Lyme Disease Foundation (2018). No tick is a good tick. They all carry infectious diseases. Retrieved from https://canlyme.com/

Canadian Patient Safety Institute. (2018). *Healthcare associated infections (HAIs).* Edmonton, AB: CPSI. Retrieved from http://www.patientsafetyinstitute.ca/en/Topic/Pages/Healthcare-Associated-Infections-(HAI).aspx

The Canadian Press. (2017, March 25). *More than 200 Canadians infected by mosquitoe-borne chikungunya virus.* Toronto, ON: The Globe and Mail. Retrieved from https://www.theglobeandmail.com/life/health-and-fitness/health/more-than-200-canadians-infected-by-mosquitoe-borne-chikungunya-virus/article21208214/

Centers for Disease Control and Prevention. (2014, Updated November 2). *Ebola (Ebola virus disease).* Atlanta, GA: CDC. Retrieved from https://www.cdc.gov/vhf/ebola/symptoms/index.html

Centers for Disease Control and Prevention. (2015, Updated February 12). *West Nile virus: Clinical evaluation and disease.* Atlanta, GA: CDC. Retrieved from https://www.cdc.gov/westnile/healthcareproviders/healthCareProviders-ClinLabEval.html

Centers for Disease Control and Prevention. (2016, Updated February 18). *Ebola virus disease.* Atlanta, GA: CDC. Retrieved from https://www.cdc.gov/vhf/ebola/about.html

Centers for Disease Control and Prevention. (2017a, Updated December 6). *Sudden acute respiratory syndrome (SARS).* Atlanta, GA: CDC. Retrieved from https://www.cdc.gov/sars/about/fs-sars.html

Centers for Disease Control and Prevention. (2017b, Updated January 10). *Tetanus: Symptoms and complications.* Atlanta, GA: CDC. Retrieved from https://www.cdc.gov/tetanus/about/symptoms-complications.html

Centers for Disease Control and Prevention. (2017c, Updated November 27). *World map of areas with risk of Zika.* Atlanta, GA: CDC. Retrieved from https://wwwnc.cdc.gov/travel/files/zika-areas-of-risk.pdf and/or https://wwwnc.cdc.gov/travel/page/world-map-areas-with-zika

Centers for Disease Control and Prevention. (2017d, Updated July 14). *Zoonotic diseases.* Atlanta, GA: CDC. Retrieved from https://www.cdc.gov/onehealth/basics/zoonotic-diseases.html

Chai, C. (2016, February 3). *Zika virus: Don't donate blood for 3 weeks after returning home from travel.* Toronto, ON: Global News. Retrieved from http://globalnews.ca/news/2495745/zika-virus-dont-donate-blood-for-3-weeks-after-returning-home-from-travels/

Chan, P. K. (2002, May 1). Outbreak of avian influenza A (H5N1) virus infection in Hong Kong in 1997. *Clinical Infectious Disease, 34*(Suppl. 2), S58–S64. doi:10.1086/338820. Retrieved from https://www.ncbi.nlm.nih.gov/pubmed/11938498

Chhabra, M., Mittal, V., Bhattacharya, D., Rana, U. V. S., & Lal, S. (2008). Chikungunya fever: A re-emerging viral infection. *Indian Journal of Medical Microbiology, 26*(1), 5–12.

Cooke, R. A. (2008). *Infectious diseases: Atlas, cases, text.* Toronto, ON: The McGraw-Hill Companies.

Cordinale, M., Kaiser, D., Lueders, T., Schnell, S., & Egert, M. (2017). Microbiome analysis and confocal microscopy of used kitchen sponges reveal massive colonization by *Acinetobacter, Moraxella* and *Chryseobacterium* species. *Scientific Reports, 7.* doi:10.1038/S41598-017-060555.9. Retrieved from https://www.nature.com/articles/s41598-017-06055-9

CTV News. (2015, December 9). *Canadian cases of chikungunya virus spiked in 2014: PHAC.* Toronto, ON: Author. Retrieved from https://www.ctvnews.ca/health/canadian-cases-of-chikungunya-virus-spiked-in-2014-phac-1.2181366

Cunhn, B. A. (2006, November). Antimicrobial therapy of multidrug-resistant *Streptococcus pneumoniae,* vancomycin-resistant enterococci, and methicillin-resistant *Staphylococcus aureus. Medical Clinics of North America, 90*(6), 1165–1182. Retrieved from https://www.ncbi.nlm.nih.gov/pubmed/17116442

Cyranoski, D. (2017, December 1). News: Bat cave solves mystery of deadly SARS virus and suggests new outbreak could occur. *Nature—International Journal of Science, 552*(7683), 15–16. doi:10.1038/d41586-017-07766-9

Davis, C. P. (1996). Normal flora (Chapter 6). In S. Baron (Ed.), *Medical microbiology* (4th ed.), Galveston, TX: University of Texas Galveston Medical Branch. Retrieved from https://www.ncbi.nlm.nih.gov/books/NBK7617/

de Vrese, M., & Marteau, P. R. (2007). Probiotics and prebiotics: Effects on diarrhea. *Journal of Nutrition, 137*(3 Suppl. 2), 803S–811S.

Dominguez-Bello, M. G., Costello, E. K., Contrevas, M., Magda, M., Hidalgo, G., Fierer, N., & Knight, R. (2010, June 21). Delivery mode shapes the acquisition and structure of the initial microbiota across multiple body habitats in newborns. *Proceedings of the National Academy of Science, USA, 107,* 11971–11975. Retrieved from https://www.ncbi.nlm.nih.gov/pmc/articles/PMC2900693/

Donatelle, R. J., Johnson-Munroe, A., Munroe, A., & Thompson, A. M. (2008). *Health: The basics* (4th Canadian ed.). Toronto, ON: Pearson Benjamin Cummings.

Drebot, M. A., Lindsay, R., Barker, I. K., Buck, P. A., Fearson, M., & Artrob, H. (2003, March–April). West Nile virus surveillance and diagnostics: A Canadian perspective. *Canadian Journal of Infectious Diseases, 14*(2), 105–114. Retrieved from https://www.ncbi.nlm.nih.gov/pmc/articles/PMC2094912/

Epstein, P. R. (2001, July). Climate change and emerging infectious diseases. *Microbes and Infection, 3*(9), 747–754. Retrieved from http://www.sciencedirect.com/science/article/pii/S1286457901014290

Ferguson, R. (2016, February 19). *Ontario has first confirmed case of Zika.* Toronto, ON: The Star.com (Queen's Park Bureau). Retrieved from https://www.thestar.com/news/canada/2016/02/19/ontario-has-first-case-of-zika-virus-in-person-who-travelled-to-colombia.html

Furness, J., Wolfgang, A. A., & Kunze, N. C. (1999, November). The intestine as a sensory organ: Neural, endocrine and immune responses. *American Journal of Physiology, Gastrointestinal and Liver Pathology, 277*(5), G922–G928. Retrieved from http://ajpgi.physiology.org/content/277/5/G922

Gasmi, S., Ogden, N. H., Lindsay, L. R., Burns, S., Fleming, S., & Kaffi, J. R. (2017). Surveillance for Lyme disease in Canada: 2009–2015. *Canadian Communicable Disease Report, 43*(10), 194–199. Retrieved from https://www.canada.ca/en/public-health/services/reports-publications/canada-communicable-disease-report-ccdr/monthly-issue/2017-43/ccdr-volume-43-10-october-5-2017/surveillance-surveillance-lyme-disease-canada-2009-2015.html

Goldin, B. R., & Gorbach, S. L. (2008, February 1). Clinical indicators for probiotics: An overview. *Clinical Infectious Diseases, 46*(Suppl. 1), S96–S100. Retrieved from https://www.academic.oup.com/cid/article/46/Supplement_2/S96/278134

Government of Canada. (2006). *Public Health Agency of Canada Act S.C. 2006-12-12.* Ottawa, ON: Author. Justice laws website. Retrieved from http://lois-laws.justice.gc.ca/eng/acts/P-29.5/FullText.html

Government of Canada. (2008). *Understanding influenza.* Ottawa, ON: Author. Retrieved from https://www.canada.ca/en/health-canada/services/healthy-living/your-health/diseases/avian-influenza-bird-flu.html

Government of Canada. (2012, November). Statement on personal protective measures to prevent arthropod bites. *Canadian Communicable Disease Report, 38*(ACS-3). ISSN: 1481–8531. Retrieved from https://www.canada.ca/en/public-health/services/reports-publications/canada-communicable-disease-report-ccdr/monthly-issue/2012-38/statement-on-personal-protective-measures-prevent-arthropod-bites.htmlGovernment of Canada. (2013, November 23).

The chief public health officer's report on the state of public health in Canada 2013—Healthcare-associated infection: Due diligence. Ottawa, ON: Author. Retrieved from https://www.canada.ca/en/public-health/corporate/publications/chief-public-health-officer-reports-state-public-health-canada/chief-public-health-officer-report-on-state-public-health-canada-2013-infectious-disease-never-ending-threat/healthcare-associated-infections-due-diligence.html

Government of Canada. (2016a). *A–Z infectious diseases.* Ottawa, ON: Author. Retrieved from https://www.canada.ca/en/public-health/services/infectious-diseases/a-infectious-diseases.html#wnv

Government of Canada. (2016b). *Background: Public health agency of Canada.* Ottawa, ON: Author. Retrieved from https://www.canada.ca/en/public-health/corporate/mandate/about-agency/background.html

Government of Canada. (2016c, March 1). *Blastomycosis.* Ottawa, ON: Author. Retrieved from https://www.canada.ca/en/public-health/services/diseases/blastomycosis.html

Government of Canada. (2016d). *Human health issues related to avian influenza in Canada.* Ottawa, ON: Author. Retrieved from https://www.canada.ca/en/public-health/services/reports-publications/human-health-issues-related-avian-influenza.html

Government of Canada. (2016e, September 9). *Zika virus infection: Global update.* Ottawa, ON: Author. Retrieved from https://travel.gc.ca/travelling/health-safety/travel-health-notices/152?_ga=1.148763134.855139244.1484067758

Government of Canada. (2017a). *Causes of Ebola virus disease.* Ottawa, ON: Author. Retrieved from https://www.canada.ca/en/public-health/services/diseases/ebola/health-professionals-ebola.html

Government of Canada. (2017b). *For health professionals: Flu (Influenza).* Ottawa, ON: Author. Retrieved from https://www.canada.ca/en/public-health/services/diseases/flu-influenza/health-professionals-flu-influenza.html

Government of Canada. (2017c, March 08). *Prevention of Zika virus.* Ottawa, ON: Author. Retrieved from https://www.canada.ca/en/public-health/services/diseases/zika-virus/prevention-zika-virus.html

Government of Canada. (2017d, December 20). *Surveillance of Zika virus.* Ottawa, ON: Author. Retrieved from https://www.canada.ca/en/public-health/services/diseases/zika-virus/surveillance-zika-virus.html

Government of Canada. (2017e). *Surveillance of West Nile virus.* Ottawa, ON: Author. Retrieved from https://www.canada.ca/en/public-health/services/diseases/west-nile-virus/surveillance-west-nile-virus.html

Grice, E. A., & Segre, J. A. (2011, April). The skin microbiome. *National Review of Microbiology, 9*(4), 244–253. Retrieved from https://www.ncbi.nlm.nih.gov/pmc/articles/PMC3535073/

Hahn, D. B., Payne, W. A., Gallant, M., & Fletcher, P. C. (2006). *Focus on health* (2nd ed.). Toronto, ON: McGraw-Hill Ryerson.

Hatchette, T. F., Davis, I., & Johnston, B. L. (2014). Lyme disease: Clinical diagnosis and treatment. *Canadian Communicable Disease Report, 40,* 194–208. Retrieved from https://www.canada.ca/en/public-health/services/reports-publications/canada-communicable-disease-report-ccdr/monthly-issue/2014-40/ccdr-volume-40-11-may-29-2014/ccdr-volume-40-11-may-29-2014.html

Health Canada. (2003). *Summary of severe acute respiratory syndrome (SARS) cases: Canada and international.* Ottawa, ON: Author. Retrieved from www.hc-sc.gc.ca/pphb-dgspsp/sars-sras/eu-ae/index.html

HealthLinks, B. C. (2017, November 27). *Insect repellents.* Vancouver, BC: Author. Retrieved from https://www.healthlinkbc.ca/health-topics/uf4815

Heymann, D. L. (2015). *Control of communicable diseases manual: An official report of the American public health association* (20th ed.). Washington, DC: American Public Health Association.

Hooper, L. V., & Gorden, J. I. (2001, May). Commensal host-bacterial relationship in the gut. *Science, 292*(5519), 1115–1118. Retrieved from http://science.sciencemag.org/content/292/5519/1115.full

Hu, B., Zeng, L. P., Ge, X. Y., Zhang, W., Li, B., & Shi, Z. L. (2017, November 30). Discovery of a rich gene pool of bat SARS-related coronaviruses provides new insights into the origin of SARS coronavirus. *PLOS Pathogens, 13*(11), e1006698. Retrieved from http://journals.plos.org/plospathogens/article?id=10.1371/journal.ppat.1006698

Infection Control and Prevention Canada. (2018). *Information about Ebola virus.* Winnipeg, MB: Author. Retrieved from https://ipac-canada.org/ebola-virus-resources.php

Insel, P. M., Roth, W. T., Irwin, J. D., & Burke, S. M. (2016). *Core concepts in health* (2nd ed.). Toronto, ON: McGraw-Hill Ryerson.

International Society of Travel Medicine. (2018). *GeoSentinel: The global surveillance network of the ISTM in partnership with the CDC.* Dunwoody, GA: Author. Retrieved from http://www.istm.org/geosentinel

Kandel, C., Simor, A. E., & Redelmier, D. A. (2014, July 8). Elevator buttons as unrecognized sources of bacterial colonization in hospitals. *Open Medicine, 8*(3), e81–e86.

Keaton, J., & Chang, M. (2016, February 1). *WHO declares Zika virus as international emergency.* Toronto, ON: CTV News and The Associated Press. Retrieved from https://www.ctvnews.ca/health/who-declares-zika-virus-an-international-emergency-1.2759788

Li, W., Wong, S. K., Li, F., Kuhn, J. H., Huang, C., Choe, H., & Farzan, M. (2006, May). Animal origins of SARS coronavirus: Insights from ACEZ-protein interactions. *Journal of Virology, 80*(9), 4211–4219. Retrieved from http://jvi.asm.org/content/80/9/4211.full

Liang, L., & Gong, P. (2017, June). Climate change and human infectious disease: A synthesis of research findings from global and spatial–temporal perspectives. *Environmental Health, 103,* 99–103. Retrieved from http://www.sciencedirect.com/science/article/pii/S0160412016309758

Lind, M. (2018). *Lyme disease: The four stages of Lyme disease.* New York, NY: Organic Daily Post. Retrieved from https://organicdailypost.com/stage-1-lyme-disease/

Lior, L. Y., & Njoo, H. (2015, December 17). Ready to go! Canada's new rapid response team. *Canada Communicable Disease Report (CCDR), S15–S16,* 9–13. Retrieved from http://publications.gc.ca/collections/collection_2015/aspc-phac/HP3-1-41S6-eng.pdf

Litvinjenko, S., & Lunny, D. (2017). Blastomycosis hospitalizations in northwestern Ontario: 2006–2015. *Canadian Communicable Disease Report, 43*(10), 200–205. Retrieved from https://www.canada.ca/en/public-health/services/reports-publications/canada-communicable-disease-report-ccdr/monthly-issue/2017-43/ccdr-volume-43-10-october-5-2017/surveillance-blastomycosis-hospitalizations-northwestern-ontario-2006-2015.html

Lyme Disease Association of Australia. (2018). *Late stage Lyme disease.* GPO Box 5108, Melbourne VIC 3001. Available at: http://www.lymedisease.org.au/. Retrieved from http://www.lymedisease.org.au/about-lyme-disease/late-stage-lyme-disease/

Lyme Disease Association, Inc. (2018). *Cases, stats, maps & graphs: Lyme in 80+ countries worldwide.* Jackson, NJ: Author. Retrieved from https://www.lymediseaseassociation.org/about-lyme/cases-stats-maps-a-graphs/940-lyme-in-more-than-80-countries-worldwide

Manitoba Health Communicable Disease Control Unit. (2015). *Communicable disease management protocol: Blastomycosis.* Winnipeg, Manitoba: Author. Retrieved from https://www.gov.mb.ca/health/publichealth/cdc/protocol/blastomycosis.pdf

Manning, D. (2017). *Germs in the kitchen.* Atlanta, GA: WebMD. Retrieved from https://www.webmd.com/food-recipes/features/germs-in-kitchen#1

Maunder, R., Hunter, J., Vincent, L., Bennett, J., Peladeau, N., & Mazzulli, T. (2003, May 13). The immediate psychological and occupational impact of the 2003 SARS outbreak in a teaching hospital. *Canadian Medical Association Journal, 168*(10), 1245–1251. Retrieved from https://www.ncbi.nlm.nih.gov/pmc/articles/PMC154178/

McFarland, L. V. (2007). Meta-analysis of probiotics for the prevention of traveler's diarrhea. *Travel and Medical Infectious Disease, 5*(2), 97–105.

Murgue, B., Murri, S., Zientara, S., Durand, B., Durand, J. P., & Zeller, H. (2001). West Nile outbreak in horses in southern France, 2000: The return after 35 years. *Emerging Infectious Diseases, 7,* 692–696.

Murgue, B., Zeller, H., & Duebel, V. (2002). *The ecology and epidemiology of West Nile virus in Africa, Europe, and Asia.* In J. S. Mackenzie, A. D. T. Barrett, & V. Deubel (Eds.). *Japanese encephalitis and West Nile viruses* (pp. 195–222). New York, NY: Springer-Verlag.

National Institute of Allergy and Infectious Disease. (2017, November 14). *Three decades of responding to infectious disease outbreaks. NIAID director Anthony S. Fauci, M.D., highlights lessons from AIDS to Zika.* Bethesda, MD: National Institutes of Health. Retrieved from https://www.niaid.nih.gov/news-events/three-decades-responding-infectious-disease-outbreaks

National Institute of Allergy and Infectious Disease. (2018). *Emerging infectious diseases/pathogens.* Bethesda, MD; National Institutes of Health. Retrieved from https://www.niaid.nih.gov/research/emerging-infectious-diseases-pathogens

National Institutes of Health. (2012, Updated September). *Emerging and re-emerging infectious diseases. National Institutes of Health in collaboration with National Institute of Allergy and Infectious Disease.* Colorado Springs, CO: BSCS. Retrieved from https://science.education.nih.gov/supplements/nih_diseases.pdf

Nebehay, S. (2016, February 3). *Concerned by report of sexual spread of Zika virus.* Toronto, ON: *The Globe and Mail.* Available at: https://www.theglobeandmail.com/canada/. Retrieved from http://www.theglobeandmail.com/news/world/who-concerned-by-report-of-sexual-spread-of-zika-virus/article28531722/

O'Connor, A. (2009, December 14). The claim: Flu viruses live longer on surfaces than cold viruses .*New York Times*, D5. Retrieved from http://www.nytimes.com/2009/12/15/health/15real.html

Ogden, N. H., Abdel-Malik, P., & Pulliam, J. R. C. (2017, October 5). Commentary-emerging infectious diseases: Prediction and detection. *Canadian Communicable Disease Report (CCDR), 43*(10), 206–211. Retrieved from https://www.canada.ca/en/public-health/services/reports-publications/canada-communicable-disease-report-ccdr/monthly-issue/2017-43/ccdr-volume-43-10-october-5-2017/commentary-emerging-infectious-diseases-prediction-detection.html

Ogden, N. H., Koffi, K. J., Pelcat, Y., & Lindsay, L. R. (2014). Environmental risk from Lyme disease in central and eastern Canada: A summary of recent surveillance information. *Canadian Communicable Disease Report, 40*(5), 74–82. Retrieved from http://www.phac-aspc.gc.ca/publicat/ccdr-rmtc/14vol40/dr-rm40-05/assets/pdf/14vol40_05-eng.pdf

Oregon State University. (2013, September 16). Gut microbes closely linked to proper immune function and other health issues. *Science Daily.* Retrieved from https://www.sciencedaily.com/releases/2013/09/130916122214.htm

Pan American Health Organization. (2014, June 13). Number of reported cases of Chikungunya fever in the Americas, by counts or territory with autochthonous transmission 2013–2014 (to week noted). Cumulative cases. *Epidemiological week? EW24.* Washington, DC: Author. Retrieved from file:///C:/Users/100241938/Downloads/2014-jun-13-cha-CHIKV-authoch-imported-cases-ew-24.pdf

Pan American Health Organization. (2017). *Chikungunya.* Washington, DC: Author. Retrieved from http://www.paho.org/hq/index.php?option=com_topics&view=article&id=343&Itemid=40931&lang=en

Patz, J. A., Epstein, P. R., Burke, T. A., & Balbus, J. M. (1995). Global climate change and emerging infectious diseases. *JAMA, 275*(3), 217–223. Retrieved from https://www.researchgate.net/profile/John_Balbus2/publication/14596729_Climate_change_and_emerging_diseases/links/5892448e458515aeac945bf1/Climate-change-and-emerging-diseases.pdf

Payne, E. (2016a, September 6). *The deadly history of Ebola.* Ottawa, ON: Ottawa Citizen. Retrieved from http://ottawacitizen.com/news/world/the-deadly-history-of-ebola

Payne, E. (2016b, September 2). *The story of the Canadian vaccine that beat back Ebola.* Ottawa, ON: Ottawa Citizen. Retrieved from http://ottawacitizen.com/news/national/the-canadian-vaccine-how-scientists-in-a-country-without-a-single-case-of-ebola-wrestle-the-deadly-disease-to-the-gorund

Peiris, J. S., Guan, Y., & Yuen, K. Y. (2004). Severe acute respiratory syndrome. *National Medicine, 10*, S88–S97 (PMID:15577937).

Powers, A. M., & Logue, C. H. (2007). Changing patterns of chikungunya virus: Re-emergence of a zoonotic arbovirus. *Journal of General Virology, 88*(9), 2363–2377.

Public Health Agency of Canada. (2007, September). *Core competencies for public health in Canada: Release 1.1.* Ottawa, ON: Author. Web-Based link: http://www.phac-aspc.gc.ca/core_competencies or http://www.phac-aspc.gc.ca/php-psp/ccph-cesp/pdfs/cc-manual-eng090407.pdf

Public Health Agency of Canada. (2010). *Pathogen safety data sheets: Infectious substances—Blastomyces dermatitidis.* Ottawa, ON: Author. Retrieved from https://www.canada.ca/en/public-health/services/laboratory-biosafety-biosecurity/pathogen-safety-data-sheets-risk-assessment/blastomyces-dermatitidis.html

Public Health Agency of Canada. (2012a). *The Canadian Nosocomial Infection Surveillance Program* (CNISP). Ottawa, ON: Author. Retrieved from http://www.phac-aspc.gc.ca/nois-sinp/survprog-eng.php

Public Health Agency of Canada. (2012b). *Infectious disease outbreaks: Progress between SARS and pandemic influenza H1N1.* Ottawa, ON: Author. Retrieved from http://www.phac-aspc.gc.ca/ep-mu/rido-iemi/index-eng.php#the

Public Health Agency of Canada. (2013). *The chief public health officer's report on the state of public health in Canada, 2013, infectious diseases, the never-ending threat.* Ottawa, ON: Author. Retrieved from http://www.phac-aspc.gc.ca/cphorsphcrespcacsp/2013/assets/pdf/2013-eng.pdf

Public Health Agency of Canada. (2016, January 15). *Zika virus infection in the Americas. Travel health notice.* Ottawa, ON: Author. Retrieved from https://www.canada.ca/en/public-health/services/public-health-notices/2016/public-health-notice-zika-virus.html

Public Health Agency of Canada. (2017a). *Case definition for communicable diseases under national surveillance*. Ottawa, ON: Author. Retrieved from https://www.canada.ca/en/public-health/services/reports-publications/canada-communicable-disease-report-ccdr/monthly-issue/2009-35/definitions-communicable-diseases-national-surveillance/lyme-disease.html

Public Health Agency of Canada. (2017b). *Lyme disease in Canada—A federal framework*. Ottawa, ON: Author. Retrieved from https://www.canada.ca/en/public-health/services/publications/diseases-conditions/lyme-disease-canada-federal-framework.html

Public Health Agency of Canada. (2017c). *The plague*. Ottawa, ON: Author. Retrieved from https://www.canada.ca/en/public-health/services/chronic-diseases/plague.html

Public Health Agency of Canada. (2017d). *Surveillance of West Nile virus*. Ottawa, ON: Author. Retrieved from https://www.canada.ca/en/public-health/services/diseases/west-nile-virus/surveillance-west-nile-virus.html

Public Health Ontario. (2013, August). *Guide for public health units: Considerations for adult mosquitoe control*. Toronto, ON: Queen's Printer for Ontario. Retrieved from https://www.publichealthontario.ca/en/eRepository/Guide_Considerations_Mosquitoe_Control_2013.pdf

Public Health Ontario. (2017, Updated October 17). *West Nile virus*. Toronto, ON: Author. Retrieved from https://www.publichealthontario.ca/en/BrowseByTopic/InfectiousDiseases/Pages/IDLandingPages/West-Nile-Virus.aspx

Rerksuppaphol, S., & Rersuppaphol, L. (2012). Randomized controlled trial of probiotics to reduce common cold in schoolchildren. *Pediatrics International, 54*(5), 682–687.

Salazar, R., Castillo-Neyra, R., Tustin, A. W., Borrini-Mayori, K., Naquira, C., & Levy, M. Z. (2015, February). Bed bugs (*Cimex lectularius*) as vectors of trypanosoma cruzi. *The American Journal of Tropical Medicine, 92*(2), 331–335. Retrieved from http://www.ajtmh.org/content/journals/10.4269/ajtmh.14-0483

Scutti, S. (2013, July 18). The four best bug repellents: DEET, IR 3533, Picaridin, oil of lemon eucalyptus most effective says EWG. *Consumers News*. Environmental Working Group Publications. Retrieved from http://www.medicaldaily.com/four-best-bug-repellents-deet-ir3535-picaridin-oil-lemon-eucalyptus-most-effective-says-ewg-247785

Seitz, A. E., Adjemian, J., Steiner, C. A., & Prevots, D. R. (2015, June). Spatial epidemiology of blastomycosis hospitalizations: Detecting clusters and identifying environmental risk factors. *Medical Mycology, 53*(5), 447–454. doi:10.1093/mmy/myv014

Semeniuk, I. (2017, March 24). *Canadian vaccine for Ebola virus proves highly effective in guinea trial*. Toronto, ON: The Globe and Mail. Retrieved from https://www.theglobeandmail.com/technology/science/canadian-vaccine-for-ebola-virus-proves-extremely-effective-in-clinical-trial/article33416753/

Shapiro, E. D. (2014, May 5). Lyme disease. *New England Journal of Medicine, 4*(370), 1724–1730. Retrieved from https://web.archive.org/web/20161019142422/http://portal.mah.harvard.edu/templatesnew/departments/MTA/Lyme/uploaded_documents/NEJMcp1314325.pdf

Snacken, R., Kendal, A. P., Haaheim, L. R., & Wood, J. M. (1999, April). Lessons from Hong Kong, 1997. *Emerging Infectious Diseases, 5*(2). Retrieved from https://wwwnc.cdc.gov/eid/article/5/2/99-0202_article

Steere, A. C., Coburn, J., & Glickstein, L. (2004, April 15). The emergence of Lyme disease. *The Journal of Clinical Investigations, 113*(8), 1093–1101. Retrieved from https://www.ncbi.nlm.nih.gov/pmc/articles/PMC385417/

Todor, K. (2012). The normal bacteria flora of humans. In *Todor's online textbook of bacteriology*, Madison, WI: Author. Retrieved from http://textbookofbacteriology.net/normalflora_3.html

Torresi, J., & Leder, K. (2009). Defining infections in international travellers through the GeoSentinel surveillance network. *National Review of Microbiology, 7*(12), 895–901.

Tortora, G. J., Funke, B. R., & Case, C. L. (2016). *Microbiology: An introduction* (15th ed.). Toronto, ON: Pearson.

Vector Disease Control International. (2013). *West Nile virus: What is West Nile virus and how does it spread?* Little Rock, AR: Author. Retrieved from http://www.vdci.net/vector-borne-diseases/west-nile-virus-education-and-mosquitoe-management-to-protect-public-health

Vighi, G., Marcucci, F., Sensi, C., Di Cara, G., & Fratti, F. (2008, September 15). Allergy and the gastrointestinal system. *Allergy & Experimental Immunology, 153*(Suppl. 1), 3–6. doi:10.111/j.1365-2249.2008.03713x. Retrieved from https://www.ncbi.nlm.nih.gov/pmc/articles/PMC2515351/

Wang, L. F., & Cramer, G. (2014). Emerging zoonotic viral diseases. *Revue scientifique et technique/Office international des épizooties, 33*(2), 569–581. Retrieved from https://www.oie.int/doc/ged/D14089.PDF

Weaver, S. C. (2006). Alphavirus Infections. In R. L. Guerrant, D. H. Walker, & P. F. Weller (Eds.), *Tropical infectious diseases: Principles, pathogens, and practice*. (2nd ed., pp. 831–838). Philadelphia, PA: Elsevier Churchill Livingston.

Webber, R. (2016). *Communicable diseases: A global perspective* (5th ed.). Boston, MA: C.A.B. International.

World Health Organization. (2003). *SARS outbreak contained worldwide*. Geneva, Switzerland: Author. Retrieved from http://www.who.int/mediacentre/news/releases/2003/pr56/en/

World Health Organization. (2011). *Report on the burden of endemic health care-associated infection worldwide: Clean care is safer care*. Geneva, Switzerland: Author (ISBN: 978 92 4 1501507). Retrieved from http://apps.who.int/iris/bitstream/10665/80135/1/9789241501507_eng.pdf

World Health Organization. (2015). *Global vaccine action plan. Monitoring evaluation and accountability. Secretariat annual report 2014*. Geneva, Switzerland: Author. Retrieved from http://www.who.int/immunization/global_vaccine_action_plan/gvap_secretariat_report_2014.pdf

World Health Organization. (2016a). *Health topics: Zika virus*. Geneva, Switzerland: Author. Retrieved from http://www.who.int/topics/zika/en/

World Health Organization. (2016b, May). *Tool for influenza pandemic risk assessment (TIPRA): Version I*. Geneva, Switzerland: Author. Retrieved from http://apps.who.int/iris/bitstream/10665/250130/1/WHO-OHE-PED-GIP-2016.2-eng.pdf?ua=1

World Health Organization. (2016c, June 10). *World Health Organization situation report: Ebola virus disease 10 June 2016*. Geneva, Switzerland: Author. Retrieved from http://apps.who.int/iris/bitstream/10665/208883/1/ebolasitrep_10Jun2016_eng.pdf?ua=1

World Health Organization. (2017a). *Cumulative number of confirmed human cases for avian influenza A (H5N1) reported to WHO, 2003–2017*. Geneva, Switzerland: Author. Retrieved from http://www.who.int/influenza/human_animal_interface/2017_12_07_tableH5N1.pdf?ua=1 and http://www.who.int/influenza/human_animal_interface/H5N1_cumulative_table_archives/en/

World Health Organization. (2017b). *Emergency preparedness, response*. Geneva, Switzerland: Author. Retrieved from http://www.who.int/csr/en/

World Health Organization. (2017c). *Fact sheet: Antibiotic resistance*. Geneva, Switzerland: Author. Retrieved from http://www.who.int/mediacentre/factsheets/fs194/en/

World Health Organization. (2017d). *Health topics: Emerging diseases*. Geneva, Switzerland: Author. Retrieved from http://www.who.int/topics/emerging_diseases/en/

World Health Organization. (2017e). *Health topics: International health regulations (IHR)*. Geneva, Switzerland: Author. Retrieved from http://www.who.int/topics/international_health_regulations/en/

World Health Organization. (2017f). *The history of Zika virus*. Geneva, Switzerland: Author. Retrieved from http://www.who.int/emergencies/zika-virus/timeline/en/

World Health Organization. (2017g). *Immunization, vaccines and biologicals: The expanded programme on immunization*. Geneva, Switzerland: Author. Retrieved from http://www.who.int/immunization/programmes_systems/supply_chain/benefits_of_immunization/en/

World Health Organization. (2017h). *Plague. Fact sheet*. Geneva, Switzerland: Author. Retrieved from http://www.who.int/mediacentre/factsheets/fs267/en/

World Health Organization. (2017i). *WHO toolkit for the care and support of people affected by complications associated with Zika virus*. Geneva, Switzerland: Author. (ISBN: 978-92-4-151271-8). Retrieved from http://www.who.int/mental_health/neurology/zika_toolkit/en/

World Health Organization. (2017j). *WHO Zika podcast episodes—Evidence in action*. Geneva, Switzerland: Author. Retrieved from http://www.who.int/mediacentre/multimedia/podcasts/2017/en/

World Health Organization. (2017k, March 10). *Zika situation report*. Geneva, Switzerland: Author. Retrieved from http://www.who.int/emergencies/zika-virus/situation-report/10-march-2017/en/

World Health Organization. (2017l). *Zika virus: Fact sheet*. Geneva, Switzerland: Author. Retrieved from http://www.who.int/mediacentre/factsheets/zika/en/

World Health Organization. (2018a). *70 years of influenza control: Into the history of influenza control*. Geneva, Switzerland: Author. Retrieved from http://www.who.int/influenza/gip-anniversary/en/

World Health Organization. (2018b). *Avian influenza A (H7N9) virus.* Geneva, Switzerland: Author. Retrieved from http://www.who.int/influenza/human_animal_interface/influenza_h7n9/en/

World Health Organization. (2018c). *Chikungunya.* Geneva, Switzerland: Author. Retrieved from http://www.who.int/denguecontrol/arbo-viral/other_arboviral_chikungunya/en/

World Health Organization. (2018d). *Chikungunya: Fact sheet.* Geneva, Switzerland: Author. Retrieved from http://www.who.int/mediacentre/factsheets/fs327/en/

World Health Organization. (2018e). *Director-generals office: Health emergencies represent some of the greatest risk to global economy and security. Remarks delivered by Dr Tedros Adhanom Ghebreyesus to G20 8 July 2017 (Hamburg, Germany, July 8th, 2017).* Geneva, Switzerland: Author. Retrieved from http://www.who.int/dg/speeches/2017/g20-summit/en/

World Health Organization. (2018f). *Ebola outbreak 2014–2015.* Geneva, Switzerland: Author. Retrieved from http://www.who.int/csr/disease/ebola/en/

World Health Organization. (2018g). *Ebola virus disease fact sheet No. 103.* Geneva, Switzerland: Author. Retrieved from http://www.who.int/mediacentre/factsheet

World Health Organization. (2018h). *Emergency preparedness response: Severe acute respiratory syndrome (SARS).* Geneva, Switzerland: Author. Retrieved from http://www.who.int/csr/sars/en/

World Health Organization. (2018i). *Emergency preparedness, response: Summary of probably SARS cases with onset of illness from 1 November 2002 to 31 July 2003.* Geneva, Switzerland: Author. Retrieved from http://www.who.int/csr/sars/country/table2004_04_21/en/

World Health Organization. (2018j). *Emergency preparedness, response: Update 95-chronology of a serial killer.* Geneva, Switzerland: Author. Retrieved from http://www.who.int/csr/don/2003_07_04/en/

World Health Organization. (2018k). *Executive summary: Insect-borne diseases.* Geneva, Switzerland: Author. Retrieved from http://www.who.int/whr/1996/media_centre/executive_summary1/en/index9.html

World Health Organization. (2018l). *FluNet.* Geneva, Switzerland: Author. Retrieved from http://www.who.int/influenza/gisrs_laboratory/flunet/en/

World Health Organization. (2018m). *Human infection with Asian influenza A (H7N9) virus-China.* Geneva, Switzerland: Author. Retrieved from http://www.who.int/csr/don/15-march-2017-ah7n9-china/en/

World Health Organization. (2018n). *Influenza: Avian and other zoonotic influenza.* Geneva, Switzerland: Author. Retrieved from http://www.who.int/influenza/human_animal_interface/en/

World Health Organization. (2018o). *Influenza: Frequently asked questions on human infection caused by avian influenza A (H7N9) virus.* Geneva, Switzerland: Author. Retrieved from http://www.who.int/influenza/human_animal_interface/faq_H7N9/en/

World Health Organization. (2018p). *Media centre: Final trial results confirm Ebola vaccine provides high protection against disease.* Geneva, Switzerland: Author. Retrieved from http://www.who.int/mediacentre/news/releases/2016/ebola-vaccine-results/en/

World Health Organization. (2018q). *Middle East respiratory syndrome coronavirus (MERS-CoV).* Geneva, Switzerland: Author. Retrieved from http://www.who.int/mediacentre/factsheets/mers-cov/en/

World Health Organization. (2018r). *SARS-sudden acute respiratory syndrome.* Geneva, Switzerland: Author. Retrieved from http://www.who.int/ith/diseases/sars/en/

World Health Organization. (2018s). *Vector-borne diseases: Lyme disease.* Geneva, Switzerland: Author. Retrieved from http://www.who.int/mediacentre/factsheets/fs387/en/index10.html

World Health Organization. (2018t). *Zoonoses and veterinary public health. Global early warning systems for major animal diseases including zoonoses (GLEWS).* Geneva, Switzerland: Author. Retrieved from http://www.who.int/zoonoses/outbreaks/glews/en/index1.html

Wu, X., Lu, Y., Zhou, S., Chen, L., & Xu, B. (2016, January). Impact of climate change on human infectious diseases: Empirical evidence and human adaptation. *Environmental International, 86,* 14–23. Retrieved from http://www.sciencedirect.com/science/article/pii/S0160412015300489

Zhong, N. S., Zheng, B. J., Li, Y. M., Poon Xie, Z. H., & Chan, K. H., (2003). Epidemiology and cause of severe acute respiratory syndrome (SARS) in Guangdong, People's Republic of China, in February, 2003. *Lancet, 362,* 1353–1358 (PMID:14585636).

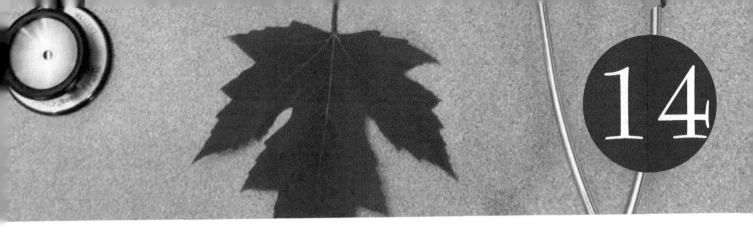

Major Noncommunicable Diseases: Current and Future Challenges

The question is not how to get cured, but how to live!
(Joseph Conrad—born Józef Teodor Konrad Korzeniowski, December 3, 1857–August 3, 1924)

Learning Objectives

After completion of this chapter, the student will be able to:

- Describe the prevalence and impact of major non-communicable diseases (NCDs) in Canada and globally.
- List and describe the impact of the four major types or groupings of NCDs on public health systems in Canada, including heart disease, cancer, diabetes, and respiratory diseases.
- List and describe key social determinants of health and risk factors associated with the development of NCDs.
- Describe the impact of living with a chronic NCD and the role of self-management.
- List and describe the four targeted behavioural risk factors for the development of NCDs and so-called "best buy" public health interventions.
- List and describe certain vulnerable populations in Canada (e.g., indigenous people, older adults) who are at increased risk of developing NCDs.
- Discuss the impact of looking after a family member or significant other with a chronic NCD, including the concept of caregiver burden.
- Critically examine population trends, including the growing incidence of older adults, and the current and future predicted impacts of NCDs on public health systems in Canada.

Core Competencies for Public Health Addressed in Chapter 14

Core Competencies	Competency Statements
1.0 Public Health Sciences	1.1, 1.2, 1.3,
2.0 Assessment and Analysis	2.2, 2.3, 2.4, 2.5, 2.6
3.0 Policy and Program Planning, Implementation, and Evaluation	3.1, 3.2, 3.6, 3.7
4.0 Partnerships, Collaboration, and Advocacy	4.1, 4.2, 4.3
5.0 Diversity and Inclusiveness	5.1, 5.2, 5.3
6.0 Communication	6.2
7.0 Leadership	7.1, 7.2

Note: Please see the following document or web-based link for a detailed description of these specific competencies. Public Health Agency of Canada (PHAC, 2007).

Introduction

A **non-communicable disease (NCD)** is defined as a chronic disease not typically caused by an infectious agent (i.e., non-infectious or non-communicable) that often has complex aetiologies, has an insidious onset, often characterized by multiple associated risk factors, long latency periods and is normally incurable in nature. Historically, when a disease was transmittable via an organism (e.g., virus, bacteria, protozoa), it was deemed to be *communicable* (or infectious) in nature; otherwise the disease was labelled *non-communicable* (or non-infectious). However, this simple distinction is becoming less clear-cut and defined as we continue to learn more about the nature, evolution, epidemiology, and aetiology of various NCDs, especially in regards to the development of certain cancers. For examples, the links between hepatitis B virus and the development of hepatocellular cancer, and human papilloma virus (HVP) and cervical cancer are now well established and documented; whereas, both can now be prevented via routine vaccinations (e.g., Clifford, Smith, Plumber, Munoz, & Franceschi, 2003; Cooke, 2008; El-Serog, 2012; Webber, 2016). We shall examine cancer as one of the major NCDs facing Canadians is greater detail later.

We argue that few pandemics have resulted in as much suffering, premature deaths, functional impairments, disability, and decreased health-related quality of life as NCDs (Bartfay & Bartfay, 2015). NCDs are the leading cause of death in Canada and globally; which require complex responses from clients, their families, and our public health systems because chronic illness often incorporates multiple physical and/or psychosocial-related health problems that have a protracted and unpredictable course (Public Health Agency of Canada [PHAC], 2016; WHO, 2017a, 2017b). Moreover, treatment for one chronic condition may adversely affect and/or complicate other conditions. For example, furosemide (i.e., Lasix) is a common diuretic prescribed to help reduce the presence of edema (i.e., excess fluid retention) caused by chronic conditions such as heart failure, liver disease, and kidney disease. Although furosemide is effective in managing edema, certain clients may also experience undesirable and/or potential dangerous side effects including vertigo and dizziness, muscle weakness, drowsiness, nausea and vomiting, headaches, and blurred vision.

In Canada, more than one in five Canadian adults live with one of these NCDs (i.e., cardiovascular disease [CVD], cancer, chronic respiratory disease [CRD], diabetes); and two-thirds of all deaths each year are caused by these major NCDs (PHAC, 2016). For example, in 2011/2012, an estimated 2.3 million of Canadians were living with ischemic heart disease; almost 2 million were living with COPD, and 700,000 were living with the after effects of a stroke. The PHAC (2016) reports that over 800,000 Canadians had been diagnosed with cancer within the past 10 years, and nearly 90% of all newly diagnosed cancers cases occurred in adults aged 50 years or older (Table 14.1).

Table 14.1 Mortality Rates for Major NCDs in Canada. Probability of dying between the ages 30 and 69 years from one of the major chronic diseases noted above was 10.4%.

Type of NCD	Mortality Rates
Cancer	213.7 per 100,000
Cardiovascular disease (CVD, e.g., ischemic heart disease, acute myocardial infarction, stroke)	194.7 per 100,000
Chronic respiratory disease (CRD, e.g., COPD, asthma)	44.7 per 100,000
Diabetes	20.0 per 100,000
Total combined (i.e., cancer, CVD, CRD, and diabetes)	473.0 per 100,000

Source: Adapted from Canadian Chronic Disease Indicators (CCDI) Steering Committee. (2017).

NCDs such as CVDs, cancer, diabetes and CRDs, are leading causes of death, and are responsible for 70% of premature deaths worldwide for both men and women (N = 15 million) between the ages 30 to 70 years annually (World Health Organization [WHO], 2017a, 2017b). CVDs account for most NCD deaths (N = 17.7 million); followed by cancers (N = 8.8 million); CRDs (N = 3.9 million), and diabetes (N = 1.6 million) each year. These four groups of diseases also account for over 80% of all premature NCD deaths globally (WHO, 2017a, 2017b). Although a discussion on all NCDs is beyond the scope and purpose of this chapter, we shall concentrate our discussion to these four aforementioned conditions.

As necessitated at the 64th World Health Assembly (resolution WHA 64.11), the Secretariat has developed a global action plan for the prevention and control of NCDs for the period of 2013 to 2020 (WHO, 2011a, 2011b, 2013, 2017a). The action plan provides a road map with a menu of policy options for all member states and other stakeholders, to take coordinated and coherent action, at all levels (i.e., local community-based to global), to attain nine voluntary global targets. One of the major targets includes a 25% relative reduction in premature mortality from CVDs, cancer, diabetes, or CRDs by 2025 (WHO, 2011a, 2011b, 2013, 2017a).

According to WHO's (2013) projections, the total annual number of deaths from NCDs will increase to 55 million by 2030 if "business as usual" continues (NCDs). Indeed, CVDs, cancer, diabetes, and CRDs are already the leading global causes of death worldwide (WHO, 2017a, 2017b). For all countries, the cost of inaction far outweighs the cost of taking action on NCDs as recommended in this action plan. Continuing "business as usual" will result in loss of productivity and an escalation of healthcare costs in all countries. It is widely recognized that the conditions in which people live and work and their lifestyles influence their health and quality of life. The four shared behavioural lifestyle risk factors with the largest contribution to morbidity and mortality due to NCDs involve (i) tobacco use; (ii) unhealthy diet; (iii) physical inactivity; and (v) harmful use of alcohol (WHO, 2013, 2017a).

The NCD pandemic is driven by poverty, globalization of marketing and trade of health-harming products, rapid urbanization, and changing population trends including a growing incidence of older adults. For example, nearly one in six Canadians (5.8 million) are 65 years or older, and this age group is growing four times faster than overall population (PHAC, 2016). Indeed, at the time of Confederation in 1867, the average life expectancy (LE) for Canadians was only 42 years, and by 1921 this had increased to 60 years (Roberts, Clifton, Ferguson, Kampen, & Langlois, 2004). Statistics Canada (2017) reports that LE has been steadily increasing for Canadians over the decades, and is currently 82 years. Age is a major predictor for the development of NCDs in Canada and internationally. As of 2015, the number of adults aged 65 years or older outnumbered those aged 14 and younger. With the first of the baby boom generation turning age 65 years in 2011, older adults will account for an increasingly larger proportion of the Canadian population; which is predicted to reach approximately 25% (or 1:4 Canadians) by the year 2036 (Canadian Institute for Health Information [CIHI], 2011, 2017, 2018).

For example, vulnerable and socially disadvantaged clients get sicker and die sooner than people of higher social and economic status; especially because they are at greater risk of being exposed to harmful products such as tobacco, or unhealthy dietary practices, and often have limited access to health services (GBD 2015 Risk Factors Collaborators, 2016; WHO, 2017a, 2017b). For individuals with low social and economic status, healthcare costs for NCDs often quickly drain household resources and savings. Hence, the exorbitant costs associated with chronic management and care of NCDs often force millions of people worldwide into poverty annually and stifle national growth and development services (GBD 2015 Risk Factors Collaborators, 2016; WHO, 2017a, 2017b).

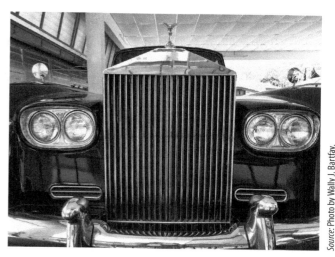

Source: Photo by Wally J. Bartfay.

Photo 14.1 Does poverty play a role in the development of NCDs? Poverty is a major social determinant of health which has far reaching negative effects both on the development, access to healthcare services, and treatment of NCDs in Canada and internationally. Individuals with higher incomes and social status are consistently better-off in terms of their health status and the probability of developing a NCD in Canada and abroad.

Prevention of NCDs in the 21st Century: Four Targeted Behavioural Risk Factors

From a public health perspective; which is supported by decades of research, it may be rightfully argued that prevention is the best way to tackle the global pandemic of NCDs. Although not all NCDs are preventable per se, four modifiable behavioural risk factors are considered key to the development of NCDs in Canada and globally (GBD 2015 Risk Factors Collaborators, 2016; PHAC, 2016; WHO, 2011a, 2011b, 2017a, 2017b).

> NCDs are caused, to a large extent, by four behavioural risk factors that are pervasive aspects of economic transition, rapid urbanization and 21st-century lifestyles: tobacco use, unhealthy diet, insufficient physical activity and the harmful use of alcohol (WHO, 2011a, p. 9).

It is noteworthy that approximately four in five Canadian adults have at least one modifiable risk factor for the development of an NCD (self-reported tobacco smoking, physical inactivity, unhealthy eating, and harmful use of alcohol) (PHAC, 2016). We shall examine these four major modifiable risk factors in greater detail later.

Decades of public health practice and research have identified targeted population-based NCD prevention strategies known as "best buys," which have been documented to be cost effective and appropriate for nations to engage in NCD prevention (GBD 2015 Risk Factors Collaborators, 2016; PHAC, 2016; WHO, 2011a, 2011b, 2017a, 2017b). **Best buys** are defined by WHO (2011) as population-based actions that should be undertaken immediately to produce accelerated results in regards to NCD prevention, decreasing associated morbidities and mortalities, and decreasing associated healthcare costs and burden. Improved access to healthcare services (especially in rural and remote regions), early detection and screening, and timely diagnosis and treatments are other effective approaches for reducing the impact of NCDs (WHO, 2017a, 2017b, 2017c). Table 14.2 provides a list of "best buys" as highlighted by WHO (2011).

Table 14.2 "Best Buys" for Population-Based Prevention of NCDs

- Protecting people from the harmful effects of tobacco smoke, and banning smoking in all public places (e.g., work environments, shopping malls, restaurants, public transport)
- Warning and educating the public about the dangers of tobacco use (e.g., product health risk disclosures on packages)
- Raising taxes on tobacco products
- Restricting access to retailed alcohol

- Enforcing bans on alcohol advertising (e.g., print, mass and social media)
- Raising taxes on alcohol products (e.g., beer, wine, liquor)
- Reduce salt intake and content of food (e.g., especially highly processed foods)
- Replace trans fat in food products with polyunsaturated fat
- Promote public awareness about the importance of diet and physical activity for the prevention of NCDs (e.g., through mass and social media)

Source: Adapted from World Health Organization (2011).

A major reduction in the healthcare burden associated with NCDs in Canada may be achieved, in part, from these population-based "best buy" interventions; which are cost effective and may even be revenue generating (e.g., tobacco and alcohol tax increases, implementation of a sugar tax). Nonetheless, both a social and political will is required, and it is critical for public health professionals and workers, and researchers to educate public health policy and law makers about the best available evidence and practice standards.

For example, the *WHO Framework Convention on Tobacco Control* was, in fact, the first treaty negotiated under the auspices of the WHO (2003, 2011). It is noteworthy that approximately 4.7 billion people (or 63% of the world's population) are currently covered by at least one comprehensive tobacco control measure; which has quadrupled since 2007 when only 1 billion people (or 15% of the world's population) were covered (WHO, 2017c). Moreover, more than half of the top reported performers were from low- and middle-income countries, which validate the claim that population-based interventions are effective regardless of income or social economic status (WHO, 2017c). This example highlights the effectiveness of "best-buys" population-based public health interventions. Nonetheless, the control and use of tobacco products remain a major global public health challenge in the 21st century due to increased globalization; direct foreign investment in tobacco companies; transnational tobacco advertising and marketing; self-promotion and sponsorship (e.g., national or regional social or sporting events), and the growing "black-market" related to contraband and/or counterfeit cigarettes have all contributed to the continued use of tobacco products. We shall examine this major modifiable risk factor in greater detail later from a Canadian context.

1. *Tobacco Use and Smoking*

   Since the year 2001, there has been a decrease in the age-standardized rate (ASR) of daily or occasional smokers in Canada. Specifically, the ASR in 2001 was 25.1% compared to 17.8% in 2014, representing a 2.1% annual decrease (PHAC, 2016). Nonetheless, 7.8% of youth (12–19 years old) reported daily or occasional smoking. Smoking rates were highest among young adults aged 20 to 34 years (24.3%); followed by adults aged 35 to 64 years at approximately 20% (or 1:5) (PHAC, 2016; Figure 14.1).

2. *Physical Inactivity and Sedentary Lifestyles*

   It is recommended that children and youth engage in moderate-to-vigorous physical activity for at least 60 min each day (Tremblay et al., 2011b). It is noteworthy that a significant proportion of both girls (94.1%) and boys (86.9%) do not meet the level of activity recommended by current national guidelines. The most recent data shows that the proportion of 5- to 11-year olds who do not meet the guidelines is 86.5%, while it climbs to 94.4% for 12- to 17-year olds (PHAC, 2016). In adults,

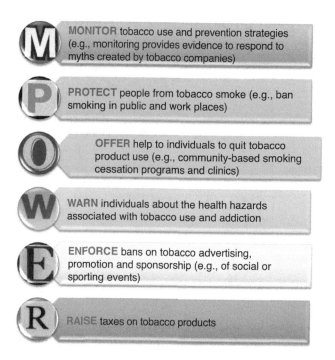

Figure 14.1 MPOWER Acronym for the Control and Prevention of Tobacco Related NCDs

Source: Courtesy of Wally J. Bartfay. Adapted from World Health Organization (2017c).

adherence to the guidelines diminishes with age. Hence, Canadian youth who are currently inactive are at increased risk at developing an NCD as an adult. For adults, 150 min of moderate-to-vigorous physical activity each week is recommended, performed in bouts of 10 min or more (Tremblay et al., 2011b). The proportion of men and women who do not obtain enough physical activity to meet the guidelines does not differ significantly: 76.5% for men and 79.1% for women. A greater proportion of younger adults (aged 18–34 years) achieve the recommended amount of moderate-to-vigorous physical activity, in comparison with older adults. Alarmingly, more than four in five adults aged 35 years or older are inactive: 82.0% for 35- to 49-year olds, 83.3% for 50- to 64-year olds and 88.2% for adults aged 65 years and over (PHAC, 2016).

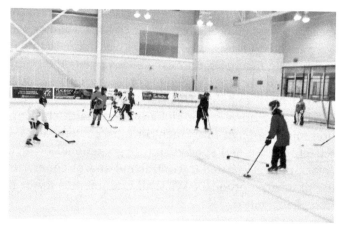

Photo 14.2 Despite Our Love for Sports Such as Hockey, an Alarming Growing Number of Canadian Youth and Adults Are Physically Inactive. More than three quarters (77.8%, or 20.1 million) of Canadian adults 18 years of age and over and 90.7% of children and youth aged 5–17 years are not meeting current recommended Canadian Physical Activity Guidelines (PHAC, 2016; Tremblay et al., 2011b).

The Canadian Society for Exercise Physiology (2012) recommends that parents, guardians, and caretakers limit screen time to 0 min per day for children under 2 years of age; less than 1 hour per day for children aged 2 to 4 years, and less than 2 hours per day for children aged 5 to 11 years. There are currently no national guidelines for children aged 12 years or older or for adults. Sedentary behaviour related to use of technologies involving video display terminals (VDTs), such as smartphones, laptop computers, and tablets is a relatively new public health issue. Sedentary behaviours, which are generally characterized by long periods of sitting, such as streaming movies online, playing passive video games, social media and texting, have been associated with health risks, including obesity and decreased fitness. There is strong evidence that this association is independent of physical activity (PHAC, 2016).

The Canadian Society for Exercise Physiology, with the support of PHAC, released Canada's first evidence-based sedentary behaviour guidelines in 2011 (Tremblay et al., 2011a). In 2012 to 2013, 51.8% of children and youth aged five to 17 years failed to meet the Canadian Sedentary Behaviour Guidelines. The trend was stable for the years 2007 to 2009 with 48.7% not meeting the guidelines, and 49.6% in 2009 to 2011. In 2012 to 2013, 49.8% of the girls and 53.8% of boys failed to meet the guidelines. In general, younger children spend less time being sedentary than older children and youth: 7.4 hours per day among children aged 5 to 9 years compared to 8.8 hours per day among those aged 10 to 14 years, and 9.5 hours per day among those aged 15 to 17 years. With rapidly changing mobile technology,

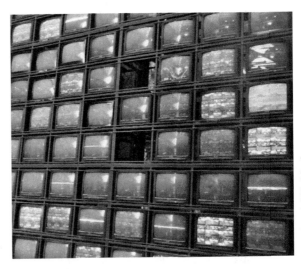

Photo 14.3 Does Our Increased Reliance and Addiction to Technology Contribute to Sedentary Behaviours in Canadians. Growing habit and use of screen-based technologies (e.g., smartphones and smart televisions, computers, mobile devices) is a growing public health concern for both youth and adults, since it negatively impacts health via the promotion of sedentary lifestyles. In fact, Canadians are amongst the most active Internet users globally, and spend on average approximately 43.5 hours per week online, compared to the global average of 23.1 hours (Canadian Broadcasting Corporation [CBC], 2011).

Source: Photo by Wally J. Bartfay.

increasing Internet usage, and the popularity of social media, developing consistent measures to monitor trends in sedentary behaviour can be expected to be a public health focus for the short-to-medium term in Canada (PHAC, 2016).

1. *Unhealthy Diet*

Current trends suggest that Canadians are eating significantly less fresh fruit and vegetables deemed essential to proper nutrition and health. In fact, 60.3% (or 17.1 million) of Canadians aged 12 years and older consume fruits and vegetables less than five times per day (PHAC, 2016). It is interesting to note that significantly more men than women consume fruits and vegetables less than five times per day (67.6% vs. 53.3%). Unhealthy eating varies across age groups: from 56.4% in youth aged 12 to 19 years to 63.6% in people aged 50 to 64 years, followed by a decline in the older age groups (PHAC, 2016).

Obese individuals are at an increased risk for the development of certain chronic conditions including hypertension, type 2 diabetes, CVDs, some cancers, and even premature death (Reilly, Methven, & McDowell, 2003). One in four adults (26.4%), one in six youth aged 12 to 17 years (16.5%) and one in 11 children aged 5 to 11 years (8.8%) are obese (PHAC, 2016). [T]Moreover, the strongest predictor of being obese as an adult is being obese as a child. Obesity rates have dramatically increased in the last few decades, while only 13.8% of adults and 6.3% of children and youth were obese during 1978 to 1979 (Bancej et al., 2015; Roberts, Shields, de Groh, Aziz, & Gilbert, 2012). Rates among men (26.5%) and women (26.2%) were comparable. Among children and youth aged five to 17 years, boys (14.7%) have a higher rate of obesity than girls (10.3%). In adults, rates were highest in the 35 to 49 and the 50 to 64 age groups, with 29.2% and 29.6% of them being obese, respectively (PHAC, 2016). In fact, more than 90% of Canadian children are not meeting current physical activity guidelines in Canada, and we rank amongst the worst of OECD countries for adult obesity rates (PHAC, 2016).

The Heart and Stroke Foundation (Heart and Stroke Foundation of Canada, 2003) report entitled *The Growing Burden of Health Disease and Stroke* reported that indigenous people were particularly at increased risk for the development of CVD, including heart disease and stroke. Findings from this report indicated that indigenous people were more likely to have major risk factors associated with the development of CVD; including being overweight or obese, consuming large amount of highly processed foods high in saturated and trans fats, salt, and sugar, were more likely to be smokers and also have diabetes. The *2002–2003 First Nations Regional Longitudinal Health Survey* found that indigenous women aged 20 to 34 years were more likely to be obese or morbid obese, in comparison to non-indigenous women (National Indigenous Health Organization, 2006). The reader is referred to Chapter 4 for a detailed discussion on Indigenous health and associated risk factors for the development of NCDs.

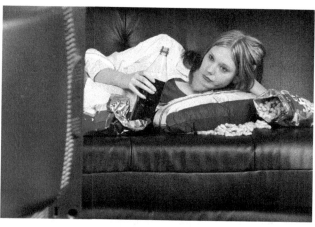

Photo 14.4 Canadian children are bombarded with over 25 million junk food and drink ads online every year, and over 90% are highly processed in nature with high sugar, fat, and salt contents (Choi, 2017). It is estimated that 4.1 million deaths per year globally are attributed to excess salt/sodium intake (GBD 2015 Risk Factors Collaborators, 2016; WHO, 2017a, 2017b). In addition, two-thirds of all packaged foods sold in Canada are loaded with sugar (Choi, Vuchnich, & Tang, 2017). Canadian children consume approximately 33 teaspoons of sugar per day (or 33 cubes of sugar).

(i) Harmful use of alcohol

More than half of the 3.3 million annual deaths, including cancer and other NCDs, are attributable to alcohol use (GBD 2015 Risk Factors Collaborators, 2016; WHO, 2017a, 2017b). *Canada's Low-Risk Alcohol Drinking Guidelines* were developed in 2011 to help Canadians moderate their alcohol consumption and reduce immediate and long-term alcohol-related harms. Immediate health risks are associated with "binge" or heavy drinking, which is characterized by the consumption of four or more drinks for women and five or more drinks for men on a single occasion. Long-term excessive alcohol consumption has been associated with an increased risk of chronic disease, including chronic liver disease, certain cancers, CVDs and premature death (Butt, Beirness, Gliksman, Paradis, & Stockwell, 2011; PHAC, 2016).

It is noteworthy that currently one in six (15.7%) Canadians aged 15 years and over exceed the Low-Risk Drinking Guidelines (2013, CADUMS). Between 2001 and 2014, the age-standardized proportion of Canadians who reported heavy drinking increased from 14.9% ASR to 17.9% ASR, representing an annual increase of 1.4%. The proportion of males that reported exceeding the

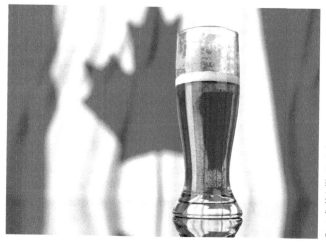

Photo 14.5 Alcohol Consumption Has Been Linked to the Development of Various NCDs, Including Cancer. More than one in six (17.9%, or over 5.2 million) Canadians aged 12 years and over reported that they engaged in heavy drinking on at least one occasion per month in the past year (PHAC, 2016).

Web-Based Resources Box 14.1   Additional Resources Related to NCDs and Their Prevention and Management From a Public Health Perspective

Learning Resource	Website
Chronic Disease Prevention—Program Planning and Evaluation (Toronto Public Health) -This website provides public healthcare professionals and workers with numerous guides and resources related to program planning and evaluation for the prevention and management of communicable and non-communicable diseases.	http://www.toronto.ca/health/chronicdiseaseprevent.htm or http://www1.toronto.ca/wps/portal/contentonly?vgnextoid=a253ba2ae8b1e310VgnVCM10000071d60f89RCRD
World Health Organization (WHO). (2011). *Global status report on preventing noncommunicable diseases 2010.* **Geneva, Switzerland: Author. ISBN: 978-92-4-068645-8.** -This report highlights so-called "best buys"; which are actions that should be immediately undertaken to produce accelerated results in terms of decreased mortality and morbidity, non-communicable disease (NCD) prevention, and decreased associated healthcare costs.	http://www.who.int/nmh/publications/ncd_report_full_en.pdf
WHO. (2013). *Global action plan for the prevention and control of NCDs 2013–2020.* **Geneva, Switzerland.: Author. ISBN: 978-92-4-150623-6.** - This action plan provides a road map for all member states and other stakeholders to take coordinated action at all levels to attain the nine voluntary global targets. -This includes a 25% targeted reduction in premature deaths from cardiovascular diseases, cancer, diabetes, and/or chronic respiratory diseases (CRDs) by 2025.	http://www.who.int/nmh/publications/ncd-action-plan/en/ or http://apps.who.int/iris/bitstream/10665/94384/1/9789241506236_eng.pdf?ua=1
WHO. (2017b). *Noncommunicable diseases: Progress monitor 2017.* **Geneva, Switzerland: Author. ISBN: 978-92-4-151302-9.** - This report is based on the latest data tracked against 10 progress indicators to chart progress in developing national responses. -It also highlights achievements and challenges faced by all developing countries in fulfilling promises made since the first United Nations High-level Meeting on NCDs in 2011.	http://apps.who.int/iris/bitstream/10665/258940/1/9789241513029-eng.pdf?ua=1

low-risk alcohol drinking guidelines for chronic drinking is higher in comparison to their female counterparts (18.8% vs. 12.7%). This difference is even greater for heavy drinking in males compared to females (22.6% vs. 13.3%) (PHAC, 2016).

In short, tobacco use, unhealthy diet, physical inactivity, and harmful use of alcohol are the most critical to target from a public health perspective in Canada and internationally for the prevention of NCDs (GBD 2015 Risk Factors Collaborators, 2016; WHO, 2013). In reality, the major causes of NCDs are these four noted risk factors, and if they were eliminated at least 80% of all heart diseases, stroke, over 40% of cancers, and type 2 diabetes would be prevented (WHO, 2005a).

Premature Mortality and HALE Trends in Canada

In Canada, as in the other developed countries, the majority of deaths occur in the older population. Consequently, the usual mortality measures reflect mainly the outcomes of the diseases occurring among the elderly. On the other hand, premature mortality refers to deaths that occur at a younger age than expected and, therefore, reflect the potential for avoidable deaths. Approximately Ten percent (10.7%) of 30-year-old

Canadians are expected to die before their 70th birthday from either a CVD, cancer, diabetes, or CRD (PHAC, 2016). The probability of dying between ages 30 and 69 years from any of the four main chronic diseases was higher in males (12.7%) than in females (8.8%). This was also true for each of these diseases, particularly for CVDs which were 2.5 times (PHAC, 2016). It is notable that the population of Nunavut had a rate more than two times greater than the national Canadian average. This territory displayed very high premature mortalities for CRDs (eight times greater) and cancer (two times greater) (PHAC, 2016). In addition, the Northwest Territories, Yukon and Newfoundland and Labrador presented a risk of premature mortality that was at least 20% higher than for Canada as a whole.

LE at birth is 83.0 years in Canada; where females currently have a LE at birth of 85.2 years, and males of 80.8 years in Canada (PHAC, 2012, 2016). The health-adjusted life expectancy (HALE), which reflects the number of years lived in "full health," is 72.6 years at birth (PHAC, 2012). **HALE** is defined as a composite measure of a population heath status that belongs to a defined family of health expectancies, and summarizes the expected number of year's equivalent to a state of so-called full health and well-being (Bartfay & Bartfay, 2015). The reader is referred to Chapter 9 for a detailed discussion of HALE and other global burden of disease measures. When taking health-related quality of life (HRQOL) measures into consideration, females have a HALE at birth of 73.7 years and males 71.4 years (PHAC, 2016). Nunavut, the Northwest Territories and Yukon had the lowest HALE (66.4 years), while Quebec had the highest (73.9 years; Figure 14.2).

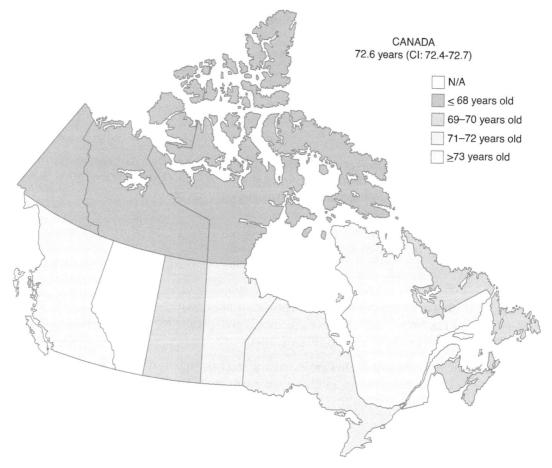

Figure 14.2 Live expectancies have been slowly increasing over the past five decades in Canada. Health-Adjusted Life Expectancy (HALE) by Province and Territory, Canada (2008/2009–2010/2011)

Chronic Disease Multi-Morbidity in Canadians

The recognition that people may have two or more chronic diseases or conditions concurrently, referred to as *multi-morbidity*, adds another layer of complexity to prevention and management by public healthcare professionals and workers. Indeed, these individuals are at a greater risk of adverse health outcomes and have increased healthcare needs (Guh et al., 2009; Roberts, Rao, Bennett, Loukine, & Jayaraman, 2015). More than one in 30 (3.6% or over 975,000) Canadian adults aged 20 years and older and nearly one in eight (11.7%) of Canadians aged 65 years and older have at least two of the four major chronic diseases—CVD, cancer, CRD, and diabetes (PHAC, 2016; Roberts et al., 2015). Females aged 65 years and older had significantly higher rates (13.1%) than males (10.3%). Among Canadian adults aged 20 years and older, 3.6% have at least two of the four major "physical" chronic diseases. This proportion increases dramatically with age, ranging from 0.3% in those aged 20 to 34 years; and 0.9% in those aged 35 to 49 years; to 3.7% in those aged 50 to 64 years; 11.0% in those aged 65 to 79 years, and up to 13.9% in those aged 80 years and over (PHAC, 2016). The highest age-standardized prevalence rates among Canadians aged 65 years and over were in Yukon (14.7% ASR) and Alberta (14.4% ASR), and the lowest rates where present in British Columbia (9.5% ASR) and Manitoba (8.8%) (PHAC, 2016).

Major NCDs: A Canadian Perspective

The prevention of NCDs will increase the number and proportion of people who are healthy and avoid high associated healthcare costs in the future. Approximately 15% of the population experiences disability, and the increase in NCDs is having a profound effect on disability trends in Canada and internationally. For example, NCDs are estimated to account for about two-thirds of all years lived with a disability in low-income and middle-income countries (GBD 2015 Risk Factors Collaborators, 2016; WHO, 2013). NCD-related disability (e.g., amputation, blindness, or paralysis) puts significant demands on social welfare and health systems; lowers national growth and productivity, and impoverishes families. Rehabilitation needs to be a central health strategy in NCD programs in order to address risk factors (e.g., obesity and physical inactivity), as well as loss of function due to associated complications (e.g., blindness due to diabetes, immobility due to stroke). Access to rehabilitation services can decrease the effects and consequences of disease, hasten discharge from acute care hospitals that are not equipped, proficient or suited to provide care for NCDs, slow or halt deterioration in the health of clients, and improve HRQOL (WHO, 2013).

We also argue that it is also critical to examine the impact of NCDs from a HRQOL perspective. **HRQOL** is a multidimensional concept that includes domains related to physical, mental, emotional, and social functioning. This concept goes beyond direct measures of population health, life expectancy, and causes of death, and focuses on the impact health status has on overall quality of life (Ferrans, 2005; Moriarity, Zack, & Kobau, 2003; WHO, 2005b). At the personal level, HRQOL includes the client's perceptions of their own physical and mental health and well-being, available social supports, functional ability, and socioeconomic status. At the community level, HRQOL includes resources, policies, access to healthcare services, and various social and economic conditions. Hence, from a public health context, HRQOL enables public health professionals, workers, and agencies to examine broader areas related to evidence-informed public health practice and policy that concentrates on specific common themes or conditions. The reader is referred to Chapter 9 for a further discussion on measures of disease burden associated with NCDs including the disability-adjusted life year (DALY); healthy life years (HeaLY) lost measure; HALE; and quality-adjusted life year (QALY). We shall examine the following four major NCDs facing Canadians across the lifespan: (i) cancer; (ii) CVDs; (iii) CRDs; and (iv) diabetes.

1. **Cancer**
   Cancer is a collective term used to describe a group of diseases characterized by uncontrolled cell growth and division or the loss of the cell to perform normal apoptosis. It is a neoplasm clinically characterized by uncontrolled cell growth of anaplastic cells which typically invade surrounding

tissues and may also metastasize to other surrounding or distant tissues or organs in the body. In fact, cancer is not just one disease, but a large group of almost 200 diseases (Canadian Cancer Society's Advisory Committee on Cancer Statistics, 2017; DeVita, Lawrence, & Rosenberg, 2011; Harris, 2013). Its two main characteristics are uncontrolled growth of the cells in the human body, and the ability of these cells to migrate from the original site and spread to distant sites. Cancers (i.e., malignant neoplasms) can arise from virtually any tissue and are conventionally named by their site of origin (e.g., prostate cancer, breast cancer, colon cancer, lung cancer). Cancer cells first invade contiguous tissues, and may then spread through lymphatic channels and blood vessels to other tissue or organs of the body. Cancer cells cause death by metastasizing (i.e., spreading) from their primary site to other sites or vital organs (e.g., brain, lungs, liver, kidneys); and subsequently overwhelm the normal cellular constituency, which eventually results in the collapse of their vital life-sustaining functions. Hence, early detection (e.g., screening for breast and prostate cancer) and treatment are critical in preventing its spread and proliferation (Canadian Cancer Society's Advisory Committee on Cancer Statistics, 2017; DeVita, Lawrence, & Rosenberg, 2011; Harris, 2013; Table 14.3).

Increasingly cancers, including some with global impact such as cancer of the cervix, liver, oral cavity, and stomach, have been shown to have an infectious aetiology. In developing countries, infections are known to be the cause of about one-fifth of cancers. High rates of other cancers in developing countries that are linked to infections or infestations include herpes virus and HIV in Kaposi sarcoma, and liver flukes in cholangiocarcinoma (GBD 2015 Risk Factors Collaborators, 2016; WHO, 2013).

Although major advances in cancer treatment and survival occurred in the last few decades, cancer has been the leading cause of death in Canada since 2006 (Canadian Cancer Society Advisory Committee, 2017; PHAC, 2016;). It is estimated that 45% of women and 49% of men in Canada will develop cancer during their lifetime. The number of new cancer cases continues to rise steadily as the Canadian population continues to grow and age (Government of Canada, 2017). The five-year survival rates for cancer is approximately 60% in Canada, although this rate varies greatly in terms of the stage and type of cancer diagnosed. For examples, the five-year survival rates for thyroid (98%) and testicular cancer (98%) are excellent; whereas the rates for esophageal (14%) and

Table 14.3 Screening and Secondary Prevention Activities of Canadians for Cancer. A major goal of public health practice is to implement an intervention to alter the adverse consequences of the natural history of disease and health-related events. Screening is defined as a population-based public health strategy employed to identify the possible presence of an as-yet-undiagnosed condition (e.g., breast, cervical, or colon cancer) in clients without known signs or symptoms. Secondary prevention activities and measures enable early detection of cancers and the delivery of prompt evidence-informed interventions for the client.

Specific Screening or Prevention Activity	Percentage of population
Women aged 50–74 years who report having mammogram at least once in past five years.	83.5%
Women aged 25–69 years who report having at least one Papanicolaou smear or "Pap smear" in short, done in past three years.	79.7%
Percentage of adults aged 50–74 years who report having at least one fecal occult blood test, colonoscopy, or sigmoidoscopy done in recommended period.	51.1%

source : Adapted from CCDI Steering Committee (2017).

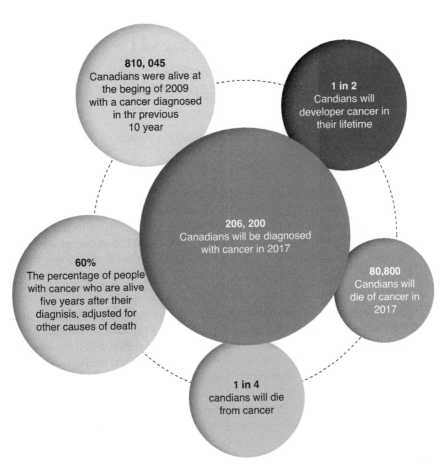

Figure 14.3 Canadian Cancer Statistics at a Glance. Cancer is the leading cause of death among Canadian adults, and the leading cause of death among children aged 15 years or younger as of 2012.

Source: Canadian Cancer Society's Advisory Committee on Cancer Statistics (2017, p. 6). Available at: cancer.ca/Canadian-Cancer-Statistics-2017-EN.pdf.

pancreatic (8%) are poor by comparison (Canadian Cancer Society Advisory Committee, 2017; Government of Canada, 2017; Figure 14.3).

One-in-two Canadians will develop cancer in their lifetime and one-in-four will die from this disease. In 2017, it is estimated that 206,200 Canadians will develop cancer and 80,000 will die from this disease (Canadian Cancer Society Advisory Committee, 2017). Moreover, although an estimated 90% of all cancers cases in Canada develop over the age of 50 years, it has been a leading cause of death for young children aged 15 years or younger since 2012 (Canadian Cancer Society Advisory Committee, 2017). Prostate, breast, and colorectal cancers account for over half of all prevalent cases in Canada. Over 800,000 (2.4%) Canadians have been diagnosed with cancer in the past 10 years, and approximately two in five Canadians are expected to be diagnosed with cancer in Canada in their lifetime, and one in four will die from cancer (Canadian Cancer Society Advisory Committee, 2017; PHAC, 2016). In general, cancer incidence rates are higher in Eastern Canada and lower in Western Canada. In 2013, the lowest incidence rate ASR was observed in Yukon (397/100,000) (PHAC, 2016).

Exposure to carcinogens such as asbestos, diesel exhaust gases, and ionizing and ultra-violet radiation in both living and working environments can increase the risk of developing cancer. Similarly, indiscriminate use of agrochemicals in agriculture and discharge of toxic products from unregulated chemical industries may cause cancer and other NCDs such as kidney and liver diseases. These exposures have their greatest potential to influence NCDs early in life, and thus special attention must be paid to preventing exposure during pregnancy and childhood (GBD 2015 Risk Factors Collaborators, 2016; WHO, 2013).

Research Focus Box 14.1

**Exposure to Pesticides and Risk of Childhood Cancer:
A Meta-Analysis of Recent Epidemiological Studies**

Study Aim/Rationale

The authors performed a meta-analysis of case–control and cohort studies to clarify the possible relationship between exposure to pesticides and childhood cancers.

Methodology/Design

Two cohort and 38 case–control studies were selected for the first meta-analysis. After evaluating homogeneity among studies using the Cochran Q test, the authors calculated a pooled meta-odds ratio (OR) stratified on each cancer site. The authors then constructed a list of variables believed to play an important role in explaining the relation between parental exposure to pesticide and childhood cancer, and performed a series of meta-analyses. The authors also performed a distinct meta-analysis for three cohort studies with relative risk (RR) data.

Major Findings

Meta-analysis of the three cohort studies did not show any positive links between parental pesticide exposure and childhood cancer incidence. However, the meta-analysis of the 40 studies with OR values showed that the risk of lymphoma and leukaemia increased significantly in exposed children when their mother was exposed during the prenatal period (OR = 1.53; 95% confidence interval [CI]: 1.22–1.91 and OR = 1.48; 95% CI: 1.26 1.75). The risk of brain cancer was correlated with paternal exposure either before or after birth (OR = 1.49; 95% CI: 1.23–1.79 and OR = 1.66; 95% CI: 1.11–2.49). The OR of leukaemia and lymphoma was higher when the mother was exposed to pesticides (through household use or professional exposure). Conversely, the incidence of brain cancer was influenced by the father's exposure (occupational activity or use of household or garden pesticides).

Implications for Public Health

Despite some limitations in this study, the incidence of childhood cancer does appear to be associated with parental exposure during the prenatal period.

Source: Vinson, Merhi, Baldi, Raynal, and Gamet-Payrastre (2011).

In 2015, the International Agency for Research on Cancer, an arm of the WHO, declared that *glyphosate*, the world's most widely employed weed killer often sold under the trade names of "Roundup" and "Vision"; is a probable carcinogen (Cressey, 2015; Food and Agricultural Organization (FAO) of the United Nations and World Health WHO, 2016); Spector, 2015. In 2015 to 2016, the Canadian Food Inspection Agency (CFIA) tested a total of 3188 food samples for glyphosate. Glyphosate residues was found in 29.7% of food samples it tested; which included infant foods, and 1.3% were above the acceptable limit (CBC News, 2017; CFIA, 2017).

Is There a Relationship Between Sugar Consumption and Cancer?

There is also a growing body of research which shows that it is sugar's relationship to higher insulin levels and related growth factors that may impact cancer cell growth most significantly, and also increase the risk for the development

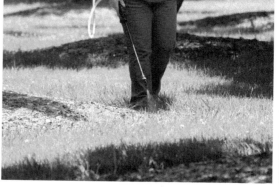

© ND700/Shutterstock.com

Photo 14.6 "Cosmetic" and Agricultural Pesticide Use and Cancer. Many "cosmetic" (e.g., for home lawn use to combat dandelions and grab grass) and agricultural pesticides are known as probable carcinogenic agents (e.g., Chiu, Weisenburger, & Zahm, 2004; Jaga & Dharmani, 2005; Liang et al., 2016; Vinson et al., 2011). In 2013, 59% of Canadian households that had a lawn or garden reported using cosmetic pesticides (Statistics Canada, 2017).

of other NCDs (e.g., type 2 diabetes, heart disease, non-alcoholic fatty liver disease [NAFLD]) (Klement & Kammereer, 2011). Indeed, many types of cancer cells (e.g., squamous cell carcinoma) have plenty of insulin receptors, making them more responsive than normal cells to insulin's ability to promote growth. According to the 2004 Canadian Community Health Survey, approximately one-in-five calories consumed by Canadians comes from sugar (Langlois & Garriguet, 2015). On average in 2004, Canadians consumed 110.0 g of sugar a day; the equivalent of 26 teaspoons, and 21.4% of their total daily caloric intake (Langlois & Garriguet, 2015). This dietary sugar may occur naturally (e.g., from fruit and milk), or it may have been added to foods and beverages to improve palatability, for instance, in soft drinks, salad dressings, syrup, and candy. This is notable from a public health perspective because it is estimated that Canadian's consume the equivalent of 20 1 kg bags of sugar per year, and consumption of sugar has been steadily increasing over the decades. Moreover, 66% of packaged foods and beverages sold in Canada contain added sugars, and sales for energy drinks (which contain 84 g of sugar on average) and sports drinks (which contain 40 g of sugar on average) have increased 579% since 2005 (Acton, Vanderlee, Hobin, & Hammond, 2017; Schmidt, 2017).

Palliative Care, End-of-Life Care (EOLC), and Community-Based Hospice Services

The special needs of clients dying with cancer and other terminal illnesses are now widely acknowledged, and are no longer viewed as taboo topics in Canadian society. The time from diagnosis of a terminal type of cancer to death varies considerably, depending on the stage and type of cancer, the extent of the disease, and the client's overall state of well-being and fortitude. **Palliative care** is an approach that seeks to improve the quality of life of clients and their families facing problems associated with life-threatening illness, through the prevention and relief of suffering by means of early identification and impeccable assessment and treatment of pain and other problems, physical, psychosocial, and spiritual (WHO, 2018c).

EOLC is a term used to describe care provided in the last days or weeks of life (Subcommittee of the Standing Senate Committee on Social Affairs, Science and Technology, 2000). The principle goals of EOLC are to: (i) Provide comfort and supportive care during the dying process; (ii) improve the quality of life remaining for the client; and (iii) help to ensure a dignified death. The Senate of Canada report entitled *Quality End-of-Life Care: The Right of Every Canadian* declares that EOLC must be an unshakeable core value of Canada's health-care systems (Subcommittee of the Standing Senate Committee on Social Affairs, Science and Technology, 2000). Currently, it is estimated that 259,000 Canadians die each year, and only 5% of Canadians receive

---

Group Activity-Based Learning 14.1

How Can Public Health Professionals and Workers Better Help to Convey the Wishes of the Clients to Their Family Members and Loved Ones?

This Group Activity-Based Learning Box highlights the importance of effective communication and being an advocate for your client in the community. Consider the following case involving a 68-year women who was diagnosed with stage 4 breast cancer with metastasis to the liver, colon, and bone, and has less than two months to live. The client has requested that no future medical treatments be undertaken and that a "do-not-resuscitate" (DNR) should be part of her plan of care. She has requested to be referred to hospice care in her community. The client is competent and is legally and ethically the decision maker regarding her own care and treatment options. Working in small groups of three to five students, discuss and answer the following questions.

1. The family asks the public health nurse why their mother is no longer receiving chemotherapy or radiation in hospital. How should the public health respond and best advocate the wishes of the client?

2. If this client was in your community, how would you facilitate referral to a hospice care facility?

integrated and interdisciplinary EOLC (Quality of Life Care Coalition, 2010). By 2036, the number of Canadians dying will increase to 425,000 per year and a larger proportion of these will require EOLC and/or palliative care services due to our ageing population and the growing number of associated NCDs.

Hospice is a concept of care that provides compassion, concern, and support for dying clients and their families. The objective of hospice care is to provide community-based support and care for clients and their families during the last stages of an incurable disease so they might live as fully and as comfortably as possible in their home and/or homelike setting. Although 96% of Canadians support the concept of hospice care, only 16% to 30% receive hospice services in Canada, depending on their place of residence (Canadian Hospice and Palliative Care Association, 2014). To be eligible, a client's anticipated LE is typically three months or less; and they agree with the hospice's philosophy of care that seeks to address their physical, emotional, social, and spiritual needs, and to also provide support to family caregivers and significant others. The majority of Canadians (73%) surveyed feel that provincial governments place too little priority on palliative EOLC (Canadian Hospice

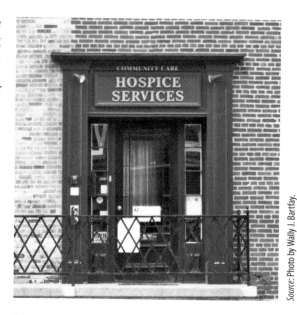

Source: Photo by Wally J. Bartfay.

Photo 14.7 There is a growing need in Canada for community-based hospice care services. Hospice is a type of palliative care provided in a home and/or specialized care facility for those facing a life-limiting illness such as cancer.

Palliative Care Association, 2014). Clients experiencing the inevitability of death are in need of public healthcare professionals and workers who are knowledgeable about their personal needs, issues, and attitudes toward that affect their end of life journey. As a multicultural society, we must also be aware and respectful of diverse cultural differences and religious beliefs and how they might influence the dying experience.

1. **Cardiovascular Disease**

    CVD is defined as a class of diseases that involve the heart or blood vessels and include: coronary heart disease; disease of the blood vessels supplying the heart muscle, and cerebrovascular disease which are disease of the blood vessels supplying the brain. CVD is the leading cause of death globally and the second leading cause of death in Canada (Heart Research Institute, 2018; WHO, 2018a). An estimated 17.7 million people died from CVDs in 2015, representing 31% of all global deaths. Of these deaths, an estimated 7.4 million were due to coronary heart disease and 6.7 million were due to stroke (WHO, 2018a). In Canada, someone dies from heart disease or stroke every 7 min; it accounts for 29% of all deaths in Canada; Aboriginal people are 1.5 to 2 times more likely to development CVD, and the associated healthcare costs are in excess of $20.9 billion in Canada. Most CVDs can, in fact, be prevented by addressing behavioural risk factors such as tobacco use, unhealthy diet and obesity, physical inactivity and harmful use of alcohol using population-wide strategies. We shall examine some of the most common forms of CVD in greater detail.

Ischemic Heart Disease

Ischemic heart disease is a chronic condition in which the heart muscle is damaged or works inefficiently because of the absence or relative deficiency of its blood supply. Moreover, IHD is the number one cause of years of life lost (YLLs) due to premature mortality and the second leading cause of DALY lost. About 2.3 million (8.4%) Canadians aged 20 years and older are living with diagnosed ischemic heart disease (PHAC, 2016). It is noteworthy that 9.8% men over the age of 20 years were living with a diagnosed IHD, while 7.1% women 20 years and older were living with the same condition (PHAC, 2016).

Hypertension

Hypertension, also known as high blood pressure (HBP), is defined as a sustained elevation of systemic arterial blood pressure and if often a chronic condition. Hypertension is one of the most important risk factors for death and disability, and is predicted to become the leading cause of death and disability worldwide by 2020 (Sliwa, Stewart, & Gersh, 2011). It is notable the 91% of clients diagnosed with hypertension have at least one additional risk factor for the development of CVD (Campbell et al., 2011). In terms of attributable deaths, the leading metabolic risk factor globally is elevated blood pressure (to which 19% of global deaths are attributed); followed by being overweight and/or obesity, and elevated blood glucose levels (GBD 2015 Risk Factors Collaborators, 2016; WHO, 2017a, 2017b). Approximately 6.9 million (24.9%) Canadians aged 20 years and older are living with diagnosed hypertension (PHAC, 2016). Prevalence rates were similar in females (25.6%) and in males (24.2%). In 2011/2012, the prevalence of diagnosed hypertension increased with increasing age, with over 70% of adults aged 65 years and older being affected (PHAC, 2016).

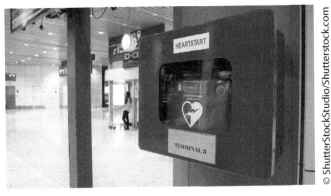

Photo 14.8 Community-Based First-Aid Defibrillator. Defibrillators placed in various strategic community locations, including shopping centres, airports, schools, community, and recreational centres, libraries, restaurants and workplaces can significantly increase the chance of survival of a heart attack victim. Public health legislation and policies can help to ensure that first-aid defibrillators are readily available when needed.

Stroke

Stroke, also known as a "brain attack," is a sudden loss of brain function that occurs when blood flow supplying oxygen to a part of the brain is interrupted. A stroke may occur when there is ischemia present (i.e., inadequate blood flow) to a part of the brain, or it may result from hemorrhage into the brain that results in damage or death of brain cells. A **thrombotic stroke** is caused by a thrombus (i.e., blood clot) that forms in a cerebral artery that has been narrowed or damaged by atherosclerosis. An **embolic stroke** is cause by an embolus (i.e., wondering blood clot) that is carried in the blood stream and may become wedged in a cerebral artery. Several embolic strokes are linked to *atrial fibrillation*, where blood may pool in an atrium and form a clot. In Canada, stroke is the third leading cause of death, after cancer and heart disease, and the fourth leading cause of YLLs due to premature mortality and the tenth largest contributor to disability adjusted life years (DALYs) (PHAC, 2016; WHO, 2018a).

Stroke is a major public health concern because more than 50,000 Canadians suffer a

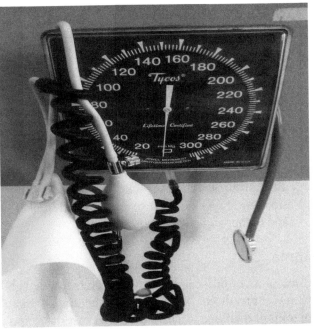

Photo 14.9 Hypertension or High Blood Pressure Is a Major Risk Factor for the Development of CVD. Increasing rates of sedentary behaviours, obesity, and sodium consumption amongst Canadian youth and adults are likely to further contribute to the hypertension burden (Dasgupta et al., 2014; Padwal, Bienek, McAlister, & Campbell, 2015).

stroke annually; a stroke occurs in Canada approximately every 10 min; 14,000 die as a consequence; approximately 300,000 are currently living with the after effects of stroke (e.g., paralysis, memory loss, mobility issues), and stroke costs the Canadian economy $3.6 billion a year in physician services, hospital costs, lost wages, and decreased productivity (Government of Canada, 2011; Ontario Stroke Network, 2017). For every minute delay in treating a stroke, the average client loses 1.9 million brain cells, 13.8 billion synapses, and 12 km of axonal fibres (Ontario Stroke Network, 2017). Hence, early recognition of the typical symptoms (see Figure 14.4 for F.A.S.T. acronym) and clinical intervention are critical for victims suffering from a stroke.

Studies have shown that the burden is increasing among younger adults, with the proportion of all strokes in those aged less than 55 years increasing over time, while the mean age of stroke is decreasing. The prevalence of diagnosed stroke increases with age, and approximately 10% of adults aged 65 years and older

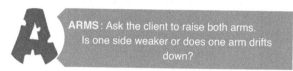

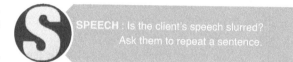

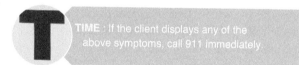

Figure 14.4 F.A.S.T. Acronym for the Recognition of Stroke

Source: Courtesy of Wally J. Bartfay.

being affected (PHAC, 2016). As a result, the burden of stroke is likely to increase even further in the decades to come due to our ageing Canadian population.

1. **Chronic Respiratory Diseases**

   CRDs are diseases of the airways and other parts of the lung that affect all ages and include asthma, chronic obstructive pulmonary disease (COPD), lung cancer, cystic fibrosis, sleep apnea, and occupational lung diseases (Government of Canada, 2014). CRDs not only affect the client with on the disease, but their family and loved ones, community, and the healthcare system. The two most important risk factors associated with the development of CRDs are exposure to tobacco smoke (through personal smoking and/or exposure to second-hand smoke) and indoor and outdoor air quality.

Asthma

Asthma is a chronic condition characterized by cough, shortness of breath, chest tightness and wheezing. Asthma symptoms and attacks usually occur after exercise, exposure to allergens or irritants, or viral respiratory infections (PHAC, 2015). Despite the increase in adherence to appropriate care strategies and awareness of asthma attack triggers, two out of three Canadians with active asthma do not have good control of their condition. Asthma is the tenth leading cause of years lived with disability (YLDs; PHAC, 2016).

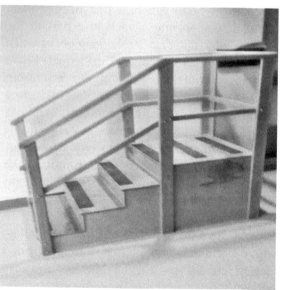

Source: Photo by Wally J. Bartfay.

Photo 14.10 Rehabilitation, Which Includes Physiotherapy, Is Critical for the Recovery Process Following a Stroke. Learning to walk both up and down stairs is often a major component following a stroke that result in alterations to the client's motor, balance, and/or coordination.

Approximately 3.8 million (10.7%) Canadians aged one year and older are living with asthma; which represents 9.5% of adults aged 20 years and older and 15.3% of children aged 1 to 19 (PHAC, 2016). The prevalence of asthma was 11.3% among females and 10.2% among males. The prevalence rates were highest in the 1 to 19 (15.3%) age group followed by the 20 to 34 (11.4%) age group, after which they declined until age 65. The rate among those aged 80 years and older was 10.3% (PHAC, 2016).

Chronic Obstructive Pulmonary Disease

Chronic Obstructive Pulmonary Respiratory Disease (COPD) is a chronic and progressive condition characterized by gradual airway obstruction, shortness of breath, cough and sputum production. Cigarette smoking is the main cause of COPD. Cardinal symptoms experienced by clients with COPD include dyspnea, difficulty breathing or shortness of breath, and limitations in activity (Global Initiative for Chronic Obstructive Lung Disease [GOLD], 2016; O'Donnell et al., 2007).

Exposure to tobacco smoke is the primary cause of COPD accounting for between 80% and 90% of all cases, and significant airway obstruction develops in 15% to 20% of self-reported smokers (Health Canada, 2010). Quitting smoking has been associated with improved lung function, reduced chronic cough and airway mucus production, and decreased mortality from COPD. COPD may also develop in clients with intense or prolonged exposure to various chemicals, dusts, vapours, irritants, or fumes in the home or workplace (GOLD, 2016). COPD may also result from recurring infections involving organism such as *Haemophilus influenza, Strepto-coccus pneumoniae*, and *Moraxella catarrhalis* (Sethi & Murphy, 2008).

COPD is the seventh leading cause of YLLs due to premature mortality and the ninth largest contributor to DALYs (PHAC, 2016). The prevalence rates of COPD were very similar for males (9.6%) and females (9.5%) aged 35 and older. The prevalence rates steadily increased from 2.8% in the 35 to 49 age group, and climbing to 25.4% in the 80 and older age group (PHAC, 2016). It is notable that the age-standardized prevalence of COPD among adults 35 years and older ranged from 8.4% ASR in Prince Edward Island to 23.3% ASR in Nunavut. Nova Scotia and the three territories all had rates that were more than 20% higher than the average Canadian rate (PHAC, 2016).

1. **Diabetes**

   Diabetes (DM) is regarded as a multisystem chronic disease that involves abnormal hormone insulin production, and/or impaired insulin utilization, which results in abnormal metabolism of carbohydrates and elevated levels of glucose in the blood and/or urine. Insulin is a hormone produces by the pancreas that regulates blood glucose (sugar); which is released from pancreatic ß cells as its precursor, proinsulin, and is then routed through the liver (Canadian Diabetes Association, 2018; PHAC, 2011; WHO, 2018b). **Hyperglycaemia** (i.e., elevated blood glucose levels) is a common manifestation of uncontrolled DM; which over time can lead to serious damage to many of the body's systems, especially the nerves and blood vessels. **Hypoglycaemia** (i.e., low blood glucose levels) occurs when there is too much insulin in proportion to the available circulating blood glucose (i.e., <4 nmol/L), and often results from a mismatch in the timing of food intake and the peak action of insulin or OHAs that increase endogenous insulin secretion. Common symptoms of hypoglycaemia include confusion, stupor, irritability, visual disturbances, difficulty speaking, and even coma in extreme cases. Hypoglycaemia can be treated via the administration of a fruit juice (e.g., orange) or by ingesting 15 to 20 g of a simple fast-acting carbohydrate (e.g., 6 Life Savers candies). Treatment via foods containing fat (e.g., ice cream bars, cookies, chocolate bars) should be avoided given that fat hinders the absorption of glucose and will delay response times.

Diabetes can lead to many complications which includes CVD, eye disease (e.g., retinopathy); vision loss/blindness, kidney failure, nerve damage, problems with pregnancy, amputations of limbs, oral disease, erectile dysfunction in males, and depression (PHAC, 2011; WHO, 2018b). It is noteworthy from a public health perspective that almost half of all deaths attributable to high blood glucose levels occur before the age of 70 years (WHO, 2018b).

Insulin Metabolism

In brief, insulin facilitates the transport of glucose from the bloodstream across cell membranes to their cytoplasm. The release of insulin subsequently causes cells to take in glucose to use as energy or to store as fat. This causes blood glucose levels to go back down to normal levels. Adipose and skeletal tissues have specific receptors for insulin and are considered *insulin-dependent tis*sues; whereas other tissues (e.g., blood cells, brain, liver) do not directly depend on the hormone insulin for glucose transport, but nonetheless require an adequate supply for normal function and metabolism. Interestingly, although the liver is not considered an *insulin-dependent tissue* per se; insulin receptor sites in the liver help to facilitate the hepatic uptake of glucose and its conversion to glycogen. Conversely, other hormones (e.g., glucagon, epinephrine, cortisol, growth hormone); which are known as *counter-regulatory hormones*, work to oppose the effects of insulin by increasing blood levels by stimulating glucose production and output by the liver, and by decreasing the movement of insulin into cells.

Prevalence of DM

Currently worldwide, DM is the tenth leading cause of YLLs to premature death (PHAC, 2016). However, the WHO (2018b) projects that DM will be the seventh leading cause of death by 2030 worldwide. The WHO (2018b) reports that the number of people with DM has risen from 108 million in 1980 to 422 million in 2014, and the global prevalence of DM among adults over 18 years of age has risen from 4.7% in 1980 to 8.5% in 2014. Moreover, an estimated 1.6 million deaths were directly caused by DM in 2015 alone (WHO, 2018b).

There are approximately 11 million Canadians living with DM or prediabetes, and every 3 min another Canadian is diagnosed with the condition (Canadian Diabetes Association, 2018). Specifically, more than 2.7 million (7.7%) Canadians aged one year and older are living with diagnosed DM (type 1 and type 2 combined); which represents 9.8% of adults aged 20 years and older and 0.3% of children aged 1 to 19 years (PHAC, 2016). Moreover, 7.2% of females and 8.3% of males aged one year and older were living with diagnosed DM (type 1 and type 2 combined) in Canada. Diabetes has seen the second highest annual percent increase since 2000/2001 among all diseases studied in Canada (PHAC, 2011, 2016).

The prevalence rates for DM increased by age group, starting at 0.3% for those aged one to 19 years; rising slowly to 4.5% among those 35 to 49 years, and then climbing more steeply with age among those in the 65 to 79 age group (24.6%) and 80 and older (26.1%) age groups (PHAC, 2016). The increase in diabetes prevalence rates is likely attributable to the high rates of obesity and overweight in Canadian population as well as changing demographic due to our ageing population involving the Baby Boomer generation. The number of prevalent cases for diagnosed diabetes is projected to be over four million people by 2020 (PHAC, 2016). Indigenous people are three to five times more likely than the general population to develop type 2 DM, and an estimated 25% of First Nations peoples living on reserves who are aged 45 years or older have DM (Canadian Diabetes Association, 2018; PHAC, 2011, 2016). We shall examine the major types of DM in greater detail later.

Prediabetes

Prediabetes, which is also known as *impaired glucose tolerance* (IGT) and *impaired fasting glucose* (IFG), occurs when a client's fasting or a 2-hour plasma glucose level is higher than normal, but lower than is considered necessary for a diagnosis of DM. The clinical range for these glucose levels are 6.1 to 6.9 nmol/L for IFG and 7.1 to 11 nmol/L for IGT. It is estimated that up to 6 million Canadians have prediabetes, and approximately 50% of these will progress to develop type 2 DM (described later) (Canadian Diabetes Association, 2018; Gillies et al., 2007). Clients with prediabetes are often asymptotic, but long-term damage to various organs (e.g., heart) and blood vessels may be occurring. Public health professionals and workers should encourage clients with prediabetes to maintain a healthy weight, engage in regular physical activity and exercise, eat a balanced diet, and take prescribed medications when indicated (Canadian Diabetes Association, 2018; Gillies et al., 2007).

Impaired Glucose Tolerance and Impaired Fasting Glycemia

IGT and **IFG** are intermediate conditions that are regarded in transition between normality and DM (Canadian Diabetes Association, 2018; WHO, 2018b). People with IGT or IFG are at high risk of progressing to type 2 diabetes, although this is not inevitable (Canadian Diabetes Association, 2018). Clients identified as having an IGT or IFG may be able to prevent diabetes through a combination of increased physical activity and exercise, eating a healthy and balanced diet, and reduction of body weight. Regular exercise, for example, increases insulin sensitivity and can have a direct effect on lowering blood glucose levels. Furthermore, it can contribute to weight loss, which also helps to decrease insulin resistance.

Type 1 DM

Type 1 DM, previously known as *insulin-dependent, juvenile or childhood-onset DM*, results from a progressive destruction of pancreatic ß cells owing to an autoimmune process in susceptible clients, and is therefore characterized by a deficient insulin production that requires daily administration of insulin (Canadian Diabetes Association, 2018; PHAC, 2011, 2016; WHO, 2018b). Symptoms of type 1 DM include excessive excretion of urine (polyuria), thirst (polydipsia), constant hunger, weight loss, vision changes, delays or alterations in wound healing, and fatigue. Approximately 5% to 10% of all clients have type 1 DM; and it most often occurs in individuals less than 30 years of age, with a peak onset between the ages of 11 and 13 years (Canadian Diabetes Association, 2018; PHAC, 2011, 2016; WHO, 2018b). A subclass of type 1 DM, known as *latent auto-immune diabetes mellitus in adults* (LADA), is the clinical term employed to describe a small number of clients who also appear to have immune-related loss of pancreatic ß cells (Canadian Diabetes Association, 2018).

Although the exact cause of type DM is not known, it is believed to be associated with human leukocyte antigens (e.g., HLA-DR3 and HLA-DR4); where in theory if a client is exposed to a viral infection, ß cells in the pancreas are destroyed either directly or indirectly through an autoimmune response (Morahan, 2012; Nguyen, Varney, Harrison, & Morahan, 2013). Type 1 DM is always managed via the injection of exogenous insulin administered via an infusion pump or by injection. Without insulin, the client is at risk of developing a potentially fatal condition known as *diabetic ketoacidosis* (DKA). Meal planning also helps with keeping blood glucose at the desired levels.

Type 2 DM

Type 2 DM, formerly known as *non-insulin-dependent* or *adult-onset DM*, results from the body's ineffective use of insulin. Type 2 DM occurs when the body can no longer properly use the insulin that is released, termed *insulin insensitivity*, and/or does not make enough insulin per se. As a result, glucose levels quickly rise in the blood instead of being used as energy source. Type 2 DM comprises the majority of clients (i.e., 90%) with DM around the world who are typically 35 years or older, and the prevalence increases with age with approximately 50% of clients being diagnosed at age 55 years and older. It is noteworthy from a public health perspective that between 80% and 90% of clients are deemed overweight or obese (especially abdominal and visceral adiposity), and self-report to be physically inactive at the time of diagnosis (Canadian Diabetes Association, 2018; PHAC, 2011, 2016; WHO, 2018b). Although type 2 DM most often develops in adults, overweight, obese, and inactive children can also be affected.

The following four metabolic abnormalities have been shown to play a role in the development of type 2 DM: (i) Insulin resistance in terms of glucose and lipid metabolism in which tissues do not respond to the action of insulin; (ii) a marked decrease in the ability of the pancreas to produce insulin, as the ß cells become fatigued from the compensatory overproduction of insulin or when ß cells mass is lost; (iii) inappropriate glucose production by the liver; and (iv) alteration in the production of hormones and cytokines by adipose tissue (i.e., *adipocytokines*). Symptoms are often similar to those of type 1 DM, but are often less marked or pronounced in nature. As a result, the disease may be diagnosed several years after onset, once damage to organs (e.g., heart) and blood vessels have already occurred. Depending on the severity of type 2 DM, it may be managed through physical activity and exercise regimes, and meal planning. It may also require prescription medications and/or insulin to control blood glucose levels more effectively (Canadian Diabetes Association, 2018; PHAC, 2011, 2016; WHO, 2018b).

Gestational Diabetes

Gestational DM is defined as any degree of glucose intolerance with onset or first recognition occurring during pregnancy; and is clinically employed whether insulin or only diet modification is used for treatment, and whether or not the condition persists after pregnancy. Gestational DM is a temporary condition that occurs during pregnancy and is clinically regarded as a state of hyperglycaemia with blood glucose values that are above normal values, but below those use for diagnosis of DM (Buchanan & Xiang, 2005; Canadian Diabetes Association, 2018; WHO, 2018b). It affects approximately 2% to 4% of all pregnancies in non-indigenous women and approximately 8% to 18% of indigenous women in Canada, and involves an increased risk of developing DM in both the mother and child (Canadian Diabetes Association, 2018). It is typically detected between 24 and 28 weeks of gestation, which usually involves a gestational diabetes screen (GDS) involving a 50 g glucose load that is assessed 1-hour post-plasma glucose. Treatment of gestational DM is critical to reduce the incident of prenatal death and neonatal complications (e.g., hyperbilirubinemia, respiratory distress syndrome, hypoglycaemia). Nutritional counselling is often considered the first-line of therapy, and physical activity should also be encouraged as tolerated by the client. Although most women diagnosed with gestational DM will have normal glucose levels within six weeks of giving birth, their risk for developing type DM in five to 10 years is significantly higher than the general population (Buchanan & Xiang, 2005; Canadian Diabetes Association, 2018).

Importance of Influenza Vaccination for Clients with CRDs and CVDs

The elderly and those with chronic diseases are at increased risk of developing complications and/or death due to influenza infection. Moreover, influenza infection may trigger an exacerbation and deterioration of their pre-existing conditions, particularly for CRDs (COPD and asthma) and CVDs (e.g., heart failure and IHD) (Centers for Disease Control and Prevention, 2016; Heart and Stroke Foundation of Canada, 2018). Therefore, annual vaccination is the cornerstone of influenza prevention and acts as both primary and secondary prevention strategies for these high risk clients with CRDs and CVD.

Currently, about half (48.2%) of Canadians with a chronic disease receive the recommended annual influenza vaccine (PHAC, 2016; Schanzer, Langley, & Tam, 2008). The vaccination rate for females with a chronic disease (50.0%) was slightly higher than that of males (46.8%). The immunization rate among individuals with a chronic disease generally increased with age from 23.0% in those aged 20 to 34 years to a high of 66.5% in those aged 65 to 79 years. More than a quarter of the children and youth (12–19 years old) with a chronic disease had been vaccinated (PHAC, 2016).

Future Directions and Challenges

Canadians are living longer than ever before, and the LE gap is closing between men and women. Nearly one in six Canadians (5.8 million) are 65 years or older, and this age group is growing four times faster than the overall population (PHAC, 2016). Furthermore, rates of smoking continue to decrease in Canada, and mortality from major chronic conditions (especially that related to CVDs, CRDs, and certain cancers) has also declined. By contrast, the high rates of physical inactivity, sedentary behaviours and obesity rates, especially among Canada's children and youth, are a major concern. While Canadians are living longer, it is important that they live longer in good health.

Care for clients with an NCD should be ideally embedded within a healthcare system that promotes client empowerment and decision making. Unfortunately, healthcare systems in Canada are principally built around the acute episodic model of care based largely in hospitals; which are not designed to address or manage the complex physical, social, psychological, or financial needs of clients living with NCDs who reside in their community (Bartfay & Bartfay, 2015). It is critical to point out that receiving a clinical diagnosis alone does not predict healthcare needs, individual levels of care required, functional outcomes, or how the client and their family will ultimately respond to the actual NCD diagnosed.

The PHAC developed the *Canadian Chronic Disease (CCDI) Indicator Framework* in 2012 in order to improve access to current surveillance data by providing up-to-date, consistent, reliable, and ongoing information on chronic disease and associated risk and protective factors (RPFs) (CCDI Steering Committee, 2017). In 2014, the Framework was expanded to include injury, and was renamed *Chronic Disease and Injury Indicator Framework* (CDIIF). The CDIIF includes indicators based on six main domains: social and environmental determinants, maternal, and child health RPFs, behaviour RPFs, risk conditions, disease prevention practices, and health outcomes/status (CCDI Steering Committee, 2017).

There is increasing concern that Canada's healthcare systems will be unable to meet the growing healthcare needs of this ageing population, especially in regards to NCDs. Over the past few decades, population ageing has contributed relatively modestly to rising public-sector healthcare spending each year (i.e., <1% annually). These findings may appear counterintuitive when we consider that older adults are proportionately higher users of acute care hospital and physician services, home and continuing care, and prescription drugs. In fact, since 1997, acute care hospitals have accounted for the most significant share of health spending, followed by drugs and physician services (CIHI, 2017, 2018). In 2017, hospitals (28.3%), drugs (16.4%), and physician services (15.4%) continued to use the largest share of health dollars, and total health expenditure was over $242 billion ($6604 per person or 11.5% of GDP) (CIHI, 2017, 2018). If we assume that population ageing will contribute approximately 1% point per year to total health expenditure in the near future; ageing trends in Canada alone will add an additional $2 billion to healthcare spending costs annually (CIHI, 2017, 2018; Figure 14.5).

As the population continues to age, decision-makers will be faced with the challenge of determining the level of care (hospital, long-term institutional and community) for older Canadians that balances access to and quality and appropriateness of care with the cost of care (CIHI, 2017, p. 28).

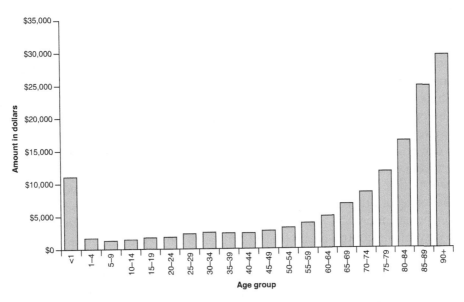

Figure 14.5 Provincial and Territorial Government Health Expenditure per Capita, by Age Group, Canada (2015). Adults aged 65 years and older are major drivers of healthcare spending in Canada. In 2015 (the latest available year for data broken down by age group), per-person spending for older adults increased significantly with age: $6607 for those aged 65 to 69 years, $8495 for those aged 70 to 74 years, $11,570 for those aged 75 to 79 years, and $21,407 for those aged 80 and older (CIHI, 2017, 2018).

Source: Canadian Institute for Health Information (CIHI, 2017, p. 23). Copyright © 2015 by Canadian Institute for Health Information. Reprinted by permission.

In terms of formal support, an estimated 1 million Canadians receive home care at any given time; about eight out of every 10 are Canadians aged 65 years and older (CIHI, 2011). The services provided to them vary by age and need and include both home health and home support services. In contrast, approximately 80% of all informal and unpaid care provided in Canada comes from lay family members (i.e., 75% are female spouses or daughters), friends and/or neighbours (Canadian Association for Retired Persons [CARP], 2014; CIHI, 2011). Informal caregiver provide unpaid assistance with tasks such as transportation and personal care, and help ageing Canadians to remain in their homes; thereby reducing direct costs and demands on healthcare systems.

According to the *2008/2009 Canadian Community Health Survey (CCHS)–Healthy Aging*, an estimated 3.8 million (or 35%) Canadians aged 45 years or older (35%) were providing informal care to an older family member for a health condition (Turner & Findlay, 2015). Moreover, three-quarters of caregivers reported that the person whom they assisted was at least 75 years old, and one-third were caring for a loved one aged 85 years or older (Turner & Findlay, 2015). Data shows that 32% of informal lay caregivers who provide more than 21 hours of direct care per week report distress in this role (CIHI, 2011). Without a doubt, the impacts of informal caregiving provided by an estimated 6.1 million Canadians are not confined to the home, but are also felt in the workplace in terms of reduced productivity. Specifically, the burden of informal caregiving translates into 2.2 million hr of reduced effort in the workplace every week, and an estimated $1.3 billion in lost productivity annually (Bernmier, 2015).

Despite ageing and NCD trends in Canada and globally, we must remember as public health professional and workers that many chronic diseases are, in fact, largely preventable. Indeed, the WHO estimates that at least 80% of heart disease, stroke, diabetes, and 40% of all cancers are preventable.

Exposure to environmental and occupational hazards, such as indoor and outdoor air pollution, with fumes from solid fuels, ozone, airborne dust, and allergens may cause CRD and some air pollution sources including fumes from solid fuels may cause lung cancer, indoor and outdoor air pollution, heat waves and chronic stress related to work, and unemployment are also associated with CVDs.

In reality, the major causes of chronic diseases are known, and if these risk factors were eliminated, at least 80% of all heart disease, stroke, and type 2 diabetes would be prevented; over 40% of cancer would be prevented (WHO, 2005a). Although effective interventions exist for the prevention and control of NCDs, their implementation is inadequate worldwide. Comparative, applied, and operational research, integrating both social and biomedical sciences, is required to scale up and maximize the impact of existing interventions and should include "needs driven" population-based research (WHO, 2013).

These NCDs share key modifiable behavioural risk factors like tobacco use, unhealthy diet, lack of physical activity, and the harmful use of alcohol, which in turn lead to overweight and obesity, raised blood pressure, and raised cholesterol, and ultimately disease (WHO, 2017a, 2017b). Effectively tackling NCDs and their associated social determinants of health (e.g., poverty, unemployment, lower education levels). Feasible and cost effective interventions exist to reduce the burden and impact of NCDs now and in the future. Tracking national implementation of a key set of tracer actions linked to these interventions allows for global benchmarking and monitoring of progress being made against NCDs. It also serves to highlight challenges and areas requiring further attention. Since the 2011 High-level Meeting, governments have made many political commitments to prevent and control NCDs (WHO, 2017a, 2017b). Progress, however, has been insufficient and highly uneven.

Advance the implementation of multisectoral, cost-effective, population-wide interventions in order to reduce the impact of the common non-communicable disease risk factors, namely tobacco use, unhealthy diet, physical inactivity and harmful use of alcohol, through the implementation of relevant international agreements and strategies, and education, legislative (WHO, 2013). Encourage the development of multisectoral public policies that create equitable health-promoting environments that empower individuals, families, and communities to make healthy choices and lead healthy lives. Develop, strengthen, and implement, as appropriate, multisectoral public policies and action plans to promote health education and health literacy, including through evidence-based education and information strategies and programs in and out of schools and through public awareness campaigns (WHO, 2013). Promote the development and initiate the implementation, as appropriate, of cost-effective interventions to reduce salt, sugar, and saturated fats. Consider producing and promoting more food products consistent with a healthy diet, including by reformulating products to provide healthier options that are affordable and accessible and that follow relevant nutrition facts and labelling standards, including information on sugars, salt, and fats and, where appropriate, trans-fat content (WHO, 2013).

We must recognize and acknowledge where health disparities exist between indigenous and non-indigenous populations in the incidence of non-communicable diseases and their common risk factors, and that these disparities are often linked to historical, economic, and social factors, and encourage the involvement of indigenous peoples and communities in the development, implementation, and evaluation of non-communicable disease prevention and control policies, plans, and programs (WHO, 2013).

Group Review Exercise

Cholesterol Confusion, Statistical Deception and the Statin Controversy

About these articles

Statins are cholesterol-lowering drugs widely marketed and prescribed in Canada and internationally to prevent heart attacks and strokes. Although statins produce a dramatic reduction in cholesterol levels, they have failed to substantially improve cardiovascular outcomes. The following two articles address this controversial issue and examine how pharmaceutical companies employ statistical deception to inflate claims about the effectiveness and safety of statins to healthcare professionals and the general public.

Instructions

This assignment may be done alone, in pairs, or in groups of up to five people (note: if you are doing this assignment in pairs or groups, please only submit one hard or electronic copy to your instructor). The assignment should be type-written and no more than four to six pages maximum in length (double-spaced please). Read and critically analyze the following two articles and answer the following questions.

- Diamond, & Ravnskov(2015, February 12). How statistical deception created the appearance that statins are safe and effective in primary and secondary prevention of cardiovascular disease. *Expert Review of Clinical Pharmacology, 8* (2). doi:10.1586/17512433.2015.1012494
- Dubroff, R., & de Lorgeril, M. (2015, July 26). Cholesterol confusion and statin controversy. *World Journal of Cardiology, 7*(7): 404–409. ISSN: 1949-8462 (online), doi:10.4330/wjc.v7.i7.404

1. Provide a brief overview of the cholesterol hypothesis in the development of coronary heart disease. Is there sufficient evidence to support this hypothesis, and the proposed roles of statins?

2. Describe how large pharmaceutical companies use statistical deception to inflate claims regarding the effectiveness of statins with special reference to the statistical terms *relative risk* and *absolute risk and* overall reductions in *mortality*. Justify your answer based on the best available scientific evidence provided.

3. Describe some of the major side effects, complications, and/or risk factors associated with statin use and other conditions that have been linked to their prolonged use?

4. Describe alternative theories of atherosclerosis which are independent of cholesterol metabolism, and which may provide the key to future public health prevention strategies.

5. Describe the proven benefits of adopting a healthy and active lifestyle and the Mediterranean diet for the prevention of coronary heart disease.

Summary

- A NCD is defined as a chronic disease not typically caused by an infectious agent (i.e., non-infectious or non-communicable) that often has complex aetiologies, has an insidious onset, often characterized by multiple associated risk factors, long latency periods and is normally incurable in nature.
- More than one in five Canadian adults live with one of these NCDs (i.e., CVD, cancer, CRD, diabetes); and two-thirds of all deaths each year are caused by these major NCDs.
- Four in five Canadian adults have at least one modifiable risk factor for the development of an NCD (self-reported tobacco smoking, physical inactivity, unhealthy eating, and harmful use of alcohol).
- A major reduction in the healthcare burden associated with NCDs in Canada may be achieved, in part, from these population-based "best buy" interventions; which are cost effective and may even be revenue-generating (e.g., tobacco and alcohol tax increases, implementation of a sugar tax).
- Cancer is a collective term used to describe a group of diseases characterized by uncontrolled cell growth and division or the loss of the cell to perform normal apoptosis.
- It is estimated that 45% of women and 49% of men in Canada will develop cancer during their lifetime.
- Palliative care is an approach that seeks to improve the quality of life of for client's and their families facing problems associated with life-threatening illness, through the prevention and relief of suffering by means of early identification and impeccable assessment and treatment of pain and other problems, physical, psychosocial, and spiritual.
- EOLC is a term used to describe care provided in the last days or weeks of life.
- Hospice is a concept of care that provides compassion, concern, and support for dying clients and their families.
- CVD is defined as a class of diseases that involve the heart or blood vessels and include: coronary heart disease; disease of the blood vessels supplying the heart muscle, and cerebrovascular disease which are disease of the blood vessels supplying the brain.
- CVD is the leading cause of death globally and the second leading cause of death in Canada.
- CRDs are diseases of the airways and other parts of the lung that affect all ages and include asthma, COPD, lung cancer, cystic fibrosis, sleep apnea, and occupational lung diseases.
- The two most important risk factors associated with the development of CRDs are exposure to tobacco smoke (through personal smoking and/or exposure to second-hand smoke) and indoor and outdoor air quality.
- DM is regarded as a multisystem chronic disease that involves abnormal hormone insulin production, and/or impaired insulin utilization, which results in abnormal metabolism of carbohydrates and elevated levels of glucose in the blood and/or urine.
- There is increasing concern that Canada's healthcare systems will be unable to meet the growing healthcare needs of this ageing population, especially in regards to NCDs.

Critical Thinking Questions

Diabetes and Heart Disease in a First Nations Client

Mr Diabo is a 48-year-old First Nations male who has no previous history of hypertension or heart disease. Mr Diabo resides at a First Nations reserve with his wife and two children. At a community-based screening clinic, his blood pressure was found to be 182/120 mmHg. Mr Diabo states that he is not a "stressed individual." His father died from a stroke six years ago and his mother and sister both have been previously diagnosed with type 2 diabetes. He was previously diagnosed with type 2 DM five years ago, and is non-adherent to his diabetic treatment regime, and does not take his medications (i.e., hydrochlorothiazide (HCTZ) 12.5 mg daily orally and Enalapril sodium (Vasotec) 5 mg daily orally) because he believes it interferes with his sexual function. Mr Diabo admits to being inactive and is moderately obese. He smokes a half pack of cigarettes daily and enjoys drinking a six-pack of beer on Friday and Saturday nights with his friends at a local sports bar. His electrocardiogram shows left ventricular hypertrophy; urinalysis reveals the presence of protein (0.4 g/L), and his serum creatinine level is 143 nmol/L.

1. What specific risk factors does Mr Diabo have for the development of diabetes and heart disease?
2. Is there evidence of target-organ damage present? Justify your answer.
3. As a public health professional and worker, what would be your priorities for managing Mr Diabo's DM and hypertension? Discuss the importance of cultural safety in developing a plan of care for Mr Diabo in his community.
4. What resources and/or agencies are available in your community to assist Mr Diabo?

References

Acton, R. B., Vanderlee, L., Hobin, E. P., & Hammond, D. (2017). Added sugar in packaged foods and beverages available at a major Canadian retailer in 2015: A descriptive analysis. *Canadian Medical Association Journal (CMAT) Open, 5*(1), E1–E6. Retrieved from http://davidhammond.ca/wp-content/uploads/2014/12/2017-Added-Sugar-in-Pre-packaged-Foods-CMAJ-Open-Acton-et-al.pdf

Bancej, C., Jayabalasingham, B., Wall, R. W., Rao, D. P., Do, M. T., de Groh, M., . . . Jayaraman, G. C. (2015, September). Evidence Brief – Trends and projections of obesity among Canadians. *Health Promotion and Chronic Disease Prevention Canada, 35*(7), 109–112.

Bartfay, W. J., & Bartfay, E. (2015). *Public health in Canada*. Boston, MA: Pearson Learning Solutions. ISBN: 13: 978-1-323-01471-4.

Bernmier, N. F. (2015, June 5). *The real costs of informal caregiving in Canada*. Montreal, QC: Policy Options Politiques. Retrieved from http://policyoptions.irpp.org/2015/06/05/the-real-costs-of-informal-caregiving/

Buchanan, T., & Xiang, A. H. (2005, March). Gestational diabetes mellitus. *Journal of Clinical Investigations, 115*(3), 485–491. Retrieved from https://www.jci.org/articles/view/24531

Butt, P., Beirness, D., Gliksman, L., Paradis, C., & Stockwell, T. (2011, November). *Alcohol and health in Canada: A summary of evidence and guidelines for low-risk drinking*. Ottawa, ON: Canadian Centre on Substance Abuse.

Campbell, N. R. C., Poirier, L., Tremblay, G., Lindsay, R., Reid, D., & Tobe, S. W. (2011).The science supporting new 2011 CHEP recommendations with an emphasis on health advocacy and knowledge translation. *Canadian Journal of Cardiology, 27*(4), 407–414.

Canadian Association for Retired Persons. (2014, February). *CARPs new vision for caregiver support*. Toronto, ON: Author. Retrieved from http://www.carp.ca/wp-content/uploads/2014/02/Caregiver-Brief-Feb-2014.pdf

Canadian Broadcasting Corporation. (2011, March 9). *Canadians lead world Internet use: A report*. Toronto, ON: CBC. Retrieved from http://www.cbc.ca/news/technology/canadians-lead-world-in-internet-use-report-1.1063588

Canadian Broadcasting Corporation (CBC) News. (2017, April 13). Nearly a third of food samples in CFIA testing contains glyphosate residues. Toronto, ON: CBC. Retrieved from http://www.cbc.ca/news/health/cfia-report-glyphosate-1.4070275

Canadian Cancer Society's Advisory Committee on Cancer Statistics. (2017, June). *Canadian cancer statistics 2017*. Toronto, ON: Canadian Cancer Society. ISBN: 0835-2976. Retrieved from http://www.cancer.ca/en/cancer-information/cancer-101/canadian-cancer-statistics-publication/?region=on.

Canadian Chronic Disease Indicators (CCDI) Steering Committee. (2017, August). At-a-glance. Canadian chronic disease indicators report. *Health Promotion and Chronic Disease Prevention in Canada. Research, Policy and Practice, 37*(8), 248–251. Retrieved from https://www.canada.ca/content/dam/phac-aspc/documents/services/publications/health-promotion-chronic-disease-prevention-canada-research-policy-practice/vol-37-no-8-2017/ar-03-eng.pdf

Canadian Diabetes Association. (2018). *WHO, 2018*. Toronto, ON: Author. Retrieved from https://www.diabetes.ca/about-diabetes/types-of-diabetes

Canadian Food Inspection Agency. (2017). *Safeguarding with science: Glyphosate testing in 2015–2016*. Ottawa, ON: Author. Retrieved from http://static.producer.com/wp-content/uploads/2017/04/CFIA_ACIA-9123346-v1-FSSD-FSSS-Glyphosate-Final-Report-15-16_0184101.pdf#_ga=1.196489061.892407858.1492107204

Canadian Hospice and Palliative Care Association. (2014, March). *CHPCA fact sheet—Hospice palliative care in Canada*. Retrieved from http://www.chpca.net/media/330558/Fact_Sheet_HPC_in_Canada%20Spring%202014%20Final.pdf

Canadian Institute for Health Information. (2011). *Health care in Canada, 2011. A focus on seniors and aging*. Ottawa, ON: CIHI. Retrieved from https://secure.cihi.ca/free_products/HCIC_2011_seniors_report_en.pdf

Canadian Institute for Health Information. (2017). *National health expenditure trends, 1975 to 2017*. Ottawa, ON: Author. ISBN: 978-1-77109-649-2 (PDF). Retrieved from https://www.cihi.ca/sites/default/files/document/nhex2017-trends-report-en.pdf

Canadian Institute for Health Information. (2018). *Health spending*. Ottawa, ON: CIHI. Retrieved from https://www.cihi.ca/en/health-spending

Canadian Hospice Palliative Care Association. (2014, March). *CHPCA fact sheet: Hospice palliative care in Canada*. Ottawa, ON: Author. Retrieved from http://www.chpca.net/media/330558/Fact_Sheet_HPC_in_Canada%20Spring%202014%20Final.pdf

Canadian Society for Exercise Physiology. (2012). *Canadian sedentary behaviour guidelines. 2012 scientific statement*. Ottawa, ON: Author. Retrieved from http://www.csep.ca/CMFiles/Guidelines/CanadianSedentaryGuidelinesStatements_E_2012.pdf

Centers for Disease Control and Prevention. (2016). *Flu and heart disease*. Atlanta, GA: Author. Retrieved from https://www.cdc.gov/flu/heartdisease/index.htm

Chiu, B. C., Weisenburger, D. D., & Zahm, S. H. (2004). Agricultural pesticide use, familial cancer, and risk of non-Hodgkin lymphoma. *Cancer Epidemiology, Biomarkers and Prevention, 13*(4), 525–553.

Choi, C. (2017, February 1). *Canadian kids bombarded with more than 25M junk food and drink ads online every year*. Toronto, ON: Global News. Retrieved from https://globalnews.ca/news/3217654/canadian-kids-are-bombarded-with-more-than-25-million-online-ads-for-junk-food-and-sugary-drinks-each-year/

Choi, C., Vuchnich, A., & Tang, V. (2017, January 12). *Two-thirds of packaged foods in Canada are full of sugar: Canadian study*. Toronto, ON: Global News. Retrieved from https://globalnews.ca/news/3175339/most-packaged-foods-you-eat-are-full-of-added-sugar-canadian-study/

Clifford, G. M., Smith, J. S., Plumber, M., Munoz, N., & Franceschi, S. (2003, January 13). Human papillomavirus types in invasive cancer worldwide: A meta-analysis. *British Journal of Cancer, 88*, 63–71. Retrieved from https://www.nature.com/articles/6600688.

Cooke, R. A. (2008). *Infectious diseases: Atlas, cases, text*. Toronto, ON: The McGraw-Hill Companies.

Cressey, D. (2015, March 23). Widely used herbicide linked to cancer. *Scientific American and Nature Magazine, 312*(2), 23–28. Retrieved from https://www.scientificamerican.com/article/widely-used-herbicide-linked-to-cancer/

Dasgupta, K., Quinn, R. R., Zarnke, K. B., Rabi, D. M., Ravani P., Daskalopoulou, S. S., … Rabkin, S. W. (2014, May). The 2014 Canadian Hypertension Education Program recommendations for blood pressure measurement, diagnosis, assessment of risk, prevention, and treatment of hypertension. *Canadian Journal of Cardiology, 30*(5), 485–501.

DeVita, V. T., Lawrence, T. S., & Rosenberg, S. A. (Eds.). (2011). *DeVita Hellman and Rosenberg's cancer: Principles and practice of oncology* (9th ed.). Toronto, ON: Williams & Wilkins.

Diamond, D. M., & Ravnskov, U. (2015, February 12). How statistical deception created the appearance that statins are safe and effective in primary and secondary prevention of cardiovascular disease. *Expert Review of Clinical Pharmacology, 8*(2), 201–210. doi:10.1586/17512433.2015.1012494

Dubroff, R., & de Lorgeril, M. (2015, July 26). Cholesterol confusion and statin controversy. *World Journal of Cardiology, 7*(7), 404–409. ISSN: 1949-8462 (online), doi:10.4330/wjc.v7.i7.404

El-Serog, H. B. (2012, May). Epidemiology of viral hepatitis and hepatocellular carcinoma. *Gastroenterology, 142*(6), 1264–1273.

Ferrans, C. E. (2005). Definitions and conceptual models of quality of life. In: J. Lipscomb, C. C. Gotay, & C. Snyder (Eds.). *Outcomes assessment in cancer* (pp. 14–30). Cambridge, UK: Cambridge University.

Food and Agricultural Organization (FAO) of the United Nations and World Health Organization. (2016, May). *Joint FAO/WHO meeting on pesticide residues: Summary report, May 9–13, 2016*. Geneva, Switzerland: Author. Retrieved from http://www.who.int/foodsafety/jmprsummary2016.pdf?ua=1

GBD 2015 Risk Factors Collaborators. (2016). Global, regional, and national comparative risk assessment of 79 behavioural, environmental and occupational, and metabolic risks or clusters of risks, 1990–2015: A systematic analysis for the Global Burden of Disease Study 2015. *Lancet, 388*(10053), 1659–1724.

Global Initiative for Chronic Obstructive Lung Disease. (2016). *Global strategy for the diagnosis, management and prevention of COPD.* Retrieved from http://goldcopd.org/global-strategy-diagnosis-management-prevention-copd-2016/

Gillies, C., Abrams, K., Lambert, P., Cooper, N. J., Sutton, A. J., Hsu, R. T. & Khunti, K, (2007). Pharmacological and lifestyle interventions to prevent or delay type 2 diabetes in people with impaired glucose tolerance: Systematic review and meta-analysis. *British Medical Journal, 334,* 1–9. doi:10.1136/bmj.39063.689375.55

Government of Canada. (2011). *Tracking heart disease and stroke in Canada: Highlights 2011.* Ottawa, ON: Author. Retrieved from https://www.canada.ca/en/public-health/services/chronic-diseases/cardiovascular-disease/tracking-heart-disease-stroke-canada-stroke-highlights-2011.html

Government of Canada. (2014). *Chronic respiratory diseases.* Ottawa, ON: Author. Retrieved from https://www.canada.ca/en/public-health/services/chronic-diseases/chronic-respiratory-diseases.html

Government of Canada. (2017). *Cancer.* Ottawa, ON: Author. Retrieved from https://www.canada.ca/en/public-health/services/chronic-diseases/cancer.html

Guh, D. P., Zhang, W., Bansback, N., Amarsi, Z., Birmingham, C. L., & Anis, A. H. (2009, March). The incidence of co-morbidities related to obesity and overweight: A systematic review and meta-analysis. *BMC Public Health, 25*(9), 88–95.

Harris, R. E. (2013). *Epidemiology of chronic disease: Global perspectives.* Toronto, ON: Jone & Bartlett Learning.

Health Canada. (2010). *Canadian tobacco use monitoring survey (CTUMS).* Ottawa, ON: Author. Retrieved from http://publications.gc.ca/site/eng/9.504355/publication.html

Heart and Stroke Foundation of Canada. (2003). *The growing burden of heart disease and stroke in Canada, 2003.* Chapter 1—Risk factors. Toronto, ON: Author. Retrieved from www.cvdinfobase.ca/cvdbook/CVD_En03.pdf

Heart and Stroke Foundation of Canada. (2018). *Flu season is coming. How you can protect your heart this winter.* Ottawa, ON: Author. Retrieved from http://www.heartandstroke.ca/articles/flu-season-is-coming

Heart Research Institute. (2018). *Facts about heart disease.* Toronto, ON: Author. Retrieved from http://www.hricanada.org/about-heart-disease/facts-about-heart-disease.

Jaga, K., & Dharmani, C. (2005). The epidemiology of pesticide exposure and cancer: A review. *Review of Environmental Health, 20*(1), 15–38.

Klement, R. J., & Kämmerer, U. (2011). Is there a role for carbohydrate restriction in the treatment and prevention of cancer? *Nutrition and Metabolism, 8,* 75–81.

Langlois, K., & Garriguet, D. (2015). Sugar consumption among Canadians of all ages. *Health Reports, 22,* 5 (82-003X). Ottawa, ON: Statistics Canada. Retrieved from http://www.statcan.gc.ca/pub/82-003-x/2011003/article/11540-eng.htm

Liang, Z, Wang, X., Xie, B., Zhuy, Y., Wu, J., Li, S., … Meng, S. (2016, October 11). Pesticide exposure and risk of bladder cancer: A meta-analysis. *Oncotarget, 7*(4), 66959–66969. Retrieved from https://www.ncbi.nlm.nih.gov/pmc/articles/PMC5341850/

Morahan, G. (2012). Insights into type 1 diabetes provided by genetic analyses. *Current Opinion in Endocrinology, Diabetes and Obesity, 19,* 263–270. PMID: 22732486.

Moriarity, D. G., Zack, M. M., & Kobau, R. (2003, September 2). The Centers for Disease Control and Prevention Healthy Days Measures—population tracking of perceived physical and mental health over time. *Health and Quality of Life Outcomes, 1,* 37. Retrieved from https://hqlo.biomedcentral.com/articles/10.1186/1477-7525-1-37

National Indigenous Health Organization. (2006). *2002–2003 First nations regional longitudinal health survey.* Ottawa, ON: Author. Retrieved from http://fnigc.ca/sites/default/files/ENpdf/RHS_2002/rhs2002-03-technical_report.pdf

Nguyen, C., Varney, M. D., Harrison, C. C., & Morahan, G. (2013, June). Definition of high risk Type 1 diabetes HLA-DR and HLA-DQ types using only three single nucleotide polymorphisms. *Diabetes, 62*(6), 2135–2140. Retrieved from http://diabetes.diabetesjournals.org/content/62/6/2135

O'Donnell, D. E., Aaorn, S., Bourbeau, J., Herhandez, P., Marciniuk, D. D., Balter, M., … Ford, G. (2007). Canadian Thoracic Society recommendations for management of chronic pulmonary disease—2007 update. *Canadian Respiratory Journal, 14*(Suppl. B), 5B–32B.

Ontario Stroke Network. (2017). *Stroke stats and facts.* Toronto, ON: Author. Retrieved from http://ontariostrokenetwork.ca/information-about-stroke/stroke-stats-and-facts/

Padwal, R. S., Bienek, A., McAlister, F. A., & Campbell, N. R. (2015, August 15). Outcomes research task force of the Canadian hypertension education program. Epidemiology of hypertension in Canada: An update. *Canadian Journal of Cardiology, 32*(5), 687–694.

Public Health Agency of Canada. (2007, September). *Core competencies for public health in Canada: Release 1.1.* Ottawa, ON: Author. Web-based link: http://www.phac-aspc.gc.ca/core_competencies or http://www.phac-aspc.gc.ca/php-psp/ccph-cesp/pdfs/cc-manual-eng090407.pdf

Public Health Agency of Canada. (2011). *Diabetes in Canada: Facts and figures from a public health perspective.* Ottawa, ON: Author. 2011. Retrieved from www.phac-aspc.gc.ca/cd-mc/publications/diabetes-diabete/facts-figures-faits-chiffres-2011/pdf/facts-figures-faits-chiffres-eng.pdf

Public Health Agency of Canada. (2012). *Health-adjusted life expectancy (HALE) in Canada 2012.* Ottawa, ON: Author. Retrieved from http://publications.gc.ca/collections/collection_2012/aspc-phac/HP35-32-2012-eng.pdf

Public Health Agency of Canada. (2015). *Fast facts about asthma: Data compiled from the 2011 Survey on living with chronic diseases in Canada.* Ottawa, ON: Author. Retrieved from www.phac-aspc.gc.ca/cd-mc/crd-mrc/asthma_fs_asthme-eng.php

Public Health Agency of Canada. (2016, December). *How healthy are Canadians? A trend analysis of the health of Canadians form a healthy living and chronic disease perspective.* Ottawa, ON: Author. ISBN: 978-0-660-06582-3. Retrieved from https://www.canada.ca/content/dam/phac-aspc/documents/services/publications/healthy-living/how-healthy-canadians/pub1-eng.pdf

Reilly, J. J., Methven, E., & McDowell, Z. C. (2003). Health consequences of obesity. *Archives of Disease in Childhood, 88*(9), 748–752.

Roberts, K. C., Rao, D. P., Bennett, T. L., Loukine, L., & Jayaraman, G. C. (2015, August). Prevalence and patterns of chronic disease multimorbidity and associated determinants. *Canada Health Promotion and Chronic Disease Prevention in Canada Research, Policy and Practice,, 35*(6), 87–94.

Roberts, K. C., Shields, M., de Groh, M., Aziz, A., & Gilbert, J. A. (2012, September). Overweight and obesity in children and adolescents: Results from the 2009 to 2011 Canadian Health Measures Survey. *Health Reports, 23*(3), 37–41.

Roberts, L. W., Clifton, R. A., Ferguson, B., Kampen, K., & Langlois, S. (2004). *Recent social trends in Canada 1960–2000.* Montrèal, QC: University Press.

Schmidt, L. A. (2017, September). Experts fear sugar will kill you sooner. *Readers Digest,* 34–39.

Sethi, S., & Murphy, T. F. (2008). Infection in the pathogenesis and course of chronic obstructive pulmonary disease. *New England Journal of Medicine, 359*(22), 2355–2365. doi:10.1056/NEJMra0800353

Sliwa, K., Stewart, S., & Gersh, B. (2011). Hypertension: A global perspective. *Circulation, 123,* 2892–2896. doi:10.1161/CIRCULATIONAHA.110.992362

Spector, M. (2015, April 10). Roundup risk assessment. *The New Yorker.* Retrieved from https://www.newyorker.com/news/daily-comment/roundup-and-risk-assessment

Statistics Canada. (2017). *Canadians and nature: Fertilizers and pesticides, 2013.* Ottawa, ON: Author. (16-508-X). Retrieved from http://www.statcan.gc.ca/pub/16-508-x/16-508-x2015007-eng.htm

Statistics Canada. (2017). *Life expectancy.* Ottawa, ON: Author. Retrieved from https://www.statcan.gc.ca/eng/help/bb/info/life

Subcommittee of the Standing Senate Committee on Social Affairs, Science and Technology. (2000). *Quality end-of-life care. The right of every Canadian.* Ottawa, ON: Senate of Canada. Retrieved from https://sencanada.ca/content/sen/committee/362/upda/rep/repfinjun00part1-e.htm

Tremblay, M. S., LeBlanc, A. G., Janssen, I., Kho, M. E., Hicks, A., Murumets, K., ... Colley R. C. (2011a, January). Canadian sedentary behaviour guidelines for children and youth. *Applied Physiology, Nutrition, and Metabolism, 36*(1), 59–64.

Tremblay, M. S., Warburton, D. E., Janssen, I., Paterson, D. H., Latimer, A. E, ... Rhodes, R. E., Kho, M. E. (2011b, February). New Canadian physical activity guidelines. *Applied Physiology, Nutrition, and Metabolism, 36*(1), 36–46.

Turner, A., & Findlay, L. (2015). *Informal caregiving for seniors.* Ottawa, ON: Statistics Canada. Retrieved from http://www.statcan.gc.ca/pub/82-003-x/2012003/article/11694-eng.htm

Vinson, F., Merhi, M., Baldi, I., Raynal, H., & Gamet-Payrastre, L. (2011). Exposure to pesticides and risk of childhood cancer: A meta-analysis of recent epidemiological studies. *Occupational and Environmental Medicine, 68,* 694–702. Retrieved from https://www.ncbi.nlm.nih.gov/pubmed/21606468

Webber, R. (2016). *Communicable diseases: A global perspective* (5th ed.). Boston, MA: C.A.B. International.

World Health Organization. (2003). *WHO framework convention on tobacco control.* Geneva, Switzerland: Author. ISBN: 9241591013. Retrieved from http://www.who.int/fctc/text_download/en/

World Health Organization. (2005a). *Preventing chronic diseases: A vital investment WHO global report.* Geneva, Switzerland: Author. Retrieved from: https://www.who.int/chp/chronic_disease_report/part1/en/index11.html

World Health Organization. (2005b). The World Health Organization quality of life assessment (WHOQOL): Position paper from the World Health Organization. *Social Science and Medicine, 41*(10), 1403–1409.

World Health Organization. (2011a). *Global status report on preventing noncommunicable diseases 2010.* Geneva, Switzerland: Author. ISBN: 978-92-4-068645-8. Retrieved from http://www.who.int/nmh/publications/ncd_report_full_en.pdf

World Health Organization. (2011b). *Sixty-forth world health assembly.* Geneva, 16–14 May, 2011. Resolutions and decisions. Annexes. Geneva, Switzerland: Author. Retrieved from http://apps.who.int/gb/ebwha/pdf_files/WHA64-REC1/A64_REC1-en.pdf

World Health Organization. (2013). *Global action plan for the prevention and control of NCDs 2013–2020.* Geneva, Switzerland: Author. ISBN: 978-92-4-150623-6. Retrieved from http://www.who.int/nmh/publications/ncd-action-plan/en/ or http://apps.who.int/iris/bitstream/10665/94384/1/9789241506236_eng.pdf?ua=1

World Health Organization. (2017a). *Noncommunicable diseases: Fact sheet.* Geneva, Switzerland: Author. Retrieved from http://www.who.int/mediacentre/factsheets/fs355/en/

World Health Organization. (2017b). *Noncommunicable diseases: Progress monitor 2017.* Geneva, Switzerland: Author. ISBN: 978-92-4-151302-9. Retrieved from http://apps.who.int/iris/bitstream/10665/258940/1/9789241513029-eng.pdf?ua=1

World Health Organization. (2017c). *WHO on the global tobacco epidemic 2017: Monitoring the growth and use and prevention policies.* Geneva, Switzerland: Author. Retrieved from http://apps.who.int/iris/bitstream/10665/255874/1/9789241512824-eng.pdf?ua=1&ua=1

World Health Organization. (2018a). *Cardiovascular disease. Fact sheet.* Geneva, Switzerland. Author. Retrieved http://www.who.int/mediacentre/factsheets/fs317/en/

World Health Organization. (2018b). *Diabetes fact sheet.* Geneva, Switzerland. Author. Retrieved from http://www.who.int/mediacentre/factsheets/fs312/en/

World Health Organization. (2018c). *WHO definition of palliative care.* Geneva, Switzerland: Author. Retrieved from http://www.who.int/cancer/palliative/definition/en/

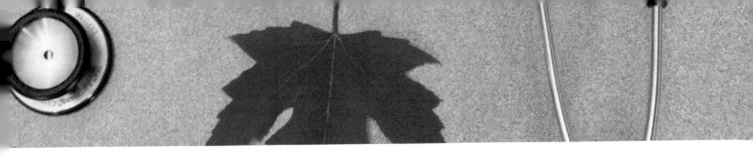

Appendix A: 36 Core Competencies (Public Health Agency of Canada)

Core Competency Statements

The core competency statements are not designed to stand alone, but rather to form a set of knowledge, skills, and attitudes practiced within the larger context of the values of public health.

Attitudes and Values

All public health professionals share a core set of attitudes and values. These attitudes and values have not been listed as specific core competencies for public health because they are difficult to teach and even harder to assess. However, they form the context within which the competencies are practiced. This makes them equally important.

Important values in public health include a commitment to equity, social justice, and sustainable development, recognition of the importance of the health of the community as well as the individual, and respect for diversity, self-determination, empowerment, and community participation. These values are rooted in an understanding of the broad determinants of health and the historical principles, values, and strategies of public health and health promotion.

Statements In Seven Categories

The 36 core competencies are based on the core functions of public health: population health assessment, health surveillance, disease and injury prevention, health promotion, and health protection. They are organized under seven categories: public health sciences; assessment and analysis; policy and program planning, implementation, and evaluation; partnerships, collaboration, and advocacy; diversity and inclusiveness; communication; and leadership.

ONE...

Public Health Sciences

This category includes key knowledge and critical thinking skills related to the public health sciences: behavioural and social sciences, biostatistics, epidemiology, environmental public health, demography, workplace health, and the prevention of chronic diseases, infectious diseases, psychosocial problems, and injuries. Competency in this category requires the ability to apply knowledge in practice.

A Public Health Practitioner is Able to . . .

1.1 Demonstrate knowledge about the following concepts: the health status of populations, inequities in health, the determinants of health and illness, strategies for health promotion, disease and injury prevention, and health protection, as well as the factors that influence the delivery and use of health services.

1.2 Demonstrate knowledge about the history, structure, and interaction of public health and health care services at local, provincial/territorial, national, and international levels.

1.3 Apply the public health sciences to practice.

1.4 Use evidence and research to inform health policies and programs.

1.5 Demonstrate the ability to pursue lifelong learning opportunities in the field of public health.

TWO . . .

Assessment and Analysis

This category describes the core competencies needed to collect, assess, analyze, and apply information, including data, facts, concepts, and theories. These competencies are required to make evidence-based decisions, prepare budgets and reports, conduct investigations, and make recommendations for policy and program development.

A Public Health Practitioner Is Able To . . .

2.1 Recognize that a health concern or issue exists.

2.2 Identify relevant and appropriate sources of information, including community assets and resources.

2.3 Collect, store, retrieve, and use accurate and appropriate information on public health issues.

2.4 Analyze information to determine appropriate implications, uses, gaps, and limitations.

2.5 Determine the meaning of information, considering the current ethical, political, scientific, sociocultural, and economic contexts.

2.6 Recommend specific actions based on the analysis of information.

THREE . . .

Policy and Program Planning, Implementation, and Evaluation

This category describes the core competencies needed to effectively choose options and to plan, implement, and evaluate policies and/or programs in public health. This includes the management of incidents such as outbreaks and emergencies.

A Public Health Practitioner Is Able To . . .

3.1 Describe selected policy and program options to address a specific public health issue.

3.2 Describe the implications of each option, especially as they apply to the determinants of health and recommend or decide on a course of action.

3.3 Develop a plan to implement a course of action taking into account relevant evidence, legislation, emergency planning procedures, regulations, and policies.

3.4 Implement a policy or program and/or take appropriate action to address a specific public health issue.

3.5 Demonstrate the ability to implement effective practice guidelines.

3.6 Evaluate the action, policy, or program.

3.7 Demonstrate an ability to set and follow priorities, and to maximize outcomes based on available resources.

3.8 Demonstrate the ability to fulfill functional roles in response to a public health emergency.

FOUR . . .

Partnerships, Collaboration, and Advocacy

This category captures the competencies required to influence and work with others to improve the health and well-being of the public through the pursuit of a common goal. Partnership and collaboration optimizes performance through shared resources and responsibilities. Advocacy—speaking, writing, or acting in favour of a particular cause, policy, or group of people—often aims to reduce inequities in health status or access to health services.

A Public Health Practitioner Is Able To . . .

4.1 Identify and collaborate with partners in addressing public health issues.

4.2 Use skills such as team building, negotiation, conflict management, and group facilitation to build partnerships.

4.3 Mediate between differing interests in the pursuit of health and well-being, and facilitate the allocation of resources.

4.4 Advocate for healthy public policies and services that promote and protect the health and well-being of individuals and communities.

FIVE . . .

Diversity and Inclusiveness

This category identifies the sociocultural competencies required to interact effectively with diverse individuals, groups, and communities. It is the embodiment of attitudes and practices that result in inclusive behaviours, practices, programs, and policies.

A Public Health Practitioner Is Able To . . .

5.1 Recognize how the determinants of health (biological, social, cultural, economic, and physical) influence the health and well-being of specific population groups.

5.2 Address population diversity when planning, implementing, adapting, and evaluating public health programs and policies.

5.3 Apply culturally relevant and appropriate approaches with people from diverse cultural, socioeconomic, and educational backgrounds, and persons of all ages, genders, health status, sexual orientations, and abilities.

SIX . . .

Communication

Communication involves an interchange of ideas, opinions, and information. This category addresses numerous dimensions of communication including internal and external exchanges; written, verbal, nonverbal, and listening skills; computer literacy; providing appropriate information to different audiences; working with the media and social marketing techniques.

A Public Health Practitioner Is Able To . . .

6.1 Communicate effectively with individuals, families, groups, communities, and colleagues.

6.2 Interpret information for professional, nonprofessional, and community audiences.

6.3 Mobilize individuals and communities by using appropriate media, community resources, and social marketing techniques.

6.4 Use current technology to communicate effectively.

SEVEN . . .

Leadership

This category focuses on leadership competencies that build capacity, improve performance, and enhance the quality of the working environment. They also enable organizations and communities to create, communicate, and apply shared visions, missions, and values.

A Public Health Practitioner Is Able To . . .

7.1 Describe the mission and priorities of the public health organization where one works, and apply them in practice.

7.2 Contribute to developing key values and a shared vision in planning and implementing public health programs and policies in the community.

7.3 Utilize public health ethics to manage self, others, information, and resources.

7.4 Contribute to team and organizational learning to advance public health goals.

7.5 Contribute to maintaining organizational performance standards.

7.6 Demonstrate an ability to build community capacity by sharing knowledge, tools, expertise, and experience.

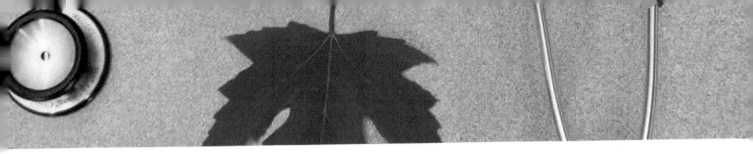

Glossary of Key Terms

aboriginal. Indigenous peoples who are and remain the earliest or initial inhabitants of a place or land.

accessibility. This criterion of the Canada Health Act declares that no individual can be discriminated against in terms of receiving health care services based on their age, lifestyle or present health status or condition.

acculturative stress. Is defined as difficulties faced by new immigrants in adapting to their new host country and society.

acquired (passive) immunity. Occurs when there is a transfer of antibodies from the mother to the infant or child via the placenta or through routine breast feeding, or may come from already-produced antibodies by another host (e.g., immune globulin).

action (cooperative/ participatory) research. A qualitative research methodcharacterized by the systematic study of the reported needs of individuals, groups or entire communities and the empowerment and implementation of a planned change to mutually and cooperativelysolve real-life problems.

active immunity. Occurs through vaccination and is present when the body develops its own antibodies against a pathogen or antigenic substance.

active surveillance. Is defined as the collection of health related data via sentinel public health tracking systems, screening tools and interviews in order to identify the occurrence of disease in a defined community or geographical region when individuals present with suggestive clinical signs and symptoms.

acute diseases. Are defined as those disorders or conditions that are relatively severe in nature with a sudden onset, but have a short duration of clinical signs and symptoms.

adaptive emergence Is defined as a genetic change in a microorganism that results in a phenotype that is capable of invading a new ecosystem, particularly via jumping to a new host species, which includes humans.

agent. Is defined as a toxic substance, microorganism, or environmental factor, such as radiation or a lifestyle, that must be present (or absent) for the problem to occur.

airborne or respiratory transmission. Occurs when microorganisms or pathogens become suspended in droplet nuclei or aerosols in the air (e.g., via coughing, sneezing) and enter a susceptible host through a port of entry (e.g., nose or mouth) (Jo Damazo and Bartfay, 2010).

air quality index (AQI). Which is also commonly referred to as the *"Index of the Quality of Air"* (IQUA) has been developed to help inform the general public, public health care professionals and workers, and researchers of the prevailing air quality in their communities.

allergies and inflammatory disease. Allergies are caused by the body's reaction to an invading foreign agent, substance or allegen and which results in the development of antibodies. Subsequent exposure causes the release of chemical mediators and a variety of signs and symptoms (e.g., anaphylaxis bronchospasm, dyspnea, eczema, laryngospasms, rhinitis, sinusitis, urticaria). Inflammations are protective responses by body tissues to an irritation or injury and may be acute or chronic in nature and histamine, kinins and other various substances mediate the inflammatory process. Cardinal signs and symptoms of inflammation are redness (rubor), heat (calor), swelling and pain (dolor), which may result in loss of function.

allostatic load. Is defined asthe "wear and tear on the body" which accumulates as a function of time due to chronic or repeated episodes of stress that result in fluctuating or heightened neural or neuroendocrine responses.

allostasis. The process by which the body responds to stressors in order to regain stability or homeostasis.

amyotrophic lateral sclerosis (ALS). Also known as *Lou Gehrig's disease*, is defined as a progressive motor neuron disease that involves both the upper and lower motor neurons and is characterized by wasting of the muscles of the body resulting from the destruction of motor neurons in the brain stem and anterior gray horns of the spinal cord and degeneration of the pyramidal tracts.

analytical epidemiology. Seeks to identify risk factors and/or determinants of health that help to explain the causation or etiology of a health-related state, event or condition.

anorexia nervosa Is a mental health disorder characterized by a refusal to maintain a body weight at a minimally health level; a distorted view of one's body shape or weight; intense pathological fear of getting fat or gaining weight; unnecessary influence on self-evaluation; denial of the seriousness of their low body weight, and amenorrhea in female clients of childbearing age (for at least three consecutive mental cycles.

antigenicity. Refers to the ability of the antigen system to have the required strength, activity, and effectiveness to respond to a disease threat where the antigens stimulate the immune system to make the body think it has the disease, and the immune system responds appropriately by developing the necessary antibodies.

applied research. Here defined as public health investigations that focus on finding solutions to existing problems, and to generate knowledge that will directly influence practice.

arthropod-borne viruses or arboviruses. Are viruses that are spread by arthropods which include insects and arachnids (e.g., ticks, mites, spiders), and include yellow fever, dengue fever and Venezuelan equine encephalitis.

asthma. Is a chronic condition characterized by cough, shortness of breath, chest tightness and wheezing.

attributable risk or risk difference. Is defined as a measure of association that provides information about the effect of the absolute effect of the exposure or the excess risk of disease or health condition in those exposed compared to those unexposed.

attributable risk percentage. Is defined as the proportion of the disease or health condition of interest in the population being investigated that could be prevented by eliminating the exposure.

autonomic nervous system (ANS). Is the part or component of the nervous system that controls basic body processes such as your heart rate, breathing, blood pressure and hundreds of other involuntary process, and consists of the sympathetic and parasympathetic divisions.

avian influenza. Often called *"Avian flu"* or *"Bird flu"* in the mass and social medias, is a contagious viral infection that can affect several species of food producing birds (e.g., chickens, turkeys, quails, guinea fowl) as well as pet birds and wild birds. Type A's (e.g., H5N1, H7N9) are the greatest concern to public health because it can infect humans and cause pandemics.

avoidable or amendable mortalities. Are defined as untimely and premature deaths that should not have occurred with the presence of timely and effective primary health care services or other public health interventions, practices, programs, policy interventions and/or health related legislations.

basic ro (transmissibility index or reproductive number). Of an infectious disease agent, gives an indication of the transmissibility of the known agent, and can also be employed to estimate the vaccine coverage (if available) in an otherwise susceptible population to prevent person-to-person spread in a community or geographical area.

basic research. Here defined as activities undertaken to extend the base of knowledge in public health or to formulate or refine an existing conceptual model or theory.

best buys. Are population-based actions that should be undertaken immediately to produce accelerated results in regards to NCD prevention, decreasing associated morbidities and mortalities, and decreasing associated health care costs and burden.

Big Mac Index. First published by Pam Woodall in the September edition of *The Economists* as an informal and light-hearted guide for assessing the purchasing power parity (PPP) between two different currencies, and provides a guide to test the extent to which market exchange rates result in goods costing the same in different countries (Jacobsen, 2008; Tough & Preece, 2015).

bimaadiziwin. This concept incorporates a belief by First Nations people of a path to the good life (spiritual and physical health and well-being) via a reciprocal and balanced relationship between themselves and Mother Earth (environment).

Binge-Eating Disorder (BED). Is characterized by uncontrollable binge-eating sessions, usually followed by feelings of guilt and shame with associated weight gain

binge-eating/purging type of anorexia nervosa. Is less recognized and common in nature where an individual restricts their caloric intake of food items, but also regularly engage in binge-eating and/or purging behaviours (at least weekly).

Bill C-31 of 1985. Bill permits Aboriginal women who choose to marry non-Aboriginal men can now apply for status and be registered.

bioterrorism. The use of a microorganism with the deliberate intent of causing infection in order to achieve certain goals (PHAC, 2001).

bipolar disorder. Which was previously known as manic depressive illness, is characterized by altering and unusual periods or cycles of depression followed by elevated mood that can last for days, weeks or even months in duration (APA, 2013). The elevated mood component is known as mania or hypomania, depending on its severity, and/or whether or not symptoms of psychosis are present.

blastomycosis. Is defined as an invasive fungal disease caused by the organism *Blastomyces dermatitidis*, and whose natural reservoir is found in decaying wood, leaves and soil.

British North America Act (Constitution Act, 1867). Established Canada as a nation. Sections 91 and 92 of the Act specify the federal and provincial governments' responsibilities, respectively.

building related illness" (BRI). The term is employed when signs and symptoms are present for a specific clinically diagnosable illness which can be directly attributed to airborne building contaminates.

Canada Health Act (1982). Replaced HIDSA and the Medical Care Act and was based on five founding criteria's: Public administration, comprehensiveness, universality, portability and accessibility.

Canada Health Act Dispute Avoidance and Resolution (2004). Involves a formal process to help settle disputes between Provincial and Territorial governments and Federal penalties for violations of the Canada Health Act.

Canada Health and Social Transfer (1996). Federal funding system which merged EPF transfers for health and post-secondary education with the Canada Assistance Plan.

cancer. Collective term used to describe a group of diseases characterized by uncontrolled cell growth and division or the loss of the cell to perform normal apoptosis. It is a neoplasm clinically characterized by uncontrolled cell growth of anaplastic cells which typically invade surrounding tissues and may also metastasize to other surrounding or distant tissues or organs in the body.

cardiovascular disease. Is defined as a class of diseases that involve the heart or blood vessels and include: coronary heart disease: disease of the blood vessels supplying the heart muscle; cerebrovascular disease which are disease of the blood vessels supplying the brain.

case control study. A non-experimental quantitative research design that seeks to compare and contrast a "case" (i.e., a person or patient with a specific diagnosis or condition under investigation) with a matched control (i.e., a person without the condition or diagnosis).

case study. An in-depth description and analysis of a single individual, patient or group presenting with a specific health related condition or phenomenon of interest.

chemical agents. Consist of a variety of chemicals, solvents and compounds (e.g., pharmaceuticals, acids, alkali compounds, heavy metals, poisons and some enzymes) that can result in the development of disease or alterations to health.

chemical toxicity. Occurs when a chemical agent or substance produces detrimental effects on living organisms in the environment, including humans.

chronic diseases. Are defined as those disorders or conditions which tend to be relatively less severe in nature but are continuous in duration, and which can last for long periods of time including an entire lifetime.

Chronic Obstructive Respiratory Disease (COPD). Is a chronic and progressive condition characterized by gradual airway obstruction, shortness of breath, cough and sputum production

Chronic Respiratory Diseases (CRDs). Are diseases of the airways and other parts of the lung that affect all ages and include asthma, chronic obstructive pulmonary disease (COPD), lung cancer, cystic fibrosis, sleep apnea and occupational lung diseases.

classification of disease. Consists of a standardized system and terminology used for the purposes of categorizing diseases by their clinical nature, and permits the statistical compilation of group of cases of disease by arranging disease entities into categories that share similar clinical manifestations.

climate change. Is defined as significant and dramatic changes in the frequency, intensity, spatial extent, duration, and timing of extreme weather (e.g., hurricanes, tornadoes) and climate associated events (e.g., draught, ice storms, flooding), which can result in unprecedented extreme weather and climatic events that threaten human societies, infra-structures, health and human survival.

clinical trial. A clinical study designed to assess the safety, efficacy and effectiveness of a new pharmaceutical agent, therapy or clinical intervention that involves 4 main phases: (i) Phase I: Occurs after the initial development of the medication or therapy and seeks to determine issues surrounding safety and tolerance; (ii) Phase II: Seeks preliminary evidence of related to the effectiveness and desirable clinical outcomes of the medication, therapy or clinical intervention; (iii) Phase III: Involves a full experimental test which seeks to determine efficacy and includes randomization of subjects and a control group and is often referred to a "randomized clinical trial (RCT)". The RCT is utilized to establish approval of the experimental medication, therapy or clinical intervention for use; and (iv) Phase IV involves long-term monitoring for unknown side effects and possible hazards related to the medication, therapy or intervention in general populations. This phase also seeks to determine the cost-effectiveness and clinical utility post approval.

cohort study. A quantitative trend or time-dimensional study that focuses on a specific subpopulation which is often an age-related subgroup from which different samples are selected at different points in time.

colonization. The process of establishing a colony or group of settlers in a new land or territory, whether previously inhabited or not, during which the settlers are either partially or fully subject to or accountable to their mother country of origin.

communicability of the disease. Is the ability of a disease to be transmitted from one individual to another or from one group or population to another.

communicable disease. Defined as an illness caused by a specific agent or its toxic products that arise through transmission of that agent or its products from an infected person, animal, or reservoir to a susceptible host, either directly or indirectly through an intermediate plant or animal host, vector, or the inanimate environment (Health Canada, 2003).

comprehensiveness. This criterion of the Canada Health Act declares that the specific provincial and territorial health care insurance plans must cover all insured health services provided by hospitals, physicians or dental surgeons performing necessary procedures in hospitals.

compulsions. Are defined as defined as repetitive actions, behaviours or mental acts that are difficult to resist or control by the individual, and which are often performed rigidly in response to an obsession in an attempt to prevent or reduce anxiety and stress.

concern for welfare. Is the second principle of the TCPS2 which addresses all aspects of an individual's life as well as the welfare of groups and communities, which requires a favourable balance between the actual or potential risks and benefits of the research investigation.

concussion. Is a type of brain injury caused by the brain moving inside of the skull which often causes damage and/or results in changes of how brain cells function leading to symptoms that can be physical (headaches, dizziness); cognitive (problems remembering or concentrating), and/ or emotional (feeling depressed) in nature.

congenital or familiar diseases. A group of diseases caused by familiar genetic tendencies by which particular traits or conditions are genetically transmitted from the parents to their offspring's.May also result due to injury to the fetus or embryo in utero caused by environmental, biological or chemical agents.

contact tracing. Is the process of identifying relevant contacts of a person with an infectious disease and ensuring that they are aware of their exposure and occurs in response to a communicable disease report made to a local health authority and consists of interviewing the infected individual regarding their social, work or professional contacts of people they may have come into contact with during the known incubation period of the disease.

coping. Is defined as an individual's cognitive and/or behavioural attempts and resources to manage specific physiological or emotional/ psychological stressors they are confronted with.

coping resources. Are defined as internal and external assets, characteristics, behaviours, problem solving skills and/or actions that can be employed by an individual to manage a stress response.

community. Is defined as a permeable collection of citizens who interact with each other and their environment, and who share common traits, culture, qualities, features, social structures, and/or geographical boundaries (i.e., specific neighbourhoods) (Hitchcock, Schubert, Thomas and Bartfay, 2010). Members of the community gain their personal and social identity by sharing common beliefs, values and norms which have been developed by the community in the past and may be modified in the future. They also exhibit some awareness of their identify as a group or collective, and share common needs and a commitment to meeting them (WHO, 1988).

community health. Is a discipline within public health which concerns itself with the study and improvement of the health characteristics of communities that tend to focus on geographical areas or boundaries, rather than on populations with shared characteristics (Goldman, Brunnell and Posner, 2014; WHO, 2004).

correlational study. A non-experimental quantitative study which seeks to examine the nature of relationships between two or more variables in a single clearly defined group or population.

cortisol. Also called hydrocortisone, is a primary corticosteroid secreted by the cortex of the adrenal gland that produces a number of physiological responses to the threat stressor such as increasing blood glucose levels, potentiating the action of epinephrine and norepinephrine on blood vessels and inhibiting inflammatory responses *in-vivo*.

Cottage Hospital Medical Care Plan (1934). This plan was developed by Newfoundland and Labrador and took into account the unique geography of the region.This plan provided out-port care by having registered nurses and physicians regularly visit remote communities by the sea.

critical infrastructures. Defined as physical or information technology facilities, networks, services, and/or assets that are deemed vital and essential for the health, safety or economic well-being of Canadians across the lifespan, and for the effective functioning of governments.

cross-sectional study. Are quantitative studies that involve the collection of data at one point in time to examine and describe the status of specific phenomena or relationships among phenomena from different age or developmental groups at a fixed point in time.

cultural safety. Is based on a broad definition of culture care and on the public health care professional's interpretations and analyses of their own cultural selves and the impact of these on providing health care, and requires the mutual empowerment of both the client and the public health care professional or worker.

cumulative Index. Is defined as the proportion of people who become diseased during a specified time period, and provides an estimate of the probability or risk that an individual will develop a disease or condition during this specified time period.

cytokines. Are soluble proteins or glycoprotein chemical messengers secreted by lymphocytes and help regulate and coordinate the immune responses.

degenerative disease. A disease or group of diseases characterized by the progressive deterioration of the structure or function of tissue, organ or body part over time and result in mental or physical alterations to function.

dementia. Is defined as a chronic and often progressive neurological disorder that results in a progressive deterioration of mental processes and is clinically characterized by memory disorders, personality and behavioural changes, emotional and mood disturbances, and impaired cognition, concentration, judgment and/or reasoning.

depression. Is a common type of mood disorder characterized by the loss of interest, feelings of sadness, melancholy, dejection, worthlessness, emptiness, hopelessness, changes to libido, appetite, sleep disturbances and other physical symptoms that are inappropriate and out of proportion to reality.

descriptive statistics. Are used to describe and synthesis data (e.g., means, medium, mode, ranges, percentages).

descriptive study. Studies that have as their main objectives the accurate portrayal and/or account of characteristics of persons; events, or groups in real-life situations in order to develop a better understanding of these as well as the frequency with which these phenomena occur.

descriptive epidemiology. Involves the identification, description, observation, measurement, interpretation, and dissemination of health related states, events, patterns, trends and/or injury differentials by person, place and time.

diabetes. Is a multisystem chronic disease related to abnormal hormone insulin production, and/or impaired insulin utilization, which results in abnormal metabolism of carbohydrates and elevated levels of glucose in the blood and urine.

disability. Is defined as any degree of physical infirmity, impairment, malformation or disfigurement that is caused by a bodily injury, birth defect, illness or disease that may be physical, cognitive, mental, sensory, emotional, developmental, or some combination of these.

discourse analysis. A qualitative research method that seeks to development an understanding of the rules, mechanisms, and structure of human communication and conversations.

disease. Is here defined as an interruption, cessation or disorder either mental or physical in nature that may arise from a single or combination of factors such as an infectious agent or a determinant of health (e.g., genetic predisposition, biochemical imbalance, lifestyle, environment) that is characterized by a recognizable set of clinical signs and symptoms.

distress. Is regarded as negative stress that consists of unpleasant situations or experiences (e.g., death of a loved one, job loss, loss of a home due to fire or a natural disaster, being diagnosed with a life threatening health condition).

dose-response. Is defined as a quantitative estimate between the relationship between a suspected chemical and the observed toxic effect (e.g., cancer slope factor or weight-of-the-evidence classification for carcinogenicity).

eating disorders. Are characterized by severe disturbances in perceptions of one's body shape, negative body image, unhealthy eating patterns and behaviours, and unhealthy efforts to control one's body weight and/or fat.

Ebola virus disease (EVB). Which is also called *ebola haemorrhagic fever* is a disease which affects humans and other primates, and is caused by the Ebola virus. EVB was first identified in 1976 in Nzara, South Sudan and in Yambuku, the Democractic Republic of Congo (formally Zaire). Signs and symptoms of EVB include high fever, sore throat, skin rash, muscle aches and pain, headaches, nausea and vomiting, diarrhea, and decreased liver and kidney function. Death is usually attributed to low blood pressure and severe loss of body fluids or blood.

ecological psychology. A qualitative research method that seeks to development an understanding of the environment's influence on human behaviour and attempts to identify principles that explain the interdependence of humans and their environmental context.

ecosystem. Is defined as a local or regional community or area of living organisms which include humans and other animals, plants and microorganisms and the physical settings in which they occupy and live within.

editing analysis style. The qualitative researcher acts as an interpreter who critically reads and examines the subjective data in an attempt to discover meaningful segments or categorization schemes that can be subsequently employed to sort and organize the data. The researcher then searches for emerging patterns and structures.

embolic stroke. Is cause by an embolus (i.e., wondering blood clot) that is carried in the blood stream and may become wedged in a cerebral artery

emergencies act. Replaced the War Measures Act as the source of the federal's government's authority to act during a national crisis or emergency to ensure the safety and security of all Canadians.

Emergency Management. Is defined as a critical component of all public health systems in Canada and abroad which involves a diverse group of highly skilled professionals and government officials to protect the health and safety of the public at large during a crisis or emergency that requires immediate and coordinated action.

Emergency Management Act. Which defines the specific roles and responsibilities for all federal ministers, and provides direction for critical infrastructure protection which is a major challenge during a major disaster or national emergency (Ministry of Justice, 2014c). This Act also replaces specific sections of the Emergency Preparedness Act and enhances and promotes communication and information exchange between various levels of government.

Emergency Preparedness Act. Which provides a basis for the planning and programming to deal with disasters, and addresses the need for co-operation between the provinces and territories and the federal government. This Act also addresses the need for public awareness, and provides a structure or legislative framework for the necessary training and education of public health professionals and workers and first responders to disasters and emergencies (Ministry of Justice, 2014b).

emerging infectious diseases. Are defined as one that has appeared in a population for the first time, or that may have existed previously but is rapidly increasing in incidence or geographic range.

emotion focused coping. Involves positively managing and dealing with the emotions that arise when a stressful life event occurs.

Employment and Social Insurance Act (1935). R.B. Bennett proposed that the federal government collect taxes in order to fund certain Canada-wide social benefits, including health. This was rejected by the provinces and in 1937; the British Privy council ruled the proposal was ultra vires.

endemics. Are defined as those diseases or illnesses which tend to always be present at low levels in populations in a defined geographical area or region (e.g., Chicken Pox, seasonal influenza).

end-of-life care (EOLC). Is a term used to describe care provided in the last days or weeks of life (Subcommittee of the Standing Senate Committee on Social Affairs, Science and Technology, 2000).

environment. Is more than one's physical or geographical location, but is currently regarded as a critical social determinant of health that consists of interdependent and interconnected components of one's physical, biochemical, social-political, cultural and spiritual milieus and situations.

environmental health. Is defined as a branch of public health which examines both positive and negative factors and influences in the environment and ecosystem on human health.

environmental and occupational risk assessment for public health. Is here defined as a formalized process for characterizing and estimating the impact or magnitude of harm to human health and/or damage to natural or artificial ecosystems resulting from exposure to one or more hazardous chemicals or substances on a specific target population or community, and are intended to provide objective information to help establish or inform public health policy and planning decisions.

epidemic. A number of cases of an infectious agent or disease (outbreak) which is clearly in excess of the normally expected frequency of that disease in a defined population.

epidemiology. Is defined as the scientific study of the distribution and determinants of health-related states or events in human populations across the lifespan and the application of this study to maintain, control and prevent alterations to health and well-being.

epp report (1986). Expanded on Mark Lalonde's (1974) definition of health promotion by including the tenets of primary care, and by refining the role of various broad socio-political and environmental determinants of health. This Framework also cautioned about *"blaming the victim"*, and denounced strategies that concentrated on the individual solely (e.g., lifestyle) without consideration for these broad aforementioned determinates of health.

eradication. Is defined and achieved when there is no risk of infection or disease globally even in the absence of immunization and/or other public health disease control measures, and when the agent is no longer present in nature.

ethnographic research. A qualitative anthropological research method that seeks to study the evolution, meanings, patterns and experiences of a defined cultural group in a holistic fashion, and which seeks to develop conceptual models and theories of cultural behaviour.

ethnomethodology. A qualitative research method that seeks to develop a better understanding of how individuals make sense of everyday activities, their social group's norms and assumptions,and how they interpret their social world to behave in socially acceptable ways.

ethology. Is a qualitative research method that seeks to develop a better understanding of human behaviour as it evolves in its natural setting or context.

etiology. Is the scientific study of all known and suspected risk factors, causes and/or social determinants of health that may be involved with the development of a health-related state, event or condition and includes the susceptibility of the individual and the nature of disease agents.

eukaryote organisms. Have a complex cell or cells that have a membrane-bound nucleus and include fungi, plants and animals.

eustress. Is regarded as positive stress that presents the opportunity for personal growth, satisfaction and new and desirable life experiences (e.g., getting married, starting university, learning a new language or musical instrument, beginning a new career).

evidence. Includes, but is no limited to, published quantitative and qualitative research reports from a variety of disciplines; current best-practice guidelines; legislations and policies, observations and experiences, and both expert and lay opinions and perspectives for all stakeholders concerned.

evidence-based medicine (EBM). Is defined as the conscientious, explicit, and judicious use of current best evidence in making decisions about the care of individual patients, and the practice of EBM means integrating individual clinical expertise with the best available external evidence from research studies.

evidence based practice. Involves the critical appraisal and utilization of current and sound scientific research and data to develop health policies, determine health outcomes and trends in diverse populations across the lifespan, and evaluate the effectiveness of public health care initiatives and interventions.

evidence-informed public health (EIPH). Is the process of distilling and disseminating the best available evidence from research, practice and experience and using that evidence to inform and improve public health policy and practice (National Collaborating Centres for Public Health (2011, p.1).

experimental study. A study in which the investigator intentionally manipulates the independent variable; randomly assigns subjects to either experimental (treatment or intervention) group and to control groups (do not receive treatment or intervention), and controls for experimental conditions in an attempt to decrease the possibility of error and increase the probability that the study's findings are an accurate reflection of reality. Hence, all true or classical experiments must have the following 3 conditions present: (i) random assignment; (ii) manipulation, and (iii) control.

fecal/oral transmission. Of an infectious microorganism or pathogen can occur directly by physical contact with hands or other contaminated objects with organisms from human or animal feces and then placed in the mouth (Jo Damazo and Bartfay, 2010).

Federal-Provincial Fiscal Arrangement and Established Programs Financing Act (1977). This Act altered the previous 50/50 cost sharing formula and replaced it with a per capita block grant.

fight-fight-or-freeze response. Describes how an individual ultimately reacts to a threat stressor.

first Nations. Refers to peoples who occupied land prior to the arrival of European explorers and colonizers, and is a term that is generally used to refer to Indians in Canada.

follow-up study. A quantitative study undertaken to determine the outcomes of individuals or groups with a specified condition, diagnosis or who have received a specified treatment, therapy or intervention.

gender. Is defined as the array of socially, politically and/or culturally constructed roles, relationships, attitudes, personality traits and characteristics, behaviours, values and power structures between males and females.

general adaptation syndrome model. Developed by Selye (1974, 1983) describes how the human body moves through three stages when confronted by stressors: (i) alarm reaction; (ii) resistance, and (iii) exhaustion.

generalized anxiety disorder (GAD). Is defined as a psychological disorder that can affect both children and adults and is characterized by a chronic and exaggerated anxiety, tension and/or worry about an impending disaster related to some aspect of life or daily living, which may include work or career matters, social relationships, and/or financial matters even when, in fact, nothing seems to be provoking it (APA, 2013; Statistics Canada, 2015c).

geometric mean. Is a type of average that is less influenced by extreme values, in comparison to the traditional arithmetic mean and provides a better estimate of central tendency for highly skewed data, and is a common measure employed in the measurement of environmental chemicals found in human blood or urine (Statistics Canada, 2011c).

gestational diabetes. Is defined as any degree of glucose intolerance with onset or first recognition occurring during pregnancy; and is clinically employed whether insulin or only diet modification is used for treatment, and whether or not the condition persists after pregnancy.

gini index. Is a measure of the inequality in the distribution of incomes within a given country (Jacobsen, 2008). A country with a Gini Index of zero (0 or perfect equality) means that everyone in that country has the same income, whereas an index of 100 would indicate perfect inequality.

glascow coma scale (GCS). Is a relatively quick, practical and standardized neurological scale widely employed around the world for assessing the degree to which consciousness is impaired via 3 main clinical indicators: (i) best eye opening response; (ii) best verbal response, and (iii) best motor response. Grading = Severe head injury/ trauma, GCS < 8–9; Moderate head injury/ trauma, GCS 8 or 9–12, and Minor head injury or trauma, GCS ≥ 13.

global warming. Is defined as the increase in the earth's overall temperature as a result of both human and natural causes including greenhouse gas emissions through carbon-based fuel combustion, industrial pollution, depletion of the protective ozone layer, deforestations and volcanic emissions into the atmosphere.

greenhouse effect. Is defined as the trapping of infrared radiation from the earth by greenhouse gases in the earth's atmosphere, which results in the warming of the surface temperature of the earth.

grey matter. A component of the brain that contains the cells bodies that are responsible for voluntary motor neurons and preganglionic autonomic motor neurons, along with cells bodies for association neurons (internerons).

grounded theory. An inductive qualitative research approach based on symbolic interaction theory that seeks to discover the meaning of problems that exist in a real-life social context and the process that individuals employ to handle them, and it also involves the formulation and redevelopment of propositions until a theory is developed.

health. Health is not a single state or goal, but a process that involves various interconnected and interdependent factors and dynamic states of existence across the lifespan. Health is not a single lineal destination. It is a dynamic and complex interactive journey through one's physical, biochemical, social-political, cultural and spiritual environments. The ability to identify and to realize aspirations, to satisfy needs, and to change or cope with the environment. Health is therefore a resource for everyday life, not the objective of living. Health is a positive concept emphasizing social and personal resources, as well as physical capacities (Canadian Public Health Association and WHO, 1986, p. 426).

health behaviours. Those behaviours exhibited by persons that affect their health either positively (e.g., exercise) or negatively (e.g., smoking), which may be consciously selected, although unconscious needs may thwart the individual's ability to carry-out conscious intentions.

health care system. Is a collective term employed to describe all the health care services (e.g., client education, consultations, conducting clinical assessments, surgery) provided by health care professionals (e.g., physicians, nurses, dieticians, dentists) in a variety of clinical and community-based settings (e.g., community clinics, school-based immunization programs, stroke rehabilitation units, emergency rooms, surgical clinics).

health determinant. A factor or known variable or lifestyle that helps to either create or diminish states of health and well-being across the lifespan.

health indicators. Are measures of health and factors that can affect health and are employed to measure, monitor, and compare important factors that influence the health of Canadians across the lifespan and health care systems (Health Council of Canada, 2011).

health promotion. Activities or interventions that identify the risk factors associated to disease; the lifestyle changes related to disease and illness prevention; the process of enabling individuals, families, groups or entire communities to increase their control over and improve their health; these activities and strategies are directed toward developing resources of clients to maintain or enhance their physical, social, emotional and spiritual well-being.

health protection. A term used to describe important activities of public health, in food hygiene, water purification, environmental sanitation, drug safety and other activities that eliminate as far as possible the risk of adverse consequences to health attributable to environmental protection (PHAC, 2007, p. 12).

Health-related Quality of Life (HRQOL). Is a multi-dimensional concept that includes domains related to physical, mental, emotional, and social functioning. This concept goes beyond direct measures of population health, life expectancy, and causes of death, and focuses on the impact health status has on overall quality of life.

health surveillance. Is defined as "the tracking and forecasting of any health event or health determinant through the continuous collection of high-quality data, the integration, analysis and interpretation of those data into reports, advisories, alerts, and warnings, and the dissemination to those who need to know" (Kirby, 2003, p. 26).

health system. Encompasses a broader concept which is defined as all activities whose primary purpose is to promote, restore and/or maintain health across the lifespan.

helminthes. Are endoparasitic worms that live inside the body of a host human or animal (e.g., pinworms, hookworms, flatworms, roundworms, tapeworms).

herd immunity. Is based on the notion that if a significant percentage (e.g., 80%) of a given population has been immunized against an infectious agent, this can protect the whole population, including the non-immunized individuals, by severely limiting its ability to spread.

hermeneutics. A qualitative research approach which utilizes interpretive phenomenology to develop a better understanding of the lived experiences of humans and how they interpret those experiences in the social, cultural, political and/or historical context.

herpetophobia. Is the the general fear (or phobia) of reptiles and/or amphibians.

historical research. Is a qualitative research approach that seeks to systematically discover and critically analyze remote or recent past events, causes or trends and to shed light on present behaviours, practices or phenomenon.

holism. This concept incorporates an emphasis on the interconnectedness between the mind, body, spirit, culture, and environments.

holistic health. Health from this perspective directly challenges the mechanistic biomedical model which asserts that ill health results from a biological breakdown of a component of the human body that results from disease. Although there are numerous definitions of health based on this perspective, the most widely utilized and quoted definition is the WHO definitions (1948, 1986).

holistic health paradigm. Incorporates the belief that human beings are more than the sum of their mind and body parts, but are dynamic and interrelated wholes that include their mind, body, spirit, culture, and environments.

homogeneity. Refers to the degree to which subjects in the study are similar, equivalent or consistent in nature with respect to the extraneous variables included in the study.

Hospital Insurance and Diagnostic Services Act (1957). The federal government agreed to reimburse provinces for a portion of the costs associated with providing health care insurance.

horizontal transmission. Involves the direct transport of an infectious agent or pathogen from person-to-person.

hospice. Is a concept of care that provides compassion, concern and support for dying clients and their families.

host. Refers to the animal and/or human on which the agent acts to create disease or altered states of health and well-being.

huntington's disease. Is defined as a genetically transmitted autosomal dominant disorder that affects both men and women equally, and is characterized by chronic, devastating loss of all neurological functions resulting in dementia.

hyperglycaemia. (i.e., elevated blood glucose levels) is a common manifestation of uncontrolled diabetes; which over time can lead to serious damage to many of the body's systems, especially the nerves and blood vessels.

hypertension. Also known as high blood pressure (HBP), is defined as a sustained elevation of systemic arterial blood pressure and if often a chronic condition.

hypoglycaemia (i.e., low blood glucose levels) occurs when there is too much insulin in proportion to the available circulating blood glucose (i.e., <4 nmol/L), and often results from a mismatch in the timing of food intake and the peak action of insulin or OHAs that increase endogenous insulin secretion.

hypothesis. Is a prediction statement made by the researcher regarding the expected relationships between two or more variables.

iatrogenic. Literately means "doctor generated", but it's definition has been expanded to include all adverse effects associated with diagnostic procedures; medical, surgical, nursing or other allied health interventions, and the over prescription of medications.

impaired glucose tolerance (IGT) and impaired fasting glycaemia (IFG). Are intermediate conditions that are regarded in transition between normality and diabetes.

incident command system (ICS). Is a management system that is employed by first responders for on-site emergencies and consists of a formalized command structure with specific areas of responsibility assigned to individuals as needed.

incident management system (IMS). Is a standardized function-driven model employed throughout North America to manage and response to emergencies, crisis and disasters, and provides the framework for all levels of government in Canada to develop emergency response plans regardless of the nature of the incident or its level of complexity. The basis IMS structure consists of five components: (i) Command; (ii) operations; (iii) planning; (iv) logistics, and (v) finance and administration.

incubation period. Is defined as the time that elapses between inoculation and infection by a pathogen in the host and the appearance of the first clinical signs or symptoms of the disease.

infection. Is defined as an invasion of the body caused by a pathogen (e.g., bacteria, viruses, fungi, protozoa, prion) that results in specific signs and symptoms that develop in response to the pathogen which may be localized or systemic in nature.

injury. Is defined as an act, either intentional or unintentional in nature that results in a wound, damage and/or trauma to an individual.

illness. Is defined as a subjective or psychological state experienced by an individual who feels aware of not being well or their experience with a disease, and it is a social construct fashioned out of transactions between health care professionals and affected individuals in the context of their common culture (Porter, 2008).

immersion/crystallization style. Is a subjective and interpretive style that requires the total immersion and reflection of the text materials, which eventually leads to an intuitive crystallization of the data.

immune system. Is defined as a complex system that is responsible for distinguishing a host from everything foreign and for protecting the body against a host of infectious agents and foreign substances.

immunological competence. Is defined as the body's ability to defend itself against pathogens and includes factors such as age, heredity, temperature, nutritional status, presence of other diseases (e.g., diabetes, AIDS, Cooley's anemia) and environmental conditions.

immunity. Is defined as the specific amount of resistance to disease by an individual.

incidence. Quantifies the number of new events or cases of a disease or condition that develop in a population of individuals at risk during a specified time period.

incidence rate or incidence density (ID). Determines the impact of exposure in a defined population and is a measure of the instantaneous rate of development of a disease or condition in a population.

indian. Is both acquired via a birth status who is born to First Nations parents, and legislated by the Canadian Indian Act of 1876.

Indian Act of 1867. First to define who First Nation (Indian) was versus those who were note. This Act also provided a vehicle to legislate over First Nation's peoples and the lands reserved for them.

indian agents. Were hired by the Department of Indian Affairs (DINA) and were responsible for enforcing and carry-out the specific terms of the treaties signed nationally.

infectious agents. Are defined as pathogens that can lead to the development of a disease and include bacteria, fungi, viruses (e.g., West Nile virus), metazoan (e.g., hookworm) and protozoa (e.g., malaria).

inferential statistics. Are based on the laws of probability and provide a means for drawing conclusions about a population based on quantitative data derived from a sample.

inflammatory response. Occurs when the body in injured or infected resulting in the release of histamine and other substances that cause blood vessels to dilate and fluid to flow-out of capillaries into the surrounding tissue.

injury. Is defined as an act, either intentional or unintentional in nature that results in hurt, damage and/or trauma to an individual.

interval/continuous data. There is a specified rank ordering on a defined attribute and the distance between those objects are assumed to be equivalent in nature along a continuum, but there is no true zero.

inuit. Refers to Aboriginal peoples who are distinct from Indians, but are treated in the same manner as registered Indians by the Federal Government in Canada. The term Inuit has replaced the former term "Eskimo" which is regarded as offensive by some individuals because of its connotation with the descriptor "eaters-of-raw-meat."

ischemic heart disease. Is a chronic condition in which the heart muscle is damaged or works inefficiently because of the absence or relative deficiency of its blood supply.

isolation. Is defined as the separation of an infectious individual for defined period of time (e.g., 30 days) to prevent or limit the direct or indirect transmission of an infectious agent.

Jakarta Declaration of Health Promotion (1997). Advanced the notion that various prerequisites for health were required including inter alia: peace, shelter; education; social security and relations; income, nutrition; sustainable resources and ecosystems; social justice, and respect for human rights including equality and the empowerment of women.

justice. Is the third principle of the TCPS2 which requires that individual's be treated fairly and equitably, so that no specific group, community or segment of the population bears an undue burden of risk associated with the study, and no part of society at large is excluded from the potential benefits that the research study may bestow.

knowledge utilization. Relates to the process for formally applying and utilizing research findings to guide EIPH in the public and health care sciences.

lalonde report (1974). Was the first strategic policy directive related to health promotion as a critical component for our publicly funded health care system in Canada. It outlined four critical elements that determine the health of Canadians: (i) human biology; (ii) environment; (iii) lifestyle, and (iv) the health care organization.

levels of prevention. A five-level model of intervention (primordial, primary, secondary, tertiary and quarternary) used in the epidemiological approach and which is designed to prevent, halt and/or reverse the process of pathological change as early as possible in order to prevent damage.

listeria. A potentially life threatening food-borne illness caused by the bacteria *Listeria monocytogenese* which may be present in the soil, vegetation, water and/or processed meats including deli cold cuts, hot dogs, soft cheeses, raw meat and unpasteurized milk products.

lyme disease. Is a multisystem infection that is manifested by progressive stages and is caused by the spirochete *Borrelia burgdorferi* sensu stricto transmitted by blacklegged deer ticks.

matching. Involves the deliberate pairing of subjects in one group with those in another comparison group based on their similarity on one or more diagnosis, characteristic, trait or dimension in order to enhance the comparability of groups.

measures of association. Are defined as statistical measures used to investigate the degree of dependence between two or more events or variables.

Medical Care Act (1966). This Act and HIDSA collectively established a formula for federal transfer payments to the provinces' to cover the cost of public health insurance plans utilizing a formula of 50 cents to the dollar.

medical model of health. This perspective of health comprehends the human body as a contraption or apparatus, in which all the components or parts or interconnected, but are capable of being separated and therefore individually treated by specialists (e.g., cardiologists treats the malfunctioning heart; nephrologists treat malfunctioning kidneys, etc.). Health is achieved when all the biological (machine) components of the body function properly.

medicare. A collective term to refer to Canada's publicly administered and funded national health care insurance systems.

medicine wheel. Is regarded as a powerful and sacred symbol of the universe depicting the circularity of life and encourages the balance between us through the four aspects of self: (i) physical; (ii) mental; (iii) emotional, and (iv) spiritual.

mental health. Is defined the capacity of each and all of us to feel, think, and act in ways that enhance our ability to enjoy life and deal with the challenges we face (PHAC, 2006 & 2012). Is further defined as a state of well-being in which every individual realizes his or her own potential, can cope with the normal stresses of life, can work productively and fruitfully, and is able to make a contribution to her or his community (WHO, 2014).

meta-analysis. Is a statistical technique for integrating and pooling completed and published numerical (quantitative) research findings on a select topic or area of inquiry, and treats the findings as a single summary piece of information.

metabolic diseases. Are caused when glands or organs in the body fail to maintain or secrete adequate amounts of hormones or other biochemical's necessary to maintain homeostasis and result in dysfunction or malfunction of certain organs, physiologic or metabolic processes that result in disease states.

meta-summaries. Are interpretative summaries of primary qualitative research investigations that provide a synthesis of these studies to produce a narrative about selected phenomenon or a specific topic.

meta-synthesis. Is a scholarly synthesis of primary qualitative research studies and is conducted to provide a critical analysis and synthesis of the collective findings into a new conceptual model, framework or theory on a select topic or problem of interest.

métis. Are individuals born of marriages between Aboriginal and non-Aboriginal parents. They are legally considered the same as non-status Indians in Canada.

mixed methods (hybrid) research. Consists of a blending of both qualitative and quantitative approaches and methods.

mode of disease transmission. Is defined as the mechanism or means by which an infectious agent or pathogen is transferred from an infected or diseased host to an uninfected and susceptible non-immunized host.

mode of transmission. Is the fourth required link in the chain of infection and refers to the way the pathogen is passed from a reservoir to a susceptible host, and involve two principle methods: (i) Direct transmission, and (ii) indirect transmission.

mood disorder. Is defined as an emotional disturbance that is intense and persistent enough in nature to affect normal daily functions and routines.

morbidity rate. Is defined as the incidence of non-fatal cases of a disease or health condition in the total population at risk during a specified point in time.

mortality rate. Is defined as the incidence of death in a defined population during a specified period of time and is calculated by dividing the total number of fatalities (deaths) during that period by the total population.

multiple sclerosis (MS). Is defined as a chronic and progressive degenerative autoimmune disorder of the CNS characterized by disseminated and demyelination of nerve fibres of the brain, spinal cord, and optic nerves and inflammation and gliosis (scarring) in the CNS.

myasthenia gravis (MG). Is defined as a chronic disease of the neuromuscular junction in which an autoimmune process slowly destroys acetylcholine (ACh) receptors at the postsynaptic muscle, and is characterized by fatigability and fluctuating muscle weakness of selected voluntary muscle distribution, especially those innervated by motor nuclei of the brain stem (e.g., extraocular, mastication, facial, swallowing and speech).

National Ambient Air Quality Objectives" (NAAQOs). Are dynamic national goals for improving outdoor air quality and reducing air pollution.

national emergency. Defined by the Emergencies Act of Canada as "an urgent and critical situation of a temporary nature that seriouslyendangers the lives, health or safety of Canadians and is of such proprotions or nature as to exceed the capacity of a province to deal with it, or seriously threatens the sovereignty, security and territorial integrity of Canada, and cannot be effectively dealth with under any other law of Canada" (Ministry of Justice, 2014a, p. 8).

National Health Grants Act (1948). Marked the beginning of the federal government's role in partially subsiding public provincial and territorial health care systems via taxed-based funds.

natural history of a disease. Is defined as the unaltered course that a disease would take without any intervention such as therapy or lifestyle changes…[and] can be understood by viewing the concept as a continuum, with exposure to the agent suspected of causing the disease or condition at one end, through the development of signs and symptoms of illness in a progression of severity, to the ultimate outcome of the disease, whether that be disability or death, at the other end.

natural immunity. Is defined as an innate resistance to a specific antigen or toxin by the individual that results from the development of antibodies as a result of the host's having acquired the primary infection and which protects against acquiring subsequent infections by the same toxin or antigen.

nervous system. Is a highly complex and specialized system responsible for the control and integration of the body's many functions and activities, and consists of two main divisions: (i) Central nervous system (CNS), and (ii) peripheral nervous system (PNS).

neurological disorders. Are defined as diseases of the central and peripheral nervous system, which include the brain, spinal cord, cranial nerves, peripheral nerves, nerve roots, autonomic nervous system, neuromuscular junction, and muscles (WHO, 2016).

nomenclature. Is defined as a set of highly detailed and precise collection or set of terms that are utilized by public health professionals and workers for both recording and describing clinical diagnoses for the purposes of classifying ill persons into defined groups.

nominal/continuous data. The lowest level of measurement which involves the assignment of characteristics into mutually exclusive and collectively exhaustive categories.

nomophobia. The fear of being without a mobile phone or device; being beyond contact, or not being able to be in contact with or be connected to a mobile telecommunications provider

noncommunicable diseases (NCDs). Is defined as a chronic disease not typically caused by an infectious agent (i.e., non-infectious or non-communicable) that often has complex etiologies, has an insidious onset, often characterized by multiple associated risk factors, long latency periods and is normally incurable in nature.

non-status indian. Recognized as First Nations person, but the tribe to which they belong did not sign a treaty to become registered per se.

non-therapeutic research. Is conducted to generate new knowledge about an intervention, therapy or treatment. However, it will unlikely benefit the subject/ patient partaking in the investigation, but may benefit future subjects or patients.

norepinephrine. Which is also known as noradrenaline, is a neurotransmitter released by the sympathetic division and targets specific tissues (e.g., muscles) and organs (e.g., heart) to enable the individual to quickly handle situation, and it also increases alertness, awareness and attention.

nunavut. Was formally established and recognized as a territory in 1999, and is located in the Eastern Arctic region of Canada.

nutritive agents. Consists of nutritional substances that are deficient or excessive within a host.

obsessions. Are defined as unwanted thoughts or impulses.

Obsessive Compulsive Disorder (OCD). Is characterized by obsessions or compulsions that are recurrent and persistent in nature, and thoughts that are intrusive and inappropriate and result in high levels of anxiety and/or distress (APA, 2013; Statistics Canada, 2015c).

occupational health and safety. Is a branch or subspecialty of public health which examines both positive and negative health outcomes that are influenced or associated with exposure to general work conditions and/or specific known hazards that are encountered in work environments, and which seeks to preserve, promote and/or restore the health and safety of workers.

odds ratio. Is typically calculated for case-control studies and provides a measure of the strength of the association between exposure and the disease or health condition under investigation.

ordinal/ranked data. Attributes are ordered according to a defined criterion which captures information about equivalence and its relative rank. However, they do not inform us about how much greater one rank or category is in comparison to the other.

ophidiophobia (or ophiophobia). Is a specific phobia associated with the abnormal fear of both venemous and non-venemous snakes.

Ottawa Charter of Health Promotion (1986). Health was viewed as a resource for the first time and it directly challenged the medical model of health. The Charter outlined five broad strategies for global health promotion: (i) Build healthy public policies; (ii) create supportive environments; (iii) strengthen community action; (iv) develop personal skills, and (v) re-orientate health services.

outcomes research. Research designed to critically and objectively examine and document the effectiveness of health care policies and services and the end results of patient care.

palliative care. Is an approach that seeks to improve the quality of life of for client's and their families facing problems associated with life-threatening illness, through the prevention and relief of suffering by means of early identification and impeccable assessment and treatment of pain and other problems, physical, psychosocial and spiritual. (WHO, 2018).

pandemic. Is defined as a massive epidemic that involves populations in widespread geographic areas or regions of the world (e.g., HIV/AIDS, SARS).

panic attack. Is defined as a sudden and intense acute form of anxiety that often results in intense disabling physical reactions and feeling of dread or terror.

panic disorder. Is defined as a syndrome of severe surges in anxiety, accompanied by physical symptoms such as tachycardia, shortness of breath, loss of physical balance or equilibrium, and a feeling of losing mental control.

panel study. Are similar to follow-up studies, however the same individuals, patients or group of people (i.e., the panel) are employed to examine changes related to data, clinical outcomes and/or phenomenon at two or more points in time.

paradigm. Is defined as a specific worldview or perspective; way of thinking, and/or methodology of practice in the health sciences.

parasites. Are defined as eukaryotic organisms that are capable of causing illness or disability and survive by living off a host (animal or human).

parkinson disease (PD). Is defined a progressive neurodegenerative disease of the CNS (basal ganglia) characterized by a constellation of clinical manifestations including a slowing down in the initiation and execution of movement (bradykinesia), increase muscle tone rigidity, mild tremors at rest, slowness of movement, and impaired and decreased balance, muscle coordination and postural reflexes.

passive surveillance. Is defined as the notification of health authorities by public health care professionals of individuals who have clinical signs and symptoms, and this relies on laboratory tests for confirmation of the diagnosis of the disease on the reportable disease list for the respective province or territory in Canada.

pathogen. Is defined as any microorganism (e.g., virus, bacteria) or other matter (e.g., prion) that can cause disease in humans or animals and/ or result in a morbid process or state.

peripheral nervous system. Consists of cranial nerves III through XII, the spinal nerves, their associated ganglia (groupings of cell bodies) and the peripheral components of the autonomic nervous system (ANS).

personality. Is defined as the sum of all cognitive, behavioural and emotional tendencies of a specific individualthat are formed and developed over-time due to personal memories, social relationships, interactions with one's environment (i.e., physical, social, environmental, occupational), values, attitudes, habits and skill sets.

personality trait. Refers to enduring personal characteristics that are revealed in particular patterns of behaviour in a variety of social situations and interactions.

pesticides. Include various biochemical classes of agents and substances that are employed for killing or destroying insects or other organism harmful to plant species or animals and include insecticides, herbicides, fungicides, rodenticides, algaecides, and slimicides.

phenomenology. An inductive and descriptive qualitative research approach that seeks to describe and develop a better understanding of the lived experiences of humans.

phobia. Is a profound and persistent fear of a specific object, event, activity, or situation that results in a compelling desire to avoid that specific source of fear. Phobias are reported to be more prevalent in women than in men.

physical agents. Include natural forces, forms of energy or mechanical agents that may negatively affect the health and well-being of humans (e.g., radiation, excessive exposure to ultraviolet waves, excessive heat or noise).

population-attributable risk (PAR). Provides a measure of a disease or health condition in a population attributed to the exposure, and is typically expressed per 10^n.

population-attributable risk percent (PAR%). Provides a measure of the percentage of the disease or health condition in the population that can be attributed to the exposure.

portal of entry. Where pathogenic agents enter the bodies of susceptible hosts.

portal of exit. The third required link on the chain of infection where pathogenic agents leave their reservoirs, and include the blood, and urinary, respiratory, reproductive, and/or digestive systems.

Post-Traumatic Stress Disorder (PTSD). Is a disorder caused by a traumatic event that is outside the normal realm of human experience, such as rape, assault, torture, being kidnapped or held captive, military combat, severe car accidents, and natural or manmade disasters that results in emotional and/or social impairments due to anxiety, depression, recurrent flashbacks, difficulty sleeping and concentrating, and feelings of guilt of having survived when others may not have (APA, 2013; Statistics Canada, 2015c).

portability. This criteria of the Canada Health Act declares that residents must continue to be covered who are temporarily out of province or territory, and also applies to individuals who have moved to another region and are required to undergo a waiting period in this new region.

prediabetes. Which is also known as *impaired glucose tolerance* (IGT) and *impaired fasting glucose* (IFG), occurs when a client's fasting or a 2-hour plasma glucose level is higher than normal, but lower than is considered necessary for a diagnosis of diabetes.

prevalence. Is defined as the proportion (percentage) of individuals in a given population who have the disease or altered states of health at a given point in time, and provides an estimate of the probability (or risk) that an individual will be ill at a stated point in time.

prevention. Is defined as actions, measures, interventions, programs, policies and/or legislations which seek to avert the development or progression of disease or possible harm, injury, disability, or death and improve, maintain and/or restore health related quality of life across the lifespan.

primary care. Is what an individual receives when they visit their health care provider for advice or treatment of a disorder or aliment.

primary health care approach. Is defined as a model of health care that emphasizes equity, accessibility, full participation by individuals and communities, the use of universally acceptable and affordable technologies and methods, intersectoral collaboration,and is based on practical, scientifically sound and socially acceptable health care approaches and interventions which embrace the following five types of health care: (i) Promotive; (ii) preventive; (iii) curative; (iv) rehabilitative, and (v) supportive/ palliative.

primary health care model. This model addresses the social-determinants of health and its services are centred on defined principles and values, and includehealth care services that are equitable, accessible, collaborative in nature, and based the use of appropriate technologies and methods.

primary prevention. Consists of preventative approaches and interventions that seek to avert the occurrence of alterations to health. For example, immunization of a child with the measles, mumps and rubella (MMR) vaccine.

primordial prevention. Consists of conditions, actions, and measures that minimize hazards to health and that inhibit the emergence and establishment of process and factors known to increase disease, alterations to health, injury, and/or death.

prion. Is defined as a self-replicating, protein-based pathogenic agent that can infect humans and animals.

private. Refers to out-of-pocket health care services paid for by an individual or private insurance plan or benefit (e.g., employee health benefits).

privately funded. Refers to *out-of-pocket* health care services that are paid for by an individual and/or private insurance plan or benefit (e.g., employee health benefits).

probiotics. Are defined as living microorganisms (e.g., bacteria) which when administered in adequate amounts confer a positive health benefit to the host.

program planning. Is defined as an organized and structured systematic decision-making process which attempts to meet specific primary health care aims or objectives through the application of currently available, and competing or needed resources in the future based on identified priorities or projected needs.

prospective design study. A quantitative study design that commences with an examination of presumed causes or independent variables (e.g., inactivity, obesity, high levels of low density lipoproteins (LDLs) and then goes forward in time to observe the presumed effects of these on the dependent variable which may include clinical outcomes, diagnosis or conditions (e.g., cardiovascular disease).

psychoanalysis. Is defined as a theory first developed by Sigmund Freud during the 1890s and is a form of therapy that seeks to treat mental health disorders by analyzing the interaction of conscious and unconscious elements in the mind and bringing repressed fears and conflicts into the conscious mind.

psychoanalytic techniques. Includes the interpretations of dreams and free association treatment sessions during which the client is encouraged to talk freely about personal experiences, and especially about early childhood conflicts.

psychotherapy. Also known as "talk therapy", is defined as a process whereby mental health issues and concerns are treated through communication and relationship factors between a client and a trained mental health professional.

psychoneuroimmunology (PNI). Is a current field of research examining the interactions and critical relationships between the nervous, endocrine and immune systems.

public. A term employed to denote health care services that are funded primarily via legislated tax-based or derived funds and processes.

public administration. This criterion of the Canada Health Act declares that health care is the responsibility of territorial and provincial governments, and therefore must be subject to regular public audits of how it is administered.

publicly funded. Refers to a taxed-based system to support health care services rendered in public hospitals, community clinics or institutions in Canada.

public health. A holistic and evidence-informed discipline that seeks to promote, maintain and/or restore the health and the quality of life of individuals, families, communities and/or entire populations over the lifespan through health promotion and prevention and various primary health care initiatives, activities, policies and/or legislations. It is also the art and science of "persuasion" for advancing and promoting the health of society at large.

public health professionals. Include physicians, nurses, public health inspectors, health promoters, epidemiologists, nutritionist and dentist.

public health workers. Are regional or community-based health advocates who seek to promote health and well-being in its broadest form.

puerperal fever. Also known as *"childbed fever"* is a syndrome associated with a systemic bacterial infection and septicemia that occurs after childbirth and usually results from unsterile obstetrical techniques and/or contaminated instruments. It is characterized by endometritis, high fever, tachycardia, uterine tenderness, foul lochia and may result in bacteremic shock and mortality.

purging behaviours. Include self-induced vomiting, misuse of laxatives or diet pills, diuretics and/or enemas and excessive amounts of exercise to combat weight gain.

quasi-experimental design study. An intervention-based study with a control group, however the subjects or comparative groups (e.g., schools, communities, regions, etc.) are not randomly assigned to treatment conditions.

quaternary prevention. Consists of a group of actions and measures which seek to prevent, monitor, decrease and/or alleviate possible harm or adverse effects (a.k.a. iatrogenic effects) caused by health interventions, treatments, diagnostic procedures, medications and/or programs.

qualitative research. Involves a holistic and subjective process used to describe and to promote a better understanding of human experiences and phenomena via the collection of rich narrative data, and to develop conceptual models and theories that seek to describe these experiences and phenomenon.

quantitative research. Is a formal, precise, systematic and objective process in which numerical data are used to obtain information on a variety of health-related phenomenon of interest or concern.

quasi-statistical/ manifest content analysis style. Consists of an accounting-type of frequency inventory or system used to determine the number of times an underlying word, phrase, insight, phenomenon, construct or theme appears in a qualitative data set.

quarantine. Is defined as the restriction of activities of individuals who remain disease or symptom free but who have been exposed to an infectious agent.

ratio data. Is the highest level of measurement which provides information about the ordering and exact magnitude between the levels of the critical attribute due to a clearly defined and ratio zero.

reduction. Refers to any strategy that will result in fewer animals being used for scientific investigations, in accordance with CCAC (2013) guidelines.

re-emerging infectious diseases. Are defined as diseases that were once regarded as major public health problems globally or in a particular country, and then declined dramatically, but have subsequently re-emerged as a public health concern for a significant proportion of the population.

refinement. Refers to the modification of husbandry (i.e., care and housing of animals) and/or experimental procedures to minimize pain and distress (e.g., administration of analgesics) (CCAC, 2013).

relative risk or risk ratio. Is defined as the ratio between the rates in the exposed and unexposed groups.

relaxation response. Defined as the counterpart to the fight-or-flight response where the body is no longer in perceived danger, and the autonomic nervous system functioning returns to a normal state.

replacement. Refers to methods which avoid or replace the use of animals in an area where animals would otherwise have been used, in accordance with CCAC (2013) guidelines.

research. A systematic and purposeful method of scientific inquiry into the nature of phenomena of interests to public health care professionals and scientists in an attempt to develop new knowledge and practice standards, test existing hypotheses and for the development conceptual models and theories.

research control. Seeks to eliminate the effects of possible extraneous influences on the dependent variable so that the true relationship between the independent and dependent variables can be understood.

research design. Is a detailed plan or blueprint for the research methods and strategies that will be employed by the researcher in order to answer the research question or hypothesis.

respect for persons. Is the first principle of the TCPS2 that stipulates that an individual's autonomy and their freedom to choose what will happen to them must be ensured. This principle also means that consent must be ongoing in nature. Hence, participants must be allowed to withdraw from the study at any time if they so choose to.

research process. Is here defined as a series of 9 steps and techniques used to structure a study and to gather, analyze, interpret, disseminate and apply data and information in a systematic and formularized fashion.

research question. Is a clear statement of scientific inquiry that the investigator wants to answer through a specific study.

reserve system. Established by the Indian Act of 1876, this legislated over First Nations populations and which established specific lands reserved for them.

reservoir. Is defined as the natural environment in which a pathogen typically resides, and may be a person, animal or environment (e.g., soil, water).

restricting type of anorexia nervosa. Is the most common form whereby an individual severely restricts their food intake via dieting and/or fasting.

ripple effect. Is defined as a public health situation, interaction or intervention and is similar to the ever expanding ripples across a static body of water when an object is dropped into it where an effect from an initial state can be followed incrementally. These public health situations, interactions or interventions can directly or indirectly affect and impact individuals, groups or entire communities.

sacred Tree. Embodies the common Aboriginal belief that spiritual life consists of a harmonious union or connectedness with all natural things symbolized by a sacred tree.

schizophrenia. Is defined as a mental disorder characterized by abnormal social behaviour(s), marked disturbances in thinking and cognition, and perceptions of reality.

screening. is defined as a population-based public health strategy employed to identify the possible presence of an as-yet-undiagnosed condition (e.g., breast, cervical, or colon cancer) in clients without known signs or symptoms.

seasonal affective disorder (SAD). Is a type of depression which affects approximately 2% to 6% of Canadians, especially during the fall and winter months and is characterized by irritability, apathy, carbohydrate cravings, weight gain, sleep disturbances, apathy, fatigue, and general feelings of sadness.

secondary prevention. Consists of activities that are aimed at early detection of an altered state of health, and interventions which are aimed at stopping or reversing further processes with this altered state of health. For example, screening sexually active teenagers for the presence of sexually transmitted infections (STI's).

semi-structured interviews. Consist of a list of predetermined probing topics or questions that are fluid in nature and therefore can be elaborated on by the researcher to seek additional information or clarification as so desired.

sex. Is defined one's biological and physiological characteristics that distinguish males and females in binary terms, and incorporate multi-dimensional characteristics and traits such as hormones, genes and one's anatomical make-up.

sexting. The act of sending sexually explicit images, which include pictures, photos or videos via a mobile information or communications device (e.g., smartphone, tablet, laptop).

sick building syndrome (SBS). Affected occupants of these certain buildings have subjective complaints of feeling ill or sick. Signs and symptoms including irritation of the eyes, nose or throat; dry cough; dizziness and nausea; difficulty concentrating and generalized fatigue; neurotoxic or general health problems; skin irritations and rashes; nonspecific hypersensitivity reactions, headaches; odor, and altered taste sensations. These signs and symptoms typically fade or disappear once the individual leaves the particular room, zone or building affecting them.

sickness. Is defined as a state of social dysfunction of an individual with a disease or the result of being defined by others in one's culture as unhealthy, and the expected role that the individual should assume when ill (Porta, 2008).

sick role. Is defined as a behavioural pattern in which an individual accepts and readily adopts the signs and symptoms of a physical or mental disorder in order to receive care, seek sympathy and/or be protected from the demands and stresses of life in their defined culture.

signs. Are defined as manifestations of an illness that an individual can see (e.g., rash on extremities, edema in the feet, blood in the urine).

social-determinants of health. The structural determinants and conditions of daily life responsible for a major part of health inequities between and within countries. They include the distribution of power, income, goods and services, and the circumstances of people's lives, such as their access to health care, schools and education; their conditions of work and leisure; and the state of their housing and environment. The term "social determinants" is thus shorthand for the social, political, economic, environmental and cultural factors that greatly affect health status (WHO, 2008, p.1).

social justice. The entitlement of all Canadians to basic necessities, including adequate income and health protection, and the acceptance of collective action and obligation to make such possible in our society.

Social Union Framework Agreement (1999). Merely requires that the provinces and territories to promise to spend the money on health care and to measure its outcomes.

somatogenic theories. Of mental illness or disorders identify disturbances in physical functioning resulting from either illness, genetic inheritance, brain damage, or chemicalor force of nature imbalance.

statistical control. Involves the use of various statistical procedures to control for extraneous or possible confounding influences on the dependent (outcome) variable under investigation.

statistical hypothesis testing. Provides an objective means for determining whether or not the stated hypotheses were supported by the data collected, and permits researchers to make decisions about whether the results likely reflect chance sample differences or true population differences.

status indian. A First Nations individual who is a member of a band with a treaty number.

stress. Is defined as a unique and subjective perception or reaction to a specific current existing or imminent situation or condition that results in emotional and physiological responses resulting from various demands, expectations and/or unpredictable circumstances experienced in our daily lives. Stress can also be defined as any physical, social, political, economic, or cultural force which creates an imbalance and which can have either negative or positive influence on an individual or group.

stressor. Is defined as any situation or event that triggers an emotional or physiological response by an individual.

stress response. Is defined as the individual's reaction to a specific stressor.

stroke. Also known as a "brain attack", is a sudden loss of brain function that occurs when blood flow supplying oxygen to a part of the brain is interrupted.

structured interviewed. Consists of predetermined and fixed questions or categories of information (e.g., fixed response options) that are specified in advance by the researcher and which cannot be deviated from.

Sudden Acute Respiratory Syndrome (SARS). Is defined as a potentially life-threatening coronavirus (SARS-CoV) infection that affects the respiratory system with an average incubation period of six days, and which is spread by close person-to-person contact by infected individuals, most often via droplets expelled into the air during coughing or sneezing episodes.

surveys, questionnaires and self-reports. Non-experimentalresearch that seeks to obtain quantitative information about people's actions, behaviours, knowledge, intentions, opinions or attitudes and helps to provide knowledge related to the prevalence, distribution and interrelationships of variables within a population.

survival rate. The percentage of individuals who are alive 5 years after being diagnosed or after commencement of a treatment regime, or the number of living cases per number of cases of the disease.

sustainable development. Encompasses environmental, economic, cultural and socio-political sustainability for resource extraction and use by humans that seeks to meet current needs while being cognizant for the importance of preserving these limited and finite resources for use by subsequent future generations.

S.W.O.T. Is an acronym for Strengths, Weaknesses, Opportunities, and Threats. A S.W.O.T analysis can be employed to identify both internal and external strengths and analysis or your proposed program along with potential barriers, gaps, challenges and opportunities.

symptoms. Are defined as those aspects of the illness that an individual experiences, feels or perceives (e.g., shortness of breath, fatigue, headaches, abdominal pain).

systemic infection. Is defined as an invasion by a microorganism that spreads through the blood or lymphatic system to large portions of the host's body or tissues.

systematic review. A narrowly focused synthesis of research investigations on a select topic, field of inquiry, practice intervention and/or related research problem.

telehealth or e-health. Is defined as "the use of telecommunications technologies and electronic information to exchange healthcare information and to provide and support services such as long distance clinical healthcare to clients" (Hebda & Czar, 2013, p. 505).

template analysis style. The qualitative researcher develops a rudimentary analysis guide or template to which narrative data units are applied (e.g., behaviours, events, linguistic expressions), and these templates undergo constant revision as more subjective data are gathered and interpreted.

terra nullius. Refers to unoccupied, uninhabited and vacant land.

territorial formula financing. Was introduced during the mid-1980's in an attempt to replace a system comprised of annual grants provided by the federal government to the three territories (Yukon, Northwest Territory and Nunavut).

tertiary prevention. Consists of activities that are aimed at preventing further deterioration or progress of an altered state of health. For example, providing health education by public health nurses related to home-based monitoring of blood glucose levels and insulin administration for individuals with diabetes.

therapeutic research. Provides subjects/ patients with an opportunity to receive an experimental treatment that may have beneficial results.

threshold dose. Is defined as the highest dose at which no toxic effects are observed.

thrombotic stroke. Is caused by a thrombus (i.e., blood clot) that forms in a cerebral artery that has been narrowed or damaged by atherosclerosis.

time component. Helps to establish the required incubation periods for communicable agents, the life expectancy of the host or pathogen, and the duration and course of the disease or altered health condition.

time series design study. A type of quasi-experimental study which seeks to establish patterns and involves the collection of quantitative data over an extended time period and one with multiple data collection points both prior to and after an intervention, therapy or treatment to examine changes in a variable or variables across time.

tommy douglas. Regarded as the *"father of Medicare"*, since he is credited as being the first in Canada to introduce a universal hospital-based insurance plan for residents of Saskatchewan in 1948.

toxicology. Is defined as the study of the adverse effects of synthetic chemical substances and products and natural toxins, which includes their cellular, biochemical and molecular mechanisms of action, and the actual or potential ability of these chemicals to cause harm, harm, ill effects, disease and/or mortality in living organisms including humans.

traumatic brain injury (TBI). Is defined as is an insult or injury to the brain, not of a degenerative or congenital nature, but caused by external physical force that may produce a diminished or altered state of consciousness resulting in an impairment of cognitive abilities and/or physical functioning.

treaty indian. An individual born to First Nations parents who are both treaty or registered members of a recognized band in Canada, and whose parents must register them under their specific treaty number.

trend study. A study in which samples from a general population are studied over time with respect to some characteristic or phenomenon; and where different samples are selected at specified repeated intervals, but the samples are always drawn from the same population.

trephination. AKA trepanning or burr holing is a surgical intervention where a hole is drilled, incised or scraped into the skull using simple tools, and is an example of one of the earliest treatments and supernatural explanation for mental illness (i.e., madness or insanity) and epilepsy.

type 1 diabetes. Previously known as *insulin-dependent, juvenile or childhood-onset DM*, results from progressive destruction of pancreatic ß-cells owing to an autoimmune process in susceptible clients, and is therefore characterized by a deficient insulin production that requires daily administration of insulin.

type a personality. Individuals are highly controlling in nature, ultracompetitive in nature, impatient, aggressive, cynical, confrontational, verbally, emotionally and/or physically hostile or abusive.

type b personality. Individuals are generally relaxed, laid-back, easy going, and contemplative. These individuals tend to be better at relaxing without feeling guilty and working without becoming overly anxious or agitated.

type c personality. Individuals with this personality type are characterized by the suppression of anger and feelings. These individuals appear to lack emotions, often have feelings of hopelessness, suppress their wants, needs or desires, do not usually assert themselves, and prefer to pacify others.

type d personality. This is a relatively new personality construct where individuals tend to have a joint tendency towards negative affectivity (e.g. worry, irritability, gloom) and social inhibition (e.g. reticence and a lack of self-assurance). These individuals often possess a negative outlook on life, are gloomy, socially inept, and anxious worriers who live with a constraint fear of rejection by others.

typhoid fever. Is a highly infectious disease clinically characterized by a high fever, rose-coloured spots on the chest or abdomen, electrolyte imbalance due to diarrhea, mental depression, physical weakness, and occasional intestinal hemorrhage and perforation of the bowel.

universality. This criterion of the Canada Health Act declares that all residents in Canada are entitled to insured health services, and that it should be administered on uniform terms and conditions.

unstructured interviews. Are informal in nature and consists of general or broad questions posed by the researcher that are not predetermined or planned in nature regarding their content or specific nature of the data sought to be collected.

variable. Is a defined attribute of a person or object that varies and/or takes on different values (e.g., age, heart rate, income).

variolation. Is defined as a prophylactic intervention that was widely practiced prior to the development of vaccines that involved the intentional and planned inoculation of an uninfected individual with content consisting of pustule matter (containing the virus) derived from an infected person to protect against the more severe form of smallpox.

vector-borne diseases. Are caused by infectious agents that are transmitted by a vector or carrier, such as an insect (e.g., fly, tick, mosquitoe).

vertical transmission. Occurs when an infectious disease is transmitted between a parent and child or offspring via sperm, placenta, breast milk or contact with the vaginal canal at birth (e.g., sexually transmitted infections such as HIV/AIDS, herpes, syphilis).

waterborne mode of transmission. Occurs via contract or consumption of contaminated water supplies, and includes contamination of water supplies from fecal contamination from humans or animals which result in enteric illness or disease.

wellness. A positive sense of well-being and/or a deliberate lifestyle choice characterized by personal responsibility and enhancement of one's physical, mental, spiritual, cultural, environmental and social-political health.

west nile virus (WNV). Is a mosquitoe-borne arbovirus that was first discovered in 1927 and isolated in 1937 from the blood of a febrile client in the West Nile province of Uganda, Africa, and is a member of the flavivirus genus (Family *Flaviviridae*).

white matter. A component of the brain that contains the axons of the ascending sensory and descending (suprasegumental) motor fibres, and the myelin surrounding these fibres gives them the characteristic white appearance.

white Paper. This policy document attempted to abolish the Indian Act of 1867 and promote self-government of Aboriginal peoples, but was never passed by Parliament.

Workplace Hazardous Materials Information System" (WHMIS). Is a comprehensive federally legislated system to ensure the safe use and handling of hazardous materials and substances in Canadian workplaces.

Yerkes-Dodson Law. A bell-shaped curve which demonstrates graphically the theoretical association between optimal levels of stress and peak performance.

zika virus. Is spread by the Aedes mosquitoe and was first detected in rhesus monkeys in Uganda, Africa in 1947. Typical symptoms of exposure include fever, headaches, conjunctivitis, rash and joint and muscle pain and last for a duration of 2 to 7 days. Complications for pregnant females include miscarriages and birth defects (e.g., microcephaly).

zoonotic mode infections. Are defined as diseases which are transmissible between animals and humans, and which do not necessarily require a human host to maintain their life cycles.